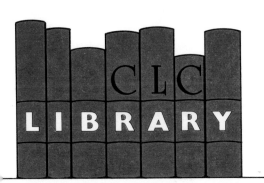
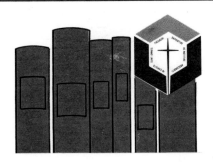

Human
Neuroanatomy

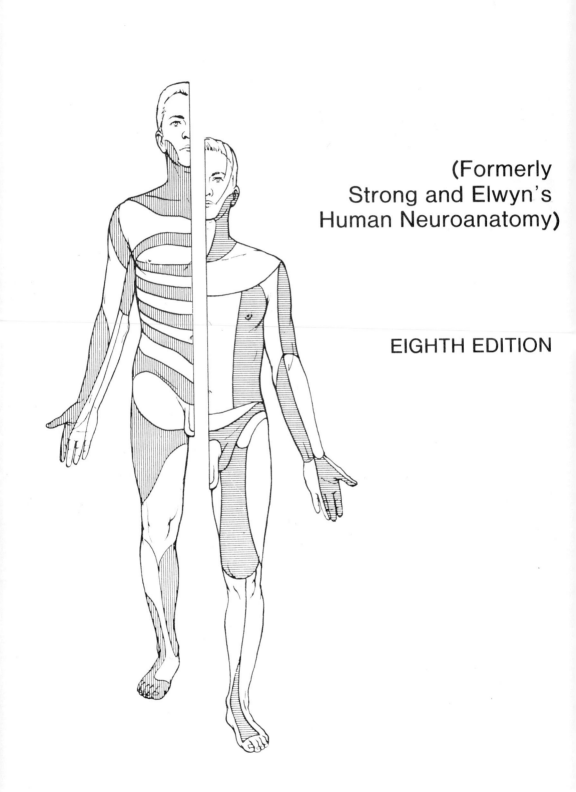

(Formerly
Strong and Elwyn's
Human Neuroanatomy)

EIGHTH EDITION

Human Neuroanatomy

MALCOLM B. CARPENTER, M.D.

Professor and Chairman, Department of Anatomy,
Uniformed Services University of the Health Sciences,
Bethesda, Maryland

JEROME SUTIN, Ph.D.

Professor and Chairman, Department of Anatomy,
School of Medicine, Emory University,
Atlanta, Georgia

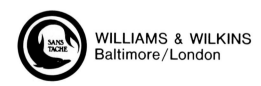

WILLIAMS & WILKINS
Baltimore/London

Copyright ©, 1983
Williams & Wilkins
428 East Preston Street
Baltimore, Maryland 21202 U.S.A.

Made in the United States of America

First Edition, May 1943
  Reprinted December 1943
  Reprinted December 1945
  Reprinted December 1946
Second Edition, 1948
  Reprinted June 1951
Third Edition, 1953
Fourth Edition, 1959
  Reprinted October 1960
  Reprinted August 1962
Fifth Edition, 1964
  Reprinted July 1965
Sixth Edition, 1969
  Reprinted April 1970
  Reprinted June 1971
  Reprinted May 1973
Seventh Edition, 1976
  Reprinted August 1976
  Reprinted June 1977
  Reprinted July 1978
  Reprinted October 1979
  Reprinted April 1981

Library of Congress Cataloging in Publication Data

Carpenter, Malcolm B.
  Human neuroanatomy.

  Bibliography: p.
  Includes index.
  1. Neuroanatomy. I. Sutin, Jerome. II. Title. [DNLM: 1. Nervous system—Anatomy and histology. WL 101
QM451.T7 1983   611'.8   82-4897
ISBN 0-683-01461-7 AACR2

38,837

Composed and Printed at
Waverly Press, Inc.
Mount Royal and Guilford Avenues
Baltimore, Maryland 21202 U.S.A.

Preface to the Eighth Edition

The last decade has witnessed a tremendous expansion of knowledge in the neurosciences due to a series of fundamental conceptual advances, the development of sophisticated new research technics and the recognition of the overwhelming importance of the nervous system in all branches of medicine. The interdependence of the biomedical sciences is nowhere more evident than in the neurosciences. A significant advance in neuroanatomy, neurochemistry, neuropharmacology or neurophysiology contributes to our understanding in all of these fields. Fundamental correlations of structure and function constitute the centerpiece which unites the neurosciences. These multifaceted developments in expanding fields make it difficult to write a neuroanatomy text for medical students. Neuroanatomical data must be related to information from other disciplines in a meaningful way. Newer research methods, particularly those derived from the field of cell biology, have made it possible to resolve a variety of old problems and to embellish established concepts with important new details. In the midst of these changes, the authors have attempted to provide the medical student with a reasonable guide to the structural and functional organization of the nervous system that will be useful in all the neurosciences and have clinical application. It is recognized that few neuroscience courses in American medical schools are identical, even though similar material is presented. The text represents a reasonably comprehensive treatment of the subject and attempts to meet the requirements of a broad spectrum of medical students.

We believe that a textbook should present data as well as conclusions and provide documentation from the literature. The complexity of the nervous system, rapid progress in the neurosciences and the desire to fit experimental data into a conceptually satisfactory framework have sometimes led to the premature formulation of generalizations. We have tried to balance the presentation of facts and their interpretation, recognizing that the former are more enduring and the latter are changing. The student must appreciate that information from many species and specialized neurons has been used to develop general concepts. The application of these concepts to the solution of specific problems in humans must be tempered by an awareness of the sources of knowledge and constancy of neural mechanisms among species.

While this textbook is entitled *Human Neuroanatomy*, and emphasizes information about the human and infrahuman primate nervous system, it draws upon neurobiological studies in both vertebrates and invertebrates which provide sources of new information about the brain. This is a multilevel textbook which we hope will be of value to both beginning and advanced students. It is important that the instructor guide the beginning student in the selection of topics and depth of coverage expected in an introductory course.

The eighth edition of *Human Neuroanatomy* has undergone extensive revisions in all chapters, although it has retained the format of the last edition. Considerable new material has been added concerning the cerebrospinal fluid and the blood-brain barrier, the neuron, axoplasmic flow and neurotransmitters. The chapter on the autonomic nervous system has been expanded

v

and revised in the light of new basic concepts. New concepts concerning pain mechanisms and descending autonomic pathways have emerged from immunohistochemical and physiological studies of the spinal cord. As experience has amply demonstrated, a good understanding of the spinal cord is essential if the student is to fully appreciate the more complex brain stem. Chapters on the medulla, pons and midbrain have been re-worked and include data on cell groups associated with specific neurotransmitters. Attempts have been made to simplify the complex organization of cerebellar input and output systems which characterize this structure. New data concerning the multiple divisions of the diencephalon have contributed greatly to our understanding of the somatosensory, auditory and visual systems and the role of brain peptides and neurotransmitters in the regulation of endocrine functions. The relationships between the amygdala and other centers of visceral function have been updated. The chapter on the cerebral cortex provides new data on relationships with thalamic nuclei and the manner in which the cell columns and laminae within the cortex process information. Particularly impressive studies of the visual system have received special attention. The final chapter deals with the blood supply of the central nervous system. In each chapter dealing with the central nervous system a section on "Functional Considerations" attempts to synthesize information especially pertinent to clinical problems. Over 100 new illustrations have been added, many in color. The atlas section at the back of the book consists of 24 full color plates which students have found useful. Responsibility for the revisions of various chapters has been divided. Professor Carpenter took major responsibility for Chapters 1, 2, 7, 9, 10, 12, 13, 14, 15, 17, 19 and 20 while Professor Sutin assumed the editorship of the remaining chapters. The nomenclature of the *Nomina Anatomica*, published in 1977, has been used as a guide. As is well known, this nomenclature is incomplete with respect to many commonly used neuroanatomical terms.

The new illustrations for this edition of the text have been done largely by Robert J. Demarest, Director of the Audiovisual Department of the College of Physicians and Surgeons, Columbia University. Marty Nau of the Department of Anatomy at the Uniformed Services University has also contributed many excellent drawings. The superb illustrations of the late Ivan Summers from Professor Mettler's *Neuroanatomy* (1948) continue to be used. Antonio B. Pereira, who has worked with the senior author for more than twenty years, prepared new histological material and did all of the new photographs. The authors are most grateful for these important contributions. The drawings of Robert J. Demarest are well known for their clarity and innovative nature.

Colleagues at many medical schools have offered valuable suggestions for improving the book and have given generously of their time. They have also complied with our requests for illustrations which seem particularly useful in understanding cardinal concepts. While the names of all individuals who have supplied illustrations are cited in the figure legends, particular gratitude is expressed to the following: Dr. Fred A. Mettler, Uniformed Services University; Dr. Joe Hanaway, Washington University; Drs. Jacqueline McGinty and Floyd E. Bloom, Salk Institute; Drs. Leslie L. Iversen and Stephen Hunt, Cambridge University; Dr. George K. Aghajanian, Yale University; Dr. Jerzy E. Rose, University of Wisconsin; Dr. Konrad Akert, Institut für Hirnforschung der Universitat Zurich; Dr. Ralph Norgren, Rockefeller University; Dr. Ray Guillery, University of Chicago; Dr. Charles R. Noback, Columbia University, Dr. Terry L. Hickey, University of Alabama; Drs. David H. Hubel, Torsten N. Wiesel and Simon LeVay, Harvard University; Dr. Edward G. Jones, Washington University; Dr. Madhu Kalia, Hahnemann Medical College; Dr. Andrew Shally, Tulane University and Veterans Administration Hospital; Dr. Roger Gorski, University of California at Los Angeles; Dr. O. E. Millhouse, University of Utah; and Dr. Michael Gershon, Columbia University. As all who are familiar with *Human Neuroanatomy* know, there are many contributions to this text which were made over a long period of time by the late Professor Raymond C. Truex, not all of which can now be readily identified.

Special acknowledgment must go to Mrs.

Doris Lineweaver at Pennsylvania State University and Mrs. Trudy Levy at Emory University who cheerfully provided secretarial and editorial assistance. The authors also greatly appreciate the many contributions made by Mrs. Lillian Magruder of the Uniformed Services University and Mrs. Geraldine Luttrell of Emory University. We particularly want to thank our wives, Carly Carpenter and Avril Sutin, for many hours of editorial assistance. Finally, the authors are grateful to the Publishers, and especially to Ms. Sara A. Finnegan, President of Williams & Wilkins, for their confidence and encouragement.

Malcolm B. Carpenter
Jerome Sutin

Preface to the First Edition

Neurology, more perhaps than any other branch of medicine, is dependent on an accurate knowledge of anatomy as a basis for the intelligent diagnosis and localization of neural disturbances. This book, the result of many years of neuroanatomical teaching, is intended to supply this basic anatomical need, to give the student and physician a thorough and clear presentation of the structural mechanisms of the human nervous system together with some understanding of their functional and clinical significance. It is an attempt to link structure and function into a dynamic pattern without sacrificing anatomical detail.

The book is a human neuroanatomy sufficiently rich in content to obviate the necessity of constantly consulting larger anatomical texts. It may be conveniently divided into two parts. The first part (Chapters I–VIII) is concerned with the general organization and meaning of the nervous system, its embryology and histological structure, and with some fundamental neurological problems as they apply to man. This is followed by a discussion of the organization and segmental distribution of the peripheral nerve elements, including an analysis of the functional components of the spinal nerves and of the various receptors and effectors. If these earlier chapters are perhaps more extensive than in most other texts, it is due to the conviction that the book should be complete in itself, and also that a knowledge of these preliminaries is essential for an understanding of the complex machinery of the spinal cord and brain.

The second and larger part (Chapters IX–XX) is devoted to the architectonics of the central nervous system and may be regarded as "applied neuroanatomy." Special features of this part are the many fine photographs, both gross and microscopic, of the human brain and spinal cord, the great wealth of anatomical detail, and the discussion of the structural mechanisms in the light of clinical experience. While the individual portions of the nervous system are treated separately, an attempt has been made to achieve organic structural continuity by judicious repetition and overlapping and by constant reference to related topics already familiar to the student from previous chapters. The plan of exposition is substantially the same for each topic. The gross structure and relationships are concisely but thoroughly reviewed with the aid of clear and graphic illustrations. The internal structure is then presented in detail, usually based on a carefully graded series of fine and clearly labeled microphotographs of human material. At each level the student is familiarized with the exact location, extent and relationships of the various structures seen in the section. Finally the anatomical features of each part are reviewed more comprehensively as three-dimensional structural mechanisms, with a full discussion of their connections and clinical significance. We believe that this treatment will make the complicated structural details alive and interesting to the student. The illustrations are not segregated in the back of the book in the form of an atlas but are scattered in the text, in proper relation to the levels studied.

Besides the many original illustrations, a number of others selected from various and duly acknowledged sources have been completely redrawn and relabeled for the sake of clarity and simplicity. All the illustrations, whether original or borrowed, have been executed by Frances H. Elwyn to whose skill and patience the authors are deeply indebted. We are also indebted to Dr. H. Alsop Riley for the use of several microphotographs; to Drs. R. C. Truex and Benjamin Salzer for the reading of several chapters; and especially to Dr. Otto Marburg for his many stimulating discussions and suggestions and for his critical reading of the chapters on the mesencephalon, diencephalon, and cerebral hemispheres.

Thanks are also due to Rosette Spoerri for her competent help in preparing the manuscript and bibliography.

The authors cannot express too strongly their obligation to the publishers for their continuous courtesy and cooperation in all matters, and for their infinite patience in waiting for a manuscript long overdue.

Adolph Elwyn
Oliver S. Strong

Contents

CHAPTER 1

Meninges and Cerebrospinal Fluid

The brain and spinal cord are delicate semisolid structures requiring protection and support. The brain is invested by various membranes, floated in a clear fluid and encased in a bony vault. Three membranes surround the brain. The most external is a dense connective tissue envelope known as the *dura mater* or *pachymeninx*. The innermost connective tissue membrane is the *pia mater*, a thin translucent membrane, adherent to the surface of the brain and spinal cord, which accurately follows every contour. Between these membranes is a delicate transparent layer of reticular fibers, the *arachnoid*. The pia mater and arachnoid have a similar structure and collectively are called the *leptomeninges*.

DURA MATER

The cranial dura consists of: (a) an outer *periosteal layer* adherent to the inner surface of the cranium which is rich in blood vessels and nerves and (b) an inner *meningeal layer* lined with flat cells. At certain sites these layers are separated and form large venous sinuses (Fig. 1-1). The meningeal layer gives rise to several septa which divide the cranial cavity into compartments. The largest of these is the sickle-shaped *falx cerebri* which extends in the midline from the crista galli to the internal occipital protuberance (Fig. 1-2). Posteriorly this septum is continuous with other transverse dural septa arising from the su-

perior crest of the petrous portion of the temporal bone. These septa form the *tentorium cerebelli* which roofs over the posterior fossa. The free borders of the tentorium form the *tentorial incisure* (Figs. 1-2 and 1-3), the only opening between these compartments. Thus these dural reflections divide the cranial cavity into paired lateral compartments for the cerebral hemispheres, and a single posterior compartment for the cerebellum and hindbrain. The brain stem passes through the tentorial notch (Fig. 1-4). The occipital lobes lie on the superior surface of the tentorium. A small midsagittal septum below the tentorium forms the *falx cerebelli* (Fig. 1-2) which partially separates the cerebellar hemispheres. The *diaphragma sellae* roofs over the pituitary fossa and is perforated by the infundibulum. The dural sinuses are discussed in relationship with the cerebral veins in Chapter 20.

The major blood supply for the dura is provided by the middle meningeal artery, a branch of the maxillary artery, which enters the skull via the foramen spinosum (Figs. 1-3 and 20-4). The ophthalmic artery gives rise to anterior meningeal branches and the occipital and vertebral arteries provide posterior meningeal branches. Skull fractures lacerating these meningeal arteries produce space occupying epidural hemorrhages between the skull and the dura that require prompt surgical intervention.

1

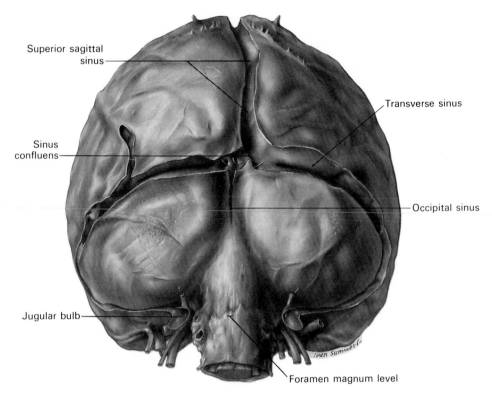

Superior sagittal
sinus

Transverse sinus

Sinus
confluens

Occipital sinus

Jugular bulb

Foramen magnum level

Figure 1-1. Posterior view of the dura surrounding the brain. Prominent dural sinuses have been opened. The periosteal layer of the dura has been cut at the margins of the foramen magnum. (Reproduced with permission from F. A. Mettler: *Neuroanatomy*, Ed. 2, The C. V. Mosby Co., St. Louis, 1948.)

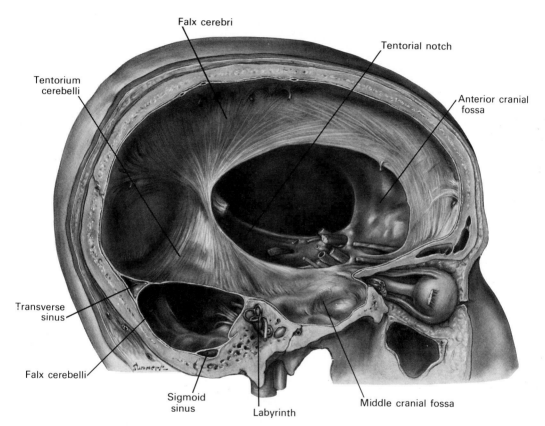

Figure 1-2. Sagittal section of the head showing the falx cerebri, the tentorium cerebelli and the falx cerebelli. (Reproduced with permission from F. A. Mettler: *Neuroanatomy*, Ed. 2, The C. V. Mosby Co., St. Louis, 1948.)

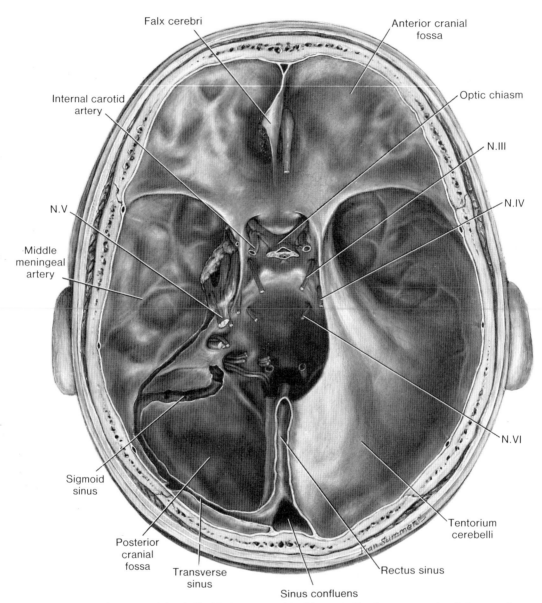

Figure 1-3. View of the base of the skull with dura mater. The falx cerebri has been removed and the tentorium cerebelli has been cut away on the left to expose the posterior fossa. (Reproduced with permission from F. A. Mettler: *Neuroanatomy*, Ed. 2, The C. V. Mosby Co., St. Louis, 1948.)

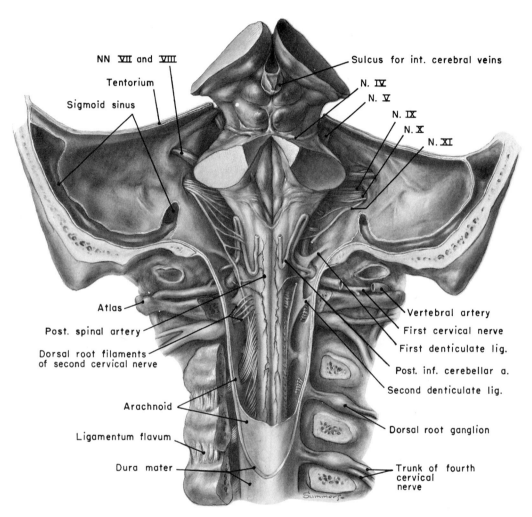

Figure 1-4. Posterior view of the brain stem, upper cervical spinal cord and meninges. (Reproduced with permission from F. A. Mettler: *Neuroanatomy*, Ed. 2, The C. V. Mosby Co., St. Louis, 1948.)

The supratentorial dura is innervated by branches of the trigeminal nerve (1966), while the infratentorial dura is supplied by branches of the upper cervical spinal nerves and the vagus nerve (1314, 1315).

The innermost layer of the dura is composed of flattened mesothelial cells with a dense cytoplasm. This layer usually is in close contact with the arachnoid, suggesting that the *subdural space* is a potential space rather than an actual space (601).

The *spinal dura* is a continuation of the meningeal layer of the cranial dura (Figs. 1-4 and 1-5). The periosteum of the vertebrae corresponds to the outer (periosteal) layer of the cranial dura. Inner and outer surfaces of the spinal dura are covered by a single layer of flat cells, and the dense membrane is separated from the periosteum by a narrow *epidural space*. The spinal epidural space contains areolar tissue and the internal vertebral venous plexuses (Fig. 20-3). This actual space is largest at the level of the second lumbar vertebra where it is nearly half the diameter of the spinal canal. Clinically the epidural space is used to inject a local anesthetic to produce an extensive paravertebral nerve block, known as *epidural anesthesia*. The epidural space can be distinguished because it has a negative pressure. *Caudal anesthesia*, used in obstetrics, is a form of epidural anesthesia in which the local anesthesia is introduced into the epidural space via the sacral canal.

The spinal dura extends as a closed tube from the margins of the foramen magnum to the level of the second sacral vertebra (Fig. 1-6). At the caudal termination of the dural sac the dura invests the filum terminale to form a thin fibrous cord, the *coccygeal ligament* (Fig. 1-6). This ligament extends caudally to the coccyx where it becomes continuous with the periosteum. The spinal cord ends at the lower border of the first lumbar vertebra. Extensions of the dura passing laterally around the spinal nerve roots form dural root sleeves (Figs. 1-5 and 1-7).

PIA MATER

This vascular membrane is composed of: (a) an inner membraneous layer, the *intima pia* (1306), and (b) a more superficial *epipial layer*. The intima pia, adherent to underlying nervous tissue, follows its contours closely and is composed of fine reticular and elastic fibers (Figs. 1-8 and 1-9). Where blood vessels enter and leave the central nervous system, the intima pia is invaginated forming a perivascular space (Fig. 1-14). The intima pia, like the arachnoid, is avascular and derives its nutrients by diffusion from the cerebrospinal fluid and the underlying nervous tissue (601, 1702, 1703). The epipial layer is formed by a meshwork of collagenous fiber bundles continuous with the arachnoid trabeculae. The blood vessels of the spinal cord lie within the epipial layer. Over the convex surface of the cerebral cortex, the epipial layer is absent and the large cerebral vessels lie on the intima pia where they are anchored by fine arachnoid trabeculae (Fig. 1-10). The pia mater is made up of a sheet of leptomeningeal cells virtually indistinguishable from those of the arachnoid except that they form a single layer and do not overlap (601, 1958). Subpial astrocytes form a continuous sheath of underlying cytoplasm; between the pia and subpial astrocytic layer is an osmiophilic basement membrane separated from the plasma membranes.

The spinal cord is attached to the dura mater by a series of lateral flattened bands of epipial tissue known as the *denticulate ligaments* (Figs. 1-4, 1-5 and 1-7). Each triangular-shaped ligament is attached medially to the lateral surface of the spinal cord midway between the dorsal and ventral roots. The bases of these ligaments arise in the pia mater, and their apices are firmly attached to the arachnoid and the inner surface of the dura. The denticulate ligaments alternate with the dural evaginations which mark the exits of the cervical, thoracic and first lumbar spinal nerves. On each lateral surface of the spinal cord 18 to 24 denticulate ligaments anchor the spinal cord to the dura. In the region of the conus medullaris epipial tissue forms a covering of the filum terminale (Fig. 1-6).

Certain regions of the pia mater deserve special attention. The epipial layer surrounding the brain and spinal cord is interrupted at the filamentous attachments of the cranial and spinal nerves. As the individual nerve fibers enter or leave the brain and spinal cord they pierce the intima pia from which they derive an investment of

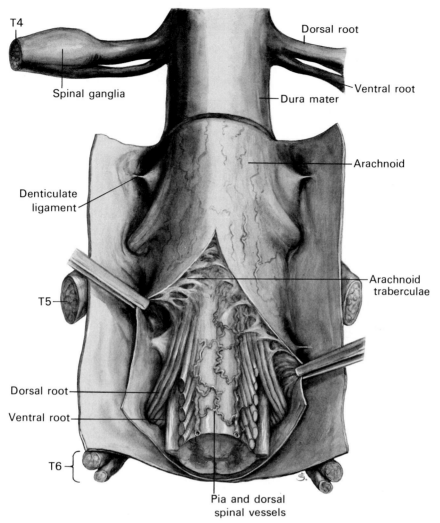

T4

Dorsal root

Spinal ganglia

Ventral root

Dura mater

Arachnoid

Denticulate
ligament

Arachnoid
trabeculae

T5

Dorsal root

Ventral root

T6

Pia and dorsal
spinal vessels

Figure 1-5. Posterior view of part of the upper thoracic spinal cord. The dura and arachnoid have been split at the midline to expose the spinal cord and pial vessels. Above the intact dura covers the spinal cord and spinal nerve roots. (Reproduced with permission from F. A. Mettler: *Neuroanatomy*, Ed. 2, The C. V. Mosby Co., St. Louis, 1948.)

squamous cells and fine reticular fibers (Fig. 1-8). The more fibrous intima pia is firmly anchored to the surface of the spinal cord by a thin but distinct *superficial glial membrane* (Fig. 1-9). The latter is composed of fine processes of more deeply located fibrous astrocytes. Cell bodies of astrocytes can be observed in the glial membrane and many of the glial fibers possess bulbous expansions. The glial fibers and astrocytes are particularly prominent in regions where the dorsal and ventral spinal roots penetrate the pia mater. In the region of the posterolateral sulcus such glial ele-

ments constitute a barrier to the regeneration of avulsed nerve fibers or injured dorsal roots.

In the region of the ventricles the brain wall is formed by a single layer of ependymal cells, the outer surface of which is firmly adherent to the pia mater. In the roof of the third ventricle (Figs. 1-11 and 2-28*B*), in the lower part of the roof of the fourth ventricle (Figs. 1-11 and 11-14) and on the medial wall of the inferior horn of the lateral ventricle (choroid fissure; Fig. 18-10), the intima pia blends with the ependymal layer to form the *tela choroidea*

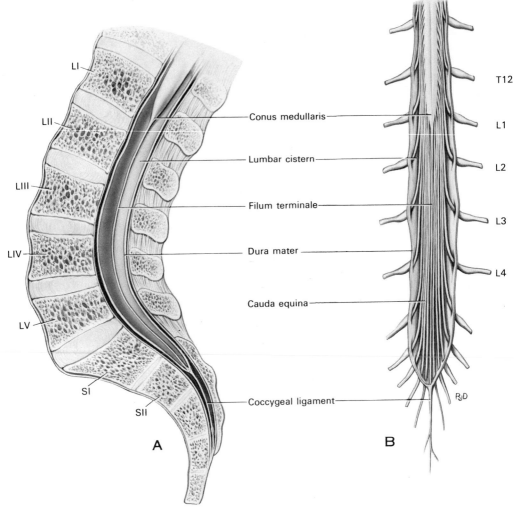

Figure 1-6. Diagrammatic representation of the caudal part of the spinal cord and lumbar cistern. (*A*) Sagittal view of the conus medullaris, lumbar cistern and lumbosacral vertebrae. (*B*) Posterior view of the cauda equina and nerve roots.

(Fig. 5-17). The tela choroidea anchors the choroid plexuses to the walls of the ventricles. It has a triangular shape in the roof of the third and fourth ventricles, while the tela choroidea of the lateral ventricle (Fig. 2-28) is horseshoe-shaped as it follows the choroidal fissure (Figs. 18-9 and 18-10). The two layers of the pia mater in the transverse cerebral fissure, below the splenium of the corpus callosum and above the pineal body, form the *velum interpositum* (Fig. 2-28). The internal cerebral veins, branches of the posterior cerebral artery, and arteries to the choroid plexuses of the third and lateral ventricles lie between these two layers (Figs. 20-23 and 20-24).

ARACHNOID

The arachnoid is a delicate nonvascular membrane between the dura and the pia mater which passes over the sulci without following their contours (Figs. 1-5, 1-8, 1-10, 1-12 and 1-14). This membrane also extends along the roots of the cranial and spinal nerves. Arachnoid trabeculae extend from the arachnoid to the pia. The space between the arachnoid and the pia mater, filled with cerebrospinal fluid, is called the *subarachnoid space* (Figs. 1-11 and 1-14). Certain cranial nerves, the olfactory, the optic and the vestibulocochlear, are surrounded by a subarachnoid space (601,

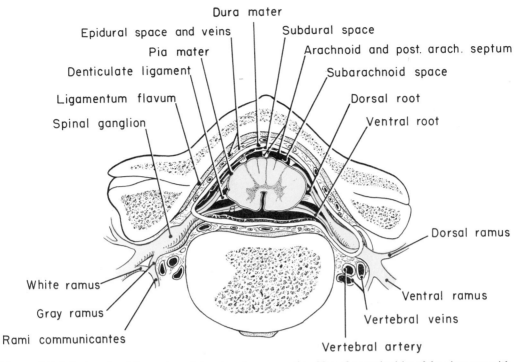

Figure 1-7. Spinal cord and its meningeal coverings in cross section. Note the continuities of the pia mater with the denticulate ligament, and of the dura mater with the epineurium of the spinal nerves. (Modified from Corning (537).)

2310). A small subarachnoid space also surrounds the spinal nerve roots in the root sleeves (Fig. 1-7). In the spinal regions fewer arachnoid trabeculae are concentrated into several subarachnoid septa; hence the spinal subarachnoid space is a more continuous cavity and the spinal arachnoid a more distinct membrane (Figs. 1-7 and 1-8). The arachnoid membrane is made up of leptomeningeal cells with a watery cytoplasm which forms long, irregular pseudopods that interdigitate with those of adjacent cells. These cells form a protoplasmic layer which may be several cells thick and exhibit great irregularity. When certain substances are injected into the subarachnoid space, these cells may swell and participate in phagocytic activity by ingesting particles of the foreign material. They may also become detached and form free macrophages.

The subarachnoid space is filled with cerebrospinal fluid and is in direct communication with the fourth ventricle of the brain by means of three apertures, one median and two lateral. The median aperture, or *foramen of Magendie* (Fig. 2-20), is lo-

cated in the caudal part of the thin ventricular roof; the lateral apertures, or *foramina of Luschka* (Figs. 2-20 and 11-2), open into the pontine subarachnoid cistern posterior to the emerging fibers of the ninth cranial nerve (Fig. 1-10).

The extent of the subarachnoid space surrounding the brain shows local variations. Over the convexity of the cerebral hemisphere this space is narrow, except in the depths of the sulci. At the base of the brain and around the brain stem the pia and the arachnoid often are widely separated, creating *subarachnoid cisternae* (Figs. 1-10 and 1-11). The largest cistern is found between the medulla and the cerebellum. This is the *cerebellomedullary cistern* (cisterna magna) into which the foramina of the fourth ventricle open (Figs. 1-10 and 1-11). Cerebrospinal fluid from the fourth ventricle passes into the cerebellomedullary cistern via the median foramen of Magendie and the two lateral foramina of Luschka. Other cisterns of considerable size are the *pontine cistern*, the *interpeduncular cistern*, the *chiasmatic cistern* and the *superior cistern* (Figs. 1-10 and 1-11).

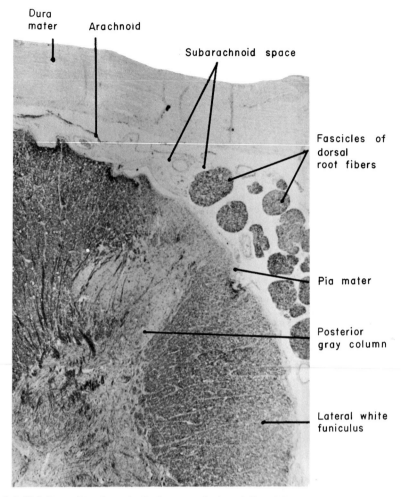

Figure 1-8. Relations of meninges to the human spinal cord (Luxol-fast blue stain, photograph, ×28).

The superior cistern, surrounding the posterior, superior and lateral surfaces of the midbrain, is referred to clinically as the *cisterna ambiens* (595, 2520). This cistern is of great importance because it contains the great vein of Galen, and the posterior cerebral and superior cerebellar arteries. Most of these cisterns can be visualized by special radiographic technics (e.g., pneumoencepholography or computerized tomography).

The *lumbar cistern* extends from the conus medullaris (lower border of the first lumbar vertebra) to about the level of the second sacral vertebra (Fig. 1-6). It contains the filum terminale and nerve roots of the cauda equina. It is from this cistern that cerebrospinal fluid is withdrawn in a lumbar spinal tap.

Arachnoid Granulations. In regions adjacent to the superior sagittal sinus (Figs. 1-1, 20-19 and 20-22) the cerebral pia-arachnoid gives rise to tufted prolongations which protrude through the meningeal layer of the dura into the superior sagittal sinus (Fig. 1-12). These granulations are variable in number and location and each consists of numerous arachnoid villi. These villi have a thin outer limiting membrane beneath which are bundles of collagenous and elastic fibers (Fig. 1-13). Cells similar to those of the pia-arachnoid are scattered among the fibers, and small oval epithelial cells cap the surface of the villi. Arachnoid granulations frequently are surrounded by a venous lacuna along the margin of the superior sagittal sinus. At advanced age the arachnoid granulations become larger and more numerous and tend to become calcified. The structure of a small granulation

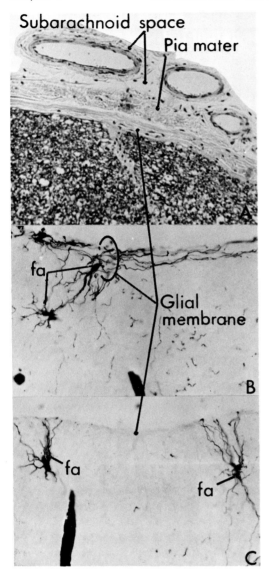

Subarachnoid space
Pia mater

Glial membrane

fa

fa

fa

A

B

C

Figure 1-9. Photographs of human spinal cord that demonstrate the structure and relations of pia mater and external glial membrane. These layers form the covering of the spinal cord. (*A*) Note that the glial membrane is closely adherent to inner surface of pia mater (Luxol-fast blue-cresyl violet stain, ×143). In *B* and *C*, the processes and terminal enlargements of fibrous astrocytes (*fa*) are identified as they enter into the formation of the glial membrane (Golgi stain, ×263).

along the optic nerves (2310). In both the spinal and cerebral arachnoid, cell clusters are sometimes formed which become attached to the dura. These growths may become calcified or, under abnormal conditions, form the sites where tumors arise.

Arachnoid granulations and villi are the major site of fluid transfer from the subarachnoid space to the venous system. The dural sinuses cannot collapse and the pressure within them is negative in the upright position. Venous pressure is therefore less than the hydrostatic pressure of the cerebrospinal fluid so that fluid moves from the subarachnoid space to the venous dural sinuses. Arachnoid granulations appear to function as passive, pressure-dependent, one-way-flow valves whose membranes are readily permeable to metabolites, Prussian blue reagents and even large molecular weight substances. For example, if plasma proteins, serum albumin or inulin are injected into the subarachnoid space, they rapidly appear in the venous blood (600, 2585). These valves are spongy tissue containing a series of interconnecting tubes approximately 6 μm in diameter. The tubes remain open only when the cerebrospinal fluid (CSF) flows from the subarachnoid space into venous blood under a pressure head (917, 918, 1214, 1215). When the pressure of venous blood exceeds that of the CSF, the tubes collapse (2694). The surface of an arachnoid villus has a layer of overlapping endothelial cells (2114). In the absence of pressure differences between the CSF and venous blood, the membranes of these cells are folded and have numerous microvilli. When CSF pressure exceeds venous pressure, the microvilli disappear, the cells are stretched and CSF flows into the venous sinuses. Bulk volume flow of CSF occurs through the arachnoid tubular system and between stretched endothelial cells. Flow of CSF into the venous sinuses is proportional to the increase in CSF pressure but does not begin until it exceeds venous pressure by 3 to 6 cm of water.

PIA-GLIA AND THE PERIVASCULAR SPACES

The intima pia or pia-glia is regarded as the external limiting membrane of the central nervous system (CNS). If the intima pia is considered the external limiting membrane of the CNS, the ependyma must con-

within a lateral lacuna of the superior sagittal sinus is shown in Figure 1-13. Although arachnoid villi are most numerous in relation to the superior sagittal sinus, they are found also along the other intracranial venous sinuses. Arachnoid villi also have been described in the spinal arachnoid (701) and

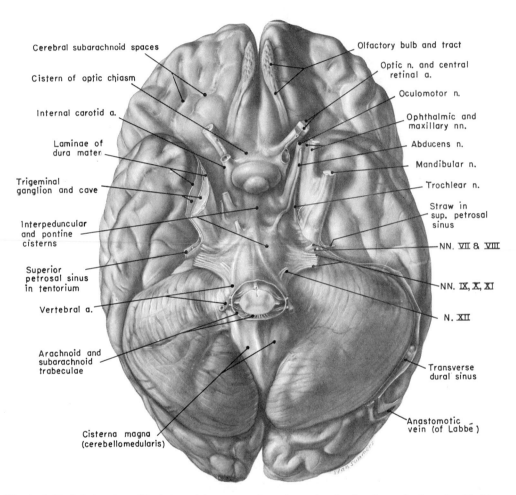

Cerebral subarachnoid spaces

Cistern of optic chiasm

Internal carotid a.

Laminae of
dura mater

Trigeminal
ganglion and cave

Interpeduncular
and pontine
cisterns

Superior
petrosal sinus
in tentorium

Vertebral a.

Arachnoid and
subarachnoid
trabeculae

Cisterna magna
(cerebellomedularis)

Olfactory bulb and tract

Optic n. and central
retinal a.

Oculomotor n.

Ophthalmic and
maxillary nn.

Abducens n.

Mandibular n.

Trochlear n.

Straw in
sup. petrosal
sinus

NN. VII & VIII

NN. IX, X, XI

N. XII

Transverse
dural sinus

Anastomotic
vein (of Labbé)

Figure 1-10. Inferior view of brain, cranial nerves and meninges showing locations of subarachnoid cisterns. (Reproduced with permission from F. A. Mettler: *Neuroanatomy*, Ed. 2, The C. V. Mosby Co., St. Louis, 1948.)

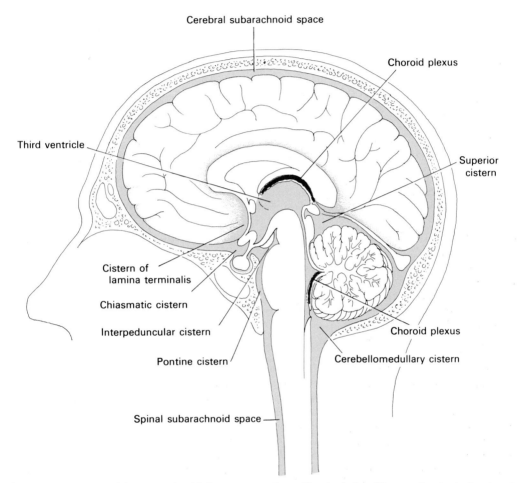

Figure 1-11. Diagram of the subarachnoid cisterns as seen in a midsagittal view. The superior cistern is referred to clinically as the cisterna ambiens. The choroid plexus in the roof of the third ventricle and in the fourth ventricle is shown in *red*.

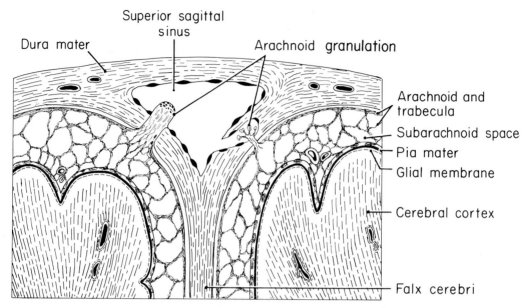

Superior sagittal
sinus

Dura mater

Arachnoid granulation

Arachnoid and
trabecula

Subarachnoid space

Pia mater

Glial membrane

Cerebral cortex

Falx cerebri

Figure 1-12. Diagram of meningeal-cortical relationships. Arachnoid granulations may penetrate dural sinuses or terminate in a lateral lacuna of a sinus. The pia is firmly anchored to cortex by the glial membrane.

stitute the internal limiting membrane. It has been suggested that the intima pia arises from ectoderm (1702). The arachnoid membrane which represents the principal physiological barrier that protects the CNS and separates it from surrounding connective tissue also has been considered to be of ectodermal origin (601, 1958). Thus the parenchyma of the CNS, the glia, the ependyma and the leptomeninges arise from ectoderm, while the blood vascular system and the dura mater are of mesodermal origin. As blood vessels enter and leave nervous tissue, they carry with them arachnoid and pia-glia which form a cuff around the vessel (Fig. 1-14). The space between the blood vessel and its "adventitial sheath" has been called the *Virchow-Robin space*. It was suggested that these spaces might permit the flow of cerebrospinal fluid from the subarachnoid spaces into the depths of the tissue. Electron microscopic studies indicate that as blood vessels penetrate neural tissue from the subarachnoid space, reflections of the intima pia and arachnoid which form the "adventitial sheath" are carried with it (1648, 1703). However in the central nervous system these two layers become continuous and there is no real space between them. Thus the concept that cerebrospinal fluid flows down to the smallest branches of the vascular tree is not

sustained. When the smallest veins and capillaries are reached no adventitial elements surround them. Only processes of astrocytes surround the basement membranes of the capillary endothelium (Fig. 1-15).

CEREBROSPINAL FLUID

The CSF is a clear, colorless liquid containing small amounts of protein, glucose and potassium and relatively large amounts of sodium chloride. There are no substances normally found in CSF which are not also found in blood plasma. No cellular component is found in CSF, although 1 to 5 cells/mm^3 are considered to be within normal limits. The CSF serves to support and cushion the central nervous system against trauma. The buoyancy of CSF is indicated by the fact that a brain weighing 1500 g in air weighs only 50 g when immersed in CSF (1502). Buoyancy reduces the momentum and acceleration of the brain when the cranium is suddenly displaced, thereby reducing concussive damage (1886). The CSF also removes waste products of neuronal metabolism, drugs and other substances which diffuse into brain from the blood. As the CSF streams over the ventricular and pial surfaces of the brain, it drains away solutes and carries them through the arachnoid villi into venous blood. In addition

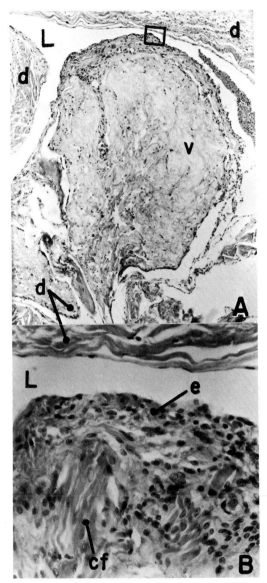

Figure 1-13. (*A*) Section of a human arachnoid granulation (*V*) in a lateral lacuna of a dural sinus (*L*). Relations of the dura (*d*) and area of enlargement are identified (×28). (*B*) Magnified area to demonstrate epithelial cap (*e*) and connective tissue fibers (*cf*) of granulation (Luxol-fast blue-cresyl violet stain, photograph, ×270).

some drugs such as penicillin and certain neurotransmitters like serotonin and norepinephrine are rapidly removed from the CSF by the choroid plexus (110). The 30% of the CSF derived from extrachoroidal sources may contribute to the bulk volume movement within normal brain parenchyma (2114). The CSF also plays an im-

portant role in integrating brain and peripheral endocrine functions in that hormones or hormone-releasing factors from the hypothalamus are secreted into the extracellular space or directly into the CSF. These hormones, which include hormone-releasing factors, are carried via CSF to the median eminence in the floor of the third ventricle, from which site they are transported by ependymal cells (i.e., tanycytes) into the hypophysial portal system (Figs. 16-12 and 16-13). The CSF also influences the microenvironment of neurons and glial cells because there is no diffusion barrier between CSF at either the ependymal lining of the ventricles or at the pia-glial membrane (2114). Changes in CSF calcium, potassium and magnesium ion concentrations may affect blood pressure, heart rate, vasomotor reflexes, respiration, muscle tone and the emotional state of animals (1469).

Because the brain is nearly incompressible within the cranium, the combined volumes of brain, CSF and intracranial blood must be maintained at a constant level. The volume of any one of these components can be increased only at the expense of one or both of the others. Any space-occupying lesion, such as a tumor or hematoma, usually results in an increase in CSF pressure. In the recumbent position the normal CSF pressure measured at the lumbar cistern is about 100 to 150 mm H_2O; in the sitting position the pressure measured at the same site varies between 200 and 300 mm H_2O.

The CSF has been regarded as an ultrafiltrate of the blood plasma because of their resemblance, except for huge differences in protein concentration (plasma, 6500 mg/100 g; CSF, 25 mg/100 g). Approximately 70% of the CSF is produced by secretion at the choroid plexus, located in the walls of the lateral ventricles and in the roof of the third and fourth ventricles (Figs. 1-11, 2-20 and 2-28). The remaining 30% of the CSF is derived from the capillary bed of the brain and metabolic water production (2030, 2114; 2246, 2259). Estimates of metabolic water production, based on the assumption of complete oxidation of glucose for a 1500-g human brain, suggests a net contribution of about 12% of the total CSF. Thus approximately 18% of the CSF is derived from extrachoroidal sources, presumable as a capillary ultrafiltrate. In man the total volume of CSF has been estimated to

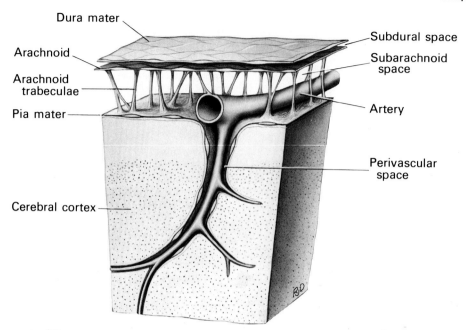

Dura mater

Arachnoid

Arachnoid
trabeculae

Pia mater

Cerebral cortex

Subdural space

Subarachnoid
space

Artery

Perivascular
space

Figure 1-14. Diagram of the meninges showing relationship of the membranes to the subarachnoid and perivascular spaces.

be about 140 ml of which 23 ml are contained within the ventricles (601). The net production of CSF in man has been estimated to be between 0.35 and 0.37 ml per minute which indicates the formation of over 400 ml per day (601, 2114). These data indicate a CSF turnover rate of 0.25% per minute (581). The CSF is formed at a hydrostatic pressure head of 15 ml of H_2O which is sufficient to drive it through the ventricular system and into the subarachnoid spaces surrounding the brain and spinal cord (601). Pulsations of the choroid plexus also probably contribute to the movement of CSF within the ventricular system.

The characteristic distribution of the number of ions and nonelectrolytes in CSF and plasma, however, is such that the CSF cannot be described as a simple filtrate or dialysate of the blood plasma. In general the CSF has higher Na^+, Cl^- and Mg^{2+} concentrations and lower K^+, Ca^{2+} and glucose concentrations than would be expected in a plasma dialysate. Finally the osmotic pressure relationships are not sufficient to produce a virtually protein-free fluid from the blood plasma (601).

The choroid plexus is a villous structure extending from the ventricular surface like coral fronds into the CSF. The plexus consists of a single layer of cuboidal epithelium with basal infoldings on the choroidal stroma and apical microvilli in contact with the CSF. The cuboidal epithelial cells of the plexus rest on a basement membrane enclosing an extensive capillary network embedded in a connective tissue stroma (see Fig. 1-18). The barrier to passive exchange of proteins and hydrophilic solutes between blood and CSF is not located in the choroidal capillaries. The capillaries are porous and have endothelial fenestrations. The barrier is formed by tight junctions surrounding and connecting apical regions of the epithelial cells (Figs. 1-18 and 5-19). Blood-borne horseradish peroxidase (HRP) passes through the capillary fenestrations and diffuses into the connective tissue stroma but does not pass beyond the tight junctions into the CSF (252). The choroid plexus regulates a large part of the production, as well as, the composition of the CSF. A Na^+-K^+ exchange pump, catalyzed by Na^+-K^+-ATPase, drives Na^+ toward the ventricular surface of the plexus and K^+ in the opposite direction. Thus the concentration of K^+ is lower and the concentration of Na^+ is higher in the choroidal secretion than in serum or in an ultrafiltrate of the

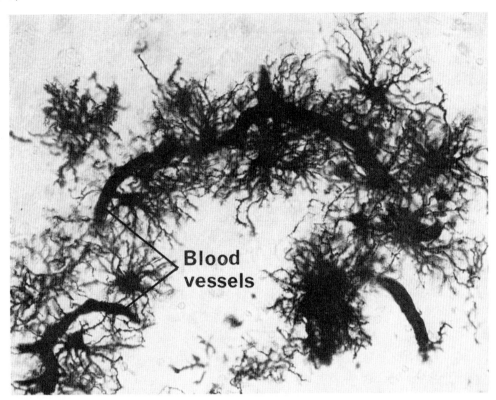

Figure 1-15. Astrocytes and perivascular processes on blood vessels in the human cerebral cortex (Golgi stain, ×450).

plasma (1711). These data suggest that K^+ is transported out of the CSF, while Na^+ is actively transported into it. The choroid plexus also plays a role in the regulation of Mg^{2+} and Ca^{2+} in the CSF. Fluid secreted by the choroid plexus contains a higher concentration of Mg^{2+} and a lower concentration of Ca^{2+} than does an ultrafiltrate of the plasma. Considerable controversy concerns the manner in which water, the largest constitutent of the CSF, moves across the choroidal eipthelium. The hypothesis based upon hydrostatic pressure is supported by data indicating that modifications of choroidal blood flow can increase or decrease the CSF secretion rate (2693). Approximately 25% of the volume of blood flowing to the choroid plexus normally is secreted as CSF. The other theory concerning the water content of the CSF suggests that water moves across the choroidal epithelium under a standing osmotic gradient established by the active transport of Na^+. This hypothesis is based upon the observation that movement of water into the

CSF is quantitatively coupled to the active transport of Na^+ (2606). Water secretion is reduced proportionally to the inhibition of the enzyme Na^+-K^+-ATPase which catalyzes the Na^+ pump.

CSF formed in the lateral and third ventricles passes via the cerebral aqueduct into the fourth ventricle. The fluid enters the cerebellomedullary cistern via the medial and lateral apertures of the fourth ventricle. From this site the fluid circulates in the subarachnoid spaces surrounding both the brain and the spinal cord. The bulk of the CSF is passively returned to the venous system via the arachnoid villi. The hydrodynamic permeability of the arachnoid villi is large compared with that of peripheral capillaries. Large protein molecules leave the CSF by passage through the arachnoid villi at roughly the same rate as smaller molecules. The rate of exit of CSF via the arachnoid villi is pressure-dependent and begins when CSF pressure exceeds venous pressure by 3 to 6 cm of water. The arachnoid villi serve as one-way valves. If the

CSF pressure is greater than venous pressure, the leaflike valves open and CSF enters the dural sinuses. When venous pressure exceeds CSF pressure, the valves close and blood cannot enter the CSF. Small amounts of CSF may be taken up by the ependyma, arachnoid capillaries and perivascular tissues.

An excessive amount of CSF produces an elevated pressure and in infants can cause hydrocephalus with enlargement of the ventricles, damage to neural tissue and changes in the neural cranium. Such increases in CSF may result from an overproduction of fluid, an obstruction to its flow or inadequate absorption. In most instances hydrocephalus results from obstruction within the ventricular system. Removal of the choroid plexus from one lateral ventricle usually causes that ventricle to collapse, while obstruction of one interventricular foramen causes dilatation of the ipsilateral lateral ventricle.

BARRIERS RELATED TO THE BRAIN

The functional capacity of all neurons of the brain and spinal cord is dependent upon the nature of the chemical milieu which surrounds them. To maintain the physiochemical composition of the microenvironment of neurons, axons and glia within the narrow limits of neuron survival requires a unique regulatory mechanism. The system that regulates the transport of chemical substances between arterial blood, the CSF and brain tissue is the blood-brain barrier, a series of regulatory interfaces between blood and the nervous system (601, 783, 2114). The blood-brain barrier separates the two major compartments of the central nervous system, the brain and the CSF, from a third compartment, the blood. The sites of the barrier are the interfaces between the blood and these two compartments of the CNS. These interfaces regulate diffusion at cerebral capillaries and the exchange of metabolites and metabolic products between blood and brain. Two separate barriers, a "blood-CSF barrier" and a "blood-brain barrier" have been distinquished in order to explain why intravascular substances enter the CSF and the brain at different rates (601). When substances, such as glucose or urea, are in-

jected intravascularly they diffuse rapidly and come to equilibrium with extracellular, or interstitial, fluids of most tissues. The observation that the transport of substances from the blood to the CSF requires hours instead of minutes gave rise to the concept of the blood-CSF barrier. Injections of certain dyes, such as trypan blue, into the blood stains most body tissue quickly but does not enter the CSF. Early studies indicated important differences between CSF and the interstitial fluid of most body tissues and further established that this barrier is not absolute, but selectively permeable. The kinetic aspects of the passage of substances from blood into brain are included under the term blood-brain barrier, by analogy with the blood-CSF barrier. The concept of the restriction of the passage of dissolved substances from blood to brain dates from the studies of Ehrlich (693) who demonstrated that intravenous injections of many vital dyes stained practically all body tissues, except the brain. These two barriers differ greatly in surface area. The surface area of the blood-brain barrier has been estimated to be 5000 times greater than that of the blood-CSF barrier (1939).

The brain barriers develop at the time when blood vessels invade the brain (953). Additional evidence suggests that the adult barriers react differently to the electrical charges of various vital dyes (102, 813). According to these authors the blood-brain barrier is more permeable to basic (positively charged) dyes, whereas the blood-CSF barrier is more permeable to acid (negatively charged) dyes. Such interfaces are structural and functional entities which dynamically control the transfer of chemical substances into and out of the three fluid compartments of the brain (i.e., extracellular (interstitial), intracellular and CSF).

The ependyma surfaces of the cerebral ventricles and the pia-glial membrane on the surface of the brain do not impede the exchange of substances between the CSF and brain and do not constitute a sub-barrier (2114). The walls of the cerebral ventricles and the spinal canal are lined by a single layer of epithelial cells whose cilia beat synchronously to cause local mixing of CSF. Ependymal cells are not connected by tight junctions and do not hinder macro-

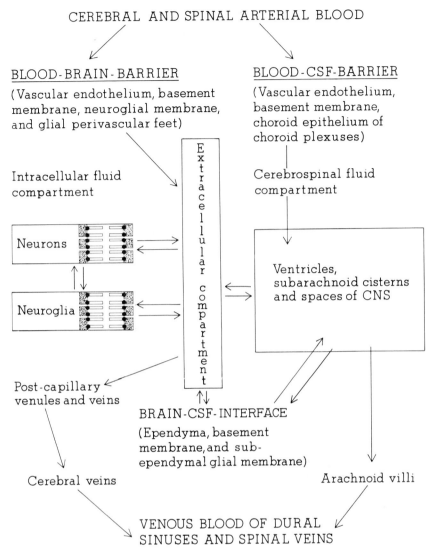

Figure 1-16. Schematic diagram of the blood-brain barrier, the blood-CSF barrier and the brain-CSF interface that separate the brain and CSF from the cerebral vascular compartment. The blood-brain barrier is a series of interfaces between arterial blood, CSF and neural tissue that regulate the transport of chemical substances. Tight junctions between endothelial cells (Fig. 1-17) of cerebral capillaries (the blood-brain barrier) and a paucity of pinocytosis restrict the passage of solutes from the blood into the extracellular compartment (i.e., interstitial fluid). The blood-CSF barrier is formed by tight junctions surrounding apical regions of the cuboidal epithelium of the choroid plexus (see Figs. 1-18 and 5-19). The brain-CSF interface, consisting of the ependymal lining of the cerebral ventricles and the pia-glial membrane on the external surface of the brain, does not impede the exchange of solutes between the CSF and the brain. The extracellular compartment has been estimated to constitute about 18% of wet brain weight (741).

molecular exchange between the CSF and the brain. Ferritin and HRP injected into CSF of the ventricles diffuse between ependyma cells and enter the extracellular space of the brain (249). In addition these tracers are found in pinocytotic vesicles within ependyma cells. Drugs injected into the cerebral ventricles easily cross the ependymal lining and produce immediate pharmacological and behavioral effects (739). A schematic diagram of relationships between the blood-brain barrier, the blood-CSF barrier and the brain-CSF interface is shown in Figure 1-16. Excellent reviews of the brain barriers consider this subject in depth (600–602, 783, 1703, 1939, 2114, 2283, 2562, 2585).

Blood-Brain Barrier. Arteries of the brain and spinal cord are invested with pia-arachnoid as they lie in the subarachnoid space (Fig. 1-14). The pia and subjacent glial membrane blend with the vessel wall before it penetrates into the substance of the brain or spinal cord. The smaller branches of the arterial tree, within the nervous tissue, have only thin neuroglial membrane investments which persist down to the capillary level. The capillary endothelium, its continuous and homogeneous basement membrane and the numerous processes of the astrocytes are all that separate the plasma in the vessel from the extracellular (i.e., interstitial) space within the central nervous system (Fig. 1-15). These are the structures that have been equated with the blood-brain barrier.

In all parts of the body the exchanges between blood and tissue take place in the capillary bed. The brain is no exception to this generalization, but there are some significant differences. A capillary is distinguished from an arteriole and a venule by the absence of a well defined muscular coat. The wall of a capillary consists only of flattened endothelial cells resting on a basement membrane surrounded by a thin adventitial layer made up of cells and fibers; these latter cells, referred to as *pericytes*, are often enclosed within parts of the basement membrane (601). Capillaries within the CNS contain a continuous inner layer of endothelial cells connected by tight junctions. Similar capillaries are found in the retina, the iris, the inner ear and within the endoneurium of peripheral nerves (2114). Tissue with capillaries of this type are derived totally or partially from neuroectoderm (1012, 1881). The morphological and enzymatic properties of capillaries in tissue derived from neuroectoderm are controlled by specific angiogenic substances released by neural tissue (774). When iris tissue is transplanted to brain it is vascularized with capillaries that do not contain monoamine oxidase or dopa-decarboxylase; embryonic brain tissue transplanted in the anterior chamber of the eye is vascularized from the iris but the capillaries contain these brain enzymes (2114). The tight junctions between endothelial cells of cerebral capillaries restrict intercellular diffusion (Fig. 1–17). The presence of high resistance tight junctions between adjacent brain endothelial cells and the paucity of pinocytosis or capillary fenestrations means that circulating substances in the cerebral vascular system can enter the brain only via: (a) carrier mediation or (b) lipid mediation (1939). The tight junctions that connect capillary endothelial cells in essence form a continuous cell layer that has the permeability properties of a plasma membrane. The basement membrane surrounds the endothelial cells and approximately 85% of its surface is covered by glial cells (1648). The tight junctions between endothelial cells prevent the transfer of La (OH)$_3$, microperoxidase, HRP and ferritin (251, 252, 2124). The capillary surface area in one g of brain has been estimated to be 240 cm^2 (569).

Cerebral blood vessels have neither a well-developed small pore system for diffusion nor a vesicular transport system. Pinocytotic vesicles are rare in endothelial cells of cerebral capillaries or venules, but are occasionally seen in arterioles. In addition endothelial cells of cerebral vessels do not contain contractile protein as seen in peripheral capillaries, and capillary permeability does not increase in response to histamine, serotonin or norepinephrine (2698). The capillary endothelial cells in the central nervous system are metabolically active with respect to both oxidative and hydrolytic enzymes. Enzymes within these cells regulate the transport of amines and amino acids. An example of this regulation is seen in Parkinson's disease (paralysis agitans) in which there is a deficiency of dopamine, a neurotransmitter synthesized in the substantia nigra and conveyed by axons to specific portions of the corpus striatum. Because dopamine cannot cross the blood-brain barrier, L-dopa is given to correct this metabolic defect. L-Dopa crosses the blood-brain barrier and is decarboxylated in the capillary endothelium to dopamine, a biogenic amine that is therapeutically effective (Fig. 1-17). Although it has been suggested that active transport mechanisms exist across cerebral capillaries, their precise role in active transport is difficult to distinguish from that of the choroid plexus.

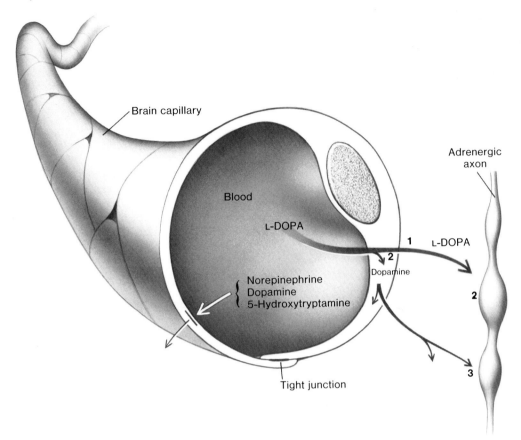

Figure 1-17. Diagrammatic drawing of a brain capillary demonstrating a tight junction between endothelial cells that constitute the blood-brain barrier. Endothelial cells of brain capillaries contain enzymes that regulate the specific transport of biogenic amines (norepinephrine, dopamine and 5-hydroxytryptamine) and amino acids. L-Dopa passes the blood-brain barrier (*1*), is decarboxylated to dopamine in the capillary endothelium (*2*) and enters neural tissue (*3*), where it is degraded by monamine oxidase. Decarboxylation of L-dopa to dopamine (2) also take place after its incorporation into axonal varicosities of aminergic neurons (2114).

Capillaries in skeletal and cardiac muscle contain endothelial cells separated by 10-nm clefts that provide a system of small pores for solute exchange. In addition, these capillaries have abundant pinocytotic vesicles for the transport of macromolecules and contain contractile protein (2114). Although tight junctions between endothelial cells are occasionally seen in muscle capillaries they are not uniformly present as in brain capillaries.

The blood-brain barrier in the central nervous system is not everywhere complete. In certain regions of the brain the continuous capillary endothelia are replaced by capillaries with fenestrated endothelia. These regions with capillary fenestrations provide specific sites for the transfer of proteins and solutes irrespective of molecular size and lipid solubility. Regions of the brain devoid of a blood-brain barrier include the pineal body, the neurohypophysis, the area postrema, the subfornical organ, the organum vasculosum of the lamina terminalis (or supraoptic crest) and the median eminence of the hypothalamus. All of these regions are highly vascular, and many are known or suspected of having a secretory function. Thus the blood-brain barrier, except in the special regions noted above, functions as a differential filter that permits the selective exchange of many substances from blood to the *extracellular compartment* (i.e., interstitial fluid). It appears to be impermeable to many substances (e.g., vital dyes).

Certain regions outside of the CNS have neural tissue in direct contact with the ex-

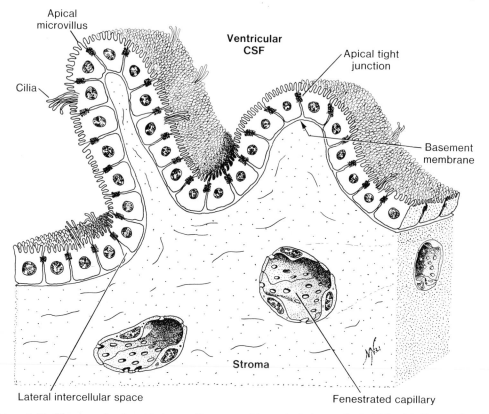

Apical
microvillus

Ventricular
CSF

Apical tight
junction

Cilia

Basement
membrane

Stroma

Lateral intercellular space

Fenestrated capillary

Figure 1-18. Diagram of a choroid plexus villus covered by a single layer of cuboidal epithelium with apical microvilli protruding into the ventricular CSF. The base of these cells rests upon a basement membrane. Tight junctions connecting apical regions of the epithelial cells constitute the blood-CSF barrier (see Fig. 5-19). The underlying connective tissue stroma contains capillaries with fenestrations.

tracellular fluid. Regions without an intervening barrier include: (a) the terminals of peripheral nerves, (b) sensory ganglia, (c) the olfactory epithelium and (d) the optic nerve where it penetrates the sclera (2114). The absence of a barrier at these sites represent loci where protein, including toxins and viruses, may enter the extracellular space.

Neurons and neuroglial cells comprise the *intracellular fluid compartment* of the brain (Fig. 1-16). Passage of substances into, and out of, glial cells and neurons takes place from the extracellular space through cell membranes. Estimates of the total extracellular space between neurons, neuroglia and capillaries of the brain vary widely. Electron micrographic studies suggest that neurons, neuroglial cells and their processes take up essentially all the available room except for a fairly constant space of 20 nm between adjacent cellular elements (617, 735, 2289). Neurochemical studies, on the other hand, assume that the

chloride ion is distributed mainly in the extracellular fluid and have used brain chloride as a measure of the extent of the extracellular volume in the brain. Such values for brain extracellular space range between 25 and 40% (700, 2766). More recent data suggest that the extracellular space equals approximately 18% of wet brain weight (741).

Blood-Cerebrospinal Fluid Barrier. The epithelium and adnexia of the choroid plexuses of the lateral, third and fourth ventricles actively secrete CSF (Fig. 1-16). Evidence that they are an effective barrier is attested to by the relatively higher concentration of sodium and chloride ions in CSF than in the plasma. In composition the CSF is the same as that of the interstitial fluid of the brain. The barrier to passive exchange of proteins and small hydrophilic solutes between blood and CSF is not at the choroidal capillaries. Capillaries of the choroid plexus have fenestrated endothelia that permit exchange of solutes (Fig. 1-18).

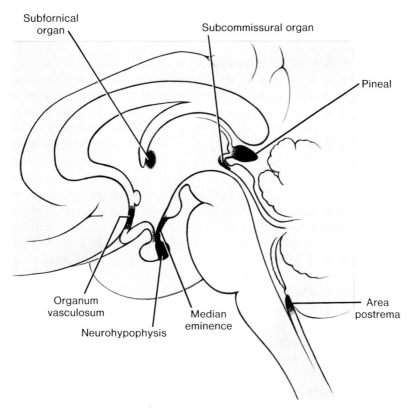

Figure 1-19. Drawing of a midsagittal section of the human brain indicating the locations of the circumventricular organs. All of these structures, except the *area postrema*, are unpaired, are situated in the midline and are related to diencephalic structures. All, except the *subcommissural organ*, are highly vascularized and lack a blood-brain barrier. Neuropeptides have limited transport across the blood-brain barrier but can enter and leave the brain, via the CSF, in regions of the circumventricular organs. The *organum vasculosum of the lamina terminalis* (OVLT) resembles the median eminence but its function has not yet been clarified; this structure, particularly prominent in rodents, is also designated as the supraoptic crest. The *median eminence* serves as a neuroendocrine transducer and the final common pathway by which releasing factors are discharged into the hypophysial portal system. (Modified from Weindl and Safroniew (2689).)

The blood-CSF barrier is located at tight junctions which surround and connect the cuboidal epithelial cells on the surface of the choroid plexus. Protein tracers like Evans blue-albumin injected intravascularly stain the stroma of the choroid plexus but do not enter the CSF. HRP passes through pores of choroidal capillaries to fill the connective tissue stroma but does not pass beyond the tight junctions which surround the apical regions of epithelial cells of the choroid plexus (252). The surface area of the blood-CSF barrier is only about 0.02% of the surface area of the blood-brain barrier (179). In spite of great quantitative differences in surface area, it is probable that some circulating substances enter the brain via the blood-CSF barrier (1939). Available evidence suggests that some circulating peptides (e.g., insulin) and plasma

proteins (e.g., prealbumin) may be selectively transported into the CSF via the blood-CSF barrier. The ependymal surface of the cerebral ventricles and the pia-glial membrane on the surface of the brain do not impede exchanges between the CSF and the brain. Molecules with a relatively high plasma/CSF ratio (compared with inulin) are transported cross the blood-CSF barrier in a selective and limited fashion.

Circumventricular Organs. The circumventricular organs are areas of specialized tissue located at strategic positions in the midline ventricular system (Fig. 1-19). Included under this designation are the following: (a) the subfornical organ, (b) the organum vasculosum of the lamina terminalis, (or supraoptic crest), (c) the median eminence, (d) the neurohypophysis, (e) the pineal, (f) the subcommissural organ and

(g) the area postrema (32, 1677, 2689). With the exception of the area postrema, located along the caudal margins of the fourth ventricle (Figs. 1–19 and 11–12), all of these structures are unpaired and all occupy midline positions related to portions of the diencephalon. All of these structures, except the subcommissural organ, are highly vascularized and contain fenestrated capillary loops surrounded by perivascular connective tissue spaces. The circumventricular organs, with the exception of the subcommissural organ, lack a blood-brain barrier. The absence of this barrier, demonstrated by permeability to horseradish peroxidase, suggests that these tissues are permeable to proteins and peptides.

The *neurohypophysis* is a well known target of various peptidergic neuroendocrine neurons. Fibers from the magnocellular hypothalamic nuclei terminate in the neural lobe of the hypophysis around fenestrated capillaries. These terminal fibers contain neurophysin, vasopressin and oxytocin, which are stored and released into the general circulation from the neural lobe of the hypophysis. The *organum vasculosum of the lamina terminalis* (OVLT) appears to be a vascular outlet for luteinizing hormone releasing hormone (LHRH) and somatostatin, which inhibits the release of somatotropin (growth hormone) (2689). The OVLT may serve not only as a neurohemal outlet for hypothalamic peptides, but may also serve a hemo-neural function whereby certain peptides, proteins and amines in the blood are sensed by neurons with receptor properties. The *median eminence*, recognized as a circumventricular organ, serves as a neuroendocrine transducer that translates bioelectrical activity in the central nervous system into blood-borne signals in the form of releasing factors (2302). The final common pathway of neuroendocrine control of the anterior pituitary by the hypothalamus has been postulated to be a pool of neurosecretory neurons whose axons terminate upon fenestrated portal capillaries in the median eminence and discharge releasing factors into the hypophysial portal system (Fig. 16-12) (1338). The *subfornical organ*, located between the interventricular forminia, has connections with the choroid plexus and its vascular permeability suggests that it may regulate body fluids (2469, 2689). The *pin-*

eal body contains specialized cells known as pinealocytes and produces melatonin under the influence of light deprivation (see p. 497). The *subcommissural organ* (SCO) is located beneath the posterior commissure at the junction of the third ventricle and the cerebral aqueduct (Fig. 13-13). Cells of SCO are not highly vascularized, but secrete a mucopolysaccharide into the CSF which forms filaments that converge as Reissner's fiber. This curious fiber can be traced from the cerebral aqueduct through the fourth ventricle to the caudal end of the central canal of the spinal cord. The function of this structure is unknown. The *area postrema* located at the junction of fourth ventricle and spinal canal has a structure similar to that of the subfornical organ (Fig. 11-12). It is surrounded by fields of terminal fibers containing neurophysin, oxytocin and vasopressin, although none of these peptides can be identified within the area postrema. The area postrema is considered a chemoreceptor that triggers vomiting in response to circulating emetic substances (i.e., apomorphine and digitalis glycosides) (218, 219).

Recent evidence of the widespread distribution of peptides in the CNS suggests that the CSF may be a conduit by which these substances modulate neuronal function in different regions of the brain (1195). Although neural peptides have limited access to the CNS across the blood-brain barrier, in the circumventricular organs hypothalamic hormones have been detected in high concentrations. The peptides which have been identified in the CSF include: (a) thyroid releasing hormone, (b) luteinizing hormone releasing hormone, (c) somatostatin, (d) opioid peptides, (e) cholecystokinin, (f) angiotensin II, (g) substance P, (h) adenohypophysial hormones and (i) neurohypophysial hormones. There is some evidence that neural peptides in the CSF may be altered by neurological disease. These data raise the interesting possibility that measurements of neural peptides in the CSF might provide a sensitive "marker" for the anatomical localization of pathological processes in specific regions of the CNS (1195).

Blood-Brain Barrier in the Newborn. It has been suggested that the blood-brain barrier in the fetus and newborn is immature because blood-borne dyes stain these brains more extensively than adult brains (103, 742). Electron microscopic evidence indicates that tight junctions surrounding epithelial cells of the choroid plexus of the rat at early developmental stages do not differ qualitatively from the adult (1938). However, the water content of the cerebral cortex and white matter of the brain of the rhesus monkey progressively diminishes during fetal development and postpartum maturation (2307). An expanded extracellular space in the brains of the newborn appears to provide a greater volume for the distribution of extracellular markers (e.g., inulin). This increased extracellular space appears to account for the observation that trypan blue given intravenously stains the brain of an immature animal. Although the dye enters the brain only at the nonbarrier sites, it extends further in the extracellular space than in the mature brain (144, 145).

Unconjugated bilirubin, a breakdown product of hemoglobin, can stain the brain of the newborn if severe jaundice results from accelerated destruction of red cells, as occurs in erythroblastosis fetalis associated with Rh incompatibility. This condition, known as *kernicterus*, results in a yellow staining of the brain, especially the nuclei of the corpus striatum. Unconjugated bilirubin is very lipid-soluble and crosses the lipoid membranes of capillary endothelia in both the adult and immature brain. In the adult bilirubin is bound to serum albumin and does not enter the brain. The immature liver of the neonate cannot conjugate large quantities of bilirubin and unconjugated bilirubin passes the blood-brain barrier to stain the brain nuclei yellow (2114). The mortality in kernicterus is high and infants that survive have a high incidence of motor disorders and mental retardation (1670).

CHAPTER 2

Gross Anatomy of the Brain

The nervous system is composed of two parts, the central nervous system and the peripheral nervous system. The *peripheral nervous system* consists of the spinal and cranial nerves, while the *central nervous system* is represented by the brain and spinal cord. The autonomic nervous system, often considered as a separate functional entity, is part central and part peripheral.

The human brain is a relatively small structure weighing about 1400 g and constituting about 2% of the total body weight. The brain is regarded as the organ solely concerned with thought, memory and consciousness, but these are only a few of its complex and varied functions; there are many others. All information we have concerning the world about us is conveyed centrally to the brain by an elaborate sensory system. Receptors of many kinds act as transducers which change physical and chemical stimuli in our environment into nerve impulses which the brain can read and give meaning to. The ability to discriminate between stimuli of the same and different types forms one of the bases for learning. Attention, consciousness, emotional experience and sleep are all central neural functions. Such higher functions as memory, imagination, thought and creative ability are poorly understood but must be related to complex neuronal activity. The brain is also concerned with all kinds of motor activity, with the regulation of visceral, endocrine and somatic functions and with the receptive and expressive use of symbols and signs that underlie communication. While the gross features of the human brain are not especially impressive, its versatility, potential capabilities, efficiency and self-programming nature put it in a class beyond any "electronic brain."

The brain consists of three basic subdi-

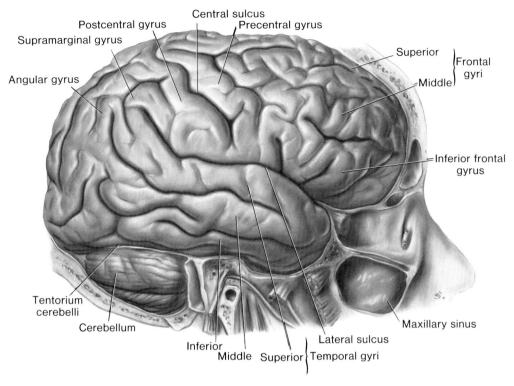

Supramarginal gyrus
Postcentral gyrus
Central sulcus
Precentral gyrus
Superior
Frontal gyri
Middle
Angular gyrus
Inferior frontal gyrus
Tentorium cerebelli
Cerebellum
Maxillary sinus
Inferior
Middle
Superior
Lateral sulcus
Temporal gyri

Figure 2-1. Lateral view of the brain exposed in the skull to show topographical relationships. (Reproduced with permission from F. A. Mettler: *Neuroanatomy*, Ed. 2, The C. V. Mosby Co., St. Louis, 1948.)

visions, the cerebral hemispheres, the brain stem, and the cerebellum (Figs. 2-1–2-3, 2-8, 2-24–2-26 and 2-29). The massive paired *cerebral hemispheres* are derived from the *telencephalon*, the most rostral cerebral vesicle. The brain stem consists of four distinct parts: (a) the *diencephalon*, (b) the *mesencephalon*, (c) the *metencephalon* and (d) the *myelencephalon*. The diencephalon, the most rostral brain stem segment (Figs. 2-24 and 2-25) is the part of the brain stem most intimately related to the forebrain (i.e., telencephalon). The mesencephalon, or midbrain, is the smallest and least differentiated division of the brain stem. The metencephalon (pons) and myelencephalon (medulla) together constitute the *rhombencephalon* or hindbrain. The cerebellum is a derivative of the metencephalon that develops from ectodermal thickenings about the rostral borders of the fourth ventricle, known as the rhombic lip (Figs. 2-26, 2-29, 2-30, 3-11*A* and 3-14).

THE CEREBRAL HEMISPHERES

The paired cerebral hemispheres are mirror image duplicates consisting of a highly convoluted gray cortex (pallium), an underlying white matter of considerable magnitude and a collection of deeply located neuronal masses, known as the basal ganglia (Figs. 2-3–2-6, 2-8 and 2-9). The cerebral hemispheres are partially separated from each other by the *longitudinal fissure*. This fissure *in situ* contains the falx cerebri (Fig. 1-2). In frontal and occipital regions the separation of the hemispheres is complete, but in the central region the fissure extends only to fibers of the broad interhemispheric commissure, the corpus callosum (Figs. 2-3–2-6, 2-8 and 2-9). Each cerebral hemisphere is subdivided into lobes by various sulci (Figs. 2-1–2-3). The major lobes of the brain are named for the bones of the skull overlying them. Although the boundaries of the various lobes as seen in the gross

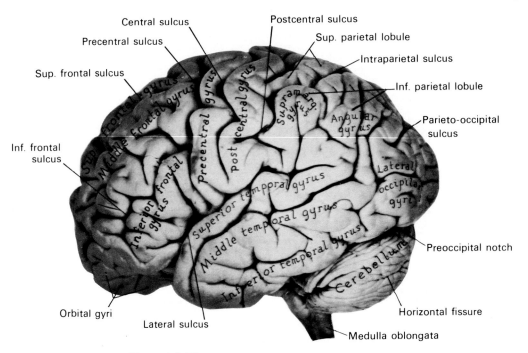

Figure 2-2. Photograph of the lateral surface of the brain.

specimen are somewhat arbitrary, multiple cortical areas in each lobe are histologically distinctive. The gray cellular mantle of the cerebral cortex in man is highly convoluted. The crest of a single convolution is referred to as a *gyrus; sulci* separate the various gyri, producing a pattern with more or less constant features. On the basis of the more constant sulci and gyri, the cerebrum is divided into six so-called lobes: (a) frontal, (b) temporal, (c) parietal, (d) occipital, (e) insular and (f) limbic. Neither the insula nor the limbic lobe is a true lobe. The insula is a cortical area buried in the depths of the lateral sulcus (Figs. 2-7, 2-9, 2-10 and 2-13). The limbic lobe is a synthetic lobe on the medial aspect of the hemisphere consisting of portions of the frontal, parietal, occipital and temporal lobes which surround the upper part of the brain stem (Fig. 18-17).

Lateral Surface

The two most important sulci for topographical orientation on the lateral convexity of the hemisphere are the lateral and central sulci (Figs. 2-1 and 2-2). The *lateral sulcus* begins inferiorly in the Sylvian fossa and extends posteriorly, separating the frontal and temporal lobes. Caudally this sulcus separates portions of the parietal and temporal lobes. The terminal ascending ramus of the sulcus extends into the inferior part of the parietal lobe. Portions of the frontal, parietal and temporal lobes, adjacent to the lateral sulcus, which overlie the insular region are referred to as the *opercular portions* of these lobes (Fig. 2-7). The *central sulcus* is a prominent sulcus running from the superior margin of the hemisphere downward and forward toward the lateral sulcus (Figs. 2-1 and 2-2). Usually this sulcus is bowed in two locations and superiorly it does not extend onto the medial surface of the hemisphere for any distance. The depths of the sulcus constitute the boundary between the frontal and parietal lobes.

Frontal Lobe. This, the largest of all the lobes of the brain, comprises about one-third of the hemispheric surface. The frontal lobe extends rostrally from the central sulcus to the frontal pole; its inferior lateral boundary is the lateral sulcus. The convexity of the frontal lobe has four principal convolutions: (a) a *precentral* gyrus that

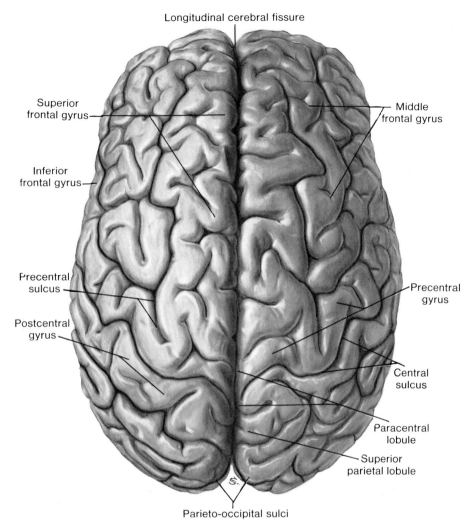

Longitudinal cerebral fissure

Superior
frontal gyrus

Middle
frontal gyrus

Inferior
frontal gyrus

Precentral
sulcus

Precentral
gyrus

Postcentral
gyrus

Central
sulcus

Paracentral
lobule

Superior
parietal lobule

Parieto-occipital sulci

Figure 2-3. Superior view of the brain indicating the main sulci and gyri. (Reproduced with permission from F. A. Mettler: *Neuroanatomy*, Ed. 2, The C. V. Mosby Co., St. Louis, 1948.)

parallels the central sulcus and (b) three horizontally oriented convolutions, the *superior, middle* and *inferior frontal gyri* (Figs. 2-1 and 2-2). The anterior boundary of the precentral gyrus is the *precentral sulcus*, which extends onto the medial surface of the hemisphere. The precentral gyrus and the anterior bank of the central sulcus comprise the *primary motor area*, where all parts of the body are represented in a distorted but topographical manner (Fig. 19-12). Regions of the frontal lobe rostral to the primary motor area are referred to as *premotor* and *prefrontal* areas. The broad middle frontal gyrus often is

divided by a shallow horizontal sulcus into upper and lower tiers (Figs. 2-1 and 2-2). The inferior frontal gyrus is divided by anterior ascending rami of the lateral sulcus into three parts: (a) *pars orbitale,* (b) *pars triangularis* and (c) *pars opercularis.* The pars triangularis and opercularis in the dominant hemisphere (usually the left in right-handed individuals) are referred to as *Broca's speech area,* a region concerned with the motor mechanisms of speech formulation.

The inferior surface of the frontal lobe lies on the superior surface of the orbital part of the frontal bone and is concave

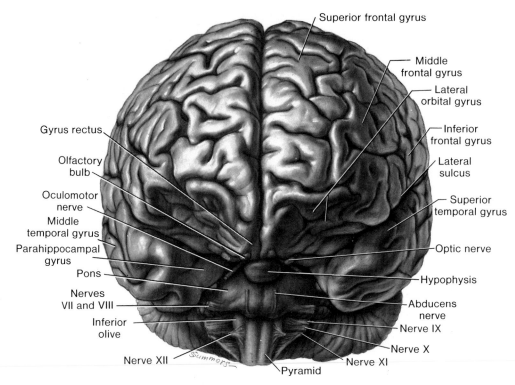

Superior frontal gyrus

Middle frontal gyrus

Lateral orbital gyrus

Gyrus rectus

Inferior frontal gyrus

Olfactory bulb

Lateral sulcus

Oculomotor nerve

Middle temporal gyrus

Superior temporal gyrus

Parahippocampal gyrus

Optic nerve

Pons

Hypophysis

Nerves VII and VIII

Abducens nerve

Inferior olive

Nerve IX

Nerve X

Nerve XII

Nerve XI

Pyramid

Figure 2-4. Frontal view of the rostral aspect of the brain. (Reproduced with permission from F. A.Mettler: *Neuroanatomy*, Ed. 2, The C. V. Mosby Co., St. Louis, 1948).

(Figs. 2-4, 2-8 and 2-9). The olfactory bulb and tract lie in a sulcus near the medial margin of the hemisphere known as the *olfactory sulcus*. The *gyrus rectus* lies medial to the olfactory sulcus and the medial orbital gyrus lies lateral to this sulcus. The orbital gyri occupy the concave lateral area.

Parietal Lobe. The boundaries of the parietal lobe are not precise, except for its anterior border on the lateral convexity formed by the central sulcus, and its posterior border on the medial aspect of the hemisphere (*parieto-occipital sulcus*) (Figs. 2-2 and 2-5). On the convexity of the hemisphere the posterior boundary is arbitrarily considered as an imaginary line projected from the superior limit of the parieto-occipital sulcus to the small indentation on the inferior surface known as the *preoccipital notch* (Fig. 2-2). Three parts of the parietal lobe are distinguished: (a) a *postcentral gyrus* running parallel and caudal to the central sulcus, (b) a *superior parietal lobule* and (c) an *inferior parietal lobule*. The postcentral gyrus, usually not continuous, but broken up into superior and inferior segments, lies between the central and postcentral sulci. The *postcentral sulcus* extends over the superior margin of the hemisphere and demarcates the caudal limit of the paracentral lobule (Fig. 2-5). The posterior bank of the central sulcus and the postcentral gyrus constitute the *primary somesthetic area*, the cortical region where impulses concerned with tactile and kinesthetic sense from superficial and deep receptors converge and are somatotopically represented. The majority of cortical neurons in the postcentral gyrus are concerned with fixed receptive fields on the contralateral side of the body that are place-specific, modality-specific and related to discriminative aspects of sensation. The *intraparietal sulcus*, a horizontally oriented sulcus, divides portions of the parietal lobe caudal to the postcentral gyrus into superior and inferior parietal lobules (Fig. 2-2). The *inferior parietal lobule* consists of two gyri, the *supramarginal*, about both banks of an ascending ramus of the lateral

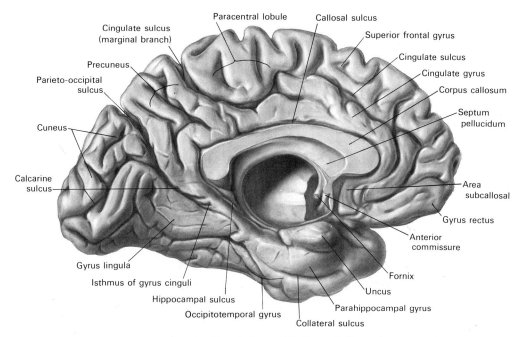

Figure 2-5. Medial surface of the cerebral hemisphere with diencephalic structures removed. (Reproduced with permission from F. A. Mettler: *Neuroanatomy,* Ed. 2, The C. V. Mosby Co., St. Louis, 1948.)

sulcus, and the *angular,* which surrounds the ascending terminal part of the superior temporal sulcus (Figs. 2-1 and 2-2). The inferior parietal lobule represents a cortical association area where various multisensory perceptions of a higher order from adjacent parietal, temporal and occipital regions overlap. This region is especially concerned with mnemonic constellations that form the basis for understanding and interpreting sensory signals. This is one region of the cortex where different disturbances occur as a consequence of lesions in the dominant and nondominant hemisphere.

Temporal Lobe. This large lobe lies ventral to the lateral sulcus and on its lateral surface displays three obliquely oriented convolutions, the *superior, middle* and *inferior temporal gyri* (Figs. 2-1 and 2-2). The *superior temporal sulcus* courses parallel with the lateral sulcus and its ascending ramus terminates in the angular gyrus. On the inner bank of the lateral sulcus several short, oblique convolutions form the transverse gyri of Heschl; these gyri constitute the *primary auditory cortex* in man (Figs. 2-7 and 2-10). The inferior

surface of the temporal lobe which lies in the middle fossa of the skull reveals part of the *inferior temporal gyrus,* the broad *occipitotemporal gyrus* and the *parahippocampal gyrus* (Figs. 2-8 and 2-9). The parahippocampal gyrus and its most medial protrusion, the *uncus,* are separated from the occipitotemporal gyrus by the collateral sulcus (Fig. 2-5). The rostral part of the parahippocampal gyrus, the uncus and the lateral olfactory stria constitute the pyriform lobe, parts of which constitute the *primary olfactory cortex* (Figs. 2-5, 2-8 and 2-9).

Occipital Lobe. The small occipital lobe rests on the tentorium cerebelli (Figs. 2-1 and 2-6). The rostral boundary of this lobe is the parieto-occipital sulcus on the medial aspect of the hemisphere (Fig. 2-5). The lateral surface of the occipital lobe is poorly delimited from the parietal lobe and is composed of a number of irregular *lateral occipital gyri* which are separated into groups by the *lateral occipital sulcus.* (Figs. 2-2 and 2-6).

On the medial aspect of the hemisphere the occipital lobe is divided by the *calcarine sulcus* into the cuneus and the *lingual*

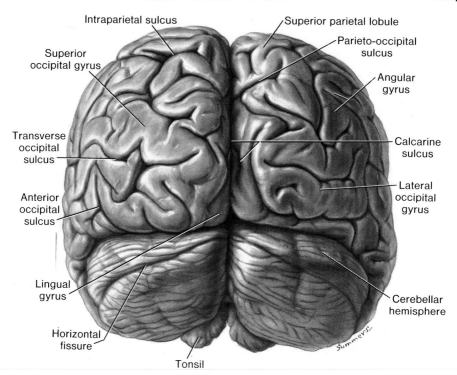

Figure 2-6. Posterior view of the cerebral hemispheres and cerebellum. (Reproduced with permission from F. A. Mettler: *Neuroanatomy*, Ed. 2, The C. V. Mosby Co., St. Louis, 1948.)

gyrus (Figs. 2-5 and 2-6). The calcarine sulcus joints the parieto-occipital sulcus rostrally in a Y-shaped formation. The cortex on both banks of the calcarine sulcus represents the *primary visual cortex* (i.e., striate). The visual cortex in each hemisphere receives impulses from the temporal half of the ipsilateral retina and the nasal half of the contralateral retina and is concerned with perception from the contralateral half of the visual field.

The Insula. This cortical area lies buried in the depths of the lateral sulcus and can be seen only when the temporal and frontal lobes are separated. This so-called lobe is a triangular cortical area, the apex of which is directed forward and downward to open into the lateral fossa (Figs. 2-7, 2-10 and 2-13). The surface is covered by the *gyri breves* and *longus* which course nearly parallel to the lateral sulcus. The relationships of this region can be appreciated in transverse and horizontal sections of the hemisphere (Figs. 2-12–2-15). The opening leading to the insular region is called the *limen*

insula. The temporal, frontal, and parietal opercular regions cover the insula.

Medial Surface

In a hemisected brain convolutions on the medial surface can be studied. The convolutions on the medial surface of the hemisphere are somewhat flatter than those on the convexity. The most prominent structure on the medial surface is the massive interhemispheric commissure, the *corpus callosum* (Figs. 2-5, 2-10, 2-19, 2-21 and 2-27). This structure, composed of myelinated fibers, reciprocally interconnects broad regions of the two hemispheres. Different parts of the corpus callosum are referred to as the *rostrum, genu, body* and *splenium* (Figs. 2-10 and 2-19). Fibers in this structure spread out as a mass of radiations to nearly all parts of the cortex. Callosal fibers, projecting to parts of the frontal and occipital lobes, form the so-called *anterior* and *posterior forceps*, which are best appreciated in horizontal sections of the brain (Fig. 2-10). The corpus callosum

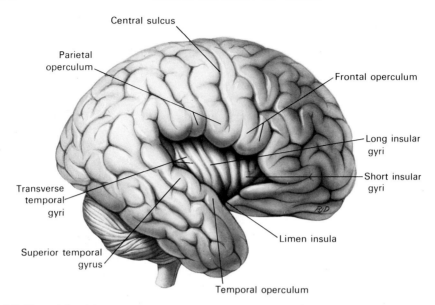

Figure 2-7. View of the right cerebral hemisphere with the banks of the lateral sulcus drawn apart to expose the insula.

forms the floor of the longitudinal fissure, as well as a good part of the roof of the lateral venticle. The corpus callosum plays an important role in interhemispheric transfer of learned discriminations, sensory experience and memory. Although surgical section of the corpus callosum in man produces little disturbance of ordinary behavior, temperament or intellect, information received exclusively by the nondominant hemisphere (usually the right) cannot be communicated in speech or writing (856–858). In these same patients there was no impairment of speech or writing when information was processed in the dominant hemisphere (left). These studies conclude that linguistic expression and analytical functions are organized almost exclusively in the dominant hemisphere. The nondominant hemisphere is concerned with spatial concepts, recognition of faces and some musical ability.

The *callosal sulcus* separates the corpus callosum from the cingulate gyrus; posteriorly this sulcus curves around the splenium to be continued into the temporal lobe as the *hippocampal sulcus* (Fig. 2-5). The *cingulate gyrus*, dorsal to the callosal sulcus, encircles the corpus callosum and consists of two tiers. The *cingulate sulcus*, dorsal to the cingulate gyrus, runs parallel to the callosal sulcus, but near the splenium turns dorsally as the *marginal sulcus*. The anterior portion of cortex dorsal to the cingulate gyrus is the medial surface of the superior frontal gyrus. The *paracentral lobule* is formed by the precentral and postcentral gyri which extend onto the medial surface of the hemisphere, and is notched by the central sulcus (Fig. 2-5). The *paracentral sulcus*, continuous with the precentral sulcus, forms the rostral border of this lobule, while the *marginal sulcus*, continuous with the postcentral gyrus, forms the caudal border. The portion of the parietal lobe caudal to the paracentral lobule is known as the *precuneus*; this lobule lies immediately rostral to the parieto-occipital sulcus previously discussed.

Limbic Lobe. This is a synthetic lobe, consisting of large cortical convolutions on the medial aspect of the hemisphere which surround the rostral part of the brain stem and the interhemispheric commissure (Fig. 18-17). According to Broca (257) the limbic lobe includes the *subcallosal, cingulate* and *parahippocampal gyri*, as well as primitive cortical derivatives, the *hippocampal formation* and the *dentate gyrus*, which in the course of development have become invaginated within the temporal lobe (Fig. 2-9). The parahippocampal gyrus is directly

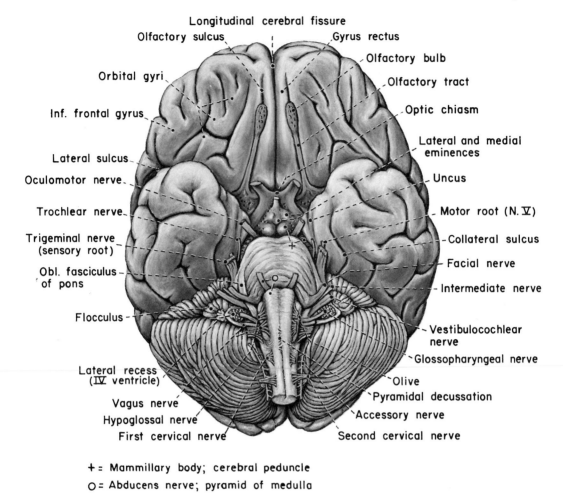

Longitudinal cerebral fissure
Olfactory sulcus
Gyrus rectus
Olfactory bulb
Orbital gyri
Olfactory tract
Inf. frontal gyrus
Optic chiasm
Lateral and medial eminences
Lateral sulcus
Oculomotor nerve
Uncus
Trochlear nerve
Motor root (N. Ⅴ)
Trigeminal nerve (sensory root)
Collateral sulcus
Obl. fasciculus of pons
Facial nerve
Intermediate nerve
Flocculus
Vestibulocochlear nerve
Glossopharyngeal nerve
Lateral recess (Ⅳ ventricle)
Olive
Pyramidal decussation
Vagus nerve
Hypoglossal nerve
Accessory nerve
First cervical nerve
Second cervical nerve

+ = Mammillary body; cerebral peduncle

O = Abducens nerve; pyramid of medulla

Figure 2-8. Inferior surface of the brain showing the cranial nerves. (Reproduced with permission from R. C. Truex and C. E. Kellner: *Detailed Atlas of the Head and Neck.* Oxford University Press, New York, 1948.)

continuous with the cingulate gyrus by a narrow strip of cortex, posterior and inferior to the splenium, known as the *isthmus of the cingulate gyrus* (Fig. 2-5). The parahippocampal gyrus, the most medial convolution of the temporal lobe, is bounded laterally by the *rhinal* and *collateral sulci* and superiorly and medially by the *hippocampal sulcus* (Figs. 2-8 and 2-9). Rostrally the parahippocampal gyrus hooks around the hippocampal sulcus to form a medially protruding convolution, the *uncus.* The proximity of the uncus to the cerebral peduncle should be noted.

There are differences of opinion concerning what should be lumped together as the so-called "limbic lobe" (270). While all of these structures appear early in phylogenesis, physiological evidence suggests that wide functional differences exist between various components and separate functions are expressed by distinctive neural mechanisms.

The Inferior Surface

The inferior surface of the hemisphere consists of two parts: (a) a larger posterior portion, representing the inferior surfaces of the temporal and occipital lobes, and (b) the orbital surface of the frontal lobe (Figs. 2-4, 2-8 and 2-9). The inferior surface of the occipital lobe and the posterior part of the temporal lobe lie on the tentorium cerebelli (Figs. 1-2 and 2-1), while rostral parts of the

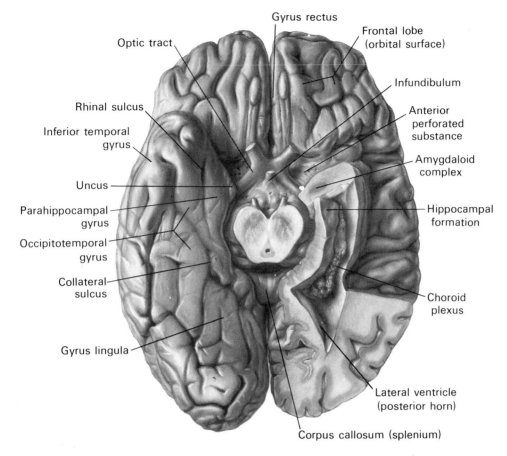

Figure 2-9. View of the inferior surface of the brain following transection of the midbrain. The inferior and posterior horns of the left lateral ventricle have been opened and portions of the temporal and occipital lobes have been removed. (Reproduced with permission from F. A. Mettler: *Neuroanatomy*, Ed. 2, The C. V. Mosby Co., St. Louis, 1948.)

temporal lobe lie in the middle cranial fossa. Gyri present in this posterior part include: (a) the lingual gyrus, (b) the extensive occipitotemporal gyrus and (c) the parahippocampal gyrus and uncus (Fig. 2-9). Part of the inferior temporal gyrus may be seen lateral to the occipito-temporal gyrus. A small part of the isthmus lies medially posterior to the splenium of the corpus callosum (Fig. 2-5).

The orbital surface of the frontal lobe has a deep, straight sulcus medially, the olfactory sulcus, which contains both the olfactory bulb and tract (Figs. 2-4, 2-8 and 2-9). The *gyrus rectus* lies along the ventromedial margin of the hemisphere medial to the olfactory sulcus. The region lateral to the olfactory sulcus contains the orbital gyri whose convolutional patterns are vari-

able (Figs. 2-4 and 2-9). Posteriorly to the olfactory tract divides into *medial* and *lateral olfactory striae* (Figs. 2-8 and 2-9). Caudal to this is the olfactory trigone and the *anterior perforated substance*, a region studded with small openings through which numerous small blood vessels pass to deep regions (Figs. 2-8, 2-9, 2-23 and 20-10).

The White Matter

The massive white matter of the cerebral hemisphere forms the medullary core of the cortical convolutions and contains basically three types of fibers in prodigious quantity. Fibers within the white matter are classified as: (a) *projection fibers* that convey impulses either from the cortex to distant loci, or from distant loci to the cortex, (b) *association fibers* that interconnect various

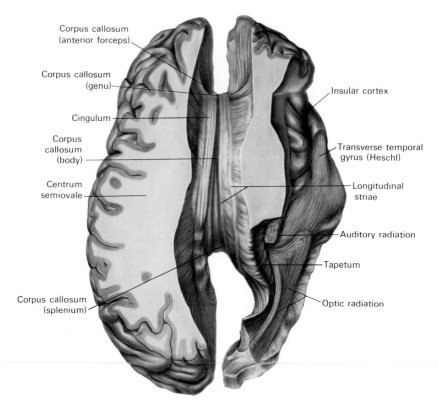

Corpus callosum
(anterior forceps)

Corpus callosum
(genu)

Cingulum

Corpus
callosum
(body)

Centrum
semiovale

Corpus callosum
(splenium)

Insular cortex

Transverse temporal
gyrus (Heschl)

Longitudinal
striae

Auditory radiation

Tapetum

Optic radiation

Figure 2-10. Dissection of the superior surface of the hemispheres exposing the corpus callosum, cingulum, longitudinal striae and the optic and auditory radiations. (Reproduced with permission from F. A. Mettler: *Neuroanatomy*, Ed. 2, The C. V. Mosby Co., St. Louis, 1948.)

cortical regions of the same hemisphere and (c) *commissural fibers* that interconnect corresponding cortical regions of the two hemispheres. The white matter extends from the cortex to the basal ganglia and the ventricular system. The common central mass of the white matter, containing commissural, association and projection fibers, has an oval appearance in horizontal sections of the brain and is termed the *semioval center* (Fig. 2-10).

Projection Fibers. Afferent and efferent fibers conveying impulses to and from the entire cerebral cortex enter the white matter and are arranged as radiating bundles that converge toward the brain stem (Figs. 2-11 and 2-18). These radiating projection fibers are known as the *corona radiata*. Near the upper part of the brain stem these fibers form a compact band known as the *internal capsule*, which is flanked medially and laterally by nuclear masses (Figs. 2-12, 2-14, 2-15 and 2-18). Two

distinct parts of the internal capsule are evident in horizontal sections of the hemispheres: (a) an anterior limb and (b) a posterior limb (Fig. 2-12). The *anterior limb* of the internal capsule partially separates two of the largest components of the basal ganglia, the caudate nucleus and the putamen (Figs. 2-12, 2-13 and 2-14). Fibers in the anterior limb of the internal capsule are directed horizontally, obliquely, laterally and upwards toward the frontal lobe, and in horizontal sections of the hemisphere appear to be cut in the longitudinal axis of the fiber bundles (Figs. 2-11, 2-12, 2-13 and 2-18). In horizontal sections of the hemisphere the anterior and posterior limbs of the internal capsule meet at an obtuse angle with the apex directed medially. The larger and longer *posterior limb* of the internal capsule is flanked medially by the diencephalon and laterally by a part of the basal ganglia known as the lentiform nucleus (Figs. 2-12, 2-15 and 2-18). The

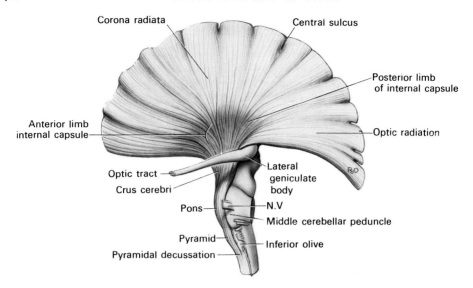

Figure 2-11. Drawing of a dissection demonstrating the continuity and relationships of the corona radiata, the internal capsule, the crus cerebri and the medullary pyramid.

region of junction between the anterior and posterior limbs of the internal capsule is referred to as the *genu*. Fibers in the posterior limb of the internal capsule course in nearly a vertical plane toward the brain stem, and in horizontal sections fibers appear to be cut transversely (Fig. 2-12). The most posterior component of the posterior limb of the internal capsule contains fibers, radiating toward the calcarine sulcus, known as the *optic radiation* (Figs. 2-10, 2-11, 2-18 and 2-35). Afferent fibers in the internal capsule arise mainly from the thalamus and project to nearly all regions of the cortex; these fibers are referred to as *thalamocortical radiations* (Fig. 2-18). Efferent fibers in the internal capsule arise from cells in various regions of the cerebral cortex and project to specific nuclear masses in the brain stem and spinal cord. These fibers are categorized as corticothalamic, corticopontine, corticobulbar and corticospinal. Cortical fibers projecting to the brain stem and spinal cord traverse the internal capsule and enter the crus cerebri, its equivalent at midbrain levels (Figs. 2-11, 2-13, 2-23 and 2-25). The continuity of projection fibers in the internal capsule, the crus cerebri and the medullary pyramid is shown in Figure 2-11.

Association Fibers. Fibers interconnecting various cortical regions within the same hemisphere are divided into long and short groups. *Short association fibers* arch through the floor of each sulcus to connect adjacent convolutions; these fibers course transversely to the long axis of the sulci (Fig. 2-16). *Long association fibers*, interconnecting cortical regions in different lobes within the same hemisphere, form three main bundles: (a) the uncinate fasciculus, (b) the arcuate fasciculus and (c) the cingulum (Figs. 2-17 and 2-19).

The *uncinate fasciculus* is a compact bundle between the limen insula which connects the orbital frontal gyri and parts of the inferior and middle frontal gyri with anterior portions of the temporal lobe (Figs. 2-17 and 2-18). A deep placed part of this fasciculus is thought to connect the frontal and occipital lobes (i.e., inferior occipitofrontal fasciculus). The *arcuate fasciculus* sweeps dorsally around the insular region and its fan-shaped ends connect the superior and middle frontal gyri with parts of the temporal lobe. A group of superiorly situated fibers in this bundle, extending caudally into portions of the parietal and occipital lobe, is known as the *superior longitudinal fasciculus* (Fig. 2-17).

The *cingulum*, the principal association bundle on the medial aspect of the hemisphere, lies in the white matter of the cingulate gyrus (Fig. 2-19). This bundle con-

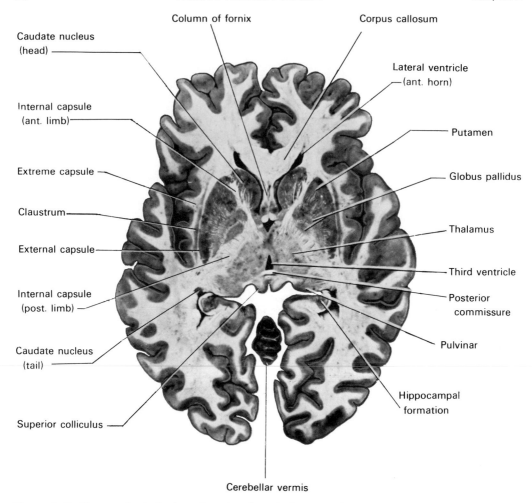

Figure 2-12. Photograph of a horizontal section through the cerebral hemispheres showing relationships of internal structures to the internal capsule.

tains fibers of variable length which connect regions of the frontal and parietal lobes with parahippocampal gyrus and adjacent temporal cortical regions (Figs. 2-10 and 2-19).

The cortical area deep to the insula contains association fibers in the *extreme* and *external capsules* (Figs. 2-12, 2-14 and 2-15). These capsules are two thin layers of white matter separated by a sheet of gray matter, known as the *claustrum*. All three of these structures overlie the lateral aspect of the corpus striatum.

Commissural Fibers. Fibers interconnecting corresponding cortical regions of the two hemispheres are represented by two structures: (a) the corpus callosum and

(b) the anterior commissure. The *corpus callosum* is a broad thick plate of dense myelinated fibers that reciprocally interconnect broad regions of the cortex in all lobes with corresponding regions of the opposite hemisphere (Figs. 2-5, 2-10 and 2-19). These fibers traverse the floor of the hemispheric fissure, form most of the roof of the lateral ventricles and fan out in a massive callosal radiation as they are distributed to various cortical regions (Fig. 2-21). The parts of the corpus callosum are designated as: (a) rostrum, (b) genu, (c) body and (d) splenium. The genu contains fibers interconnecting rostral parts of the frontal lobes; fibers from the remaining parts of the frontal lobe and the parietal lobe traverse the

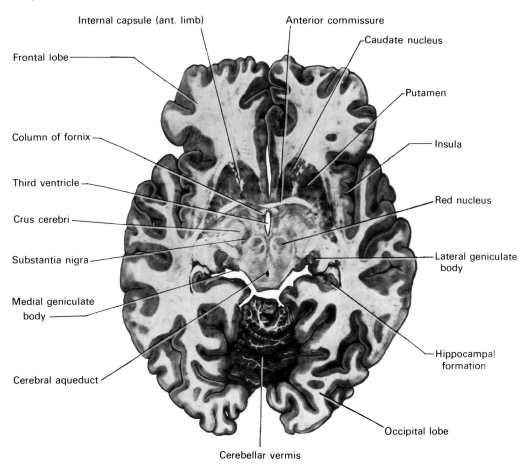

Figure 2-13. Photograph of a horizontal section through the cerebral hemispheres passing through the anterior commissure and the crus cerebri.

body of the corpus callosum. Fibers transversing the splenium relate regions of the temporal and occipital lobes. Fibers in the splenium of the corpus callosum, which sweep inferiorly along the lateral margin of the posterior horn of the lateral ventricle and separate the ventricle from the optic radiation, form the *tapetum* (Figs. 2-10 and 2-21).

The *anterior commissure* is a small compact bundle which crosses the midline rostral to the columns of the fornix (Figs. 2-5, 2-13, 2-14, and 2-19). This commissure has a general shape not unlike bicycle handlebars and consists of two parts that cannot be distinguished in the gross specimen (Fig. 18-9). A small anterior part of the commissure interconnects olfactory structures on the two sides (Fig. 18-4), while the larger posterior part mainly interconnects regions

of the middle and inferior temporal gyri (791, 2705).

THE BASAL GANGLIA

The basal ganglia are large subcortical nuclear masses derived from the telencephalon (Figs. 2-12–2-15). Structures composing the basal ganglia are the *caudate nucleus*, the *putamen*, the *globus pallidus* and the *amygdaloid nuclear complex*. The caudate nucleus, putamen and globus pallidus constitute the *corpus striatum*. The term *lentiform nucleus* (lenticular nucleus) refers to the putamen and the globus pallidus. The lentiform nucleus, with the size and shape of a Brazil nut, appears in transverse sections as a wedge with the apex directed medially. This nuclear mass lies between the internal and the external capsules. A

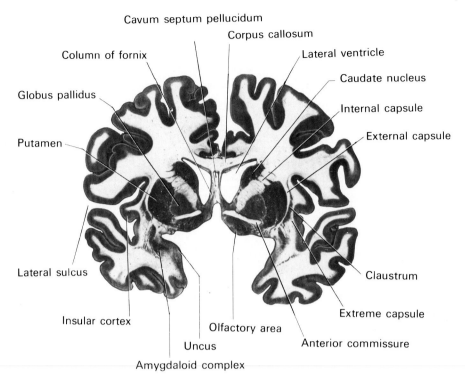

Cavum septum pellucidum

Corpus callosum

Column of fornix

Lateral ventricle

Caudate nucleus

Globus pallidus

Internal capsule

Putamen

External capsule

Lateral sulcus

Claustrum

Insular cortex

Extreme capsule

Olfactory area

Uncus

Anterior commissure

Amygdaloid complex

Figure 2-14. Photograph of a frontal section of the brain passing through the columns of the fornix and the anterior commissure.

slightly curved vertical lamina of white matter divides the lentiform nucleus into an outer portion, the putamen, and an inner portion, the globus pallidus.

The Putamen. This is the largest and most lateral part of the basal ganglia; it lies between the lateral medullary lamina of the globus pallidus and the external capsule (Figs. 2-12–2-15). It is traversed by numerous fascicles of myelinated fibers directed ventromedially toward the globus pallidus, but these are seen clearly only in stained sections. The rostral part of the putamen is continuous with the head of the caudate nucleus (Fig. 17-4).

The Globus Pallidus. The globus pallidus, forming the most medial part of the lentiform nucleus, consists of two segments separated by the medial medullary lamina of the globus pallidus (Figs. 2-12, 2-14 and 2-15). The globus pallidus appears pale and homogeneous in freshly sectioned brains. Its medial border is formed largely by the fibers of the posterior limb of the internal capsule.

The Caudate Nucleus. This is an elongated arched gray mass related throughout its extent to the lateral cerebral ventricle (Figs. 2-12–2-15 and 17-4). It consists of an enlarged rostral part, called the *head* of the caudate nucleus, which protrudes into the anterior horn of the lateral ventricle. The *body* of the caudate nucleus lies dorsolateral to the thalamus near the lateral wall of the lateral ventricle. The *tail* of the caudate nucleus follows the curvature of the inferior horn of the lateral ventricle and enters the temporal lobe (Fig. 2-12). The tail of the caudate nucleus terminates in the region of the amygdaloid nuclear complex (Fig. 2-15).

The Amygdaloid Nuclear Complex. This is a gray mass in the dorsomedial part of the temporal lobe which underlies the uncus (Figs. 2-9, 2-14 and 2-15). This complex lies dorsal to the hippocampal formation and rostral to the tip of the inferior horn of the lateral ventricle. The amygdaloid complex gives rise to fibers of the *stria terminalis*, which arch along the entire medial border of the caudate nucleus and are especially evident near the junction of the caudate nucleus and thalamus (Figs. 2-24 and 2-28*B*). The terminal vein lies near the stria terminalis.

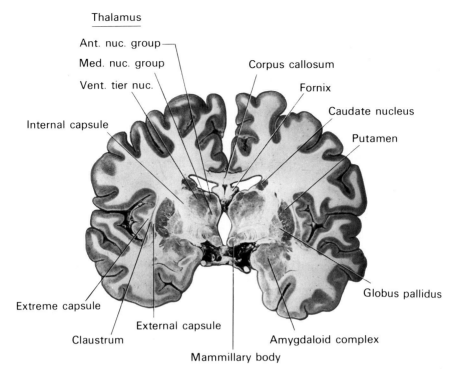

Figure 2-15. Photograph of a frontal section of the brain at the level of the mammillary bodies. In this section the main nuclear groups of the thalamus are identified and portions of all components of the basal ganglia are present. The amygdaloid nuclear complex lies in the temporal lobe internal to the uncus and ventral to the lentiform nucleus.

THE LATERAL VENTRICLES

The ependymal-lined cavities of the cerebral hemisphere constitute the lateral ventricles. The arched-shaped lateral ventricles contain cerebrospinal fluid and conform to the general shape of the hemispheres (Fig. 2-20). The lateral ventricles can be divided into five parts: (a) the anterior (frontal) horn, (b) the ventricular body, (c) the collateral (atrium) trigone, (d) the inferior (temporal) horn and (e) the posterior (occipital) horn. Each lateral ventricle communicates with the slit-shaped, midline third ventricle by two short channels, known as the interventricular foramina (Monro). These foramina serve as a basic reference point and are of great importance in radiographic studies.

The Anterior Horn. The anterior horn of the lateral ventricle lies rostral to the intraventricular foramen, has a triangular shape in frontal section and extends forward, laterally and ventrally to end in a rounded termination in the white matter of the frontal lobe (Figs. 2-12, 2-14 and 2-20). The roof and rostral wall of this horn are formed by the corpus callosum, while its medial wall is the *septum pellucidum* which separates the ventricles of the two hemispheres (Fig. 2-5). The lateral wall of the ventricle is formed by the head of the caudate nucleus whose surface bulges convexly into the cavity (Figs. 2-12–2-14 and 2-28A).

The Body of the Lateral Ventricle. This extends caudally from the interventricular foramen to an ill-defined point near the splenium of the corpus callosum. This narrower arched part of the ventricle continues until the ventricle begins to widen into the collateral trigone (referred to by neuroradiologists as the atrium). The *collateral trigone* composes that part of the lateral ventricle near the splenium of the corpus callosum where the body of the lateral ventricle is confluent with the temporal and occipital horns (Fig. 2-20).

The Inferior Horn. The inferior horn of the lateral ventricle curves downward and forward around the posterior aspect of the

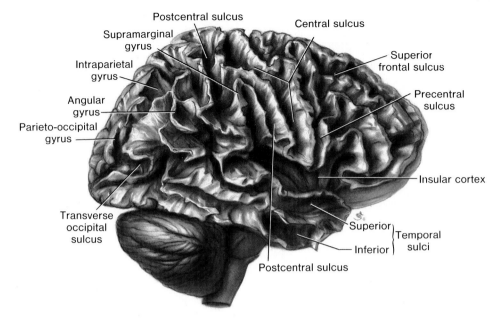

Figure 2-16. Lateral view of the brain after removal of the cortical gray matter. The medullary laminae and short association fibers of major gyri are indicated. (Reproduced with permission from F. A. Mettler: *Neuroanatomy*, Ed. 2, The C. V. Mosby Co., St. Louis, 1948.)

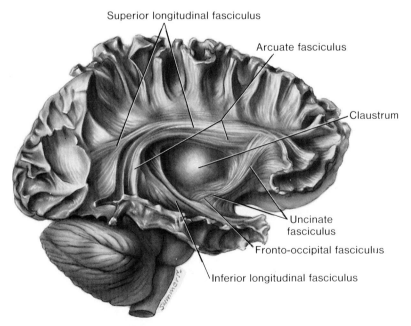

Figure 2-17. Dissection of the lateral surface of the hemisphere revealing the long association fibers interconnecting cortical regions in different lobes. (Reproduced with permission from F. A. Mettler: *Neuroanatomy*, Ed. 2, The C. V. Mosby Co., St. Louis, 1948.)

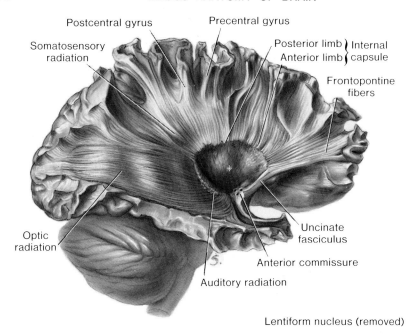

Figure 2-18. Dissection of the lateral aspect of the cerebral hemisphere to reveal the corona radiata and the optic radiation. The lentiform nucleus (*, asterisk) has been removed. (Reproduced with permission from F. A. Mettler: *Neuroanatomy*, Ed. 2, The C. V. Mosby Co., St. Louis, 1948.)

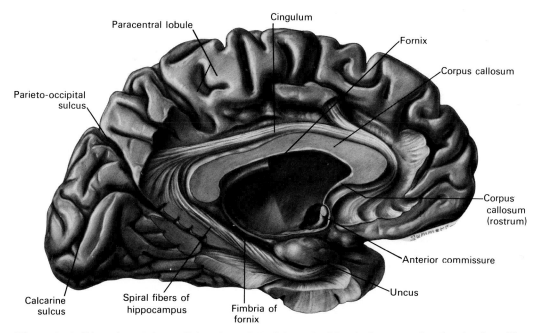

Figure 2-19. Dissection of the medial surface of the left cerebral hemisphere exposing the cingulum. The diencephalon has been removed. (Reproduced with permission from F. A. Mettler: *Neuroanatomy*, Ed. 2, The C. V. Mosby Co., St. Louis, 1948.)

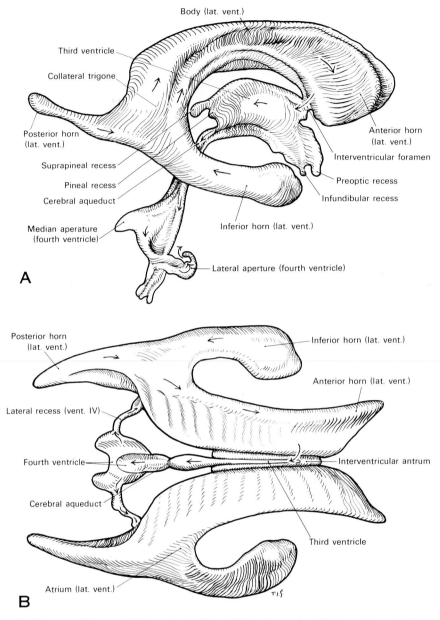

Figure 2-20. Diagrams of the ventricular system in lateral (*A*) and superior (*B*) views. *Arrows* indicate directon of CSF flow. (After Bailey (97)).

thalamus, and extends rostrally into the medial part of the temporal lobe to end approximately 3 cm from the temporal pole (Fig. 2-9). The roof and lateral wall of this horn are formed by the tapetum (Figs. 2-10 and 2-21) and the optic radiation; the floor contains the *collateral eminence* caused by the deep collateral sulcus (Fig. 2-9). The inferior horn of the lateral ventricle contains the *hippocampal formation* in the

medial wall of the horn which extends from the region of the splenium to the temporal tip of the ventricle (Figs. 2-9, 2-12 and 2-13). The hippocampal formation, representing the phylogenetically oldest type of cortex, has become folded into the ventricle along the hippocampal sulcus. Along the superior and medial surfaces of the hippocampus is a flattened band of fibers, known as the fimbria, which extends from the re-

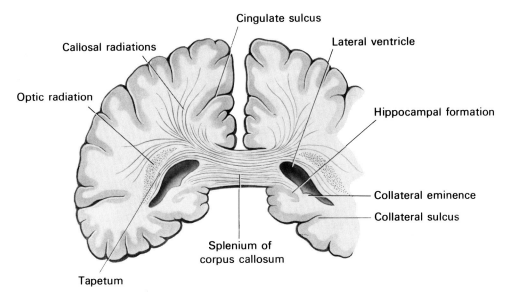

Cingulate sulcus

Callosal radiations

Lateral ventricle

Optic radiation

Hippocampal formation

Collateral eminence

Collateral sulcus

Splenium of
corpus callosum

Tapetum

Figure 2-21. Drawing of a frontal section at the level of the splenium of the corpus callosum. Callosal fibers lateral to the ventricle are known as the tapetum. The optic radiations lie lateral to the tapetum.

gion of the uncus toward the splenium of the corpus callosum. The fimbria extends under the corpus callosum and becomes the fornix (Figs. 2-9, 2-19, 2-26 and 2-27).

The Posterior Horn. The posterior horn of the lateral ventricle extends from the collateral trigone into the occipital lobe. This horn exhibits a high degree of variability in appearance and is often rudimentary. Often the occipital horn has the appearance of a small finger-like projection with a rounded tip. The roof and lateral wall of this horn are formed by tapetal fibers of the corpus callosum, while its floor is the white matter of the occipital lobe (Fig. 2-21). The *calcar avis*, a longitudinal prominence, is produced by the deep penetration of the calcarine sulcus.

Portions of the lateral ventricles contain *choroid plexus*, formed by the invagination of the ependymal roof plate into the ventricular cavities. Choroid plexus develops at sites where ependyma and pia mater containing blood vessels come together. This plexus is present in the body, collateral trigone and in the inferior horn of the lateral ventricle, and extends through the interventricular foramen to lie in the roof of the third ventricle (Fig. 2-28).

THE BRAIN STEM

In the intact brain only the anterior surface of the brain stem can be seen through-

out its extent, because the cerebral hemispheres and cerebellum overlap the lateral and posterior surfaces. On the anterior surface of the brain stem the medulla, pons, midbrain and part of the *hypothalamus* (diencephalon) can be identified (Figs. 2-4, 2-8 and 2-23). The most rostral portion of the brain stem, the diencephalon, is surrounded by hemispheric structures on all sides except for a small region between the *optic chiasm* and the *mammillary bodies*. The midbrain appears very small, but root fibers of the oculomotor nerve can be seen emerging between two massive fibers bundles, the *crura cerebri* (Figs. 2-8, 2-9 and 2-23). The ventral surface of the pons produces a convex protrusion covered by transversely coursing fiber bundles which disappear laterally in the substance of the cerebellum. The medulla, caudal to the pons, reveals the large *medullary pyramids* medially and the oval *olivary eminences* dorsolaterally. The transition from medulla to spinal cord is characterized by the disappearance of the medullary pyramids, the development of the anterior median fissure of the spinal cord, a conspicuous reduction in size and the appearance of paired spinal nerves.

Removal of the cerebral hemispheres and cerebellum reveals the posterior and lateral surfaces of the brain stem (Figs. 2-24 and 2-25). The expanded diencephalon appears as

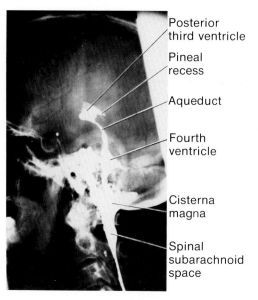

Posterior
third ventricle

Pineal
recess

Aqueduct

Fourth
ventricle

Cisterna
magna

Spinal
subarachnoid
space

Figure 2-22. Positive contrast ventriculography clearly outlining the fourth ventricle, cerebral aqueduct and the posterior part of the third ventricle. In this lateral view radiopaque material also fills part of the cisterna magna and part of the spinal subarachnoid space.

paired oval nuclear masses on each side of a vertical slitlike third ventricle (Fig. 2-24). The *thalamus* and *epithalamus*, seen in the posterior view of the brain stem, lie between the fibers of the internal capsule and are flanked dorsolaterally by the body and tail of the caudate nucleus. Along the dorsomedial margin of the thalamus is the *stria medullaris*, a band of fibers coursing posteriorly toward the habenula and the base of the pineal gland. The most caudal part of the thalamus, the pulvinar, overlies part of the midbrain (Fig. 2-24).

The dorsal aspect of the midbrain reveals the *superior* and *inferior colliculi* and their *brachia*, which relate these structures to particular parts of the thalamus. The trochlear nerve emerges from the dorsal part of the midbrain caudal to the inferior colliculus (Figs. 2-24 and 2-25).

The dorsal aspects of the hindbrain are revealed by removing the cerebellum (Fig. 2-24). This discloses the rhomboid fossa, an unpaired symmetrical ventricle that overlies the pons and medulla. The rhomboid-shaped fourth ventricle is surrounded by three paired cerebellar peduncles, which relate the three lowest brain stem segments to the cerebellum. The fourth ventricle contains several eminences which overlie nuclear masses, the most evident of which are the *facial colliculus* and the *hypoglossal eminence*. Caudal to the fourth ventricle on the dorsal surface of the medulla are nuclear masses related to ascending spinal systems, namely, the *cuneate* and *gracilis tubercles* (Fig. 2-24).

Structurally the midbrain and hindbrain consist of three distinctive parts: (1) a roof plate dorsal to the ventricular system, (2) a central core of cells and fibers beneath the ventricular system known as the tegmentum, and (3) a massive collection of ventrally located fibers derived from cells of the cerebral cortex (Figs. 2-26 and 2-27). The *roof plate* of the midbrain is represented by the *tectum* or *quadrigeminal plate*, consisting of the superior and inferior colliculi; in the hindbrain the roof plate is more elaborate and is presented by the *cerebellum* and the *tela choroidea*. The *tegmentum* of the midbrain, pons and medulla represents the brain stem *reticular formation*, a large collection of cells and intermingled fibers that subserve multiple functions. The *cortically derived ventral fiber system* forms the *crus cerebri* at midbrain levels, one of the principal constituents of the *ventral* or *basilar part* of the pons, and the *medullary pyramids* of the medulla (Fig. 2-25). Both the reticular formation and the cortically derived ventral fiber system are continuous within the brain stem, but undergo change and modification at various levels (Fig. 2-11).

The Medulla

The medulla (myelencephalon), the most caudal basic subdivision of the brain stem, extends from the level of the foramen magnum to the caudal border of the pons. The transition from spinal cord to medulla is gradual and characterized by: (a) the obliteration of the anterior median fissure ventrally and the decussation of the medullary pyramids, (b) the appearance of the gracilis and cuneate tubercles dorsally, (c) the disappearance of spinal nerves and the appearance of cranial nerves and (d) the development of the fourth ventricle (Figs. 2-22–2-25). The full development of the medullary pyramids, the appearance of the inferior olivary eminence, the widening of the fourth ventricle and the gradual increase in

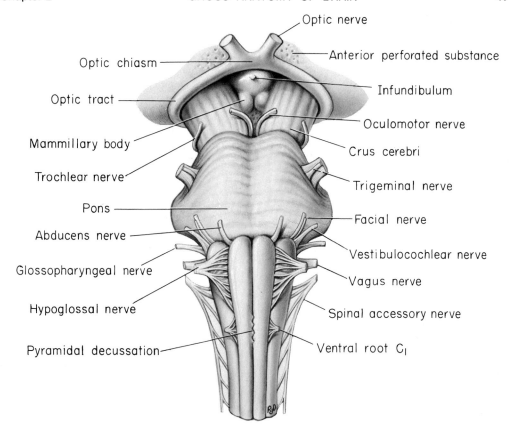

Optic nerve

Optic chiasm

Anterior perforated substance

Infundibulum

Optic tract

Oculomotor nerve

Mammillary body

Crus cerebri

Trochlear nerve

Trigeminal nerve

Pons

Facial nerve

Abducens nerve

Vestibulocochlear nerve

Glossopharyngeal nerve

Vagus nerve

Hypoglossal nerve

Spinal accessory nerve

Pyramidal decussation

Ventral root C₁

Figure 2-23. Drawing of the anterior surface of the medulla, pons and midbrain.

size of the inferior cerebellar peduncle give the medulla its characteristic configuration (Figs. 2-23 and 2-24). Cranial nerves associated with the medulla are: (a) the hypoglossal (N. XII) whose fibers emerge ventrolaterally between the pyramid and the inferior olivary complex, (b) the accessory (N. XI), the vagus (N. X) and the glossopharyngeal (N. IX) whose fibers emerge from the postolivary sulcus and (c) the vestibulocochlear nerve (N. VIII) whose separate components enter the brain stem at the junction of the pons and medulla (Fig. 2-25). Auditory fibers are most dorsal and caudal and partially arch over the lateral aspect of the inferior cerebellar peduncle.

The Fourth Ventricle

The fourth ventricle is a broad shallow rhomboid-shaped cavity overlying the pons and medulla that extends from the central canal of the upper cervical spinal cord to the cerebral aqueduct of the midbrain (Figs.

2-20, 2-22 and 2-24). Its roof is the cerebellum and the *superior* and *inferior medullary veli*, which extend toward an apex within the cerebellum known as the *fastigium* (Figs. 2-20, 2-26, 2-27 and 2-32). The superior medullary velum forms the roof of the pontine part of the ventricle, while the inferior medullary velum and the *tela choroidea* form the roof over the medullary part of this ventricle. *Choroid plexus* from the tela choroidea projects into the caudal part of the ventricle. The widest part of the fourth ventricle is immediately caudal to the *middle cerebellar peduncles*. In this region there is a *lateral recess* on each side, which extends over the surface of the inferior cerebellar peduncle to open into the *cerebellomedullary* (magna) *cistern* (Figs. 1-10 and 1-11). These small lateral recesses contain choroid plexus that protrudes through the *foramina of Luschka* into the subarachnoid space (Figs. 2-8 and 2-20). A small median aperture in the caudal part of the ventricle is known as the *foramen of*

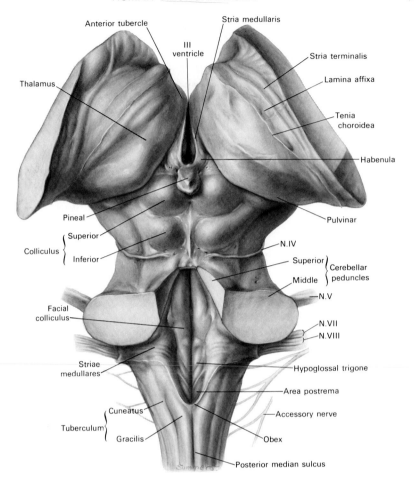

Figure 2-24. Posterior aspect of the brain stem with the cerebellum removed. (Reproduced with permission from F. A. Mettler: *Neuroanatomy*, Ed. 2, The C. V. Mosby Co., St. Louis, 1948.)

Magendie. Through these three apertures cerebrospinal fluid flows from the ventricular system into the subarachnoid spaces. Using positive contrast ventriculography the fourth ventricle, cisterna magna and cerebral aqueduct can be viewed in detail (Fig. 2-22).

The *rhomboid fossa* which forms the floor of the fourth ventricle is divided by the *median sulcus* into symmetrical halves. The sulcus limitans divides each half into a *medial eminence* and a lateral region known as the *vestibular area* (Fig. 11-17). The vestibular nuclei lie beneath the vestibular area. The *facial colliculus* and the *hypoglossal trigone* lie within the medial eminence, with the latter near the caudal border of the ventricle. Transversely coursing fibers of the *striae medullares* run from

the region of the lateral recess toward the midline and disappear in the median sulcus (Fig. 2-24); these strands of myelinated fibers lie rostral to the hypoglossal trigone. The *vagal trigone* lies lateral to the hypoglossal trigone. The most caudal end of the rhomboid fossa resembles a pen and is called the *calamus scriptorius.* The point of caudal junction of the walls of the fourth ventricle is known as the *obex* (Fig. 2-24). Immediately rostral to the obex on each side of the fourth ventricle is a slightly rounded eminence, the *area postrema.*

The Pons

The pons (metencephalon), representing the rostral part of the hindbrain, is well delimited on the anterior surface of the

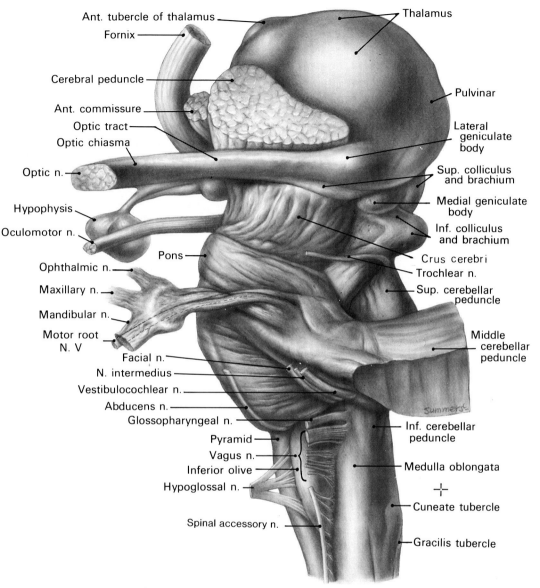

Figure 2-25. Lateral view of the brain stem with the cerebellum removed showing the sites of emergence and entrance of most of the cranial nerves. (Reproduced with permission from F. A. Mettler: *Neuroanatomy*, Ed. 2, The C. V. Mosby Co., St. Louis, 1948.)

brain stem (Figs. 2-23, 2-25 and 2-26). The massive pontine protuberance covered by broad bands of transversely oriented fibers is separated from the crus cerebri of the midbrain by the superior pontine sulcus and from the anterior surface of the medulla by the inferior pontine sulcus. The predominantly transverse fibers in the ventral part of the pons form the *middle cerebellar peduncle* (Figs. 2-25 and 2-31). An

anterior median depression, the *basilar sulcus*, indicates the position occupied by the basilar artery (Figs. 2-23 and 20-10).

Transverse sections of the pons reveal the basic organization (Fig. 12-1). The pons consists of a massive *ventral part* composed of: (a) longitudinal descending fiber bundles, (b) pontine nuclei (c) transversely oriented fibers projecting to the cerebellum, and a smaller dorsal part, known as the

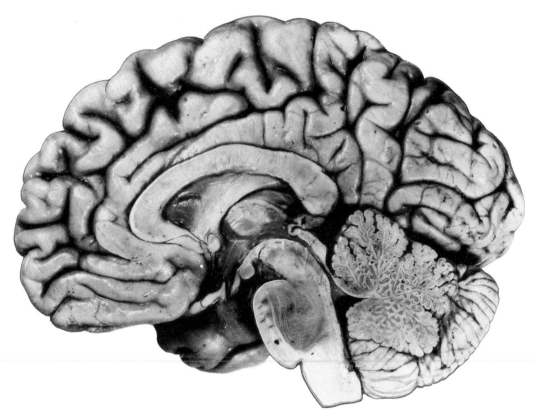

Figure 2-26. Photograph of a midsagittal section of the brain stem. Structures are identified in Figure 2-27.

tegmentum. The tegmental portion contains aggregations of cells and fibers which form a central core known as the reticular formation. The pontine tegmentum is continuous with the reticular formation of the medulla and midbrain. Cranial nerve nuclei, ascending sensory systems and older descending motor pathways are found within the tegmentum. Cranial nerves associated with the pons are the trigeminal (N. V), abducens (N. VI), facial (N. VII), and the two components of the vestibulocochlear nerve (N. VIII). The *abducens nucleus* lies in the floor of the fourth ventricle and is partially encircled by fibers of the facial nerve. Facial nerve fibers and cells of the abducens nucleus underlie the *facial colliculus* seen in the floor of the fourth ventricle (Fig. 2-24). Fibers of the abducens nerve emerge from the ventral surface of the brain stem at the junction of the pons and medulla (Fig. 2-25). The facial and vestibulocochlear nerves emerge and enter the lateral surface of the pons at the *cerebellopon-*

tine angle, formed by the junction of pons, medulla and cerebellum (Figs. 2-25 and 12-6). The trigeminal nerve, consisting of motor and sensory fibers, passes through rostral parts of the middle cerebellar peduncle to reach nuclei in the dorsolateral pontine tegmentum (Fig. 2-25).

The *middle cerebellar peduncle* consists of a large number of fibers, arising from the pontine nuclei, which project to the cerebellum; this is the largest of the three cerebellar peduncles (Figs. 2-24 and 2-25).

The Midbrain

The midbrain (mesencephalon) is the smallest and least differentiated part of the brain stem (Figs. 2-9, 2-24–2-26). It consists of: (a) the *tectum*, represented by the superior and inferior colliculi, (b) the *tegmentum*, ventral to the cerebral aqueduct and (c) the massive *crura cerebri* (Figs. 2-23, 2-25 and 13-1). The tegmentum and *crura cerebri* are separated by a large pigmented

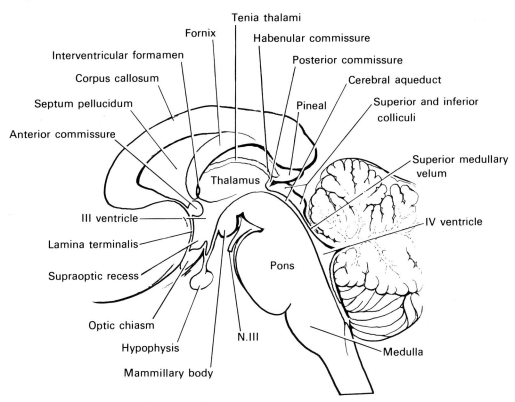

Figure 2-27. Drawing of a midsagittal section of the brain stem identifying some of the structures shown in Figure 2-26.

nuclear mass, the *substantia nigra* (Fig. 2-13). The superior colliculus and a region immediately rostral to it, known as the *pretectum*, are important relays in the visual system. The inferior colliculus relays auditory impulses to thalamic nuclei that in turn project to specific cortical areas.

Two cranial nerves are associated with the midbrain, the oculomotor (N. III) and the trochlear (N. IV). The oculomotor nerve emerges from the *interpeduncular fossa*, between the massive crura cerebri (Figs. 2-8, 2-9, and 2-25). The slender trochlear nerve exits from the dorsal surface of the brain stem, caudal to the inferior colliculus; fibers of this nerve cross in the superior medullary velum and course anteriorly around the brain stem (Figs. 2-24 and 2-25). The fibers of the *superior cerebellar peduncle*, seen on each side of the upper part of the fourth ventricle (Figs. 2-24 and 2-25), decussate completely in the caudal midbrain tegmentum. Crossed fibers of this peduncle traverse and surround a discrete nuclear mass in the tegmentum called the

red nucleus (Fig. 2-13).

Crus Cerebri. The crus cerebri on the ventral surface of the midbrain are collections of fibers originating in broad areas of the cerebral cortex that pass through the internal capsule (Figs. 2-11 and 2-23). These fibers project to: (a) spinal cord (i.e., corticospinal), (b) pontine nuclei (i.e., corticopontine) and (c) specific regions of the lower brain stem (i.e., corticobulbar). A large part of the corticobulbar fibers project to parts of the reticular formation.

Substantia Nigra. The pigmented substantia nigra, rich in dopamine and other neurotransmitters, is the largest single nuclear mass in the midbrain. It has connections with parts of the corpus striatum, thalamus and superior colliculus and is considered to subserve a motor function (Fig. 2-13).

The Diencephalon

The diencephalon, the most rostral part of the brain stem, is a paired structure on each side of the third ventricle (Figs. 2-12,

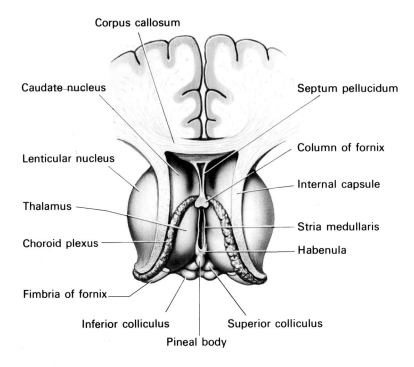

Corpus callosum

Caudate nucleus

Septum pellucidum

Column of fornix

Lenticular nucleus

Internal capsule

Thalamus

Stria medullaris

Choroid plexus

Habenula

Fimbria of fornix

Inferior colliculus   Superior colliculus

Pineal body

A

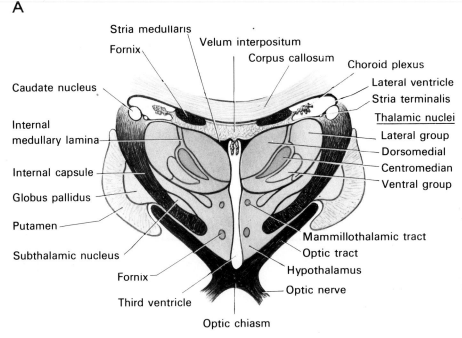

Stria medullaris

Fornix

Velum interpositum

Corpus callosum

Choroid plexus

Caudate nucleus

Lateral ventricle

Stria terminalis

Thalamic nuclei

Internal
medullary lamina

Lateral group

Dorsomedial

Centromedian

Internal capsule

Ventral group

Globus pallidus

Putamen

Mammillothalamic tract

Subthalamic nucleus

Optic tract

Hypothalamus

Fornix

Optic nerve

Third ventricle

Optic chiasm

B

Figure 2-28. (*A*) Posterior view of the diencephalon and related structures. (*B*) Schematic drawing of a frontal section through the diencephalon (see Fig. 15-7) and adjacent structures indicating some of the major nuclear groups of the thalamus. The hypothalamus lies on both sides of the third ventricle below the hypothalamic sulcus.

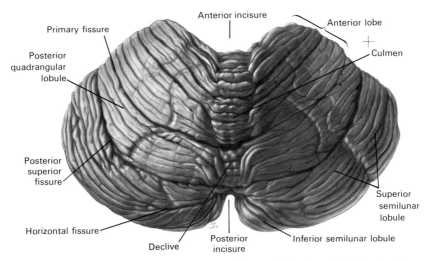

Figure 2-29. Superior surface of cerebellum. (Reproduced with permission from F. A. Mettler: *Neuroanatomy*, Ed. 2, The C. V. Mosby Co., St. Louis, 1948.)

2-15 and 2-24–2-27). The lateral ventricles, corpus callosum, fornix and velum interpositum lie superior to the diencephalon (Fig. 2-28). Fibers of the posterior limb of the internal capsule and the body of the caudate nucleus constitute its lateral border. Caudally the diencephalon appears continuous with the tegmentum of the midbrain; the posterior commissure is the junctional zone between the diencephalon and mesencephalon (Figs. 2-12 and 2-27). The rostral boundary of the diencephalon is near the interventricular foramen, but portions of the hypothalamus extend almost to the *lamina terminalis* (Figs. 2-26 and 2-27). The diencephalon consists of four parts: (a) the epithalamus, (b) the thalamus, (c) the hypothalamus and (d) the subthalamus (Figs. 2-26–2-28).

The Epithalamus. The epithalamus evident on the dorsal surface of the diencephalon, consists of: (a) the pineal body, (b) the habenular nuclei, (c) the stria medullares and (d) the tenia thalami (Fig. 2-24).

The Thalamus. The thalamus, the largest diencephalic subdivision, is an oblique egg-shaped nuclear mass at the rostral end of the brain stem (Figs. 2-12, 2-15, and 2-24–2-28). This nuclear complex lies between the interventricular foramen and the posterior commissure and extends from the third ventricle to the medial border of the

posterior limb of the internal capsule. The thalamus lies dorsal to the hypothalamic sulcus, a shallow groove on the lateral wall of the third ventricle (Figs. 2-26–2-28). The lateral and caudal parts of the thalamus overlie midbrain structures. The superior surface of the thalamus is covered by a thin layer of fibers known as the *stratum zonale.* A narrow lateral strip of the superior surface, adjacent to the body of the caudate nucleus, is covered by ependyma and forms part of the floor of the lateral ventricle. This strip is called the *lamina affixa* (Fig. 2-24). The *stria terminalis* and the *terminal vein* lie dorsally at the junction of thalamus and caudate nucleus. The *stria medullaris* extends along the dorsomedial margin of the thalamus near the roof of the third ventricle. The medial surfaces of thalami on each side of the third ventricle are partially fused in about 80% of human brains. This place of fusion is called the *interthalamic adhesion* or *massa intermedia* (Fig. 2-28).

Although most subdivisions of the thalamus are not evident in gross specimens, the *anterior tubercle* of the thalamus is discernible rostrally as a distinct swelling (Fig. 2-25). The expanded posterior part of the thalamus that overhangs part of the midbrain is known as the *pulvinar* (Figs. 2-12 and 2-24). The *medial* and *lateral genic-*

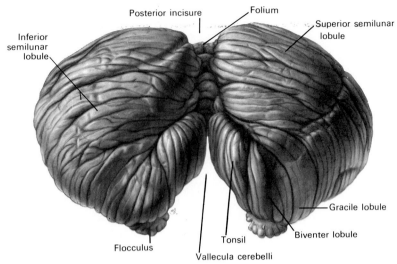

Figure 2-30. Posteroinferior view of the cerebellum. (Reproduced with permission from F. A. Mettler: *Neuroanatomy*, Ed. 2, The C. V. Mosby Co., St. Louis, 1948.)

ulate bodies, important relay nuclei concerned with audition and vision, lie ventral to the pulvinar (Fig. 2-25). Together these structures are referred to as the *metathalamus*. The thalamus is divided into anterior, lateral, medial and ventral nuclear groups by a thin layer of myelinated fibers, known as the *internal medullary lamina* of the thalamus, which can be seen grossly in transverse sections of the brain (Figs. 2-15 and 2-28). Nuclear groups within the internal medullary lamina are collectively referred to as the *intralaminar thalamic nuclei*. The largest of the intralaminar nuclei is the centromedian nucleus (Fig. 2-28*B*).

The thalamus is regarded as the neural structure whose relationship with other parts of the neuraxis provides the key to understanding the organization of the central nervous system. Like most keys it is small. This small part of the diencephalon is concerned with: (a) distributing most of the afferent input to the cerebral cortex, (b) the control of the electrocortical activity of the cerebral cortex and (c) the integration of motor functions by providing the relays through which impulses from the corpus striatum and cerebellum can reach the motor cortex. Through influences that modify electrocortical activities the thalamus plays important roles in arousal, maintaining consciousness and in mechanisms that produce various kinds of sleep.

The Hypothalamus. The hypothalamus lies ventral to the hypothalamic sulcus and forms the inferior and lateral walls of the third ventricle (Figs. 2-26–2-28 and 16-1). This subdivision of the diencephalon extends from the region of the optic chiasm to the caudal border of the mammillary bodies. The gross structures visible on the ventral surface include the *optic chiasm, infundibulum, tuber cinereum* and *mammillary bodies* (Figs. 2-8, 2-9, 2-23, 2-26 and 2-27). The hypothalamus is divided into medial and lateral nuclear groups by fibers of the fornix which mainly end in the mammillary body. Three rostrocaudal regions of the hypothalamus are recognized: (a) a supraoptic, dorsal to the optic chiasm, (b) a tuberal region centrally and (c) a mammillary region caudally (Fig. 16-1).

The hypothalamus has a rostrocaudal extent of about 10 mm. This subdivision of the diencephalon is concerned with visceral, endocrine and metabolic activity, as well as with temperature regulation, sleep and emotion.

The Subthalamus. The subthalamus is a transitional zone ventral to the thalamus and lateral to the hypothalamus. It is bounded by the thalamus above, the hypothalamus medially and the internal capsule laterally (Figs. 2-15 and 2-28). The largest discrete nuclear mass is the *subthalamic nucleus*, a lens-shaped structure on

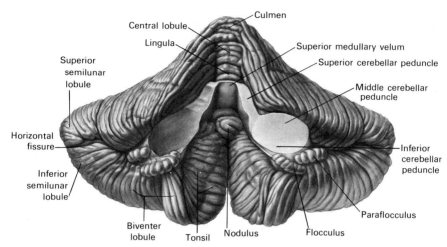

Figure 2-31. Inferior surface of cerebellum removed from brain stem by transection of cerebellar peduncles. (Reproduced with permission from F. A. Mettler: *Neuroanatomy*, Ed. 2, The C. V. Mosby Co., St. Louis, 1948.)

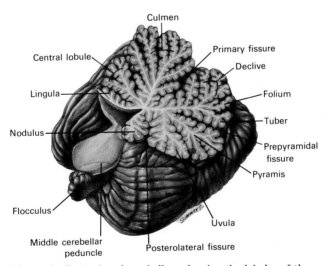

Figure 2-32. View of the sagittally sectioned cerebellum showing the lobules of the cerebellar vermis. The primary fissure is the deepest of all cerebellar vermis. (See Fig. 14-1). (Reproduced with permission from F. A. Mettler: *Neuroanatomy*, Ed. 2, The C. V. Mosby Co., St. Louis, 1948.)

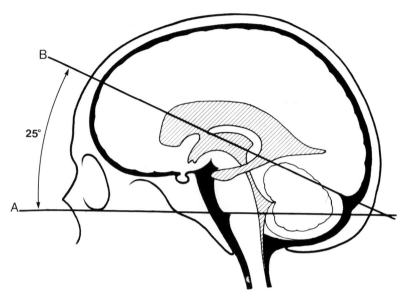

Figure 2-33. Outline drawing of the head and brain demonstrating tomographic planes. The zero degree plane (*A*) corresponds to the baseline of Reid which passes through the inferior margin of the orbit and the external auditory meatus. Tomograms taken in parallel planes at an angle of 25° to the base line of Reid (*B*) provide more information about structures in the posterior fossa. (Reproduced with permission from J. Hanaway, W. R. Scott and C. M. Strother: *Atlas of the Human Brain and the Orbit for Computed Tomography.* Warren H. Green, Inc., St. Louis, 1980.)

the inner aspect of the internal capsule (Fig. 15-7). This region is traversed by many important fiber systems in their projection to thalamic nuclei. A small, relatively clear area, known as the *zona incerta*, serves as an important landmark in distinguishing certain fiber bundles (Fig. 15-7). The subthalamic nucleus and pathways traversing this region are concerned with the integration of somatic motor function.

THE CEREBELLUM

The cerebellum overlies the posterior aspect of the pons and medulla and extends laterally under the tentorium to fill the greater part of the posterior fossa (Figs. 2-1, 2-6, 2-8 and 2-26). The superior surface is somewhat flattened, while the inferior surface is convex. A shallow *anterior cerebellar incisure* is present superiorly. A deeper and narrower *posterior cerebellar incisure* contains a fold of dura mater, the *falx cerebelli* (Fig. 1-2).

The cerebellum consists of a midline portion, the *vermis*, and two lateral lobes or *hemispheres*. This structure is essentially wedge-shaped, having a superior surface which is covered by the tentorium, a posterior surface in the suboccipital region and an inferior surface which overlies the fourth ventricle. On the superior surface the distinction between vermis and hemispheres is not sharp (Fig. 2-29). On the inferior surface two deep sulci clearly separate the vermis from the hemispheres. Inferiorly a deep median fossa, the *vallecula cerebelli*, is continuous with the posterior incisure. The floor of this fossa is formed by the inferior vermis (Fig. 2-30).

Structurally the cerebellum consists of a gray cortical mantle, the cerebellar cortex, a medullary core of white matter and four pairs of intrinsic nuclei. Three paired cerebellar peduncles connect the cerebellum with the three lower segments of the brain stem (Figs. 2-24, 2-25 and 2-31).

The cerebellar cortex consists of a large number of narrow leaflike laminae known as cerebellar folia. Cerebellar folia are nearly parallel with each other and for the most part are oriented transversely. Each lamina contains several secondary and tertiary folia.

Five transversely oriented fissures divide the cerebellum into lobes and lobules (Fig.

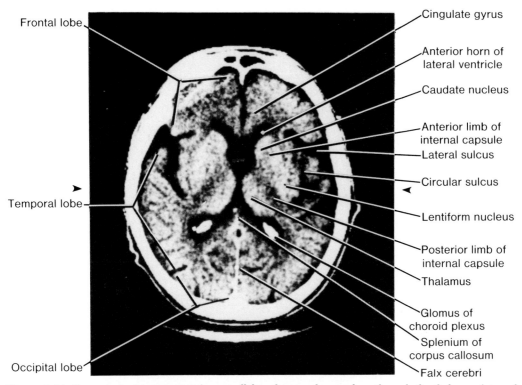

Frontal lobe

Cingulate gyrus

Anterior horn of
lateral ventricle

Caudate nucleus

Anterior limb of
internal capsule

Lateral sulcus

Circular sulcus

Temporal lobe

Lentiform nucleus

Posterior limb of
internal capsule

Thalamus

Glomus of
choroid plexus

Splenium of
corpus callosum

Occipital lobe

Falx cerebri

Figure 2-34. Computerized tomogram taken parallel to the zero degree plane through the thalamus, internal capsule and corpus striatum. (Reproduced with permission from J. Hanaway, W. R. Scott and C. W. Strother: *Atlas of the Human Brain and the Orbit for Computed Tomography.* Warren H. Green, Inc., St. Louis, 1980.)

14-1). These fissures and the various lobular subdivisions can be identified on the isolated cerebellum or in midsagittal section (Fig. 2-32). On the superior surface of the cerebellum two fissures can be identified: (1) the *primary* and (2) the *posterior superior* (Fig. 2-29). The *horizontal fissure,* one of the most distinctive, roughly divides the cerebellum into superior and inferior halves. On the inferior surface the *prepyramidal* and *posterolateral fissures* are found (Fig. 2-32).

The cerebellar vermis is the key to understanding the gross organization of the cerebellum, but in this part there is no median raphe and the midline is difficult to establish. Portions of the cerebellum rostral to the primary fissure constitute the *anterior lobe of the cerebellum* (Figs. 2-29 and 14-1). In the vermis the lobules consist of the lingula, the central lobule and the culmen (Fig. 2-32); in the hemisphere the lingula has no corresponding part, but the *alar central lobule* and the *anterior quad-*

rangular lobule correspond to the central lobule and the culmen.

The *posterior lobe* of the cerebellum, between the primary and posterolateral fissures, represents the largest subdivision of the cerebellum (Figs. 2-32 and 14-1). Vermal parts of the posterior lobe in sequence are the *declive, folium, tuber, pyramis,* and *uvula* (Fig. 2-32). The *simple lobule,* between the primary and posterior superior fissures, corresponds to the declive of the vermis (Fig. 14-1). The *ansiform lobule* is that part of the cerebellar hemisphere between the posterior superior fissure and the *gracile lobule.* The horizontal fissure divides the ansiform lobule into the *superior semilunar lobule* (crus I) and the *inferior semilunar lobule* (crus II). Vermal counterparts of the ansiform lobule are the folium and tuber. Between the prepyramidal and posterolateral fissures are the *pyramis* and *uvula* in the vermis and the *biventer lobule* and the *cerebellar tonsil* in the hemisphere (Figs. 2-31 and 2-32).

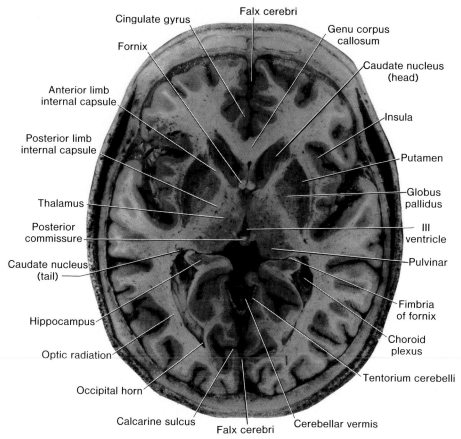

Figure 2-35. Section of the head and brain in the same horizontal plane as the computerized tomogram shown in Figure 2-34. (Reproduced with permission from J. Hanaway, W. R. Scott and C. W. Strother: *Atlas of the Human Brain and the Orbit for Computed Tomography.* Warren H. Green, Inc., St.Louis, 1980.)

The *flocculonodular lobule* lies rostral to the posterolateral fissure and consists of the vermal nodulus and the paired flocculi (Fig. 2-31). The *nodulus* lies immediately caudal to the inferior medullary velum (Fig. 2-32).

In midsagittal section the relationships of the cerebellum to the brain stem are evident (Fig. 2-26). The complex branching of the medullary core and the treelike appearance of the laminae and folia have given rise to the descriptive term, *arbor vitae* (Figs. 2-26, 2-27 and 2-32). The intrinsic deep nuclei of the cerebellum can be seen only in sections. These nuclei are the dentate (most lateral), the emboliform, the globose and the fastigial (Figs. 14-13 and 14-14). The fastigial nuclei, commonly called the roof nuclei, lie in the roof of the fourth ventricle.

Although the cerebellum is derived from the metencephalon, this portion of the neuraxis functions in a suprasegmental manner. It is concerned primarily with coordination of somatic motor function, control of muscle tone and equilibrium. The cerebellum receives inputs directly or indirectly from virtually all sensory receptors, including the organs of special sense, but this sensory information does not enter the conscious sphere. Present evidence suggests that the cerebellum functions as a special kind of computer that automatically processes, organizes and integrates sensory inputs and provides prompt responses that contribute to smooth and effective control of somatic motor function. The output systems from the cerebellum arise largely from the deep cerebellar nuclei and their influences upon motor function are mediated

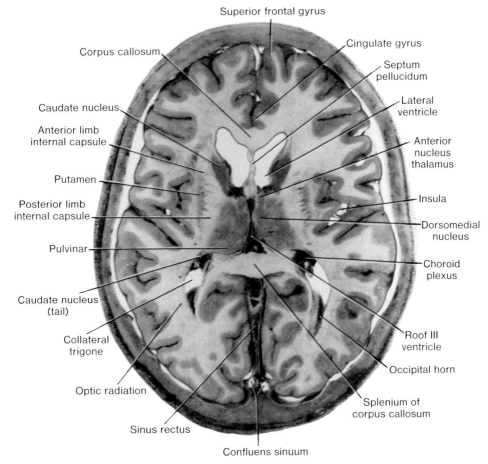

Figure 2-36. Section of the head and brain made in a plane corresponding to the 25° plane (*B*) in Figure 2-33. This section passes through dorsal regions of the third ventricle, thalamus and internal capsule, as well as through the splenium of the corpus collosum and the rectus sinus. (Reproduced with permission from J. Hanaway, W. R. Scott and C. W. Strother: *Atlas of the Human Brain and the Orbit for Computed Tomography.* Warren H. Green, Inc., St. Louis, 1980.)

through brain stem nuclei at multiple levels.

COMPUTERIZED X-RAY TOMOGRAPHY

There are several roentgenographic technics for visualizing gross structures in and around the brain for diagnostic purposes. Those which have been successfully used for many years depend upon introduction of air or contrast media into the subarachnoid space or ventricles (Fig. 2-22). The blood vessels of the brain and brain stem can be studied in detail from carotid and vertebral angiograms which depend upon injection of a water soluble contrast media

and serial x-rays which first reveal the arteries and later filling of the veins (Figs. 20-3, 20-8, 20-14 and 20-15). Under ordinary circumstances the soft tissues within the cranium are so nearly homogeneous in radiodensity that the brain is almost completely invisible on plain films of the head. All living tissues except bone fall within a narrow band of photon absorption coefficients that prevents discrimination of different tissue densities by conventional roentgenographic technics (2520). In addition, when an x-ray beam penetrates the head, it superimposes the densities of all structures in its path; the composite density is recorded on the x-ray film.

A system theoretically capable of producing a cross sectional display of discontinuities of radiodensity within an irregular object, such as the head, was described by Oldendorf (1869). He used a γ-ray source and a collimated scintillation counter to detect discontinuities in a rotating model. Computerized tomography, a technic capable of presenting an image of a cross section of the brain or body, is a remarkable method for x-ray examination of soft tissue developed by Hounsfield. This system utilizes scintillation counters as the primary detector, rather than x-ray film, and the information is fed into a computer capable of direct imaging. Using scintillation counters to detect photon attentuation (i.e., absorption coefficients) instead of x-ray film increases the sensitivity of the method by two orders of magnitude (1832). This method uses a thin x-ray beam and photon detectors (sodium iodide crystals and photomultipliers) accurately aligned with the x-ray source to provide a detailed plot of the x-ray absorption coefficients in the scanned cross section of the body. The x-ray beam and the photon detectors scan the head in a linear fashion allowing 160 readings of photon transmission. The scanning unit is then rotated 1 degree around the head and the process is repeated; 180 scans are taken, each with the apparatus rotated an additional 1 degree. This results in 28,800 readings of photon detectors which are processed by a computer which calculates 6400 absorption values for each brain slice. From the computer calculations a picture of the brain slice is constructed in the form of a matrix (80×80) of 6400 picture points each indicating an absorption coefficient value. Considerably greater definition is supplied by newer instruments using a 160×160 (25,600 picture points) or 320×320 (102,400 picture points) matrix.

Although computerized tomograms can be taken in a horixontal plane parallel to the base line of Reid (a plane established by the external auditory meatuses and the inferior orbital margin), such scans do not permit visualization of all posterior fossa structures (Fig. 2-33). An example of a computerized tomogram in the horizontal plane and a corresponding section of the head and brain in the same plane are shown in Figures 2-34 and 2-35. In order to visualize the largest number of intracranial structures, including those in the posterior fossa, computerized tomograms usually are taken in parallel planes at angles of 25° with reference to the baseline of Reid (Figs. 2-33 and 2-36).

Computerized x-ray tomography provides a pictorial cross section of the intracranial contents and brain at multiple levels which cannot be obtained by any other radiological technic. The method is entirely noninvasive and has the capacity to reveal differential densities in the components of the brain. The scanner is capable of discriminating between the absorption coefficients of gray and white matter (2520). Certain contrast agents containing iodine can be used to enhance the contrast of tomograms, especially when lesions or neoplasms show increased vascularity.

CHAPTER 3

Development and Histogenesis of the Nervous System

FORMATION OF NEURAL TUBE

The fertilized ovum undergoes a period of cell division until it reaches the uterus. At this time the spherical ball of cells develops a cavity, forming the blastula. A bilaminar layer of cells, called the embryonic disk, forms a few days after the blastula becomes implanted into the uterine wall (Fig. 3-1). During the 3rd week of development the embryonic disk becomes trilaminar and at this stage the three primary tissues of the embryo, ectoderm, entoderm and mesoderm, can be distinguished.

The central and peripheral nervous systems are derived from a thickened plate of ectoderm, known as the *neural plate*, which first appears late in the 3rd week of fetal life. The neural plate lies dorsally, rostral to the primitive streak and Hensen's node, and at first consists of a single layer of cells (Fig. 3-2). This ectoderm undergoes rapid proliferation and becomes stratified. The growth rate near the margins of the plate exceeds that in the midline, causing the formation of a *neural groove*, which is bounded on each side by an elevated *neural fold* (Fig. 3-3). As the primitive ectodermal cells proliferate, the neural groove deepens, and the neural folds thicken, become more prominent and ultimately fuse dorsally to form the *neural tube*. Closure of the neural tube begins in the region of the fourth somite (i.e., future cervical region) and proceeds in both cranial and caudal directions. During the formation of the neural tube its lumen has temporary cranial and caudal connections with the amniotic cavity via the *anterior* (*rostral*) and *posterior neuropores* (*caudal*) (Fig. 3-2). The anterior neuropore which represents the most rostral opening of the embryonic neural tube closes in embryos of 18 to 20 somites and ultimately becomes the *lamina terminalis*. The posterior neuropore usually closes later when the embryo has reached the 25 to 26 somite stage. At early stages in the formation of the neural tube, before closure is complete, rostral portions of the neural tube are enlarged and indicate the formation of primary brain vesicles. Three primary brain vesicles are evident by the time the neural tube is completely closed (Fig. 3-10). From these vesicles the brain is formed. Caudal portions of the neural tube which remain relatively small in diameter form the spinal cord.

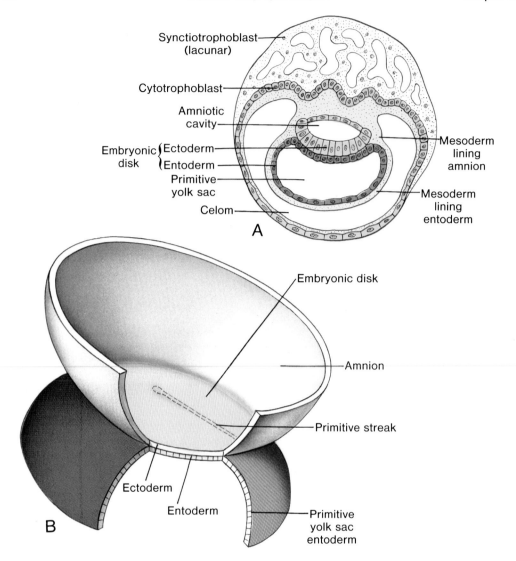

Figure 3-1. (*A*) Drawing of the embryonic disk in a blastocyst at the end of the 2nd week of development: cytotrophoblasts are *green*; mesoderm is *yellow*; ectoderm is *blue* and endoderm is *light red*. (*B*) Schematic diagram of the embryonic disk viewed from the amniotic cavity. The appearance of the primative streak indicates the start of gastrulation.

The appearance of the neural folds heralds the segmentation of bilateral strips of paraxial mesoderm into somites (Figs. 3-2 and 3-3). New somites continue to be formed in a craniocaudal sequence; at the end of the 4th week 40 somites normally are present (82).

NEURAL CREST

The lateral margins of the neural plate are thinner and continuous with the general body ectoderm. The thinned lateral margins of the neural plate (neural crest cells) are approximated as the neural folds meet and fuse. Neural crest cells form a temporary intermediate layer between the neural tube and the surface ectoderm (Fig. 3-3). This temporary layer extends from the level of the mesencephalon to the caudal somites and is for a time continuous across the midline. Neural crest cells divide in the midline, migrate laterally and become segmented into cell clusters between the neural tube and the somites (Fig. 3-3). These clusters of neural crest cells give rise to the primary sensory neurons of the dor-

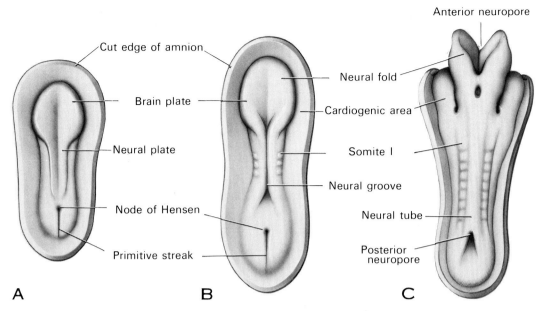

Figure 3-2. Diagrams illustrating early development of human nervous system. (*A*) Late presomite and early neural plate stage (modified from Davis (597)). (*B*) Early somite and neural groove stage (modified from Ingalls (1183)). (*C*) Eight-somite and early neural tube stage (modified from Payne (1952)).

sal root ganglia of spinal nerves. Similar cell clusters in the hindbrain give rise to sensory neurons which form cranial nerve ganglia (nerves V, VII, VIII, IX and X), but these are not segmentally arranged (Fig. 3-10).

The neural crest has a temporary existence as its cells migrate widely in the body and undergo various differentiations in different tissues (1146). All of the sensory cells and fibers of the peripheral nervous system (with a few exceptions) and most of the peripheral cells of the autonomic nervous system, are derived from the neural crest. Thus the neural crest gives rise to the unipolar spinal ganglion cells and their equivalent in the sensory ganglia of cranial nerves V, VII, IX and X. Some elements persisting as bipolar cells form the auditory nerve (1012). Other derivatives of the neural crest include: (a) the neurolemmal sheath cells of all peripheral nerves, (b) capsule cells in ganglia, (c) sympathetic ganglia, (d) chromaffin cells and (e) pigment cells (236).

Cells of the sympathetic ganglia and the chromaffin cells of the adrenal medulla produce high levels of specific amines such as norepinephrine or epinephrine. Other cells that contain high concentrations of amines are found throughout the gut and its associated glands. These have been termed APUD (amine precursor uptake and decarboxylation) cells. APUD cells can be recognized with fluorescence histochemical technics. Some of the polypeptide hormone-producing cells in the pancreas, stomach and other parts of the gut also show a fluorescence histochemical reaction, but it cannot be assumed that these cells are of neural crest origin (2008).

HISTOGENESIS OF NEURAL TUBE

The histogenetic changes whereby the columnar ectoderm is converted to nervous tissue are essentially the same in all parts of the neural tube. According to classic concepts, as the neural tube closes it is formed by a single layer of columnar cells. This epithelium proliferates forming a pseudostratified neuroepithelium several layers thick. Large ovoid cells near the central canal form a *germinal layer* in which rapid mitotic cell division takes place. Newly formed undifferentiated cells migrate peripherally so that the wall of the neural tube assumes a three-layered appearance. The three layers formed by these cells and their processes are: (a) an internal *ependymal layer* composed of columnar cells arranged radially around the central canal, and ovoid germinal cells undergoing mitosis; (b) a middle *mantle layer* of

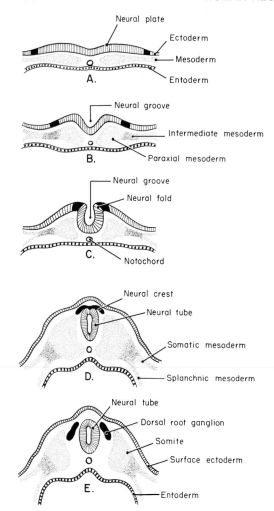

Figure 3-3. Diagrams of transverse sections of embryos at different ages to show development of the spinal cord. (*A*) Neural plate stage, (*B*) early neural groove stage, (*C*) late neural groove stage, (*D*) early neural tube and neural crest stage and (*E*) neural tube and dorsal root ganglion stage.

densely packed primitive neuroblasts derived from the germinal cells; and (c) an external *marginal layer* composed of the processes of cells in the mantle and ependymal layers (Fig. 3-4).

More recent studies based upon autoradiographic and electron microscopic studies have challenged the classic concepts described above (1426–1429, 1547, 1548). These new data indicate that the wall of the recently closed neural tube consists of only one type of cell, the *neuroepithelial cell*. Neuroepithelial cells form a pseudostratified epithelium which extends from the *internal limiting membrane* to the *ex-ternal limiting membrane*. Each neuroepithelial cell is wedge-shaped and possesses cytoplasmic processes which reach the internal limiting membrane and are attached to adjacent cells by *terminal bars* (Fig. 3-5). Nuclei of neuroepithelial cells have an oval shape and may be at variable distances from the external limiting membrane. Desoxyribonucleic acid (DNA) synthesis occurs only in nuclei near the external limiting membrane. When DNA synthesis is complete, the nucleus moves toward the lumen of the neural tube and the cell loses its contact with the external limiting membrane. Cells undergo mitosis when the nucleus has reached the innermost zone, and daughter cells remain attached by the terminal bars at the internal limiting membrane. After division the cells elongate and their nuclei migrate toward the external limiting membrane where further DNA synthesis occurs. Following closure of the neural tube, neuroepithelial cells give rise to another cell type characterized by a large round pale nucleus and dark-staining nucleolus. These cells no longer have the ability to synthesize DNA and constitute the primitive nerve cells or *neuroblasts* (Fig. 3-5). Neuroblasts, produced in increasing numbers, surround the neuroepithelial layer and form the *mantle layer*. The outermost layer containing the processes of the neuroblasts forms the *marginal layer* (Fig. 3-4).

NEURONS

Neuroblasts, arising from division of neuroepithelial cells, migrate into the mantle layer of the neural tube and increase in number as neuroepithelial cells continue to differentiate. These cells form rounded *apolar neuroblasts* (Fig. 3-6), which further differentiate into *bipolar neuroblasts* with two cytoplasmic processes on opposite sides of the cell body. One cytoplasmic process elongates to form a *primitive axon*. The other cytoplasmic process develops numerous small outgrowths which form arborizations known as *primitive dendrites*. At this stage the cell becomes a *multipolar neuroblast*. Further growth and differentiation results in the formation of an adult nerve cell or *neuron*. Neuroblasts in the lateral part of the anterior horn are formed first, and these are followed by those in the medial part of the anterior horn, the internun-

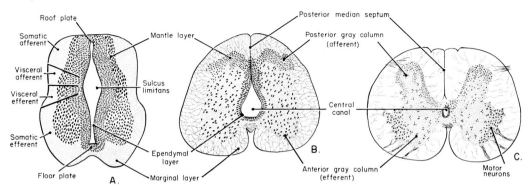

Figure 3-4. Diagrams of differentiating layers of the spinal cord. (*A*) Section through spinal cord of a 5-week human embryo, (*B*) cervical spinal cord of an 8-week human embryo and (*C*) cervical spinal cord of a 10-week human embryo (after Keibel and Mall (1274)).

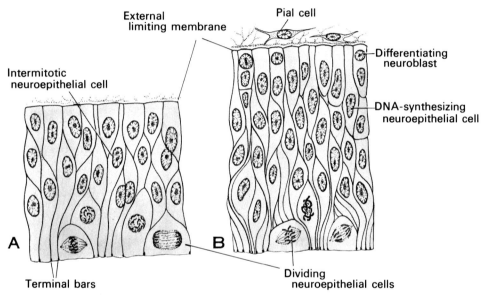

Figure 3-5. Modern concepts of the development of the recently closed neural tube indicate only one cell type, the neuroepithelial cell. (*A*) Wall of the recently closed neural tube with neuroepithelial cells which form a pseudostratified epithelium extending from the lumen to the external limiting membrane. (*B*) Cross section of the wall of the neural tube at a more advanced stage than in *A*. Neuroepithelial cells are in phases of DNA synthesis or mitosis, except near the external limiting membrane where differentiating neuroblasts are found (after Langman (1427)).

cial zone and posterior horn (1430). Neuroblasts, once formed, lose their ability to divide.

As neuroblasts mature the axonal processes do not seem to establish synapses randomly with cells that they contact. Rather, they appear to be attracted to particular groups of target cells. Sperry (2397) suggested that chemical gradients or specific chemical affinities enabled axons to establish synaptic contacts only with appropriate postsynaptic neurons. Molecular mechanisms for cellular recognition are being studied by many investigators, but the field is still in its early stages. Proteins that promote the aggregation of neurons in specific portions of the brain have been isolated (1757) and cell surface glycoproteins, such as *N*-acetyl-D-glactosamine have been implicated in adhesion between specific pre- and postsynaptic elements (928). Experiments in developing amphibi-

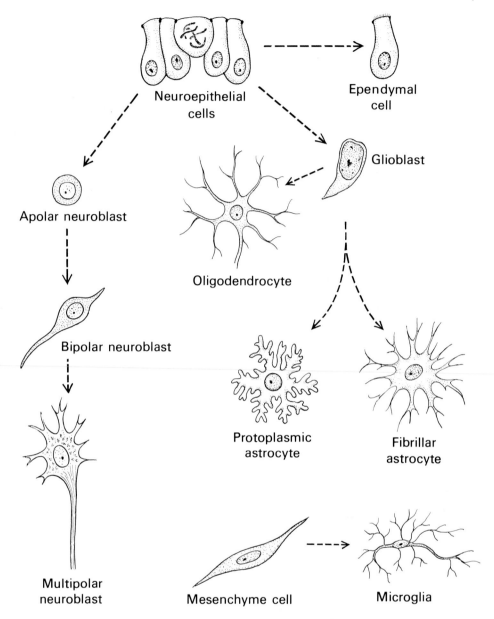

Figure 3-6. Schematic diagram of the histogenesis of neurons and neuroglial cells. Neuroblasts, glioblasts and ependymal cells originate from neuroepithelial cells. The origin of the oligodendrocyte is obscure, but both protoplasmic and fibrillar astrocytes are derived from glioblasts. The microglia are considered to arise from mesenchyme.

ans in which an eye is transplanted into the spinal cord show that factors other than cell surface recognition sites are also involved in the specification of neural connections. Axons from the ectopic (spinal) eye reach the optic tectum and form synapses only when the embryo's own eyes are removed (888), suggesting that some affer-

ent axons may mask cellular recognition sites, or render them ineffective.

GLIA CELLS

Some of the neuroepithelial cells differentiate into primitive *glioblasts* which form supporting cells. The majority of glioblasts are formed after the production of neuroblasts has ceased (1428). Glioblasts become spindle-shaped bipolar cells that extend the entire thickness of the neural tube. Their large nuclei are placed close to the lumen and their processes are attached to both the internal and external limiting membranes of the neural tube. Some glioblasts retain this position and become transformed into ependymal cells (Fig. 3-6). During maturation most ependymal cells lose their attachment to the external limiting membrane and their processes extend only a short distance from the central canal to become anchored in a subependymal glial membrane (Fig. 5-13). Ependymal cells in the adult form the lining of the central canal of the spinal cord and the ventricular surfaces of the brain. Epithelial cells of the choroid plexus (Fig. 5-15) are believed to be modified ependymal cells (i.e., of glioblast origin). Other glioblasts in the mantle layer lose their attachments with the limiting membrane and assume apolar or unipolar appearances. In later stages of development these detached stem cells send out new processes and are transformed ultimately into fibrous and protoplasmic astrocytes (Fig. 3-6). Smaller glial cells, the oligodendrocytes, are thought to be derived from glioblasts. These cells are found mainly in the marginal layer and play a role in developing myelin sheaths (Fig. 5-9) (319, 323).

In addition to the above neuroglia, the adult central nervous system contains *microglia*, considered by Rio-Hortega (2167) to be of mesodermal origin. These cells do not appear in the central nervous system until it has been invaded by blood vessels and their perivascular adventitia. Despite many descriptions of microglia in light microscopy, there is uncertainty regarding their identification in the electron microscope (1982). Microglia are considered to serve a phagocytic function and may be derived from blood histiocytes.

In tissue culture neurons develop normally only when they are embedded in dense glia (1788). Glial cells retain a measure of motility in the adult, whereas neurons are immobile beyond the neuroblast stage. Glial cells also can divide and increase in number, while neurons do not divide after birth and remain in permanent interphase throughout life (50). The latter is a significant point, for neural pathways,

reflexes and storage of learned information all require a metabolically stable and permanent system of neurons. Structural and functional features of the neuroglial elements are presented in Chapter 5.

SPINAL CORD

Continued cell proliferation produces anterior and posterior thickenings in the mantle layer. Anterior thickenings form the larger *basal plates*, from which the anterior gray horn (motor) of the adult spinal cord is formed. Smaller posterior thickenings constitute the *alar plates*, from which the future posterior gray horn (sensory) of the spinal cord is formed. A longitudinal groove, the *sulcus limitans*, marks the lateral junction of basal and alar plates (Fig. 3-4). The sulcus limitans extends the length of the primitive spinal cord and continues into the brain stem; it remains as a prominent sulcus in the floor of the fourth ventricle in the adult brain (Fig. 11-17). In transverse sections of the neural tube the lumen is rhomboid-shaped with relatively thin *roof* and *floor plates* (Fig. 3-4). The roof and floor plates furnish only glioblastic elements.

Neuroblasts of the basal plates become the efferent peripheral neurons. Their axons penetrate the marginal layer and external limiting membrane and emerge from the spinal cord as ventral root fibers (Figs. 3-7 and 3-9). Fibers of the ventral root pass directly to skeletal muscle or to autonomic ganglia for the innervation of visceral structures (Figs. 3-9 and 9-28). All axons of cells of the alar plate remain within the central nervous system. Some arch anteriorly, cross through the basal plate to the opposite side, and reach the marginal layer, where they ascend or descend for variable distances (Fig. 3-7). Other axons remain on the same side and ascend or descend in the marginal layer. These neurons, whose processes are entirely confined to the central nervous system, constitute the *central*, or *intermediate*, *cells*. Those whose axons remain on the same side are known as *association cells*; those whose axons cross to the opposite side are *commissural cells*.

As development proceeds, the proliferation of the germinal cells gradually decreases and ultimately stops altogether. As more and more indifferent cells are trans-

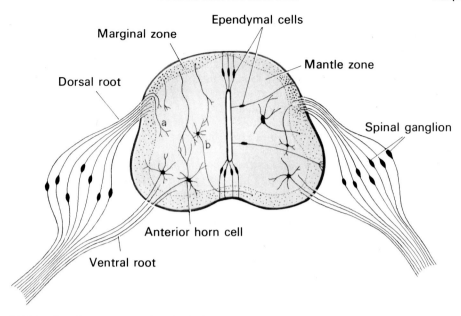

Figure 3-7. Drawing of transverse section of spinal cord and spinal ganglia of a chick embryo. The mantle zone becomes the butterfly gray of the adult spinal cord, while the marginal zone develops into the white matter containing ascending and descending fiber tracts. *a* indicates afferent fiber with collaterals; *b* represents a column cell that projects contralaterally. Based upon silver impregnation.

formed into neuroblasts, the nuclear layer progressively diminishes in size and ultimately is reduced to a single layer of columnar ependymal cells. In certain places, as in the anterior commissure of the spinal cord, some of the ependymal cells may retain their embryonal glioblastic character and extend the whole thickness of the neural wall (Fig. 3-7).

The mantle layer, on the other hand, progressively increases in size and becomes the gray matter of the spinal cord. It is surrounded by an expanding marginal layer which contains the descending and ascending axons of the central cells. At a much later period, most of the axons become myelinated and the marginal layer assumes the white, glistening appearance characteristic of the white matter of the adult spinal cord.

The expansion of the alar plates in a medial direction brings these plates into close apposition. The *posterior median septum*, formed of glial processes and intima pia, marks the line of junction in the adult (Figs. 3-4 and 9-6). In the floor plate region, an invagination forms the anterior median fissure and greatly reduces the size of the central canal (Figs. 3-4 and 9-7). As a con-

sequence of these changes, the embryonic neural tube is transformed into the spinal cord.

The spinal cord has a long cylindrical shape and is curved in the embryonic axis. There is an acute ventral flexure, *the cervical flexure*, at the junction of the spinal cord and hindbrain (rhombencephalon). Until the beginning of the 3rd month the spinal cord extends the entire length of the vertebral canal. After this time the mesodermal elements which have formed the cartilages and bones of the vertebral column grow more rapidly than the spinal cord, so that at birth the most caudal part of the spinal cord, the *conus medullaris*, lies at the level of the third lumbar vertebra. The sites of emergence of spinal nerves do not change, but there is a lengthening of root filaments between the intervertebral foramina and the spinal cord which is most marked for lumbar and sacral spinal roots. The large number of nerve roots surrounding the *filum terminale* (Fig. 1-6) constitute the *cauda equina*. In the adult the conus medullaris lies between the L1 and L2 vertebrae and the spinal cord occupies only the upper two-thirds of the vertebral canal (Fig. 9-3).

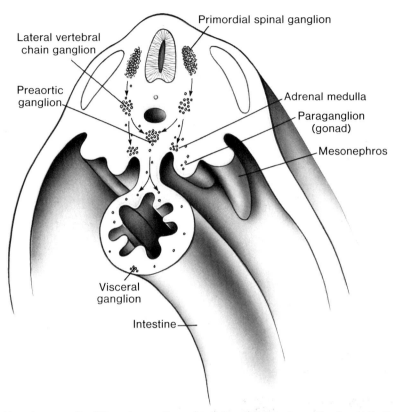

Figure 3-8. Neural crest cells differentiate to form the primordial spinal ganglia. Sympathetic neuroblasts migrate ventrally where clusters of cells differentiate further to form sympathetic ganglia, preaortic ganglia, chromaffin cells of the adrenal medulla, and autonomic neurons of the alimentary tract.

Neuron Differentiation. In the spinal ganglia, derived from the neural crest, a similar differentiation takes place. Many of the original polygonal or round cells become spindle-shaped and bipolar with the development of two neurofibrillar processes, one central and one peripheral (Figs. 3-7 and 4-7). The central processes enter the spinal cord as dorsal root fibers and there bifurcate into ascending and descending arms which contribute collaterals to the mantle layer or gray matter (Figs. 3-7 and 9-28).

In human embryos with a crown-to-rump length of 25 mm, many of the neuroblasts have attained the bipolar stage. A few neurons with greater amounts of cytoplasm and distinct neurofilaments appear transitional in shape and are referred to as pseudounipolar cells (Fig. 4-7). The cytoplasm of the cell body elongates, and the two processes become approximated. Ultimately the elongated cell cytoplasm forms the single stem of a T, while the top of the

T is formed by the thin central and thicker peripheral processes (2524, 2578). Many neurons are of the unipolar type in spinal ganglia of human 100 mm fetuses. Most of the spinal ganglia cells are true unipolar neurons in the newborn human infant. An occasional bipolar neuron or those in transitional stages may at times be observed in the adult dorsal root ganglia. It is interesting to note that a generous number of ganglionic neuroblasts may be produced initially. Thus, embryonic dorsal root and sympathetic ganglia appear to have an overabundance of neuroblasts when compared to the number of fully differentiated ganglion cells present at birth. For example, total cell counts of the submandibular ganglia in a graded series of human fetuses showed a progressive reduction from 12,128 cells at 17 weeks of gestation to 5,988 at full term (572). Cell death appears to be a normal event in the course of embryonic development, and it is estimated that 25 to 75% of the original neuron population in

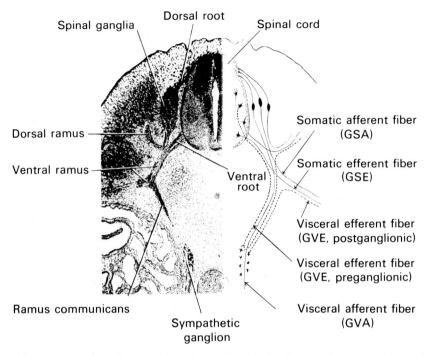

Figure 3-9. Transverse section of 14-mm pig embryo. The functional categories of spinal nerve fibers are indicated on the right (Bielschowsky's silver stain, photograph).

many parts of the neuraxis dies in neonatal life (2081).

Not all of the cells in the spinal ganglia differentiate into neuroblasts. Some develop into *capsule* or *satellite cells* which form a capsule around the bodies of the spinal ganglion cells (Fig. 4-2*A*). Others wander out along the course of the growing peripheral nerve fibers, envelop them and ultimately become Schwann cells. These play an active role in the formation of myelin and may be considered as a peripheral type of neuroglia, perhaps most closely related to oligodendrocytes.

Besides the spinal ganglia, there are other peripheral aggregations of nerve cells known as *autonomic* or *sympathetic ganglia* (Figs. 3-9 and 8-2). Arising mainly from the neural crest, these cells form two ganglionic chains on the anterolateral aspect of the vertebral column (vertebral sympathetic ganglia). Others wander further to form the ganglia of the mesenteric plexuses (collateral or prevertebral ganglia), while some actually invade the walls of the viscera, or settle close to them, as the terminal or peripheral autonomic ganglia (Figs. 3-8 and 8-1). Here, too, differentiation occurs in several directions. Some cells enlarge to

form the multipolar sympathetic ganglion cells, whose axons terminate in visceral effectors, smooth muscle, heart muscle and glandular epithelium (Fig. 4-7). Others, as in the case of the spinal ganglia, give rise to satellite cells, which envelop the bodies of one or several ganglion cells. Finally, some differentiate into the chromaffin cells found in the adrenal medulla, carotid bodies and other portions of the body.

Segmental Arrangement of Peripheral Nerve Elements. With the differentiation of the various types of nerve cells in early stages of development, a neuronal mechanism adequate for complete, if simple, reflex arcs is established. Such arcs consist of afferent, intermediate and efferent neurons and their peripheral extensions. However, the synaptic junctions of these cells, which make such reflex arcs functional, are as yet unformed.

In embryos of about 10 mm the various components of the peripheral nervous system already are laid down and may be recognized in a transverse section of any typical body segment (Fig. 3-9). The central processes of the spinal ganglion cells form the *dorsal* roots; the *ventral root* is composed of axons from cells in the anterior gray of the spinal cord (mantle layer). Distal to the ganglion, the ventral root unites with the peripheral processes of the spinal ganglion cells to form a mixed *spinal nerve* (Figs. 3-9 and 7-1). Each spinal nerve containing afferent and efferent fibers, divides into a *dorsal* and a *ventral ramus* and also sends a fiber bundle known as the *ramus communicans* to the vertebral sympathetic chain. The dorsal ramus supplies the muscles and skin of the back; the larger ventral ramus goes to the ventrolateral parts of the body wall. Four functional types of peripheral nerve fibers may be distinguished: *general somatic afferent* (GSA), *general visceral afferent* (GVA), *general somatic efferent* (GSE) and *general visceral efferent* (GVE). All of these functional types of fibers are found in both dorsal and ventral rami. The somatic efferent or "motor" fibers arise from large cells in the anterior gray matter, leave the spinal cord through the ventral roots and go directly to the skeletal voluntary muscles of the body wall. The somatic afferent or "sensory" fibers are the peripheral processes of spinal ganglion cells, which terminate as receptors in the skin and deeper portions of the body wall. The central processes enter the cord as dorsal root fibers (Fig. 9-28).

The efferent innervation of visceral structures is different from that of the somatic muscles, for two neurons always are involved in the conduction of impulses from the central nervous system to the effector organs (Figs. 3-9 and 8-2). The *preganglionic visceral efferent* fibers are axons of spinal cord neurons which pass through the ventral root and ramus communicans to terminate in a vertebral or prevertebral sympathetic ganglion. The axons of sympathetic cells form the *postganglionic visceral efferent* fibers, which course through the ramus communicans in the reverse direction, join the main branches of the spinal nerve and are distributed to the smooth muscle and glandular epithelium of the body (Figs. 8-1 and 8-2). In the adult the ramus communicans consists of white and gray portions. The former contains the *myelinated* preganglionic fibers, the latter the *unmyelinated* postganglionic fibers.

Earlier it was mentioned that cell death appears to be a normal process during development. Somewhat later in development, there is a change in synapses formed by motor neurons upon striated muscle and by parasympathetic preganglionic axons upon postganglionic cells (2081). In newborn animals both muscle fibers and ganglion cells are innervated by several different axons, but in the adult each cell is usually innervated by a single axon. In the case of ganglion cells, the number of synaptic terminals per cell may actually increase, but the number of cells innervated by a single axon decreases. It is not known whether the polyneuronal innervation represents an initial indiscriminate formation of synapses that is subsequently modified by trophic signals transmitted from the target cell to afferent axons, or whether synapse elimination is due to genetic programming of motor neurons and preganglionic neurons (621).

Finally, *visceral afferent fibers* convey impulses from the thoracic and abdominal viscera. Like the somatic afferent fibers, their cell bodies are in the spinal ganglia and their central processes enter the spinal cord via the dorsal root (Fig. 9-28).

BRAIN

As soon as the anterior neuropore is closed, the rostral cavity of the neural tube shows three dilatations or brain vesicles. These three early subdivisions are the *prosencephalon* or forebrain, the *mesencephalon* or midbrain and the *rhombencephalon* or hindbrain (Fig. 3-10*A*). The constricted region between the mesencephalon and rhombencephalon is known as the isthmus. The brain vesicles maintain many of the fundamental morphological features seen in more caudal parts of the embryonic neural tube, in that each has roof and floor plates and alar and basal plates. Although the walls of these vesicles are thin, the sulcus limitans is present at the junction of alar and basal plates in caudal brain vesicles (rhombencephalon and mesencephalon). The large dilated cavities within each brain vesicle are the forerunners of the ventricular system, although they are destined to undergo extensive alterations in size, shape and extent as a consequence of cell proliferation, growth and various brain flexures. These ventricular cavities are continuous with the central canal of the spinal cord. The lateral margins of the prosencephalon develop shallow depressions, the optic sulci, which subsequently becomes evaginated to

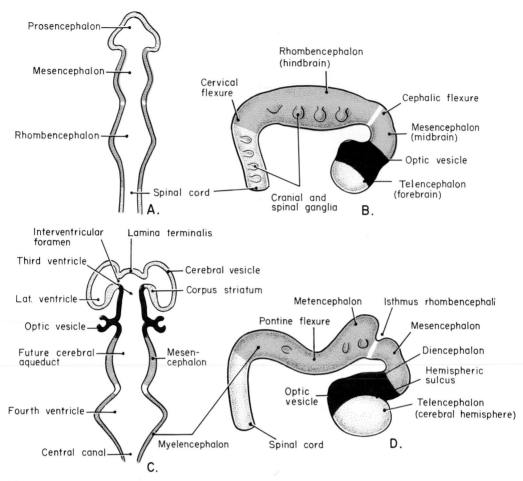

Figure 3-10. Diagrams of the developing brain vesicles and ventricular system. (*A* and *B*) Three brain vesicle stage of a 4-week embryo. (*C* and *D*) Five brain vesicle stage of a 6-week human embryo. The prosencephalon, telencephalon and spinal cord are *stippled*. The diencephalon is shown in *dark red*, while the mesencephalon is *blue*. The derivatives of the rhombencephalon (pons and medulla) are in *light red* and the isthmus is *white* (modified from Hochstetter (1108) and Langman (1427)).

form the optic vesicle (Fig. 3-10, *B* and *C*). Each optic vesicle becomes modified to form an *optic cup* which is joined to the prosencephalon by a hollow optic stalk.

Two prominent brain flexures appear at an early embryonic stage. The *cervical flexure* develops at the junction of rhombencephalon and spinal cord, with its concavity directed ventrally. A second ventral flexure, the *cephalic flexure*, occurs at the junction of mesencephalon and rhombencephalon (Fig. 3-10, *B* and *D*). Rapid changes in the brain occur in the 4th and 5th week of development. In the 6th week a third impressive flexure with a dorsal concavity develops in the rhombencephalon and divides

it into two segments, the *metencephalon* and the *myelencephalon*. This prominent *pontine flexure* creates the *transverse rhombencephalic sulcus* on the dorsal surface of the brain stem (Figs. 3-10*D* and 3-11*A*). A relatively shallow hemispheric sulcus on each side of the forebrain divides the prosencephalon into a cephalic *telencephalon*, or *endbrain*, and a caudal part, the *diencephalon*. The optic stalks and optic vesicles are attached to the diencephalon. It has been assumed that bending of the developing neural tube results from differences in the rate of cell proliferation.

In chick embryos, cyclic adenosine monophosphate can act as a stimulus for axial

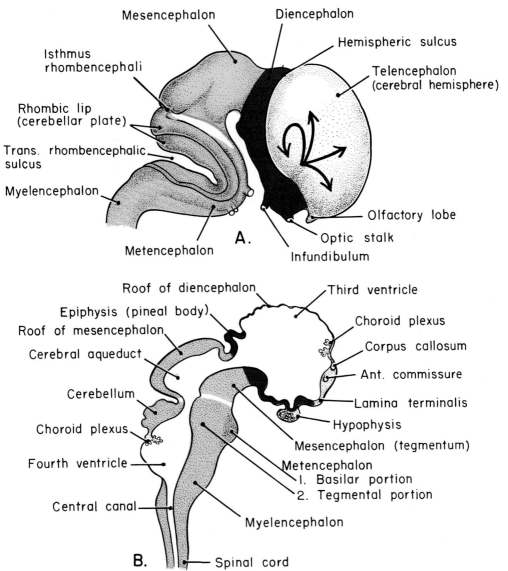

Figure 3-11. Diagrams of the developing brain vesicles and ventricular system. (*A*) Lateral view of cerebral vesicle and developing brain stem in human embryo of 8 weeks. *Arrows* indicate directions of growth and expansion of cerebral hemisphere. (*B*) Sagittal section through the brain stem of a 12-week human fetus. The telencephalon is *stippled*, the diencephalon is *dark red* and the mesencephalon is *blue*. Rhombencephalic derivatives (metencephalon and myelencephalon) are *light red*, while the isthmus is *white* (modified from Hochstetter (1108)).

bending of the embryo which is caused, at least in part, by cell movement (2179).

The basic pattern of the ventricular system of the brain is evident in early stages of development (Fig. 3-11B). The roof of the rhombencephalon is extremely thin and the underlying cavity (*fourth ventricle*) appears as a shallow, diamond-shaped depres-

sion called the *rhomboid fossa* (Figs. 2-24, 3-11-*B*, 3-14 and 3-16). With continued growth, the lumen of the midbrain will become narrowed to form the *cerebral aqueduct*. Medial growth and expansion of the diencephalon also reduce the lumen of this segment of the brain to a thin vertical cleft, the *third ventricle*. A large opening (*inter-*

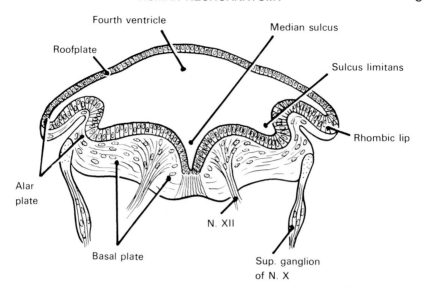

Figure 3-12. Diagram through medulla of a 5-week human embryo. Note the prominent sulcus limitans separating structures derived from the basal and alar plates.

ventricular foramen) behind the lamina terminalis provides continuity between the third ventricle and the cavity of the laterally expanding cerebral hemisphere. The primitive *lateral ventricle* within each cerebral hemisphere will become altered extensively by subsequent development (Figs. 3-10 and 3-15).

Five distinctive subdivisions of the developing brain are established at this stage, and each subdivision undergoes elaborate, and sometimes unique, development as growth continues (Fig. 3-11). The five basic subdivisions of the brain are: (a) *the telencephalon*, (b) *the diencephalon*, (c) *the mesencephalon*, (d) *the metencephalon* and (e) *the myelencephalon*. The development of each subdivision is considered separately, even though the embryological events described occur simultaneously.

Myelencephalon

The *medulla*, the most caudal brain segment, is derived from the myelencephalon. This brain segment extends from levels of the first spinal nerve of the cervical cord to the beginning of the pontine flexure (Fig. 3-11). As the future medulla oblongata, it differs from the spinal cord in that the walls are shifted laterally at higher levels by the expanding fourth ventricle. As a result the alar plate lies lateral to the basal plate. The sulcus limitans continues to mark the boundary between these two plates in both

gross and microscopic specimens (Figs. 2-24, 3-12 and 11-17). Derivatives of the basal plate form the motor nuclei of cranial nerves, and come to occupy positions in the floor of the fourth ventricle medial to the sulcus limitans (Fig. 3-12). The most medial cell column gives rise to general somatic efferent (GSE) fibers that form cranial N. XII. Intermediate cell columns are associated with special visceral efferent (SVE) fibers, issuing from the nucleus ambiguus, that form components of cranial nerves IX, X and XI (Fig. 11-17). General visceral efferent (GVE) cell columns, also medial to the sulcus limitans, and represented by the dorsal motor nucleus of the vagus nerve (N. X) and inferior salivatory nucleus (N. IX), give rise to preganglionic parasympathetic fibers that are widely distributed.

Derivatives of the alar plate form sensory relay nuclei lateral to the sulcus limitans. The most lateral of these nuclei are the auditory and vestibular (special somatic afferent (SSA) cranial nerve components), and those of the trigeminal complex (general somatic afferent (GSA)). General and special visceral afferent (GVA and SVA) cell columns, represented by the solitary nuclei, lie medial to the above group (Fig. 3-13). The most medial and caudal cell groups of the alar lamina differentiate into the nuclei gracilis and cuneatus (general somatic afferent, GSA). Some cells derived from the alar lamina migrate ventrally to

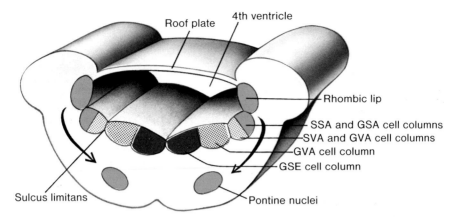

Figure 3-13. Schematic drawing of the caudal metencephalon showing the cell columns of the cranial nerve nuclei with respect to the sulcus limitans. Cell groups derived from the alar plate are shown in *blue*, while those from the basal plate are *red*. Both the rhombic lip (cerebellum) and the pontine nuclei develop from the alar plate. Cells of the pontine nuclei migrate ventrally (*arrows*). *Dark blue,* rhombic lip, special (*SSA*) and general somatic afferent (*GSA*) cell columns and the pontine nuclei; *blue stipple,* special (*SVA*) and general visceral afferent (*GVA*) cell columns; *red stipple,* general visceral (*GVE*) efferent cell column; *red,* general somatic efferent (*GSE*) cell column.

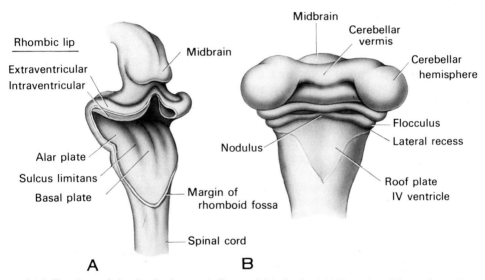

Figure 3-14. Drawings of the developing cerebellum and hindbrain. (*A*) Posterior oblique view of human embryo at 6 weeks. (*B*) Posterior view of human fetus at 4 months' gestation (after Prentiss and Arey (2066)).

form portions of the *inferior olivary complex,* the largest cerebellar relay nucleus of the medulla (Fig. 11-12). Fibers forming the medullary pyramids are cortically derived, late in appearance and occupy ventromedial regions near the midline.

In the region of the fourth ventricle, the roof plate consists of a single layer of ependymal cells covered by a thin layer of pia mater. These two layers form the tela choroidea, and prolongations project into the ventricle in the region of the transverse rhombencephalic sulcus to form the choroid plexus (Fig. 5-17). Openings in the roof plate appear (4 to 5 months) which establish continuity between the fourth ventricle and the subarachnoid space surrounding the brain stem. Two lateral apertures (foramina of Luschka) connect the lateral recesses of the fourth ventricle with the pontine cistern (Figs. 1-10 and 1-11). A single median aperture (foramen of Magendie) in the lower roof connects the fourth ventricle with the cerebellomedullary cistern.

Metencephalon

This rostral portion of the hindbrain, extending from the pontine flexure to the rhombencephalic isthmus, develops into two elaborate and distinctive components of the neuraxis. Both the pons and cerebellum are derived from the metencephalon (Figs. 3-13 and 3-14).

The *pons* consists of two parts: (1) a phylogenetically older *dorsal portion*, lying in the floor of the fourth ventricle, referred to as the pontine tegmentum, and (2) a more recently acquired *ventral portion*, in which some cortical efferent fibers terminate while others continue to more caudal regions. The pontine tegmentum is derived from the basal plate (Fig. 3-13). A medial general somatic efferent (GSE) cell column gives rise to fibers of the abducens nerve (N. VI). An intermediate and interrupted cell column of typical motor neurons gives rise to special visceral efferent (SVE) fibers that form cranial nerves V and VII, and respectively innervate the musculature of the first and second branchial arches. General visceral efferent (GVE) cells contained in the superior salivatory nucleus supply preganglionic parasympathetic innervation for the submandibular, sublingual and lacrimal glands. Cells of the basal plate also contribute to the pontine reticular formation (Fig. 3-13).

Ventromedial portions of the alar plate form cell groups similar to those described for the medulla (1427, 1428). These cell groups are concerned with: (a) the vestibulocochlear nerve (SSA), (b) the trigeminal nuclear complex (GSA) and (c) the solitary nucleus (SVA and GVA). The *pontine nuclei* which form massive cell collections in the newer ventral portion of the pons originate from the alar plate of both the metencephalon and myelencephalon (Fig. 3-13). Corticofugal fibers which develop later end, in part, upon these nuclei. The pontine nuclei give rise to a massive collection of fibers which cross the midline and enter the opposite cerebellar hemisphere; fibers in this bundle form the *middle cerebellar peduncle* (Figs. 2-25 and 2-31).

The *cerebellum* is derived from the dorsolateral portions of the alar plates which bend posteriorly and medially to form the rhombic lips (Figs. 3-11 and 3-14). The rhombic lips are at first widely separated from each other, and each lip projects partly into the fourth ventricle (intraventricular portion) and partly on the surface of the metencephalon above the roof plate. Further deepening of the transverse rhombencephalic sulcus at the pontine flexure causes the cerebellar rudiments of both sides to fuse in the midline caudal to the roof of the mesencephalon (1012). Fusion of the rhombic lips forms the transverse *cerebellar plate*. At 3 months these cerebellar primordia have a dumbbell-shaped appearance (Fig. 3-14) in which the unpaired central part represents the *vermis* and the two large lateral knobs represent the *hemispheres*. Near the end of the 4th month fissures begin to develop on the cerebellar surface. The first fissure to appear is the *posterolateral* (prenodular) *fissure* which separates the *nodulus* from other parts of the vermis and the *flocculus* from the rest of the cerebellar hemisphere. The *flocculonodular lobe* (*archicerebellum*), phylogenetically the oldest part of the cerebellum, has the most extensive connections with the vestibular system (280, 645, 1437). The portion of the cerebellar plate between the posterolateral fissure and the isthmus represents the rudiment of the *corpus cerebelli*. The first fissure to become visible in the corpus cerebelli is the *primary fissure*. The primary fissure is the deepest of all cerebellar fissures, and it separates the anterior and posterior lobes (Figs. 2-32 and 14-1). All parts of the cerebellum rostral to the primary fissure constitute the *paleocerebellum* (anterior lobe) while the *neocerebellum* (posterior lobe) lies between the primary and posterolateral fissures. The neocerebellum is subsequently divided into lobules by three transverse fissures, the prepyramidal, the horizontal and the posterior superior.

Cerebellar primordia initially consist of the three layers (ependymal, mantle and marginal) which characterize the primitive neural tube. With development neuroblasts migrate through the mantle and marginal layers to the surface where they form the *external granular layer* (1021, 1700, 2602). Cells of the external granular layer retain their ability to divide, thus forming a proliferative zone on the surface of the cerebellum. Cells of the external granular layer eventually migrate inward and ultimately form the innermost cellular layer of the cerebellar cortex, the *granular layer*. *Purkinje cells* and *Golgi type II cells* are formed relatively early; Purkinje cells, representing the principal discharge element of the cerebellar cortex, form a distinctive layer along the outer margin of the granular layer. Although cells of the transient external granular layer migrate inward, their processes, the *parallel fibers*, remain in the *molecular layer* where synaptic contacts are established with Purkinje cell dendrites.

The *deep cerebellar nuclei* are considered to be derived from neuroblasts located close to the ventricular surface of the cerebellum. The largest and most lateral of these nuclei, the *dentate nucleus*, has a convoluted appearance (Fig. 14-13) which becomes evident during the 5th month (1437). The *roof nuclei* (the fastigial nuclei) develop near the midline and have profuse connections with the vestibular nuclei. In lower forms the *globose* and *emboliform nuclei* are not clearly separated and are referred to as the *interposed nuclei*. Cranial and caudal portions of the thin metencephalic roof plate persist in the adult as the superior and inferior medullary veli (Figs. 2-26 and 2-27).

Mesencephalon

The *mesencephalon* is the most primitive of the brain vesicles and ultimately forms the smallest, least differentiated division of the brain stem. The alar and basal plates are separated by a well defined sulcus limitans (Fig. 3-11). The cavity of this vesicle is greatly reduced during development and ultimately becomes the cerebral aqueduct. The portion of the midbrain ventral to the aqueduct consists of the *midbrain tegmentum*, dorsally, and the *crus cerebri* ventrally; these structures are separated by the *substantia nigra* (Fig. 13-1). The tegmentum is derived from the basal and floor plates. Motor neurons derived from the basal plates form the general somatic efferent (GSE) cell columns that compose the oculomotor complex (N. III) and what must be regarded as a caudal appendage to it, the trochlear nuclei (N. IV). These cranial nerves, and the abducens nerve, innervate the extraocular muscles derived from the preotic somites. A smaller lateral cell group from the basal plate migrates dorsal to the

somatic cell columns of cranial N. III to form the visceral nuclei (GVE) of this complex. The marginal layer of each basal plate eventually is invaded by massive collections of corticofugal fibers which form the crus cerebri. These are corticospinal, corticopontine and corticobulbar fibers largely destined for more caudal regions of the neuraxis.

The alar plates of the mesencephalon proliferate and produce two longitudinal eminences separated by a median depression dorsal to the aqueduct. These eminences form the *quadrigeminal plate* (Fig. 3-16); a later developing transverse depression divides each longitudinal eminence into a *superior* and *inferior colliculus* (Fig. 2-24). Neuroblasts forming the inferior colliculus produce a central homogeneous cell mass surrounded by a narrow cortical rim. The superior colliculus is a more complex stratified structure formed by waves of migrating neuroblasts. Its development resembles that of the cerebral cortex in that cell migrations follow an "inside-out" sequence (819), which means that cells forming the deeper layers appear first and those destined for the superficial layers must pass through the deep layers. The inferior colliculus serves as a major relay complex in the auditory system, while the superior colliculus serves as a subcortical integrative center for the visual system.

The *midbrain reticular formation* and that specialized portion of it known as the *red nucleus* are considered to be derived from the alar plate (1012, 1428). The formation of the *substantia nigra* appears poorly understood. Some authors (1428) consider it to be derived from cells of the alar plate, while others (517, 2308, 2309) suggest that the substantia nigra arises relatively l e from cells that migrate ventrally from the basal plate. Cells of the pars compacta of the substantia nigra do not contain melanin pigment at birth; appreciable pigmentation does not develop until the 4th or 5th year. In the rabbit neurons of the substantia nigra have been found to contain dopamine on the 19th day of gestation (2526).

Diencephalon

The prosencephalon which divides into the diencephalon and the telencephalon

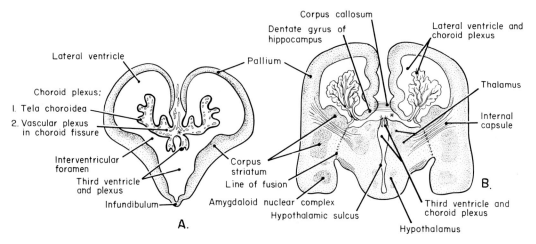

Figure 3-15. Diagrams of frontal sections through diencephalon, ventricular system and choroid plexuses of the developing brain. (*A*) Invagination of choroid plexuses into lateral and third ventricles. (*B*) Choroid plexuses and secondary fusion of telencephalon with diencephalon. The transverse cerebral fissure is indicated in both *A* and *B* by an *asterisk* (*) (modified from Hamilton et al. (1011)).

gives rise to the entire central nervous system rostral to the midbrain (Fig. 3-10).

The *diencephalon* develops from the thickened lateral walls of the caudal portion of the original prosencephalic vesicle, which is considered to be formed only by the alar plates. The prosencephalon is caudally continuous with the mesencephalon, and at an early embryonic stage optic cups, formed from the optic vesicles, are attached to the lateral walls of the diencephalon. The cavity of the prosencephalon becomes narrowed to form the third ventricle. The *posterior commissure* is considered to mark the caudal limit of the diencephalon (Fig. 2-12), while the *interventricular foramen* represents its boundary with the telencephalon (Fig. 3-15). The *lamina terminalis*, representing the membrane formed by the closure of the anterior (rostral) neuropore, is a telencephalic derivative, but its ventral part forms a matrix in which the *optic chiasm* ultimately develops.

The roof plate of the diencephalon becomes very thin and rostral parts of it invaginate to form the *choroid plexus* of the third ventricle (Figs. 3-11 and 3-15). Caudal portions of the roof plate thicken medially and evaginate posteriorly to form the *pineal gland*. This gland, which develops about the 7th week, ultimately becomes solid and lies in the midline dorsal to the posterior commissure. The roof plate of the diencephalon may form another evagination in the region of the interventricular

foramen, known as the *paraphysis*. This epithelial sac may persist into adult life as a paraphysial cyst and produce intermittent blockages in the flow of cerebrospinal fluid (317, 591). Other epithalamic structures, considered to be derived from the roof plate, or adjacent parts of the alar plate, are the *habenular nuclei* and *habenular commissure* (1382). These structures lie dorsally, immediately rostral to the posterior commissure. The habenular nucleus, which receives fibers of the *stria medullaris* and gives rise to the *fasciculus retroflexus*, links the septal nuclei with the midbrain reticular formation.

The alar plates forming the lateral walls and floor of the prosencephalon develop distinct longitudinal sulci on the surfaces facing the lumen. This depression is the *hypothalamic sulcus* which serves to divide the major part of the diencephalon into the *thalamus* and *hypothalamus* (Figs. 3-15 and 15-7). Some authors have suggested that the hypothalamic sulcus may be the diencephalic equivalent of the sulcus limitans, but this seems unlikely since it does not mark the division of alar and basal plates, or the boundary between sensory and motor regions. Active proliferation and cell differentiation produces an expansion of thalamic regions dorsal to the hypothalamic sulcus which greatly narrows the third ventricle. The thalamic nuclear masses of each side approach the midline and fuse in an *interthalamic adhesion* in about 80% of

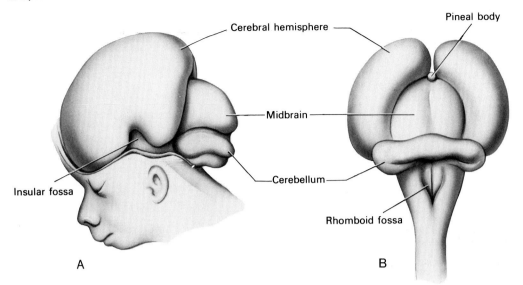

Figure 3-16. Drawings of the cerebral vesicle and brain stem in the 12-week human fetus. (*A*) Lateral view, (*B*) posterior view.

human brains. Cell growth in the thalamus proceeds rapidly and results in the formation of thalamic nuclear groups, some of which are clearly separated by medullary laminae (Figs. 2-15 and 2-28). The *principal nuclear groups* of the thalamus are: (1) the anterior, (2) the medial, (3) the ventral and (4) the dorsal. The *medial* and *lateral geniculate bodies* (metathalamus) represent a caudal extension of the ventral nuclear group which function in part as relay neurons. The dorsal nuclear group, in general, serves as association neurons. Thalamic nuclear groups, readily detectable in gross specimens, include the anterior, the medial, the geniculate bodies and the pulvinar.

The part of the alar plate inferior to the hypothalamic sulcus (Figs. 3-11 and 3-15) on both sides of the third ventricle forms the hypothalamus. Cells in this region differentiate into a number of separate nuclear groups which subserve visceral, endocrine and regulatory functions. The most prominent nuclear group forms the *mammillary body*, a rounded protuberance on the ventral surface of the hypothalamus (Figs. 2-8 and 2-9). A small evagination in the floor of the diencephalon caudal to the optic chiasm forms the primordium of the *infundibulum*, which gives rise to the *neurohypophysis*. The *anterior lobe* of the *hypophysis* forms from an ectodermal diverticulum of stomodeum known as *Rathke's pouch*, which

superiorly comes in contact with the infundibulum; Rathke's pouch loses its pharyngeal attachment and differentiates into the anterior lobe of the hypophysis (Fig. 3-11).

Telencephalon

This most rostral segment of the developing brain is composed of the two evaginating *cerebral vesicles* and their median connection, the *lamina terminalis* (Figs. 3-10 and 3-11). Each cerebral vesicle is in wide communication with the third ventricle via the interventricular foramen (Fig. 3-15) and expands upward, forward and backward. Through this caudal expansion the telencephalic vesicles cover the diencephalon dorsally and laterally. The region where the cerebral vesicle is attached to the roof of the diencephalon becomes very thin. Here the single layer of ependymal cells and the vascular mesenchyme in the roof of the third ventricle become continuous with similar layers in the lateral ventricle that form the choroid plexus. The line of invagination which first appears at the level of the interventricular foramen is called the *choroidal fissure*. Thus the choroid plexus of the third and lateral ventricles is continuous through the interventricular foramina along the line of vesicle evagination, the choroid fissure. A small horizontal cleft persists between the cerebral vesicle and the diencephalon (Fig. 3-16). This narrow tri-

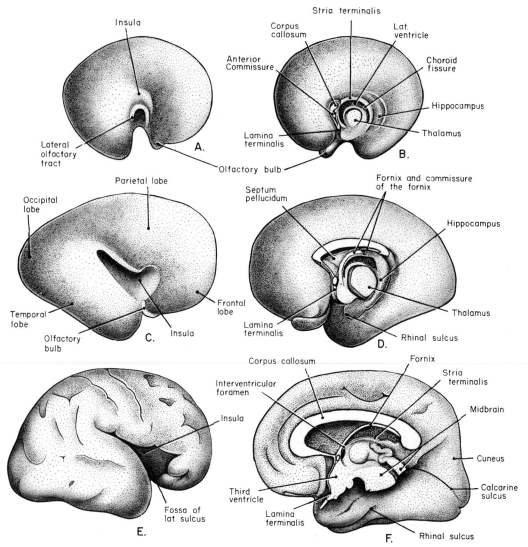

Figure 3-17. Development of human cerebral hemisphere. (*A* and *B*) Lateral and medial surfaces of the hemisphere in a fetus of 3 months. (*C* and *D*) Lateral and medial surfaces of the hemisphere in a fetus at beginning of the 5th month. (*E* and *F*) Lateral and medial surfaces of the hemisphere at the end of the 7th month (modified from Keibel and Mall (1274)).

angular space dorsal to the thalamus is lined with a double layer of pia mater and filled with loose mesenchyme (velum interpositum, Fig. 2-28). This space represents the most rostral extension of the *transverse cerebral fissure*. The small *asterisk* (*) in Figure 3-15*A* and *B* is located within the transverse cerebral fissure. The lower pial layer of this fissure, as observed in frontal section, forms the roof of the diencephalon and becomes invaginated as the choroid plexus of the third ventricle (Figs. 2-28 and 3-15). The adult cerebral hemisphere also

is separated from the cerebellum by the transverse cerebral fissure. The tentorium cerebelli occupies part of the transverse fissure and separates the inferior surfaces of the hemispheres from the superior surface of the cerebellum (Fig. 2-1).

Immediately above the choroid fissure the medial wall of the cerebral vesicle becomes thickened and forms the *hippocampal ridge* (Figs. 3-15 and 3-17). This ridge bulges into the lateral ventricle as a longitudinal elevation, the *hippocampal formation*. The hippocampal formation expands posteriorly and is carried downward into the temporal lobe. The medial surface of the hemisphere develops a corresponding groove, the *hippocampal fissure*, which runs parallel to the choroid fissure throughout its extent. The hippocampal formation and the dentate gyrus together constitute the *archipallium*, phylogenetically the oldest cortex.

The walls of the primitive telencephalic vesicle consist of ependymal, mantle and marginal layers and represent only the alar plates. The mantle layer ventrolaterally undergoes relatively rapid thickening as a consequence of cell proliferation and creates a cell mass that protrudes into the lumen of the vesicle. This thickened basal region is known as the *striatal portion* because it ultimately gives rise to the *corpus striatum* (Fig. 3-15). The thinner, more dorsal wall of the brain vesicle is referred to as the *suprastriatal portion*. The suprastriatal portion is the primordium of the *cerebral cortex*.

Corpus Striatum and Internal Capsule. The thickened basal striatal region appears in the telencephalon at the level of the interventricular foramen (Fig. 3-15) (1012). With the expansion of the cerebral hemispheres back over the diencephalon, part of the striatal ridge is carried in the wall of the lateral ventricle dorsal to the lateral border of the thalamus and down into the roof of the inferior horn of the lateral ventricle. Large numbers of developing corticofugal and corticopedal fibers projecting from, and to, the developing cerebral cortex incompletely divide the corpus striatum into a dorsomedial portion which bulges into the lateral ventricle and a ventrolateral portion medial to the insular region. The paraventricular striatal tissue medial to these fibers forms the *caudate nucleus* which throughout most of its extent is closely related to the lateral ventricle (Figs. 2-12, 2-13 and 2-28). The *amygdaloid nuclear complex* arises from the same medial primordium. The portion of the corpus striatum lateral to these cortical fiber systems, which collectively form the *internal capsule*, constitutes the *lentiform nucleus* (Fig. 3-15). The lentiform nucleus is divided into two parts: (a) a larger lateral part known as the *putamen* and (b) a smaller inner part, the *globus pallidus*. Although

the basal ganglia are classically regarded as subcortical telencephalic nuclei, some authors (1381, 1385, 2149) consider parts, or all, of the globus pallidus to be derived from portions of the hypothalamus. The *subthalamic nucleus*, a small nucleus with connections mainly with the globus pallidus, also is considered a hypothalamic derivative. The internal capsule, formed by fibers projecting to and from the cerebral cortex, has a complex development (1093), but ultimately forms two major limbs: (a) an *anterior limb* which partially separates the head of the caudate nucleus and the putamen and (b) a larger *posterior limb* between the thalamus and the globus pallidus (Figs. 2-12 and 2-13).

The *cerebral hemispheres* grow and expand rapidly, first forward to form the frontal lobe area, then laterally and upward to form the future parietal lobe (*arrows* in Figs. 3-11 and 3-16). Posterior and inferior expansions soon produce the occipital and temporal lobes. The expansions of the cerebral hemispheres cover the diencephalon and posterior surface of the midbrain. The anterior, posterior and inferior expansions during development explain the curved shape and the relations of several internal telencephalic structures in the adult brain (e.g., lateral ventricle, choroid plexus, caudate nucleus and fornix). The cortex covering the lenticular nucleus remains as a fixed area, the insula (Fig. 3-18). This region becomes buried in the floor of the lateral sulcus by the subsequent overgrowth of adjacent lobes (Fig. 3-17).

Cerebral Cortex. The early evolution of the forebrain is similar in all mammals, and has been reviewed (89, 169, 1175, 2122, 2432). The suprastriatal portion of the early telencephalic vesicle appears to be composed of three concentric zones during its smooth-surfaced (lissencephalic) stage. A *germinal* or *matrix zone* surrounds the lateral ventricle. Most of the cells of this zone migrate outwards to become nerve and glial cells upon maturation. However, some cells remain in this zone to form the internal limiting membrane, ependyma and the subependymal glial layer. The pale *intermediate zone* becomes the white matter of the cerebral hemispheres. It has many radiating fibers and is traversed by neuroblasts and glioblasts migrating from the

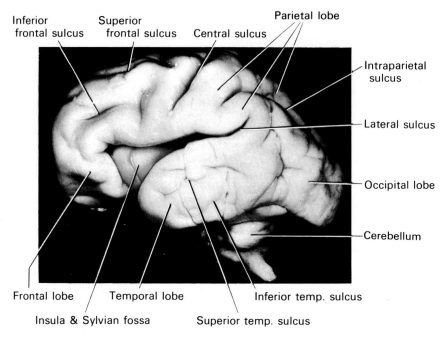

Figure 3-18. Lateral view of the brain of a 7-month human fetus. Note the primitive sulcal pattern and the exposure of the insular cortex (photograph).

matrix zone to the more superficial layer. An outer *cortical zone* or *plate* represents the prospective neopallium (isocortex). This zone has two distinct layers. The deeper pyramidal layer has many cells and will form layers II to VI of the adult six-layered cortex (Fig. 19-1). The marginal layer is composed mostly of fibers and becomes the molecular (plexiform) or most superficial layer (I). In areas of the olfactory cortex (allocortex) the six layers are not present. In these regions the migrant neuroblasts and glioblasts enter the cortical zone and form a thin nuclear layer close to the surface.

There is evidence that the neuroblasts invade the cortical zone to form a primitive pyramidal layer before the glial cells arrive (1528). It also has been shown that cells formed at the same time remain in the same part of the pyramidal layer; and that newly formed cells migrate beyond those already present (77). Hence, cells in the deeper strata of the pyramidal layer were formed earlier and are older than more superficially located cells. In man the cortical zone becomes highly cellular due to massive neuroblast migrations in the 12th week. At birth the human neopallium has assumed

a stratified appearance as a result of neuron differentiation and laminae formation by the incoming and outgoing nerve fibers.

Although the hippocampal formation appears early in development (see p. 621), its constituent cells are not organized into the characteristic adult arrangement until late embryonic life (74, 1012). The superior and rostral portions of the hippocampal formation undergo regressive changes in association with development of the corpus callosum, but these parts persist in the adult as the indusium griseum or supracallosal gyrus (Figs. 2-10 and 18-8).

In the early weeks of gestation the surfaces of the cerebral hemispheres are lissencephalic (smooth). The developing commissures form conspicuous bundles on the cut medial surfaces (Figs. 3-15 and 3-17). During the 6th and 7th months, the surfaces of the hemispheres grow rapidly and develop convolutions (*gyri*) separated by shallow or deep furrows (*sulci*). As a result of such surface folds, two-thirds of the cerebral cortex becomes buried in the walls and floor of the sulci when the brain attains its adult size. Fetal sulci appear in an orderly sequence; the phylogenetically older sulci appear first, and more recently acquired sulci

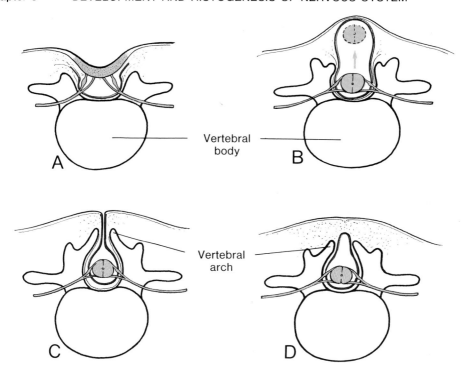

Vertebral
body

Vertebral
arch

Figure 3-19. One type of spinal malformation is called *spina bifida*. In this condition there is a failure of closure of the posterior arch of one or more vertebrae and in some types there is a failure of development of the neural tube. *A* diagrammatically illustrates failure of closure of both the neural tube and the vertebral arch. In *B*, the neural tube develops normally, but the meninges and subarachnoid space extend dorsally through the defect in the vertebrae to produce a *meningocele*. If the spinal cord forms part of the subcutaneous herniation (*arrow*), it is called a *myelomeningocele*. *C* represents a minor defect in the vertebral arch in which a dermal sinus extends from the skin to the subarachnoid space. This sinus may close secondarily. *D* represents *spina bifida occulta*, in which the meningeal herniation does not extend far above the defect in the vertebral arch. Skin overlying the vertebral defect may contain a dense tuft of hair. Nerves and neural tissue are in *blue*; the meninges are in *red*. [Modified from Tuchmann-Duplessis et al. (2589).]

appear later (Figs. 3-17*E*, 3-17*F* and 3-18). The principal sulci and gyri that form the characteristic pattern of the human cerebral cortex all can be identified in the full-term infant.

Commissures. The medially placed *lamina terminalis* represents the cephalic end of the early neural tube and extends from the roof plate of the diencephalon to the optic chiasm (Figs. 3-11 and 3-17). This primitive midline telencephalic structure thus provides the only bridge whereby nerve fibers can pass from one cerebral hemisphere to the other. The first fibers to cross between the two hemispheres (*commissural fibers*) are within the *anterior commissure*. This structure appears in the lower portion of the lamina terminalis by the 3rd month. It connects the olfactory bulb and portions of the temporal lobe of

one side with the same structures of the opposite hemisphere (Figs. 18-4 and 18-9). The small *commissure of the fornix* (psalterium) is the second to appear in the lamina terminalis close to the roof of the diencephalon (Fig. 3-17*D*). Its fibers connect portions of the hippocampal formation with each other.

The largest and most important commissure to cross in the lamina is the *corpus callosum*. The first of these commissural fibers, connecting nonolfactory cortical areas of the two hemispheres, appears as a small bundle rostral to the commissure of the fornix. The size of the corpus callosum parallels the rapid growth and expansion of the neopallium. It first extends anteriorly to connect the frontal lobes and then enlarges posteriorly as the parietal lobes develop. As the constituent fibers increase in number, the corpus callosum arches back over the thin roof of the diencephalon (Figs. 3-17 and A-29). The area between the corpus callosum and the fornix becomes very thin and forms the septum pellucidum. The above commissures and septum pellucidum thus develop within, and represent prolongations of, the embryonic lamina terminalis. The fibers of the *optic chiasm* cross in the junctional zone between the lamina terminalis and the rostral wall of the diencephalon (Figs. 2-27 and 3-17).

After the neural tube has been formed, it lies deep to the overlying ectoderm and is surrounded on all sides by primitive mesoderm (mesenchyme). This embryonic relationship is shown in Figure 3-9. Here the more darkly stained mesenchyme is seen to the left of the spinal nerve and neural tube. From the surrounding mesoderm the muscles, blood vessels, cartilage, bone and connective tissue of the body are derived. The mesoderm thus gives rise to several supporting structures of the nervous system (e.g., skull, vertebrae, meninges (dura mater), intervertebral discs, ligaments, sheaths of peripheral nerves, blood vessels and microglia). These mesodermal structures are of paramount importance, for they provide not only support, but protection and nourishment, to the nervous system.

Supporting tissues are, under some circumstances, responsible for serious damage to the nervous system. For example, an artery may rupture with extensive hemorrhage, or the lumen of a vessel may be occluded suddenly and produce anoxia in the area of its neural distribution. Tumors commonly arise from the meninges, from the connective tissue sheaths along peripheral nerves or from glioblasts. An intervertebral disc may rupture posteriorly into the vertebral canal and compress the spinal cord or spinal nerves; also fractures of the skull and vertebrae often compress the underlying brain or spinal cord.

CONGENITAL ANOMALIES

A detailed discussion of malformations of the developing neural tube or changes in brain development resulting from malnutrition are beyond the scope of this textbook. An example of malformations involving both the developing neural tube and the vertebral column will serve as an example. Defects in the development and fusion of the dorsal arch of the vertebra may result in herniation of the dura and arachnoid membranes dorsally, forming a cystlike expansion of the subarachnoid space. This is called a meningocele (Fig. 3-19B). When the spinal cord is displaced dorsally into the cyst, it is termed a meningomyelocele. If the dural sac does not extend far enough into the subcutaneous tissue to form a cyst, there may be no protrusion of the overlying skin (Fig 3-19D). This condition is termed spina bifida occulta and is often marked by a tuft of hair on the overlying skin. In some cases, the caudal neuropore may not close completely, forming a channel or fibrous cord extending from a dimple on the surface of the skin to the meninges (Fig. 3-19C).

A more serious defect involves failure of the neural plate to close and form the neural tube. The neural plate remains exposed to the outside, and the subsequent differentiation of neurons is arrested. This is termed spina bifida with myeloschisis (Fig. 3-19A).

CHAPTER 4

The Neuron

The tissue of the central nervous system is made up of two classes of cells that may be broadly categorized as neurons and neurologia. Neuroglia will be discussed in Chapter 5. Neurons have processes, called dendrites, radiating from a central portion of the cell, known as the soma or perikaryon. Another process, the axon, extends for variable distances from the soma and establishes specialized junctional contacts, called synapses, upon the dendrites and cell bodies of other neurons. The processes and synapses are a reflection of cellular specialization for long distance intracellular communication and unique forms of intercellular interaction.

Intracellular communication is accomplished through two mechanisms: electrical and chemical (Fig. 4-1). Electrical intracellular communication is a property of the neuronal surface membrane. While in this chapter the detailed biophysical or chemical aspects of cellular communication in the nervous system will not be considered, some introduction to general concepts is provided for students who have not yet studied cellular physiology. In a "resting" neuron the interior of the cell is 70 to 90 mV negative with respect to the extracellular fluid. This electrical potential reflects steady-state ionic concentration gradients resulting from the selective permeability properties of the cell membrane. There is a high potassium concentration inside the cell relative to the outside, and a high sodium concentration outside the cell relative to the inside. Potassium ions move freely through the membrane, and the resting potential is due largely to the distribution of potassium ions needed to balance the charge of impermeant anions. In the resting neuron, the surface membrane is effectively impermeable to sodium ions because of a unidirectional transport mechanism called the sodium pump. When a neuron becomes active, the permeability of the membrane to sodium and other ions changes. This movement of ions, termed conductance, is inversely proportional to the resistance of the membrane. In axons the conductance change has a duration of approximately 1 msec and is called an action potential. In

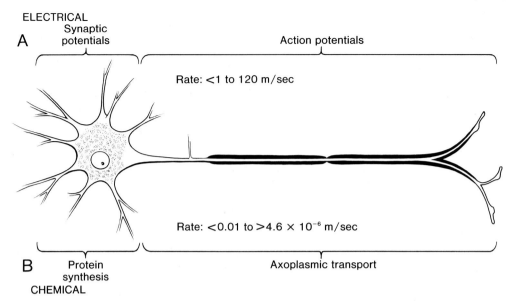

ELECTRICAL
Synaptic
A potentials   Action potentials

Rate: <1 to 120 m/sec

Rate: <0.01 to >4.6 × 10⁻⁶ m/sec

B Protein   Axoplasmic transport
synthesis
CHEMICAL

Figure 4-1. Diagrammatic comparison of major types of *intra-* and *intercellular* communication in neurons. The dendrites and soma of the cell are shown toward the left, the axon and synaptic terminals toward the right. In (*A*) two regions of the neuron concerned with intracellular electrical communication are shown. One zone sustains graded, nonpropagated synaptic potentials and the other all or none, propagated action potentials. (*B*) The rates of chemical (axoplasmic) transport between the soma and synaptic terminals are shown for comparison with rates of electrical communication by action potentials.

dendrites and soma, the conductance change has a duration varying from a few to more than 100 msec. These longer duration changes are called synaptic potentials and are graded in amplitude. In contrast to synaptic potentials, action potentials are always of the same amplitude once the threshold has been exceeded. A potential change which causes the inside of a cell to become less negative with respect to the extracellular fluid is termed a depolarizing potential. An increased negativity of the interior of the cell is termed a hyperpolarizing potential. Synaptic potentials may be either depolarizing or hyperpolarizing, while action potentials are always depolarizing. Action potentials are usually generated in the soma at the region of the emergence of the axon and propagated along the axonal membrane to its terminal (Fig. 4-1). At the terminal the depolarization of the surface membrane as it is invaded by the action potential leads to an influx of calcium ions, which in turn causes the release of a chemical called a neurotransmitter. The action potential can be regarded as a means of transferring a signal from the soma, along the axon, to the synaptic ter-

minals, where the process of intercellular communication is initiated (see Kuffler and Nicholls (1376) for review). The rate of propagation of action potentials depends upon the diameter of the axon and its associated myelin sheath and can range from less than 1 to about 120 m/sec (Fig. 4-1).

In addition to action potentials, there is a second type of intracellular communication which is chemical in nature. Many of the neurotransmitter substances are synthesized and stored in the synaptic terminals of the axon. However, their synthesis depends upon enzymes which are synthesized in the cell body and moved by a process called axoplasmic transport along the axon to the terminal (Fig. 4-1). In contrast to the rapid rate of propagation of action potentials, rates of axoplasmic transport range from less than 0.01 to more than 4.6×10^{-6} m/sec.

Intercellular communication, for the most part, is accomplished through the release of a neurotransmitter at the synapse (Fig. 4-30). The transmitter diffuses across the small extracellular space between the membrane of the synaptic terminal and the surface membrane of the adjacent neuron.

The membrane of the dendrite and soma of the postsynaptic cell contains specific molecular binding sites for the transmitter. When these binding sites can be shown to be associated with a response in the postsynaptic neuron, they are called receptors. These receptors may be part of an ion conductance channel, so that the transmitter-receptor interaction results in an opening or closing of a channel for a specific ion. In some cases, the transmitter-receptor interaction leads to the activation of enzymes and a sequence of chemical reactions in the postsynaptic cell. When these reactions result, over time, in changes in the number of receptors or transmitter synthetic enzyme molecules in the postsynaptic cell, it is said to be a trophic effect (Fig. 4-29).

The *neuron doctrine*, popularized by Waldeyer (2648), had its foundation in the extensive studies of Cajal (348), which were based upon the Golgi method (913, 916). This doctrine states that the individual nerve cell (i.e., neuron) constitutes the genetic, anatomic, trophic and functional unit of the nervous system. All neural pathways, circuits and reflex arcs are composed of individual neurons arranged in simple or complex patterns.

A variety of staining technics have revealed the principal features of the neuron and the manner in which individual neurons are inter-related. The electron microscope and cytochemical technics have provided new insight into the fine structure and the functional roles of specific organelles. Recent data, acquired with these technics, all support the neuron doctrine.

NEUROANATOMICAL METHODS

Histological Technics

Although unstained fresh nerve tissue, or nerve tissue grown in tissue culture, may be studied with the phase microscope, the customary method is to use stained preparations. It is essential that fresh nerve tissue be fixed in a solution which kills bacteria, inactivates autolytic enzymes and produces minimal shrinkage, swelling or distortion. Appropriate fixatives also make components of the nerve cell receptive to suitable dyes or permeable to colloidal solutions. The most common fixatives for neural tissue are aldehydes and alcohols. These fixatives often are used in conjunction with a variety of chemicals, such as chloral hydrate, ammonia, pyridine, glacial acetic acid and mercuric chloride. In experimental studies in animals excellent fixation of neural tissue is achieved by perfusion technics, but this is not possible in man. Since several hours usually intervene between death and autopsy, it is rarely possible to obtain perfectly fixed human neural tissue. Appropriate fixation renders many components of the nerve cell, such as chromatin, receptive to suitable dyes (i.e., cresyl violet; Fig 4-2E) or neurofilaments more permeable to colloidal silver solutions (Fig. 4-2 A and B).

Formalin fixation followed by a mordanting in potassium dichromate preserves the normal lipids of myelin, and enhances the appearance of the myelin sheaths when stained with hematoxylin (e.g., Weigert method, Fig. 9-20). Primary fixation in potassium dichromate, followed by an osmic acid solution, selectively stains the fatty acids of degenerating myelin black, while the normal myelin remains a yellow-brown color (Marchi method, Fig. 10-4) When the initial fixative contains solvents (e.g., alcohol, ether, chloroform), lipids of myelin are removed and only a clear space remains (Fig. 4-3, A and B). If such solvents are avoided the lipids of the normal myelin sheath are readily stained by osmic acid (Fig. 4-3, C–E) and Luxol fast blue (Fig. 4-3, F and H).

Nerve tissue has a strong affinity for weak silver solutions (i.e., argyrophilia). Blocks of nerve tissue are impregnated with silver salts for several days, and then placed in suitable reducing solutions. This action results in the deposition of silver particles within the nerve cell and its processes. The reduced silver particles in nonneural tissue are removed by subsequent solutions, so that the neurons and their processes appear golden brown or black against a light yellow background. The Cajal (351) and Ranson (2107) technics both permit bulk staining of tissue blocks and are used to elucidate the structural features of the central and peripheral nervous system. Figure 4-2C shows sympathetic ganglion cells and axons of a peripheral nerve stained by the Cajal silver nitrate method.

Other methods have been developed which permit the staining of mounted sections. In the Bodian (203, 204) method the

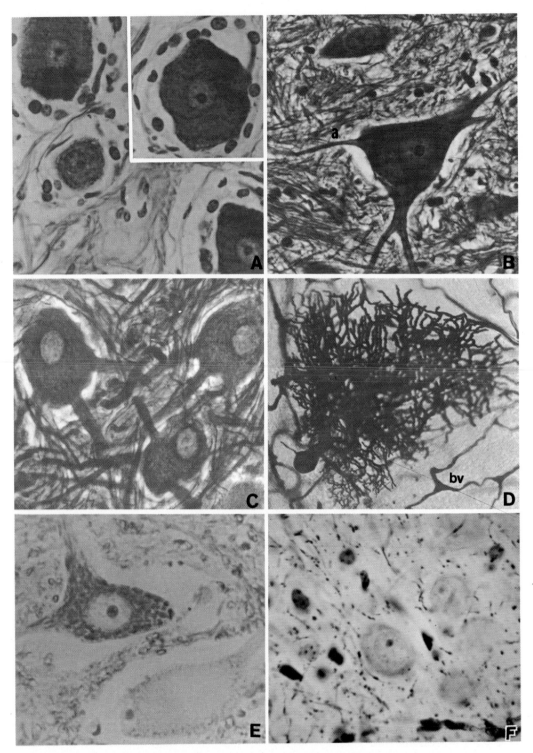

Figure 4-2.   Shape, size and appearance of nerve cells stained by different technics. (All photographs are ×370 except (*D*) which is ×125.) (*A*) Unipolar neurons of dorsal root ganglion. Three larger cells contain melanin granules (silver protargol technic). (*B*) Multipolar neuron of reticular formation. An area of cytoplasmic lipofuscin pigment appears between the nucleus and axon (*a*) of the large cell (silver protargol technic). (*C*) Multipolar neurons of sympathetic ganglion with interlacing of dendrites and small axons (Cajal silver nitrate

slides are placed in a silver protein solution (protargol) with metallic copper and incubated at 37°F (3°C). Again, the silver is reduced as in the bulk method. The silvered sections are then passed through a solution of gold chloride. Since gold has a higher atomic number and atomic weight than silver, the gold replaces the silver particles in the nerve tissues of the section. The sections then are developed in oxalic acid, and the non-neural gold particles are removed. Nerve cells, their nuclei and processes are all beautifully visualized by this method as shown in Figures 4-2, *A* and *B*, and 4-3*A*. The Holmes' (1135) silver technic is another useful silver modification giving consistently excellent results (see Fig. 4-3, *F* and *H*).

For many years gold chloride was used to demonstrate the motor nerve endings in skeletal muscle, and the myenteric plexus of the intestine. Garven's modification (852) of Ranvier's gold chloride method is still a useful procedure for the successful demonstration of motor nerve endings in teased muscle fiber preparations (Fig. 4-3*G*).

The Golgi silver technics are one of the oldest and most widely used methods for studying neurons and neuroglia (913). These technics produce a black deposit which literally fills the cell bodies and processes of many neurons. Although only a fraction of the total number of neurons and neuroglia are stained black, these often are revealed in great detail against a nearly colorless background (Fig. 4-2*D*). In addition to neurons and neuroglia the blood vessels also may be stained (Fig. 1-15). The method is empirical and the results are uncertain, but magnificient neuronal and neuroglial details are revealed in successful preparations (Figs. 5-2 and 14-6).

The illustrations of nerve tissue shown in Figures 4-2 and 4-3 represent a few of the traditional methods used to study the neuron. Basic information and procedural steps in the classical neurological stains can be found in text references edited by Adams et al. (6), Ambrogi (52), Baker (105), Culling (578), Gasser (854), Humason (1172), McManus and Mowry (1572) and Windle (2747).

Much of our recent knowledge of neuron cytology has resulted from the use of the electron microscope and the freeze-etch apparatus. The short wave length of a beam of electrons from a high voltage source permits a greater resolution of biological structures than that obtained from electromagnetic radiation in the visible spectrum. Electron microscopy requires very thin tissue sections, less than 50 nm. The preparation of such sections requires special attention to fixation and embedding but reveals great detail about cellular structure (Fig. 4-10).

Histochemistry

In addition to the general morphology of neurons, it is important to be able to study the cellular localization of specific chemical substances. In recent years a number of histochemical and immunocytochemical techniques (730, 1524) have been developed to permit visualization of neurotransmitters and neurosecretory products. In general, these methods are based upon formation of (a) a colored, insoluble precipitate, (b) a compound with characteristic fluorescence when excited by ultraviolet light or (c) a complex with a labeled antibody.

Axon Tracing

The study of connectivity, or the relation of one part of the nervous system with another, requires tracing of the long axonal processes of neurons. This was first done by placing lesions in the brain and visualizing the degenerating axons with specific stains (Fig. 4-2*F*). One method which proved valuable in the past, the Nauta and Gygax (1821, 1822) technic, results in a

---

technic.) (*D*) Purkinje cell of cerebellar cortex whose dendritic branches are studded with small gemmules. Adjacent blood vessels (*bv*) are identified in this preparation (Golgi technic). (*E*) Cytoplasmic chromatin and nuclear appearances of normal (above) and injured (below) anterior horn cells of spinal cord. The small eccentric nucleus and depleted chromatin pattern (chromatolysis) resulted from earlier axonal destruction (Luxol-fast-blue and cresyl-violet technic). (*F*) Terminal degeneration in the ventral lateral nucleus of the thalamus following a localized lesion in the medial segment of the globus pallidus. Degenerated pallidothalamic fibers appear as black beaded strands and dots near the soma and dendrites of thalamic neurons (Wiitanen (2721) silver technic).

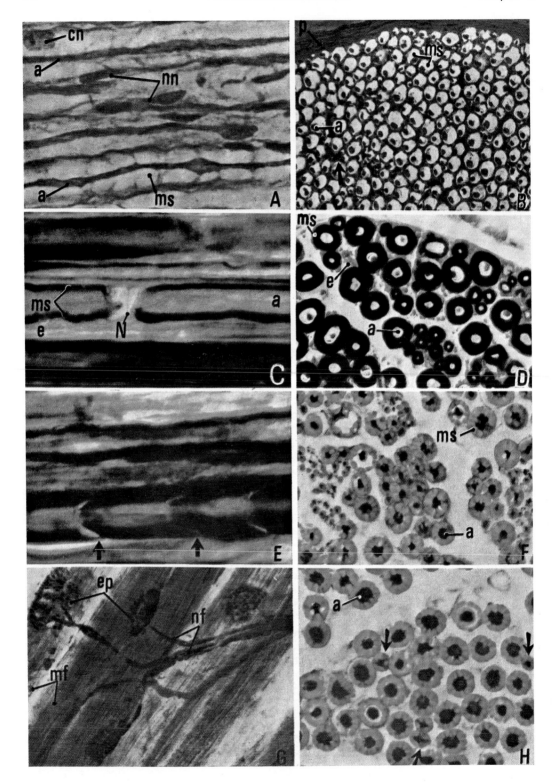

selective silver impregnation of degenerating axons. Staining of normal nerve fibers and endings is suppressed and these have a golden yellow appearance (Fig. 9-30). Thick, as well as thin, degenerating axons of injured neurons appear as discontinuous black droplets or beaded segments arranged in an orderly linear fashion (degeneration "en passage"). Arborizing degenerating axons, observed in close proximity to nerve cells, represent "terminal" fiber degeneration. The Nauta procedure has been evaluated in detail by Eager and Barrnett (668). Selective staining of the terminal end feet of nerve processes (synaptic knobs, bouton termineaux) upon the dendrite or cell body of another neuron also is accomplished by the use of modified silver methods (Fig. 4-24). The technics of Barr (123), Glees (890), Rasmussen (2119a), Fink and Heimer (750) and Wiitanen (2721) have all been used in numerous studies to localize terminal fibers of pathways within the central nervous system (Fig. 4-2F).

More recently, several methods have been introduced that are based upon the intracellular movement of substances along the axon. Radioactively labeled amino acids injected into a small region of the brain are taken up by neuron cell bodies where they are incorporated into cellular protein and transported in an orthograde direction from the cell body to the axon terminal. Autoradiographs are prepared by coating the slides with a nuclear emulsion. After several weeks of exposure, the emulsion is developed and fixed to reveal tracks of silver grains overlying labeled axons and terminals (555, 686).

Another way of studying neuronal interconnections utilizes the retrograde transport of materials from axon terminal to cell body. When the glycoprotein enzyme horseradish peroxidase (HRP) is injected into nervous tissue, it is incorporated into neurons by the process of micropinocytosis. This is most marked at axon terminals, and the HRP is transported back to the cell body where it is ultimately degraded. By reacting the tissue with an appropriate substrate such as tetramethyl benzidine, an insoluble polymer is formed wherever the enzyme is located (1453, 1456, 1678, 2474).

The principle of retrograde axonal transport has also been used with several fluorescent dyes. When different dyes are injected into parts of the brain, cells which have branched axon projections to different regions can be identified by the double labeling which occurs (159).

Metabolic Methods

There is a general correlation between glucose metabolism and functional activity of neurons. A method has been developed to study regional variations in energy metabolism based upon the autoradiographic analysis of $[^{14}C]$-2-deoxyglucose (2-DG) incorporation (2377). 2-DG is an analogue of glucose which is transported from blood to neurons where it is phosphorylated to 2-deoxyglucose-6-phosphate. 2DG-6P is not metabolized further, and its accumulation in neurons is related to the rate of glucose utilization of the cell. This method has proved useful in studying cellular and synaptic regions active following specific forms

Figure 4-3. Size and appearance of nerve fibers stained by different technics. (*A*) Longitudinal section of femoral nerve stained with silver protargol. Axons (*a*), Schwann cell (*nn*) and connective tissue (*cn*) nuclei are identified. The myelin sheath (*ms*) is dissolved and remains as a clear space in such silver preparations (×370). (*B*) Cross section of sciatic nerve stained with silver nitrate. Axons (*a*), myelin space (*ms*) and connective tissue of perineurium (*p*) are identified. Small black dots between larger fibers are axons of nonmyelinated fibers (*arrow*) (×130). (*C*) Longitudinal section of myelinated nerve fiber and node of Ranvier (*N*) stained with osmic acid and light green. Myelin sheath (*ms*) stained black, axon (*a*) is unstained, and connective tissue of endoneurium (*e*) is green (×370). (*D*) Cross section of lumbar nerve in cauda equina with osmic acid and light green. Endoneurium (*e*) derived from pia mater is green, myelin (*ms*) is black, while axons (*a*) are unstained (×270). (*E*) Longitudinal section of two myelinated nerve fibers with osmic acid and light green. Lower fiber with thicker myelin sheath exhibits Schmidt-Lantermann clefts (*arrows*) (×370). (*F*) Cross section of intradural dorsal root sensory fibers with combined Holmes' silver and Luxol blue technics. Axons (*a*) appear dark brown, and myelin sheath (*ms*) is blue. Note variation in size of myelinated and non-myelinated axons (×270). (*G*) Longitudinal section of nerve fibers (*nf*) terminating as motor-end plates (*ep*) on extrafusal skeletal muscle fibers (*mf*) (gold chloride technic, ×145). (*H*) Cross section of intradural ventral root motor fibers tained as in (*F*) above. Larger fibers (*a*) terminate as motor-end plates on extrafusal muscle fibers, while smaller γ-efferent axons (*arrows*) end on intrafusal muscle fibers of neuromuscular spindle (×270).

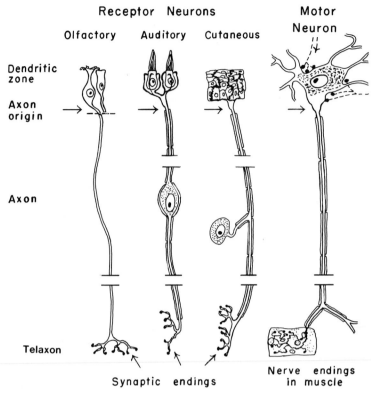

Figure 4-4. Diagram of three sensory neurons and a motor neuron based on the site of impulse origin rather than location of the cell body. Dendritic zone is concerned with the generator potential in a receptor, as well as excitatory or inhibitory input of synaptic endings (*dotted lines* on motor neuron) on another nerve cell. The axon and its terminals are related to conduction and synaptic transmission of the generated nerve impulse. The perikaryon of a neuron is the trophic center primarily concerned with the outgrowth and maintenance of processes, and their metabolic functions other than membrane activity. Note that the cell body may be located either in the dendritic zone of the region of the axon (after Bodian (205)).

of sensory stimulation or during repetitive movements.

FUNCTIONAL CONCEPT OF NEURONS

A generalized concept of neuron structure based upon the site of impulse origin, rather than the location of the cell body, has been proposed by Bodian (205). The term "*dendritic zone*" is used to denote the receptor membrane of a neuron (Fig. 4-4) which may be cytoplasmic extensions (i.e., dendrites), portions of the cell soma or specialized receptors which act as transducers. The cell body (perikaryon) remains the focal point of embryonic outgrowth of dendrites and axon and of axonal regeneration; and it also maintains the trophic aspects of neuronal activity. The position of the perikaryon is irrelevant as far as the major electrochemical functions of the neuron are concerned. Its position is related to the

outgrowth of processes and to metabolic maintenance rather than to the polarized conduction of the neuron.

This functional concept recognizes the site of impulse origin as the pivotal position in the neuron. This site may not necessarily be a fixed point in a particular neuron. Furthermore all surfaces bearing synapses (dendrites, cell body and axon) are related to response-generating functions. In these functional terms, the axon may be said to arise from any response-generating structure, such as a dendrite, the cell body or a sensory receptor. The functional role of the axon is to conduct signals away from the response-generating region. In peripheral sensory neurons, the response-generating zone is the distal tip of the axon which is usually associated with a connective tissue capsule or other receptor of epithelial or mesodermal origin. Impulse origin, or the physiological action potential ("spike"), generally occurs at or near the origin of the axon and conducts the nerve impulse away from the "dendritic zone." Axons are ensheathed by neuroglial or Schwann cells. Both axon diameter and sheath differentiation are related to the rate of impulse conduction. The branched and variously differentiated terminals of axons are called *"telaxons."* They may show membrane and cytoplasmic differentiation related to synaptic transmission or neurosecretory activity (Fig. 8-7). Mitochondrial concentrations, synaptic vesicles or secretory granules are commonly present in their bulblike terminals which release chemical compounds known as neurotransmitters. The telaxons transmit electrical or chemical signals capable of producing generator potentials in the dendritic zones of other neurons and in muscle, or they can induce stimulatory effects in innervated glands. The terms axon, dendrite and cell body, used in this text, are in accordance with functional concepts described above.

VARIETIES OF NEURONS

Neurons show wide variations in size and an infinite variety in the arrangement of their processes. However, nerve cells serving a similar function or located in a given region of the nervous system often resemble each other structurally (Figs. 4-2, 4-5 and 4-7). Thus the *bipolar* neurons are sensory in function and transmit impulses generated by olfactory, visual, vestibular and auditory receptor endings (Fig. 4-7A). The T-shaped *unipolar neurons* are characteristic of the spinal ganglia and mesencephalic nucleus of the trigeminal nerve (Figs 4-2A and 4-7, B–D).

Such sensory neurons convey nerve impulses from a variety of specialized and nonspecialized receptors. *Multipolar neurons* transmit both sensory and motor nerve impulses, and are characteristic of the brain, spinal cord and peripheral autonomic nervous system (Figs. 4-2, B–F, 4-5 and 4-7). The primary, secondary and tertiary dendritic branches of some multipolar neurons may be elaborate and enormously increase its synaptic surface (Figs. 4-5 and 4-6). A Purkinje cell of the cerebellar cortex serves as an illustrative example. Such dendrites are wide at the base, and taper rapidly. The primary, secondary and tertiary branches have a smooth surface, while the more distal dendritic branches are best with great numbers of fine spines or *gemmules* (Fig. 4-6). Fox and Barnard (790) reported the length of the spiny terminals of a single Purkinje cell to be 40,700 μm. The dendritic branchlets with their 61,000 spines have a combined synaptic surface area of 222,000 sq μm. These estimates of the spiny branchlets are now believed to be too conservative, and probably should be doubled (792).

Arborizations of neurons in other parts of the CNS are less extensive, yet they reveal a characteristic pattern of branching. For example, nerve cells of the inferior olivary nuclear complex in the medulla (Fig. 4-5A) have radiating dendrites with curly branches, whereas neurons of the thalamus (Fig. 4-5K) have long radiating dendrites with numerous branches. The cells of the *substantia gelatinosa* of the spinal cord, best seen in stained longitudinal sections, demonstrate only a few large dendrites that issue chiefly from one side of the cell (Fig. 4-5G). Smaller branches of these dendrites form a compact zone of fine parallel fibers.

It is instructive to compare the profuse dendritic branches of the central sensory and integrating neurons (Fig. 4-5, A, B, D, E, and G–K) with the robust dendrites of motor neurons (Figs. 4-5, C, F and L, and 4-7, M–O). This comparison is even more striking if one contrasts the two principal cell types of the cerebellar and cerebral cortex (Fig. 4-6). The brushlike spread of dendrites of the Purkinje cell is similar to that of other central integrating neurons (Fig. 4-5 A and I–K); yet each has individual characteristics. The large pyramidal cell (Fig. 4-6) also has an extensive dendritic spread and tiny gemmules. However, its basic structure more closely resembles that of a motor neuron (Fig. 4-5, F and L, and 4-7, I and M–O). Successful Golgi preparations permit one to follow the processes of a neuron for considerable distances. Studies using this method (787, 789, 790, 2275) provide clearer concepts of neuron structure, dendritic ramification and axonal distribution within the cerebellar cortex, and brain stem reticular formation.

The somatic and visceral neurons of the central and peripheral nervous systems of man can be compared in Figure 4-7. The

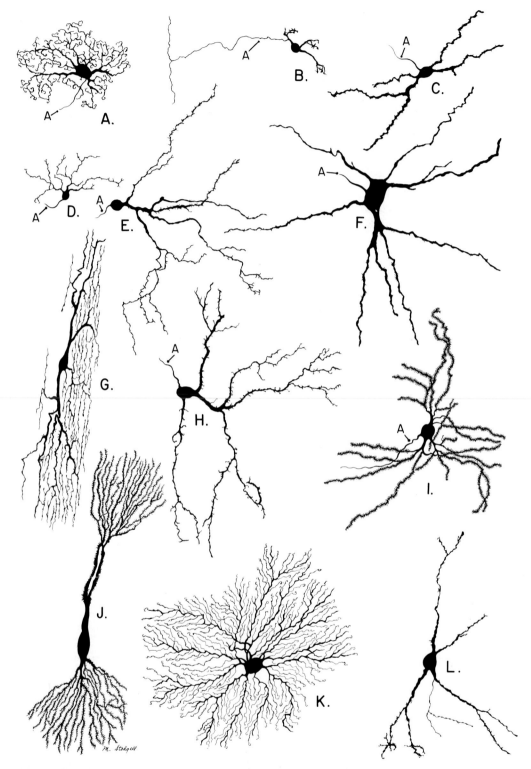

Figure 4-5. Scaled drawings of some characteristic neurons whose axons (*A*) and dendrites remain within the central nervous system. (*A*) Neuron of inferior olivary nucleus. (*B*) Granule cell of cerebellar cortex. (*C*) Small cell of reticular formation. (*D*) Small gelatinosa cell of spinal trigeminal nucleus. (*E*) Ovoid cell, nucleus of tractus solitarius. (*F*) Large cell of reticular formation. (*G*) Spindle-shaped cell, substantia gelatinosa of spinal cord. (*H*), Large cell of spinal trigeminal nucleus. (*I*) Neuron, putamen of lentiform nucleus. (*J*) Double pyramidal cell, Ammon's horn of hippocampal cortex. (*K*) Cell from thalamic nucleus. (*L*) Cell from globus pallidus (Golgi preparations, monkey). (Courtesy of the late Dr. Clement Fox, Wayne State University.)

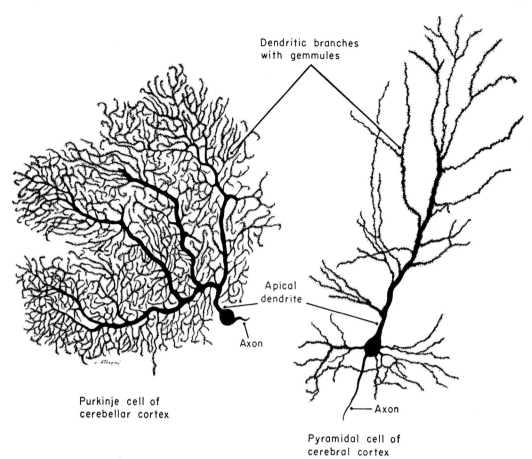

Dendritic branches
with gemmules

Apical
dendrite

Axon

Purkinje cell of
cerebellar cortex

Axon

Pyramidal cell of
cerebral cortex

Figure 4-6. Scaled drawings of two principal cell types in cerebellar and cerebral cortex. Dendritic branches provide extensive area for synaptic terminals of many other cortical and subcortical neurons (Golgi preparations, monkey). Courtesy of the late Dr. Clement Fox, Wayne State University.)

peripheral processes and axons of such neurons form the peripheral, cranial and spinal nerves. Nerve cells of the sensory and autonomic ganglia are surrounded by a thin nucleated capsule. Although nerve cells in most regions of the CNS do not undergo mitotic division after birth, they probably increase in size, as their axons and dendrites grow in length. According to the length of axon, Golgi (915) classified all nerve cells into long axon (type I) and short axon (type II) neurons. Golgi type II axons break up into extensive terminal arborizations in the immediate vicinity of the cell body.

The length of some nerve axons is quite remarkable. Giant pyramidal cells of the cerebral cortex may send axons to the caudal tip of the spinal cord, i.e., from the top of the head to the lumbar region of the

spinal cord (Fig. 10-13). Axons of motor neurons in the spinal cord may extend the length of the lower extremity to terminate in muscle fibers of the toes. A sensory unipolar neuron situated in the first sacral spinal ganglion may send a peripheral fiber to one of the toes, while its central fiber may ascend the length of the spinal cord and terminate in the medulla (Fig. 10-1). The total length of such a neuron would be from the toe to the nape of the neck. In a giraffe, such a fiber would reach the astounding length of over 15 feet.

The size of the perikaryon fluctuates within wide limits, from a diameter of 4 μm in the smallest granule cells of the cerebellum (Fig. 4-5B) and cerebral cortex to well over 100 μm in the largest motor cells of the spinal cord. In general, the size of the cell

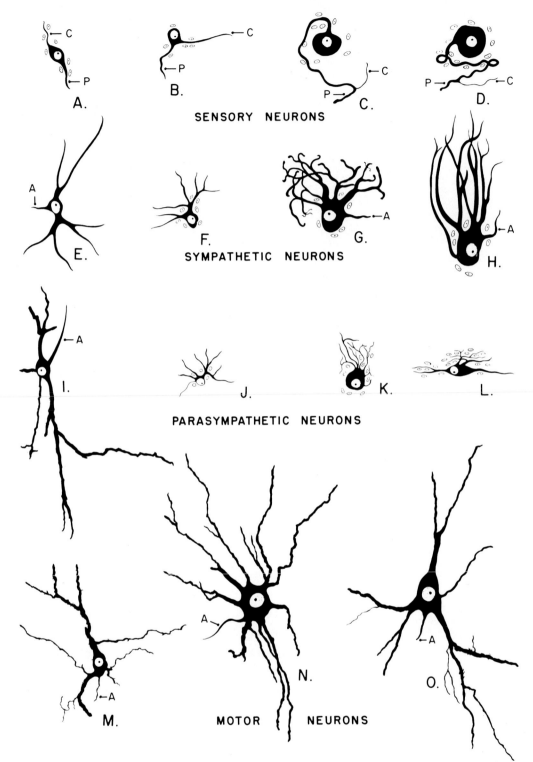

Figure 4-7. Scaled drawings of representative neurons whose axons (A) are distributed in the peripheral nervous system of man. Capsular nuclei are shown about all ganglion cells. The central (C) and peripheral (P) processes of the sensory neurons are identified. (A) Bipolar neuron, nodose ganglion (newborn). (B) Pseudounipolar neuron, nodose ganglion (newborn). (C) Unipolar neuron, dorsal root ganglion (newborn). (D) Unipolar neuron, trigeminal ganglion. (E) Multipolar neurons of intermediolateral nucleus of spinal cord. (F) Superior cervical ganglion (newborn). (G and H) Stellate ganglion. (I) Dorsal motor nucleus N. X. (J) Ciliary ganglion (newborn). (K) Intracardiac ganglion. (L) Myenteric ganglion. (M) Nucleus ambiguus. (N) Motor nucleus N. XII. (O) Anterior horn cell.

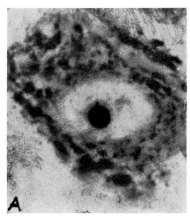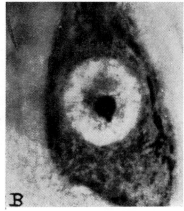

Figure 4-8. Nucleolar satellite in motor cell of spinal cord (*A*) and Betz cell of motor cortex (*B*) (female cat, cresyl violet, ×1200). (Reproduced with permission from M. L. Barr et al.: *Anatomical Record*, (124).

body is proportional to the length, thickness, richness of branchings and terminal aborizations of its dendrites and axon.

NERVE CELL BODY

The neuron body consists of a nucleus surrounded by a mass of cytoplasm whose surface layer forms a delicate plasma membrane. It appears as a fine structure in stained sections when viewed with the light microscope (Figs. 4-2 and 4-8). As observed with the electron microscope, the plasma membrane (*PM* in Fig. 4-10) has a three-layered appearance similar to that of most tissue cells. It delimits sharply the cytoplasm of the neuron (neuroplasm) from adjacent processes of other nerve cells and from neuroglial and connective tissue cells and fibers.

The cytoplasm of a neuron in a routinely stained section appears basophilic and has a large, pale nucleus with a prominent nucleolus. After appropriate staining procedures, one also can demonstrate within the cytoplasm of nerve cells neurofibrils, chromophil substance (Nissl bodies), Golgi apparatus, mitochondria, at times a central body, and various inclusions such as pigment, and lipids (Fig. 4-9). Neurofibrils are uniquely characteristic of nerve cells, whereas the other cytoplasmic constituents are observed in other tissue cells. The cytoplasm extends throughout the confines of the cell and all of its processes and, in the axon, is often called axoplasm. As observed by light microscopy, the cytoplasm appears open and somewhat dispersed, whereas it has a compact and crowded appearance in

electron micrographs (Fig. 4-10). Many of the neuronal structures seen by light microscopy require specifc stains (e.g., neurofibrils, mitochondria, Golgi apparatus, Nissl bodies and lipids), while most of these constituents are visualized simultaneously with the electron microscope.

Nucleus. This spherical structure varies in size from 3 to 18 μm, is generally proportional to cell size and is usually centrally located (Fig. 4-9). Small aggregates of desoxyribonucleic acid (DNA) are scattered in a somewhat homogeneous nucleoplasm and account for the pale appearance of the nucleus (Figs. 4-2 and 4-10). Usually one deeply staining nucleolus occupies a prominent position in the nucleus. The nuclear membrane seen with the light microscope appears sharp and continuous, while electron micrographs reveal it as a double-layered membrane, periodically interrupted by nuclear pores (*Nuc. m.* in Fig. 4-10). The nuclei of Purkinje cells have a nuclear membrane that is wrinkled or puckered on the side facing the origin of the dendritic tree (1920). This irregular depression in the nucleus, stuffed with granular endoplasmic reticulum (Fig. 4-11), has been called the nuclear cap region. This region appears to contain more nuclear pores (65 nm in diameter) than smooth portions of the nuclear membrane. For a more detailed description of nuclear ultrastructure, the student is referred to the studies of Wischnitzer (2753), Hay and Revel (1055), Peters et al. (1982) and Palay and Chan-Palay (1920).

Nucleolus. This basophilic structure

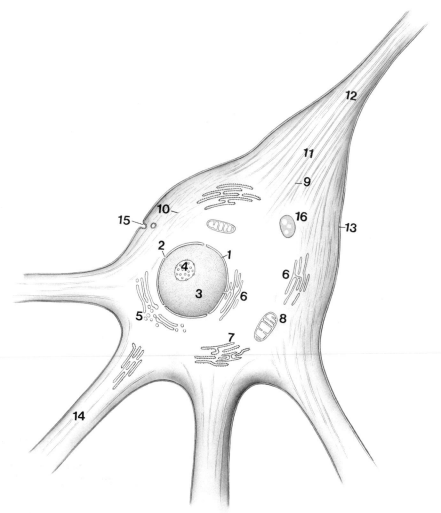

Figure 4-9. Drawing of a neuronal cell body showing major organelles as seen in electron micrographs. (*1*) nuclear membrane, (*2*) pores in nuclear membrane, (*3*) interior of nucleus, (*4*) nucleolus, (*5*) Golgi apparatus, (*6*) smooth endoplasmic reticulum, (*7*) granular endoplasmic reticulum, (*8*) mitochondrion, (*9*) microtuble (neurotubule), (*10*) microfilament (neurofilament), (*11*) axon hillock, (*12*) initial segment of axon, (*13*) soma (perikaryon) of cell, (*14*) dendrite, (*15*) pinocytotic vesicle, (*16*) lipofuschin granule.

contains a large amount of RNA as well as a diffuse coating of DNA. It is known to have positive histochemical reactions for several enzyme systems associated with respiration, energy production and the synthesizing functions of the cell. It is particularly related to the production of nucleic acid and protein in nerve cells. In most electron micrographs the nucleolus shows no limiting membrane and the structure has a dense granular appearance. A "nucleolar satellite" 1 μm or less in diameter may be found closely apposed to the nucleus in nerve cells from female specimens (124) as shown in Figure 4-8.

Chromophil Substance. There are two main types of nucleic acid in the cell: (a) ribonucleic acid [the sugar of the nucleotide is ribose (pentose)] and (b) desoxyribonucleic acid [the sugar is desoxyribose (desoxypentose)]. Cytochemical methods indicate that nucleoproteins of the desoxyribose type are found chiefly in the chromatin, which forms the spireme and chromosomes in mitosis and, during the intermitotic period, is partly represented by chromatin bodies known as karyosomes. Desoxyribonucleic acid also is found in the nucleolar satellite and in small quantities within the mitochondria (Fig. 4-9). On the other hand,

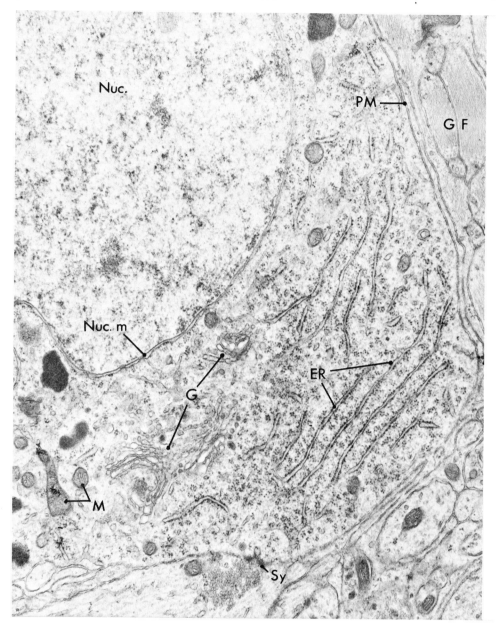

Figure 4-10. Electron micrograph showing part of a neuron in the posterior gray column (cat). The plasma membrane (*PM*) separates cytoplasmic structures from glial fibers (*GF*) and a synapse (*sy*) which are identified in the adjacent neuropil. Part of the pale nucleus (*Nuc.*) and the nuclear membrane (*Nuc.m*) appear to the upper left. The cytoplasm demonstrates pouches and vesicles of the Golgi complex (*G*), mitochondria (*M*), and an array of individual ribonucleoprotein particles. Some appear as clumps or rosettes, while some ribosomes are attached to the outer surface membranes. The parallel stacks of cisternae of the granular endoplasmic reticulum (*ER*) are characteristic of Nissl bodies (osmium fixation, ×75,000). (Courtesy of H. J. Ralston III, University of California School of Medicine, San Francisco.)

the true nucleolus is as rule a dense, spherical, optically homogenous body that is rich in ribonucleic acid. Similar ribonucleoproteins are found in the cytoplasm, and there is good evidence for the assumption that the nucleolus plays an important part in cytoplasmic protein formation (428).

In preparations stained with basic aniline dyes, the *chromophil substance* appears in the form of deeply staining granules or

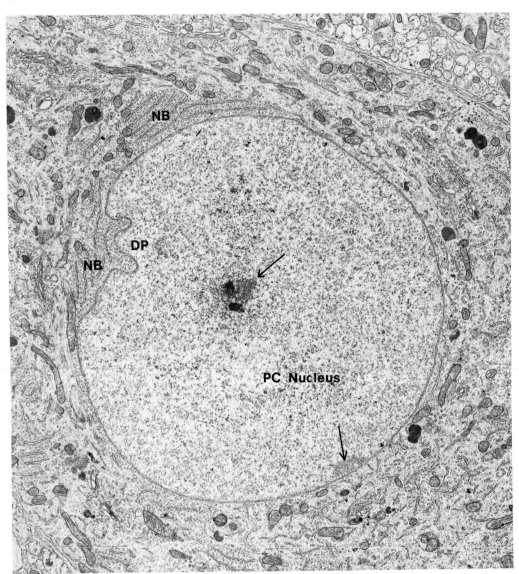

Figure 4-11.   Electron micrograph of a Purkinje cell nucleus of the rat. The nuclear chromatin is thinly and uniformly distributed throughout the nucleus, except for two sites indicated by arrows. The dendritic pole (*DP*) of the nucleus is wrinkled and capped by a small Nissl body (*NB*) (×14,000). (Courtesy of Dr. Sanford L. Palay and Victoria Chan-Palay, Harvard Medical School; from *Cerebellar Cortex: Cytology and Organization*, Springer-Verlag, Berlin, (1920).)

clumps of granules known as *Nissl (tigroid) bodies* (Fig. 4-2E). They are found in the cell bodies and dendrites of all large and many of the smaller cells, but are absent in the axon and in the axon hillock from which that process arises. They are most abundant and sharply defined in the larger cells, whose clear vesicular nucleus contains practically no basichromatin (Figs. 4-2 and 4-8).

The Nissl bodies are larger in motor than in sensory cells, and attempts have been made to distinguish the many neuron types by the size, shape, distribution and staining capacity of the chromophil granules.

The electron microscopic study of Palay and Palade (1921), identified Nissl bodies as masses of granular endoplasmic reticulum. Clusters of punctate ribonucleic acid granules 10 to 30 nm in diameter, called

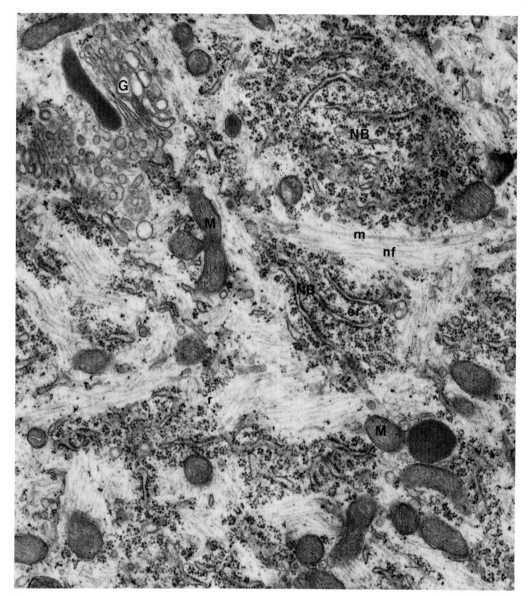

Figure 4-12. Electron micrograph of the cytoplasm of a rat dorsal root ganglion cell. The cytoplasm contains well-defined Nissl bodies (*NB*) separated by spaces containing microtubules (*m*) and neurofilaments (*nf*). Some ribosomes in the Nissl bodies are arranged in rows attached to the outer surfaces of cisternae of the granular endoplasmic reticulum (*er*) while others lie free (*r*) in the cytoplasmic matrix. Free ribosomes appear in rosettes of six or more members. *G* in the upper left indicates part of the Golgi apparatus (×46,000). (Courtesy of Drs. Alan Peters, Henry de Webster and Sanford Palay; from *The Fine Structure of the Nervous System: The Neurons and Supporting Cells*, W. B. Saunders Co., Philadelphia, (1982).)

ribosomes, were oriented upon and between the cisterns, tubules and vesicles to form a series of flattened, anastomosing, parallel-arranged sheets or membranes (Figs. 4-10 and 4-12). Dispersed free ribosomes also can be observed within the neuron cytoplasm.

Free and membrane bound ribosomes are loci for protein synthesis (Fig. 4-9). Neurons, like most cells, produce proteins which are used within the cell for both structural and metabolic purposes. A number of brain-specific proteins have been isolated biochemically, purified, and their cellular localization studied by immunohisto-chemical techniques (1501). In addition, some neurons synthesize peptide hormones or transmitters which are secreted at the axon terminal.

Following section of the axon, alterations in the discrete structure of the Nissl bodies can be demonstrated when stained by basic dyes and viewed with light microscopy (Fig. 4-2*E*). Nissl bodies in the cytoplasm about the nucleus appear dispersed or dissolved, a phenomenon termed *chromatolysis* (see pp. 126).

Neurotubules and Neurofilaments. Investigators have observed fibrillar material in the axon, dendrites and perikaryon formed by long tubular elements 20 to 30 nm in diameter (1984). Such *neurotubules* have a smooth contour and are of variable length. Neurotubules contain tubulin, a 110,000 dalton protein dimer subunit. Tubulin is not confined to the neurotubules and may also be recovered with the soluble protein fraction in brain (2326). The neurotubule consists of a ring of 13 filamentous structures with a clear lumen. The lumen has a rodlike structure in its center (1982). In the axoplasm of peripheral and central nerves one usually can see neurotubules, as well as strands of canaliculi, vesicles of endoplasmic reticulum and a few ribosomes (Fig. 4-19). In addition to neurotubules there are finer axial components called *neurofilaments* which are about 10 nm in diameter (see Fig. 4-36). A single protein subunit, filarin, has been isolated from neurofilaments derived from invertebrate nerves. A filamentous protein of somewhat lower molecular weight has been isolated from mammalian brain (1982). The neurotubules and neurofilaments observed in electron microscopy become aggregated during some types of fixation and form the neurofibrils observed with the light microscope (944, 1982) (Fig. 4-13). Nerve action potential conduction takes place at the surface membrane of the axon, and neurotubules seem to have no role in this process. Neurotubules are probably involved in axon growth, and the transport of enzymes, but detailed mechanisms remain unresolved.

Mitochondria. Granular or filamentous mitochondria are scattered throughout the entire cell body, dendrites and axon (Figs. 4-10, 4-14 and 4-23). These organelles occur even in the smallest ramifications and ter-

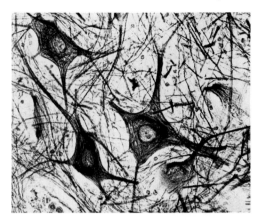

Figure 4-13. Large motor neurons from infant spinal cord showing neurofibrillar structures. Portions of dendrites and axons of other neurons fill the field (Cajal silver method, photograph).

minals of the neuron and are prominent electron microscopic features wherever intense metabolic activity occurs, such as at synapses and at sensory and motor endings (616, 1040, 1921). These widely distributed cytoplasmic organelles are involved in glycolysis, biosynthesis and cell respiration, but their most important function is to serve as a source of energy for the cell. During cell respiration the enzymatic breakdown of carbohydrates and amino acids yields CO_2, water and energy. The energy, bound in adenosine triphosphate (ATP), is utilized in the transport of ions across cell membranes and protein synthesis. The mitochondria (*M* in Figs. 4-10, 4-11, 4-12, 4-23 and 4-26) are recognized easily in most electron micrographs. The growing tips of dendrites often exhibit varicosities or swellings which are filled with mitochondria (2386). Mitochondria in these varicosities are long and slender and are arranged either parallel to the long axis of the dendrite or form gentle swirls (Fig. 4-14). Their accumulation and breakdown at the nodes of Ranvier have been observed during the early stages of Wallerian degeneration (2681).

Centrosome. A microcentrum often is demonstrated in neuroblasts. It consists of one or two granules surrounded by a clear cytoplasmic area. In some instances, fine wavy fibrils may radiate from the clear area of cytoplasm. The significance of the centrosome is puzzling, for adult neurons are

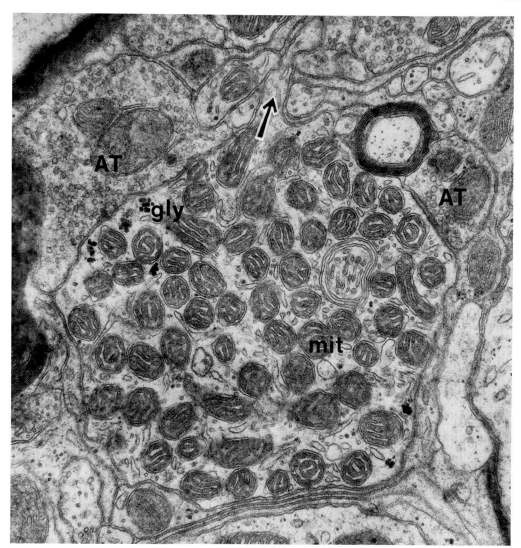

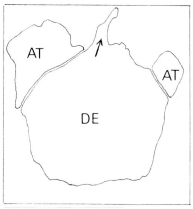

Figure 4-14. Electron micrograph of a dendritic expansion (*DE*) filled with mitochondria (*mit*) and glycogen (*gly*) granules. This growing dendritic tip shows a filopodia-like expansion (arrow) and has two axonal terminals (*AT*) synapsing upon its surface. Dendritic profiles of this type are abundant in the dorsal part of the lateral vestibular nucleus in the rat (×39,000). (Courtesy of Dr. C. Sotelo, Laboratoire d'Histologie Normale et Pathologique de Systeme Nerveux, Paris; from C. Sotelo and S. L. Palay: *Journal of Cell Biology* (2386).)

incapable of cell division. However, Murray and Stout (1789) and Murray (1786) have demonstrated that adult human sympathetic ganglia could survive, migrate and occasionally divide mitotically in tissue culture.

Golgi Apparatus. The Golgi complex, a specialization of the agranular endoplasmic reticulum, is highly developed in nerve cells (Fig. 4-9). In electron micrographs the Golgi apparatus appears as stacks of closely packed agranular membraneous cisternae associated with vacuoles and vesicles. Their close packing (*G* in Fig. 4-12) and the absence of ribosomes, either free or attached, distinguish the Golgi apparatus from the agranular endoplasmic reticulum and the Nissl substance (1982). In glandular epithelial cells the Golgi apparatus is involved in the segregation of secretory proteins into membrane bound vesicles. In the region of the Golgi apparatus sugars are added to protein to form glycoproteins. It is possible that different cisternae within the Golgi complex may perform different functions. The innermost Golgi cisternae contain acid phosphatase and the "alveolate vesicles" of this region are full of hydrolytic enzymes (814, 1982). Thus the Golgi apparatus may be associated with the production of lysosomes, which contain hydrolases that break down protein, carbohydrates and nucleic acids (1136).

Inclusion Bodies. In addition to the organelles described above some nerve cells demonstrate dense cytoplasmic bodies and pigment granules. Most of the larger adult nerve cells contain a yellowish auto-fluorescent pigment known as *lipochrome* or *lipofuscin*. The amount found within nerve cells increases with age, and appears in the form of granules which are usually aggregated in a dense mass in some part of the cell body (Fig. 4-2*B*). Occasionally they may be dispersed throughout the cell. They are insoluble in the usual lipoid solvents, are blackened by osmic acid and stained with Scharlach R. The cells of the newborn do not contain the pigment. It appears about the 6th year in the spinal ganglia, a few years later in the spinal cord and after the 20th year in the cerebral cortex. It increases in amount with advancing years, and during senescence it may occupy a large part of the cytoplasm of some neurons (2579). Both histochemical and ultrastructural evidence suggest that lipofuscin granules are a form of lysosome (718). The lipofuscin in the autonomic ganglia was thought to be related to ceroid (2467, 2468). Other histochemical studies indicate there are really three types of granules in the autonomic cells, namely, pigmented, non-

pigmented and neurosecretory (1791).

Granules of a blackish pigment known as *melanin* are found in the substantia nigra, locus ceruleus and certain pigmented cells scattered through the brain stem. It also is found in spinal and sympathetic ganglion cells (Fig. 4-2*A*). Melanin appears at the end of the 1st year and increases in amount until puberty, after which it apparently remains constant through senescence. Incubation of brain tissue in tritiated norepinephrine followed by radioautography reveals a heavy binding of norepinephrine at the surface membranes of pigmented cells of the substantia nigra, locus ceruleus and the dorsal motor nucleus of the vagus nerve (1187).

NEUROTRANSMITTERS AND NEUROSECRETION

One of the characteristics of all nerve cells is that they synthesize their own proteins. Synaptic neurosecretion of acetylcholine and norepinephrine in some neurons has been known for many years. Sensitive histochemical methods are available, at both the light and electron microscopic levels, for visualizing the intraneuronal distribution of a group of biogenic monoamines suspected of acting as neurotransmitters or modulators (1124). The biogenic monoamines are classified according to their ring structure as catecholamines (norepinephrine, dopamine) or indolamines (5-hydroxytryptamine) and can be identified with fluorescence histochemical methods (730, 1497). The cell body of monaminergic neurons usually contains low to medium concentrations of transmitter, while such concentrations are low in the axon, except for the terminal axonal enlargement (i.e., nerve endings) where amine levels are high (Fig. 4-15). Comparisons of norepinephrine neurons in the central and peripheral nervous system indicate that fluorescence is localized mainly in the perinuclear region and roughly corresponds to the position of the Golgi apparatus; in peripheral neurons the most intense fluorescence is seen in peripheral regions of the cytoplasm. At the ultrastructural level the distribution of granular vesicles closely parallels the distribution of fluorescence (1128). Both small and large granular vesicles are present in

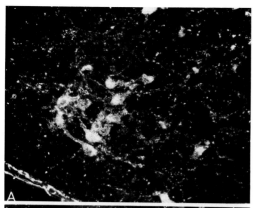

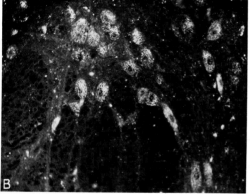

Figure 4-15. Neurons containing biogenic amines in the squirrel monkey as demonstrated by fluorescence microscopy. (*A*) Catecholamine-containing neurons located dorsolateral to the lateral reticular nucleus of the medulla. The background shows fine, beadlike varicosities containing catecholamines (×400) (*B*) Indoleamine-containing neurons in the dorsal nucleus of the raphe of the mesencephalon (×400). (Courtesy of Dr. David Felten, Indiana University School of Medicine.)

monoamine neurons. Catecholamine neurons can serve as an example to illustrate the general features of neurotransmitter biosynthesis. The amino acid tyrosine is a precursor for the transmitters norepinephrine and dopamine. The amino acid is transported across the surface membrane to the interior of the cell where it is hydroxylated to form dihydroxyphenylalanine (DOPA) by the enzyme tyrosine hydroxylase (TH). TH is the rate limiting step in transmitter synthesis and is found both in the cytoplasm of the cell body and synaptic terminals (2004) (Fig. 4-29). DOPA is converted to dopamine by the enzyme DOPA decarboxylase, and the dopamine is stored in

synaptic vesicles. In noradrenergic neurons, dopamine is converted to norepinephrine by the enzyme dopamine β-hydroxylase (DβH). DβH has been localized to the cytoplasm, Golgi apparatus and endoplasmic reticulum of the cell body. In synaptic terminals DβH is associated with the membrane of the synaptic vesicles. Certain amino acids are suspected to be neurotransmitters. Those suspected of serving this function are gamma (γ)-aminobutyric acid (GABA), glycine and glutamate; immunohistochemical methods are available by which they can be visualized in the light or electron microscope. However, enzymes essential for the synthesis of some of these putative transmitters have been isolated and used to prepare antibodies which can be labeled. In addition, autoradiographic studies of the uptake of isotopically labeled transmitter or its precursors have permitted identification of cell bodies and terminals containing the transmitter.

In recent years a large number of peptides have been identified and localized in the brain. Some of these are listed in Table 4-1. Peptides such as substance P and enkephalin may act as neurotransmitters in some locations. Other peptides may act to increase or decrease the effectiveness of other chemical transmitters, and are called neuromodulators (185, 729, 1121, 1523, 2375, 2596, 2597).

In addition to the above examples, investigators have demonstrated the existence of certain glandlike neurons in both the invertebrate and vertebrate nervous systems (1916, 2269, 2271, 2272, 2392). The hypothalamo-hypophysial system of the vertebrate brain is the classical example of this neuroendocrine mechanism. These interrelationships have been reviewed by Ortmann (1897), Bern and Knowles (166) and Gabe (832); see Chapter 16. Neurosecretory neurons constitute a link in the chain that unites the neural and endocrine systems. They represent the final pathway in which action potentials lead to the release of hormones.

Neurosecretory neurons are "specialized" in a sense, yet they have retained all of the light and electron microscope characteristics of ordinary neurons. They demonstrate all of the cytoplasmic organelles discussed above including filaments, tu-

Table 4-1
Some Brain Peptides[a]

Brain Peptides	No. of Amino Acids	Putative Function(s)
Met-Enkephalin	5	
Leu-Enkephalin	5	Analgesia
Substance P	11	Pain-nociceptive mechanisms
Neurotensin	13	
β-Endorphin	31	
ACTH	39	Stress
Angiotensin II	8	Thirst
Oxytocin	9	Parturition, milk let down
Vasopressin (ADH)	9	Fluid regulation, memory?
Vasoactive intestinal polypeptide (VIP)	28	
Somatostatin	14	
Thyrotropin releasing hormone (TRH)	3	
Leuteinizing hormone releasing hormone (LHRH)	10	Reproduction
Bombesin	14	Feeding suppression
Carnosine	2	
Cholecystokinin-like peptide	8	Feeding suppression

General Classification of Brain Peptides

Neurohypophyseal Peptides
  Vasopressin (ADH)
  Oxytocin
Adenohypophysiotropic Peptides
  Gonadotropin releasing hormone (LHRH)
  Thyrotropin releasing hormone (TRH)
  Somatostatin (GH-RIH)
Neurotransmitter or Neuromodulator Peptides
  Substance P
  Enkephalins
  Vasoactive intestinal peptide

[a] A partial list of peptides isolated from, or that act upon, the brain. In some cases the functions mentioned have been established in only one or two species and caution must be exercised in generalizing too broadly. A more detailed discussion will be found in the text of this chapter and also Chapter 16.

bules and the proximodistal transport of axoplasm. However, the neurofilaments appear to be different in nature along the axon and in its preterminal region. The neurotubules may be 30 to 50 nm in diameter, and the axons also may demonstrate multilamellate bodies (166). These neurons have unusually electron-dense material as-

sociated with the Golgi membranes, and a prominent endoplasmic reticulum. The secretory protein is synthesized by the endoplasmic reticulum which then passes it to the Golgi apparatus where it is conjugated to a carrier protein called neurophysin. The hormone and its carrier protein are enclosed in dense core vesicles which pass from the perikarya distally along the axon and may be concentrated in the preterminal regions of the fibers. Large masses of secretory material (Herring bodies) are observed along the course of these axons. The axon terminals containing neurosecretory vesicles are unique in that they abut upon a perivascular space rather than another neuron or effector cell. Their secretory product is released into the perivascular space by exocytosis of the secretory vesicles, transported into the lumen of the vessel and carried via the blood to appropriate organs whose activity it can modify (1982). The neurosecretory material produced by the supraoptic and paraventricular hypothalamic nuclei (Fig. 16-12) contains the nonapeptides vasopressin and oxytocin (115, 2353) (see also Figs. 16-2 and 16-4).

Inclusions of secretory material can be visualized by several histochemical stains and viewed with the light microscope (e.g., chromhematoxylin-phloxine stain). However, the refined cytological criteria established by electron microscopy provide the most meaningful features for identifying neurosecretory neurons. The supraoptic and paraventricular hypothalamic nuclei (Figs. 16-2, 16-5 and A-22) are the best known neurosecretory neurons in the human brain.

In mammals there is another peptide system in the hypothalamus represented by the arcuate nucleus and the median eminence. Nerve fibers originating from the arcuate nucleus course into the median eminence and terminate in relationship to the perivascular spaces, as described for the supraopticohypophysial neurosecretory system (Figs. 16-1 and 16-12). Granule-containing vesicles in these nerve endings are smaller and of at least two types. The median eminence is considered to be involved in the elaboration and control of various releasing hormones which regulate the adenohypophysis. Some of the small clear vesicles containing dense granules resemble

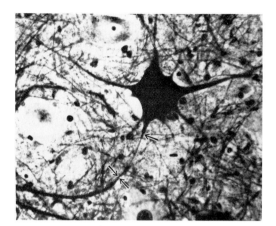

Figure 4-16. Larger motor neuron in the anterior gray horn of infant's spinal cord revealing several dendrites and the origin of the axon. The axon arises from the lower side of the cell body, tapers to thin thread for a short distance and thickens at the point where the myelin sheath develops. Small neuroglial nuclei are stained black (modified Weigert's stain, photograph).

those found in adrenergic nerve terminals. This system is discussed further in Chapter 16.

THE AXON

The axon is a slender, usually long process which arises from a conical mass of specialized protoplasm known as the axon hillock. It is distinguished from the cell body and dendrites by the complete absence of Nissl bodies, which also are lacking in the axon hillock. In smaller neurons an axon hillock is not easily identified in light microscopic preparations. The reason suggested by electron microscopy is that in these small cells there is little difference between the cytoplasm of the axon hillock and that of the neuronal cell body (1982). As the axon hillock narrows into the initial axonal segment, there is a gradual diminution in the number of ribosomes, but no abrupt change as suggested by light microscopic descriptions. Beyond the initial segment the axon contains mitochondria, neurofilaments, microtubules, agranular endoplasmic reticulum, vesicles and multivesicular bodies; no granular endoplasmic reticulum or ribosomes are present. Distally each axon breaks up into simple or extensive terminal arborizations, the telaxon. The later may be synaptic endings on other

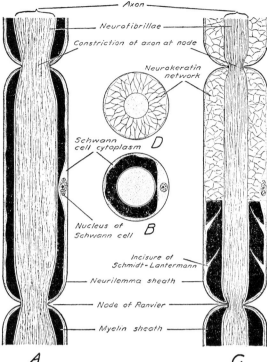

Figure 4-17. (*A* and *B*) Schematic drawings of peripheral myelin sheaths are based on de Renyl's studies of living nerve fibers. (*C* and *D*) sheaths as seen in many fixed preparations. The cross membrane is not shown. [Reproduced with permission from W. M. Copenhaver et al: *Bailey's Textbook of Histology*, Ed. 16, Williams & Wilkins, Baltimore (534)].

neurons (e.g., sensory neurons), or effector endings in muscle and glands (Figs. 4-3*G*, 4-4 and 5 in Fig. 9-28).

In the central nervous sytem, axons may be *myelinated* or *unmyelinated*. The former possess a sheath of myelin for at least a portion of their course. The oligodendrocyte forms and maintains the myelin sheath within the brain and spinal cord. In the unmyelinated fibers, the sheath is lacking. In the peripheral nervous system both myelinated and unmyelinated fibers have, in addition, an outer delicate nucleated membrane, the *sheath of Schwann*.

The *peripheral myelinated fiber* is structurally the most differentiated, consisting of axon (axis cylinder), myelin and sheath of Schwann. The myelin sheath is not continuous, but is interrupted at fairly regular intervals; the parts of the fiber free from myelin appear as constrictions known as the *nodes of Ranvier* (Figs. 4-3C and 4-17). In the fresh condition the semifluid axon is broad and homogeneous in appearance, and it occasionally shows faint longitudinal striations. In silver stained preparations, it consists of closely packed, parallel-running neurofibrils imbedded in a scanty amount of homogeneous axoplasm (Fig. 4-3A). In most fixatives the axon usually shrinks to a thin axial thread. With special methods of fixation and tissue embedding its normal size may be more nearly approximated.

Between the axon and myelin sheath there is a delicate layer or membrane known as the axolemma (Fig. 4-18). Although difficult to demonstrate histologically, the membrane may be seen in ultraviolet photographs of the living nerve fiber, since the axolemma shows a much greater ultraviolet absorption than the axon or the myelin sheath. The axolemma is part of the neuron plasma membrane, and possesses a similar structure and specialized properties. It can be identified easily in high magnification electron micrographs as a delicate membrane surrounding the axon (Figs. 4-18 and 4-19).

Myelin. The myelin sheath is acquired a short distance from the cell body (Fig. 4-16). The proximal portion of the axon is as a rule unmyelinated. The sheath is of varying thickness and is composed of a semifluid, doubly refracting substance known as *myelin*, which in the fresh state has a glistening white appearance. Physical technics have provided data concerning the orderly arrangement of lipoproteins that form myelin (2284, 2347). Studies based upon polarized light, x-ray diffraction and electron microscopy have yielded a high degree of correlation and indicate that the myelin sheath is composed of concentric layers in which protein and lipid alternate. Lipid molecules are radially oriented in their layers while protein molecules are arranged tangentially. Myelin is composed of a fundamental, radially arranged repeating unit membrane with a spacing of 17 to 18.5 nm. The repeating unit membrane is composed of two subunits each consisting of a bimolecular lipid leaflet sandwiched between monolayers of protein. Each of these subunits corresponds to a single layer of plasma membrane derived from the myelin-forming cell (Figs. 4-20 and 4-23).

With the limited magnification of light microscopy, it was presumed that peripheral myelinated nerves were enclosed by two separate layers, the myelin and Schwann cell sheaths. The histological appearances of myelinated nerves in cross section, when stained by the osmic acid and

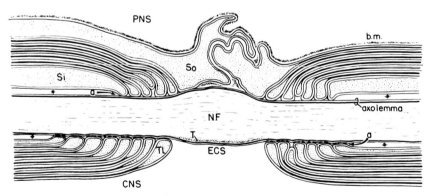

Figure 4-18. Nodal regions from PNS (*above*) and CNS (*below*). In the PNS the Schwann cell provides both an inner collar (*Si*) and an outer collar (*So*) of cytoplasm in relation to the compact myelin. The outer collar (*So*) is extended into the nodal region as a series of loosely interdigitating processes. Terminating loops of the compact myelin come into close apposition to the axolemma in region near the node, apparently providing some barrier (*arrow at a*) for movement of material into or out of the periaxonal space (marked by *). The Schwann cell is covered externally by a basement membrane. In the CNS the myelin ends similarly in terminal loops (*tl*) near the node, and there are periodic thickenings of the axolemma where the glial membrane is applied in the paranodal region. These may serve as diffusion barriers and thus confine the material in the periaxonal space (marked *) so that movement in the direction of the *arrow at "a"* would be restrained. At many CNS nodes there is considerable extracellular space (*ECS*). Compare with CNS node shown in Figure 4-17. [Courtesy of Dr. R.P. Bunge and the American Physiological Society; from *Physiological Reviews*, (322)].

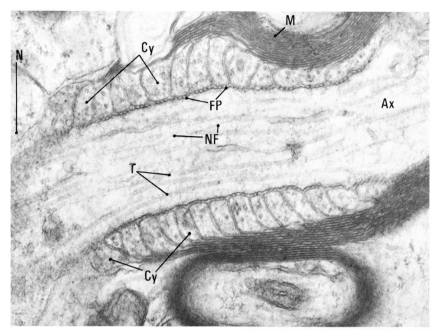

Figure 4-19. Electron micrograph of node of Ranvier on nerve fiber of spinal cord (cat). The oligoglial cytoplasm (*CY*) forms loops of myelin (*M*) around the axon (*Ax*) at the node (*N*). Fusion points (*FP*) between the myelin and axon membranes are shown also. Neurotubules (*T*) and neurofilaments (*NF*) are identified in the axoplasm (osmium fixation, ×70,000). (Courtesy of H. J. Ralston III, University of California School of Medicine, San Francisco.)

silver nitrate methods, are shown in Figure 4-3, *B* and *D*. Electron microscopy studies have revealed that myelin was formed primarily by a double-layered infolding of the Schwann cell membrane, which became wrapped spirally around the axon in concentric layers (864, 2181, 2183).

Four stages in the "jelly-roll theory" of myelin formation are depicted in Figure 4-21. In the peripheral nervous system the myelin sheath represents concentric layers of the Schwann cell, while the oligodendrocyte assumes the role of myelin formation within the central nervous system (322). In the latter case one oligodendrocyte may form a myelin layer on more than one axon (Fig. 5-9). It will be noted that the inner surfaces of the plasma membranes come into apposition and fuse to form *major dense lines* which are approximately 3 nm thick. Between each major dense line is a less dense *intraperiod line* formed by the union of the outer surfaces of the plasma membranes (Fig. 4-21). This fusion of membranes, accompanied by a reduction in cell cytoplasm, results in the repeating series of light and dark lines observed in electron micrographs (Figs. 4-20 and 4-23). Cytoplasmic remnants of the Schwann cell infolding may at times be identified at the axon-myelin junction (*S* in Fig. 4-23*A*). The primary infolding of the Schwann cell membrane often is present as an *internal mesaxon* (*Im* in Fig. 4-20). Continuity between the most superficial lamellae of the myelin sheath and the Schwann cell plasma membrane forms the *external mesaxon* (*Em* in Fig. 4-20).

These intimate relations of Schwann cell and myelin are further amplified by the tissue culture observations of Chu (455), Peterson and Murray (1987) and Ross et al. (2226). They found that myelination began in isolated segments near the Schwann cell nucleus and extended along the fiber to a node of Ranvier. Remyelination of experimentally injured axons of the cat spinal cord appears to resemble the mechanism of myelination observed along peripheral nerves and in tissue culture (321).

Nodes of Ranvier. The myelin sheath is interrupted by constrictions at varying intervals on both central and peripheral axons. These areas can be identified in both

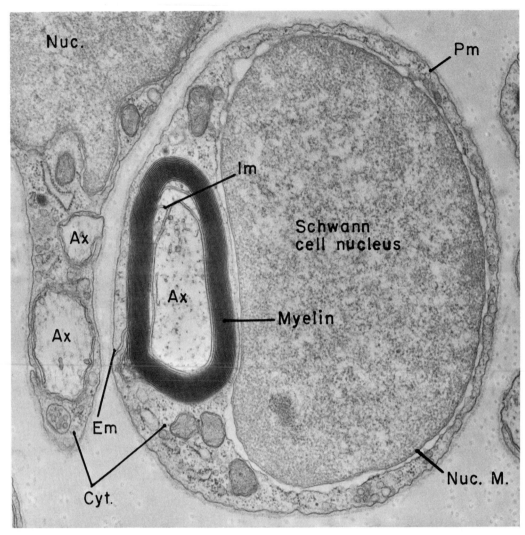

Figure 4-20. Electron micrograph of a small myelinated nerve fiber from rat dorsal root ganglion matured in tissue culture. The infolding plasma membrane (*PM*) of the Schwann cell forms an external mesaxon (*Em*) continuous with the outermost lamella of the myelin sheath. An internal mesaxon (*Im*) surrounds the axon (*Ax*) and is continuous with the most internal lamella of the myelin sheath. Note the small amount of Schwann cell cytoplasm (*Cyt.*) between the nuclear (*Nuc. M.*) and plasma membranes. At the left are two unmyelinated axons associated with another Schwann cell (osmium tetroxide fixation, Epon, lead citrate stain, ×27,000). (Courtesy of Drs. M. B. Bunge and R. P. Bunge, Washington University School of Medicine, St. Louis.)

the light and electron microscopes as regions where the myelin sheath is deficient (Figs. 4-3C and 4-19). At the nodal gap of peripheral nerves the axolemma is ensheathed by a fine basement membrane and small finger-like processes of the Schwann cell. As shown in Figure 4-18 there are some characteristic differences between the nodes of central and peripheral axons. The internodal distance and nodal gap are both shorter on central axons. Such nodes

also lack both interdigitating glial processes and a basement membrane. Thus nodes of Ranvier in the central nervous sytem have a greater extracellular space in the nodal region. The blunt spiral ends of the glial processes appear to fuse with the axolemma adjacent to a central node as shown in Figures 4-18 and 4-19. Paranodal terminations of myelin loops, on each side of the node, provide close apposition of plasma membranes rather than complete oblitera-

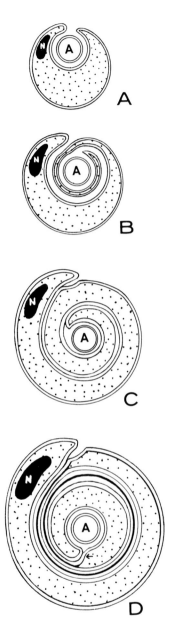

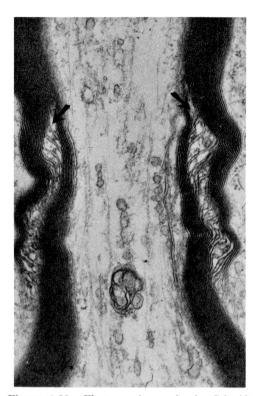

Figure 4-22. Electron micrograph of a Schmidt-Lantermann cleft (*arrows*). Clear areas consist of Schwann cell cytoplasm. (Courtesy of Dr. R. P. Bunge, and Rockefeller University Press.)

Figure 4-21. Diagram of stages in the development of the myelin sheath about an axon (*A*). Cytoplasm of the Schwann cell is stippled and its nucleus is indicated (*N*). As additional layers of cell cytoplasm become wrapped around the axon (*B* and *C*), the cytoplasm is reduced in amount and the double layered plasma membranes come into apposition (*D*). The outer membrane unit of the Schwann cell will become the future *intraperiod line* of myelin. The *dark line (major dense line)* represents the apposition of the inner (cytoplasmic) surface of the unit membrane as shown in (*D*). The internal mesaxon is also indicated (*arrow in D*).

tion of the extracellular space about the axon (* in Fig. 4-18). Electron microscopy has provided essential information on the fine structure of the node, and the following studies should be consulted for additional details (322, 1695, 1979, 1980, 1982, 2184, 2601). The length of the internodal segment varies considerably and is proportional to the diameter of the fiber, the thinner fibers having the shorter internodes. In the peroneal nerve of the rabbit the internodes on fibers 3 to 18 μm in diameter range from 400 to 1500 μm (2622), and these figures probably pertain for other mammals and man.

In unmyelinated axons the propagation of the action potential is a continuous process. In peripheral myelinated axons with regularly spaced nodes of Ranvier, the action potential appears to "jump" from node to node rather than proceed at a uniform velocity along the axon membrane between nodes. This is called "saltatory" conduction and is the result of the electrical resistance

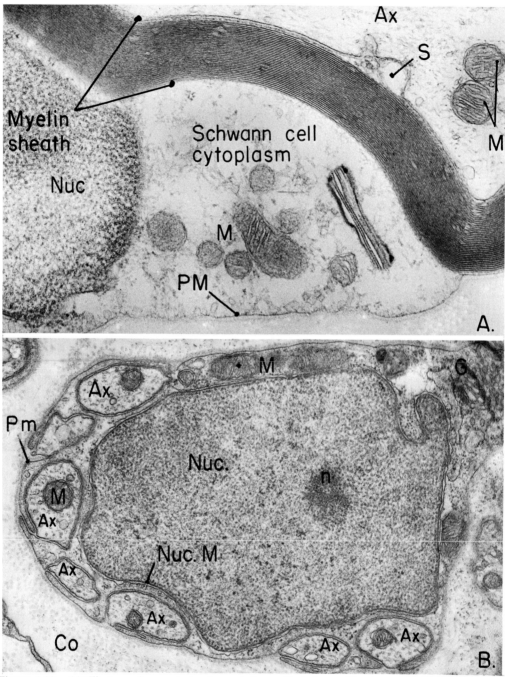

Figure 4-23. (*A*) Electron micrograph showing part of a myelinated nerve fiber in cross section. The Schwann cell cytoplasm and axoplasm (*Ax*) both contain mitochondria (*M*). Note the alternation of dense lamellae with less dense intermediate layers in the myelin sheath. This sheath is composed of thinned out Schwann cell cytoplasm wrapped concentrically around the axon (*Ax*). The innermost layer of the myelin sheath displays a local swelling (*S*). The plasma membrane (*PM*) of the Schwann cell envelops the entire structural complex (mouse sciatic nerve, ×39,000). (*B*) Electron micrograph showing the relationship of several unmyelinated axons (*Ax*) to the plasma membrane (*Pm*) of a Schwann cell. The nuclear membrane (*Nuc. M*) nucleus (*Nuc.*) and nucleolus (*n*) are identified. Mitochondria (*M*) and the Golgi complex (*G*) can be seen within the cytoplasm, while fine collagen fibrils (*Co*) surround the Schwann cell (mouse sciatic nerve, phosphate-buffered osmium tetroxide, Epon, lead tartrate, ×26,000). (Preparations by Dr. J. Rhodin, School of Medicine, University of South Florida, Tampa.)

and capacitance properties of the myelin sheath. The basic conductance mechanism of the action potential conduction along the surface membrane of myelinated and unmyelinated axons is the same.

Schmidt-Lantermann Clefts. The myelin sheath of each internode is divided at intervals into conical segments by oblique, funnel-shaped clefts, which extend to the axon (Fig. 4-3E). These are best seen in preparations treated with osmic acid but also are visible in the living fiber, when it is viewed in polarized light. Several cone-shaped indentations may occur in a myelin segment between two nodes, while the myelin sheaths of adjacent axons may be devoid of such clefts for long distances. Although long regarded as artifacts, the clefts have been observed in electron microscopic studies as shearing defects in the lamellae of the myelin sheath (320, 2183). Such clefts were shown to be areas of local separation of the spirally wrapped myelin lamellae which are nevertheless continuous across the incisure (fig. 4-22). The light appearing regions between the lamellae consist of Schwann cell cytoplasm. In other preparations, the myelin sheath may exhibit a delicate trabecular reticulum, the *neurokeratin network* (Fig. 4-17). The network probably represents a precipitated protein residue of the myelin sheath rather than a true cytoplasmic reticulum. The myelin sheath ends at or near the point where the terminal aborizations are given off. No structure similar to the Schmidt-Lantermann clefts has been identified in myelin sheaths in the central nervous system.

Sheath of Schwann. This sheath of flattened cells forms the myelin of larger fibers. It also provides a thin attenuated cytoplasmic investment on nonmyelinated fibers of the cranial and spinal nerves (Figs. 4-20 and 4-23). Schwann cells, like the neurons, are of ectodermal origin (neural crest and neural tube). Each Schwann cell has a flat, oval nucleus surrounded by a thin rim of cytoplasm which contains a Golgi complex and mitochondria (Fig. 4-20). The Schwann cells of both myelinated and nonmyelinated nerve fibers are surrounded by a typical basement membrane approximately 25 nm in thickness (*bm* in Fig. 4-18). This is separated from the plasma membrane of the Schwann cell by an interval of 25 nm. Ultrastructural studies indicate that

the Schwann cell plasma membrane, with its surrounding basement membrane, represents the older term *"neurolemma sheath"* observed in light microscopy (437, 2542). Nathaniel and Pease (1810) regard only the granular basement membrane surrounding the Schwann cell as equivalent to the neurolemma.

One Schwann cell may have extensive cytoplasmic processes as it presides over, and maintains the integrity of, the segment of myelin between two nodes of Ranvier. If an ultrathin section were cut through a small myelinated nerve fiber to include the nucleus of a Schwann cell, it would reveal ultrastructural relations similar to those shown in Figure 4-20. A longitudinally cut nerve fiber with a thicker myelin sheath is shown in Figure 4-23A. Electron micrographs of adult unmyelinated nerves may reveal several axons lying within recesses of one Schwann cell (Figs. 4-20 and 4-23B). The plasma membrane of the Schwann cell is closely applied to the axon except for a small periaxonal space of 15 to 20 nm (322). However, at some point around the circumference of each unmyelinated axon, the plasma membrane is reflected and extends superficially to form the mesaxon (Fig. 4-23B).

Endoneurium. In addition to the above described structures, each peripheral nerve fiber is surrounded by a re-enforcing sheath of delicate connective tissue, the *endoneurium (sheath of Henle,* or *of Key and Retzius).* It is composed of delicate collagenous fibers disposed longitudinally for the most part, a homogeneous ground substance and an occasional flattened fibroblast. A close contact between the endoneurial collagen and the basement membrane of Schwann cells is an inevitable consequence of the ensheathing of nerve fibers in collagen. Actual "collagen pockets" surrounded by Schwann cells have been observed along nonmyelinated axons. Thin bundles of collagen usually can be observed within the typical basement membrane surrounding a Schwann cell (844). The endoneurium is continuous with the more abundant connective tissue of the perineurium, which envelops both small and large bundles of fibers within a peripheral nerve trunk (Fig. 4-3B).

Perineurium. The outermost layers of the perineurium are composed of dense concentric layers of mostly longitudinally arranged strands of collagen. A few fibroblasts and macrophages also are present among the strands. Perineural tissue is somewhat unique in that it consists of fibroblasts and smooth lamellae that resemble mesothelium (622). The deeper concentric layers of flattened cells have prominent basement membranes, often with closed contacts. The flattened cells also have a slightly granular cytoplasm with scattered mitochondria and rough-walled vesicles.

Large molecular dyes, silver nitrate, toxins and ^{131}I-labeled proteins have been used to investigate the blood-nerve barrier in animals (2630). The peripheral nerve of the rabbit has an effective nerve barrier, interpreted as due to the vascular endothelium rather than the mesothelial cells that accompany the endoneurial connective tissue.

Epineurium. This dense, collagenous layer forms an external connective tissue ensheathment for all peripheral nerve trunks. It is continuous centrally with the dura mater of cranial and spinal nerves. Its fibrous nature reinforces the toughness of peripheral nerve trunks. The collagen strands are disposed mainly longitudinally, and the component fibers have diameters between 70 and 85 nm. A few elastic fibers and fibroblasts with elongated processes are scattered throughout the epineurium. Axial arteries to peripheral nerves are derived from the large arteries adjacent to nerve trunks. Arteries that provide nourishment to a peripheral nerve penetrate the epineurium and give off several branches. The smaller arterioles pursue proximal or distal courses within the perineurium of the nerve trunk. Most of the capillaries supplying the peripheral nerve fibers are located in the endoneurium.

UNMYELINATED PERIPHERAL NERVE FIBERS

These slender axons are enveloped by the thin Schwann cell sheath, its basement membrane and fine strands of collagen (Figs. 4-20 and 4-23B). The critical point for fiber myelination of an axon in tissue culture is reported to be a diameter of 1 μm (320). Axons of thicker diameters always are invested with a myelin sheath. The peripheral axons of most postganglionic sympathetic neurons and many cells of the spinal ganglia are unmyelinated (698). Numerous unmyelinated fibers also are found in the gray and white matter of the spinal cord and brain. Here they appear as fine naked axons embedded in glial cell processes with relationships similar to that of the Schwann cells on the peripheral unmyelinated fibers (321, 1543, 1544).

Fiber Size. Myelinated fibers vary greatly in size. The fine fibers have a diameter from 1 to 4 μm; those of medium size from 5 to 10 μm; and the largest from 11 to 20 μm (Fig. 4-3).

Collaterals or branches are given off by most fibers of the central nervous system. They are usually of finer caliber than the parent stem, extend at right angles and often arise from the proximal unmyelinated part of the axon. In the myelinated portion they are given off at the nodes of Ranvier and become myelinated themselves. In the peripheral nervous system, the fibers of somatic motor neurons, which supply skeletal muscle, branch repeatedly at acute angles before reaching the muscle (Fig. 4-3G). Within the latter the branching may be very extensive, and a single nerve fiber may furnish motor terminals to many muscle fibers. Sensory fibers probably branch in a similar manner since their terminal arborizations extend over a considerable area. A single myelinated fiber may supply sensory endings to more than 300 hair follicle groups (2684).

Myelinated fibers conduct more rapidly than unmyelinated ones. Speed of conduction is proportional to the diameter of the fiber and, more especially, to the thickness of the myelin sheath. The myelin sheath may be regarded as insulation, while the extracellular space at the nodes of Ranvier and the periaxonal space provide ready avenues for ionic diffusion.

PHYSICAL AND PHYSIOLOGICAL GROUPING OF NERVE FIBERS

When an axon is excited, a finite length of the axonal membrane is depolarized. This zone of depolarization is propagated along the length of the axon and is known as a nerve impulse or action potential. An impulse consists of a large negative voltage deflection of short duration, the *spike potential*, which is usually followed by two longer but much smaller voltage shifts known as the *negative and positive after-potentials.* The speed with which the spike potential travels over the nerve fiber constitutes the *conduction velocity* of the nerve impulse, and the number of successive potentials traversing the fiber per unit time represents the frequency of the impulses (Fig. 4-1).

Erlanger and Gasser (716) demonstrated that different fibers in a nerve trunk conduct at varying velocities. The speed of conduction is proportional to the diameter of the fiber and of the myelin sheath. Each nerve has a characteristic pattern of velocities corresponding to an analogous pattern of fiber diameters in the nerve trunk. As a result of extensive physiological investigations supported by histological studies, nerve fibers have been grouped into three main classes, A, B and C (Table 4-2). The A group includes several subdivisions, designated A_α, A_β and A_δ. Criteria for the classification are fiber diameter, conduction velocity, threshold to electrical stimulation and nature of the electrical record (184, 855, 975, 976, 1071, 1504, 1949, 2085).

The A fibers are myelinated, range in diameter from 1 to 20 μm and conduct at rates of 5 to 120 m/sec. The more finely myelinated B fibers have a diameter up to 3 μm and a conduction rate of about 3 to 15 m/sec, although a higher velocity has been observed in some fibers of this group. The C fibers are unmyelinated and conduct very slowly, about 0.6 to 2 m/sec. There is a certain amount of overlap so that a fiber of 2 μm could belong to either the A or B group, but certain features of the electrical record permit a definite classification. Thus the duration of the spike potential is always much longer in B fibers than in an A fiber, and the B fibers lack a negative afterpotential.

Studies on various types of nerves (muscular, cutaneous and autonomic) indicate a general functional grouping of the three fiber types. This grouping must not be regarded as rigid, since many fibers serving the same function may have widely different calibers. The A fibers include several subdivisions. The largest and most rapidly conducting fibers (conduction velocity 60 to 120 m/sec in man) transmit motor impulses to skeletal muscles, while other A fibers convey afferent impulses from stretch

Table 4-2
Nerve Fiber Classification

Sensory Classification Group	Conduction Velocity Classification	Function
Ia	A_α	Primary muscle spindle afferents
Ib	A_α	Golgi tendon organ afferents
II	A_β	Mechanoreception: discriminative touch, pressure, joint rotation, secondary muscle spindle afferents
III	A_δ	Mechanoreception: touch Nociception: discriminative pain
IV	C	Nociception: inflammatory or visceral pain, thermal sense

receptors in muscle. The rest of the A fibers, varying considerably in diameter and speed of conduction, carry afferent impulses from cutaneous receptors. Fibers of intermediate size are related to touch and pressure. The finest fibers transmit impulses associated with pain, and some of these fibers conduct thermal and tactile impulses.

The B fibers are associated mainly with visceral innervation and are both efferent and afferent. All the preganglionic autonomic fibers belong to this group, as well as the postganglionic fibers from the ciliary ganglion, which are partly or wholly myelinated. The more rapidly conducting B fibers transmit afferent impulses from viscera. The unmyelinated C fibers comprise the efferent postganglionic autonomic fibers and afferent fibers which are believed to conduct impulses of poorly localized pain from the viscera and the periphery (Table 4-2).

The classification of axons in peripheral nerves on the basis of conduction velocity reveals, as mentioned above, certain correlations with function. When sensory physiologists studied the organization of dorsal root fibers activated by natural stimuli, it was convenient to use a classification that applied specifically to sensory neurons, and they identified axons as belonging to groups I, II, III and IV. Each group is activated by particular types of sensory stimulation and contains fibers of a particular size range.

These are shown in Table 4-2 along with the corresponding conduction velocity classification.

THE SYNAPSE

The simplest segmental reflex requires at least two neurons (Fig. 9-29). The nerve impulse, initiated in a peripheral sensory nerve ending, passes centrally along the axon of a dorsal root ganglion cell into the spinal cord. There it activates a motor neuron, whose impulse travels along the motor fiber and causes a group of muscle fibers to contract (Fig. 9-28). Even simple reactions have, as a rule, a third or *central* neuron interposed between the afferent and efferent cells (Fig. 9-29). In the more complicated neural circuits the number of such intercalated, or *internuncial*, central neurons may be multiplied. All neural pathways therefore consist of chains of neurons related to each other so as to make possible the continuity of signal transfer over the complete circuit. The point of junction of neurons, i.e., where the axonal arborizations of one neuron come in contact with the cell body or dendrites of another, is known as the *synapse*. The synapse is not a site of cytoplasmic continuity between neurons, but an interface of which they are functionally related. Axons terminating upon the dendrite of another neuron form *axodendritic synapses*, whereas axons terminating upon the cell soma or perikaryon form *axosomatic synapses*. Less frequently axon terminals of one neuron may be located directly on other axonic terminals, or on the initial segment of the axon of another neuron (*axoaxonic synapses*). The term "synapse" may be expanded to include not only the functional contacts between two neurons, but also those between neurons and effector cells, such as muscle cells.

Synaptic junctions show many structural variations (Fig. 4-24). Most commonly, the axon terminals end in small bulblike expansions (*end feet, boutons terminaux*). Each terminal consists of a neurofibrillar loop imbedded in perifibrillar substance; sometimes there are simply small neurofibrillar rings. A large motor neuron in the spinal cord may receive several thousand such endings, most of them 1 to 2 μm in diameter. In another type of synapse, the delicate axon terminals do not form end feet but come in lengthwise apposition with the dendrites or cell body, often for considerable distances. The most striking examples are the climbing fibers of the cerebellum (Figs. 14-4 and 14-5). In some cases, unmyelinated axons run at right angles to the dendrites and come in contact with the spiny excrescences or *gemmules* with which the dendrites are beset (Fig. 4-6). Thus one axon may convey impulses to many neurons, and conversely one neuron (e.g., anterior horn cell) may receive impulses from many neurons, some of which are widely separated in the neuraxis.

Numerous electron microscopy studies have shown that synapses of the vertebrate nervous system possess the following basic similarities: (a) discontinuity between the cytoplasm of the two apposed membranes of a synapse; (b) close apposition of the presynaptic (plasma membrane of an axon terminal) and postsynaptic membranes, which are separated by a minute synaptic cleft, usually 10 to 20nm in width (Figs. 4-26 and 4-27); and (c) the presence of mitochondria, neurofilaments and numerous synaptic vesicles on the presynaptic side of the synapse (943, 1569, 1921, 1982, 2173, 2174). The vesicles of the presynaptic terminals contain chemicals by which transmission across the synaptic cleft is effected (2174–2177, 2709). In the case of cholinergic neurons each synaptic vesicle is considered to contain a quantum of acetylcholine which is released when an impulse arrives at the synapse (1270, 2799). At the neuromuscular junction quanta of acetylcholine, released a few at a time during quiescence, are associated with miniature end plate potentials. The "chemical synapse" involving the release of transmitter substance is the most common type in the mammalian central nervous system. In lower vertebrates (e.g., fish) and at some locations in the mammalian CNS "electrical synapses" function without a chemical transmitter; in these synapses there is a close contact between pre- and postsynaptic membranes, called *gap junctions*.

The most commonly occurring synaptic vesicles are about 40 nm in diameter, are roughly spherical and have clear centers (Figs. 4-26 and 4-27). Vesicles of this type are found in axon terminals at neuromuscular junctions, throughout the central

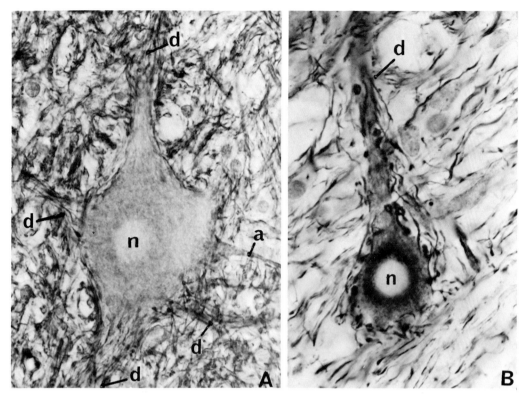

Figure 4-24. Synaptic endings on human CNS neurons after silver impregnation and observed by light microscopy. Note numerous terminal boutons on the dendrites (*d*, axodendritic synapses) and some of the cell body (axosomatic synapses). The axon (*a*) and nucleus (*n*) are identified in (*A*), which is a photograph of ×650 magnification. The smaller neuron shown in (*B*) is magnified ×920.

nervous system and in some sympathetic nerve endings. Circumstantial evidence suggests that these clear vesicles contain acetylcholine in cholinergic neurons (2175, 2709).

In cholinergic autonomic neurons each synaptic vesicle contains an estimated 1600 molecules of acetylcholine (2743). The vesicles also contain 1 mole of ATP for each 4 moles of transmitter.

As the nerve impulse invades the terminal, there is an influx of Ca^{2+} ions which leads to the exocytosis of synaptic vesicles and the release of transmitter into the synaptic cleft (Fig. 4-25). The transmitter molecules diffuse across the cleft and bind to receptor molecules in the postsynaptic membrane. The membrane of the discharged vesicles becomes incorporated into the surface membrane of the presynaptic terminal. New synaptic vesicles are generated in the terminals, partly through a process of micropinocytosis and partly from

the endoplasmic reticulum (1092). New acetylcholine (ACh) is synthesized by a soluble cytoplasmic enzyme, choline acetyltransferase (CAT), acting upon the substrate acetyl coenzyme A and choline. The newly synthesized transmitter then becomes incorporated into synaptic vesicles.

Once released into the cleft, ACh binds to receptors in the postsynaptic membrane. At least two types of cholinergic receptors can be distinguished on the basis of their pharmacology and physiology. *Nicotinic ACh receptors* are normally found at subsynaptic sites in skeletal neuromuscular junctions while *muscarinic ACh receptors* are most commonly found in the central nervous system and in peripheral autonomic neurons. A slightly larger vesicle about 50 nm in diameter containing a dense granule, 28 nm in diameter, is found in axon terminals of autonomic nerve fibers (194). Synaptic vesicles of this type are considered to be associated with catecholamines, es-

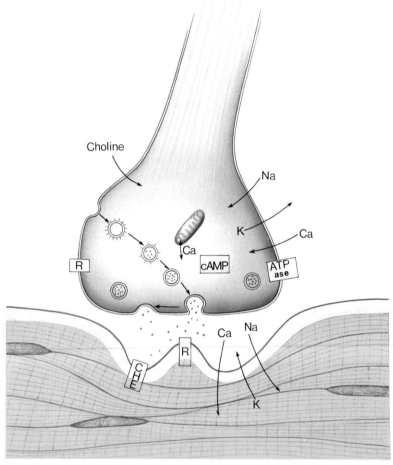

Figure 4-25. Schematic representation of a motor nerve terminal and muscle end plate showing the major biochemical and biophysical events in neuromuscular transmission. (*ATPase*) adenosine triphosphatase, (*cAMP*) cyclic adenosine monophosphate, (*CHE*) acetylcholine esterase, (*Ca*) calcium ions, (*Na*)sodium ions, (*K*) potassium ions, (*R*) transmitter receptor. (Modified from Standaert and Dretchen (2418).)

pecially norepinephrine. This type of synaptic vesicle appears in terminals of adrenergic nerve fibers, and may be seen in regions of the brain known to have a high amine content when tissue is fixed in potassium permanganate (1114, 1115).

Many specific physiological features are associated with the synapse. While an activated nerve fiber conducts equally well in either direction (orthodromic and antidromic conduction), impulses are transmitted over the reflex arc, i.e., across the synapse, in one direction only. Thus the impulse travels from the axon of one neuron to the cell body, the dendrites or more rarely the axon of another neuron. An exception to this generalization occurs at dendro-dendritic contacts exhibiting reciprocal synapses (2125). In this case, synapses of opposite polarity lie side by side. While there is electrophysiological evidence for reciprocal synapses, there is some question about their identification at the electron microscopic level (2104). Hence synapses ensure that nerve fibers normally are used for one-way signal transmission. Some of the other ways in which conduction across the synapse differs from that in a nerve fiber may be briefly mentioned. Over a reflex arc (a) conduction is slower; (b) the response may persist after cessation of the stimulus (after-discharge); (c) the rhythm of stimulus and the rhythm of response correspond less closely; (d) repetition of a given stimulus may produce a response where a single stimulus will not (summa-

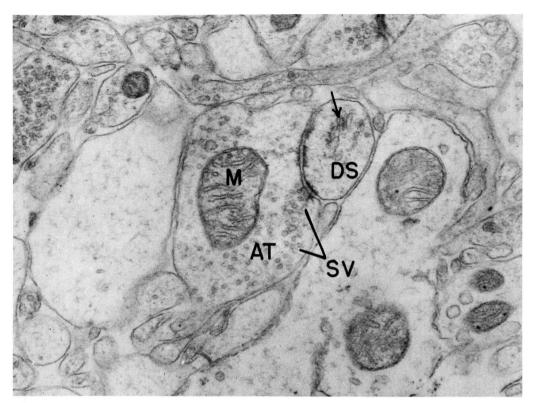

Figure 4-26. Electron micrograph of an axodendritic synapse in the human cerebral cortex. The saclike enlargement comprising the axon terminal (*AT*) contains a mitochondrion (*M*) and numerous synaptic vesicles (*SV*). The axon terminal is indented by the dendritic spine (*DS*). Profiles of the spine apparatus (*arrow*) are seen *above*, while *to the left* of the postsynaptic membrane of the dendritic spine is thickened in three places. Compare with synapse shown in Figure 4-24 (buffered osmium fixation, Epon, ×38,500). (Courtesy of Dr. J. Francis Hartmann, Presbyterian—St. Luke's Hospital, Chicago.)

tion); (e) there is greater variability in the threshold value of a stimulus, i.e., the ease with which responses can be elicited; (f) there is much greater fatigability; (g) there is greater dependence on oxygen supply and greater susceptibility to anesthetics and drugs; (h) there is a longer refractory period and (i) there is re-enforcement or inhibition of one reflex by another.

Synapses control impulse traffic, the amount and pattern of information input, and consequently the behavior of a neuron or groups of neurons. Synapses are the units that provide mutual neuronal interdependence. This interdependence involves trophic mechanisms in addition to transmission of information as electrical events in surface membranes. An example of trophic interactions is a change in the number of transmitter receptor molecules in soma or dendritic membrane of the postsynaptic neuron following denervation.

When catecholamine transmitters, such as norepinephrine or dopamine, bind to the postsynaptic membrane receptor the enzyme adenylate cyclase is activated. Adenylate cyclase catalyzes the conversion of adenosine triphosphate (ATP) to 3'5'-adenosine monophosphate (cyclic AMP). In the cytoplasm cAMP may activate one or several protein kinases which in turn may regulate phosphorylation of either plasma membrane proteins (784) or acidic nuclear protein (Fig. 4-28). The latter results in synthesis of new protein and may be the mechanism by which the formation and degradation of receptor molecules are regulated.

Denervation or pharmacological block of transmitter release in adrenergic axons leads to an increased number of adrenergic receptors in postsynaptic cells (1715). This probably accounts for the phenomenon of denervation supersensitivity, or increased

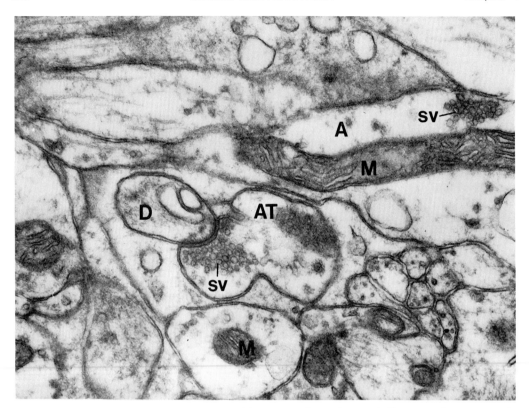

Figure 4-27.   Electron micrograph of an axodendritic synapse in monkey cerebellar cortex. Synaptic vesicles (*SV*) are present in the axon terminal (*AT*) and in the axon (*A*) in the upper right. Other organelles are: *D*, dendrite with spine apparatus, and *M*, mitochondria (×48,000). (Courtesy of Dr. Ray C. Henrikson, Albany College of Medicine of Union University.)

response to a given concentration of transmitter when compared to a normally innervated neuron or smooth muscle.

Another form of trophic interaction is the activation and changes in the amount of the rate limiting enzyme available for the synthesis of new transmitter in the postsynaptic cell (Fig. 4-29). In the case of catecholaminergic neurons, denervation results in lowered levels of cAMP in the postsynaptic cell. This decrease in cAMP leads to an increase in the amount of tryosine hydroxylase (3). These trophic changes appear to be a mechanism by which neurons attempt to adjust the sensitivity of their input and their output to compensate for a reduced number of catecholaminergic afferent axons.

The concentration of a different "2nd messenger" may be controlled by cholinergic presynaptic axons (Fig. 4-30). An example is found in the ganglia of a mollusc, *Aplysia californica*, where the release of acetylcholine from the afferent axon terminal results in an increase in 3'5'-guanosine monophosphate (cGMP) in the postsynaptic cell. Another cell (*B* in Fig. 4-30) forms an axoaxonic synapse and facilitates transmitter release by increasing cAMP in the presynaptic terminal, resulting in an increased Ca^{++} permeability and increased synaptic vesicle exocytosis (1264). In the vertebrate superior cervical ganglion both cholinergic and dopaminergic afferent axons form synapses upon the postsynaptic neuron. Dopamine increases cAMP and acetylcholine increases cGMP levels in the postsynaptic cell. The specific effects of cAMP and cGMP are not known, but it is hypothesized that each cyclic nucleotide phosphorylates different membrane proteins (963).

In recent years there has been great interest in the role of a calcium binding protein called "calmodulin." The calmodulin-Ca^{++} complex may regulate some of the

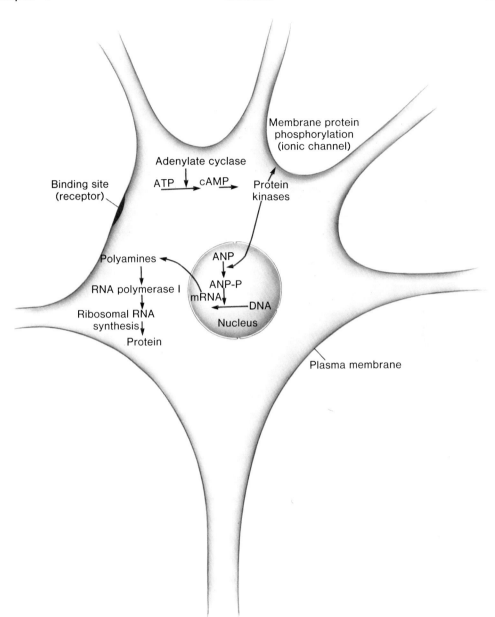

Figure 4-28. Diagram showing how cyclic AMP may participate in synaptic transmission and also initiate trophic changes. (Based upon Greengard (964, 965).) A transmitter receptor site in the surface membrane is shown at the *upper left*. When the catecholamine transmitter binds to the receptor, adenylate cyclase becomes available to form cyclic adenosine monophosphate (cAMP). cAMP activates protein kinases, some of which phosphorylate surface membrane proteins presumed to be associated with ionic channels. Other protein kinases may migrate to the nucleus initiating a chain of events ultimately resulting in increased protein synthesis. (*ATP*) adenosine triphosphate, (*ANP*) acidic nuclear protein, (*ANP-P*) phosphorylated acidic nuclear proteins, (*DNA*), desoxyribonucleic acid, (*mRNA*) messenger ribonucleic acid.

enzymes related to cyclic nucleotide formation or degradation (451). Although there is little specific information on calmodulin regulated mechanisms in synaptic terminals, it has been shown to be present in brain homogenates. For additional details on the synaptic complex the reader is referred to the articles by Eccles (671), Pap-

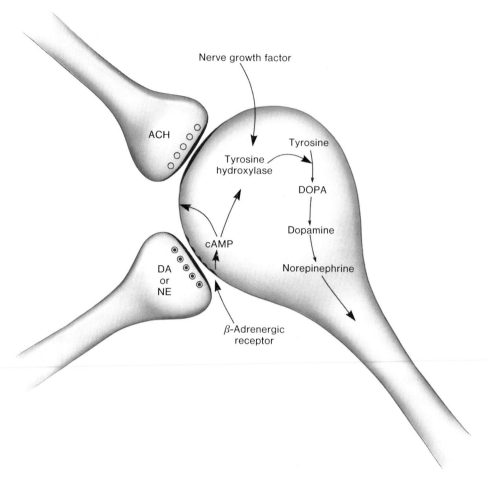

Figure 4-29. A diagram of a cholinergic (Ach) and catecholaminergic (DA or NE) synapse upon a noradrenergic cell of the superior cervical ganglion. The level of the enzyme tyrosine hydroxylase, important in the synthesis of the transmitters dopamine and norepinephrine, is regulated by the level of cAMP. Prolonged periods of increased cAMP levels result in reduced amounts of tyrosine hydroxylase.

pas (1937), de Robertis (2174), Nathaniel and Nathaniel (1808), Katz (1270), Guillery (982) and Peters et al. (1982).

AXOPLASMIC TRANSPORT

Axoplasmic transport refers to the movement of proteins and other substances along the axon. The movement occurs in both directions: *anterograde*, from cell body toward axon terminal, and *retrograde*, from terminal toward cell body (Fig 4-36). Even large particles, such as vesicles, and complex macromolecules, such as neurotropic viruses, move along the axon. Two early observations led to the concept of axoplasmic flow. It was found (2690, 2691) that constriction of an axon by a ligature

led to a buildup of material on the proximal side, and that proteins migrated along axons in both the peripheral and central nervous system (652) (Fig 4-37*B*). Isotopically labeled amino acids injected near the cell body are transported into the cell and become incorporated into newly synthesized proteins. The movement of the labeled proteins along the axon can be measured by either scintillation counting or autoradiographic methods. A method has also been devised which permits direct labeling of cellular protein (749). Anterograde transport has been found to occur at three different rates, termed fast, intermediate and slow. Fast transport consists predominantly of membrane bound vesicles derived from the Golgi apparatus and endoplasmic retic-

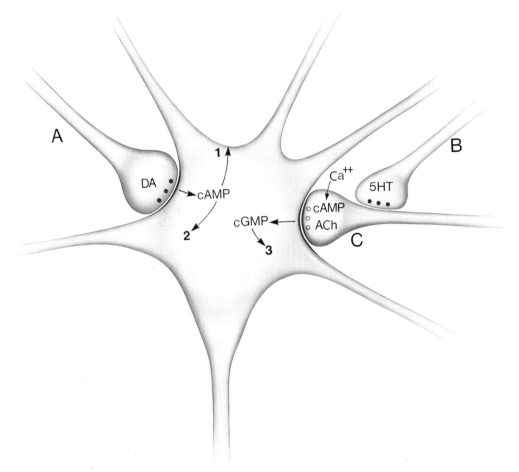

Figure 4-30. Diagram showing ways in which synaptic actions might be mediated by a "second messenger." This model is based upon observations in invertebrate (1264) and vertebrate (963) nervous system. *Cell A* is *dopaminergic* and controls the level of 3′5′-adenosine monophosphate (cAMP) in the postsynaptic cell. cAMP may (1) phosphorylate a membrane protein to alter membrane ionic permeability and/or (2) alter synthesis of a rate limiting enzyme for transmitter synthesis. *Cell B* is *serotonergic* and increases cAMP in the presynaptic terminal of cell C, resulting in an increased Ca^{++} permeability and transmitter exocytosis. *Cell C* is *cholinergic* and increases 3′5′-guanosine monophosphate (cGMP) in the postsynaptic cell. Increased cGMP (3) may phosphorylate a different specific membrane protein.

ulum, including membrane bound neurotransmitters (Fig. 4-36) (584, 934, 1440, 1862). This component has a mean rate of about 400 mm/day (653, 1861). Slow transport occurs at rates of 1 to 5 mm/day and involves soluble enzymes and filamentous proteins that make up neurotubules and neurofilaments (Table 4-3). (See Grafstein (932) for review.) The mechanisms of fast and slow transport differ, but details are not well understood. Fast transport can be blocked by the alkaloids colchicine or vinblastine which bind to tubulin and disrupt microtubules, while slow transport is much less impaired.

Table 4-3
Axoplasmic Transport[a]

Rate (mm/day)	Substances Transported
200–400 (fast)	Peptides, acetylcholinesterase, glycoproteins, glycolipids
50 (intermediate)	Mitochondrial proteins
15	Unidentified proteins
2–4 (slow)	Actin, creatine phosphokinase, enolase
0.21	Neurofilament proteins, tubulin

[a] Biochemical studies show that identified proteins are transported at specific rates. (Based upon the work of Lassek (1441).)

Virtually all of the protein synthesis in neurons occurs in the cell body, with only minor amounts detected in axons, terminals and distal dendrites. The growth and subsequent maintenance of long axonal and dendritic processes must require some mechanisms for moving newly synthesized structural protein and enzymes throughout the neuron.

In addition to orthograde axoplasmic transport from cell body to distal processes, it has been found that some substances can be taken up by axonal terminals or distal dendrites and transported back to the cell body (Fig. 4-36). Retrograde axoplasmic transport carries some neurotropic viruses, such as herpes simplex, to the neuronal cell bodies. Micropinocytosis seems to be an important mechanism for incorporating within the axon terminal vesicles which are transported to the cell body and degraded within the system of lysosomal organelles (256). Retrograde transport may be studied by placing the glycoprotein horseradish peroxidase (HRP) in the vicinity of nerve endings. The enzyme marker adheres to membrane of the axon terminal which is pinocytosed and transported back to the cell body for lysosomal degradation (1454). The enzyme can be visualized by histochemical treatment using a substrate that is converted into a colored insoluble polymer.

The mechanisms of orthograde and retrograde transport are not yet fully understood. [For review, see Schwartz (2293).] Retrograde transport does not seem to involve the agranular reticulum (1455).

DEGENERATION OF NERVE FIBERS

The cell body is the trophic center of the neuron, and any process detached from it disintegrates. Crushing injuries or interruption of an axon produces detectable changes in the cell body (chromatolysis), as well as in the central and distal stumps of the injured fiber. When an axon is divided, degenerative changes of a traumatic character first affect the cut edges. In the proximal portion of the fiber, which is attached to the cell body, the degenerative changes (retrograde degeneration) extend only a short, although variable distance, depending on the nature of the injury. In a clean cut only one or two internodes may be involved. In more severe injuries, such as gunshot wounds or inflammatory processes, the retrograde degeneration may extend as much as 2 or 3 cm. However, the degeneration is soon succeeded by reparative processes leading to the formation of new axonal sprouts from the central stump.

In the distal portion, the axon and myelin sheath completely disintegrate, and degeneration occurs throughout the length of the fiber, including its terminal arborization. This process is known as *secondary* or *Wallerian degeneration* (Figs. 4-31 and 4-32). The changes as a rule appear simultaneously along the length of the nerve fiber distal to the injury. Functional failure of the nerve also is abrupt down the length of the distal nerve trunk (1852, 2250). In these studies muscle responses to distal nerve stimulation ceased 54 to 72 hr after sciatic nerve section, depending on whether nerve injury occurred in the thigh or at the level of the knee.

Axonal changes begin almost at once. Electron micrographs of the sciatic nerve following crush injury demonstrate that the initial change is an accumulation of mitochondria in the axoplasm at the nodes of Ranvier (Fig. 4-37A). This is followed by a breakdown of the axoplasm and mitochondria (2681). Twelve hours after injury the axon is swollen and irregular in shape. Within a few days it begins to break up into fragments. However, the breaking up process may continue for a considerable time in some fibers, and fragments of degenerating axons have been found as late as 3 or 4 weeks after the injury. The synaptic terminals are affected similarly. The myelin sheath likewise degenerates. Two or 3 days after section, constrictions appear which break the myelin into elongated ellipsoid segments, which in turn fragment into smaller ovoid or spherical droplets or granules (Figs. 4-31 and 4-32). The whole process resembles the breakup of a liquid column under surface tension and is ascribed to the fact that the fiber is no longer kept in a turgid condition by neuroplasmic pressure emanating from the cell body (2786).

The myelin changes, at first purely physical, are followed by chemical changes as well; the myelin breaks down into simpler intermediate substances, which react to the Marchi stain.

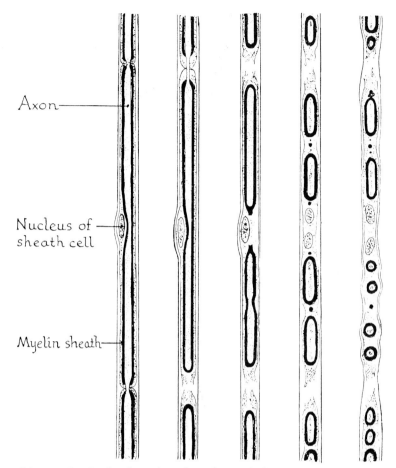

Axon

Nucleus of sheath cell

Myelin sheath

Figure 4-31. Diagram showing breakup of myelin and axon during nerve degeneration. Note increase in sheath cell protoplasm and division of the nucleus [Reproduced with permission from J. Z. Young: *Physiological Reviews* (2785).]

Ultrastructural studies provide information about the degenerative process. Nineteen hours after peripheral nerve injury there is a loosening of the myelin lamellae (1463). Myelin disintegration is evident at 4 days in Schwann cells and well advanced 96 hr after crushing dorsal roots of the cauda equina (1809). These authors have elucidated the key roles of the Schwann cell and its basement membrane in both degeneration and regeneration. Schwann cells undergo hypertrophy, demonstrate unusual numbers of ribosomes, multiply in number, become mobile and form elaborate basement membranes. These cells are almost exclusively responsible for the removal of axon remnants and autodigestion of disintegrated myelin. There is no connective tissue response in the endoneurium,

and leucocytes do not appear to participate in the phagocytosis of neuronal debris. The only endoneurial response is a slow accumulation, and slight increase, in the amount of collagen adjacent to the basement membranes. Newly formed and hypertrophied Schwann cells have extensive tapering and overlapping cytoplasmic processes, which in light microscopy formerly were interpreted as multinucleated syncytial cords (band fibers).

Nuclear division of the Schwann cells begins around the 4th day and continues actively to about the 25th, mitosis occurring over the whole length of the fiber. The increase in the number of nuclei is considerable, in some instances as much as 13 times the original population (2).

During degeneration the Schwann cell

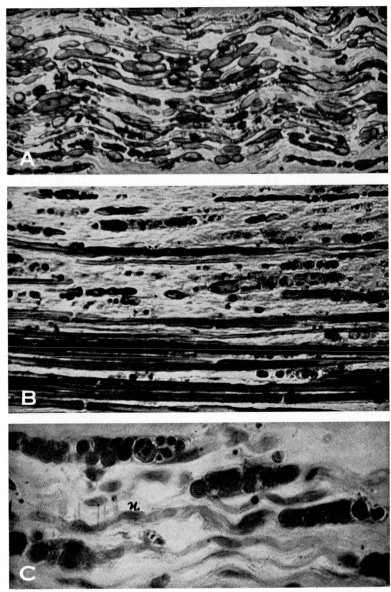

Figure 4-32. (*A*) Distal stump of a nerve cut 3 to 5 days previously (osmic cid). (*B*) Distal stump of a nerve partly cut 12 to 15 days previously (osmic acid). Normal fibers and two nodes of Ranvier are shown at the *bottom*. (*C*) Distal stump of a nerve cut 12 to 15 days previously (osmic acid and iron hematoxylin). In addition to the clumps or islands of degenerating myelin, several band fibers and their nuclei (*n*) are shown (photographs).

plasma and basement membranes become separated from each other to markedly increase the extent and complexity of the extracellular spaces (1809). The reactive Schwann cells form new elaborately folded and successive basement membranes one inside the other. These Schwann cells and basement membranes thus form numerous extracellular compartments or tubes surrounded by collagen of the endoneurium.

Regenerating axonal sprouts from regions above the injury later enter these extracellular compartments or "tubes" between the basement membrane and Schwann cell. If no axonal sprouts enter the tube, it shrinks considerably and the walls thicken, due to the increase in the collagen content of the endoneurium.

Retrograde Degeneration. The neuronal body whose axon is injured likewise

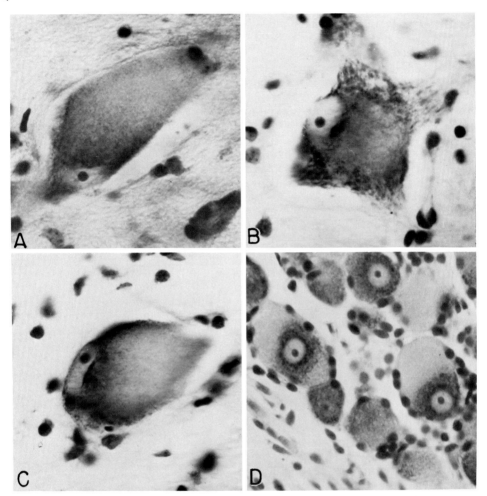

Figure 4-33. Four examples of central chromatolysis in the monkey. (*A* and *B*) Neurons in the brain stem reticular formation following section of the reticulospinal tracts (cresyl violet, ×600, ×500). (*C*) Retrograde cell change in lateral vestibular nucleus (cresyl violet, ×500). (*D*) Retrograde cell changes in the superior vagal ganglion (cresyl violet, ×500).

shows marked degenerative changes (Figs. 4-2*E* and 4-33). The cell body swells and becomes distended, the nucleus is displaced toward the periphery and the Nissl bodies undergo dissolution. Nissl body breakdown begins in the center of the cell and spreads outward (central chromatolysis). With light microscopy the fixed Nissl material appears to undergo lysis (Fig. 4-33). Cytochemical and electron microscopic studies indicate that there is an increase in the total quantity of RNA in the perikaryon, and suggest that the cisternae and ribosomes are dispersed and less concentrated. The fact that these cells imbibe water results in tremendous increases in cell volume. Ultrastruc-

tural changes also have been observed in many neuronal organelles (e.g., mitochondria, endoplasmic reticulum, Golgi apparatus, ribosomes and lysosomes) following nerve section or x-irradiation of ganglion cells in tissue culture (1136, 1321, 1634). Histochemical changes occur in a number of oxidative and hydrolytic enzymes within chromatolytic and regenerating neurons (1798). Such changes reflect a reduction, or an increase, in glucose metabolism, a breakdown of Golgi bodies or increased RNA and nucleoprotein synthesis.

The extent and rapidity of these changes depend on the type of neuron involved, on the nature of the lesion and especially on the location of the injury. A lesion of the axon near the cell body produces a greater central effect than one more distant. The effect depends upon the percentage of the neuron destroyed. If the lesion is near the cell body, the latter may ultimately die and the proximal portion of the nerve fiber attached to it degenerates. Chromatolysis in the cell body reaches its maximum 12 to 14 days following injury to the axon. This retrograde alteration of Nissl material (axon reaction) has been employed extensively in neuroanatomical research to locate the cells of origin of axons in central tracts, or in a peripheral nerve (Figs. 4-2E and 4-33).

REGENERATION

If the neuron survives injury, *regeneration* takes place. Recovery in the cell body begins about the 3rd week and is characterized by the appearance of Nissl bodies around the nuclear membrane. The swelling of the perikaryon gradually subsides, the nucleus returns to its central position and the Nissl bodies are restored to the

normal amount and distribution. Full recovery may take from 3 to 6 months, the time depending on the mass of axon to be reconstituted. While this is going on, regenerative processes appear in the axons of the central stump. As early as the 10th hr the axonal terminals begin to swell. Each axon splits into numerous fine strands or fibers (Figs. 4-34 and 4-35) which traverse the scar formed at the site of the injury and reach the Schwann tubes of the degenerating stump. Many of these fibers enter a single tube where they are disposed peripherally (Fig. 4-35). Later some of them move to a more central position and become completely surrounded by the plasma membrane of the sheath cells (Fig. 4-35). Along or within the bands, the regenerating axons grow distally for long distances to their peripheral destinations. Nathaniel and Pease (1810) have found that regenerating axonal sprouts reach the extracellular spaces of the membrane envelope as early as 4 days after a lesion. Although many sprouts initially may occupy the spaces and

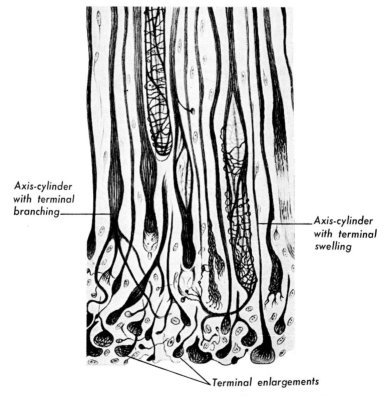

Axis-cylinder with terminal branching

Axis-cylinder with terminal swelling

Terminal enlargements

Figure 4-34. Regenerating axons in the central stump of a cat's sciatic nerve 2½ days after section of the nerve (after Cajal (348)).

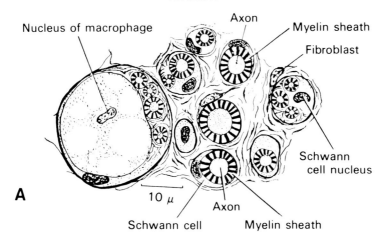

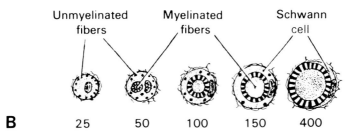

Figure 4-35. (*A*) Transverse section of peripheral stump of rabbit peripheral nerve severed 150 days previously. The stumps were left unsutured, but union was established by outgrowth. Most of the tubules contain one or more myelinated nerve fibers which are surrounded by protoplasm of the Schwann cells. (*B*) Diagram of the progress of regeneration within the Schwann tubule distal to a good nerve suture at different time intervals (days). At 25 days there are many fibers near the edge of the tube; at 50 days one or two fibers are enlarged and surrounded by Schwann cell cytoplasm; at 100 days one large myelinated fiber occupies the center of the tube, while other smaller fibers are peripheral. At approximately 400 days excess fibers disappear and a single large fiber attains its normal diameter. [Reproduced with permission from J. Z. Young: *Advances in Surgery*, (2786).]

gutters of the Schwann tube, only one persists and becomes remyelinated. This is usually the largest one (Fig. 4-35). The elimination of excess fibers may take considerable time, and some of them still may be seen in tubes 3 or 4 months after section. The enlargement of one fiber and the elimination of the others occur only if the regenerating axons make sensory or motor contact with appropriate receptor or effector endings in the periphery.

The thin regenerating axons, at first about 0.5 to 3 μm in diameter, gradually enlarge; the increase in diameter advances progressively down the tube, as if propelled by some centrifugal force from the central stump. When the fiber reaches the periphery, growth in length ceases, but the increase in diameter continues until the orig-

inal thickness is approximated. Myelination may occur as early as the 2nd or 3rd week in some fibers. It likewise advances in a proximodistal direction, and the process becomes somewhat slower in the more distal regions of the fiber. The myelin is at first laid down as a thin continuous sheath which subsequently becomes broken up into short internodal segments, about 150 to 700 μm in length. In fully regenerated nerve fibers, the internodes are shorter and more numerous, and there is no longer any definite relation between internodal length and diameter because fibers of varying thickness may possess similar internodal lengths. The time course of the events in degeneration and regeneration overlap each other. As noted above, regeneration of new axonal sprouts occurs before the disintegration of the axon and myelin sheath is completed in the distal segments of injured nerves. In a similar fashion regenerating axonal sprouts may traverse Schwann tubes which still contain degeneration debris (1810).

The growth processes observed during regeneration are remarkable. A slender axonal filament ultimately is transformed into a mature fiber whose volume in some instances may be several hundred times the volume of the original filament (Fig. 4-37A).

The manner in which this new axoplasm is formed has been investigated by Weiss and Hiscoe (2691) in a series of ingenious experiments. They fashioned small arterial rings which, when distended, could be slipped over the end of a cut nerve and placed in the desired position. The subsequent contraction of these rings produced localized constrictions with consequent reduction in the diameter of the individual fiber tubes (Fig. 4-37B). The reduction in the lumen of the tube does not at first interfere with the

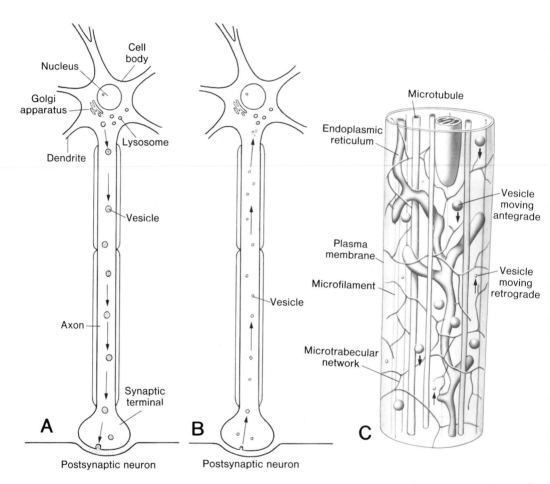

Figure 4-36. A diagram illustrating some of the major features of anterograde and retrograde axonal transport. The major components of anterograde axonal transport (A) are filamentous proteins and vesicles originating from the Golgi apparatus and endoplasmic reticulum. Retrograde axonal transport (B) involves movement toward the cell body of smaller vesicles formed by micropinocytosis at the synaptic terminal. In the cell body the vesicles coalesce and become incorporated into lysosomes for degradation. C shows organelles which are thought to be associated with axoplasmic transport. While the mechanisms are not fully understood, substances that move in an anterograde direction at slow rates seem to be associated with microtubules. Particles or reticulum-like profiles that move in a retrograde fashion become associated with agranular reticulum-like profiles which are not part of the continuous channels of the agranular endoplasmic reticulum system.

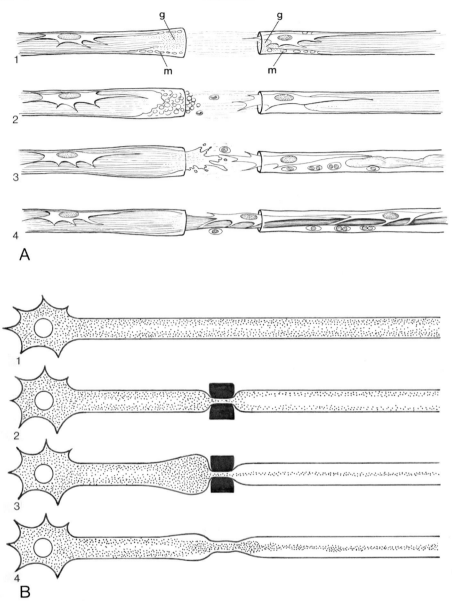

Figure 4-37. Diagrams of the stages of nerve regeneration (A) and the consequences of nerve constriction (B). Following severance of a nerve (A-1) a fibrin clot forms a bridge between the cut ends, and for a short distance in both stumps, the myelin (m) breaks into droplets and the axon breaks into granules (g). During the first few days following nerve section, the axon forms multiple sprouts (A-2, A-3) which later enter the distal Schwann cell tube (A-4). B-1 depicts a normal nerve fiber, and B-2 and B-3, show the proximal accumulation of cytoplasm which occurs gradually over a period of several weeks following application of a constricting cuff. After removal of the cuff (B-4) the swelling of the axon diminishes as axoplasmic transport is restored in the distal segment of the fiber. [Based on Young (2786) and Weiss and Hisloe (2691).]

advance of the slender regenerating axon, which passes through the constricted zone and makes contact with the periphery. "But when the fiber, as it continues to enlarge, attains the dimensions of the constricted zone, a remarkable difference appears between those parts lying at the distal and at the proximal sides of the narrow neck. The distal segment ceases to grow and remains permanently undersized, while the proximal segment not only continues to enlarge, but near the entrance of the constricted zone, enlarges excessively." It was concluded that the axoplasm exerting pressure in a distal direction and becomes dammed up where the channel narrows (Fig. 4-37). The damming increases in intensity with time, and varies with the amount of constriction and the size of the fiber. Morphologically it is expressed in several ways, such as ballooning, beading, telescoping and coiling of the fibers. On release of the constriction, some of the dammed axoplasm flows into the distal portion, which consequently increases in thickness (Fig. 4-37). The authors concluded that the formation of new axoplasm, i.e., growth in volume, occurs only in the cell body and that this axoplasm maintains a constant proximodistal motion that causes the elongation and enlargement of the regenerating fiber.

A knowledge of the mode of nerve regeneration is important as a basis for surgical treatment. If a nerve is severed, it is desirable to surgically approximate the cut ends promptly. If some time has elapsed since the injury, it is necessary to resect surrounding scar tissue and the neuroma on the proximal nerve stump before the nerve can be sutured. This subject is discussed further on p. 206.

Fiber degeneration in the CNS is similar to that observed in the peripheral nerves. However, the degeneration proceeds at a slower pace, and the removal of neural debris by glial cells takes a longer time. It is known that the large fibers of the corticospinal tract and optic nerve degenerate faster than the fibers of small size (566, 567). Such studies indicate that fibers of equal size tend to possess equal resistance to secondary degeneration. The large fibers degenerate faster, but are resorbed more slowly. Hence the debris of total degeneration in the CNS is in evidence for several months.

Regeneration within the central nervous system of mammals has been studied with both anatomical and physiological technics (304, 358, 359, 802, 2301, 2464, 2749). Such studies indicate that the central axons of injured nerve cells make abortive attempts to regenerate across an experimental gap in the spinal cord. Factors that influence and often hamper central regeneration are similar to those influencing regeneration in the peripheral nervous system (e.g., length of gap between severed stumps, hemorrhage and scar formation). Central regeneration is further thwarted by the absence of sheath cells to guide the regenerating axonal sprouts. Sugar and Gerard (2464) found evidence of functional regeneration in adult rats whose thoracic spinal cords had been transected with care to prevent injury to the blood supply. No significant return of function has been noted in the higher mammals following complete transection of the spinal cord. It has been shown that remyelination of experimentally injured axons of the spinal cord can take place in the cat (321).

Over the years various chemical compounds have been used in an attempt to stimulate the growth of the neurons and their processes. Bueker (315) noted that a fragment of mouse sarcoma 180 implanted in the body wall of a 3-day chick embryo became invaded by sensory nerve fibers from the adjacent spinal ganglia. After 4 or 5 days the ganglia appeared to be considerably enlarged. This overall increase resulted from both the number and the size of the sensory neurons, while motor neurons remained unaffected. These observations were confirmed by Levi-Montalcini and Hamburger (1476), who also noted that the sympathetic nervous system contributed more fibers to the tumor graft than did sensory ganglia. Tissue cultures of chick spinal and sympathetic ganglia, when confronted with explants of a tumor at a distance of a few millimeters, produced an exceedingly dense outgrowth of fibers on the side of the ganglia facing the tumor (1477). An extract prepared from the mouse salivary glands also promoted exuberant nerve growth *in vitro* on chick ganglia, as well as on ganglia from the mouse and rat (1472, 1473, 1475). Some of the chemical properties of this *nerve growth factor* were identified by Cohen (502). It was nondialyzable, heat-labile, destroyed by acid, stable to alkali, and had an ultraviolet absorption peak at 279 nm. Nerve growth factor has been chemically characterized as a molecule of 29,000 MW existing as a dimer of two protein subunits, which together with another protein subunit form a native molecule with a molecular weight greater than 100,000 (73).

The subunit with sensory and sympathetic neuron growth promoting properties resembles in some respects the insulin molecule in both molecular structure and cellular action. However, nerve growth factor and insulin bind to separate receptor sites on the cell surface.

An antiserum to this nerve growth factor was produced in rabbits. The antiserum, when injected into young mice, selectively destroyed the sympathetic chain ganglia, especially if administered at birth (1474). Attempts to promote neuron regeneration with the use of nerve growth factor after injury to the cat spinal cord were inconclusive (2300). For a more complete discussion of regeneration in the central nervous system, the reader is referred to Windle (2746).

CHAPTER 5

Neuroglia

Neuroglia
  Astrocytes
  Oligodendrocytes
  Microglia

Ependyma
Choroid Epithelium

The non-neural elements which form the interstitial tissue of the nervous system are known as neuroglia (i.e., "nerve glue," Virchow (2621)). Early investigators recognized that neuroglia separated neural elements from blood vessels and regarded neuroglia as an interstitial material in which characteristic stellate and spindle-shaped cells were suspended. Although peripheral nerves have a connective tissue supporting framework, this is lacking in the central nervous system. In the brain and spinal cord connective tissue is limited to the membranes which surround and envelop them (i.e., the meninges) and small extensions of these membranes which accompany blood vessels that penetrate neural tissue. The meninges form a container in which the brain and spinal cord are "floated" in the cerebrospinal fluid. At the light microscopic level the structural features of neuroglia are difficult to demonstrate except by complex selective staining methods. In ordinary preparations stained with basophilic dyes usually only the nuclei are seen. Sections impregnated by the metallic technics of Golgi (913), Cajal (349, 350) and Rió Hortega (2166, 2167) reveal the different cell types, their processes and their relationships to neurons and blood vessels (Figs. 5-1, 5-2, 5-3, 5-4 and 5-7). The morphological characteristics of neuroglia as observed in the light microscope have been described by several authors (Penfield (1961), Rió Hortega (2169), Glees (891),

Scheibel and Scheibel (2274), Windle (2748) and Polak (2028). Electron microscopic studies indicate that the interstitial material of the central nervous system is composed only of neuroglia (1982). Thus the central nervous system is composed almost entirely of two elements, neurons and neuroglia, which are separated from each other by extracellular fluid contained in a space 10 to 20 nm in width (617, 1921).

In contrast with other epithelial tissues, there is relatively little extracellular space in the central nervous system. Electron microscopic studies indicate that neurons and neuroglia are tightly packed in the central nervous system with spaces no greater than 20 nm wide between individual cells. Measurements of the extracellular space based upon equilibration with sucrose suggest a volume of 10 to 15% (603). Information concerning the volume, the nature of the fluid filling the extracellular space and the possibilities for controlling both its composition and volume is of great practical significance in relation to cerebral edema. Electron microscopic investigations suggest that experimental and clinical edema in the gray matter of the brain may be due to swelling of glial cells, particularly astrocytes (2172). In the white matter where edema is more severe, the enlargement is primarily in the extracellular region with marked widening of the 20 nm extracellular space (2533). It is apparent that cerebral edema is not a uniform reaction in neural tissue.

In mammals neuroglial cells greatly out-number nerve cells and they may comprise almost half of the total volume of the human brain. Their counterparts also are a constant feature of the peripheral nervous system. Similar supportive cells are present in all vertebrate nervous systems and in some invertebrate nervous tissue as well (318, 492). The stability of this class of cells phylogenetically suggests that their functional role must be of great importance. Glial cells of the mammalian brain are difficult to study because of their inaccessibility. For this reason information has been sought concerning neuroglia in invertebrates and lower vertebrates (1377, 1378) and in tissue culture studies (1787, 1788, 2032). Membrane electrical properties of glia cells have been investigated most extensively in the optic nerve of the mudpuppy, *Necturus*, and in the leech. The glia membrane has a high specific membrane resistance and is selectively permeable to K^+. Glia membranes also have an electrogenic Na^+/K^+ pump, but it does not contribute significantly to the normal resting potential. Glia cells may be depolarized by external K^+ and by glutamate, but have no voltage sensitive Na^+ channels. Studies in lower forms show that glia are electrically coupled to each other, and both tight and gap junctions have been observed in electron micrographs (1894).

Although numerous hypotheses have been advanced concerning the functions of neuroglial cells, most of these are unconfirmed. Among the most widely accepted functions of neuroglia is the role of oligodendrocytes and the Schwann cells in the formation of myelin sheath (322). It has been suggested that neuroglia play an important role in isolating functionally distinct groups of neuronal elements which prevent axon terminals from influencing neighboring and unrelated receptive neuronal surfaces (1919, 1981). Neuroglia may also participate actively in maintaining ionic homeostasis and thereby influence the composition of the surrounding extracellular fluid. It appears fairly well established that astrocytes play a role in the repair of injuries in the brain and that by proliferation can wall off damaged areas (1644, 2290).

Two categories of supporting cells are recognized in the central nervous system, macroglia and microglia (Fig. 5-3). The *macroglia*, astrocytes and oligodendrocytes, are derived from ectoderm, have only one type of cytoplasmic process, do not generate action potentials (1377) and have not been observed to provide or receive synapses. A third neuroglial cell type that has neither the filaments and glycogen particles characteristic of astrocytes nor the microtubules typical of oligodendrocytes has been observed in the cerebral cortex and optic nerve. These cells resemble a type of glia seen in fetal and early postnatal stages of nervous system development, and may represent a glial stem cell which is retained in the adult (2607).

Unlike neurons, neuroglia retain the ability to divide throughout life. Proliferation of macroglia occurs particularly in response to injury in the nervous system (2290). *Microglia* are considered to be of mesodermal origin and enter the embryonic brain and spinal cord when these developing structures are penetrated by blood vessels (Fig. 5-3). No morphological classification of neuroglia is entirely satisfactory, for there may be many intermediate forms between oligodendrocytes and astrocytes (891, 1543, 1545, 2103, 2180, 2289), and some authors do not consider microglia to be true neuroglial cells (see Peters et al. (1982)). In the broadest sense neuroglia, often referred to simply as glia, should include the ependyma, the neurilemma cells (Schwann cells) and the satellite cells of peripheral sensory ganglia in addition to the macroglia and microglia. Ependymal, neurilemma and satellite cells are all derived from ectoderm; neurilemma and satellite cells are derivatives of the neural crest (Fig. 3-3).

Astrocytes. These cells are the largest, most numerous and most elaborate of all the glial elements. Astrocytes are recognized by their stellate-shaped cells and their many processes which extend into the surrounding neuropil (Figs. 5-1 and 5-2). Some of the long, branched processes from each cell form expansions that are applied to the surface of blood vessels, where they form the so-called "end feet" or "sucker processes." Processes of astrocytes extending to the surface of the central nervous system form similar expansions that constitute the superficial glial membrane beneath the pia

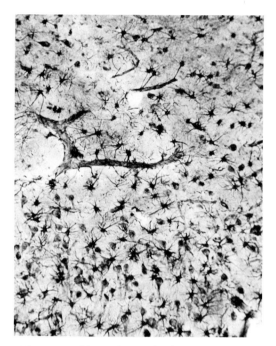

Figure 5-1. Photomicrograph of astrocytes showing their radially arranged processes and "end feet" (Cajal gold-sublimate method, ×150). (Reproduced with permission from D. Bodian: *The Neurosciences. A Study Program*, pp. 6–24, G. C. Quarton et al. (Eds.), Rockefeller University Press, New York, 1967.)

mater (Fig. 1-9). Each neuron has a specific relationship with the astrocytic processes in its vicinity, ranging from complete encapsulation to none at all (1919). They form most of the "packing tissue" of the neuropil of the nervous system (Fig. 5-2), and reduce the extracellular space to a series of irregular and interlacing small clefts. With the Golgi stain these glial cells show a delicate but pervasive framework in which the neural elements appear to be suspended (Fig. 5-2). In sharp contrast to this somewhat rigid configuration, astrocytes in tissue culture show flowing veil-like expansions in all directions, and migrate with a slow, gliding motion (1788).

A number of brain specific proteins have been biochemically isolated, purified and immunohistochemically localized. An acidic protein, with a molecular weight of 24,000 and termed S-100 because of its solubility in saturated ammonium sulfate, is found mainly in glial cells in the adult rat (1731).

Glial fibrillary acidic protein (GFAP) differs from S-100 in amino acid sequence and electrophoretic mobility and also differs from the fibrillar proteins tubulin and filarin found in neurons. GFAP is associated with fibrous astrocytes in both normal and pathological brain tissue (178) and with embryonic radial glial cells (1483).

When dissociated rat embryonic brain cells are cultured under conditions that remove neuroblasts, the remaining cells have an epithelial-like morphology. The addition of dialyzed brain extract to the medium causes astrocyte-like morphological changes and increased synthesis of GFAP. The dialysate contains a protein, called glia maturation factor (GMF), which promotes chemical as well as morphological differentiation of glial cells (1493).

Two main types of astrocytes can be distinguished in both light and electron microscopy. The *fibrous astrocyte* (spider cell) is characterized by its thin, less branched processes which radiate from the cell body for considerable distances. These glial elements often are interposed between neurons and adjacent blood vessels and have prominent perivascular "end feet" (Figs. 5-3 and 5-4). Fibrous astrocytes are most numerous in the white matter (Fig. 5-2). With appropriate stains the cell body and processes are seen to contain many delicate fibrils. Each intracellular gliofilament is 6 nm in width and of indeterminate length. Such filaments correspond to the thicker fibrils observed in muscle and epithelial cells (i.e., myofibrils and tonofibrils). In the larger processes they are arranged in straight parallel bundles and can be followed for considerable distances. Such gliofibrils also are present in the protoplasmic astrocytes to be described below. Another feature common to both types of astrocytes are small granular swellings along the processes called *gliosomes* (Figs. 5-3 and *g* in 5-4). They occur in the cell body as well, and in electron micrographs they are seen to be clumps of mitochondria which contain a more dense matrix material.

The *protoplasmic astrocytes* (mossy cells) are most numerous and easy to identify in the gray matter (Fig. 5-2). They have numerous freely branching processes, perivascular "end feet," and often are observed

Protoplasmic astrocytes of gray matter

Fibrous astrocytes of white matter

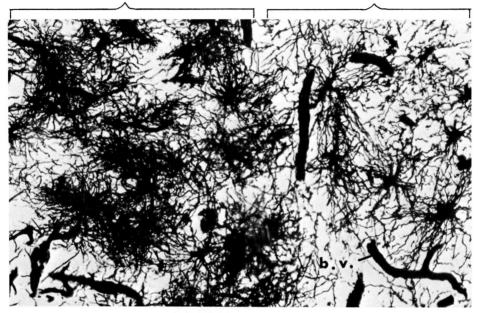

Figure 5-2. Distribution and appearance of astrocytes in gray and white matter of human spinal cord. Smaller nerve cell bodies often are obscured by profuse branches of protoplasmic astrocytes. Blood vessels (*b.v.*) also are stained in such preparations and receive vascular end feet from adjacent astrocytes (Golgi stain, photograph, ×175).

in close proximity to neuronal perikarya and dendrites. If fibrous and protoplasmic astrocytes are examined in Golgi preparations (Fig. 5-4) one can find sharp distinctive cells in each category. In the same sections one also can observe a host of intermediate and transitional cells that defy a precise morphological classification. Electron micrographs suggest the reason: they may represent different forms of the same cell (1644, 1982). Variations in cell type may in part be a reflection of the cytoarchitectural differences that exist between the gray and white matter of the brain and spinal cord. Electron microscopic features common to both types of astrocytes (Fig. 5-5) are the usual cytoplasmic organelles (dense mitochondria, scanty granular and agranular endoplasmic reticulum, gliofilaments and an abundant watery cytoplasm). The nucleus is finely granular and only moderately dense, and nuclear pores have been identified (1644, 1918). Fine structural char-

acteristics which identify the astrocyte alone were described by the latter authors. These include a watery cytoplasm that contains gliofilaments, and dense glycogen granules 15 to 40 nm in diameter.

Astrocytes demonstrate a wide variety of enzymes which suggests they may be involved in transport mechanisms between the blood and brain (5). Disruption of neurons, whether by trauma or disease, leads to hypertrophy of perineuronal glial cells (Fig. 5-6). Astrocytes in particular show a marked hyperplasia and may form a glial scar (2348).

Oligodendrocytes. The term oligodendroglia was introduced to describe small neuroglial cells with relatively few processes (2168). The delicate slender processes radiate only a short distance from a spherical or pear-shaped cell body (Figs. 5-3 and 5-7). In sections stained with basic dyes the nuclei of oligodendrocytes are smaller, more regular and more chromo-

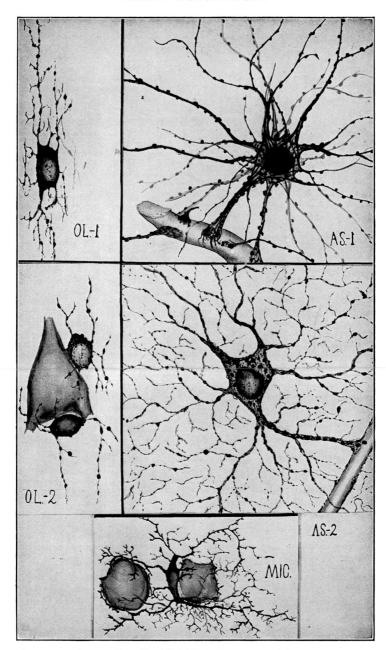

Figure 5-3. Various types of neuroglia cells. *AS-1,* Fibrous astrocyte with one or two processes forming foot plates against a neighboring blood vessel; *AS-2,* protoplasmic astrocyte with foot plate containing gliosomes (dark granules) in its body and processes; *MIC,* microglia cell whose delicate spiny processes embrace the bodies of two neurons; *OL-1,* oligodendrocyte in the white matter (interfascicular form); *OL-2,* two oligodendrocytes lying against a nerve cell (perineuronal satellites). (Reproduced with permission from the late W. Penfield: *Cytology and Cellular Pathology of the Nervous System,* Paul B. Hoeber, New York, 1932.)

philic than astrocytic nuclei. These glial cells differ from astrocytes in that: (a) their nuclei are smaller, rounder and more dense, (b) the cell body is smaller and gives rise to fewer processes and (c) their cytoplasm is more dense, containing chiefly ribosomes, mitochondria and microtubules. The dense chromatin of the nucleus has light patches

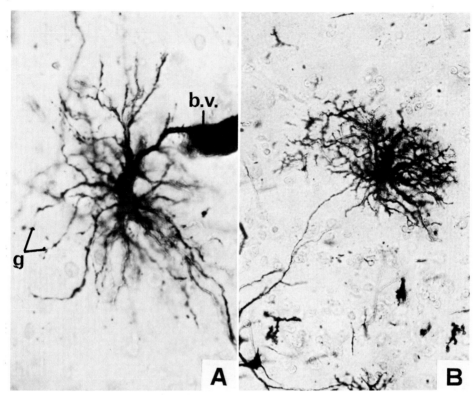

Figure 5-4. Fibrous (*A*) and protoplasmic (*B*) astrocytes in white matter of adult cerebral cortex. Note numerous gliosomes (*g*) in the processes of the fibrous astrocyte and vascular end foot on blood vessel (*b.v.*) (Golgi stain, photograph, ×550).

adjacent to numerous nuclear pores, while the cytoplasm has a crowded appearance, due to large quantities of free ribosomes and rough-surfaced endoplasmic reticulum. Other distinguishing features of their cytoplasm are prominent microtubules, dark and light multivesicular bodies and granular inclusions. The cytoplasm has mitochondria and a Golgi apparatus, but contains neither fibrils nor glycogen granules (322, 1369, 1775). The plasma membrane of the oligodendrocyte makes close contacts with adjacent myelin sheaths and the processes of adjacent glial cells (Fig. 5-8).

Three principal types of oligodendroglia can be identified by their location and relationships. *Perineuronal satellite cells* are closely apposed to neuron perikarya or their dendrites in the gray matter. This type is the most easily identified in adult material (*OL-2* in Fig. 5-3 and 5-7). *Interfascicular cells* occur in the white matter and often appear in rows between the my-

elinated fibers (*OL-1* in Fig. 5-3). The *interfascicular* oligodendrocytes are numerous in the white matter of the fetus and newborn. However, they rapidly diminish in number as myelination progresses. After the myelin sheath is formed, only the nucleus remains, so that in adult material their processes rarely are observed (Fig. 5-7B). The third type, *perivascular cells*, are observed less frequently. Oligodendrocytes whose delicate processes terminate as end feet upon adjacent blood vessels have been demonstrated by several authors (355, 1546).

Oligodendrocytes form myelin sheaths in the central nervous system (Fig. 5-8). The fine structural continuity of the plasma membrane with the myelin sheath (Fig. 5-9), and their active participation in remyelination has been reported in detail (321, 322, 1082). These cells are present in great numbers prior to myelin formation, and at this time there is a marked increase in glial

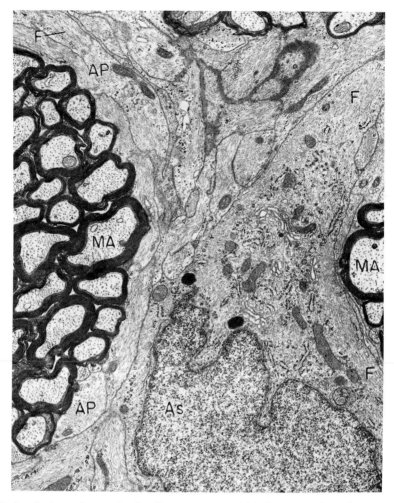

Figure 5-5. An electron micrograph of a fibrous astrocyte (*As*) from normal, adult rat optic nerve. The astrocytic cell body contains numerous filaments (*F*) as do the astrocytic processes (*AP*) which subdivide the myelinated axons (*MA*) of the optic nerve into bundles (×12,000). (Courtesy of Dr. James E. Vaughn, City of Hope Medical Center, Duarte, Calif.)

enzyme activity (811). In view of their cytoplasmic structure and role in myelin formation, these cells may be responsible for the high oxygen consumption so essential to the maintenance of myelin integrity (200). Astrocytes, as well, may participate in the latter function. It should be noted that in mammals the oligodendroglia react to injury by acute swelling, marked increases in a variety of osmiophilic organelles and increased acid phosphatase activity (1646). This study suggested a lysosomal intracellular breakdown of debris rather than phagocytosis by invading microgliocytes.

Specialized macroglial elements, such as the Bergmann cells of the cerebellum (see p. 469) and Müller cells of the retina, appear to play an important role during the fetal development of these structures.

The most common intracranial tumors are gliomas, i.e. neoplasms derived from glial cells. Approximately 50% of gliomas are morphologically classed as glioblastoma multiforme, a rapidly growing malignant tumor derived from astrocytes, while 25% are more slowly growing astrocytomas (2797, 2798). Oligodendroglial tumors account for only about 6% of the gliomas. The presence of immunoreactive glial fibrillary

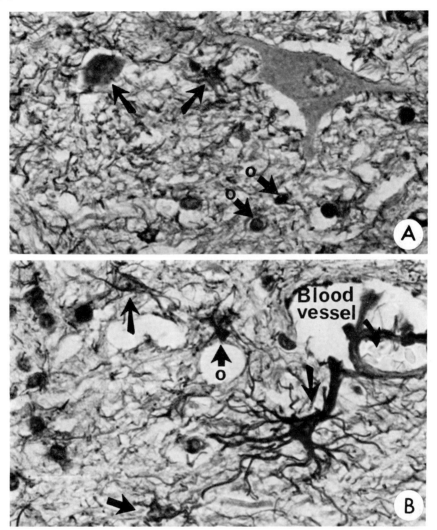

Figure 5-6. Reactive astrocytes in gray matter of adult human cord 4 weeks after a spinal stereotaxic lesion (*A*) Anterior horn cell with adjacent oligodendrocytes (*o*) and swollen astrocytes (*arrows*). (*B*) A prominent and bizarre astrocyte with enlarged vascular end foot; several smaller astrocytes with gliofibrils are indicated by *arrows*. The cell body of an oligodendrocyte (*o*) is identified for comparison of relative sizes. (Both photographs are of Holzer stained sections, ×550.)

acidic protein (GFAP) in glioblastomas and astrocytomas argues for their common origin. GFAP has also been demonstrated in some, but not all, transformed cells of ependymal tumors (658).

Microglia. Microglia were recognized as a distinctive glial element by Rió Hortega (2166, 2169) when he introduced his silver carbonate staining method (Fig. 5-3). These cells are small in comparison to astrocytes, have elongated or triangular nuclei which stain deeply with basic dyes and have wavy, branching processes that give off spinelike projections. Microglia are found in both white and gray matter, but are more abundant in gray matter (Figs. 5-10 and 5-11). These cells, presumed to be of mesodermal origin, enter the nervous system as perivascular mesenchymal cells, and there is a suggestion that such cells may be preferentially situated near blood vessels. Approximately 10% of glial cells are classified as microglia in light microscopic preparations of the cerebral cortex (307).

Although microglial cells appear inactive in normal adult brain tissue, inflammatory

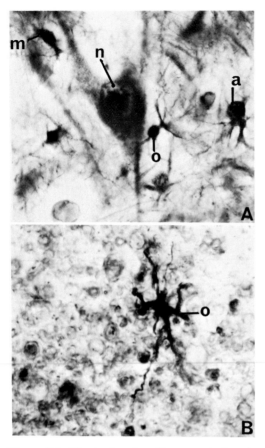

Figure 5-7. Oligodendrocytes of human spinal cord. (*A*) Newborn gray matter to demonstrate relative size of a neuron cell body (*n*), perineuronal (satellite) oligodendrocyte (*o*); astrocyte (*a*) and microglial cell (*m*) (Cajal gold sublimate stain, ×565). (*B*) Posterior white column of adult cord with oligodendrocyte (*o*) (Golgi stain, ×550).

branch then pursues an irregular and tortuous course either to adjacent neurons, or less often, to a blood vessel wall. The nucleus is ovoid or elongated, which aids in distinguishing the microglia from the oligodendrocyte. The cytoplasm is pervaded by myriads of minute vacuoles, which often gives the cell, or some of its processes, a sievelike appearance (Fig. 5-10*A*).

In spite of many descriptions of microglia in the light microscopic literature, this cell has not been identified in electron microscopic preparations (1982). Criteria for identification of microglial cells initially were arrived at by a process of elimination (735, 1081, 1775, 2289). The cell thought to correspond with the microglia was small with a dark nucleus, dark cytoplasm and compact organelles. Improved methods for fixing and handling central nervous tissue suggest that the crenated dark cells thought to be microglia were damaged cells. Explanations advanced for the failure to identify the microglia in the electron microscope suggest that: (a) oligodendrocytes and microglia may represent the same cell at the electron microscopic level, and (b) macrophages may be derived from pericytes of small vessels, rather than from neuroglial elements in the neuropil.

Microglia have long been considered the scavengers of the nervous system (i.e., the reticuloendothelial component of the nervous system). They were presumed to be pleomorphic cells capable of: (a) metamorphosis into a macrophage, (b) undergoing mitotic division and migrating at will through the already formed neuropil and (c) autolyzing or phagocytizing as a microglia cell (1961, 2169).

Great numbers of discretely arranged microglial cells have been observed in the regions of experimental injury and edema (2234). Such cellular mobilizations occur as early as 24 hr after cold injury (−50°C) and persist for days. Schultz and Pease (2290) observed a similar accumulation of microglial elements in the acute phase 24 hr after stab wounds of the cerebral cortex. The microglia underwent a remarkable transformation within this period; they exhibited a rounded appearance as the cytoplasmic volume increased and became less dense so that the nuclei became more prominent. In about 1 week these changes culminated in

or degenerative processes activate these cells which undergo rapid proliferation and migrate toward the site of injury. Histiocytes from the meninges and blood vessel walls behave similarly. Both types of cells become macrophages and phagocytize debris.

Small numbers of microglia in white matter have processes that wind along or follow myelinated fibers with a remarkable tortuosity (354, 355). A microglia cell has an irregular perikaryon and a few thick processes which often appear to take off from each pole of the cell body. These large antler-like processes divide after variable distances into many smaller branches. Each

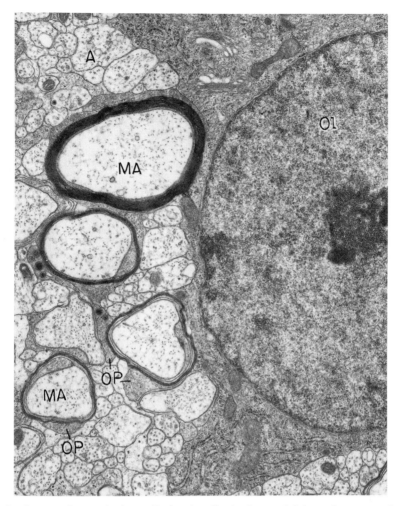

Figure 5-8. An electron micrograph of a myelin-forming oligodendrocyte (*ol*) in a 6-day postnatal rat. Specimen is taken in the ventrolateral funiculus of the spinal cord near unmyelinated axons (*A*) and axons (*MA*) exhibiting different stages of myelination. Oligodendrocytic processes (*OP*) are closely associated with several newly formed myelin sheaths (×16,000). (Courtesy of Dr. James E. Vaughn, City of Hope Medical Center, Duarte, Calif.)

the formation of typical macrophages with pale cytoplasm and no definite processes. An enlarged macrophage in the central nervous system with a foamy cytoplasmic appearance and ingested material is called a "gitter cell" (Fig. 5-11*B*). As the cytoplasm of the macrophages became packed with ingested material the nucleus was often pushed to the cell periphery. Such phagocytosed particles included myelin and lipoid droplets. Gitter cells dominated their lesions for the 1st week, then decreased in number until 90 days, at which time only an occasional phagocyte was seen (Fig. 5-11).

A similar mobilization is observed in the human nervous system after neuron injury (Fig. 5-11*A*). Three stages in the formation of a gitter cell are indicated by *arrows* in Figure 5-11*B*. These large vacuolated macrophages may assume a gigantic size and a bloated appearance. When suitable fat stains are used (e.g., osmic acid, oil red O, Sudan black, Sudan III or IV) the vacuolated gitter cells display an unusual number of fat droplets of varying size. There is much speculation, but little evidence concerning the origin of these macrophages. Some investigators consider them to be transformed microglial cells; others believe

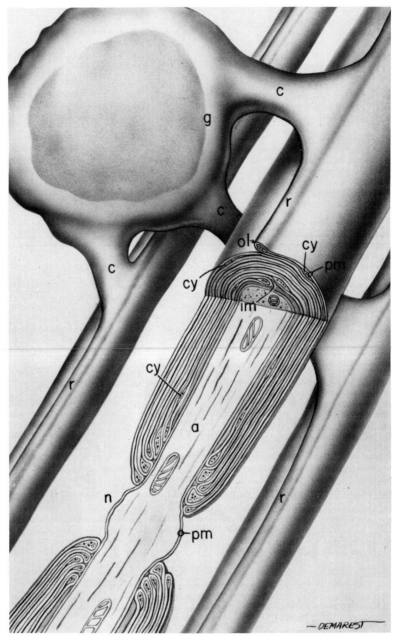

Figure 5-9. Diagram of the relationship of the oligodendrocyte to the central myelin sheath. The trilaminar plasma membrane (*pm*) is designated by two lines, separated by a space, except in the mitochondrion, where it is represented by a single line. The inner mesaxon (*im*), formed as a glial process, completes the initial turn around the axon (*a*) and starts a second turn; it is retained after myelin formation is complete. Some cytoplasm of the glial process is trapped occasionally at *cy*. A bit of glial cytoplasm also is retained on the fully formed sheath exterior. In transverse sections, this cytoplasm is confined to a loop (*ol*), but along the internode length it forms a ridge (*r*) continuous with the glial cell body (*g*) at *c*. Viewed transversely, the sheath components form a spiral with only the innermost and outermost layers ending in loops. In the longitudinal plane, every myelin unit terminates in a separate loop near a node (*n*). Glial cytoplasm is retained within these loops. (Courtesy of Dr. R. P. Bunge, from W. M. Copenhaver et al.: *Bailey's Textbook of Histology*, Ed. 16, Williams & Wilkins, Baltimore, 1971.)

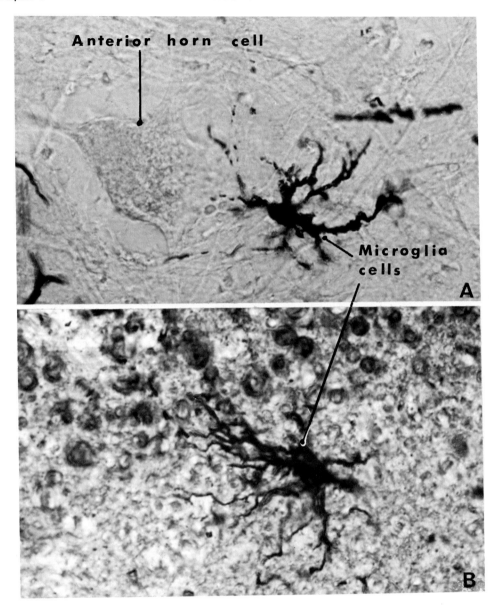

Figure 5-10. Microglial cells in gray and white matter of adult human cord 3 weeks after a spinal stereotaxic lesion. (*A*) Note thickened and stubby processes extending toward an adjacent anterior horn cell. (*B*) Note knobby angular processes of microglial cell extending into the dark zone of degenerating fibers above (Golgi stain, photographs, ×555).

them to be transformed monocytes, or undifferentiated cells of the perivascular mesenchyme. Maxwell and Kruger (1645) observed a fine structure correlation between the vascular pericyte, the microglia and the gitter cells. They believe the only cerebral element which displays macrophage activity is derived from the vascular pericyte.

EPENDYMA

The ependyma lines the central canal of the spinal cord and the ventricles of the brain. In the embryo the processes traverse the entire thickness of the neural tube to become attached to the pia mater and superficial glial membrane (external limiting

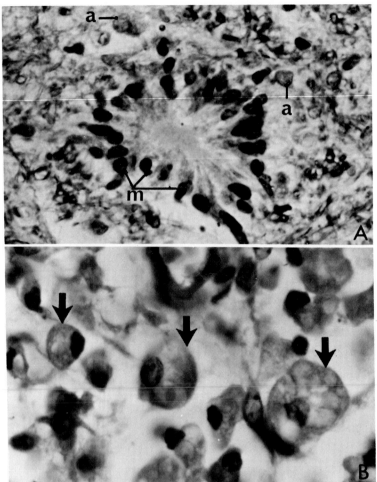

Figure 5-11. (*A*) Carousel formed by numerous microgliocytes (*m*) about a degenerating anterior horn cell 4 weeks after injury of its axon. Two astrocyte nuclei also are identified (*a*). Adult human cord (Luxol fast blue-cresyl violet stain, ×555). (*B*) Three stages (*arrows*) in the formation of a microglial phagocyte (*gitter cell*). White matter of adult human cord, 4 weeks after a stereotaxic lesion (Luxol fast blue-cresyl violet stain, ×655).

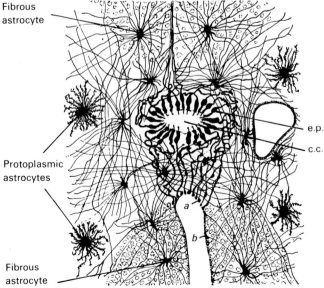

Figure 5-12. Ependyma and neuroglia in the central portion of the spinal cord of an infant 8 days old (Golgi impregnation). *a,* Terminal foot plate of ependymal cell; *b,* terminal foot plate of fibrous astrocyte; *cc,* central canal; *e.p.,* ependymal cell (after Cajal (348)).

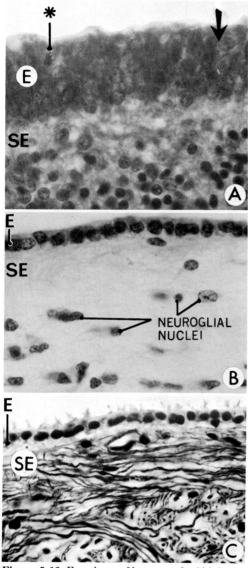

Figure 5-13. Ependyma of human and rabbit brains. (A) Ependymal cells (E) and subependymal glial membrane (SE) in a human fetus of 80 mm crown-rump (C-R) length. Mitotic figure (*) and pale germinal cell nuclei (arrow) are indicated (Luxol fast blue-cresyl violet stain). (B) Ependymal cells lining adult human third ventricle (Luxol fast blue-cresyl violet stain). (C) Ciliated ependymal cells lining adult rabbit fourth ventricle (Bodian strain) (all photographs, ×655).

consists of several layers of nuclei, and one can see the large pale nuclei of the germinal cells (arrow in Fig. 5-13A). Mitotic figures also are easy to identify (*). Cilia are observed in only the embryological stages of man, but persist in some adult animals, such as the rabbit and dog (Figs. 5-13C, 5-14 and 5-16).

Ependymal cells also have numerous microvilli on their ventricular surface (Fig. 5-16). The surface morphology of ependymal cells varies over white and gray matter. In scanning electron microscope studies of rabbit ependymal cells, those covering myelinated structures such as the corpus callosum have fewer microvilli and cilia than ependymal cells covering neuropile (1915). Additional differences are seen in the arrangement of intercellular clefts and junctional specializations of ependymal cells in two regions. These morphological differences may account for the selective changes observed in ependymal cells over periventricular white matter in experimentally induced hydrocephalus (1914).

In the human adult the single layer of ependymal cells is cuboidal, while their retracted processes are entwined in the packed astrocytic processes of the *subependymal* (SE in Fig. 5-13) or internal limiting *glial membrane*. There are few places in the nervous system where typical astrocytes and their processes are as concentrated as in this subependymal limiting membrane. During development, the pia-arachnoid pushes a layer of ependymal cells ahead of it, and invaginates into each of the primitive brain ventricles to form the tufted choroid plexuses (Figs. 3-11 and 3-15). The points of attachment, composed of pia mater and the cuboid ependymal cells, form the *tela choroidea* of the fourth, third and lateral ventricles (Fig. 5-17). These points of junction or reflection can be observed in gross brain specimens after the choroid plexus has been removed. The macroscopic torn edge of the ependyma is referred to as the *tenia choroidea* (Fig. 2-24).

Electron micrographs (Fig. 5-14) reveal that the ependymal cell cytoplasm contains small slender mitochondria, vesicles of ergastoplasm, an agranular reticulum, a Golgi complex and compact bundles of fine filaments 9 to 9.5 nm in diameter, which may be protein (1918, 2529). Histochemically,

membrane) by terminal expansions. Most of the processes retract, so that at birth these processes reach only the pia where the neural wall is thin, as in the basal plate region (Fig. 5-12). In fetal life the ependyma

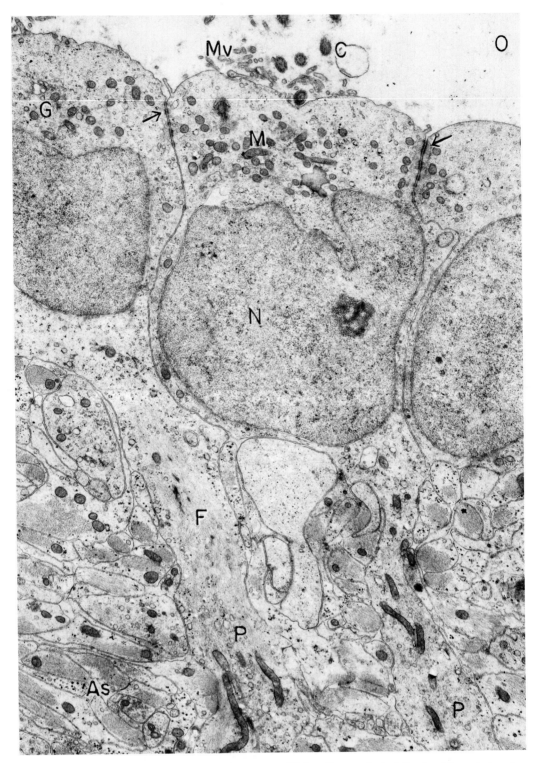

Figure 5-14. Ependymal cells with long basal processes (*P*) line the aqueduct of the dog. The apical surface may exhibit short microvilli (*Mv*) and cilia (*C*), or may be relatively smooth. Rows of desmosomal-like plaques (*arrows*) join adjacent cells apically. Most of the mitochondria (*M*) in the cells are scattered randomly, but they are also aligned in rows close to the junctions. The Golgi complex (*G*) is usually in a supranuclear position. The nucleus (*N*) may be ovoid or indented and sometimes a nucleolus is seen. Fine filaments (*F*), similar to those found in the subependymal astrocytic processes (*As*), are present in the ependymal processes (×7,800). (Courtesy of Dr. Virginia Tennyson, College of Physicians and Surgeons, Columbia University.)

the ependymal epithelium exhibits high oxidative activity as reflected by its enzyme content (i.e., acid and alkaline diphosphatase, adenosine triphosphatase). Both structural and chemical reactions reflect the secretory and absorptive functions attributed to the ependymal cells and choroid epithelium (5).

Specialized ependymal cells called *tanycytes* are found in the base of the third ventricle. Tanycyte processes extend for some distance into the neuropil where they are juxtaposed to blood vessels and neurons. Indirect evidence suggests that these cells selectively transport molecules from the cerebral spinal fluid to diencephalic neurons concerned with the regulation of gonadotropic hormone release from the anterior lobe of the pituitary gland (189, 1337).

It will be recalled that the surface layer of ependymal cells and subjacent astrocytes (i.e., subependymal glial membrane) constitute a brain-cerebrospinal fluid interface (Fig. 1-16). The lateral cell surfaces of ependymal cells are comparatively simple without elaborate folds or interdigitations. Near the apices of contiguous cells, the apposed surface membranes contribute to the formation of complex intercellular junctions which in light microscopy have been called terminal bars. Electron microscopic studies of the ependyma in the rat brain indicate that the lateral portions of the plasmalemma of contiguous cells are fused at discrete sites to form five-layered junctions, referred to as *zonulae occludens*; which obliterate the intercellular space (250). These fusions occur at some distance below the free surface (Fig. 5-15). Another type of intercellular junction, the *zonula adhaerens*, occurs near the apices of contiguous cells. Segments of the plasmalemma comprising this junction are characterized by their increased density, and the interspace of the junction contains filamentous material. This structural arrangement forms the brain-cerebrospinal fluid interface. Neither the ependymal surfaces of the cerebral ventricles nor the pial-glial membrane on the surface of the brain impede the exchange of substances between the CSF and the brain (2114). Thus the brain-CSF interface does not constitute a sub-barrier (Fig. 1-16).

CHOROID EPITHELIUM

The choroid plexuses are formed as a result of the invagination of the ependymal roof plate into the ventricular cavities by the blood vessels of the pia mater (p. 75). In human embryos the primordia of all the choroid plexuses develop during the 2nd month of gestation. A mesenchymal invagination into the thin roof area of the fourth ventricle appears first at 6 weeks. The primordia of the telencephalic choroid plexuses become visible in the 7th week, followed in the 8th week by an invagination into the roof of the third ventricle. It is not surprising that extensive structural alterations in shape and microscopic appearances accompany the different stages of choroid plexus development. Four stages have been described (2334). For our purpose, it will suffice to note that each primordium enlarges, becomes lobulated, and each lobule later demonstrates frondlike expansions (Fig. 5-17). In still later stages many villi develop on the surface. The entire lobulated, vascularized mass remains attached by a broad stalk at the point of the original invagination. The covering cells are at first pseudostratified tall epithelial cells 50 to 60 μm in thickness with a brush border on the luminal surface. At 11 weeks the choroid plexus fills 75% of the lateral ventricle, and the covering tall columnar cells have an abundance of cytoplasmic glycogen (Fig. 5-18). At this stage the mesenchyme of the underlying connective stroma becomes extremely loose and accumulates a large amount of mucin. In the interval between 15 and 17 weeks of gestation the entire plexus gradually decreases in size and the primary villi are better developed. The epithelium changes from low columnar to cuboidal and measures 15×15 μm. The loose underlying mesenchyme decreases in amount, while distinct connective tissue fibers (mostly collagen) make their appearance in the stroma. Between 29 weeks and full term the large cuboidal cells are replaced by smaller ones which are 10×10 μm. The cytoplasm loses its glycogen, while meningocytes, foamy cells and fat-laden macrophages are scattered through the stroma. Once removed, the glycogen never reappears as a normal constituent of the adult choroid epithelium. Such disappearance of glycogen after birth, or at the beginning of aerobic oxidation, suggests that the developing nervous tissue uses energy which is released by the anaerobic metabolism of glycogen. Epithelial indentations lining the interlobular clefts may become

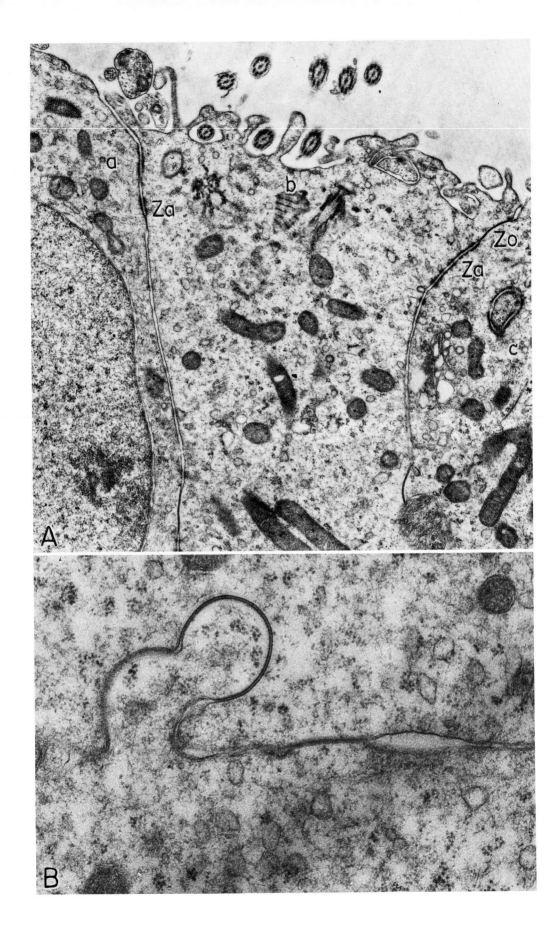

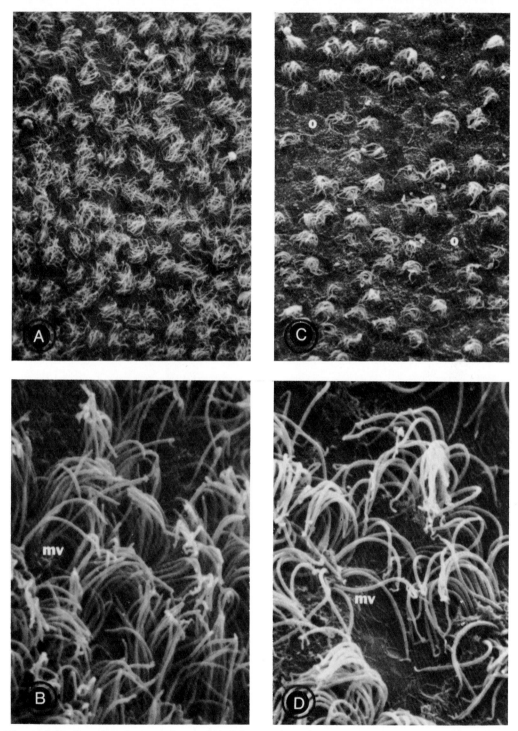

Figure 5-16. Scanning electron micrographs of the ependyma in the rabbit: (*A*) over the caudate nucleus showing clusters of surface cilia (×200); (*B*) over the caudate nucleus showing microvilli (*mv*) between ciliary clusters (×2000); (*C*) over periventricular white matter where cilia are more widely separated and nonciliated cells (*o*) are outlined by aggregates of microvilli (×200); and (*D*) over periventricular white matter where cilia arise in clusters and microvilli (*mv*) aggregate at cell boundaries (×2000). (Reproduced with permission from R. B. Page et al.: *Anatomical Record*, **194**: 67–82, 1979.)

← **Figure 5-15.** (*A*) The apical cytoplasm of three contiguous ependymal cells (*a*, *b* and *c*). The luminal surfaces of cells are joined by the *zonula occludens (zo)* which is directly continuous with a *zonula adhaerens (za)* (×21,000). In (*B*) a *zonula occludens* forms a dovetail type junction between the base of two ependymal cells. The interval between the two dense, parallel membranes can be compared with the usual intercellular space at the right (×49,000). (Reproduced with permission from M. W. Brightman and S. L. Palay: *Journal of Cell Biology*, **19**: 415–439, 1963.)

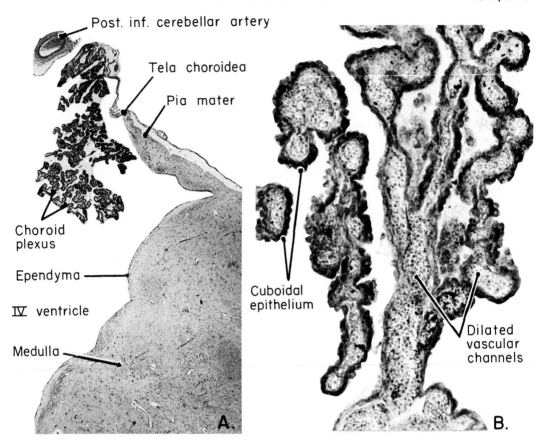

Figure 5-17. Photographs of human choroid plexus. (A) Low magnification to show topography and relations of the plexus in the fourth ventricle. (B) Higher magnification to demonstrate the epithelium and vascularity of two choroid villi.

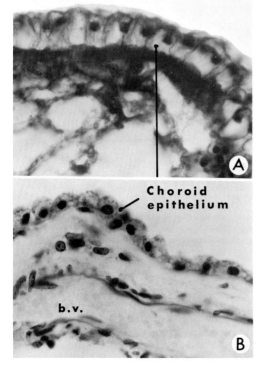

buried in the stroma during early development and form the colloid cysts observed in the adult human brain (2334). They appear red due to the blood in the stromal vessels, and the fine leaflike projections endow the choroid plexus with a shaggy surface appearance. Hardened bodies composed of concentric rings of calcium carbonate, calcium and magnesium phosphate also occur in the adult choroid plexus (psammoma bodies). They are generally spherical and originate around a group of degenerated cells (2268). Psammomatous bodies are usually of small diameter (0.01 to 0.15 mm) and appear to increase in number with age. Studies of morphological and histochemical alterations of the choroid plexus

Figure 5-18. Choroid epithelium of man. (A) Tall columnar choroid cells in a human fetus of 100 mm crown-rump length (Holmes' silver with hematoxylin counterstain). (B) Cuboidal choroid cells of adult brain. A subjacent blood vessel (b.v.) is identified (Luxol fast blue-cresyl violet stain). (Both photographs, ×655.)

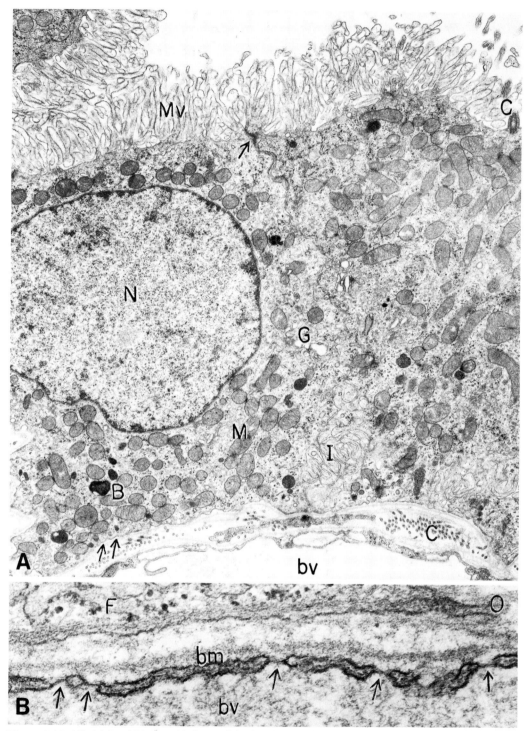

Figure 5-19. (*A*) Adult rabbit choroid plexus of the fourth ventricle. The cuboidal epithelial cells have a large nucleus (*N*). An occasional cilium (*C*) and polypoid microvilli (*Mv*) line the ventricular surface. Apically, a tight junction seals adjacent cells (*arrow*); near their base, elaborate infoldings (*I*) of the cell surfaces occur. A paranuclear Golgi complex (*G*), numerous mitochondria (*M*), heterogenous dense bodies (*B*) and vesicles are present in the cytoplasm. A basement membrane (*double arrows*) separates the choroidal epithelial cells from the connective tissue which contains collagen (*C*), processes of fibroblasts and other interstitial cells and blood vessels (*bv*). The thin wall of this choroidal capillary is typical (×8,000). (*B*) The thin capillary wall is interrupted by "pores," which exhibit a diaphragm (*arrows*) between the lumen (*bv*) and the interstitial space. A basement membrane (*bm*) coats the surface of the capillary. Fibroblast (*F*) (×66,000) (Courtesy of Dr. Virginia Tennyson, College of Physicians and Surgeons, Columbia University).

with age indicate that the height of the cuboidal epithelium gradually decreases, proliferated cells eventually desquamate and cytoplasmic vacuoles increase in number (2335). It seems likely that lipid in the cytoplasm of desquamated choroidal epithelial cells may be one source of lipids in the cerebrospinal fluid.

The histological appearance of the adult choroid epithelial cells after routine staining is shown in Figures 5-17 and 5-18*B*. They are low cuboidal cells with round and basally located nuclei. The bases of the cells are moderately smooth, while the lateral boundaries interdigitate with adjacent cells and demonstrate terminal bars. Tight junctions surrounding and connecting apical regions of epithelial cells of the choroid plexus constitute the blood-CSF barrier (Figs. 1–18 and 5–19). Small inpocketings can be seen on all surfaces of the cell (*pinocytosis*) and are regarded as a mechanism whereby surface solutes can be taken into the cell (cell drinking). An occasional cilium may occur on the apical surface of adult choroid cells. Each cell is bounded by a dense continuous cell membrane. On the ventricular surface, each cell is thrown into elaborate, finger-like extensions 80 to 90 nm in diameter which contain cytoplasmic cores (striated or brush border of light microscopy; *microvilli* in electron micrographs). Microvilli in this instance are a structural device to increase the cell surface and thereby enhance its secretory and possibly absorptive functions (Fig. 5-19). Electron microscopic studies on the developing choroid plexus of the rabbit suggest such a "dual secretory-absorptive" role (2525, 2527, 2528, 2530). Their ultrastructural observations also confirm and greatly extend the embryological data of light microscopy which were presented above. As shown in one electron micrograph (Fig. 5-19) the adult choroidal cell contains numerous mitochondria, a Golgi complex, cisternal and tubular elements of the endoplasmic reticulum, numerous small vesicles, dense bodies with a heterogeneous content and occasional cilia. These investigators also called attention to the "pores" present in the capillaries of the newborn and adult choroid plexus. They found no evidence that thorium dioxide, when injected intravenously, traversed these pores to enter the connective tissue stroma. However protein tracers (Evans blue-albumin) and HRP injected intravascularly pass through the choroid capillary pores and stain the connective tissue stroma, but do not pass beyond the tight junctions which surround apical regions of the epithelial cells of the choroid plexus (252, 2114).

Histochemical demonstration of phosphatase activity in choroid cells, particularly the intracellular location of adenosine triphosphatase and acid phosphatase, should be noted. These hydrolytic enzymes play key roles in metabolically active cells; adenosine triphosphatase participates in the ionic transport at membrane surfaces, and in oxidative phosphorylation within mitochondria. Acid phosphatase is an important constituent of the lysosomes (dense bodies of electron micrographs) which appear to play an important part in transcellular transport and digestion, as well as phagocytosis, necrosis and autolysis (5). Additional information concerning structure and function of the choroid plexus is available in reviews (574, 638).

It should be recalled that the tight junctions which surround and connect apical regions of the cuboidal epithelial cells of the choroid plexus (Fig. 5-19) act as an effective barrier which prevents large molecular substances from entering the cerebrospinal fluid (e.g., serum proteins, inulin and fluorescent dyes). However, such substances injected into the ventricles can pass through the ependyma and subependymal glia to enter the extracellular space of the brain which is guarded by astrocytes (Fig. 1-16). Thus all the neuroglial elements must be considered not only as an impressive structural skeleton, but also as dynamic units that regulate the chemical milieu of nerve cells and probably their metabolism.

CHAPTER 6

Receptors and Effectors

All information we have concerning the world about us is conveyed to the brain by an elaborate sensory system. This input, initiated from the external world, reaches the central nervous system via first order sensory nerve fibers. Sensory receptors and sensory endings act as transducers which change physical and chemical stimuli in our environment into coded nerve impulses which the brain can decode. A *sensory unit* consists of a single peripheral neuron, located in a spinal or cranial nerve ganglion, its peripheral and central ramifications, and, in certain instances, the non-neural transducer cells with which the distal end of the peripheral nerve fiber may be associated. Information conveyed centrally by sensory units provides an ongoing, constantly changing total picture of the external environment and the stimuli which it presents. From this massive barrage of sensory impulses generated in many different types of receptors and nerve endings, the central nervous system derives precise information concerning the quality, the intensity, the locus and the spatial and temporal patterns of stimuli. Stimuli in our environment elicit sensory experiences that, within certain limits, can be recognized, described and classified. Each more or less unique sensory experience is referred to as a *sensory modality*. Sensations of color compose a single modality, as do those of tones. General somatic sensibility consists of several sensory modalities which differ in quality and can be distinguished readily as touch-pressure, pain, warmth, cold and sense of position or movement of limbs at joints. Certain substances can be readily differentiated by the way they taste, and the capacity of man and animals to distinguish and discriminate a great diversity of odors is well known. The spatial position of a tactile stimulus can be located with considerable accuracy, especially on certain surfaces of the body, such as the hand or face. Certain forms of sensation arising in abdominal and thoracic viscera are poorly localized, difficult for the patient to describe and sometimes referred to false locations.

A *peripheral receptive field* is the area within which a stimulus of appropriate quality and strength will cause an afferent neuron to discharge. The receptive field may represent an area of skin in which a mechanical stimulus will excite cutaneous receptors, the angle of joint rotation necessary to excit sensory units, or an area of the visual field in which a light stimulus will evoke discharges in retinal ganglion cells. Within a peripheral receptive field the threshold for adequate stimulation varies in that it is usually lowest in the central region where the density of receptor elements is highest. Peripheral branches of one sensory unit often overlap those of adjacent sensory units, and peripheral receptive fields on the body surface vary greatly in size. Cutaneous receptive fields on the digits of the hand are small in comparison to those on proximal portions of the limbs and on the trunk, but the central representation of these densely innervated areas in the cerebral cortex is massive.

Muller's "doctrine of specific energies," interpreted in modern physiological terms, states that different sets of nerve fibers, when activated, elicit different sensations by virtue of their unique central connections (1765). A particular sensory nerve fiber provokes an identical sensation regardless of how it is excited, that is, by a natural adequate stimulus or by an artificial stimulus. Within a receptive surface, such as the skin, different sets of nerve endings and receptors are distributed in a mosaic fashion. Why a particular set of nerve fibers that terminates in an area common to other receptive elements responds selectively to a stimulus of a particular quality is unknown. The modalities and qualities of sensation seem to depend upon the temporal and spatial patterns of activation, the specificity of the sensory endings and the central connections (599).

The four elemental qualities of cutaneous sensibility are not distributed uniformly over an area of skin. Within a cutaneous area there is a local differential sensitivity to touch, warmth, cold and pain (192). Each spot receives terminal branches from several afferent nerve fibers and a single nerve fiber may innervate several sensory spots. Regardless of how a particular spot is excited, only one elementary sensory experience is evoked, if the excitation is local. Variations of the elementary sensory experience can be produced by temporal and quantitative variations of the stimulus. The wide variety of complex sensory experiences are thought to be synthesized in the central nervous system from the combinations of activities evoked in afferent nerve fibers, each of which when acting alone is associated with a sensory quality of some purity (1765).

The manner in which receptors behave in response to a continuing stimulus varies. Some receptors discharge only at the onset of a steady stimulus; these receptors are called *rapidly adapting*. Other receptors respond to a continuing stimulus with a high frequency discharge for its full duration; these receptors are called *slowly adapting*.

The transduction of mechanical, chemical or electromagnetic energy into a train of nerve impulses is accomplished by receptors that develop in three distinct ways in the embryo (Fig. 6-1). Some transducing elements, such as olfactory receptor cells in the nasal cavity, hair cells in the inner ear and taste receptors differentiate within localized thickenings of the cephalic surface ectoderm. Photoreceptors of the eye develop from the neural tube, and other sensory receptors arise from neural crest tissue. Many of the latter types of receptor cells may be in contact with a specialized ectodermal or mesodermal structure such as a layered capsule or a muscle fiber. The categorization of receptors on the basis of their embryology is important for comparative purposes, but a functional classification is most useful for the study of sensory mechanisms in mammals.

RECEPTORS

Classification

No single classification of receptors has evolved which can adequately correlate the principles of structural organization, distribution and function. The three simple categories suggested by Miller et al. (1705, 1706) are the least elaborate and restrictive. They suggested that the entire body is served by a basic triad of sensory nerve endings which are either "free," "expanded-tip" or "encapsulated." Such designations are applicable to the endings in glabrous skin and the subpapillary dermis. These terms also apply to the endings observed in fascia, tendons, ligaments, periosteum and synovial membranes (Figs. 6-2 and 6-4). However, difficulty is encountered with such categories in hairy skin and muscle spindle receptors where free nerve and expanded-tip endings are also encapsulated.

Sherrington (2325) classified all receptors into three main groups: *exteroceptors, proprioceptors* and *interoceptors* (Fig. 9-28). Exteroceptors on the external body surface receive stimuli from the outside which may, or may not, result in somatic movements. They include touch, pressure, pain and temperature, smell, sight and hearing. Some of these are *contact receptors*; others, such as smell, sight, hearing and aspects of

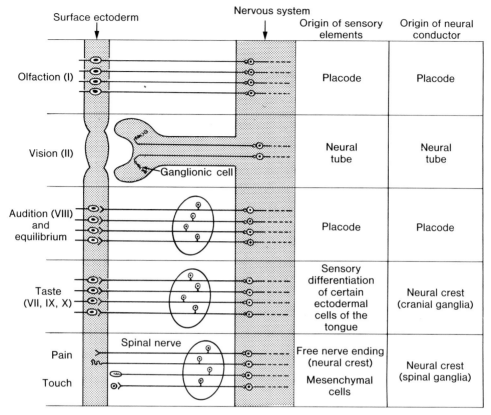

Figure 6-1. Schematic classification of sensory receptor cells according to embryonic origin. All sensory cells are derived from surface ectoderm, except those associated with vision and touch. Sensory elements in the visual system are derived from the central nervous system (neural tube), but their nature, concentration and specialization are similar to placodal cells. Touch receptors below the surface ectoderm are derived from mesenchymal cells. (Modified from Tuchmann-Duplessis et al. (2589)).

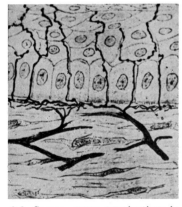

Figure 6-2. Sensory nerve terminations in corneal epithelium (from Cajal (348)).

thermal sense, are activated by distant stimuli and are known as *teloreceptors*.

The proprioceptors, which receive stimuli from the deeper portions of the body wall, especially from the joints, joint cap-

sules, ligaments and fascia, give rise to position sense and the sense of movement (i.e., kinesthesis). They are primarily concerned with the regulation of movement in response to exteroceptive stimuli. These receptors provide sensory information which is utilized in the cerebral cortex to synthesize a conscious awareness of bodily muscle activity and joint movements (*kinesthetic sense*). Most of the receptors related to the knee and temporomandibular joints are diffuse unencapsulated nerve terminals (847, 1278). Other specialized receptors (spindles) in skeletal muscle and tendon are activated by muscle contraction and stretch. Their encoded signals regulate muscular activities, either at spinal cord levels (e.g., myotatic, flexor and extensor reflexes), or they reflexly regulate muscle tone and coordination of muscle activities (i.e., synergy) via projections to specific parts of the cerebellum. Nerve endings in

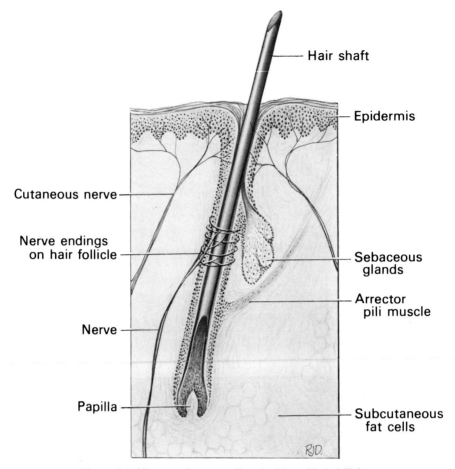

Figure 6-3. Nerves and nerve endings in skin and hair follicle.

skin, joints, fascia, muscle and tendons all transmit afferent nerve impulses from the soma or body wall. Hence exteroceptors and proprioceptors, stretch receptors in muscles and tendons, are grouped together as somatic receptors.

The interoceptors (visceroceptors) are the visceral sense organs that receive and transmit poorly localized sensory impulses related to digestion, excretion, circulation and respiration, which are primarily under the control of the autonomic system. They give rise to sensations of visceral pain and contribute to forms of visceral sensibility such as hunger, thirst and sexual feelings, and to the general feelings of well-being or of malaise. Smell, although not interoceptive, has close visceral affiliations and may be considered partly visceral.

Sensibility may also be divided into *superficial* and *deep*. The former obviously coincides with exteroceptive sense, and the latter comprises both interoceptive and proprioceptive sense, including deep pressure. A special form of sensation is the ability to recognize the vibrations of a tuning fork applied to bone or skin. This is known as *vibratory* sense, a form of mechanoreceptive sensibility dependent for its unique qualities upon the temporal pattern of the neural inputs. The perception of vibratory sense appears dependent upon two sets of primary afferents, one innervating the skin and one innervating deep tissue (1771). Cutaneous afferents probably convey impulses from Meissner's corpuscles, and deep afferents probably end in Pacinian corpuscles.

In an analysis of clinical problems related to sensation, Head (1060, 1061) proposed that there are two different kinds of sensation subserved by dual sensory mechanisms at the periphery. This dual innervation was postulated to consist of a *protopathic* sys-

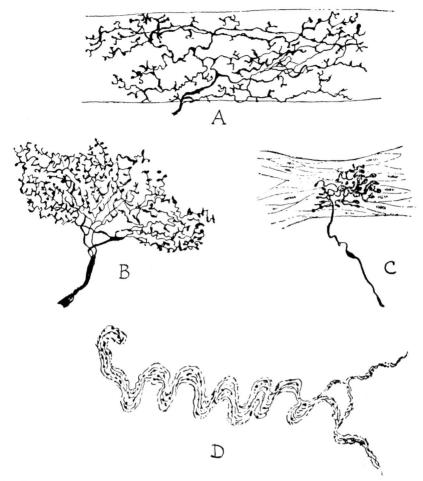

Figure 6-4. Afferent nerve endings in various visceral structures. *A*, On a large pancreatic blood vessel (after De Castro (431); *B*, in endocardium of dog (after Smirnow (2354)); *C*, in bronchial musculature of child (after Larsell and Dow (1436)); *D*, in longitudinal muscle coat of stomach of cat (after Carpenter (375)).

tem and an *epicritic* system. Protopathic sensation was considered to be mediated by a primitive system subserving pain and extreme temperature differences which yield ungraded, diffuse impressions of a marked affective character. Epicritic sensation was thought to be mediated by a phylogenetically more advanced system sensitive to smaller temperature changes and concerned with the discriminative aspects of tactile sensation (i.e., precise localization and gradation of stimulus intensity). The concept of a duality of cutaneous sensations has been severely criticized (2667), but it has been useful in studying pain in humans. It is likely that the two categories of pain reflect central rather than peripheral mechanisms. It also seems likely that the protopathic system may be anatomically related to free nerve endings of small diameter axons (2215). Affective sensations are related primarily to reactions indirectly involving bodily welfare, and neuronal activities in the limbic cortex may play an important role in this form of sensation. Discriminative sensibility forms the basis for cognitive and complex associative reactions which involve the cerebral cortex; this form of sensation is regarded as *gnostic* or *cortical*. In a general way, pain, thermal, visceral sensibility and certain aspects of touch are predominantly affective, while tactile sense, kinesthesis and teleceptive sensibilities are predominantly discriminative.

Physiologically receptors can be classified in terms of the form of energy to which they respond at the lowest stimulus intensity. *Mechanoreceptors*, responding to mechanical forces, include those that subserve touch-pressure in the skin, and position sense and kinesthesis (joints and joint capsules), as well as stretch receptors in muscle, visceral pressure receptors and hair cells in the cochlea. *Thermoreceptors*, responding separately and differentially to warmth and cold, are distributed in spot-like fashion in the skin and vary greatly in their density in different parts of the body. *Photoreceptors* subserving vision respond to light, and *chemoreceptors* initiate impulses concerned with taste and olfaction.

Pain receptors are collectively referred to as *nociceptors* since pain can be produced by different forms of energy (mechanical, chemical or thermal). Pain, frequently a frightening sensory experience, is associated with noxious stimuli that injure tissue. Because almost all descriptions of pain come from studies in man, many distinctive forms are recognized. Descriptions of particular kinds of pain guide the astute physician in his search to determine the nature and extent of the underlying pathological process. Two aspects of pain are recognized: (a) the distinct sensation and (b) the psychological reaction to pain which depends upon many variables. Certain stimuli which commonly produce pain evoke other kinds of sensory experience at weaker intensities. Melzack and Wall (1665) proposed that pain perception is modulated by both sensory feedback mechanisms and the influences of the central nervous system.

Receptors may be regarded as miniature transducers capable of responding readily to appropriate forms of energy (adequate stimulus). An appropriate external stimulus applied to a receptor gives rise to a graded electrical response, known as a "receptor potential". The term "generator potential" is used to define the electrical potential that triggers the "all or none" response in the initial segment of the sensory nerve fiber. If the receptor potential is generated in the first sensory neuron, then it is also the generator potential (599, 945). Such physiological events have been demonstrated best in the Pacinian corpuscle (1508–1511).

Receptor endings have numerous mitochondria, microvesicles, neurofilaments and even acetylcholinesterase in the case of nerve endings related to hairs. Other receptors are associated with supportive cells that demonstrate a variety of enzyme activities. Free nerve endings appear to be the receptors in fetal life, whereas encapsulated endings appear after birth (436). Throughout life receptors show a continuous cycle of breakdown, renewal and reorganization (432). This observation accounts for the variable appearance of Pacinian and Meissner's corpuscles in older individuals. Different regions and tissues of the body have marked differences in the type and number of receptors. Detailed reviews of cutaneous innervation have been published (937, 945, 2086, 2343).

Two main types of receptors are found: (a) the *free* and *diffuse endings*, which are always unencapsulated and (b) the *encapsulated* endings or corpuscles, which are enclosed in a capsule of modified supporting cells.

Free Nerve Endings. The free nerve endings are the most widely distributed receptors in the body. They are most numerous in the skin, but also are found in the mucous and serous membranes, muscle, deep fascia and the connective tissue of many visceral organs. The skin is supplied by many cutaneous nerve trunks composed of myelinated and unmyelinated fibers. Some of the large myelinated fibers are destined for the encapsulated organs described below, but the majority are of a relatively small caliber. The fibers of these small nerve trunks separate as they approach the epidermis, lose their myelin sheath, undergo branching and form extensive unmyelinated plexuses in the deeper portion of the dermis and immediately beneath the epidermis (Fig. 6-3). From this subepithelial plexus, delicate fibers penetrate the epithelium, divide repeatedly and form an end arborization of delicate terminal fibrils which wind vertically through the epidermis and end in small knoblike thickenings, upon the surface of the epithelial cells (Figs. 6-2 and 6-3). In the cornea, which has no horny layer, these intraepithelial endings may reach the surface, but in the skin they do not extend beyond the germinative layer. Intraepithelial endings also are found in mucous membranes lined by stratified epithelium, such as the esophagus and bladder. Similar endings may be seen in simple columnar epithelium as well.

Other nerve fibers form unmyelinated arborizations or terminal nets in the connective tissue of the dermis. There is some evidence that the intraepithelial endings are derived from fine myelinated fibers, while the subepidermal arborizations and plexiform nets are in the main terminals of unmyelinated nerve fibers (2768). Such terminal unmyelinated fibers are never naked, but are always invested by Schwann cells (433). Diffuse nerve endings in the form of nerve nets, or arborizations of varying complexity, are distributed widely in visceral organs. They have been described in the serous membranes, heart, bronchial tree, alimentary canal and blood vessels (Fig. 6-4). Such endings also are found in the choroid plexuses of the brain and in skeletal muscle. For the most part, they are terminals of unmyelinated fibers. Complicated arborizations have been found in the smooth muscle of the bronchi by Larsell and Dow (1436) (Fig. 6-4). These visceral receptors are endings of medium-sized or large myelinated fibers and may initiate proprioceptive bronchial reflexes.

An important type of diffuse cutaneous receptor is represented by the *peritrichial* endings of the hair follicles, which are activated by the movements of hairs (Fig. 6-3). They vary considerably in complexity and are best developed in the vibrissae of certain mammals. In the simpler forms several myelinated fibers approach the hair follicle just below its sebaceous gland, lose their myelin sheath and divide into several branches which encircle the outer root sheath (Fig. 6-3). From these branches numerous fine fibers run for a short distance upward and downward in the outer root sheath and terminate in flattened or bulbous endings. The smallest hair follicles have at least two stem nerve fibers which form an outer circular plexus and an inner palisading one formed by the longitudinally directed fibers. Larger follicles are supplied by 6 to 10 fibers, while the largest receive between 20 and 30. In the rabbit each myelinated fiber sends branches to 4 to 120 hairs, and an average of 4 different dorsal root fibers supply each hair (2685). Only free epidermal and dermal endings, and the fibers associated with hair follicles, are found in truly hairy skin.

Besides the intraepithelial endings described above, which end among or upon ordinary epithelial cells, the deeper portion of the germinative layer contains somewhat more specialized endings known as the *tactile discs* of Merkel (fig. 6-5). Each consists of a concave neurofibrillar disc or meniscus closely applied to a single epithelial cell of modified structure. A single epidermal nerve fiber may, by repeated branching, give rise to a number of such discs. These simple endings lie along the deeper sweat ridges between dermal papillae (Fig. 6-5). They are numerous at birth but gradually diminish with age. With the electron microscope the Merkel cell of man and the opossum can be distinguished from epidermal cells (1781, 1782). The Merkel cell has a lobulated nucleus and a massive accumulation of secretory granules (glycoprotein) in the cytoplasm that is apposed to the neurite. Cauna (432) believes them to be touch receptors which respond to the lever movement that results from deformation of the surface epidermis. In areas of transition to glabrous skin there is a gradual increase in the number of Merkel's discs and Meissner's corpuscles. In glabrous skin, such as the volar surface of the finger, the epidermis and dermal papillae contain a profuse array of free nerve endings, Merkel's discs and the encapsulated Meissner's corpuscle (Fig. 6-5). The subpapillary dermis under such skin contains a wide variety of endings including the end bulbs of Ruffini, and Krause and Pacinian corpuscles.

The tendency toward modification of epithelial cells receiving sensory nerve endings is exemplified in various *neuroepithelial* cells which have special forms and show staining affinities similar to nerve cells. The specific cells of the taste buds (Fig. 6-6), olfactory mucosa and hair cells in the sensory epithelia of the cochlear and vestibular apparatus are examples of such neuroepithelial cells. Such supportive cells, as well as those forming the lamellae of encapsulated endings, have surrounding basement membranes. It remains to be determined whether they are modified epithelial or transformed Schwann cells.

Diffuse Endings. The deep somatic structures of the human body have unencapsulated sensory endings that are more profuse than those observed in visceral structures (Fig. 6-4). Elaborate nerve endings have been demonstrated by Ralston et al. (2102) in the tendons, ligaments, joint capsules, deep fascia and periosteum of

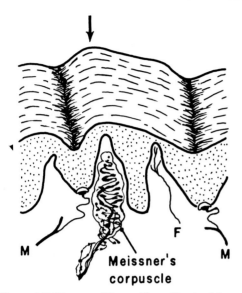

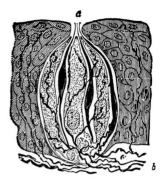

Figure 6-6. Taste bud from circumvallate papilla of tongue. *a*, Taste pore; *b*, nerve fiber entering taste bud and ending upon neuroepithelial cells. On either side are some free intraepithelial endings (from Merkel (1667)).

Figure 6-5. Diagram of the papillary ridge in glabrous skin showing Meissner's corpuscle in a dermal papilla and Merkel's discs (*M*) on the deep edges of the sweat ridges. A free nerve ending (*F*) is shown in adjacent papilla. *Arrow* indicates direction of most effective epidermal stimulation to elicit touch and tactile two point discrimination. (Modified after Cauna (432)).

man (Fig. 6-7). Ruffini (2235) originally described an encapsulated fusiform end organ in the skin and adipose tissue. Although long considered as a corpuscle, its morphology is vague and most investigators have failed to verify its abundant distribution in man. It may well represent a variation of the diffuse, expanded-tip, unencapsulated endings described by Miller et al. (1706). Encoded messages from these diffuse unencapsulated receptors appear to be an important component of impulses carried by the axons of the posterior white columns. Proprioceptive nerve impulses from these deep receptors play an important role centrally in that they make us aware of the numerous localized body changes that occur during locomotion, standing or sitting.

When recordings are made from single primary afferent neurons innervating the general body surface, cutaneous receptors sensitive to mechanical stimuli can be classified into 11 groups. The characteristics used for classification include: (a) conduction velocity, (b) distance the central axon ascends in the spinal cord and (c) pattern of action potentials generated by defined stimuli (1142) (Table 6-1).

Encapsulated Endings. These include the *tactile corpuscles of Meissner*, the *end bulbs*, the *Pacinian corpuscles*, the *Golgi-Mazzoni corpuscles*, the *neuromuscular spindles* and the *neurotendinous organs of Golgi*.

The *tactile corpuscles of Meissner* are elongated ovoid bodies, 90 to 120 μm in length, found in the dermal papillae, close to the epidermis (Figs 6-5 and 6-8). Each corpuscle is surrounded by a thin, nucleated connective tissue sheath, while the interior consists of many flattened epithelioid cells whose nuclei are placed transversely to the long axis of the corpuscle. From one to four myelinated nerve fibers supply each corpuscle. As each fiber enters, its connective tissue sheath becomes continous with the fibrous capsule. The myelin sheath disappears and the naked axon winds spirally among the epithelioid cells, giving off numerous branches which likewise spiral, show numerous varicosities and end in flattened neurofibrillar expansions. Besides the myelinated fibers, the corpuscles also may receive one or more fine unmyelinated fibers. Meissner corpuscles occur mainly in the hairless portion of the skin and are most numerous on the volar surface of the fingers, toes, hands and feet. They are found in lesser numbers in the lips, eyelids, tip of the tongue and volar surface of the forearm (1727). It is now apparent that Meissner's corpuscles are formed in excess of adult requirements, and those that survive possess a capacity for continuous growth and reorganization (432, 1706). In young persons nearly every dermal papilla contains a

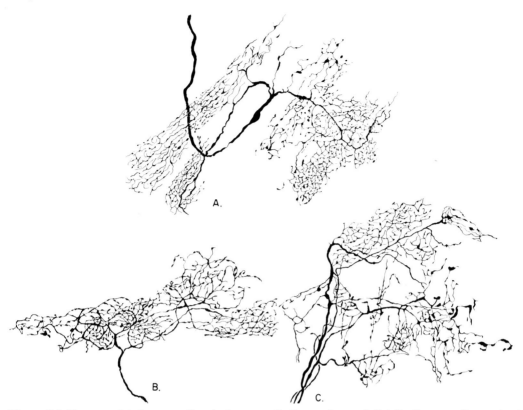

Figure 6-7. Unencapsulated nerve endings in deep somatic tissues of man. *A*, Patellar ligament; *B*, capsule of knee joint; *C*, periosteum of femur (after Ralston et al. (2102)).

small Meissner corpuscle, 25 μm in length. In older individuals, only a few papillae contain corpuscles which are larger and of more irregular arrangement. These endings always are associated with the papillary ridge which plays an essential role in their stimulation. Their relationship is designed so that the nerve endings are stimulated effectively through one surface elevation of the epidermis, which is in line with the long axis of the corpuscle (*arrow* in Fig. 6-5). This arrangement makes the Meissner corpuscle particularly suitable for tactile two-point discrimination (432).

The *end bulbs* resemble the tactile corpuscles in structure and are spherical or ovoid bodies which vary greatly in dimension. The simplest and smallest ones are found in the conjunctiva (1890); the largest in the connective tissue of the external genitalia, where they are known as *genital corpuscles.* In its simplest form (Fig. 6-9*A*), the end bulb consists of a nucleated capsule enclosing a soft gelatinous core in which nuclei may often be seen. One or more

myelinated fibers lose their myelin on entering the capsule and give off numerous lateral branches which form a complicated terminal arborization. Some end bulbs may be compound. End bulbs of various forms have a wide distribution, being found in the conjunctiva, mouth, tongue, epiglottis, nasal cavity, peritoneum (and other serous membranes), lower end of rectum and external genitalia, especially the glans penis and clitoris. They also are found in tendons, ligaments, synovial membranes and in the connective tissue of nerve trunks.

The *Pacinian corpuscles (Vater-Pacini)* are the largest and most widely distributed of the encapsulated receptors (Fig. 6-10). They are laminated, elliptical structures of whitish color, and each is supplied by a large myelinated fiber. They differ from the other encapsulated organs mainly in the greater development of their perineural capsule. This capsule is formed by a large number of concentric lamellae; each lamella of the outer bulb consists of a single continuous layer of flattened cells, and is sup-

Table 6-1

Physiological Properties of Cutaneous Axons Responding to Mechanical Stimulation of the Skin[a]

Mechano-receptor Type	Mean Peripheral Conduction Velocity (m/sec)	Level at which Most Fibers Leave the Fasciculus Gracilis	Mean Slope of Tuning Curves	Plateau Response	Type of Ramp Response; On vs. Off Sensitivity[b]	Probable or Possible Receptor Structure
C	<2	—	Does not follow above 2 Hz	<20 sec	V/D; little or no off, but has an after discharge	Free nerve endings?[c]
Aδ	20	Lower lumbar	−0.4[d]	Little or none	V; on = off	Free nerve endings in skin or around hair follicles?[c]
G₂ hair	50	½ upper lumbar, ½ nucleus gracilis	−0.2	Little	V/D; on ≫ off	
GI hair	65	Nucleus gracilis	−0.4	None	V; on ≥ off	Lanceolate, pallisade or circular endings of follicle[e]
G₁ hair	75	Nucleus gracilis	−1	None	V/A ; on = off	
F₂ field	50	½ upper lumbar, ½ nucleus gracilis	−0.15	<20 sec	V/D; little or no off	
FI field	55	½ upper lumbar, ½ nucleus gracilis	−0.25	None	V; on > off	Sparsely laminated corpuscles (such as Meissner's corpuscles, Krause end bulbs, Golgi-Mazzoni organs)?[f]
F₁ field	65	Nucleus gracilis	−0.6	None	V; on = off	
Ruffini	55	Nucleus gracilis	0	Persists	D; no off	Ruffini endings
Haarscheibe	65	Upper lumbar	0	Persists	D/V; no off	Merkel cells
Pacinian corpuscle	65	Nucleus gracilis	−2	None	A; on = off	Pacinian corpuscles

[a] A classification scheme for mechanoreceptors that is based upon the morphology or receptors in the skin of cats and their physiological properties. The scheme is derived from recordings of primary afferent neurons which ascend in the dorsal columns of the spinal cord. The free endings of Aδ axons are exquisitely sensitive to slight movement of the skin and act as velocity detectors. On hairy skin, two types of hair follicles are distinguished. Fine "down" hairs emerge in groups from a follicle and the larger "guard" hairs emerge singly. Receptors associated with guard hair follicles are designated type G. Receptors responding to stimulation of the skin between hairs or movement of clumps of hairs are field receptors (type F). F receptors are also found in glabrous skin. "Haarschiebe" is the term given to small, fairly evenly spaced protuberances on the surface of the skin. Field (F) and guard hair (G) receptors are subdivided according to their phasic (F_1, G_1), tonic (F_2, G_2) or intermediate (FI, GI) response patterns. (Reproduced with permission from K. W. Horch et al.: *Journal of Investigative Dermatology* (1142).

[b] A = acceleration response; D = displacement response; V = velocity response; FI = intermediate field receptors; GI = intermediate guard hair receptors.

[c] Receptor identification uncertain and based on supposition.

[d] Estimated.

[e] It is not known to what extent G_1 endings differ in structure from G_2, if at all. Both G_1 and G_2 neurons can innervate the same hair.

[f] Receptor identification based on reasonable likelihood.

ported by fine collagen fibrils of the interlamellar spaces. The interlamellar spaces contain a network of fine fibers, blood vessels and some free cells in a semifluid substance. Blood vessels accompany the nerve fiber to the capsule but ramify only in the outer bulb. At birth the Schwann cell and myelin sheaths are lost as the large nerve fiber enters the inner bulb. However, the capsule continues to grow and enlarge, so that in the human adult both the Schwann cell and myelin elements can at times be identified within the inner bulb (434, 435). No fine nerves enter the inner bulb with

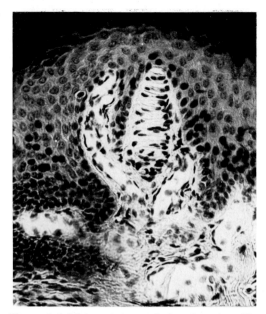

Figure 6-8. Meissner's corpuscle in a dermal papilla of human finger tip (photograph).

the large fiber. Cauna and Mannan found that the average length of the corpuscle at birth was from 500 to 700 μm. The size increases gradually throughout life to become 3 to 4 mm in length. In persons over 70 years of age the corpuscles are less numerous, show regressive changes and are smaller and more irregular. The entire length of the unmyelinated fiber within the corpuscle is sensitive to deformation, and can initiate "all or none" responses (1912, 1913). They removed the surrounding capsule and found the mechanoreceptor function was still intact. These authors concluded that the short-lasting receptor potential, obtained from intact corpuscles, must be attributed to properties of the lamellae. In addition to pressure the Pacinian corpuscle deep in the limbs may be sensitive to vibratory stimuli. The corpuscles are found in subcutaneous tissue, especially of the hand and foot, in the peritoneum, pleura, mesenteries, penis, clitoris, urethra, nipple, mammary glands and pancreas and in the walls of many viscera. They are especially numerous in the periosteum, ligaments and joint capsules, and they also occur in muscular septa and occasionally in the muscle itself.

Related to the Pacinian corpuscles are the lamellated *corpuscles of Golgi-Mazzoni*, found in the subcutaneous tissue of

the fingers and on the surface of tendons (Fig. 6-9*B*). They are ovoid bodies with lamellated capsules of varying thickness and a central core of granular protoplasm in which the single myelinated fiber forms a rich arborization with varicosities and terminal expansions.

Stretch Receptors. Among the most highly specialized encapsulated end organs are the stretch receptors, represented by the neuromuscular spindles and neurotendinous organs.

The *neuromuscular spindles* (muscle spindles) are fusiform in shape and widely scattered in the fleshy bellies of skeletal muscles. Each spindle consists of from 2 to 10 slender striated muscle fibers, enclosed within a thin connective tissue capsule, and attached at both ends to the epimysium or ordinary striated muscle (Fig. 6-11). These slender muscle fibers are known as *intrafusal fibers* and are small compared with the *extrafusal fibers* that produce contractile tension within a muscle.

In submammalian species, muscle spindles are innervated by collateral branches of axons which supply extrafusal striated muscle fibers. In the mammal, muscle spindles are largely supplied by an independent group of motor axons, called fusimotor or γ-axons. It is now recognized that mammals have a significant number of muscle spindles innervated by collaterals of axons also innervating the extrafusal muscle fibers. These axons, which show the innervation pattern previously associated exclusively with submammalian species, are called β-axons to distinguish them from exclusively skeletomotor α-axons and exclusively fusimotor γ-axons (4, 175, 1431). Fusimotor axons are of two types: dynamic and static. The dynamic γ-axons increase the sensitivity of the spindle primary endings to changes of muscle length. Static γ-axons reduce spindle afferent sensitivity to changes of muscle length, but increase spindle afferent firing at a constant length.

Intrafusal muscle fibers are of two distinct sizes: one is of smaller diameter (10 to 12μm), is shorter in length (3 to 4 mm) and has a single chain of central nuclei; the second or larger spindle fibers are about 25 μm in diameter, are 7 to 8 mm in length and in the equatorial region are enlarged to accommodate an area of numerous small nuclei ("nuclear bag" of Barker (117)). The

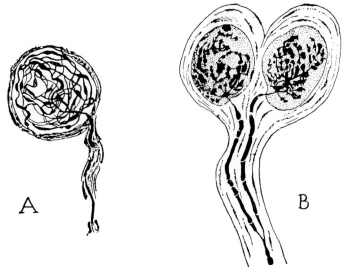

Figure 6-9. *A*, End bulb of Krause from conjunctiva (636); *B*, compound corpuscle of Golgi-Mazzoni from the subcutaneous tissue of the finger tip (from Ruffini (2235)).

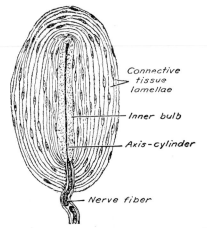

Connective tissue lamellae

Inner bulb

Axis-cylinder

Nerve fiber

Figure 6-10. Human Pacinian corpuscle (after Cajal (348)).

small intrafusal fibers are known as "nuclear chain fibers," and the larger ones are designated "nuclear bag fibers" (119, 234, 235). The ends of the nuclear chain fibers are attached to the polar parts of the longer nuclear bag fibers. There are usually two of the longer fibers and five of the smaller fibers in each spindle, but these numbers are variable. A nuclear bag fiber with its capsule and associated sensory and motor nerve endings is shown in Figures 6-11 and 6-12. Two or more myelinated afferent fibers enter each spindle. A thick primary afferent fiber forms a spiral, branching and reticulated ending within the nuclear bag area (primary, annulospiral or nuclear bag ending). Silver-stained primary

and secondary sensory endings on intrafusal muscle fibers are shown in Figure 6-13. The primary receptor has a low threshold to stretching of the muscle or its tendon, and also discharges a volley of impulses when the intrafusal fiber contracts as a result of stimulation by a γ efferent motor axon (Figs. 6-11). The neuromuscular spindle is arranged parallel to the extrafusal or contractile fibers of the muscle; hence tension on the spindle is relaxed and afferent volleys from the annulospiral endings cease during active muscle contraction (i.e., the spindle is unloaded, and its receptors are silent). The primary afferent fibers (*Ia* in Fig. 6-12*A*) are 8 to 12 μm in diameter, have fast conduction velocities and their central processes within the spinal cord participate in the monosynaptic stretch (myotatic) reflex that regulates muscle tone (Figs. 9-33 and 9-34).

The myelinated secondary afferent fibers (*II* in Fig. 6-13*B*), with diameters of 6 to 9 μm also enter the spindle to form small rings, coils and spraylike varicosities on both sides of the nuclear bag area. These are called secondary, flower-spray or myotube endings (Figs. 6-11 and 6-13*B*). Secondary endings are the principal sensory terminals associated with nuclear chain fibers (119, 234, 235). Both the primary and secondary endings are terminals of sensory fibers, for they degenerate after section of appropriate dorsal roots.

Small fusimotor fibers (γ efferents), 3 to

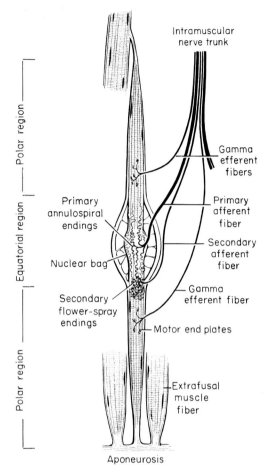

Figure 6-11. Diagram of a nuclear bag intrafusal muscle fiber within a neuromuscular spindle. The intrinsic sensory and motor nerve endings on the spindle fiber are identified, and the polar and equatorial regions are indicated on the left. Normally there are 2 to 10 small and large intrafusal fibers within each neuromuscular spindle (after Barker (117)).

7 μm in diameter, enter each spindle and terminate. Two kinds of γ fiber endings upon the intrafusal muscle fibers have been described. Some end as diffuse, multiterminal "trail fibers," while others terminate in miniature "end plates" (Fig. 6-14). Barker (118) maintains that both nuclear bag and nuclear chain muscle fibers usually receive each type of γ motor endings. Boyd (234) maintains that nuclear bag intrafusal fibers usually receive "plate endings," and nuclear chain muscle fibers usually receive "trail endings."

As noted above, the contraction of intrafusal muscle fibers by γ efferent nerves induces discharges in the afferent nerves from the spindle. The fusimotor fibers thus reset the spindle mechanism and thereby regulate the sensitivity of the receptor. Contraction of the spindle fibers contributes nothing *per se* to the contractile tension of the muscle (1948). In addition, the neuromuscular spindles receive a variable number of fine unmyelinated fibers which appear to be vasomotor to the small vessels within the spindle. Other fine nerve fibers ramify in the capsule and probably mediate pain impulses.

The recorded dimensions of human muscle spindles vary enormously, the extremes for length being 0.05 and 13 mm. The usual length is 2 to 4 mm. Spindles have been found in practically all muscles but they are most numerous in the muscles of the extremities. They are especially abundant in the small muscles of the hand and foot. Fewer muscle spindles are present in the extraocular muscles (528, 531, 962, 1669). Cells in part of the trigeminal ganglion convey afferent impulses from muscle spindles in the extraocular muscles (1599).

Information conveyed centrally from the neuromuscular spindles play a major role in the reflex regulation of muscle tonus. Ascending impulses from these receptors are conveyed via nuclei in the spinal cord and medulla mainly to the cerebellum and are secondarily concerned with conscious sensory experience. Responses of primary and secondary endings to mechanical stimuli differ in that the primary ending is more sensitive to the dynamic component of the stimulus. Thus, primary endings measure both velocity of stretching and length, while secondary endings measure mainly length. Collaterals from these sensory fibers have monosynaptic junctions with alpha (α) motor neurons (Figs. 9-28 and 9-34). More than one internuncial neuron is interposed between these collaterals and the γ efferent neurons as shown in Figure 9-28. If the primary fiber (*Ia*) from the annulospiral ending is stimulated, there is a central delay of 2 msec before the efferent fiber response is recorded. Hence the annulospiral collaterals use central internuncial neurons to influence γ efferent neurons, and such connections are polysynaptic (1642).

Neurotendinous organs (Golgi tendon organs, GTO) are encapsulated spindle shaped receptors found at the junction of muscle and tendon, and occasionally in muscular septa and sheaths. GTO have

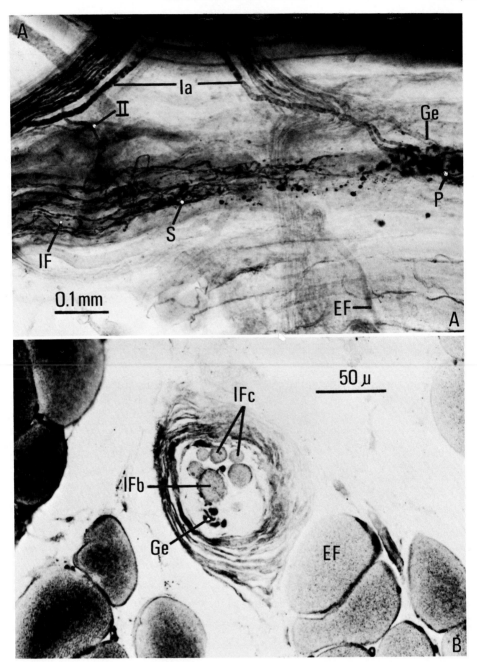

Figure 6-12. Human intercostal neuromuscular spindle. (A) Longitudinal squashed preparation showing sensory and motor neural elements related to the intrafusal muscle fibers (*IF*). Compare diameters of sensory fibers (*Ia*) related to primary (*P*, annulospiral) ending, sensory fiber (*II*) of secondary (*S*, flower-spray) ending, and γ efferent (*Ge*) fiber. An adjacent extrafusal muscle fiber (*EF*) and artery (*A*) are identified. (B) Cross section of muscle spindle demonstrating its multilayered capsule and the diameters of the nuclear bag (*IFb*) and nuclear chain (*IFc*) intrafusal fibers. Gamma efferent axons (*Ge*) and extrafusal (*EF*) muscle fibers are identified (modified De Castro silver stain). (Courtesy of Dr. W. R. Kennedy, University of Minnesota).

been demonstrated in practically all muscles. The capsule of the GTO is approximately 8 to 10 times longer than it is wide and consists of several concentric lamellae that form cytoplasmic sheets closely applied to each other (1668). Cells of one lamella extensively overlap adjacent cells in the same concentric lamella. The outer

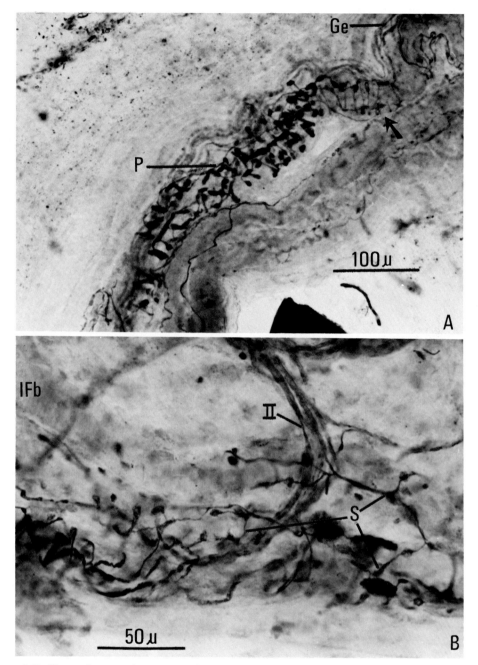

Figure 6-13. Human intercostal neuromuscular spindles with two types of sensory endings. (*A*) Primary (*P*, annulospiral) ending on each intrafusal muscle fiber has a thick axon with many side branches and terminal enlargements. The slender coil (*arrow*) is not seen on all primary endings. Adjacent efferent axons (*Ge*) are identified. (*B*) Secondary (*S*, flower-spray) endings found on both bag and chain intrafusal muscle fibers (*IFb*). Architecture is similar to that of primary ending except for the slender, delicate nature of the branches. The axon related to this secondary ending is identified (*II*) (modified De Castro silver stain). (Courtesy of Dr. W. R. Kennedy, University of Minnesota).

lamina appears as typical squamous epithelium without fenestrations, and the extensive overlap of neighboring cell processes suggests that intracapsular fluids are not easily exchanged with extracapsular fluids. The cells which form the capsule of the GTO resemble those of the perineural epithelial sheath surrounding nerve trunks,

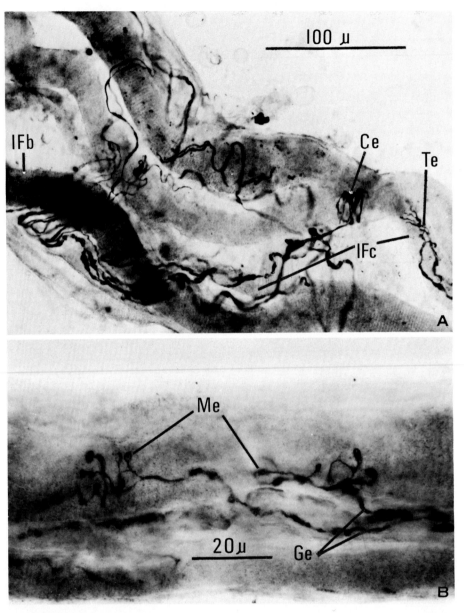

Figure 6-14. Human intercostal neuromuscular spindle. (*A*) γ efferent axons near sensory area that demonstrate trail (*Te*) and coiled (*Ce*) endings. In other sections these axons and endings are found on bag (*IFb*) and chain (*IFc*) intrafusal muscle fibers. (*B*) γ efferent (*Ge*) motor end plates (*Me*) found toward capsular pole of spindle. Pairs of end plates occur frequently. Here two end plates are seen on one bag fiber (modified De Castro silver stain). (Courtesy of Dr. W. R. Kennedy, University of Minnesota).

and the capsule is regarded as a direct continuation of the perineural sheath.

The GTO capsule exhibits four morphologically distinct levels (2286). At the proximal opening several loosely organized cellular lamellae surround entering muscle fibers. A slight distance below the capsule opening is the proximal collar, where collagen bundles of the muscle fibers are tightly enveloped by capsule cells so as to provide an effective seal between intracapsular and extracapsular fluids (Fig. 6-15). Distally there also is a capsular collar from which collagen bundles leave their capsular investments in a staggered fashion to join the central tendon. The receptor body, oc-

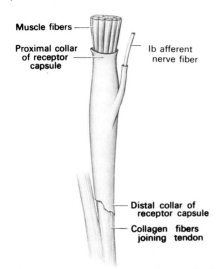

Muscle fibers

Proximal collar
of receptor
capsule

Ib afferent
nerve fiber

Distal collar of
receptor capsule

Collagen fibers
joining tendon

Figure 6-15. Schematic diagram of a Golgi tendon organ. Muscle fibers converge as they enter the proximal opening of receptor capsule, below which is a slight constriction known as the proximal collar. Ib afferent fiber emerges from the central region of the receptor capsule in a connective tissue sleeve. Near the distal collar of the capsule collagen bundles emerge, and at staggered levels join the fibrils of the central tendon. (Modified from Schoultz and Swett (2286)).

cupying nearly 80% of the length of the GTO, lies between the proximal and distal collars. The capsule wall of the receptor body is uninterrupted except for an opening near the midpoint through which the primary afferent fiber (Ib) enters the lumen of the capsule. The lumen of the receptor body is divided by thin cytoplasmic processes into longitudinally oriented compartments which in cross section have a honeycombed appearance. Cells and their processes which partition the lumen have been termed septal cells. These cells resemble fibroblasts and probably originate from lamellae of the capsule wall. In the greater part of the receptor body compartments contain a mixed assortment of collagen fibrils from muscle fibers (Fig. 6-16). A large number of collagen fibers appear to terminate within the capsule lumen in an undetermined manner.

The primary afferent fiber (Ib) enters the capsule lumen in the equatorial region of the receptor body and divides into major ascending and descending branches. Unmyelinated collaterals from the major branches project radially through openings between septal cells to penetrate periph-

erally located compartments containing longitudinal collagen bundles derived from muscle fibers. Preterminal nerve fibers branch extensively and spiral around discrete collagen bundles. Attempted serial reconstructions of the GTO indicate that collagen bundles spiral about one another like the strands of a rope and often split to entrap smaller nerve fibers and terminals (Fig. 6-16). Evidence suggests that the mechanical component of the transducer process must involve physical distortion of the axonal membranes during an increase in tensile forces along the collagen strands. It has been suggested that contraction, or passive muscle stretch, would tighten the braided strands of collagen in the GTO, reduce the size of the septal spaces and pinch nerves laced between them (2286).

The afferent nerve fibers from tendon organ receptors are large fibers of about 12 μm diameter. GTO are relatively insensitive to passive stretch because they lie in series with the contractile muscle that absorbs most of the stretch and prevents elongation of the tendon. Muscle contraction causes the tendon organs to discharge proportional to the tension developed. Contractions which shorten the muscle without developing much tension produce only weak excitation of the tendon organ. If the contraction shortens the muscle, lengthens the tendon and develops tension, the tendon organs fire vigorously (Fig. 9-33) (1076). If the stimulus is appropriate, the tendon organ is an extremely sensitive receptor. Contractions produced by stimulation of an isolated motor unit can easily cause individual tendon organs lying in series with it to discharge (1148).

Afferent nerve fibers from the muscle spindle (primary) and the GTO are large and conduct impulses centrally at rapid rates. In order to distinguish between these two subgroups, the annulospiral afferent nerves are designated as Group Ia, while the tendon organ afferents are referred to as Ib nerve fibers. While stretch receptors in muscle furnish some information which enters the conscious sphere signaling the position of a limb or joint, these receptors function mainly in the automatic control of muscle tone.

Besides the neuromuscular and neurotendinous organs, muscle and tendon have a variety of other sensory structures: free

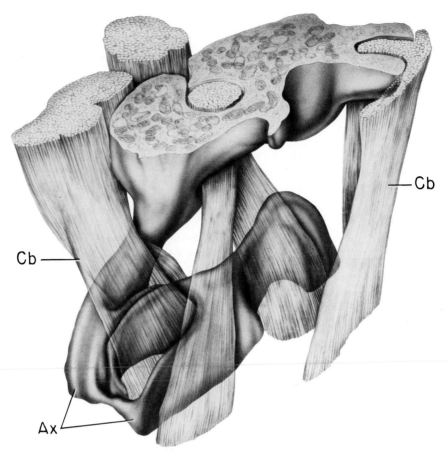

Figure 6-16. Three-dimensional reconstruction of relationships between axonal branches (*Ax*) and longitudinally oriented collagen bundles (*Cb*) in a septal cell compartment of a Golgi tendon organ (GTO). The spiraling axon threads its way through the collagen bundles. Most collagen bundles do not run a straight parallel course through the GTO lumen, but twist like the strands of a braided rope. Increasing tensile forces on the collagen strands cause them to straighten and twist which results in pinching of the axonal branches trapped between them. (Reproduced with permission from T. W. Schoultz and J. E. Swett: *Journal of Neurocytology*, (2286)).

nerve endings, end bulbs and Pacinian corpuscles. The latter are especially numerous in tendons.

Relation of Receptors to Sensory Modalities

It is generally maintained, although not proven, that each type of receptor is activated by only one kind of physical or chemical change and hence is associated with only one kind of sensory modality. The problem of relating the various receptors to specific sensory modalities has been exceedingly difficult and many important details remain unknown (2343).

It seems probable that painful stimuli are received by the diffuse, cutaneous end arborizations. Not only would their universal presence and unspecialized terminals indicate this, but also their sole presence in places where stimuli give rise only to pain (e.g., the tympanic membrane of the ear and the pulp of the teeth).

Touch is represented by the endings in hair follicles, Meissner's corpuscles, and probably by tactile discs and some other intraepithelial endings. The peritrichial endings, stimulated by movements of the hair, give rise to a delicate and discriminative sensibility with a marked affective tone. Shaving greatly reduces sensibility to touch. On the hairless part of the body tactile stimuli are received primarily by the corpuscles of Meissner, which are probably the chief sense organs of discriminative touch.

The receptors for temperature are not

well known, but they are probably end bulbs of various kinds. Possibly some are diffuse endings. It is known that the margin of the cornea is sensitive only to cold and pain, and is provided only with diffuse endings and end bulbs of Krause. Hence the latter and similar subcutaneous end bulbs are believed to be receptors for cold. In the same way, the diffuse unencapsulated nerve endings are believed to be related to warmth.

The different parts of the body surface vary considerably as to their capacity for affective and discriminative sensibility. The skin of the hand and fingers is particularly sensitive, and provides a variety of exteroceptive impulses that are integrated in the cerebral cortex. In other regions such as the back, abdomen and especially the genitalia, affective sensibility predominates, to the partial exclusion of discriminative aspects of sensation.

The Pacinian corpuscles, found in both deep subcutaneous and visceral structures, appear physiologically to be pressure transducers, but there is no evidence that they subserve steady pressure, or that pressure sensitivity is particularly acute in regions where Pacinian corpuscles are found. The rapidly adapting nature of the Pacinian corpuscle suggests that it may be particularly sensitive to vibration. This receptor may play a role in the threshold detection of tactile stimuli, despite its deep position, because it has a lower threshold for short mechanical stimuli than more superficial intracutaneous receptors (1495).

The proprioceptive senses of position and movement are initiated by the constant or varying tension states of the skeletal muscles, and their tendons, and by the movements of the joints. The changes in tension and pressure are received by the Pacinian and unencapsulated corpuscles found in the joint capsules, ligaments and periosteum (Fig. 6-7). Such afferent inputs are transmitted to cortical levels where they are utilized in the formulation of kinesthetic sense (conscious proprioception or kinesthesis). Proprioceptive impulses from neuromuscular spindles are used for regulation of the spinal myotatic reflex, or project via cerebellar pathways to regulate muscle tonus and synergy (i.e., such sensory inputs are for subcortical reflex control of skeletal

muscle). The subcortical regulation of muscle tone and posture thus provides a background of muscle tone upon which discrete cortical (voluntary) activity, such as locomotion and fine finger movements, is based.

There is much that is still obscure about visceral sensibility. It is known that the viscera are insensitive to many mechanical and chemical stimuli, yet they may be the source of intense pain as well as contribute to the sensations of hunger, thirst and so on. Visceral pain is due mainly to either distension or spasm of the muscle coats. Hence diffuse intramuscular nerve endings appear to be the receptors for these stimuli (Fig. 6-4). The blood vessels also may give rise to painful sensation, which is likewise due to spasms in their muscular walls and to the resulting stimulation of similar diffuse endings. The totality of stimuli, constantly received by these diffuse visceral receptors during normal and abnormal function, probably gives rise to the general affective sensibility of internal well-being or of malaise.

Referred Pain. One peculiarity of visceral pain is that painful visceral stimuli are often "felt" in the corresponding somatic segment, or segments, of the body wall, a phenomenon known as "referred pain." Centrally the receptive nuclei for somatic and visceral pain impulses are associated closely within the dorsal gray column of the spinal cord. Referred pain is most likely due to central mechanisms within the spinal cord, although the precise neurons involved have not been ascertained. A common explanation is that the constant bombardment of pain impulses, from a diseased viscus, lowers the threshold of stimulation of adjacent central (somatic) relay neurons. Normally these relay neurons are concerned with somatic sensations and not with transmission of visceral pain. As a result, normal incoming somatic sensory impulses that terminate in this "sensitized" neuron pool are relayed to higher centers, where they are misinterpreted as painful stimuli coming from body surfaces.

Sinclair et al. (2344) have suggested that the production of referred pain may be due to the branching of the sensory fibers which conduct pain impulses. One limb of a branched axon goes to the visceral site where the disturbance originates, while others go to the peripheral area to which the pain is referred.

Pain referred to the skin from a viscus tends to be "felt" in a relatively small circumscribed area, usually, but not always, within the dermatone of the same spinal segment that supplies the viscus. This pain rarely occupies the whole, or even the major part, of the corresponding dermatone. In the reference zone there may be changes in the quality of sensation in response to stimuli and alterations of theshold (2343). Pain is the only sensory modality commonly referred in this manner. Thus, referred pain has a dermatomal disribution corresponding to the spinal nerves. The following are some classical examples of a diseased viscus that causes pain to be referred to the overlying body wall and corresponding dermatomes: diaphragm referred to dermatome C4; heart referred to dermatomes C8 to T8; bladder referred to dermatomes T1 to T10; stomach referred to dermatomes T6 to T9; intestine referred to dermatomes T7 to T10; testes, prostate and uterus referred to dermatomes T10 to 12; kidneys referred to dermatomes T11 to L1; and rectum referred to dermatomes S2 to S4 (Figs. 7-1, 7-11 and 7-12).

EFFECTORS

The endings of the peripheral fibers in the effector organs of the body fall into two groups: somatic efferent and visceral efferent. The somatic efferent terminations represent the motor terminals of myelinated axons whose cell bodies are located in the anterior gray horn of the spinal cord. These fibers go directly to the skeletal muscles. The visceral endings are terminals of unmyelinated fibers which arise from cells of the various autonomic ganglia. These fibers supply the heart (cardiomotor), visceral muscle (visceromotor), blood vessels (vasomotor), hair (pilomotor), salivary and digestive glands (secretory) and sweat glands (sudomotor).

During development cholinergic axons form a specialized synapse, the myoneural junction, with skeletal muscle fibers which already contain acetylcholine receptors distributed over the whole of the muscle membrane. As the neuromuscular junction is formed, acetylcholine receptors cluster in the muscle membrane at the site of axon contact and gradually disappear from the extrajunctional membrane (177). In the case of sympathetic motor neurons, differentiation to become either cholinergic or noradrenergic is made relatively late in development and depends both on the local environment of the neurons and their activity (1947).

Somatic Effectors. The somatic efferent fibers terminate upon the skeletal muscle fibers in small, flattened oval expansions, the *motor end plates* or myoneural junction (Figs. 4-3G and 6-14). Motor end plates are located in narrow zones in a given muscle. Each end plate always lies in the midportion of the fiber it supplies. Larger muscle fibers have larger end plates, and in the rabbit and monkey the diameters of end plates differ in "red" and "white" muscle fibers (487). For example, in red extrafusal fibers the end plates are significantly larger. These muscle fibers are known to be slow reacting and capable of sustained contraction. According to Coers (486) the mean diameter of adult human limb motor end plates is 32.2 μm. In man most of the end plates have a length of 40 to 60 μm. The myelinated fibers, in their course to the muscle, repeatedly divide, and branch even more extensively as they spread out within the fleshy belly of the muscle. In this manner a single motor nerve fiber provides end plates to a variable number of the large extrafusal muscle fibers (Fig. 4-3G). Each terminal nerve branch loses its myelin sheath as it approaches the sarcolemma of a muscle fiber, while the Schwann cell sheath continues to invest even the smallest terminals. Electron microscopy has confirmed and elucidated many of the structural features of the motor end plate (553, 2126, 2127, 2182, 2185, 2788). The axoplasm of the small nerve branches contains numerous mitochondria, vesicles, round and oval profiles, small granular elements and tubular-appearing components of the endoplasmic reticulum. Such nerve terminals do not lie within the sarcoplasm of the muscle fiber, as believed previously, but occupy troughs which are hollowed out by infoldings of the sarcolemma (Fig. 6-17). The floor of the trough is usually corrugated by numerous secondary invaginations of the sarcoplasm (junctional folds).

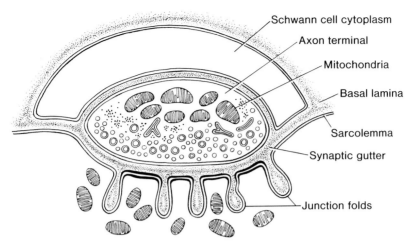

Figure 6-17. Diagram of motor ending on a skeletal muscle fiber as seen in transverse section by electron microscopy. The mitochondria are presumed to play an active role in the synthesis of acetylcholine, whereas the numerous smaller vesicles shown in this diagram represent a stored state of acetylcholine. Small clusters of dark granules also are found in the axon terminal. Note the separation of axon, Schwann cell and muscle membranes by the basal lamina. (Modified from Robertson (2182, 2185) and from Couteaux (553)).

The entire depressed area is called a "synaptic gutter." Within the gutter the axon membrane and sarcolemma remain as discrete structures separated by a gap, or synaptic cleft. The whole ending is covered over by Schwann cell cytoplasm. The membranes of the Schwann cell, axon and sarcolemma are all separated from each other by a thin layer of moderately electron dense material (basal lamina) which also extends out into the extracellular space around the entire ending.

The synaptic vesicles within the axon terminals of the end plate are presumed to represent the storage sites of acetylcholine (Fig. 6-17). With the arrival of a nerve impulse, numerous quanta of acetylcholine are released through the presynaptic membrane into the synaptic gutter. The liberated acetylcholine binds to postsynaptic receptor sites, and alters the permeability of the postsynaptic (sarcolemmal) membrane of the muscle fiber. Acetylcholine receptors and acetylcholinesterase have been localized to the sarcolemma at the apical portions of the junctional folds (747) (Fig. 6-17). Depolarization and a muscle action potential result from this series of events.

When a foreign motor nerve is implanted into an adult rat soleus muscle and the nerve normally providing innervation severed, changes in four molecular components of the newly formed neuromuscular junctions can be followed. Within 2 days, acetylcholine receptors appear in clusters in the new endplate region. The clusters continue to grow in size and receptor number over the next 30 days. About 2 weeks following reinnervation an endplate-specific form of the enzyme acetylcholinesterase is present. Specific antigens of the synaptic basal lamina appear slightly earlier and accumulate with a timecourse paralleling that for acetylcholinesterase. The maturation of the synaptic basal lamina appears to occur only after acetylcholine receptors form clusters (2687).

A large number of microscopic histochemical technics have been used to localize the enzymes of the motor end plate in man and numerous animals. These have been reviewed extensively by McLennan (1569) and Zacks (2788). If an inadequate amount of acetylcholine is produced (or it is destroyed too rapidly by acetylcholinesterase), muscle contraction is altered and the involved muscles are prone to early fatigue (Fig. 6-19). If the enzyme acetylcholinesterase is inactivated by anticholinesterase drugs (e.g., by neostigmine), the endogenous acetylcholine is preserved at the end plate for longer periods. This rationale when applied to patients with myasthenia gravis may result in some recovery of muscle strength, and the ability of a muscle to respond to repetitive nerve stimulation.

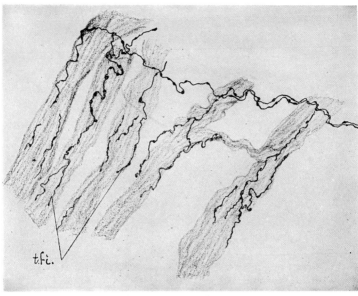

Figure 6-18. Motor nerve terminations in the smooth muscle bands of a bronchus (rabbit); *tfi*, terminal fibrils (from Larsell and Dow, (1436)).

The excitation of a striated muscle fiber by a motor neuron can be blocked in several ways by naturally occurring toxins. These toxins have been useful tools for analyzing mechanisms of nerve conduction and transmitter release (Fig. 6-19). Tetrodotoxin blocks Na^+ channels in the axon membrane and thereby prevents the generation of action potentials. Botulinum toxin blocks the release of acetylcholine from synaptic vesicles. Alpha (α)-bungarotoxin, derived from the venom of a snake, binds irreversibly to the acetylcholine receptor, blocking access of the transmitter. These three toxins block neuromuscular transmission through different mechanisms.

The axon of one motor neuron supplies a variable number of skeletal muscle fibers. In the larger back muscles (e.g., sacrospinalis, gluteus maximus), a single anterior horn cell may provide motor end plates to over 100 muscle fibers. Each motor neuron to a muscle of the thumb, or an extrinsic eye muscle, may supply only a few skeletal muscle fibers. Namba et al. (1797) have described two kinds of motor endings in the extraocular muscles of man. The superior rectus muscles had both *en plaque* and *en grappe* endings. The levator palpebrae had only *en plaque* terminals with a mean diameter of 27 μm. As many as 12 *en grappe* endings were found on superior rectus fibers 10 to 20 μm thick. *En grappe* endings had a mean diameter of only 9.6 μm. All the skeletal muscle fibers supplied by one motor neuron and its axon constitute a *motor unit*. A muscle with many motor units for a given number of muscle fibers is capable of more precise movements than a muscle with a few motor units for the same number of muscle fibers. It also follows that only a few anterior horn cells and motor units are required to maintain reflex muscle tone during periods of rest or sleep. However, many or all motor units may be called into operation when demands are made upon the muscle for maximal contraction.

Visceral Effectors. The unmyelinated autonomic fibers which supply visceral muscle either end in simple arborizations, or first form extensive intramuscular plexuses from which the terminals arise. The terminal fibrils wind between the smooth muscle cells and end in small neurofibrillar thickenings, or delicate loops on the surface of the muscle fibers (Fig. 6-18). Similar terminals arise from delicate plexuses which surround the tubules or acini of glands, pass between the cells and terminate upon the plasma membrane of the

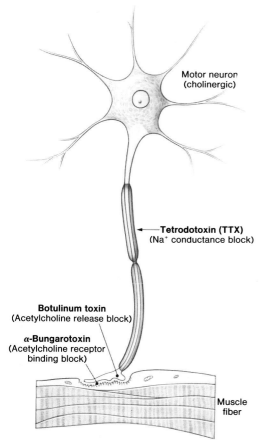

Motor neuron
(cholinergic)

Tetrodotoxin (TTX)
(Na⁺ conductance block)

Botulinum toxin
(Acetylcholine release block)

α-Bungarotoxin
(Acetylcholine receptor
binding block)

Muscle
fiber

Figure 6-19. Examples of sites of action of some animal and bacterial neurotoxins. Tetrodotoxin (*TTX*), obtained from the ovaries of the puffer fish, prevents the inward movement of Na^+ ions, thereby blocking the propagation of the action potential along the axon. Botulinum toxin, of bacterial origin, blocks the release of acetylcholine from the synaptic terminal. The venom of the Formosan krait, α-bungarotoxin, binds almost irreversibly to acetylcholine receptors at the muscle end-plate, thereby preventing acetylcholine (ACh) from initiating an action potential in the muscle fiber.

glandular cells. Terminal endings occupy small troughs in the plasma membranes of both cardiac and smooth muscle fibers, sometimes for long distances. However, no end plates, or specialized endings, have been observed on visceral muscle by either light or electron microscopy. Groups of tiny axons surrounded by Schwann cell cytoplasm do come into intimate contact with single smooth muscle cells of the small intense (multiaxonal junctions). In the large intestine (toad) single axons diverge from nerve bundles and come to lie, free of the Schwann sheath, in shallow grooves in the muscle cell. It is likely that one muscle cell has several widely separated single axon contacts (2199). Axon terminals have either a predominance of granular or agranular vesicles and numerious mitochondria. A plethora of fine nerve fibers and plexuses have been demonstrated about blood vessels and in a variety of tissues by the fluorescence technic developed by Falck et al. (731). This technic reveals an exquisite array of adrenergic nerve fibers and their terminals and has been used to study the course and relations of adrenergic nerve fibers to the smooth muscle within several organs (Fig. 8-6). The meticulous studies of Thaemert (2539, 2540) are equally informative. He has made three-dimensional montages from serial section electron micrographs to demonstrate the intricate nerve-muscle fiber relationships in both smooth and cardiac muscle. The gut contains a population of intrinsic neurons termed the "enteric nervous system." Some of these cells are serotinergic interneurons which probably act upon other cholinergic and purinergic intrinsic neurons that control smooth muscle (866).

CHAPTER 7

Segmental and Peripheral Innervation

Although the spinal cord is a long cylindrical, unsegmented structure, the 31 pairs of spinal nerve associated with localized regions produce an external segmentation. On the basis of this external segmentation the spinal cord is considered to consist of 31 segments, each of which receives and furnishes paired dorsal and ventral root filaments (Fig. 9-1). The spinal segments are divided in the following manner: 8 cervical, 12 thoracic, 5 lumbar, 5 sacral and 1 coccygeal. Thus there are 31 pairs of segmentally arranged spinal nerves which receive and distribute fibers to various parts of the body. Spinal nerves emerge from the vertebral canal via the intervertebral foramina. The first cervical nerve emerges between the atlas and the occiput (Fig. 1-4). The eighth cervical nerve emerges from the intervertebral foramen between C7 and T1; all more caudal spinal nerves emerge from the intervertebral foramina beneath the vertebrae of their same number (Fig. 9-3).

Spinal Nerve. Each spinal nerve arises from a region of the spinal cord by two roots, a dorsal afferent root and a ventral efferent root. The two roots traverse the dural sac, penetrate the dura and reach the intervertebral foramen, where the dorsal root swells into the spinal ganglion that contains the cells of origin of the afferent fibers (Fig. 4-2A and 7-1). Distal to the ganglion, the dorsal and ventral roots unite and emerge from the intervertebral foramen as a *mixed spinal nerve* or *common nerve trunk*, containing both afferent and efferent fibers. The dorsal roots are, as a rule, thicker than the ventral ones and vary with the size of their respective ganglia. The first cervical and the first coccygeal nerves represent exceptions in that the dorsal root fibers frequently are absent.

Each dorsal root is composed of myelinated and unmyelinated nerve fibers which vary in size from 0.5 to 20 μm. They are the processes of the large, medium-sized, or small dorsal root ganglion cells. The larger myelinated fibers (10 to 20 μm) convey sensory impulses to the spinal cord from elaborate receptors located in the dermis, subcutaneous connective tissue, muscles, tendons, joint capsules, ligaments, periosteum and deep fasciae. Large afferent fibers conduct rapidly (5 to 120 m/sec) and, by virtue of their several physiological properties, are classified as the *A fiber* component of peripheral nerves. Smaller myelinated nerve fibers in dorsal roots (0.5 to 10 μm) convey sensory information to the cord from less specialized receptors, and from free nerve endings in the skin, viscera, muscles and connective tissues of the body. Small, unmyelinated, slow-conducting sensory fibers of the dorsal roots are classified physiologically as *C fibers*. The diameter spectra of the fibers within a dorsal root are shown in Figure 7-6.

In recent years it has become evident that there are a large number of sensory fibers in certain ventral roots (2725). Electron microscopic studies have revealed a surprisingly large number of unmyelinated fibers in the ventral roots of several mammals including man (490). Approximately 28% of the axons in the ventral root in man are unmyelinated. In addition there are a small number of myelinated sensory fibers in the ventral root (2745). Evidence that these fibers were afferent originally was based upon the observation that following ventral root section, some fibers distal to the cut survived, while proximal root fibers degenerated (491). Retrograde transport technics provided more conclusive evidence in that horseradish peroxidase (HRP) injected into the spinal cord after dorsal root section (proximal to the ganglion) resulted in labeling of spinal ganglion neurons (1647). In addition, physiological recording from fine filaments of the ventral roots revealed unmyelinated sensory fibers (482, 495). An important question, not entirely resolved, is whether these unmyelinated sensory ventral root fibers enter the spinal cord directly, or whether they curve back and enter the spinal cord via the dorsal root. At least some of these fibers enter the spinal cord direct through the ventral root. As yet no special sensory mechanism has been demonstrated for the ventral root afferents (2725). Since their large numbers have only recently been demonstrated, their precise function is not yet established.

These observations suggest that complete deafferentation cannot be accomplished by dorsal root section (rhizotomy) alone.

The major portion of the ventral root of a spinal nerve is composed of myelinated axons that vary in diameter from 3 to 13 μm. The vast majority are the axons (9 to 13 μm) of large anterior horn cells (GSE, general somatic efferent) of the spinal cord (Figs. 7-6B and 9-24). They conduct rapidly and have functional properties similar to the large sensory A fibers of the dorsal root. Each large A(α) fiber in the ventral root enters a peripheral nerve and supplies motor impulses to a variable number of *extrafusal muscle fibers* (Fig. 4-3G). Smaller myelinated fibers, 3 to 6 μm in diameter, form a second component of the ventral root (γ efferent fibers). These finer axons arise from smaller multipolar neurons scattered among the larger cells of the anterior gray horn (Figs. 9-24 and 9-28). Such small motor axons of ventral roots and motor nerves are designated as "gamma efferents," and they innervate the *intrafusal fibers* of the neuromuscular spindle (Figs. 6-11 and 9-28). A third fiber component is found only in the ventral roots of spinal nerves T1 to L2 (Fig. 8-1). These myelinated fibers range from 3 to 10 μm in diameter and are the preganglionic axons of visceral motor neurons (GVE, general visceral efferent) located in the intermediolateral cell column of the spinal cord. Preganglionic visceral efferent fibers leave the ventral root to enter the ganglia of the sympathetic trunk through a white communicating ramus (Figs. 7-1, 8-1, 8-2 and 9-28). The preganglionic visceral components of the ventral spinal roots conduct more slowly (3 to 15 m/sec); they are concerned with visceral reflexes and are designated as *B fibers*. Similar preganglionic visceral efferent fibers (parasympathetic) are found in the ventral roots of sacral nerves (2, 3 and 4 (Fig. 8-1).

Spinal Ganglia. The spinal and autonomic ganglia are part of the peripheral nervous system. Almost all of the afferent fibers, both somatic and visceral, have their cell bodies in the spinal ganglia. These aggregations of unipolar nerve cells form spindle-shaped swellings on the dorsal roots (Figs. 1-4, 1-5, 7-1 and 9-1). Each ganglion is surrounded by a connective tissue capsule that is continuous with the epineurium

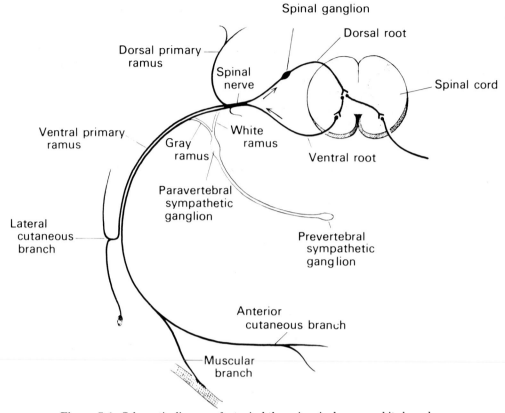

Figure 7-1. Schematic diagram of a typical thoracic spinal nerve and its branches.

of the spinal nerves. Cells of the spinal ganglia have a peripheral location beneath the capsule, and bundles of nerve fibers entering and leaving the ganglia form a central core (Fig. 7-2). In the trigeminal ganglion the cells and fibers are more loosely arranged. In spinal ganglia the interneural spaces contain large and small axons, satellite cells, Schwann cells and blood vessels. Studies of the topographic organization of cells in dorsal root ganglia of the cat indicate that cells in medial and caudal regions project processes into the most caudal rootlets, while cells in rostral parts of the ganglia project fibers into rostral rootlets (334). Cells in the trigeminal ganglion also have a topographic arrangement in that cells contributing fibers to the ophthalmic division are located anteromedially and these distributing fibers to the mandibular division are situated posterolaterally (1303).

The unipolar neurons are ovoid or spherical in shape, and often have indentations on their surface contour (Fig. 4-1A). Their

cell diameters range from 20 to over 100 μm. Sensory ganglion cells grown in tissue culture and studied by electron microscopy have all the cytoplasmic organelles possessed by other neurons (320, 2012, 2524). However, these sensory neurons have less prominent Nissl bodies and scattered cytoplasmic chromatin; the axon often is coiled to form a "glomerulus" within its capsule, and each cell has a variable number of satellite cells. On the basis of their staining properties two types of ganglion cells have been described in the light microcope. The larger cells are lighter, while smaller cells often appear dark (obscure cells; Fig. 7-3). Rapidly preserved tissue fails to demonstrate these two cell types, suggesting that such staining variations may reflect differences in cell metabolism at the moment of fixation (2012). Bunge et al. (320) observed light and dark cells in tissue culture and believed this appearance depended on the amount of cytoplasmic neurofilaments. Angular and indented surface margins of the perikaryon represent

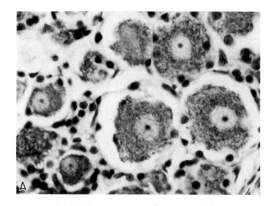

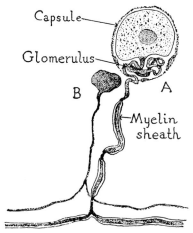

Figure 7-3. Two cells from vagus ganglion of cat. *A*, Large clear cell; *B*, small "obscure" cell with deeply staining cytoplasm (Ehrlich's methylene blue) (after Cajal (348)).

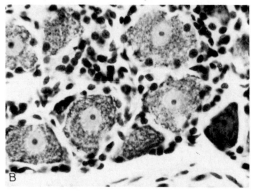

Figure 7-2. Photomicrographs of normal cells in lumbar spinal ganglion (*A*) and the superior glossopharyngeal ganglion (*B*) of the monkey. Note variations in ganglion cell size and small dark nuclei of the capsule cells (cresyl violet stain, ×500). (Reproduced with permission from P. W. Carmel and B. M. Stein: *Journal of Comparative Neurology,* **135:** 145–166, 1969.)

interdigitations with the processes of surrounding satellite cells. Such ultrastructural extensions of the perikaryon explain the surface spines and excrescences that have been observed in Golgi, silver and methylene blue preparations. These typical, and often bizarre, sensory neurons commonly are observed in ganglia from older individuals (Fig. 7-4). The numerous processes may divide repeatedly or terminate as elaborate end bulbs within the capsule. Sensory neurons with such supernumerary processes have been mistaken by some as multipolar (motor) neurons. However, no one has yet reported vesicle-containing axon terminals or morphological evidence of synaptic contacts within the spinal or trigeminal ganglia. A more detailed study of the sensory ganglia and neuronal variations that accompany senescence have been presented by Warrington and Griffith (2676), Dogiel (637), Ranson (2105), Truex (2579, 2580) and Sosa and DeZorilla (2383).

Satellite cells (capsular nuclei) are derived from the embryonic neural crest and, in the adult, form a concentric layer which closely invests the perikaryon and its unmyelinated axonic coils (2780). The round or elongated nuclei of the satellite cells are more dense than the adjacent perikaryon, and are identified easily with the light microscope (Figs. 4-2*A*, 7-2 and 7-4). They have ultrastructural features that distinguish them from Schwann cells. Satellite cells display plasma membrane redundancy in the form of folds on the surface that faces the neuron. Such folds and processes may form several layers and interdigitate with the surface evaginations of the perikaryon. The outer surface of the satellite cell is invested with a basal lamina which is continuous with that investing the myelin at the first internode (2012). The capsule of satellite cells separates the perikarya from adjacent ganglionic capillaries, and must be involved in fluid transport mechanisms. They can increase in number after birth, and may play a role in the metabolism of the ganglion cells.

Studies of cell changes in sensory ganglia, spinal and cranial, in the monkey indicate that: (a) section of the nerve proximal to the ganglia produces no cellular changes

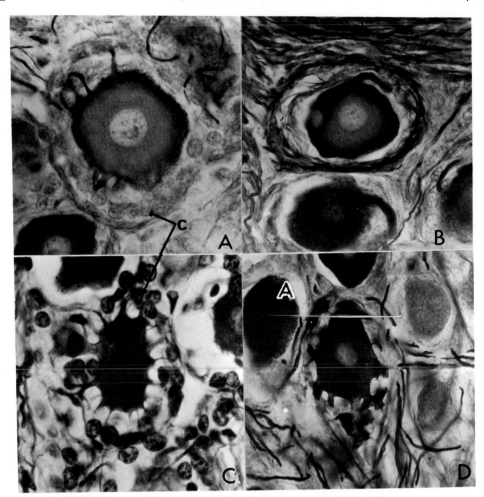

Figure 7-4. Atypical sensory neurons of adult human trigeminal ganglion. (*A*) Fenestrated cell with three looped processes on surface of perikaryon. Satellite and capsular nuclei are identified (c). (*B*) Pericellular plexus of nerve fibers surrounding unipolar ganglion cell. (*C*) Frayed cell (of Cajal) with multiple short processes most of which terminate in the surrounding capsule. Counterstained with hematoxylin to demonstrate capsular nuclei (c). (*D*) Erethized or irritated cell (of DeCastro). Note thick, palm-leaf expansions or supernumerary processes that issue from perikaryon and axon. Types shown in *A*, *C* and *D* are often observed in sensory ganglia of older individuals (Cajal silver stain, all photographs, ×650). (Reproduced with permission from R. C. Truex: *American Journal of Pathology*, **16**: 255–268, 1940.)

but causes centrally projecting fibers to degenerate and (b) section of sensory nerves distal to the ganglia produces profuse chromatolytic changes in the cells of all sizes and types within the ganglia (Fig. 7-5), but no central degeneration (374). Severance of nerve fibers distal to sensory ganglia appears to eliminate peripheral neurotrophic influences necessary for the growth and maintenance of the ganglion cell. The integrity of this influence is sufficient to sustain sensory ganglion cells after their central processes have been sectioned.

The Mixed Nerve. After union of the dorsal and ventral roots, the common nerve trunk divides into four branches or rami: dorsal ramus, ventral ramus, meningeal ramus and ramus communicans (Figs. 3-9 and 7-1). The dorsal rami supply the muscles and skin of the back; the larger ventral rami innervate the ventrolateral portion of the body wall and all the extremities. The ramus communicans connects the common spinal trunk with the sympathetic ganglia and consists of white and gray portions (Fig. 8-2). The former contains the myelin-

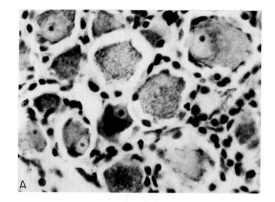

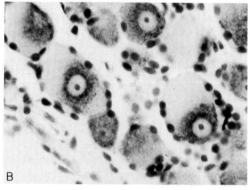

Figure 7-5. Photomicrographs of chromatolytic cells in lumbar spinal ganglion (*A*) and the superior vagal ganglion (*B*) of the monkey after section of the nerve fibers distal to the ganglia. Although lesions of this type produce classic retrograde cell changes, they produce no degeneration in the centrally projecting fibers (cresyl violet stain, ×500). (Reproduced with permission from P. W. Carmel and B. M. Stein: *Journal of Comparative Neurology*, **135:** 145–166, 1969.)

ated preganglionic fibers passing from the spinal cord to the sympathetic ganglion, while the gray rami contain the unmyelinated postganglionic fibers which rejoin the ventral rami to be distributed to the body wall. The white rami also contain afferent fibers from the viscera whose cell bodies are situated in the spinal ganglia (Fig. 9-28).

The *meningeal branch* is a small nerve trunk which usually arises as several twigs from both the common trunk and the ramus communicans (Fig. 7-1). It re-enters the intervertebral foramen to supply the meninges, blood vessels and vertebral column.

The *dorsal and ventral rami* divide into superficial (cutaneous) and deep (muscular) peripheral nerves. These nerve trunks

branch repeatedly and become progressively smaller as they extend peripherally. Ultimately these branches break up into individual nerve fibers which terminate in receptors or effectors. The cutaneous nerves are composed mainly of sensory fibers of various size, but they also contain efferent vasomotor, pilomotor and secretory fibers for the blood vessels, hair and glands of the skin. In muscle nerves there also is a mixture of sensory and motor fibers. Both somatic α and γ efferent fibers go to the skeletal muscle fibers, while numerous large (A) and small afferent fibers pass centrally from receptors in the neuromuscular spindles and tendon organs. Small pain afferents and postganglionic vasomotor (C) fibers to the blood vessels also are found in the nerves that enter each muscle. In each peripheral nerve there are fibers of various categories: myelinated and unmyelinated, large and small, visceral and somatic, sensory and motor (Fig. 7-6).

While each spinal nerve supplies its own body segment, there is considerable intermixture and "anastomosis" of adjacent nerve trunks. The dorsal rami remain relatively distinct, although interconnections between rami of adjacent segments are common in the cervical and sacral regions (1956). The ventral primary rami, however, form more extensive connections. With the exception of the thoracic nerves, which retain their segmental distribution, the cervical and lumbosacral ventral rami branch and anastomose to form the cervical, brachial and lumbosacral plexuses (Figs. 7-14, 7-15, 7-19 and 7-20). In these plexuses a regrouping of fibers occurs, so that each of the peripheral nerves which arises from the plexus contains contributions from two, three or even four ventral rami. The peripheral nerves are therefore "mixed" in a double sense; they consist not only of afferent and efferent fibers, but also of fibers which come from several spinal cord segments.

Connective Tissue Sheaths. Morphologically each peripheral nerve consists of parallel-running nerve fibers invested by a thick sheath of rather loose connective tissue, the *epineurium* (Fig. 7-7). From this sheath septa extend into the interior and divide the fibers into bundles or *fascicles* of varying size, each of which is surrounded by a fairly distinct perifascicular sheath or

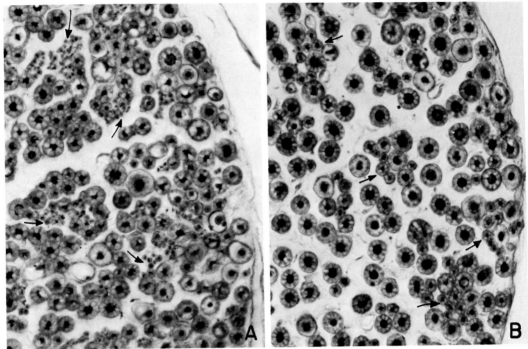

Figure 7-6. Nerve fibers of dorsal and ventral roots. (*A*) Cross section of L4 dorsal root within the dura mater. *Arrows* indicate groups of unmyelinated C fibers. (*B*) Cross section of L4 ventral root within the dura mater. *Arrows* indicate axons of smaller γ efferent neurons to spindle muscle fibers. Larger α axons supply groups of skeletal muscle fibers (Holmes' silver-Luxol fast blue stain, photograph, ×275).

perineurium. These fascicles do not run like isolated cables but repeatedly divide and join adjacent fascicles in an interchange of fibers (Fig. 7-7). As a result, the fascicular arrangement at different levels varies greatly in portions of the same nerve.

From the perineurium delicate strands invade the bundle as intrafascicular connective tissue or *endoneurium.* This tissue separates the fibers into smaller and smaller bundles and ultimately invests each fiber as a delicate tubular membrane. In the epineurial and perineurial connective tissue blood vessels and endothelial lined spaces communicate with lymph channels within smaller fascicles.

On emerging from the spinal cord, the dorsal and ventral roots receive an investment of connective tissue as they pass through the pia. This tissue is reinforced by additional connective tissue as the roots pass through the arachnoid and dura, the latter becoming continuous with the epineurium of the spinal nerve (root sleeve, Fig. 9-2).

The origin, size, course and relationships of spinal nerves to their respective vertebrae are of great clinical significance. These features of spinal nerves are described in Chapter 9 (p. 233) and illustrated in Figures 9-1 and 9-3.

SEGMENTAL INNERVATION

The external segmentation of the spinal cord produced by the spinal nerves corresponds to the general metamerism of the body. Each pair of spinal nerves innervates symmetrically arranged paired somites (metamere). The embryonic somites formed from paraxial mesoderm differentiate into: (a) a *myotome,* which gives rise to muscle and (b) a *sclerotome,* concerned with the development of the axial skeleton. Efferent fibers in the ventral roots innervate somatic musculature (myotomes) and some ventral roots contain preganglionic autonomic fibers which pass to autonomic ganglia which in turn give rise to postganglionic fibers that innervate blood vessels, smooth muscle and glandular epithelium.

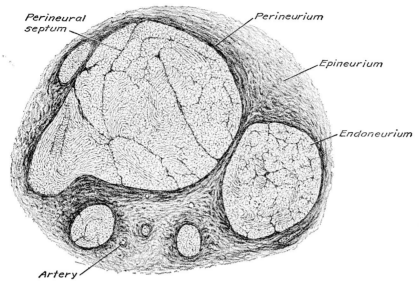

Figure 7-7. Cross section of sciatic nerve of monkey (Reproduced with permission from W. M. Copenhaver: *Bailey's Textbook of Histology*, Ed. 15, Williams & Wilkins, Baltimore, 1964.)

The dorsal roots contain most afferent fibers, somatic and visceral (Fig. 9-28). The cutaneous area supplied by fibers from a single dorsal root and its ganglion is called a *dermatome* (Figs. 7-8, 7-9, 7-11, 7-12 and 7-13).

In the adult, the correspondence between neural and body metameres is recognized readily in the trunk region, where each spinal nerve supplies the musculature and cutaneous area of its own segment. In this region the dermatomes follow one another consecutively, each forming a band encircling the body from the midposterior to the midanterior line (Figs. 7-11 and 7-12). In the extremities, the dermatomes have a more complex arrangement. During development, the metameres migrate distally into the limb buds and arrange themselves parallel to the long axis of the future limb (Fig. 7-8). In each extremity consecutive segments which have migrated peripherally are arranged about an axial line (Figs. 7-8 and 7-9). As a consequence of limb development, the fourth cervical dermatome comes to lie adjacent to the second thoracic dermatome, and the dermatomes of C5 through T1 lie in the upper extremity (Figs. 7-8, 7-9, 7-11 and 7-12). For similar reasons, the dermatomes of L2 and S3 are adjacent posteriorly (Figs. 7-9 and 7-12). The intervening segments have migrated periph-

erally to form the more distal dermatomes of the lower extremity. This migration of metameres in the formation of limbs and the rotation of the lower extremity appears to explain the more conplex arrangement of dermatomes in the extremities (Fig. 7-8). In each extremity, there is thus formed an axial line along which are placed a number of consecutive segments which have wandered out from the axial portions.

Sherrington (2322) demonstrated experimentally in the monkey the cutaneous areas supplied by the various dorsal roots. Because section of a single root did not produce a detectable anesthesia anywhere, he selected a specific root for study and cut two or three adjacent roots above and below. He found that each dermatome overlapped the sensory cutaneous areas of adjacent roots, being coinnervated by the one above and the one below (Fig. 7-10); hence at least three contiguous dorsal roots had to be sectioned to produce a region of complete anesthesia. Findings similar to those of Sherrington were obtained by irritating single roots or ganglia with strychnine and noting the resulting hypersensitive areas (661).

Dermatomes in man were first outlined by mapping the areas of cutaneous eruption and hyperalgesia occurring in association with herpes zoster (shingles), a virus which

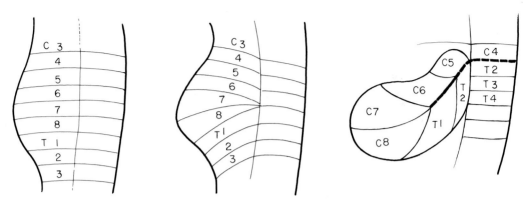

Figure 7-8. Diagram of various stages in the development of the limb bud for the upper extremity. Dermatomes C5, C6 and C7 occupy the preaxial part of the limb bud, while dermatomes C8, T1 and T2 are postaxial. The axial line is indicated by a *red* dashed line. (Modified from Haymaker and Woodhall (1059).)

often affects a single spinal ganglion (1061). Foerster (761, 762) furnished a remarkably complete map of human dermatomes based upon surgical section of various dorsal roots for the alleviation of spastic conditions, and cases of root injury due to tumors or other causes. His dermatomal maps correspond closely to those of Head (1061) and show the same overlap described by Sherrington (2322) in monkeys. Most dermatomes are supplied by fibers of three, occasionally even four, dorsal roots.

The distribution of the three principal divisions of the trigeminal nerve and the cervical spine nerves innervating cutaneous regions of the head and neck are shown in Figure 7-13. The only spinal root whose section produces an area of complete anesthesia is C2. Neither C3 nor branches of the trigeminal nerve supply cutaneous regions in the back of the head. There also is virtually no overlap in the areas supplied by the three divisions of the trigeminal nerve. This is in sharp contrast to the overlap demonstrated for spinal dermatomes. In spinal dermatomes the overlap is greater for tactile sense than for pain and thermal sense. The distribution of the human dermatomes is shown in Figures 7-11 and 7-12.

In individuals with sensory loss of the segmental type, it is important to determine the level of the lesion. Diagrams such as those shown in Figures 7-11 and 7-12 are useful for reference, but certain features of the dermatomal maps are worth remembering: (a) the nipple is located in the region of the 4th or 5th thoracic dermatome, (b) the umbilicus lies in the thoracic 9th or

10th dermatome and (c) the inguinal region corresponds to 1st lumbar dermatome. The anogenital region is supplied by the 3rd to 5th sacral nerve roots.

The segmental innervation of the skeletal musculature (myotomes) has been worked out in man and animals by: (a) selective stimulation of the ventral roots (248, 2713); (b) study of the pathological changes which occur in the anterior horn cells when a ventral root or motor nerve is cut (Figs. 4-2E, 9-1, 9-24 and 9-28); or (c) study of secondary degeneration of peripheral nerve fibers to muscle after central and peripheral lesions. As in the dermatomes, the majority of the muscles, especially those of the extremities, are innervated by two or three, and occasionally even four, ventral roots. Hence injury to a single ventral root may only weaken a muscle or have no apparent effect. Only the very short muscles of the trunk and spinal column and a few others, such as the abductor pollicis, are formed from single myotomes and retain a monosegmental innervation. The peripheral projection of fibers from individual spinal cord segments to a specific muscle thus provides a clue to the myotomic origin of skeletal muscle. The segmental motor supply to the major trunk and extremity muscles is shown graphically in Figures 7-16–7-18. Because this information is essential to a full appreciation of muscle physiology, these figures are included for reference.

Following is a list of some of the important reflex and visceral activities with the locations in the spinal cord of the anterior horn cells that carry them out.

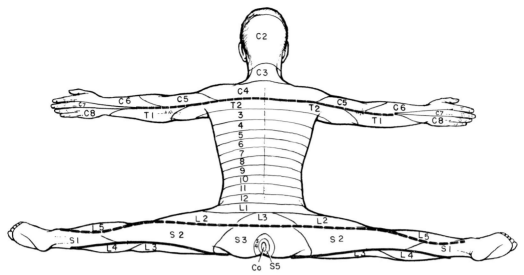

Figure 7-9. Diagram illustrating the position of the posterior (*red dashed lines*) and anterior (*red line*) axial lines. In the upper extremity the axial lines extend down the middle of the corresponding surfaces of the limb. In the lower extremity the posterior axial line (*red dashed line*) courses down the more lateral part of the leg to the region of the ankle; the anterior axial line(*red*) begins in the pubic region and winds around the inner aspect of the thigh to reach the posterior surface of the thigh. The pattern of dermatomes is shown with respect to the axial lines. (Modified from Haymaker and Woodhall (1059).)

Movements of the head (by muscles of neck), C1 to C4.

Movements of diaphragm (phrenic center), C3 to C5.

Movements of upper extremity, C5 to T1.

Biceps tendon reflex (flexion of forearm on percussion of biceps tendon), C5 and C6.

Triceps tendon reflex (extension of forearm on percussion of triceps tendon), C6 to C8.

Radial periosteal reflex (flexion of forearm on percussion of distal end of radius), C7 and C8.

Wrist tendon reflexes (flexion of fingers on percussion of wrist tendons), C8 to T1.

Movements of trunk, T1 to T12.

Abdominal superficial reflexes (ipsilateral contraction of subjacent abdominal muscles on stroking the skin of the upper, middle and lower abdomen); upper (epigastric), T6 and T7; middle T8 and T9; lower, T10 and T12.

Movements of lower extremity, L1 to S2.

Cremasteric superficial reflex (elevation of scrotum on stroking skin on the inner aspect of the thigh), T12 to L2.

Genital center for ejaculation, L1 and L2 (smooth muscle); S3 and S4 (skeletal muscles).

Vesical center for retention of urine, T12 to L2.

Patellar tendon reflex or knee jerk (extension of leg on percussion of patellar ligament), L2 to L4.

Gluteal superficial reflex (contraction of glutei on stroking skin over glutei), L4 to S1.

Plantar superficial reflex (flexion of toes on stroking sole of foot), L5 to S2.

Achilles tendon reflex or ankle jerk (plantar flexion of foot on percussion of Achilles tendon), L5 to S2.

Genital center of erection, S2 to S4.

Vesical center for evacuation of bladder, S3 to S5.

Bulbocavernosus reflex (contraction of bulbocavernosus muscle on pinching penis), S3 to S4.

Anal reflex (contraction of external rectal sphincter on stroking perianal region), S4, S5 and coccygeal.

PERIPHERAL INNERVATION

Although each spinal nerve supplies its own body segment, there is considerable intermixing and anastomosing of adjacent nerve trunks before they reach their peripheral termination. The primary dorsal rami remain relatively distinct, but interconnections are common in the cervical and sacral regions (1956). The ventral rami form more elaborate connections. Except for the thoracic nerves, which largely retain their segmental distribution, the cervical and lum-

Spinal cord   Spinal   Cutaneous
segments   ganglia   field

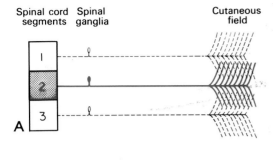

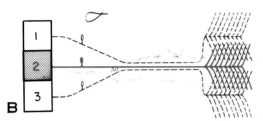

Figure 7-10. Schematic diagram illustrating the overlap of cutaneous fields of segmental innervation. In (*A*), three intercostal nerves are shown. In (*B*), the analogous arrangement is shown for a peripheral nerve in an extremity. The cutaneous distribution of fibers from the spinal ganglion associated with segment 2 of the spinal cord is shown in *red* in both *A* and *B*. Because of the extensive overlap, section of one spinal dorsal root produces virtually no loss in cutaneous sensibility. (Modified from Haymaker and Woodhall (1059).)

bosacral rami innervating the extremities anastomose and branch to form extensive plexuses in which a radical regrouping of fibers occurs. Each of the peripheral nerves arising from these plexuses contains fibers contributed by two, three, four or even five ventral rami. As a result the cutaneous areas supplied by the peripheral nerves do not correspond with the cutaneous areas supplied by the individual dorsal roots (dermatomes). The peripheral and dermatomal distributions of sensory nerve fibers are contrasted in the anterior and posterior body views in Figures 7-11 and 7-12. Similarly, several ventral roots may contribute fibers to a single muscle, and conversely several muscles may receive fibers from a single ventral root. A knowledge of the cutaneous and muscular distribution of the peripheral nerves is of importance to the neurologist in determining the level of peripheral nerve injuries; hence the more important morphological features are presented briefly. A more complete account

will be found in textbooks of anatomy and clinical neurology.

Dorsal Rami

The dorsal rami of the spinal nerves innervate the intrinsic dorsal muscles of the back and neck, and the overlying skin from vertex to coccyx (Figs. 7-1 and 7-12). These muscles constitute the extensors of the vertebral column. In the middle of the back the cutaneous area roughly corresponds to that of the underlying muscles, but in the upper and lower portions of the trunk it widens laterally to reach the acromial region above and the region of the greater trochanter below. With certain exceptions the dorsal rami have a typical segmental distribution, the field of each overlapping with that of the adjacent segments above and below (Fig. 7-10). Each ramus usually divides into a medial and a lateral branch, both of which may contain sensory and motor fibers, although the lateral branches of the cervical rami are purely motor. Deviations are found in the upper two cervical nerves (Fig. 7-13) and in the lumbosacral rami. The first or *suboccipital* nerve is purely motor and terminates in the short posterior muscles of the head (rectus capitis and obliquus capitis). The main branch of the second cervical ramus, known as the *greater occipital* nerve, ascends to the region of the superior nuchal line, where it becomes subcutaneous, and supplies the scalp on the back of the head to the vertex, occasionally extending as far as the coronal suture (Figs. 7-12 and 7-13). This nerve is joined by a filament from the third cervical ramus. The lateral branches of the upper three lumbar and upper three sacral rami send cutaneous twigs which supply the upper part of the gluteal area, extending laterally to the region of the great trochanter. These branches are known as the *superior* (lumbar) and *medial* (sacral) *clunial nerves* (Fig. 7-12).

Ventral Rami

The ventral rami of the spinal nerves supply the ventrolateral muscles and the skin of the trunk, as well as the extremities (Figs. 7-1 and 7-9). With the exception of most thoracic nerves, the ventral rami of adjacent nerves unite and anastomose to form the cervical, brachial and lumbosacral plexuses.

Cervical Plexus

The cervical plexus is formed from the ventral rami of the four upper cervical nerves. It furnishes cutaneous nerves for the ventrolateral portions of the neck and shoulder and for the lateral portions of the back of the head. The muscular branches supply the deep cervical muscles of the spinal column, the infrahyoid muscles and the diaphragm. They also contribute to the innervation of the trapezius (nerves C1 to 4) and sternocleidomastoid muscles, which are chiefly supplied by the accessory nerve (N. XI).

The *lesser occipital nerve* (C2 and C3) is distributed to the upper pole of the pinna and to the lateral area on the back of the head, overlapping only slightly the field of the greater occipital nerve (Figs. 7-12 and 7-13). The *great auricular nerve* (C2 and C3) supplies the larger, lower portion of the pinna and the skin over the angle of the mandible. The *transverse colli* (C2 and C3) innervates the ventral and lateral parts of the neck from chin to sternum (supra- and infrahyoid region). The *supraclavicular nerves* (C3 and C4), which have a variable number of branches, are distributed to the shoulder, the most lateral regions of the neck and the upper part of the breast, where their terminal branches overlap those of the second intercostal nerve (Figs. 7-11–7-13).

The chief muscular nerve, the *phrenic*, supplies the diaphragm and is derived mainly from C4, but receives smaller contributions from C3 or C5, or from both (Fig. 7-15). It frequently receives an anastomotic branch from the subclavian nerve of the brachial plexus, which enters the phrenic at a variable height. Hence in high lesions of the phrenic nerve, paralysis of the diaphragm may not be complete. The deep cervical muscles are innervated by direct segmental branches from the ventral rami, as indicated in Figure 7-16.

The hyoid muscles, except those supplied by the cranial nerves, are innervated by twigs from C1 to C3. These twigs unite into a common trunk known as the *ansa cervicalis*. The geniohyoid and thyrohyoid are supplied entirely from C1; the sternohyoid, sternothyroid and omohoid are innervated from C2 and C3, by motor twigs from the ansa cervicalis. The cervical plexus also aids in the innervation of the sternocleidomastoid and trapezius muscles. The sternocleidomastoid is supplied mainly by the spinal root of the accessory nerve, with sensory fibers that join it through a branch of C2. The trapezius receives major motor contributions from the spinal accessory nerve, and additional motor fibers from C2, C3 and C4. Brendler (248) has demonstrated that C1 may contribute motor fibers to the trapezius, while the spinal accessory nerve sends most of the motor fibers to the middle and lower portions of the muscle. These motor and sensory fibers form one or more bundles, and may be intermixed with the supraclavicular nerves.

Paralysis as a result of injury of the short segmental nerves is rare and usually associated with involvement of the spinal cord. However, the trapezius and sternocleidomastoid muscles frequently are involved as a result of penetrating stab and bullet wounds of the posterior triangle of the neck which injure the spinal accessory nerve. These muscles are superficial, and palpable so that their respective muscle actions are of diagnostic value. The sternocleidomastoid and trapezius muscles may be involved along with axial and limb muscles in diseases of the corpus striatum. One particularly troublesome disorder is the condition known as *torticollis*. Due to spasm the contracted sternocleidomastoid muscle stands out as a large cord, and the head usually is involuntarily rotated toward the opposite side. This awkward position may be maintained for long periods. Spasmodic torticollis may be associated with neuroses. In the latter cases it is often difficult to distinguish between a functional disorder and organic disease. Emotional stress usually aggravates these involuntary muscle movements.

Brachial Plexus

The nerves supplying the upper extremity and forming the brachial plexus are derived as a rule from the ventral rami of the four lower cervical and the first thoracic nerves, with a small contribution from the fourth cervical nerve (Figs. 7-14 and 7-15).

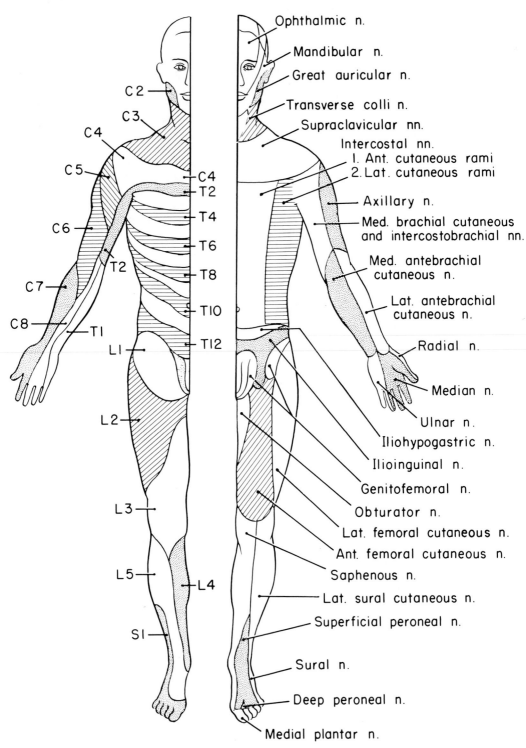

Figure 7-11. Anterior view of dermatomes (*left*) and cutaneous areas supplied by individual peripheral nerves (*right*).

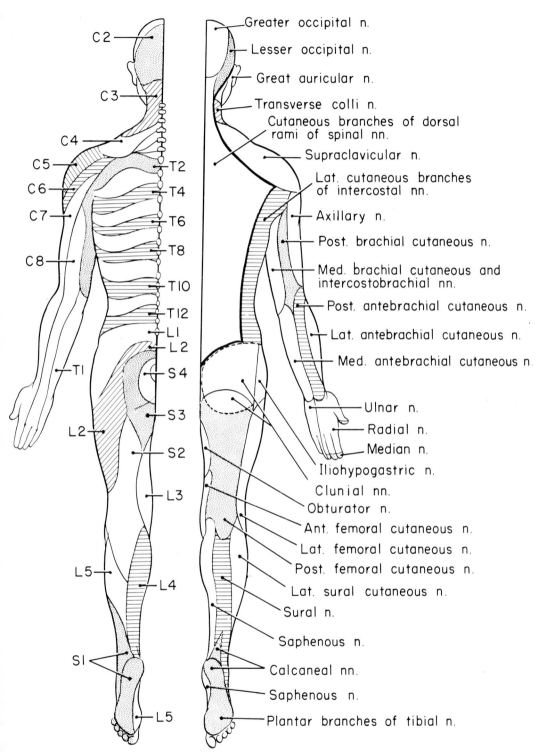

Figure 7-12. Posterior view of dermatomes (*left*) and cutaneous areas supplied by individual peripheral nerves (*right*).

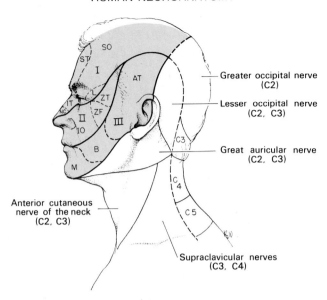

Figure 7-13. Diagram of cutaneous fields of the head and neck. The distribution of the three peripheral divisions of the trigeminal nerve are shown in *red* (*I*, ophthalmic division; *II*, maxillary division; *III*, mandibular division). Abbreviations indicate the following nerves within the trigeminal divisions: *AT*, auriculotemporal; *B*, buccal; *IO*, infraorbital; *IT*, infratrochlear; *L*, lacrimal; *M*, mental; *NC*, nasocillary (external branch); *SO*, supraorbital; *ST*, supratrochlear; *ZF*, zygomaticofacial; *ZT*, zygomaticotemporal. There is no dermatomal overlap between the three divisions of the trigeminal nerve. Branches of cervical spinal nerves innervate cutaneous regions over the back of the head and in the neck.

Considerable variations are not uncommon. If the contribution from the fourth cervical nerve is strong and that of the first thoracic negligible, the plexus is referred to as the *prefixed* type. It is called *postfixed* when the fourth cervical does not participate at all, but the first thoracic makes a strong contribution and the second thoracic sends a branch. Between these extremes there are many intermediate conditions, depending on the stronger or weaker participation of the fourth cervical, on the one hand, and the second thoracic, on the other. These variations are dependent on embryological factors. The limb buds of both arms and legs may vary in longitudinal extent and especially in their relative position to the neuraxis. The more cephalic the position of the limbs, the more cephalic will be the nerves contributing to the plexus, and vice versa.

The ventral rami supplying the plexus give rise to three *primary trunks;* C5 and C6 unite to form the *superior (upper) trunk;* C8 and T1 form the *inferior (lower) trunk;* and C7 is continued as the *middle trunk*

(Fig. 7-14). Each trunk splits into a posterior and an anterior division. The posterior divisions of all three trunks fuse to form the *posterior cord,* situated behind the axillary artery. The anterior divisions of the superior and middle trunk form the *lateral cord,* while the anterior division of the inferior trunk is continued as the *medial cord* (Fig. 7-14).

Many of the nerves supplying the shoulder muscles are given off directly from the ventral rami, or from the primary trunks and their branches before these unite to form the secondary cords. Thus the *dorsal scapular* nerve supplying the rhomboids arises from the dorsal surface of C5, and the *long thoracic* nerve to the serratus anterior arises from the dorsal surface of C5, C6 and C7. From the superior trunk the *suprascapular* nerve (C4, C5 and C6) for the supraspinatus and infraspinatus emerges dorsally, and the small nerve to the subclavius (C5 and C6) arises ventrally. The roots of the *medial and lateral pectoral* nerves (C5 to T1), which innervate the pectoralis major and minor, arise in part from the ventral surface of the superior and medial trunks, and in part from the medial cord (Fig. 7-15).

The three large peripheral nerves of the forearm (radial, median and ulnar) are formed in the following manner. The posterior cord, which receives contributions from all the plexus nerves, gives off the *thoracodorsal* (C6 to C8) and the *subscapular* nerves (C5 to C8), the former supplying the latissimus dorsi, and latter innervating the teres major and subscapularis (Fig. 7-15). Then the posterior cord splits into its two terminal branches, the larger *radial* nerve and the smaller *axillary* nerve. The lateral and medial cords each split into two branches, thus forming four nerves (Fig. 7-14). The two middle branches, one from the lateral cord and one from the medial cord, unite to form the *median* nerve. The outer branch, derived from the lateral cord, becomes the *musculocutaneous nerve*. The large innermost branch, derived from the medial cord, gives off the purely sensory *medial brachial cutaneous* and *medial antebrachial cutaneous* nerves, and its continuation becomes the *ulnar nerve* (Fig. 7-15).

A brief reference to embryology aids in explaining the formation of the plexus. During early development the primitive muscle mass of the limb is split into posterior and anterior layers, which are separated by the anlage of the humerus. The primary ventral nerve rami invading the limb split into posterior and anterior branches to supply corresponding muscles and the overlying skin. Within the primitive musculature, many simple muscles fuse to form larger and more complex ones innervated by two or more spinal nerves (Figs. 7-17 and 7-18). Such fusion usually occurs within either the posterior or the anterior musculature, and the muscles are innervated, respectively, by posterior or anterior divisions of the nerves. At the cephalic (preaxial) and the caudal (postaxial) borders of the limb, some muscles may be derived from both the posterior and the anterior musculature. These muscles are supplied by nerve fibers from both posterior and anterior divisions. A well known example is the brachialis muscle, which receives branches from the radial and musculocutaneous nerves. Thus the primitive plexus shows a division into pos-

terior and anterior plates. The posterior plate innervates the posterior or extensor half of the arm and the posterior shoulder muscles; the anterior plate supplies the volar or flexor half of the arm and the anterior muscles of the shoulder. The nerves arising from the posterior plate are the dorsal scapular, long thoracic, suprascapular, subscapular, thoracodorsal, axillary and radial (*black* in Fig. 7-15). Those from the anterior plate include the subclavius, pectoral, musculocutaneous, median and ulnar, as well as the purely sensory medial brachial and medial antebrachial cutaneous nerves.

A summary of the peripheral distribution of the principal nerves of the upper extremity follows. The cutaneous areas innervated by each nerve are shown in Figures 7-11 and 7-12. In their peripheral courses, some of the nerves of both the upper and lower extremity are particularly prone to trauma, or entrapment by fibrous tissue related to either muscles, tendons, ligaments or fascia (1346). Sensory and motor symptoms that accompany such neuropathies depend on whether the nerves are primarily motor or sensory.

Axillary Nerve. This nerve (C5 and C6) innervates the deltoid and teres minor muscles and sends the *lateral brachial cutaneous* nerve to the skin of the upper outer surface of the arm, mainly in the deltoid region. After complete section of the axillary nerve, the deltoid muscle is paralyzed and abduction without external rotation is practically impossible. In time deltoid atrophy leads to loss of the round contour normally present at the shoulder. The sensory loss is less extensive, owing to the overlap of neighboring cutaneous nerves.

Radial Nerve. This nerve (C5 to C8) supplies motor branches to the triceps muscle and all of the extensor muscles of the elbow, hands and fingers, and to the brachioradialis, supinator and abductor pollicis longus muscles. In addition, it usually sends a twig to the brachialis. Its cutaneous branches, distributed to the posterior surface of the extremity, are the *posterior brachial cutaneous nerve* to the arm, the *posterior antebrachial cutaneous* to the forearm and the *superficial radial nerve* which innervates the radial half of the dorsum of the hand and fingers as far as the distal interphalangeal joints (Fig. 7-12).

MAIN BRANCHES	CORDS	DIVISIONS	TRUNKS	VENTRAL RAMI

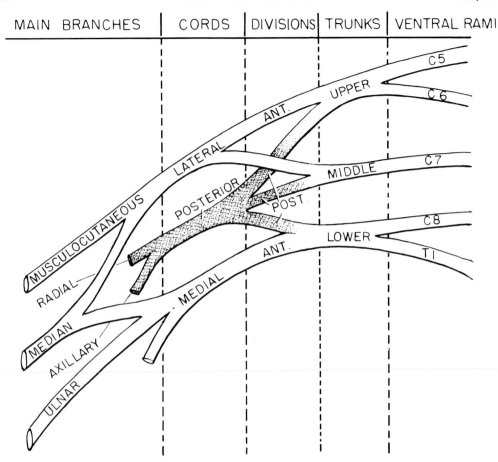

Figure 7-14. Schematic drawing of the formation of the brachial plexus, indicating ventral rami, trunks, divisions, cords and main branches. The posterior divisions and the posterior cord are shaded.

The segmental innervation of the muscles supplied by the radial nerve is indicated in Figure 7-17.

Injuries of the radial nerve give variable symptoms which depend upon the location of the lesion. Complete section of the nerve above all its branches produces inability to extend the elbow, wrist, fingers and thumb; wrist drop is the most striking feature. The sensory loss is most marked on the dorsum of the hand and thumb in the territory supplied by the superficial radial nerve. Anesthesia in the arm is negligible but usually is present in a narrow strip on the dorsal surface of the forearm from the elbow to the wrist. The limited sensory loss is due to overlap by adjacent cutaneous nerves. The most vulnerable parts of the radial nerve lie adjacent to the middle third of the humerus and over the lateral epicondyle. The radial nerve is frequently injured in fractures of the humerus and those involving the elbow.

The nerve may be compressed against the humerus during sleep, especially when the patient is anesthetized or intoxicated.

Musculocutaneous Nerve. This nerve (C5 to C7) sends muscular branches to the coracobrachialis, biceps and brachialis, and continues as the *lateral antebrachial cutaneous* nerve to supply the radial half of the forearm, on both posterior and volar surfaces (Figs. 7-11 and 7-12). In complete lesions of the nerve, flexion and supination of the forearm are weakened. The lateral portion of the brachialis may be spared since it receives, as a rule, a branch from the radial nerve, and forearm flexion can still be produced by the brachioradialis. The sensory loss is variable in extent. It is poorly defined posteriorly, due to overlap with the posterior antebrachial cutaneous nerve (a branch of the radial nerve). On the volar side, sensory loss is more extensive and approximates the territory supplied by

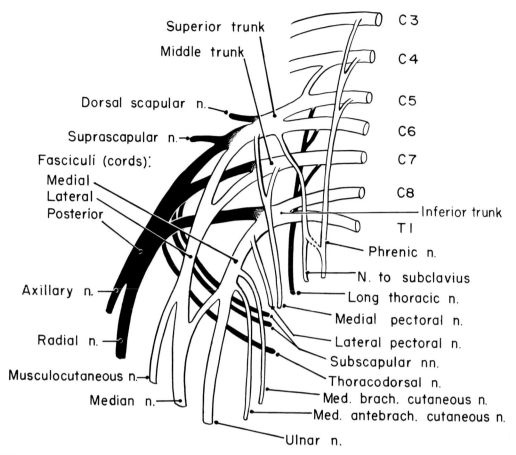

Figure 7-15. Diagram of the brachial plexus. The posterior divisions, posterior cords, and peripheral nerves formed from the posterior divisions are shown in *black*. Cords and peripheral nerves formed from the anterior divisions of the ventral primary rami are in *white*.

the lateral antebrachial cutaneous nerve (Fig. 7-11).

Median Nerve. This nerve (C6 to T1, and sometimes C5) supplies all the muscles on the volar surface of the forearm except the flexor carpi ulnaris and the ulnar head of the flexor digitorum profundis. In the hand its branches innervate the outer lumbricals (I and II) and the muscles of the thenar eminence, except for the adductor pollicis and deep head of the flexor pollicis brevis. The sensory innervation is limited to the hand; it comprises the volar surface of the thumb, index and middle fingers; the radial half of the fourth finger; and corresponding portions of the palm (Fig. 7-11). Posteriorly the nerve supplies the distal phalanx of the index and middle fingers and the radial half of the fourth finger. An inconstant *palmar* branch is distributed to

the radial half of the volar surface of the wrist, but usually this area is completely overlapped by the lateral antebrachial branch of the musculocutaneous nerve. The flexor and pronator muscles supplied by the motor branches of the median nerve have a segmental innervation, as indicated in Figure 7-17.

Injury to the nerve along its course in the arm affects all its branches. Complete interruption causes severe impairment of pronation of the forearm and weakens flexion at the wrist. The wasting of the thenar eminence and the abnormal position of the thumb give the hand a characteristic appearance after median nerve injury. Normally the thumb is partially rotated and its metacarpal bone is in a more volar plane than the other metacarpals. In injury of the median nerve this rotation is lost, and the

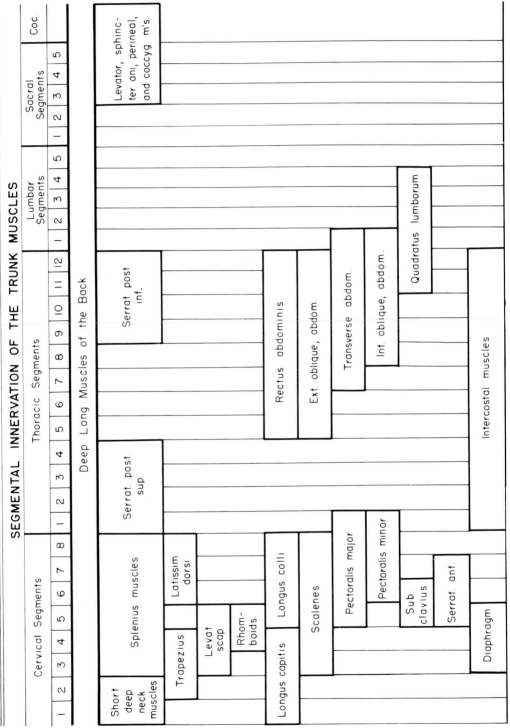

Figure 7-16. Segments of spinal cord that contribute somatic motor nerve fibers to individual trunk muscles (after Haymaker (1057)).

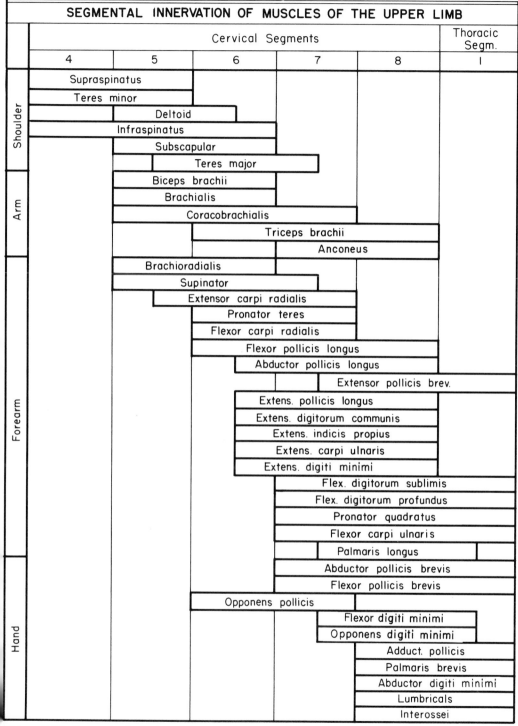

Figure 7-17. Segments of spinal cord that contribute somatic motor nerve fibers to the individual muscles of shoulder and upper extremity (after Haymaker (1057)).

thumb is extended, so that it lies in the same plane as the rest of the palm (simian hand).

Flexion of the index finger is practically abolished and is only slightly compensated by the flexor action of the interossei at the metacarpophalangeal joint. The middle finger is more variably affected. In the thumb, flexion of the terminal phalanx is completely lost, as are abduction and opposition. Makeshift movements of opposition, without abduction and rotation, can still be affected by the abductor pollicis and the deep head of the flexor brevis (pseudo-opposition). The motor defects are brought out readily in attempts to make a fist. The fourth and fifth fingers flex, but the thumb and index finger, and to a variable degree the middle finger, remain partially extended.

Sensory loss following a lesion of the median nerve is somewhat variable; usually it is less extensive than the area supplied by the nerve (Figs. 7-11 and 7-12), and it is most constant on the volar surface of the index and middle finger. Loss of appreciation of light touch generally is more constant and extensive than appreciation of pinprick, and extends from the radial border of the thumb to the base of the thenar eminence and across the palm to include the palmar aspects of the ring finger on the radial side. On the dorsum of the hand it includes the radial side of the terminal two-thirds of the ring finger and the middle and index fingers as far proximal as the middle of the proximal phalanges. Deep sensibility usually is lost in the terminal phalanges of the index and middle fingers. The median nerve is prone to injury in deep cuts at the wrist and to entrapment as it passes beneath the transverse carpal ligament with the flexor tendons (carpal tunnel syndrome). Nerve compression may follow fractures (carpal and distal radial bones) or occur without external stress. Injuries here, as well as lesions of the nerve anywhere along its course, may be accompanied by secondary autonomic system overactivity. Following incomplete regeneration of the median nerve, an intense, persistent "burning pain" may be found over one or more points in the distal course of the nerve (*causalgia*). The median nerve is the most common site of causalgia.

Ulnar Nerve. This nerve (C8 and T1) supplies the flexor carpi ulnaris and the ulnar head of the flexor digitorum profundis muscles in the forearm. In the hand, it innervates the adductor pollicis, the deep head of the flexor pollicis brevis, the interossei, the two inner lumbricals and the muscles of the hypothenar eminence. It gives off three cutaneous branches. The *palmar cutaneous* branch supplies the ulnar half of the volar surface of the wrist, an area extensively overlapped by the medial antebrachial cutaneous nerve (Fig. 7-11). The posterior branch innervates the ulnar half of the dorsum of the hand, all of the little finger and the proximal phalanx of the ulnar half of the ring finger. The *superficial volar* branch supplies the volar surface of the fifth digit, and the ulnar half of the fourth finger, and the corresponding ulnar portion of the palm (hypothenar region) (Figs. 7-11 and 7-12). The segmental innervation of muscles supplied by the ulnar nerve is indicated in Figure 7-17.

As in the case of the median nerve, injury to the ulnar nerve in the arm affects its whole distribution. Flexion of the wrist is weakened, as are flexion of the fourth and fifth fingers and adduction of the thumb. There is marked wasting of the hypothenar and interossei muscles. The paralysis of these small muscles is particularly disturbing, for it makes execution of the finger movements required for writing, sewing and other skilled activities exceedingly difficult. The interossei flex the basal phalanges and extend the middle and distal ones. Hence paralysis of the interossei results in: (a) overextension of the basal phalanges by the extensor digitorum communis and (b) flexion of the middle and distal phalanges by the flexor digitorum sublimis (claw hand).

Sensory disturbances are variable and depend upon the level of nerve injury. Total anesthesia as a rule is limited to the little finger and the hypothenar region. The ulnar nerve is prone to trauma as it crosses the medial epicondyle of the humerus, and to entrapment as it passes from the wrist to the hand.

Medial Antebrachial Cutaneous Nerve. This nerve (C8 and T1) supplies the medial half of the forearm, on both posterior and volar surfaces (Figs. 7-11 and 7-12). The extent of the sensory deficits caused by injury to this nerve varies in individual cases. On the volar side it often reaches to the middle of the arm. On the posterior surface the sensory deficit is somewhat smaller than the area of supply shown in Figure 7-12.

Medial Brachial Cutaneous Nerve. This nerve (T1) usually is associated with the *intercostobrachial* nerve derived from the second and often from the third thoracic (intercostal) nerves. These two nerves supply the axillary region and the inner surface of the arm, the area being considerably larger on the volar surface than on the posterior surface (Figs. 7-11 and 7-12). The area is overlapped extensively by adjacent cutaneous nerves. Injury to one of the nerves produces negligible symptoms. In injuries of both, the region of anesthesia is limited to the axillary region and medial surface of the upper arm.

Injuries of the Brachial Plexus

The motor and sensory deficits of the brachial plexus lesions vary considerably, depending on the extent of the injury and its location. In injury of the trunks the symptoms are segmental in character, and two main syndromes may be recognized. One syndrome affects the upper (superior) trunk and the other the lower (inferior) trunk. The upper trunk syndrome (Duchenne-Erb) involves the muscles supplied by C5 and C6, namely the deltoid, biceps, brachialis, brachioradialis, supinator, teres major, teres minor, supraspinatus and infraspinatus. In this syndrome there is difficulty in elevation and external rotation of the arm, accompanied by a severe loss of flexion and supination of the forearm. Owing to the overlap of adjacent roots, the sensory deficit is as a rule limited to the deltoid region and lateral aspect of the arm.

The lower (inferior) trunk syndrome (Klumpke or Duchenne-Aran) is relatively rare and affects primarily the small muscles of the hand innervated by C8 and T1 (Fig. 7-17). The palmaris longus and the long digital flexors usually are involved; hence the chief disabilities are in the finger and wrist movements. The sensory loss is along the medial aspects of the arm, forearm and hand. If preganglionic sympathetic fibers of the first thoracic root are included in the injury, there is drooping of the eyelid, diminution in the size of the pupil and narrowing of the palpebral fissure (Horner's syndrome, see p. 228 and Fig. 10-29).

Injuries of the cords of the brachial plexus produce symptoms similar to those of peripheral nerves, except that they are multiple and often incomplete. Thus a lesion of the posterior cord involves the radial and axillary nerves and often the thoracodorsal and subscapular nerves (Fig. 7-15). Interruption of the lateral cord affects the musculocutaneous and the lateral portion of the median nerve. Injury to the medial cord involves the ulnar and the medial portion of the median nerve, as well as the medial brachial and antebrachial cutaneous nerves.

Lumbosacral Plexus

The plexus innervating the lower extremity is as a rule formed by the primary ventral rami of L1 to S2 and the larger portion of S3; frequently there is a small contributing branch from T12 (Figs. 7-19 and 7-20). As in the case of the brachial plexus, anatomical variations occur. The plexus is *prefixed* when it is supplied by T12 to S2, and *postfixed* when it is formed from roots L2 to S4. There are also many intermediate forms, but the maximum shift in either direction rarely exceeds the extent of a single spinal nerve. These conditions are determined by the individual variations in the position of the limb buds during development. According to Foerster (759) prefixed lumbosacral plexuses are rare. The lumbosacral plexus, excluding the pudendal and coccygeal portions, which are not distributed to the leg, is conveniently subdivided into an upper *lumbar* and a lower *sacral* plexus.

The *lumbar plexus*, formed by L1, L2, L3, and the larger part of L4, usually receives a communicating branch from T12 (Fig. 7-19). The larger *sacral plexus* is supplied by the smaller portion of L4 (furcal nerve), which joins L5 to form the large lumbosacral trunk, and by S1, S2 and the greater portion of S3 (Fig. 7-20). Except for the uppermost portion supplied mainly by L1, where the conditions are somewhat obscure, both plexuses show an organization into posterior and anterior divisions and the arrangement is simpler than in the brachial plexus. The undivided lumbosacral primary rami do not form interlacing trunks but split directly into posterior and anterior divisions related, respectively, to the primitive posterior and anterior musculature of the leg. The peripheral nerves to the extremity are formed by the union of a variable number of either posterior or anterior divisions (Figs. 7-19 and 7-20). In the lum-

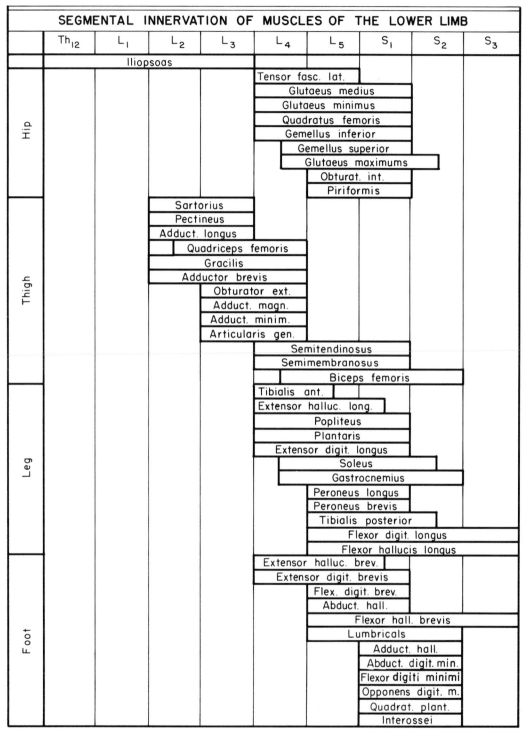

Figure 7-18. Segments of spinal cord that contribute somatic motor nerve fibers to individual muscles of hip and lower extremity (after Haymaker (1057)).

bar plexus, the anterior divisions give rise to the *iliohypogastric* (anterior branch), *ilioinguinal, genitofemoral* and *obturator nerves*. The posterior divisions give rise to

the *iliohypogastric* (posterior branch), *iliopsoas, femoral* and *lateral femoral cutaneous nerves*.

In the *sacral plexus*, the anterior divisions furnish the *tibial nerve* and the nerves to the hamstring, quadratus femoris, obturator internus and gemelli muscles; the posterior divisions form the *common peroneal* and the *superior* and *inferior gluteal nerves*. The *posterior femoral cutaneous nerve*, which supplies the back of the thigh, receives fibers from both posterior and anterior divisions. As in the case of the arm, muscles derived from both the posterior and the anterior primitive musculature are innervated by both posterior and anterior divisions. Thus the biceps femoris receives branches from the tibial, as well as peroneal portions of the sciatic nerve.

Following is a summary of the peripheral distribution of the principal nerves of the lower extremity. The cutaneous areas supplied by these nerves are shown in Figures 7-11 and 7-12.

Obturator Nerve. The obturator nerve (L2 to L4) supplies the adductor muscles of the thigh and the gracilis muscle; it sends an inconstant branch to the pectineus, which more often is innervated by the femoral nerve. Its cutaneous branch is distributed to the inner surface of the thigh (Figs. 7-11 and 7-12), the area being extensively overlapped by adjacent cutaneous nerves. The segmental innervation of the muscles supplied by the obturator nerve is indicated in Figure 7-18.

In injury of this nerve, adduction of the thigh is weakened severely but not lost, since the adductor magnus also receives some fibers from the sciatic nerve. The sensory defects usually involve only a small triangular area of the anatomical field. The obturator nerve is vulnerable to entrapment by the obturator membrane as it passes through the obturator canal.

Femoral Nerve. The femoral nerve (L2 to L4) sends motor branches to the extensors of the leg, the iliopsoas, the sartorius and also the pectineus. Occasionally a branch may go to the adductor longus. The cutaneous branches are the *anterior femoral cutaneous* nerves for the thigh and the *saphenous* nerve for the leg and foot (Figs. 7-11 and 7-12). The former supply the anterior and anteromedial surface of the thigh, comprising a relatively large autonomous sensory field. The saphenous nerve sends an infrapatellar branch to the skin in front of the kneecap and then is distributed to the medial side of the leg; the lowermost branches are distributed from the medial margin of the foot to the proximal phalanx of the great toe.

The segmental innervation of the quadriceps femoris, iliopsoas, sartorius and pectineus is shown in Figure 7-18.

Injury of the femoral nerve causes inability to extend the leg. If the lesion is high enough to involve the iliopsoas, flexion of the thigh at the hip is severely impaired. Sensory disturbances are manifested throughout the field of supply, and there are relatively large areas of total anesthesia. If the thigh nerves alone are involved the anesthesia is most extensive on the anterior surface of the thigh above the knee. In isolated lesions of the saphenous nerve, the anesthetic field extends on the inner surface of the leg from below the knee to the medial margin of the foot. The femoral nerve may become involved secondary to an abscess in the psoas muscle. The terminal sensory branch of the femoral (saphenous nerve) is subject to entrapment as it leaves the subsartorial canal.

Lateral Femoral Cutaneous Nerve. The lateral femoral cutaneous nerve (L2 and L3) supplies the lateral half of the thigh, from the lateral buttock region to the knee (Figs. 7–11 and 7-12). In spite of overlap by adjacent cutaneous nerves, injury of this nerve produces a considerable area of anesthesia on the lateral aspect of the thigh.

The cutaneous areas supplied by the *iliohypogastric* (L1), *ilioinguinal* (L1) and *genitofemoral* (L1 and L2) nerves are shown in Figures 7-11 and 7-12. The iliohypogastric and ilioinguinal nerves also send motor fibers to the internal oblique and transverse abdominal muscles. Sensory loss due to injury to one of these nerves is relatively small or may be absent, but such lesions may cause neuralgia.

Sciatic Nerve. The sciatic (ischiadic) nerve (L4 to S3), the largest nerve in the body, is the chief continuation of all the roots of the sacral plexus. It is composed of two parts, the *tibial nerve* and the *common peroneal nerve*, enclosed for a variable distance within a common sheath (Fig. 7-20). Emerging from the greater sciatic foramen, or while still within it, the nerve sends branches to the main external rotators of the thigh, namely, the obturator internus, the gemelli and the quadratus femoris muscles (L4 to S1). Lesions of these nerves are comparatively rare, and only external rotation is weakened, since other external

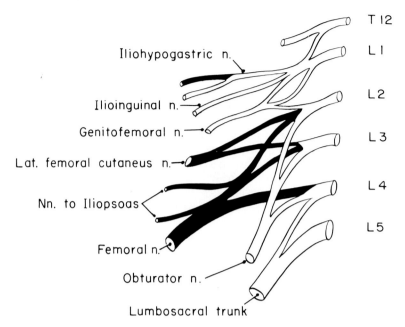

Figure 7-19. Diagram of lumbar plexus. Peripheral nerves formed by anterior divisions of ventral primary rami are *white*; nerves formed by posterior divisions of ventral primary rami are *black*.

rotators are available. In the region of the thigh, branches are given off to the flexors of the knee (hamstring muscles) and to the adductor magnus, the latter being innervated also by the obturator nerve. These branches, all derived from the tibial portion of the sciatic (ischiadic) nerve, often spring from a common trunk, which either runs independently or is loosely incorporated in the medial side of the sciatic nerve. An additional branch from the common peroneal nerve supplies the short head of the biceps femoris muscle. In injuries of the hamstring nerves flexion of the knee is impaired severely, but weak flexion still may be produced by the action of the gracilis and sartorius muscle.

The sciatic nerve splits into its two terminal nerves at varying levels in the thigh. The muscular branches of the common trunk provide motor and sensory fibers to the quadratus femoris, the obturator internus, the gemelli, the semitendinosus, the semimembranosus and the biceps femoris.

Normal peripheral nerve can be damaged by excessive stretch, as may occur in the roots and cords of the brachial plexus following undue angulation of the head and shoulder, or arm traction, during delivery. Reaction to stretch in an injured or irritated nerve with a long course, such as the sciatic, often produces pain, and paresthesias. One of the best known nerve stretching mechanisms is the straight leg-raising test (sign of Lasègue). In a person lying supine with the legs extended, elevation of one extended (straightened) leg by flexion of the thigh at the hip causes stretching of the sciatic nerve. Stretching of the sciatic nerve in the presence of meningitis, intervertebral disc disease, peripheral neuritis or nerve trauma, produces pain in the distribution of the nerve. The patient usually attempts to relieve the pain by automatically flexing the leg at the knee (Kernig's sign). This nerve is accompanied by the popliteal artery and vein, as well as a large number of postganglionic sympathetic fibers. Injuries of this nerve, like the median nerve described above, are particularly prone to be followed by causalgia.

Tibial Nerve. The tibial nerve (L4 to S3) supplies the posterior calf muscles concerned with: (a) plantar flexion and inversion of the foot and (b) plantar flexion of the toes. It also supplies the intrinsic muscles of the sole, which aid in maintaining the arch of the foot. One cutaneous branch given off in the thigh, the *sural* nerve, is distributed to the posterior and medial surface of the calf, where it is overlapped extensively by branches of the saphenous and

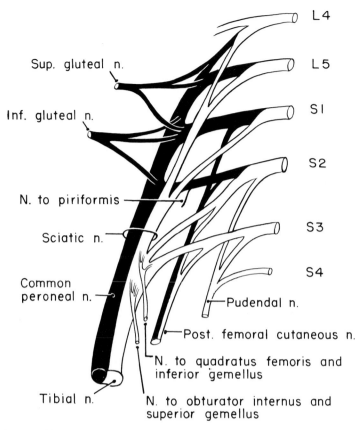

L4

Sup. gluteal n.

L5

Inf. gluteal n.

SI

S2

N. to piriformis

Sciatic n.

S3

S4

Common
peroneal n.

Pudendal n.

Post. femoral cutaneous n.

N. to quadratus femoris and
inferior gemellus

Tibial n.

N. to obturator internus and
superior gemellus

Figure 7-20. Diagram of lumbosacral plexus. Peripheral nerves formed by anterior divisions of ventral primary rami are *white*; nerves formed by posterior divisions of ventral primary rami are *black*.

lateral sural (peroneal) nerves. Terminal branches of the sural nerve (*lateral calcaneal*) supply the outer margin of the heel and a triangular area on the outer surface of the foot which extends to the lower portion of the Achilles tendon (Fig. 7-12). Other cutaneous branches of the tibial nerve (*medial calcaneal* and *plantar*) supply the back and medial margin of the heel, the plantar surface of the foot and toes and the dorsal phalanges (Figs. 7-11 and 7-12). The terminal branches of the tibial nerve are the *medial* and *lateral plantar* nerves. The segmental innervation of the calf and plantar muscles supplied by the tibial nerve is indicated in Figure 7-18.

Complete interruption of the tibial nerve above all its branches abolishes plantar flexion of the foot and toes and severely impairs inversion of the foot. Atrophy of the plantar muscles increases the concavity of the plantar arch (pes cavus). Sensory disturbances are negligible in the calf re-

gion, in which only a narrow strip may show reduced sensitivity. Total anesthesia is found on the sole of the foot, the plantar surface of the toes, the heel, and often in a triangular area on the outer surface of the foot. This nerve is vulnerable to fractures and dislocations of the medial melleolus, calcaneus and astragalus bones. It also can be compressed as it passes through the osseofibrous canal with three tendons, deep to the flexor retinaculum or deltoid ligament (tarsal tunnel syndrome).

Common Peroneal Nerve. The common peroneal nerve (L4 to S2) supplies the lateral and anterior muscles of the leg and the dorsal muscles of the foot, effecting dorsal flexion and eversion of the foot and dorsal flexion of the toes. The chief cutaneous nerves are the *lateral sural cutaneous* and the *superficial peroneal nerve* (Fig. 7-11). The former, given off in the thigh, is distributed to the outer side of the leg from the knee region to nearly the outer margin of the sole, where it invades the territories of the superficial peroneal and sural nerves. The superficial peroneal nerve supplies the dorsum of the foot and toes to the distal phalanges and a portion of the anterior surface of the leg. A small cutaneous branch of the deep peroneal nerve is distributed to the cleft between the adjacent surfaces of the great and second toe (Fig. 7-11). The common peroneal nerve divides into its superficial and deep branches as it passes to the lateral side of the neck of the fibula under cover of the peroneus longus muscle. The segmental innervation of the peronei, tibialis anterior and extensor muscles on the dorsum of the foot is indicated in Figure 7-18.

Complete section of the peroneal nerve causes paralysis of dorsal flexion and eversion of the foot and paralysis of dorsal flexion (extension) of the toes. The most striking feature is inability to elevate the foot and toes (foot drop). If the condition is prolonged, shortening of the Achilles tendon will produce a permanent plantar hyperflexion and the foot will assume an equinovarus deformity. Sensory defects will be found on the dorsum of the foot, the outer part of the leg, and between the great and second toe. The extent of the sensory loss is much smaller than the anatomical field, since cutaneous areas on both, foot and leg, are overlapped extensively by the adjacent cutaneous nerves. The common peroneal nerve is subject to injury both by compression and fracture at the neck of the fibula. A terminal branch of the deep peroneal nerve is frequently injured as it crosses the dorsum of the foot. The terminal sensory fibers of the superficial peroneal nerve may become entrapped as they pierce the deep fascia at the distal and lateral part of the leg.

Gluteal Nerves. The *superior gluteal nerve* (L4 to S1) supplies the gluteus medius, gluteus minimus and tensor fasciae latae muscles, which abduct the hip and rotate it internally. These movements are impaired by injury to the nerve.

The *inferior gluteal nerve* (L5 to S2) is distributed to the gluteus maximus, the strongest extensor of the hip. Injury causes wasting of the buttock. There is difficulty in rising from a sitting position, walking uphill or climbing stairs, where powerful contraction of the muscle is required for raising the body.

Posterior Femoral Cutaneous Nerve. The posterior femoral cutaneous nerve (S1 to S3) gives off several branches (*inferior clunial*) which supply lower portions of the buttocks. These nerves overlap branches of the lumbar and sacral dorsal rami (superior and medial clunial nerves) (Fig. 7-12). Another small branch (*perineal*) goes to the lower innermost part of the buttock, the dorsal surface of the scrotum (or labia majora) and reaches the inner surface of the thigh. The main nerve supplies the posterior aspect of the thigh, often extending below the knee and widely overlapping the territories of adjacent nerves. Injuries produce a relatively broad strip of anesthesia on the posterior surface of the thigh from the buttocks to the knee.

FUNCTIONAL CONSIDERATIONS

The origin, size, course and relations of the spinal nerves to their respective vertebrae are important factors (Figs. 9-1–9-3). Meninges, intervertebral discs, size of the intervertebral foramina and vertebral mobility often can be correlated anatomically with a variety of spinal nerve root syndromes (598). For example, a ruptured, or herniated, intervertebral disc may lead to compression of spinal nerve roots as they approach the intervertebral foramen, or the foramina may be narrowed due to osteoarthritis. Effects of stress and strain on the erect spine appear first at the weakest points. Here motion occurs and the mechanical impacts of postural strain and trauma usually are recorded (i.e., cervical and lumbar regions). Dorsal roots, except for C1, are nearly three times larger than ventral roots. However, the spinal roots vary in size in different regions. The largest nerve roots are those that participate in the formation of the nerve plexuses that supply the limbs. The sixth cervical is the largest of the cervical nerves and from this point upward the roots diminish in size. Root size in relation to bony foramina have some interesting correlations with attendant liability to mechanical irritation or compression. Cervical roots occupy only one-fourth of their respective intervertebral foramen. In contrast, from the first lumbar nerve downward the size of the nerve roots increase in relation to the size of the foramen. The first to third lumbar nerves never completely fill the foramina, and the fourth root rarely does, whereas the fifth lumbar nerve root frequently fills the intervertebral foramen. This suggests a possible explanation for the high incidence of compression of the fibers of the fifth lumbar nerve root.

Nerve compression by disease or injury can result in a variety of root symptoms, usually associated with pain of short duration. Pain often dominates the clinical picture, but not infrequently the patient complains of numbness, tingling and prickly sensations (i.e., paresthesias) localized to the dermatome supplied by the affected dorsal roots. If the ventral roots are involved, muscle spasm, weakness and vasomotor disturbances may accompany the pain. A knowledge of the radicular (segmental) distribution of the spinal nerves is helpful in evaluating root lesions which may lie in and around the vertebra of a given region.

Injury to the spinal nerves or their peripheral branches causes disturbances of both sensation and movement. Section of a dorsal root rarely produces a loss of sensation (anesthesia), although it may impair reflexes (hyporeflexia) initiated by appropriate stimuli in the areas supplied by that root. Owing to the overlapping distribution of fibers of adjacent roots, anesthesia will not be detectable unless several contiguous roots are injured or cut (Fig. 7-10). The hyporeflexia involves superficial and deep reflexes and it is associated with a diminution of tone (hypotonia) in the affected muscles.

The various activities of the central nervous system can be expressed only by impulses which impinge (i.e., synapse) upon neurons, somatic and visceral, whose axons pass peripherally to effector organs. The large α motor neurons of the anterior horn of the spinal cord give rise to axons which emerge via the ventral root and innervate striated muscle. The α motor neurons and their axons constitute anatomical and physiological units, referred to as the final common pathway or the *lower motor neuron* (2325). The concept of the lower motor neuron is not limited to the spinal cord, even though it is frequently used in that context. Cells of the motor cranial nerve

nuclei (nerves III, IV, V, VI, VII, IX, X, XI and XII) which innervate the muscles of the head and neck, also must be classified as lower motor neurons. Lesions selectively involving the lower motor neuron in the spinal cord, in the ventral root or in a peripheral nerve, produce weakness or paralysis, loss of muscle tone, loss of reflex activity and atrophy. All of these changes are confined to the affected muscles (386). Atrophy as a consequence of a lower motor neuron lesion develops gradually and in time is obvious on inspection.

Since the anterior horn cells that innervate a single muscle extend longitudinally through several spinal segments, and since several such cell columns exist at each spinal level, a lesion confined to one spinal segment will cause weakness, but not complete paralysis, in all muscles innervated by this segment. Complete paralysis will occur only when the lesion involves the column of cells in several spinal segments that innervate a particular muscle, or the ventral root fibers that arise from these cells. Because most appendicular muscles are innervated by fibers arising from parts of three spinal segments (Figs. 7-16–7-18), complete paralysis of a muscle implies a central lesion involving anterior horn cells in several spinal segments, or a lesion involving ventral root fibers from several spinal segments (Figs. 9-24 and 9-28). Since neighboring cell columns are likely to be affected at each level, such lesions usually produce paralysis in muscle groups rather than individual muscles.

The denervated muscle also shows certain changes in its reaction to electrical stimulation. Healthy muscle responds to stimulation by both the faradic (interrupted) and galvanic (continuous) current. In faradic stimulation, the response lasts as long as the stimulus is applied. In galvanic stimulation the response occurs only on closing or opening the circuit. Normally it is the application of the negative pole or cathode which produces the strongest contraction on closing the current. In the complete *reaction of degeneration*, which appears 10 to 14 days after nerve injury, the muscle no longer responds to stimulation of its motor nerve. However, the muscle still responds to direct stimulation with slow wavelike contractions, but it is the positive pole or anode which induces the strongest response on closing the circuit.

If preganglionic visceral fibers are involved by a lesion, as in the case of the thoracic and upper lumbar roots, there are sudomotor, vasomotor, and atrophic disturbances expressed by dryness and smoothness of the skin.

It becomes necessary to distinguish the deficits which occur as a consequence of lesions in spinal segments from those that occur in spinal roots, mixed spinal nerves and peripheral nerves. A lesion in ventral root fibers usually produces the same motor deficits as those resulting from destruction of anterior horn cells. However, at certain levels (i.e., thoracolumbar and sacral), section of ventral root fibers produces additional autonomic deficits which may not accompany lesions of the anterior horn cells. Section of a single ventral root, for example C5, would produce weakness in the supraspinatus, infraspinatus subscapularis, biceps brachii and brachioradialis, but not complete paralysis of any of these muscles. This pattern of distribution is unique to the C5 ventral root and different from that of any single peripheral nerve.

Lesions of mixed spinal nerves produce motor and sensory deficits that correspond to those of combined dorsal and ventral root lesions. While the motor deficits correspond almost exactly to those seen with pure lesions of the ventral root, sensory deficits follow a dermatomal distribution and tend to be less extensive because of the overlapping innervation characteristic of dermatomes. If only one mixed spinal nerve were injured, for example C5, the motor weakness would be the same as described above, but no sensory loss would be detectable. Involvement of several contiguous mixed spinal nerves would produce marked weakness or paralysis in the muscles innervated by those spinal segments and detectable sensory loss in at least one dermatome.

The above findings are in sharp contrast to the motor and sensory deficits associated with peripheral nerve lesions. With a peripheral nerve lesion the muscle paralysis and the sensory loss correspond to the peripheral distribution of the particular nerve.

In certain diseases of the lower motor neuron, the muscles exhibit small, localized spontaneous contractions known as *fascic-*

ulations. These muscle twitches, visible under the skin, represent the discharge of squads of muscle fibers innervated by nerve fibers arising from lower motor neurons. Fasciculations occur asynchronously in different parts of various muscles and are thought to be triggered by motor unit discharges that occur within the cell body of the motor neuron. Fasciculations commonly are seen in amyotrophic lateral sclerosis (Fig. 10-27), occasionally in acute inflammatory lesions of peripheral nerves and generally do not occur when the anterior horn cells are rapidly destroyed (i.e., acute poliomyelitis). The term *fibrillations*, frequently misused as the equivalent of the term fasciculations, refers to small (10 to 20 μV) potentials of 1 or 2 msec duration that occur irregularly and asynchronously in electromyograms of denervated muscle. These spontaneous discharges cannot be observed under the skin and produce no detectable shortening of muscles. These potentials represent the spontaneous activation of individual muscle fibers.

Regeneration of Injured Peripheral Nerves. Our knowledge of the processes of degeneration and regeneration has been greatly increased in recent years by investigations on mammalian nerves under various experimental conditions. Valuable information was obtained by clinical and surgical studies of the peripheral nerve injuries during the war. Seddon (2306) distinguished three types of nerve injury: (a) complete anatomical division; (b) crush or compression injuries in which the continuity of the nerve fibers is broken but the sheaths and supporting tissue remain intact; and (c) temporary impairment or nerve block. Nerve section nearly always demands surgical intervention to re-establish continuity. The recovery is more or less successful, but never complete, since many of the regenerating fibers fail to reach their respective end organs. After nerve crush there also is complete degeneration of the severed nerve fibers. Both nerve section and nerve crush are followed by loss of sensation and movement; wasting of muscles and reaction of degeneration. However, the damaged nerve fibers and their sheaths are in close anatomical contiguity after nerve crush, and subsequent regeneration usually leads to a nearly complete recovery.

In mild compression or block, there are varying degrees of paralysis, but electrical excitability remains normal. Because the nerve fibers are not severed, there is no peripheral degeneration. Recovery is more rapid; it begins in a few weeks and usually is completed within 2 or 3 months. These three types of nerve injury may appear as separate entities or in various combinations. Since the clinical symptoms after nerve section and crush are the same until regeneration is completed, surgical exploration usually is indicated to determine the nature of the injury (2441).

In a simple crush, although the continuity of the axons is interrupted, the endoneurium and other supporting tissues remain essentially intact. As a result, regenerating nerve fibers from the central stump can grow distally, traverse the minimal scar tissue between the severed axonal ends and enter appropriate Schwann cell tubes of the distal stump. After complete anatomical severance, the conditions are quite different at the site of injury. The cut ends are separated by a gap of variable extent which becomes filled with connective tissue and sheath cells, so that a scar of union is formed between the stumps. Hemorrhage and the vascular mesenchyme contribute cells to the scar tissue. These cellular elements in the lesion area seriously impede the growth of fine sprouts of regenerating axons from the proximal stump of the nerve. An enlarged heterogeneous mass at the cut end of a previously injured nerve is known as a *traumatic neuroma* (amputation or pseudoneuroma). It consists of Schwann cells, connective tissue cells and fibers, macrophages and an abundance of tangled aberrant nerve fibers. Such a skein of "lost" nerve fibers in scar tissue can be a most serious complication following peripheral nerve section or injury. Many of these fibers are "functional" processes of dorsal root ganglion cells, and these tangled ends can transmit nerve impulses into the spinal cord. Such neuromas explain why a patient may have localized "phantom pain" and/or paresthesias in a previously amputated hand or foot.

The behavior of the Schwann cells after anatomical severance is especially significant. About the 4th day, they become elongated and migrate out of the stumps into the scar, coming mainly from the peripheral stump but, to a lesser extent, also from the central one. These cells arrange themselves end to end, and form strands which traverse the fibrous tissue of the scar and establish continuity between the intact axons and the degenerating tubes of the peripheral stump. In some animals, under suitable conditions, gaps of 2 cm have been naturally bridged in this manner. In man gaps of several millimeters may be similarly bridged. Under most circumstances, however, the mass of scar tissue is too extensive to be handled by the sheath cells themselves, and surgical intervention is required. Scar tissue must be removed from both ends of the severed nerve, and these ends must be approximated and maintained by epineural sutures. The central axonal tips swell and produce a number of fine branches which enter the injured area by the 3rd day. At first they appear free in the connective tissue. Soon they apply themselves to the surface of the sheath cell strands and are led to the peripheral stump, where many of the branches enter the old Schwann cell tubes (Figs. 4-34 and 4-35). However, the number of fibers entering the distal tubes is always smaller after section of the nerve than after crush. Moreover, many nerve fibers enter tubes which are structurally unsuitable for full functional maturation. Once the fibers have entered the distal tubes, the processes of growth and maturation are the same as after crush. These are described in Chapter 4.

The rate of nerve regeneration has been studied by a number of investigators. After primary suture of the peroneal nerve in the rabbit, it takes about 7 days for the growing axon tips of the central stump to traverse the scar of the gap and reach the peripheral stump (987, 988, 2471). After crush the "scar" delay was about 5 days. Then the fastest axonal tips grew at the rate of 3.5 mm a day after suture, and 4.4 mm after a crush. Most of the axons grow distally at 3 mm a day after the peroneal nerve is crushed, and 2 mm a day after nerve section and suture. When the fine regenerated axons attain the periphery they increase in diameter and most of them ultimately become remyelinated. If a sufficient number of such fibers reach and successfully reestablish contact with appropriate sensory and motor end organs, there will be an eventual return of function. The total latent period in the rabbit between nerve regeneration and functional recovery was 20 days following nerve crush and 36 days after nerve suture.

In the longer nerves of man the process is slower, although a rate of 4.4 mm a day for growing axons was found after a crush of one of the digital nerves (226). The rate of functional regeneration falls off with the distance traversed, since increases in diameter and myelination occur more slowly in the distal portions of the fiber. A justifiable assumption for axonal growth in man under ideal conditions is about 3 mm/day. The average latent period until functional maturity after distal nerve injuries is 20 days after crush and 50 days after suture.

Regeneration can occur when two stumps are sutured after being left apart for a considerable period of time. However, it is generally agreed that functional recoveries after long-delayed sutures usually are unsatisfactory. The difficulties occasioned by long delay are due to a number of factors which interfere with the regenerative processes, and these effects become progressively more serious. Some of the factors may be briefly mentioned. After a long delay, the distal stump atrophies and the outgrowth of sheath cells is reduced or ceases. Hence good apposition of the cut nerve ends is difficult, and many axons fail to reach the degenerated atrophic Schwann cell tubes of the distal stump. The tubes themselves are greatly shrunken and receive fewer fibers, so that the chances for re-establishing appropriate peripheral connections are reduced. Myelinization is delayed and increase in diameter of the nerve fiber is restricted by the thickened endoneurium, which forms a large portion of the tube. Of special importance is the progressive atrophy of the muscles and end organs. In early stages, where the motor end plates remain intact and connected with the Schwann cell tubes, new fibers can enter directly and restore the original pattern. In later stages these channels become occluded and the end organs may completely disintegrate. The regenerating fibers often fail to enter the old sensory and motor endings or their previous locations. These fibers wander along the muscle fibers, ultimately forming new motor end plates of a more primitive character, whose distribution is irregular and different from the original pattern of innervation. All studies favor early nerve suture, perhaps 3 or 4 weeks after injury. At this time sheath cell activity is at its height and the somewhat thickened perineurium permits easier surgical apposition of the injured nerve stumps (2786). Delays of 6 months or more before suture may seriously interfere with the reparative processes but failure is not necessarily encountered in all cases. Good recovery is possible after long-delayed suture if enough axons reach appropriate Schwann cell tubes and the muscles are maintained in good condition by appropriate therapy. Sunderland (2470) has reported good restoration of function in human hand and finger muscles which had been denervated for 12 months.

CHAPTER 8

The Autonomic Nervous System

Portions of the central and peripheral nervous system concerned primarily with the regulation and control of visceral functions are termed collectively the *visceral, vegetative* or *autonomic nervous system* (Fig. 8-1).

The recognition of a vegetative nervous system is credited to Reil in 1807 (2315). Nearly 90 years later Langley introduced the term "autonomic nervous system" to include the cranial and spinal components of the vegetative nervous system and commented, "the word 'autonomic' does suggest a much greater degree of independence of the central nervous system than in fact exists, except perhaps in that part which is in the walls of the alimentary canal. But it is, I think, more important that new words should be used for new ideas than that the word should be accurately descriptive" (1424). Visceral reactions and functions are initiated mainly by internal changes that activate visceroceptors. Visceral motor responses in smooth muscle and glands are to a large extent involuntary and unconscious. Such visceral reactions as do reach conscious levels are vague, poorly localized and predominantly of an affective character. Tactile sensibility is practically absent, and temperature sense is appreciated only in certain places, such as the esophagus, stomach, colon and rectum. On the other hand, distention or spasms of the muscular walls of hollow viscera or blood vessels may produce severe distress or acute pain.

As defined by Langley (1425) the *autonomic system* was purely a visceral motor system consisting of "visceral efferent cells and fibers that pass to tissues other than the skeletal muscle." This rigid definition limited the term autonomic to a two neuron visceral efferent system, and excluded visceral afferent fibers. Yet sensory fibers accompany most visceral motor fibers and form the afferent links of most visceral reflex arcs. Visceral afferent fibers have their cells of origin in the spinal and specific cranial nerve ganglia (Figs. 8-2 and 9-28). They, like the higher brain centers, play a constant and dynamic role in the regulation of autonomic activities. In recent years the above limited concept has been liberalized to make the term "autonomic" more synonymous with "visceral," and to include both peripheral and central neural structures (1089). It behooves all concerned with visceral function to remember that central neurons and visceral afferent neurons are vital and integral parts of the autonomic system, regardless of arbitrary definitions. In similar fashion no attempt should be made to sharply delineate the nervous system into somatic and visceral portions. This is a convenient physiological subdivision, but the two are merely different parts of a single integrated neural mechanism. The higher brain centers regulate both somatic and visceral functions, and throughout most neural levels there is intermingling and association of visceral and somatic neurons. Moreover, visceral reflexes may be initiated by impulses passing through somatic afferent fibers from any receptor, and conversely visceral changes may give rise to somatic activities. Through some mechanism, as yet unexplained, stimulation of peripheral visceral efferent neurons also can alter the activity of somatic sensory receptors.

Interposed in the efferent peripheral pathway between the central nervous system and the visceral structures are aggregations of nerve cells known as the *autonomic ganglia*. The cells of these peripheral ganglia are in synaptic relation with fibers from the spinal cord or brain stem, and they send out axons which terminate in the visceral effectors: smooth muscle, heart muscle and glandular epithelium. There are fundamental differences in the innervation of striated and smooth muscle. In striated muscle, each muscle fiber is innervated by a single axon, but a single motor neuron may send axons to many muscle fibers. The nerve-muscle junction in striated fibers has a characteristic morphology and is called the motor end plate.

In smooth muscle the efferent axon has numerous swellings or varicosities which constitute sites of transmitter storage and release. There may be no specialized structure on the postjunctional membrane of the smooth muscle fiber, and not all muscle cells are innervated. Smooth muscle cells are often electrotonically coupled through gap junctions, so it is not necessary for each muscle fiber to be directly contacted by the axon (484, 2609). Peripheral autonomic neurons usually discharge at low frequencies, and may produce their maximal effect at rates of 4 to 10 Hz (997).

Pre- and Postganglionic Neurons. Unlike skeletal muscle, which is directly innervated by axons of centrally located neurons, the transmission of impulses from the central nervous system to the viscera always involves two different neurons (Figs 8-1 and 8-3). The first neuron, situated in the brain stem or spinal cord, sends a thinly myelinated *preganglionic* fiber to an autonomic ganglion, where it synapses with one or more *postganglionic* cells. Preganglionic fibers of the cranial and spinal nerves are approximately 3 μm in diameter, have slow conduction velocities (i.e., 3 to 15 m/sec) and are designated as the B fibers of peripheral nerves (1948). The usually unmyelinated axons of autonomic ganglion cells then pass as *postganglionic* fibers to visceral effectors (Fig. 9-28). Postganglionic autonomic axons have smaller diameters (0.3 to 1.3 μm), possess slower conduction velocities (0.7 to 2.3 m/sec) and are usually classified as C fibers in peripheral nerves (Table 4-2). Therefore even the simplest visceral reflex arc will involve at least three neurons: (a) visceral afferent, (b) preganglionic visceral efferent and (c) postganglionic visceral efferent (Figs. 8-2 and 9-28). Quantitative studies of mid-thoracic communicating rami in the cat show that about 10% of the axons in the white rami are sensory. About half of the sensory axons are unmyelinated. In the gray rami fewer than 1% of the axons are sensory (493, 494). While the number of afferent axons in the sympathetic rami is small, they will need to be considered in functional studies relating to visceral sensation.

The autonomic ganglia, which have a wide distribution in the visceral periphery, may be classified in three groups: (a) the *paravertebral*, (b) the *prevertebral (collateral)* and (c) the *terminal*. The paravertebral ganglia are arranged in a segmental fashion along the anterolateral surface of the vertebral column and are connected with each other by longitudinal fibers to form the two *sympathetic trunks* or ganglionated cords (Fig. 8-1). The prevertebral ganglia are irregular aggregations of cells found in the mesenteric neural plexuses surrounding the abdominal aorta and its larger visceral branches. The terminal ganglia are parasympathetic and are located within, or close to, the structures they innervate. These ganglia show extreme variations in size and compactness of organization. Some are organized into distinct anatomically encapsulated structures, as in the case of the sympathetic trunks and the autonomic ganglia of the head. Others form extensive plexuses of nerve cells and fibers, as in the intramural intestinal plexuses. Small ganglionic masses or scattered cell groups are found within, or near, the walls of visceral structures (e.g., heart, bronchi, pancreas and urinary bladder).

The outflow of preganglionic fibers from the central nervous system, which establishes synaptic connections with peripheral autonomic ganglia, arises from three well

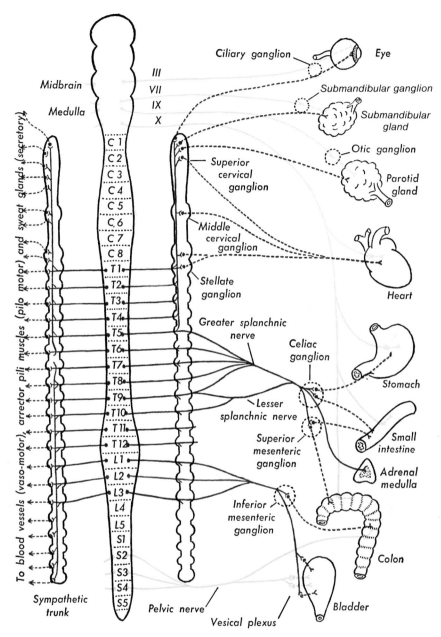

Figure 8-1. Schematic diagram showing general arrangement of the autonomic system. The sympathetic components are shown in *red*, while the parasympathetic components are in *blue*. *Solid lines* represent preganglionic fibers; *broken lines* indicate postganglionic fibers. For clearness the sympathetic fibers to the blood vessels, hair, and sweat glands are shown separately in Figure 8-2.

defined regions. The *cranial outflow* arises from visceral cell groups of the brain stem associated with the oculomotor, facial, glossopharyngeal and vagus nerves and emerges from the brain stem in association with these cranial nerves (*blue* in Fig. 8-1). Preganglionic fibers arising from these nuclei are parasympathetic and terminate

either in cranial autonomic ganglia (i.e., ciliary, pterygopalatine, submandibular or otic), or in terminal ganglia within the walls of thoracic or abdominal viscera (e.g., heart, lungs, esophagus and stomach). The *thoracolumbar outflow* arises from cells of the intermediolateral cell column in all thoracic and the upper two or three lumbar spinal

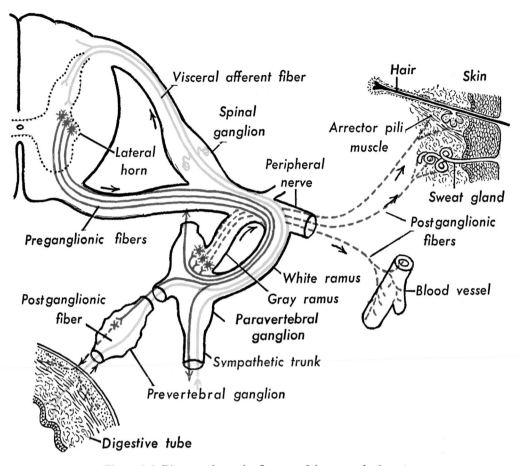

Figure 8-2. Diagram of neural reflex arcs of the sympathetic system.

segments. The peripheral processes of these cells give rise to preganglionic sympathetic fibers which emerge from the spinal cord via the ventral roots of the thoracic and upper lumbar spinal nerves (*red* in Fig. 8-1). Peripherally these fibers leave the mixed spinal nerve as the *white rami communicantes*, enter the sympathetic trunk and terminate upon cells in the paravertebral and prevertebral ganglia (Fig. 8-2). Although the thoracolumbar outflow arises from a cell column in a restricted region of the spinal cord (i.e., T1 to L3), it represents the total sympathetic output for the entire body. This is possible because some preganglionic sympathetic fibers ascend and descend in the sympathetic trunk for considerable distances before terminating upon postganglionic neurons. The *sacral outflow* arises from preganglionic visceral neurons in the second, third and fourth sacral segments of the spinal cord. These pregan-

glionic parasympathetic fibers emerge from sacral spinal segments via their corresponding ventral roots and pass to terminal ganglia within the walls of pelvic viscera (*blue* in Fig. 8-1).

Although preganglionic neurons are located in three distinct regions of the central nervous system, only two main divisions of the autonomic nervous system are recognized: (a) the *sympathetic* or *thoracolumbar system* and (b) the *parasympathetic* or *craniosacral system* (Figs. 8-1 and 8-2). In spite of the restricted central origins of preganglionic sympathetic and parasympathetic fibers, most viscera receive a double autonomic innervation. Notable exceptions are the glands of the skin and peripheral blood vessels, which receive only a sympathetic innervation. Peripherally fibers of the two divisions of the autonomic nervous system often are intermingled, but they retain their functional independence, which usually is antagonistic but closely integrated. The thoracolumbar outflow provides sympathetic innervation for all visceral structures of the body via synaptic articulations with postganglionic sympathetic neurons in peripheral autonomic ganglia. The cranial portion of the parasympathetic system supplies specific visceral structures in the head via postganglionic parasympathetic fibers from autonomic ganglia, and thoracic and abdominal viscera via the vagus nerve and postganglionic fibers from terminal ganglia. Pelvic viscera are innervated by the parasympathetic sacral outflow and postganglionic fibers from terminal ganglia. The investigation of the origin of autonomic preganglionic axons using horseradish peroxidase retrograde tracing methods is leading to some revision of the classical view. For example, there is evidence that some sympathetic fibers to the small intestine arise in the cervical sympathetic ganglia and reach the gut by traveling in the vagus nerve (1541). Where it was once thought that distinct portions of the gut were innervated by vagal and sacral parasympathetic fibers, it now appears that there is overlap in the descending colon and rectum (2260). There is some species difference in autonomic innervation of the heart and other viscera (503, 859). With further comparative studies employing newer tracing technics, it should be possible to provide a more accurate and detailed scheme of the organization of the mammalian peripheral autonomic innervation.

The Sympathetic System. The sympathetic trunks are two ganglionated cords symmetrically placed along the anterolateral aspects of the vertebral column that extend from the base of the skull to the coccyx. The cervical portion contains three ganglia formed by the fusion of the original eight segmental ganglia. The *superior cervical ganglion*, the largest of the paravertebral ganglia, is situated near the second and third cervical vertebrae. The small *middle cervical ganglion* (often absent), when present, lies near the sixth cervical vertebra. The *inferior cervical ganglion* lies at the lower border of the seventh cervical vertebra, behind the subclavian artery. This ganglion frequently fuses with the first thoracic ganglion to form the *stellate ganglion* (Fig. 8-1). In the thoracic,

lumbar and sacral regions, the ganglia are segmentally arranged. There are 11 or 12 thoracic, 3 or 4 lumbar and 4 or 5 sacral ganglia. In the sacral portion, the two trunks gradually approach each other and fuse at the coccyx in the unpaired coccygeal ganglion.

The prevertebral ganglia are irregular ganglionic masses surrounding the visceral branches of the aorta. The largest prevertebral ganglia are the paired celiac ganglia embedded in a mass of connective tissue and nerve fibers. Other prevertebral ganglia are the aorticorenal, the phrenic and the superior and inferior mesenteric. These ganglia are closely interconnected by numerous nerve fibers (Fig. 8-1) and will be described in relation to the celiac and subsidiary plexuses.

The sympathetic ganglia receive preganglionic fibers from the spinal cord through the ventral roots of all the thoracic and the upper two lumbar nerves (2003, 2316, 2317). These fibers leave the ventral roots, pass through the white rami communicantes and enter the sympathetic trunk, where they have two general destinations: (a) the paravertebral ganglia or (b) the prevertebral ganglia. Those that terminate in the paravertebral sympathetic ganglia either end in the first one entered, or pass up or down in the sympathetic trunk giving off collaterals, and finally terminate in ganglia above or below the level of their entrance (Fig. 8-1). The preganglionic fibers from the upper five thoracic nerves pass mainly upward and, in the cat, T1 contributes the smallest number of ascending fibers in the cervical sympathetic trunk (773). Those from the middle thoracic segments (T7 to T10) pass up or down, while those of the lowest thoracic and lumbar segments pass only downward. The preganglionic fibers that terminate in the prevertebral ganglia do not synapse in the paravertebral ganglia, but merely pass through them and emerge as the splanchnic nerves (Figs. 8-1 and 8-2). While the sympathetic pathway from the spinal cord to the viscera always involves two neurons, there are never more than two. Thus, synapses between pre- and postganglionic neurons occur either in the paravertebral or prevertebral ganglia, but not in both.

While the white rami communicantes are limited to the thoracic and upper lumbar nerves, each spinal nerve receives a *gray ramus communicans* from the sympathetic trunk (Fig. 8-2). The gray ramus consists of unmyelinated postganglionic fibers which innervate the blood vessels, arrector pili muscles and glands of the body wall.

The cervical sympathetic ganglia receive ascending preganglionic fibers from the white rami of the upper thoracic nerves, most of which go to the superior cervical ganglion.

The *superior cervical ganglion* gives rise to postganglionic fibers distributed as gray rami to: (a) the lower four cranial nerves, (b) the upper three or four cervical nerves, (c) the pharynx, (d) the external and internal carotid arteries and (e) the superior cervical cardiac nerve. Postganglionic sympathetic fibers passing to the external and internal carotid arteries form plexuses about these vessels and their branches (1718). From these vascular plexuses the postganglionic fibers pass through cranial autonomic ganglia to join branches of the cranial nerves. Such sympathetic postganglionic fibers supply the dilator muscle of the iris, the smooth muscle portion of the levator palpebrae, the orbital muscle of Müller, the blood vessels, sweat glands, hair of the head and face and the lacrimal and salivary glands (Fig. 8-3). The superior cervical cardiac nerve passes to the cardiac plexus.

The *middle cervical ganglion*, when present, supplies gray rami to cervical nerves C5 and C6, and sometimes also to C4 and C7. When this ganglion is absent these spinal nerves receive gray rami from the sympathetic trunk.

The *inferior cervical ganglion* furnishes gray rami to spinal nerves C7, C8 and T1 (Fig. 8-3). Thus a single ganglion may supply two or more of the lower cervical nerves, and a single nerve may be supplied by two ganglia. Potts (2050) has found that the lower four cervical nerves may each receive three gray rami derived from the sympathetic trunk and from the middle and inferior cervical ganglia. In addition, the middle and inferior cervical ganglia give off, respectively, the middle and inferior cardiac nerves, which take part in the formation of the cardiac plexus (Fig. 8-1).

The thoracic, lumbar and sacral ganglia furnish gray rami to the remaining spinal nerves. Delicate branches from the upper four or five thoracic ganglia go to the cardiac plexuses as the thoracic cardiac nerves. Other fibers from the inferior cervical ganglion reach the pulmonary plexuses to innervate the bronchial musculature and blood vessels of the lungs (Fig. 8-3). Shorter mediastinal branches from both the thoracic and lumbar ganglia form plexuses around the thoracic and abdominal aorta. In addition to these, there are two, sometimes three, important branches known as the *splanchnic nerves* which arise from the thoracic portion of the sympathetic trunk, pierce the diaphragm and terminate in the prevertebral ganglia of the mesenteric plexuses (Fig. 8-1). Although the splanchnic nerves appear to be branches of thoracic ganglia, they represent axons of preganglionic neurons which merely pass through paravertebral ganglia and the sympathetic trunk en route to the celiac and mesenteric ganglia. Thus the splanchnic nerves correspond to white rami communicantes. The *greater splanchnic nerve* arises by roots from the fifth to the ninth thoracic ganglia and goes to the celiac plexus. The *lesser splanchnic nerve* usually arises by two roots from the tenth and eleventh ganglia, and either unites with the greater splanchnic, or continues as an independent nerve to that portion of the celiac plexus which surrounds the roots of the renal arteries and terminates in the aorticorenal ganglion (1718). The *smallest splanchnic nerve*, when present, arises from the last thoracic ganglion and goes to the renal plexus. Often this nerve is represented by a branch from the lesser splanchnic nerve.

The *celiac plexus*, the largest of all autonomic plexuses, surrounds the celiac and superior mesenteric arteries. This asymmetrical paired plexus extends cranially to the diaphragm, caudally to the renal arteries and laterally to the suprarenal bodies. It becomes continuous below with the abdominal aortic plexuses. From the main plexus paired and unpaired subsidiary plexuses are given off which accompany the branches of the celiac and superior mesenteric arteries as well as other branches of the abdominal aorta. The paired plexuses include the phrenic, suprarenal and spermatic (or ovarian); the gastric, hepatic, splenic and superior mesenteric plexuses are unpaired. Within the celiac plexus are found two relatively large ganglionic

	SYMPATHETIC		PARASYMPATHETIC	
Structure Supplied	Preganglionic Cell Bodies in CNS Nuclei	Postganglionic Cell Bodies in Peripheral Ganglia	Preganglionic Cell Bodies in CNS Nuclei	Postganglionic Cell Bodies in Peripheral Ganglia
Iris of eye	intermediolateral nuc. in cord segments C8 – T2 (3)	sup. cervical ganglion and scattered along carotid plexus	Edinger-Westphal nuc. of midbrain	ciliary ganglion
Lacrimal gland	intermediolateral nuc. in cord segments T1 – 2	sup. and middle cervical symp. ganglia	sup. salivatory nuc. in pons	pterygopalatine ganglion
Submandibular and sublingual glands	intermediolateral nuc. in cord segments T1 – 3 (4)	sup. and middle cervical symp. ganglia	sup. salivatory nuc. in pons	submandibular ganglion
Parotid gland	intermediolateral nuc. in cord segments T1 – 3 (4)	sup. and middle cervical symp. ganglia	inf. salivatory nuc. in medulla	otic ganglion
Sweat glands of head and neck	intermediolateral nuc. in cord segments T1 – 3	3 cervical sympathetic ganglia		
Lungs and bronchi	intermediolateral nuc. in cord segments T1 – 5	inf. cervical and thoracic (T1 – 5) symp. ganglia	dorsal motor nuc. N. X	ganglia of pulmonary plexi
Heart	intermediolateral nuc. in cord segments T1-5 (6,7)	3 cervical and thoracic (T1-6) symp. ganglia	dorsal motor nuc. N. X	intra-cardiac ganglia of atria
Esophagus	intermediolateral nuc. in cord segments T1-6	thoracic symp. T(1-3) 4-6 ganglia	dorsal motor nuc. N. X	myenteric and submucous plexi
Stomach, small intestine; ascending and transverse colon	intermediolateral nuc. in cord segments T5-11	celiac and sup. mesenteric ganglia	dorsal motor nuc. N. X	myenteric and submucous plexi
Descending colon and rectum	intermediolateral nuc. in cord segments T12-L3	lumbar and inf. mesenteric symp. ganglia	autonomic nuc. of intermediate gray in cord segment S2-4	ganglia of hemorrhoidal myenteric and submucous plexi
Sex organs	intermediolateral nuc. in cord segments T10-L2	lumbar, sacral and inf. mesenteric symp. ganglia	autonomic nuc. of intermediate gray in cord segments S2-4	ganglia along branches of aorta and int. iliac arteries (e.g. ovarian, uterine)
Urinary bladder	intermediolateral nuc. in cord segments T12-L2	lumbar and inf. mesenteric symp. ganglia	autonomic nuc. of intermediate gray in cord segments S2-4	ganglia along vesical branches of int. iliac artery
Sweat glands and blood vessels of lower extremity	intermediolateral nuc. in cord segments L1-2	lumbar and sacral symp. ganglia		

Figure 8-3. Location of preganglionic and postganglionic autonomic neurons to important visceral structures.

masses, the *celiac ganglia,* lying on either side of the celiac artery and connected with each other by delicate fiber strands. Occasionally the two may be so close as to form a single unpaired ganglion encircling the artery. Other ganglionic masses found in the plexus include the paired aorticorenal ganglia and the *superior mesenteric ganglion* lying near the roots of their respective arteries. All these ganglia receive preganglionic fibers from the splanchnic nerves.

Caudally the celiac plexus becomes continuous with the abdominal aortic plexuses lying on either side of the aorta. From these plexuses nerve strands pass to the root of the inferior mesenteric artery and form the inferior mesenteric plexus, which surrounds that artery and its branches. Within this plexus and lying close to the root of the artery is another prevertebral ganglionic mass, the *inferior mesenteric ganglion* (Figs. 8-1 and 8-10). Further caudally, the abdominal aortic plexuses are continued into the unpaired *hypogastric* or *pelvic plexus*, which also receives strands from the inferior mesenteric plexus. On entering the pelvis the plexus breaks up into a number of subsidiary plexuses adjacent to the rectum, bladder and accessory genital organs (Figs. 8-8 and 8-10). The preganglionic fibers supplying the pelvic organs come from the white rami of the two upper lumbar nerves and from the lowest thoracic nerve. They pass through the corresponding ganglia of the sympathetic trunk, and terminate in the inferior mesenteric ganglion (Fig. 8-1). The cells of this ganglion then send their postganglionic axons by way of the inferior mesenteric and hypogastric plexuses to the pelvic viscera (Fig. 8-10).

The Parasympathetic System. The preganglionic fibers of the craniosacral division form synaptic relations with postganglionic neurons in cranial autonomic, or terminal ganglia.

Central neurons whose axons form parasympathetic preganglionic fibers of cranial nerves VII, IX and X in the rodent brain have been analyzed using retrograde tracing methods (516). The preganglionic cell bodies form a column extending from the level just below the obex to the level of the seventh cranial nerve in the pons. The column is rather compact and is located medial to the nucleus of the solitary tract and dorsolateral to the hypoglossal nucleus. At more rostral levels, the cell column is located progressively more laterally until the level of the facial nucleus; one group of cells sending axons in the greater superficial petrosal nerve (lacrimal neurons) is located lateral to the facial nucleus while neurons sending axons to the chorda tympani nerve or the otic ganglion are distributed more widely through the lateral tegmentum at the pontomedullary junction (516).

In the *cranial* region four ganglia are related topographically to the branches of the trigeminal nerve (Fig. 8-1). The *ciliary ganglion* lying against the lateral surface of the optic nerve receives preganglionic fibers from the visceral nuclei of the oculomotor complex (III) and sends postganglionic fibers (short ciliary nerves) to the sphincter of the iris and the smooth muscle of the ciliary body. The *pterygopalatine gan-*

glion, in the pterygopalatine fossa, and the *submandibular ganglion*, lying over the submandibular gland, receive fibers from the superior salivatory nucleus via the intermediate portion of the facial nerve (VII) (Figs. 8-1 and 12-20). The preganglionic fibers pass by way of the major petrosal nerve to the pterygopalatine ganglion, and by way of the chorda tympani nerve to the submandibular ganglion. The latter usually is broken up into submandibular and sublingual portions. The pterygopalatine ganglion sends postganglionic fibers to the lacrimal glands and to the blood vessels and glands of the mucous membranes of the nose and palate. Postganglionic fibers from the submandibular ganglion go to the submandibular and sublingual salivary glands and also to the mucous membranes of the floor of the mouth. The *otic ganglion* is situated medial to the mandibular nerve as it leaves the oval foramen. It receives preganglionic fibers from the inferior salivatory nucleus of the glossopharyngeal nerve (IX) by way of the minor petrosal nerve and sends postganglionic fibers to the parotid gland (Fig. 8-1). All of these cranial autonomic ganglia receive nerve filaments from the superior cervical ganglion, passing by way of the internal and external carotid plexuses. These filaments do not synapse with the ganglionic cells, but merely pass through the cranial parasympathetic ganglia to furnish sympathetic innervation to blood vessels, smooth muscle and glands.

The largest source of preganglionic parasympathetic fibers is the dorsal motor nucleus of the vagus nerve (X), which supplies practically all the thoracic and abdominal viscera except those in the pelvic region (Figs. 8-1, 8-3 and 11-24). In the thorax, these preganglionic fibers enter the pulmonary, cardiac and esophageal plexuses to be distributed to the terminal (intrinsic) ganglia of the heart and bronchial musculature. Short postganglionic fibers then go to the heart and bronchial muscle. In the abdomen, the parasympathetic fibers of the vagus nerve go to the stomach, and pass through the celiac and its subsidiary plexuses, to end in the terminal ganglia of the intestine, liver, pancreas and probably the kidneys. In the alimentary canal these terminal ganglia form the extensive ganglionated plexuses of Auerbach (myenteric) and of Meissner (submucosal). They extend the whole length of the digestive tube from the upper portion of the esophagus to the internal anal sphincter. These plexuses are composed of numerous small aggregations of ganglion cells intimately connected to each other by delicate transverse and longitudinal fiber bundles. From intramural neurons short postganglionic fibers terminate in the smooth muscle and glandular epithelium and serve motor and secretory functions. The alimentary innervation of the vagus extends as far as the descending colon (Figs. 8-1 and 8-3).

The *sacral* preganglionic parasympathetic fibers exit from the spinal cord via the second, third and fourth sacral nerves which form the *pelvic nerve* (N. erigentes) and go to the terminal ganglia of the pelvic plexuses, as well as to the myenteric and submucosal plexuses of the descending colon and rectum (Fig. 8-1). Postganglionic fibers from terminal ganglia supply the urinary bladder, descending colon, rectum and accessory reproductive organs. The sacral autonomic fibers innervate viscera not supplied by the vagus (Figs. 8-3 and 8-10).

A large number of nerve cell bodies are found in the wall of the gut. One group of cell bodies and connecting fibers is located in the submucosa, and another group lies between the layers of circular and longitudinal smooth muscle. The former is termed the submucosal plexus (of Meissner) and the latter the myenteric plexus (of Auerbach). It is currently thought that many of the autonomic cells of the gut probably do not receive synaptic input from sympathetic or parasympathetic afferents, and may constitute an independent "enteric nervous system" that represents a third division of the autonomic nervous system (865).

The enteric plexuses differ from the other autonomic plexuses in one important respect. They contain some intrinsic mechanism for local reflex action, since coordinated peristalsis occurs on stimulation of the gut after section of all the nerves which connect these plexuses with the central nervous system. The nature of this reflex mechanism is not fully understood.

It is evident from the above that all the autonomic plexuses consist of complicated intermixtures of sympathetic and parasympathetic fibers which are difficult to distinguish morphologically. It should be emphasized again that the sympathetic preganglionic fibers are interrupted in the paravertebral and prevertebral ganglia, while the parasympathetic preganglionic fibers pass by way of the plexuses to the terminal ganglia.

Visceral Afferent Fibers. There are numerous receptors in the viscera whose afferent fibers, myelinated or unmyelinated, travel centrally by way of the autonomic nerves, both sympathetic and parasympathetic. The largest myelinated fibers come principally from Pacinian corpuscles, while the smaller myelinated and the unmyelinated ones come from the more numerous diffuse visceral receptors (Fig. 6-4). Sensory fibers from the thoracic, abdominal and pelvic viscera traverse sympathetic and splanchnic nerves to reach the sympathetic trunk. They pass uninterruptedly through the trunk and white communicating rami to their perikarya of origin in the dorsal root ganglia (Figs. 8-2, 8-10 and 9-28). The parasympathetic nerves likewise contain many visceral afferent fibers. The visceral afferent fibers of the vagus nerve, whose cell bodies are in the inferior (nodose) ganglion, are distributed peripherally to the heart, lungs and other viscera. Similar fibers from the bladder, rectum and accessory genital organs pass by way of the pelvic nerves and enter the spinal cord through the second, third and fourth sacral dorsal roots (Fig. 8-10). Their cell bodies are located in corresponding sacral spinal ganglia. Visceral sensory fibers from the bladder also enter the spinal cord through the lower thoracic and lumbar spinal nerves (Fig. 8-10). The sacral visceral afferent fibers, which convey impulses from stretch receptors in the wall of the urinary bladder, play a dominant role both in reflex control and the mediation of vesical pain impulses. These afferents accompany the sacral parasympathetic outflow and convey the sensory impulses that signal bladder distension. The sensation of a distended bladder is abolished by anesthetic block of the pelvic nerves, resection of these nerves or the cutting of dorsal roots S2, S3 and S4. Visceral afferents from the bladder and adjacent viscera which ascend to the lumbar and lower thoracic dorsal root ganglia ap-

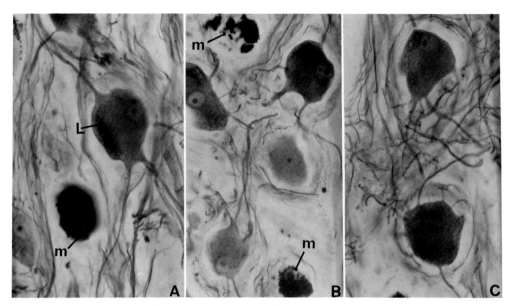

Figure 8-4. Adult human sympathetic neurons. Interdigitating dendrites often form a complex pericellular plexus. Perikarya frequently show eccentric nuclei, melanin granules (*m*), and lipofuscin granules (*L*). The nuclei of the capsule cells are not stained (Cajal silver stain, ×490).

pear to play a minor role in the regulation of the bladder. Resection of the presacral nerve and hypogastric plexus in man produces little or no alteration of vesical function.

The afferent visceral fibers are important in the initiation of various visceral and viscerosomatic reflexes mediated through the spinal cord and brain stem. Many of these reactions remain at a subconscious level, but afferent impulses also give rise to visceral pain or distress, nausea, hunger and other poorly localized visceral sensations. It is the constant stream of afferent visceral impulses that is responsible for the general feeling of internal well being, or of malaise.

Visceral pain from most abdominal and pelvic organs is carried chiefly by the sympathetic nerves. Vagal sensory fibers are concerned with specific visceromotor, vasomotor and secretory reflexes, most of which do not reach consciousness. It should be recalled that pain carried by visceral afferent fibers from diseased or inflamed organs may be "referred" to skin areas supplied by somatic afferent fibers of the same segment (see p. 173). The sense of taste is mediated by afferent fibers of the vagus, glossopharyngeal and facial nerves, while impulses giving rise to the sensation of hunger probably are carried by the vagus.

Up to 30% of the axons in lower lumbar and upper sacral ventral roots in some spinal cord segments are unmyelinated afferent fibers. The cell bodies of these axons are located in the dorsal root ganglion. Unlike most sensory fibers, the central process of these afferent neurons does not enter the cord through the dorsal root. Instead, the axon takes a recurrent course and enters the ventral root, finally terminating in the gray matter of the spinal cord. About one-third of the ventral root afferent fibers carry information from somatic structures, while the remaining two-thirds are visceral sensory afferents with receptive fields in the lower bowel and pelvis (490, 491, 2724).

Structure of Autonomic Ganglia. The autonomic ganglia are aggregations of multipolar neurons of varying size and shape, each surrounded by a connective tissue capsule. Trabeculae extending from the capsule form an internal framework which contains numerous, often pigmented perikarya, between which are irregular plexuses of myelinated and unmyelinated fibers (Fig. 8-4). Besides these ganglia, isolated autonomic cells or nonencapsulated aggregations of such cells are found widely distributed throughout the viscera.

The diameter of autonomic cells ranges from 20 to 60 μm, and the number and

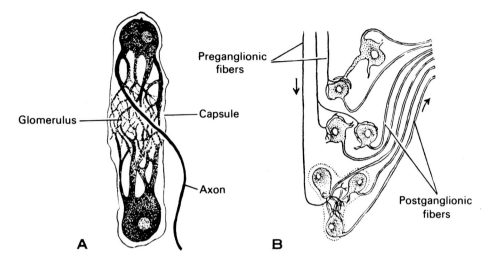

Figure 8-5. (A) Glomerulus formed by dendrites of two sympathetic ganglion cells (after Cajal, '11). (B) Diagram of the relationships between preganglionic fibers and sympathetic ganglion cells. One preganglionic fiber may come into synaptic relationships with several sympathetic postganglionic cells (after Ranson and Billingsley (2109)).

length of their branching dendrites is exceedingly variable. There may be as few as 3 or 4 on some perikarya, and as many as 20 on others. The cells have a clear ovoid and often eccentric nucleus, delicate neurofibrils and fine chromophilic bodies. Binucleated or even multinucleated cells are not uncommon. Most of the cells are surrounded by cellular capsules similar to those surrounding spinal ganglion cells (Figs. 4-7 and 7-2). Electron microscopic studies of autonomic ganglion cells reveal large pigmented granules, numerous small dense bodies and the usual perikaryonal components. Neuronal processes are readily identified as they emerge from cells or, when viewed without this continuity, by the striking number of synaptic and presynaptic junctions with which they are studded (2002). Processes filled with Nissl substance, mitochondria, large inclusion bodies and pigment particles usually are considered to be dendrites. Neuronal processes containing only neurofilaments and some smooth vesicles are regarded as axons, but the distinction between dendrites and axons on the basis of the presence or absence of Nissl substance is not easy to make. Furthermore there are no reliable morphological criteria for distinguishing between cells and fibers belonging to the sympathetic and parasympathetic systems.

Some of the cells have short dendrites which ramify within the capsules. These are numerous in the autonomic ganglia of man (Fig. 8-4). Others have long, slender dendrites which pierce the capsule and run for varying distances in the intercellular plexuses. Some cells possess both short and long processes. The intracapsular dendrites may arborize symmetrically on all sides of the cell or they may form interlocking dendritic processes between two or more cells, enclosed within a single capsule (Fig. 8-5A). Such cells probably receive common terminal arborizations of preganglionic fibers. The extracapsular dendrites have similar terminal arborizations at varying distances from the cell body.

Preganglionic fibers end in synaptic relation with the perikarya and dendrites of many postganglionic cells (Fig. 8-5B). They branch repeatedly within the ganglion and form pericellular arborizations; some of the terminals contain neurofibrillar rings or loops. More common are the axodendritic synapses where the preganglionic fibers end in diffuse arborizations about the intracapsular and extracapsular dendrites. These ganglia are not simple relays transmitting impulses between preganglionic and postganglionic neurons (1099). Small cells interpreted as internuncial neurons have been described (2722). Depending upon the species examined, these interneurons contain dopamine or norepinephrine. When treated with formaldehyde vapor or glyoxylic acid and viewed with ultraviolet illumination the catecholamine transmitter in the cell fluoresces brightly. Consequently these interneurons have become known as small intensely fluorescent, or SIF, cells (2723).

If the superior cervical ganglion (Fig. 8-1) is isolated by section of all incoming preganglionic fibers, the postganglionic perikarya do not degenerate. The isolated postganglionic perikarya may decrease slightly in diameter and show alterations of Nissl substance, endoplasmic reticulum and mitochondria, but they survive, i.e., the perikarya do not demonstrate transneuronal degeneration (126, 1013). However, following section of postganglionic axons of the cervical and ciliary ganglia, the perikarya show central chromatolysis and changes in their electrophysiological properties (126, 1177, 2679).

The capsule cells of the autonomic ganglia are known to contain a variety of enzymes (5, 2581). They have been considered as homologous to the oligodendrocytes by Schwyn (2297); to satellite and Schwann cells of dorsal root ganglia by Barton and Causey (126); or as connective tissue fibroblasts and interstitial cells. These supportive cells show a marked hyperplasia following stimulation of the preganglionic fibers for periods of 105 to 180 min (2297). Transmission through sympathetic ganglia is complex, and a detailed discussion is beyond the scope of this text. However, the student should be aware that, in addition to excitatory and inhibitory postsynaptic potentials (EPSP's and IPSP's) of short duration, the sympathetic postganglionic neurons may show very long-lasting postsynaptic responses (slow EPSP and slow IPSP). These slow PSP's, which may have a latency of many seconds and a duration measured in minutes, are generated by different ionic mechanisms than those causing the fast PSP's (659).

Chemical Mediation at Synapse. The investigations of Dale (589), Loewi (1513, 1514), Cannon (362) and many others have demonstrated that autonomic effects are mediated by chemical substances, known as *neurohumoral transmitters*, liberated at preganglionic and postganglionic nerve terminals. The neurohumoral transmitter of all preganglionic autonomic fibers, of all

postganglionic parasympathetic fibers and of postganglionic sympathetic nerve fibers innervating sweat glands is acetylcholine. Acetylcholine (ACh) also is the transmitter at somatic motor nerve terminals in skeletal muscle, and is involved in synaptic transmission at some sites in the central nervous system, although it is not the universal central transmitter. An impulse transmitted to an autonomic ganglion, or a somatic neuromuscular junction, causes the synchronous release of several hundred quanta of ACh stored in synaptic vesicles at axonal terminals. The transmitter diffuses across the synaptic cleft (20 nm) and combines with receptors on the postjunctional membrane, which may result in a localized depolarization and propagation of an impulse (see Chapter 4, p. 116). Dale (590) first proposed a functional classification of neurons: "Feeling the need of terms to describe nerve-fibres, or their impulses, in terms of a chemical function, which we can no longer regard as corresponding to their anatomical origin, I suggested the term 'cholinergic' to describe those which transmit their action by release of acetylcholine, and 'adrenergic' for those which employ a substance resembling adrenaline." At cholinergic junctions a specialized enzyme, *acetylcholinesterase* (AChE) which readily hydrolyzes free acetylcholine to choline and acetate is found in both the synaptic terminal and in the postsynaptic cell. Thus, AChE serves to terminate the transmitter action of ACh at postsynaptic sites and at effector junctions. Nerve impulses conveyed by cholinergic fibers produce rapid, localized responses of short duration in postjunctional effectors. ACh is the transmitter at various peripheral junctions but does not always have the same physiological effect on the postjunctional membrane. This is due to the existence of two different postjunctional receptor molecules to which ACh can bind to initiate a postsynaptic response. The action of ACh on one type of receptor is mimicked by the drug nicotine and on the other by the drug muscarine; hence the two receptor types are called nicotinic and muscarinic (see Chapter 4, p. 117). Atropine blocks all muscarinic responses to ACh and related cholinomimetic drugs. Nicotinic receptors in autonomic ganglia and skeletal muscle are not identical in that tetraethylammonium and hexamethonium selectively block ganglionic transmission, and *d*-tubocurarine blocks transmission at both the somatic motor end plates and at autonomic ganglia, although its action at the motor end plate predominates. Cholinergic neurons of the central nervous system also exhibit either nicotinic or muscarinic responses.

Drugs which inhibit or inactivate AChE cause ACh to accumulate at cholinergic sites and produce effects equivalent to continuous stimulation of cholinergic fibers. Physostigmine (eserine), neostigmine and edrophonium (tensilon) are "reversible" anticholinesterase drugs useful in treating myasthenia gravis, glaucoma and atony of smooth muscle. "Irreversible" anticholinesterase compounds form the basis for "nerve gases" which are among the most potent synthetic toxic agents known (1343).

The majority of postganglionic sympathetic nerves release norepinephrine as the transmitter substance and are classified as *noradrenergic*, although the older term, *adrenergic*, is widely used (364, 365, 720, 721, 1569, 1845). The widespread distribution of sympathetic nerves and the demonstration of monoaminergic neurons in the central nervous system suggest that monoaminergic mechanisms are of immense importance. The fundamental discovery (731) that certain monoamines and precursors could be made intensely fluorescent by formaldehyde gas led to the application of this principle to tissue sections (731, 732). This method permits anatomical localization of monoamines and investigations of problems related to the synthesis, storage, release and metabolism of the amines in neurons and their terminals (Figs. 4-15, 8-6, 12-32 and 13-22). Fluorescence histochemical observations indicate that in postganglionic sympathetic nerves, norepinephrine is present not only in synaptic terminals, but in the entire sympathetic neuron (720, 721, 730, 1845). Norepinephrine, as found by the fluorescence method, appears to be especially intense in enlargements of the nerve terminals referred to as varicosities. Terminal varicosities form a ground plexus in close contact with effector cells, and according to Hillarp (1098) the transmitter is released along the entire length of the terminals (Fig. 8-6). Evidence indicates that the norepinephrine content of the terminals

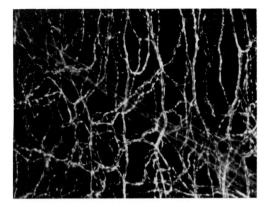

Figure 8-6. Normal rat iris. Strands of the adrenergic ground plexus over the dilator muscle are demonstrated by fluorescent histochemical technics. Several axons show pronounced varicosities (×250). (Courtesy of Dr. Torbjörn Malmfors, Karolinska Institutet, Sweden.)

can be depleted by electrical stimulation (1595, 1845). Thus there is little doubt that the varicosities are specialized structures involved in the storage and release of the transmitter. Histochemical studies have shown that the transmitter is stored in special granules within the adrenergic neurons and electron microscopic observations indicate that the storage granules and small "dense-cored" vesicles (Figs. 8-6 and 8-7) are identical (722, 2759). All parts of the sympathetic noradrenergic neuron contain norepinephrine, but the terminals contain the highest concentrations (720). Transmitter granules in adrenergic neurons are formed in the cell body, transported peripherally in the axon and stored in terminal varicosities (583, 1845) (see Chapter 4).

In the adrenal medulla the release of ACh by preganglionic sympathetic fibers and its combination with receptors on chromaffin cells is followed by the liberation of epinephrine into the extracellular fluid which ultimately enters the circulation. Osmophilic granules have been isolated from the adrenal medulla which contain high concentrations of catecholamines and collectively represent a major storage depot of epinephrine.

The adrenergic neuron also contains mechanisms for the inactivation of the transmitter substance, but these are not as rapid and efficient as those involved in the breakdown of acetylcholine. Monoamine

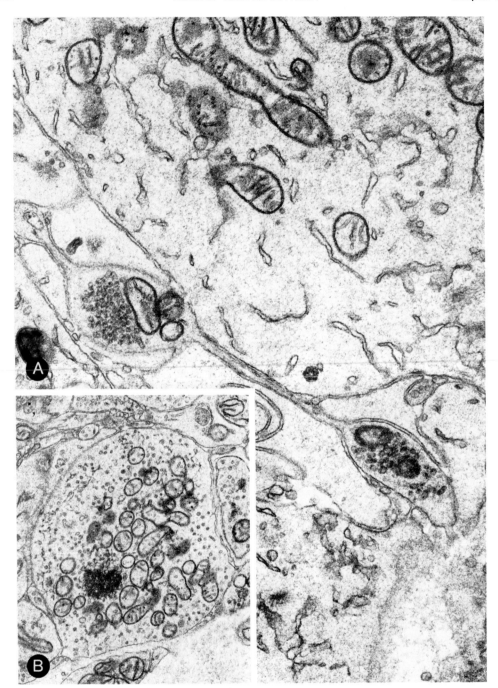

Figure 8-7. (*A*) A noradrenergic axon from the enteric nervous system of a mouse. The tissue has been fixed with NaMnO$_4$ to specifically reveal this axonal subtype. Note that the axon is varicose. Two varicosities appear in the field. Varicosities are thought to be points where neurotransmitter is released. They are distinguished by their swollen appearance and content of 50 nm synaptic vesicles that, after permanganate fixation, contain characteristic dense cores. Note that the varicosities seem to lack synaptic membrane specializations and that no preferential distribution of synaptic vesicles or an active zone can be discerned. The varicosities also contain accumulations of mitochondria. The narrow intervaricose segment between the two varicosities contains few organelles, and no synaptic vesicles or mitochondria. At the lower right, the noradrenergic terminal appears to end on the basal lamina that surrounds this portion of the enteric nervous system and that separates it from the

oxidase (MAO) is an intraneuronal enzyme considered to be involved in regulating the amine level within the neuron (367). The adrenergic transmitter released at synaptic junctions is inactivated by several mechanisms: (a) diffusion, (b) the enzyme catechol-*o*-methyl-transferase (COMT) which occurs extraneuronally and (c) binding to extraneuronal sites not involved in nerve conduction. The inactivating mechanism of greatest physiological importance is the reuptake of transmitter substance by adrenergic terminals. This uptake occurs at the neuronal cell membrane by an active mechanism called the amine pump (367, 1845). This pump in the nerve terminals has the ability to concentrate the amine more than 1,000 times.

Smooth muscle can be either excited or inhibited by norepinephrine, epinephrine and other catecholamines, depending upon the site and the concentration. Norepinephrine excites smooth muscle, isoproterenol inhibits smooth muscle and epinephrine can both excite and inhibit. Ahlquist (23) postulated two types of adrenergic receptors: (a) α receptors associated with excitatory responses and (b) β receptors associated with inhibition. There are two major exceptions to the above: (a) stimulation of β receptors in cardiac muscle produces excitatory effects and (b) stimulation of either α or β receptors in the gastrointestinal tract produces inhibitory responses that are additive. Synthetic compounds which structurally resemble naturally occurring catecholamines can combine with α or β receptors and produce sympathomimetic effects. The term *adrenergic blocking agent* is used for compounds that interfere with binding of the transmitter to postsynaptic receptors. Pharmacological studies with blocking agents have identified additional subtypes of both α- and β-adrenergic receptors (1715a, 1834).

Figure 8-7 shows autonomic axon terminals in the mouse alimentary tract. The dense core or granulated vesicles contain an adrenergic transmitter, whereas the clear, or nongranulated, vesicles are storage sites of other transmitter substances.

In early studies of the autonomic nervous system it was shown that every terminal of a given neuron released the same transmitter. This was first suggested by Sir Henry Dale and is known as Dale's principle:

It is to be noted, further, that in the cases for which direct evidence is already available, the phenomena of regeneration appear to indicate that the nature of the chemical function, whether cholinergic or adrenergic, is characteristic for each particular neurone, and unchangeable. When we are dealing with two different endings of the same sensory neurone, the one peripheral and concerned with vasodilatation and the other at a central synapse, can we suppose that the discovery and identification of a chemical transmitter of axon-reflex vasodilatation would furnish a hint as to the nature of the transmission process at a central synapse? The possibility has at least some value as a stimulus to further experiment (590).

Dale's dictum was subsequently extended to state that only one transmitter is synthesized and released from a terminal. Recent experimental evidence indicates that more than one neurotransmitter or neuromodulator is found in some neurons.

The terms "adrenergic" and "cholinergic" do not correspond completely with "sympathetic" and "parasympathetic," respectively. Thus the postganglionic fibers to the sweat glands (sudomotor fibers), although anatomically part of the sympathetic system, are cholinergic. Moreover they react to certain drugs, such as pilocarpine and atropine, in the same way as parasympathetic fibers. It should be recalled that the upper and lower extremi-

smooth muscle of the gut ×28,600). (*B*) (*inset*) A section through a noradrenergic varicosity is shown. The tissue was fixed with NaMnO$_4$ 1 hr following injection of a mouse with the neurotoxin, 6-hydroxydopamine. Noradrenergic axons actively take up and concentrate norepinephrine. 6-Hydroxydopamine is specifically taken up and concentrated by these axons because its chemical structure resembles that of norepinephrine sufficiently well for it to be subject to the norepinephrine transport mechanism. The 50 nm dense cored vesicles permit the varicosity to be identified as noradrenergic. The accumulation of dense material in the cytosol of the varicosity is an early degenerative change due to uptake of 6-hydroxydopamine. Note that the varicosity is apposed to the basal lamina. This is typical of autonomic postganglionic axon terminals and makes it necessary for the transmitter to act across a wide synaptic gap. (Courtesy of Dr. Michael D. Gershon, College of Physicians and Surgeons, Columbia University, New York.)

FUNCTION	SYMPATHETIC	PARASYMPATHETIC
Iris	dilates the pupil (mydriasis)	constricts the pupil (miosis)
Lacrimal gland	little or no effect on secretion	stimulates secretion
Salivary glands	secretion reduced in amount and viscid	secretion increased in amount and watery
Sweat glands of head, neck, trunk, and extremities	stimulates secretion (cholinergic fibers) nerve fibers	little or no effect on secretion
Bronchi	dilates lumen	constricts lumen
Heart	accelerates rate, augments ventricular contraction	decreases heart rate
GI motility and secretion	inhibits	stimulates
GI sphincters	constricts	relaxes
Sex organs	contraction of ductus deferens, seminal vesicle, prostatic and uterine musculature; vasoconstriction	vasodilation and erection
Urinary bladder	little or no effect on bladder	contracts bladder wall, promotes emptying
Adrenal medulla	stimulates secretion (cholinergic nerve fibers)	little or no effect
Blood vessels of trunk and extremities	constricts	no effect

Figure 8-8. Sympathetic and parasympathetic actions upon visceral structures.

ties have no parasympathetic nerve fibers. In these regions the sympathetic postganglionic fibers are of two distinct types: most are adrenergic, but those to the sweat glands are cholinergic (Figs. 8-8 and 8-9). There are other instances of mixed autonomic nerves. For example, the splanchnic nerves contain both adrenergic and cholinergic fibers. The latter are destined for the adrenal medulla, where acetylcholine is the transmitter substance. Overactivity of both adrenergic and cholinergic fibers is indicative of either autonomic imbalance, irritating lesions or abnormal regeneration along the course of the fibers. These may be expressed as excessive or abnormal sweating and salivation, alterations in gastrointestinal motility or increased peripheral vasoconstriction as in hypertension. Appropriate drugs can either enhance or inhibit impulses at the sympathetic and parasympathetic ganglionic synapses, or block the membrane receptor sites upon which the neurotransmitter substances produce their effects (e.g., muscle, heart, glands, blood vessels).

Denervation Sensitization. It was noted above that the postganglionic perikarya and their processes persist following section of the appropriate preganglionic fi-

bers. It is known that section of the preganglionic fibers results in increased sensitivity of the isolated neurons and the tissues they supply to circulating adrenaline. At least a part of the denervation hypersensitivity is due to an increase in adrenergic receptor sites on the postsynaptic cell membrane. The new receptor molecules are proteins and their synthesis is under genetic control, which in turn is influenced by diminished transmitter availability over a period of several weeks. This form of trophic interaction between pre- and postsynaptic neurons has been observed in many regions of the central and peripheral nervous system. It was observed that complete section of the postganglionic fibers to an organ or region resulted in far greater sensitization to adrenaline than that which followed complete preganglionic nerve section. Hampel (1019) observed the qualitative responses of the nictitating membrane of the cat to adrenaline on successive days after denervation. He found that the response reached a maximum about 8 days after preganglionic denervation. Postganglionic denervation resulted in sensitization responses that were twice as great as those that followed preganglionic section. Similar responses are observed in most other tissues supplied by

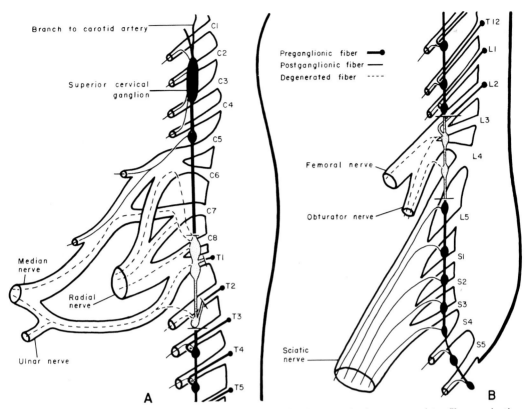

Figure 8-9. Anatomical course of preganglionic and postganglionic sympathetic vasoconstrictor fibers projecting to the upper and lower extremities. (*A*) After cervicothoracic ganglionectomy (inferior cervical ganglion, T1 and T2, *stippled*) all of the postganglionic fibers to the hand degenerate. (*B*) Resection of sympathetic ganglia L2 and L3 (*stippled*) interrupts only descending preganglionic fibers to lower lumbar and sacral sympathetic ganglia. Postganglionic fibers in the sciatic nerve to the foot region do not degenerate. (Modified from White et al. (2701).)

the adrenergic fibers. Increased sensitivity has been observed as well in structures supplied by the cholinergic fibers (e.g., lacrimal, sweat and salivary glands). The latter become sensitive to ACh, which is equally true of denervated skeletal muscle. This peculiar phenomenon often is referred to as Cannon's (363) law of denervation: "When in a series of efferent neurons a unit is destroyed, an increased irritability to chemical agents develops in the isolated structure or structures. The effect being maximal in the part directly denervated." Such denervation accounts for the increased sensitization of the superior cervical ganglion cells to acetylcholine which occurs after severance of its preganglionic fibers.

The paralysis after denervation of smooth muscle is very different from that seen in skeletal muscle where there is a persisting flaccid paralysis. Restoration of smooth muscle tone is due in part to the

sensitization of the neuroeffector mechanism to circulating epinephrine. The anatomical arrangement of the preganglionic and postganglionic sympathetic vasoconstrictor fibers to the hand and foot serves as an excellent example to illustrate this point (Fig. 8-9). In Reynaud's disease the small arteries and arterioles of the upper extremities, usually the hands, undergo episodic vasoconstriction in response to cold. As a result, the extremity demonstrates pallor and reactive hyperemia (i.e., an increased amount of blood in a part, or congestion). In chronic cases trophic changes develop with atrophy of the skin and subcutaneous tissues. Long-standing cases may develop skin ulceration or even ischemic gangrene. Removal of the inferior cervical, first and second thoracic sympathetic ganglia eliminates the vasoconstriction but destroys both the preganglionic as well as the postganglionic fibers to the forearm and hand (Fig. 8-9A). The smooth muscle of the arteries and arterioles will, in time, regain some vascular tone since the smooth muscle is also highly sensitized by removal of the postganglionic cells and fibers. Better results usually are obtained in the foot following removal of the second and third lumbar sympathetic ganglia (Fig. 8-9B). Here the partial sympathectomy interrupts the preganglionic outflow. However, it leaves intact the postganglionic cells and fibers in the lower lumbar and sacral ganglia which reach the foot through the sciatic nerve and its branches. Thus the vessels of the leg and foot regions are less sensitized to neurohumoral catecholamines.

Central Autonomic Pathways. Visceral structures innervated by the autonomic nervous system normally maintain a constant internal environment within the organism (homeostasis). Preganglionic neurons within the central nervous system (Figs. 8-1 and 8-3) are maintained in a continuous, but quantitatively variable, state of activity by a multitude of segmental and suprasegmental mechanisms. Regulation from higher levels is accomplished by multiple neuron pathways. This regulation appears to be mediated, in part, by a series of synaptic relays between several interposed neurons located at successively lower levels of the brain stem (i.e., it is a somewhat diffuse multisynaptic descending system).

The hypothalamus commonly is regarded as the principal locus of central autonomic integration (see p. 552). Simply stated, the most voluminous afferent connections of the hypothalamus originate from the hippocampal formation, the amygdaloid nuclear complex and the olfactory cortex, and indirectly from cortical regions which form portions of the limbic lobe (1820, 2090). Many of these structures are involved in neural circuitry that begins in the septal region and extends in a paramedian zone through the preoptic region and hypothalamus into the rostral mesencephalon (Fig. 16-7). In this view the hypothalamus is the central part of a continuum which suggests the term "septo-hypothalamo-mesencephalic continuum" (1820). There are a great number of reciprocal connections between structures within this subcortical continuum and phylogenetically older derivatives of the forebrain.

Investigations using silver impregnation methods for degenerating axons indicated no direct descending connections from the hypothalamus that extended beyond the mesencephalic tegmentum (980, 2090, 2757). Later studies applying newer tracing and immunohistochemical methods, showed that hypothalamic neurons project directly to medullary autonomic nuclei and the spinal cord (187, 2255, 2484) (Figs. 10-23, 11-27 and 16-11). Mesencephalic structures receive an input from the hypothalamus via: (a) a descending component of the medial forebrain bundle, (b) the mammillary bodies (mammillotegmental tract) and (c) descending projections in the periventricular gray (Fig. 16-10). Hypothalamic impulses conveyed to the mesencephalon are transmitted to more caudal parts of the neuraxis via numerous synaptic relays within the brain stem reticular formation, as well as the smaller number of direct projections (1816). It is presumed that reticular neurons convey impulses to visceral motor nuclei in the brain stem and spinal cord.

In the midbrain and upper pons, these descending tracts are located dorsally and medially near the central gray matter and floor of the fourth ventricle (237, 450, 2364, 2757). In man and most mammals that have been studied, the fibers descending into the upper midbrain stream through the prerubral field and region above the red nucleus. Stereotaxic surgery for dyskinesia in this area of the human brain has resulted in widespread autonomic deficits (372). These deficits included ptosis (drooping) of the eyelid, miosis (constriction) of the pupil and a loss of sweating (hemianhydrosis) on the same side (ipsilateral) of the body as the lesion. In man these descending fibers are uncrossed below the level of the red nucleus. These fibers are located more laterally in the pontine tegmentum and reticular formation of the medulla. Through this descending fiber system, the hypothalamus and other suprasegmental structures contribute to the regulation of a variety of visceral reflex activities (e.g., blood pressure, body temperature, sweating, secretion, eye, vesicle, rectal and sexual reflexes). Lesions of these descending central tracts can result in a complete loss, or altered control, of visceral activities at lower segmental levels. For example, lesions in the lateral reticular formation of the medulla interrupt the fibers regulating sympathetic control of the smooth muscle of the eye and may result in a Horner's syndrome (see p. 228).

A most unusual clinical entity (2151– 2154) serves as an excellent example of the disseminated and abnormal functional activities of these descending autonomic fibers. The authors originally postulated a central, possibly congenital, diencephalic origin to account for these symptoms in children of Jewish extraction: deficiency of lacrimation; transient and extreme elevation in blood pressure induced by mild anxiety; excessive sweating and drooling of saliva; and the occurrence of sharply demarcated, bilateral and symmetrical erethymatous blotches on the skin (*familial dysautonomia* or *Riley-Day syndrome*). Subsequent study has revealed other disturbances that support a diagnosis of this syndrome. These include postural hypotension, feeding difficulties from birth onward, a relative indifference to pain, erratic control of body temperature, emotional lability, absent corneal reflexes and corneal anesthesia, absent deep tendon reflexes, abnormal pupillary response to methacholine and an abnormal intradermal response to histamine. Hypotonus, poor motor coordination and developmental retardation may accompany the above findings. The precise pathological causes remain unknown, but lesions have been found in the thalamus, reticular formation of pons and medulla, spinal cord, sympathetic ganglia and the myenteric plexus (2154).

Bilateral lesions of the lateral white funiculi may result in altered sweating in regions supplied by the cord segments below the level of such lesions. Control of the bladder and rectum also may be lost. After spinal cord transection the autonomic reflexes are at first depressed (spinal shock), temperature regulation and sweating are absent and blood pressure falls profoundly. Weeks later, after spinal shock has waned, segmental reflexes caudal to the lesion reappear. Somatic segmental reflexes in time become exaggerated, but visceral reflexes usually are sluggish.

FUNCTIONAL CONSIDERATIONS

Gaskell (853) pointed out that when a visceral structure is innervated by both sympathetic and parasympathetic fibers, the effects of the two are as a rule antagonistic. The sympathetic neurons dilate the pupil, accelerate the heart, inhibit intestinal movements and contract the vesical and rectal sphincters. The parasympathetic neurons constrict the pupil, slow the heart, further peristaltic movement and relax the above named sphincters (Fig. 8-8). The apparently haphazard effects on smooth and cardiac muscle produced by each autonomic division in different organs (contraction in one, inhibition in another) are more readily explained when the *overall* activities of the two systems are taken into consideration. The parasympathetic deals primarily with anabolic activities concerned with the restoration and conservation of bodily energy and the resting of vital organs. In the words of Cannon (362):

A glance at these various functions of the cranial division reveals at once that they serve for bodily conservation; by narrowing the pupil they shield the retina from excessive light; by slowing the heart rate they give the cardiac muscle longer periods for rest and invigoration; and by providing for the flow of saliva and gastric juice, and by supplying the necessary muscular tone for the contraction of the alimentary canal, they prove fundamentally essential to the processes of proper digestion and absorption, by which energy-yielding material is taken into the body and stored. To the cranial division belongs the great service of building up reserves and fortifying the body against times of need and stress.

The sacral division supplements the cranial by ridding the body of intestinal and urinary wastes.

On the other hand, stimulation of the sympathetic component equips the body for the intense muscular action required in offense and defense. It is a mechanism that quickly mobilizes the existing reserves of the body during emergencies or emotional crises. The pupils dilate, respiration is deepened and the rate and force of the cardiac contractions are increased. The blood vessels of the viscera and the skin are constricted, the blood pressure is raised and an ample blood supply is made available to the skeletal muscles, lungs heart and brain. The peaceful activities are slowed or stopped; blood is drained from the huge intestinal reservoir, peristalsis and alimentary secretion are inhibited and the urinary and rectal outlets are blocked by contraction of their sphincters.

The two systems are reciprocal, and their dual activities are integrated into coordinated responses ensuring the maintenance of an adequate internal environment to meet the demands of any given situation. The parasympathetic activities are initiated primarily by internal changes in the viscera themselves. The sympathetic system is in considerable part activated by exteroceptive impulses that pass over somatic afferent fibers and are initiated by favorable or unfavorable changes in the external environment.

The preganglionic fibers of the sympathetic system arise from a continuous cell column in the spinal cord, and a single fiber may form synaptic relations with many cells in different paravertebral or prevertebral ganglia (Fig. 8-5B). Both types of ganglia are placed at considerable distances from the organs innervated, and from them postganglionic fibers are distributed to extensive visceral areas (Figs. 8-1 and 8-10). Such a mechanism permits a wide radiation of impulses. The norepinephrine released at most sympathetic terminals further enhances the widespread and prolonged effects of sympathetic stimulation. Thus, stimulation of a thoracic ventral root, or white ramus, causes piloerection and vasoconstriction in five, six or even more segmental skin areas.

In the parasympathetic system the preganglionic neurons are represented by more isolated cell groups whose fibers pass out in separate nerves and go directly to the terminal ganglia within or near the organs. Each preganglionic parasympathetic fiber enters into synaptic relations with fewer postganglionic neurons than is the case in the sympathetic division. Thus in the superior cervical ganglion of the cat, the ratio of preganglionic fibers to postganglionic neurons is about 1:15 or more, while in the ciliary ganglion the ratio is only 1:2 (2758). Parasympathetic action is more discrete and is limited to the portion stimulated. The liberation and rapid hydrolysis of acetylcholine by the parasympathetic postganglionic fibers is compatible with such localized autonomic responses. Thus stimulation of the glossopharyngeal nerve increases pa-

rotid gland secretion, while stimulation of the oculomotor nerve constricts the pupil, in each case without the appearance of other parasympathetic effects.

The functions of the two subdivisions of the autonomic system are most easily understood by contrasting the individual structures innervated and noting the reciprocal actions of their dual nerve supply (Fig. 8-8). The autonomic fibers to the eye provide an excellent example of this dual innervation. The sympathetic division stimulates the smooth muscle fibers of the dilator muscle of the iris, the tarsal muscle and the orbital muscle (of Müller). The tarsal muscle extends from the levator palpebrae muscle to the tarsal plate of the upper lid and aids in full elevation of the upper eyelid. The orbital muscle, at least in lower forms, keeps the ocular bulb forward in the bony orbit. Lesions in either the central or peripheral sympathetic pathways to the eye produce a triad of symptoms known as *Horner's syndrome*. As a result of sympathetic injury, the parasympathetic innervation is unopposed, and results in constriction of the ipsilateral pupil (miosis), dropping of the upper eyelid (pseudoptosis) and an apparent sinking in of the eyeball (enophthalmos). Vasodilation and dryness of the skin of the face also may be evident. Sympathetic fibers destined for the eye follow the internal carotid artery, while those to sweat glands on the face course along the branches of the external carotid artery. This dichotomy of postganglionic fibers from the cervical ganglia explains the altered patterns of autonomic function that can occur after injuries of the face, deep neck or within the skull. There may be loss of sweating on the face with preservation of sympathetic innervation to the eye or vice versa. Lesions of the cervical sympathetic trunk, inferior cervical ganglion or ventral roots of the upper thoracic nerves interrupt the fibers before they divide to follow separate courses.

Parasympathetic fibers to the eye stimulate the sphincter muscle of the iris and bring about constriction of the pupil. These axons also stimulate the ciliary muscle. Contraction of the circular fibers of the ciliary muscle causes relaxation of the ciliary zonule and thereby decreases the tension of the lens capsule. As a result of such

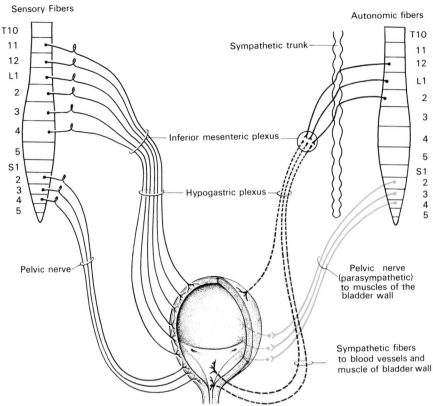

Figure 8-10. Schematic diagram of the sensory and autonomic innervation of the urinary bladder. Preganglion parasympathetic visceral motor (*blue*) fibers from S2, S3 and S4 pass to terminal ganglia which give rise to postganglionic fibers that induce contractions of the detrusor muscle. Afferent impulses from stretch receptors (*black*) in the bladder wall enter upper lumbar and lower thoracic spinal segments via the hypogastric plexus, and S2, S3 and S4 spinal segments via the pelvic nerve. Descending sympathetic fibers (*red*) in the hypogastric plexus play no essential role in micturition. Somatic motor fibers from S2, S3 and S4 spinal segments (not shown) innervate the external vesicle sphincter. Relaxation of the external sphincter and contraction of the detrusor muscle are essential for micturition.

parasympathetic activity, the pupil is constricted and the convexity of the lens is increased for near vision (accommodation).

Innervation of the salivary glands was long believed due solely to secretory fibers in the cranial parasympathetic nerves (Fig. 8-8). Many differences have been found between the several glands of the different species studied, but both parts of the autonomic system send secretory fibers to the salivary glands. Sympathetic fibers provide for vasoconstriction of blood vessels, contraction of the myoepithelial cells of the ducts and secretory fibers to the demilune gland cells (94). Stimulation of the human sympathetic trunk in the neck, or the injection of adrenaline into the salivary duct, evokes a flow of saliva from the submandib-

ular, but not from the parotid gland. The secretory response to sympathetic stimulation is of short duration when compared to the long acting response that follows parasympathetic stimulation (704). Parasympathetic fibers in cranial nerves VII and IX provide for vasodilation of the blood vessels and secretory fibers to the alveolar and acinar cells of the parotid, submandibular, sublingual and retrolingual glands. The vagus nerve contains secretory fibers to the glands of the trachea and upper digestive tract. For additional details on the innervation of the salivary glands the reader is referred to the extensive reviews by Babkin (94), Lundberg (1538), Burgen and Emmelin (328) and Emmelin (703).

The innervation of the urinary bladder

and the control of micturition represent a complex and specific autonomic function of great practical importance (Fig. 8-10). The smooth muscle of the urinary bladder exhibits two types of activity: (a) intermittent contractions which occur as the organ adapts its capacity to an increasing volume and (b) sustained contractions associated with relaxation of the external sphincter which occur during micturition.

Visceral motor fibers of S2, S3 and S4 leave the sacral nerves, and as the *pelvic nerve*, course to the lateral wall of the bladder where the fibers terminate in small vesical ganglia. Short postganglionic parasympathetic fibers to the bladder musculature induce contraction of the detrusor smooth muscle (Fig. 8-10). Somatic motor fibers from sacral spinal segments 2, 3 and 4 become incorporated in the *pudendal* (pudic) *nerve*, and via a branch of that nerve, the perineal nerve, innervate the external vesicle sphincter. Relaxation of the external sphincter (somatic nerves) and contraction of the bladder wall (sacral visceral motor) are the two events essential for micturition. The descending sympathetic fibers in the hypogastric plexus play no essential motor role in the process of urination. They innervate the vesical trigone and lower ureter, and are concerned with vasomotor control and the mechanism of ejaculation.

Afferent impulses responsible for the detrusor reflex arise from stretch receptors in the bladder wall and enter the spinal cord via the pelvic nerves (2204, 2509). If the bladder is greatly distended, afferent impulses pass via the hypogastric nerves and plexus to reach their perikarya (spinal ganglia) and spinal segments T10 to L2 (Fig. 8-10). When the intravesical pressure attains a certain value, the detrusor muscle contracts, the external sphincter relaxes and the bladder is effectively emptied. *Vesical afferents* ascending in the hypogastric nerves serve as a sensory input to the "vesical center for retention of urine" located in cord segments T12 to L2. It should be recalled that the desire to urinate is dependent upon intravesical pressure rather than fluid-volume content. The vesical capacity and frequency or urination vary with age and are influenced by reflex, psychic and local irritative factors. In chil-

dren 8 to 10 years of age the initial desire to void occurs with an intravesical pressure of 9 to 11 cm of water (bladder volume 80 to 100 ml of urine). In adults with a fluid capacity of 140 to 180 ml, an intravesical pressure of 15 to 16 cm of water induces the desire to void (360). The most essential sensory fibers from the bladder return to the spinal cord via the pelvic nerve and dorsal roots S2, S3 and S4. These afferents participate in reflexes that are integrated with the "vesical center for bladder evacuation" located in cord segments S3 to S5. The sacral afferent impulses to the spinal cord apparently reach conscious level through the long pathways which are poorly defined. It has been suggested that these pathways lie in the dorsal half of the lateral funiculus (125, 1574, 2204). Facilitating and inhibiting suprasegmental influences upon spinal mechanisms concerned with micturition suggest that regions in the pontine and midbrain tegmentum are involved (2513). In addition the cerebral cortex appears to exert some control over bladder function. Clinical studies indicate that portions of the superior frontal gyrus on the medial surface of the hemisphere may be specially concerned with control of micturition and defecation (66). Lesions in this region, involving one or both frontal lobes, may cause urgency, frequency of micturition or incontinence. Such lesions also are associated with lack of awareness of all vesical events including the sensation of the desire to micturate and the sensation that micturition is imminent. Disturbances of bladder function associated with spinal cord injury are described on p. 309.

A familiarity with the information in Figure 8-8 proves most useful in evaluating the overall functional status of the autonomic nervous system. Vital body processes such as circulation, secretion, digestion and excretion are essentially autonomic reflex responses. The autonomic nervous system also participates in many somatic-visceral and visceral-somatic reflexes which involve either cranial or spinal nerves (e.g., respiration, pupillary, lacrimal, palatal, pharyngeal, sneeze, cough, swallowing, vomiting, carotid sinus, vasomotor, sudomotor, pilomotor, vesicle, genital and emotional reflexes). Some of these reflexes will be presented as individual nerves are discussed.

Metabolic or mechanical irritations of autonomic nerve fibers in the periphery may cause exaggerations of some of the sympathetic and parasympathetic functions included in Figure 8-8. Partial or complete lesions of autonomic fibers may occur in either the central or the peripheral nervous system (Fig. 10-27). An appreciation of the nuclei, fiber pathways and resulting reflex deficits from injuries can be useful as a diagnostic aid in exploring the diffuse distribution of the autonomic system. In the periphery the postganglionic sympathetic fibers that rejoin spinal nerves (Fig. 8-2) have a distribution which compares closely to that of the sensory dermatomes (609, 2148). Hence changes in cutaneous sudomotor and vasomotor reflexes, changes in skin temperature and increased skin resistance to passage of a minute electric current implicate the involvement of sympathetic nerve fibers. A knowledge of dermatomal and peripheral nerve distributions (Figs. 7-11, 7-12, and 7-16–7-18), correlated with the segmental nuclear origins of autonomic neurons (Figs. 8-1 and 8-3), often can provide additional evidence to substantiate both the location and level of a nerve injury.

CHAPTER 9

Spinal Cord: Gross Anatomy and Internal Structure

The spinal cord is the least modified portion of the embryonic neural tube and the only part of the adult nervous system in which the primitive segmental arrangement clearly is preserved.

GROSS ANATOMY

The spinal cord is a long, cylindrical structure, invested by meninges, which lies in the vertebral canal. It extends from the foramen magnum (Fig. 1-4), where it is continuous with the medulla, to the lower border of the first lumbar vertebra (Fig. 1-6). The spinal cord has two enlargements, cervical and lumbar, each associated with nerve roots which innervate, respectively, the upper and lower extremities (Fig. 9-1). Caudal to the lumbar enlargement, the spinal cord has a conical termination, the *conus medullaris* (Figs. 1-6 and 9-1). A condensation of pia mater, extending caudally from the conus medullaris, forms the *filum terminale*; the latter structure penetrates the dural tube at levels of the second

sacral vertebra, becomes invested by dura and continues as the coccygeal ligament to the posterior surface of the coccyx (Fig. 1-6).

While the spinal cord is a continuous unsegmented structure, the 31 pairs of spinal nerves associated with localized regions produce an external segmentation (Fig. 9-1). On the basis of this external segmentation, the spinal cord is considered to consist of 31 segments, each of which receives and furnishes paired dorsal and ventral root filaments (Fig. 9-2). The spinal cord is divided into the following segments: 8 cervical, 12 thoracic, 5 lumbar, 5 sacral and 1 coccygeal. Up to the 3rd month of fetal life the spinal cord occupies the entire length of the vertebral canal, but after that time the differential rate of growth of the vertebral column exceeds that of the spinal cord. At birth the conus medullaris is located near the L3 vertebra; in the adult it is between the L1 and L2 vertebrae, and occupies only the upper two-thirds of the

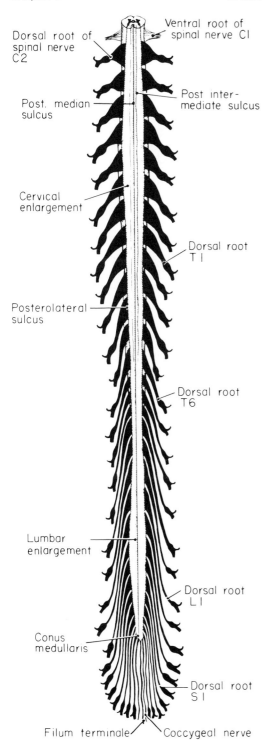

Figure 9-1. Posterior view of spinal cord showing attached dorsal root filaments and spinal ganglia. *Letters* and *numbers* indicate corresponding spinal nerves.

vertebral canal (Fig. 9-3). The sites of emergence of the spinal nerves do not change, but there is a lengthening of root filaments between the intervertebral foramina and the spinal cord; this is most marked for the lumbar and sacral spinal roots. These roots descend for a considerable distance within the dural sac before reaching their respective intervertebral foramina. The large number of lumbosacral roots surrounding the filum terminale is known as the *cauda equina* (Fig. 1-6). Spinal nerves emerge from the vertebral canal via the intervertebral foramina. The first cervical nerve emerges between the atlas and the occiput (Fig. 1-4). The eighth cervical root emerges from the intervertebral foramen between C7 and T1; all more caudal spinal nerves emerge from the intervertebral foramina beneath the vertebrae of their same number (Fig. 9-3). Dorsal root fibers usually are absent in the first cervical and the coccygeal roots, and there are no corresponding dermatomes for these segments. (Figs. 7-11–7-13).

The spinal cord, like all of the central nervous system, is derived from the embryonic neural tube. The central canal, lined by ependymal cells, represents the vestigial lumen (Fig. 9-4).

The length of the spinal cord from its junction with the medulla to the tip of the conus medullaris is about 45 cm in the male and 43 cm in the female. In contrast, the length of the vertebral column is about 70 cm. Its weight is about 35 g. In the midthoracic region, the transverse and sagittal diameters are about 10 mm and 8 mm, respectively; in the cervical enlargement (sixth cervical), 13 to 14 mm and 9 mm; in the lumbar enlargement (third lumbar), about 12 mm and 8.5 mm (see Fig. 9-5).

General Topography. When freed from its meninges, the surface of the cord shows a number of longitudinal furrows (Figs. 9-1, 9-2, 9-6 and 9-7). On the anterior surface, an *anterior median fissure*, penetrating the cord for a depth of some 3 mm, contains an epipial fold with sulcal branches of the anterior spinal artery and vein (Fig. 20-2). On the posterior surface is the shallow *posterior median sulcus*. This sulcus is continuous with a delicate glial partition, the *posterior median septum*, which extends into the cord and reaches the deep-lying gray.

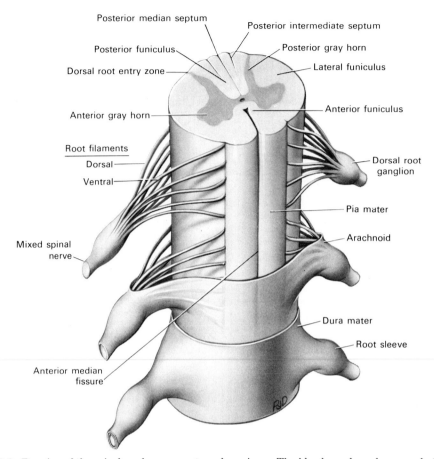

Posterior median septum
Posterior intermediate septum
Posterior funiculus
Posterior gray horn
Dorsal root entry zone
Lateral funiculus
Anterior gray horn
Anterior funiculus
Root filaments
Dorsal
Ventral
Dorsal root ganglion
Pia mater
Arachnoid
Mixed spinal nerve
Dura mater
Root sleeve
Anterior median fissure

Figure 9-2. Drawing of the spinal cord, nerve roots and meninges. The blood supply and venous drainage of the spinal cord are shown in Figures 20-1 and 20-2.

Lateral to the midline posteriorly are two less distinct sulci associated with spinal roots. The *posterolateral sulcus* is a shallow furrow into which filaments of the dorsal roots enter the spinal cord (Fig. 9-6). The *anterolateral sulcus* marks the site of emergence of ventral root fibers. Since ventral filaments emerge at less regular intervals and are less numerous than dorsal roots, the anterolateral sulcus may be more difficult to distinguish (Fig. 9-2). In cervical and upper thoracic spinal segments, the *posterior intermediate sulcus* indents the spinal cord between the posterior median and posterolateral sulci (Figs. 9-2 and 9-6). This sulcus is associated with a glial partition the *posterior intermediate septum* that extends internally toward the spinal gray (Figs. 9-2 and 9-6). The anterior median fissure and posterior median septum divide the cord into incompletely separated halves

connected by a narrow commissure, composed of gray and white matter.

Although the spinal cord is a symmetrical structure, it is not uniform in diameter. It contains two enlargements, cervical and lumbar, associated with the largest nerve roots which innervate the extremities. The *cervical enlargement*, consisting of the four lowest cervical segments and the first thoracic segment, gives rise to the nerve roots that form the *brachial plexus* (Figs. 9-1 and 9-3) and provide innervation for the upper extremity (Figs. 7-14 and 7-15). The *lumbar enlargement* (Figs. 9-1 and 9-3) gives rise to fibers that form the *lumbar plexus* (L1 to L4) and the *sacral plexus* (L4 to S2). Spinal segments vary in cross-sectional diameters and in length. Thoracic spinal segments have the greatest length while sacral segments have the shortest length. The tapered terminal portion of the spinal

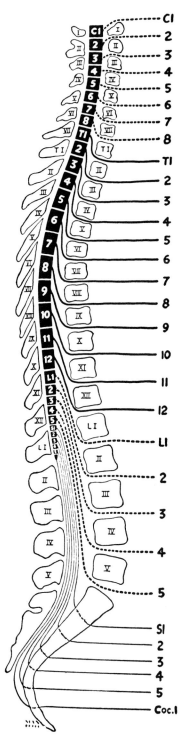

cord, the *conus medullaris*, consisting of sacral spinal segments, provides cutaneous innervation to the saddle area, motor innervation for the sphincters and parasympathetic innervation for the bladder (Fig. 8-10). The *filum terminale* extending caudally from the conus medullaris lies in the lumbar cistern surrounded by lumbosacral nerve roots forming the *cauda equina* (Figs. 1-6 and 9-1).

In transverse section the spinal cord consists of: a) a butterfly-shaped central gray substance composed of collections of cell bodies and their processes and b) a surrounding mantle of white matter composed of bundles of myelinated fibers, most of which are either ascending or descending (Figs. 9-2 and 9-7). The symmetrical butterfly-shaped gray consists of cell columns, some of which extend the length of the spinal cord and vary in configuration at different levels (Figs. 9-5 and 9-6).

Each half of the spinal cord has a *posterior gray column* or *horn* which extends posterolaterally almost to the surface near the root entry zone. An *anterior gray column* or *horn* extends anteriorly but does not reach the surface. Thoracic spinal segments are characterized by a small, pointed *lateral horn* near the base of the anterior horn (Fig. 9-7). A *gray commissure*, connecting the gray substance of the two sides, encompasses the central canal. Surrounding the central canal is a light granular area composed mainly of neuroglia, known as the central gelatinous substance (substantia gliosa). Anterior to the gray commissure is a bundle of transverse fibers, the *anterior white commissure*, composed of crossing fibers arising from nerve cells in the gray substance (Fig. 9-7).

Ascending and descending fibers occupying particular regions of the white matter of the spinal cord are organized into more or less distinct bundles (Figs. 9-6 and 9-13). Fiber bundles having the same, or similar, origin, course and termination are known as *tracts* or *fasciculi*. The white matter of the spinal cord is divided into three paired *funiculi*: posterior, lateral and anterior. The *posterior funiculus* lies between the posterior horn and the posterior median septum (Fig. 9-2). In upper thoracic and cervical regions a small *posterior intermediate septum* divides each posterior funiculus into

Figure 9-3. Diagram of the position of the spinal cord segments with reference to the bodies and spinous processes of the vertebrae (1059).

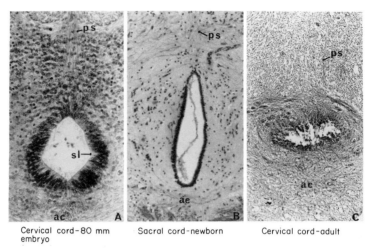

Cervical cord-80 mm   Sacral cord-newborn   Cervical cord-adult
embryo

Figure 9-4. Ependymal cells and central canal of embryonic and adult human spinal cord. The sulcus limitans (*sl* in *A*) becomes lost in the adult. Processes of the ependymal cells entering the posterior median septum (*ps*) can be seen and the fibers of the anterior white commissure are identified (*ac*) (*A*, Holmes silver stain, ×263; *B*, Luxol fast blue-cresyl violet, ×112; *C*, Holmes silver-cresyl violet, ×108).

two white columns. The *lateral funiculus* lies between the dorsal root entry zone and the site where ventral root fibers emerge from the spinal cord; the *anterior funiculus* lies between the anterior median fissure and the emerging ventral root filaments. The posterior funiculus is the largest and is composed almost exclusively of long ascending and short descending fibers that arise from cells in the spinal ganglia.

The *cervical enlargement*, consisting of the four lowest cervical segments and the first thoracic segment, gives rise to nerve roots which form the *brachial plexus* (Figs. 7-14 and 7-15). The *lumbar enlargement* (Figs. 7-19 and 7-20) gives rise to fibers that form the *lumbar plexus* (L1 to L4) and the *sacral plexus* (L4 to S2).

Although the spinal cord constitutes only 2% of the central nervous system, its functions are tremendously important since it: (a) receives afferent imputs via the dorsal roots from somatic and visceral receptors in most parts of the body, (b) gives rise to ascending pathways which transmit impulses to higher levels of the neuraxis, (c) gives rise to fibers emerging in the ventral roots that innervate somatic and visceral effectors, (d) conveys descending pathways from higher levels of the nervous system and (e) participates in a variety of somatic and autonomic reflexes. Meninges surrounding the spinal cord and nerve roots are described in Chapter 1 and the blood

supply of the spinal cord is discussed in Chapter 20.

INTERNAL STRUCTURE

The microscopic appearance of the adult spinal cord is vastly altered from the three-layered embryonic neural tube (Fig. 3-4). The incoming and outgoing processes of ganglion cells and intrinsic neurons produce marked changes in the embryonic marginal and mantle layers. The embryonic layers become longitudinal columns of gray and white matter in the adult spinal cord, each having microscopic landmarks and subdivisions (Figs. 9-2 and 9-6). Individual segments of the spinal cord show variations at different levels, for there is great variation in the size and number of fibers in the individual spinal nerves (Fig. 9-1).

Gray and White Substance

The gray and white matter are composed of neural elements supported by an interstitial neuroglial framework. The mesodermal structures comprise the blood vessels and their contents. The larger vessels are accompanied by prolongations of pial connective tissue. The gray matter contains the nerve cells, dendrites and portions of myelinated and unmyelinated nerve fibers. These fibers are axons of nerve cells located in the gray matter which pass into the white matter, or portions of the axons in the white matter which enter the gray to terminate.

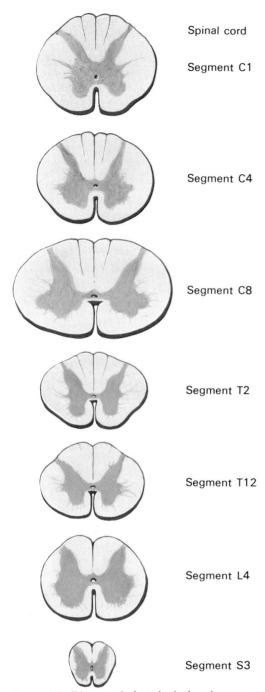

Spinal cord

Segment C1

Segment C4

Segment C8

Segment T2

Segment T12

Segment L4

Segment S3

Figure 9-5. Diagram of selected spinal cord segments at different levels showing the variations in size, shape and topography of gray and white matter.

The preponderance of neurons, neuroglia and capillaries imparts a firm consistency to the H-shaped gray substance (Fig. 9-7). This density is enhanced further by a multitude of fine glial processes, fibrils, synap-

tic terminals and dendrites, which invests neurons in an intricate meshwork, or *neuropil*. In sections stained with either hematoxylin and eosin or cresyl violet, the gray substance has a highly cellular appearance, while the fibrous elements of the neuropil are unstained (Figs. 9-12, 9-14, 9-19 and 9-21). In such sections only the neuronal perikarya, glial and endothelial nuclei are apparent. The enormous dendritic plexus of the neurons and their synaptic endings remain unstained (Fig. 4-24). Lorente de Nó (1532) has estimated that the soma of the perikaryon forms only 6% of the surface of a neuron. Hence the unstained neuropil of the gray matter in Figure 9-12 is where most dendritic plexuses are located. The central canal, surrounded by ependymal cells, is located in the cross bar of the H-shaped gray matter (Figs. 9-4 and 9-7). A sharply delineated central canal is seen only in fetal and newborn spinal cords. In the adult the ependymal lining often is discontinuous and the lumen may contain debris, round cells, macrophages and neuroglial processes (Fig. 9-4C). Surrounding the central canal are clumps of fibrous astrocytes rarely seen in other parts of the gray matter (Figs. 5-2 and 5-12). The two slender bands of gray matter above and below the central canal form the posterior and anterior gray commissures.

The white matter contains few neurons or dendrites, but is composed of ascending and descending myelinated and unmyelinated nerve fibers. The longitudinally arranged fiber bundles and their supportive neuroglial cells surround the gray matter as the posterior, lateral and anterior white funiculi. Numerous myelinated axons can be observed entering or leaving the white funiculi as dark fibers in sections stained by the Weigert method (Figs. 9-7–9-10). The structure and distribution of the glial cells are presented in Chapter 5. The processes of the astrocytes form a *superficial glial membrane* which is adherent to the deep surface of the pia mater (Figs. 1-8 and 1-9).

Spinal Cord Levels

Different levels of the spinal cord vary: (a) in size and shape, (b) in the relative amounts of gray and white matter and (c) in the disposition and configuration of the gray matter (Fig. 9-5). Cervical spinal seg-

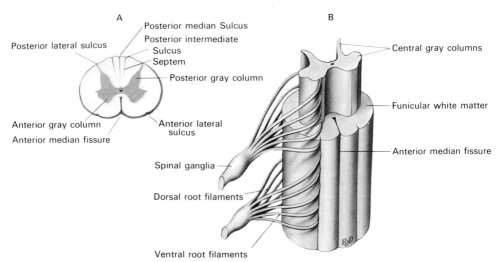

Figure 9-6. (*A*) Diagram showing internal arrangement of gray and white matter of the spinal cord. (*B*) External and internal topography of cervical spinal cord.

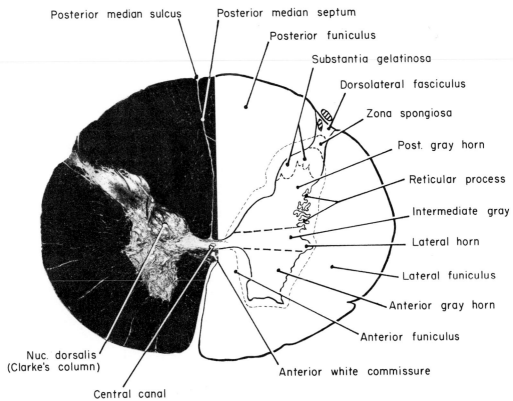

Figure 9-7. Section through a lower thoracic segment of adult human spinal cord to demonstrate subdivisions of the gray and white matter. Photograph of Weigert's myelin stain on *left* and schematic drawing on *right*. Area surrounding the gray matter, and limited peripherally by the *dotted line*, is composed of shorter ascending and descending fibers of the fasciculus proprius system.

ments contain the largest number of fibers in the white matter because: (a) descending fiber systems have not yet contributed fibers to lower segmental levels and (b) as-

cending fiber systems, augmented at each successively rostral segment, reach their maximum. The gray cell columns are maximal in the cervical and lumbar enlarge-

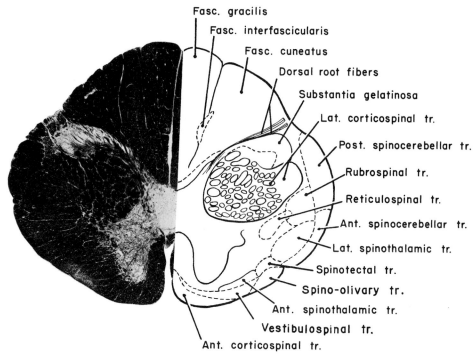

Fasc. gracilis
Fasc. interfascicularis
Fasc. cuneatus
Dorsal root fibers
Substantia gelatinosa
Lat. corticospinal tr.
Post. spinocerebellar tr.
Rubrospinal tr.
Reticulospinal tr.
Ant. spinocerebellar tr.
Lat. spinothalamic tr.
Spinotectal tr.
Spino-olivary tr.
Ant. spinothalamic tr.
Vestibulospinal tr.
Ant. corticospinal tr.

Figure 9-8. Section through upper portion of first cervical segment of adult human spinal cord. Some of the important fiber tracts are identified (Weigert's myelin stain, photograph).

ments which are associated with the larger nerves that innervate the extremities. Lumbosacral segments contain large amounts of gray matter, relative to both the size of the cord segments and the amount of white matter (Figs. 9-18 and 9-20).

Cervical Segments. These segments are characterized by their relatively large size, relatively large amounts of white matter and an oval shape (Figs. 9-5 and 9-8–9-10). The transverse diameter exceeds the anteroposterior diameter at nearly all levels. On each side the posterior funiculus is divided by a prominent posterior intermediate septum into a *fasciculus gracilis* (medial) and a *fasciculus cuneatus* (lateral).

In the lower cervical segments (C5 and below) related to the brachial plexus, the posterior horns are enlarged, and well developed anterior horns extend into the lateral funiculi (Figs. 9-11 and 9-12). Near the neck of the posterior horn is a serrated cellular area known as the *reticular process* (reticular nucleus); this process is present throughout all cervical segments. In upper cervical segments (C1 and C2) the posterior horn is enlarged, but the anterior horn is relatively small (Figs. 9-8–9-10). The

transverse diameter of the most rostral cervical spinal segment is about 12 mm, while this same diameter at C8 may be 13 to 14 mm.

Thoracic Segments. These segments show variations at different levels (Figs. 9-5, 9-7, 9-13 and 9-16). Both the fasciculi gracilis and cuneatus are present in upper thoracic segments (T1 to T6), while only the fasciculus gracilis is seen in the posterior funiculus at more caudal levels. In general the anterior and posterior horns are small and somewhat tapered; the first thoracic segment is an exception in that it forms the lowest segment of the cervical enlargement and contributes to the brachial plexus. A prominent, but small, lateral horn is present at all thoracic levels and contains the intermediolateral cell column which gives rise to preganglionic sympathetic efferent fibers (Figs. 9-13 and 9-14). At the base of the medial aspect of the posterior horn is a rounded collection of large cells, the *dorsal nucleus of Clarke* (Figs. 9-7, 9-13, 9-14 and 9-16). While this nucleus is present in all thoracic segments, it is particularly well developed at T10 through T12. The large cells of this nucleus have a characteristic appearance in that

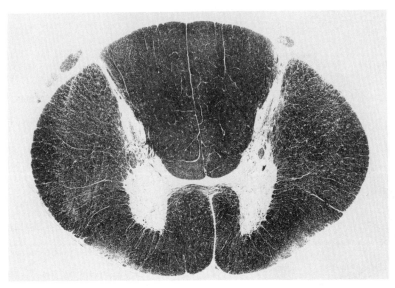

Figure 9-9. Photomicrograph of a transverse section through the second cervical segment of the adult human spinal cord. Note the narrowness of the anterior and posterior gray horns and the abundant white matter. Cell groups are identified in Figure 9-11 (Weigert's myelin stain).

their large vesicular nuclei often are eccentric, and chromophilic material is distributed peripherally in the perikaryon (Fig. 9-17).

Upper thoracic spinal nerves, except for T1, supply motor innervation only to axial musculature (i.e., the back and intercostals). Lower thoracic nerves supply the same muscles and the abdominal musculature. Thus the anterior horns of lower thoracic spinal segments are a little larger. The small diameter of the thoracic segments is due primarily to the marked reduction of gray matter (Fig. 9-13).

Lumbar Segments. These segments are nearly circular in transverse section, have massive anterior and posterior horns and contain relatively and absolutely less white matter than cervical segments (Figs. 9-5, 9-18 and 9-19). The fasciculi gracilis which compose the posterior funiculus are not as broad as at higher levels, especially near the gray commissure, and have a highly characteristic configuration (Fig. 9-18). The well developed anterior horns have a blunt process that extends into the lateral funiculi; motor cells in this process in segments L3 through L5 innervate large muscle groups in the lower extremities. Upper lumbar levels (L1 and L2) resemble lower thoracic spinal segments (Figs. 9-7 and 9-16) in that they contain the dorsal nucleus of

Clarke and the intermediolateral cell column. The dorsal nucleus of Clarke is especially well developed at L1 and L2. The transition between T12 and L1 is subtle, and these levels are difficult to identify precisely.

Sacral Segments. These segments are characterized by their small size, relatively large amounts of gray matter, relatively small amounts of white matter and a short, thick gray commissure (Figs. 9-5, 9-20 and 9-21). The anterior and posterior horns are large and thick, but the anterior horn is not bayed out laterally as in lumbar spinal segments. In caudal sequence sacral segments conspicuously diminish in overall diameter but retain relatively large proportions of gray matter. The substantia gelatinosa is particularly well developed in sacral segments, and this accounts for the thickened posterior gray column (Figs. 9-20 and 9-22A). Coccygeal segments resemble lower sacral spinal segments but are reduced in size (Fig. 9-22B). The posterior gray horn and especially the substantia gelatinosa are greatly increased in size, while the anterior gray horn becomes smaller.

Nuclei and Cell Groups

The butterfly-shaped gray matter of the spinal cord contains an enormous number of neurons of varying size and shape. Basi-

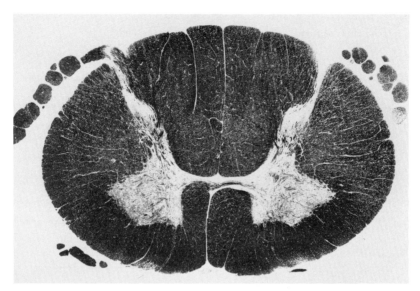

Figure 9-10. Photomicrograph of a transverse section through the fourth cervical segment of the adult human spinal cord demonstrating entering dorsal root fibers. At this level the substantia gelatinosa is larger and a well-developed lateral process of the anterior gray horn is seen. Cell groups in the spinal gray are identified in Figure 9-11 (Weigert's myelin stain).

cally these cells can be classified as root cells and column cells.

Root cells lie in the anterior and lateral horns and give rise to axons which exit via the ventral root to innervate somatic or visceral effectors through one or more peripheral nerves. *Column cells* are neurons whose peripheral processes are confined within the central nervous system. On the basis of the length, course and synaptic articulations of axons, these cells can be classified as *central, internuncial, commissural* or *association neurons.* A relatively large number of column cells give rise to fibers that enter the white matter, bifurcate and ascend or descend for variable distances. Some of these fibers form parts of intersegmental fiber systems, while other fibers have long processes which ascend to higher levels of the neuraxis and transmit impulses related to specific sensory modalities. Nerve cells are organized in the gray matter into more or less definite groups which extend longitudinally and are referred to as cell columns or nuclei. In the neuroanatomical sense, a nucleus consists of a collection of cells with common cytological characteristics whose axons can be followed to a common termination and subserve the same function. Most of our information concerning the structural organiza-

tion of the central nervous system is centered around this simple concept.

The spinal gray also contains Golgi type II cells whose short unmyelinated axons do not reach the white matter, but terminate in the gray close to their origin. Some Golgi type II cells may be commissural in that their axons cross to the gray of the opposite side, while others ascend or descend variable distances as intersegmental fibers.

Nuclear groups as well as their dendritic patterns are observed best in longitudinal sections of the cord following thionin and Golgi staining procedures. However, this plane of section is difficult for the beginning student to interpret. Transverse sections cut at 80 to 100 μm and stained with thionin, or cresyl violet, provide a more complete picture of neuronal groupings as shown in Figures 9-12, 9-14, 9-19 and 9-21. Such nuclear groups are most prominent in the human newborn. Thicker sections demonstrate more perikarya, but certain cellular details are lost or compromised.

Cytoarchitectural Lamination

A variety of eponyms and inconsistent terminologies have long been used to describe the nuclear groups in the spinal gray. Terminology has been based largely upon cytological features (i.e., cell size, shape,

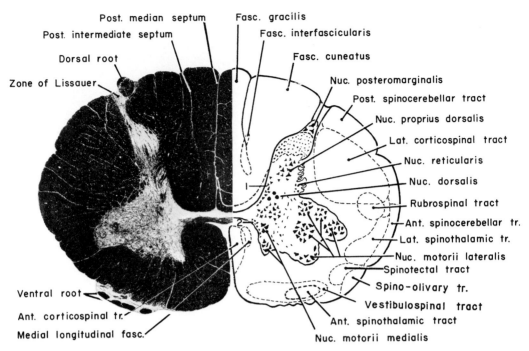

Figure 9-11. Section through eighth cervical segment of adult human spinal cord. The important cell groups and fiber tracts are identified. *1*, Nucleus cornucommissuralis posterior; *2*, nucleus cornucommissuralis anterior (Weigert's myelin stain, photograph).

processes and appearance) and the topographic location of cells within the spinal gray matter, but this scheme has been rather crude. While some believe that the terminology should be based upon synaptology (according to synaptic connections of neurons), this suggestion appears overly complex. The most satisfactory terminology is based upon the cytoarchitectural lamination of the spinal gray evident in thick sections (80 to 100 μm) of the spinal cord stained with cresyl violet. In a series of papers Rexed (2135–2137) described an architectural organization of neurons in the cat spinal cord that has proven to be valuable in research and has gradually become the accepted standard. His several zones have been corroborated and used by many investigators to describe terminal arborizations of fibers within the spinal gray. It is generally accepted that a similar lamination or zoning of the gray matter exists in all mammals. Examination of the spinal cord segments in the newborn and adult human has revealed cytoarchitectural laminae comparable to those described by Rexed in the cat (2583). This lamination of cell populations within the spinal gray has

become the most precise and most widely used method for describing cell groups within the mammalian spinal cord (Figs. 9-12, 9-14, 9-19, 9-21 and 9-23).

Studies of the *cytoarchitectonic organization* of the spinal gray recognize nine distinct cellular laminae in most regions, which are represented by Roman numerals and an area X (Fig. 9-12). Area X, the gray substance, surrounding the central canal, is present in all segments and appears fairly uniform throughout the spinal cord.

Thick frozen sections of the human spinal cord from different segmental levels are shown in Figures 9-12, 9-14, 9-19 and 9-21. They are stained to demonstrate neurons, and the boundaries of Rexed's laminae are indicated in each figure. For ease of comparison combined Weigert-Nissl stained nuclear groups are illustrated at levels near those of the laminae. There are differences in laminar configuration at various segmental levels of the spinal cord. The laminae constitute regions with characteristic properties, but their boundaries are zones of transition, where changes may occur either gradually or abruptly. Only the principal features of individual lamina are included

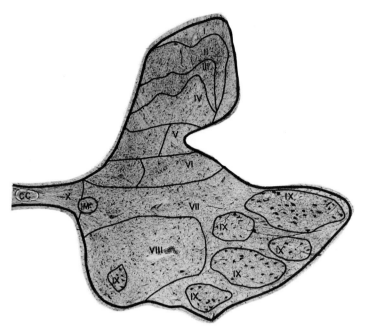

Figure 9-12. Structural lamination indicated on a thick section of human cord segment at C6. The central canal (*CC*) and intermediomedial nucleus (*IM*) are identified. Compare with Figure 9-11 (Thionin stain, photograph, ×9).

in this brief presentation. Some of the laminae correspond to recognized cell columns and nuclei, while others are regional admixtures of cells (Fig. 9-23).

Lamina I is a thin veil of gray substance that caps the surface of the posterior horn and bends around its margins. It has a spongy appearance and is penetrated by small and large fiber bundles (Figs. 9-18, 9-19 and 9-23). It contains small and medium-sized cells with scant cytoplasm and scattered fairly large spindle-shaped cells oriented parallel to the convex surface of the posterior horn (Figs. 9-15, 9-18 and 9-20). The cytoplasm of the large cells is rich in granular endoplasmic reticulum and other organelles (2098, 2099). A complex array of nonmyelinated axons, small dendrites and synaptic knobs lie within this lamina which corresponds to the *posteromarginal nucleus*. In light microscopic preparations it is best identified in sections through the lumbar enlargement (Figs. 9-18 and 9-20).

Studies in the rat, cat and monkey in which horseradish peroxidase (HRP) has been used to trace anterograde projections of dorsal root fibers into the spinal cord indicate that thin fibers of the lateral division end principally in lamina I and the outer part of lamina II (1490). The high density of terminals in lamina I (marginal zone) and in the outer part of lamina II indicate that these parts of the spinal gray receive a major afferent input (Fig. 9-15). Physiological observations further demonstrate that lamina I and the outer zone of lamina II receive direct projections from cutaneous nociceptors but have no direct input from cutaneous receptors responding to innocuous stimuli (1491). Iontophoretically injected HRP into single neurons of lamina I has revealed the dendritic arborizations, spines and terminal varicosities of these neurons (1492). No correlation could be made between cell size, configuration or dendritic arborizations and determined physiological characteristics of those neurons. Other evidence indicates that axons of fibers in the dorsolateral fasciculus of Lissauer end upon neurons in lamina I (1297). A large proportion of axons in the dorsolateral fasciculus arise from cells of the substantia gelatinosa (lamina II). An electron microscopic study has shown that axons of neurons in lamina II end axosomatically upon cells in lamina I, while primary afferent fibers terminate axodendritically (1803). Almost all evidence suggests

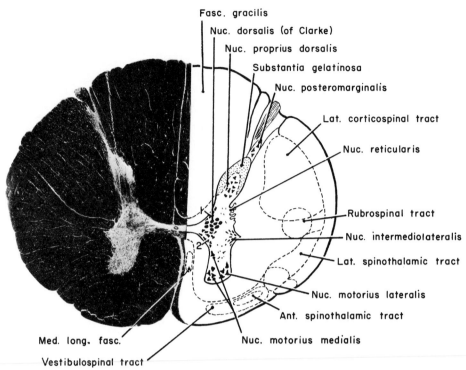

Figure 9-13. Section through fifth thoracic segment of adult human spinal cord. Important cell groups and fiber tracts are identified. *1*, Nucleus cornucommissuralis posterior; *2*, nucleus cornucommissuralis anterior (Weigert's myelin stain, photograph).

that neurons of lamina I respond specifically to nociceptive and thermal stimuli (Fig. 9-15). The suggestion that cells of lamina I contribute some fibers to the spinothalamic tract is based upon: (a) retrograde cell changes following spinothalamic tractotomies for relief of pain in man (1401) and (b) antidromic stimulation and retrograde labeling with HRP indicating that cells of lamina I project axons to the thalamus (1389, 2574, 2727, 2728). Other evidence indicates that some cells, or dichotomizing axons of cells, in lamina I give rise to descending propriospinal projections extending for 8 or more spinal segments (332). These descending fibers may influence motor neurons involved in withdrawal reflexes, or be part of an indirect input to other ascending systems.

Lamina II which forms a well delimited band around the apex of the posterior horn is readily identified in both myelin sheath and cell stains (Figs. 9-8, 9-11, 9-16, 9-18 and 9-20). This fairly broad band is covered dorsally and dorsolaterally by lamina I but its medial border is the posterior funiculus. Lamina II is composed of tightly packed small cells, corresponds to the *substantia gelatinosa* of Rolando and is the oldest cytoarchitectonic region delimited in the spinal cord (2135). Although found at all spinal levels, it is massive in the cord enlargements. Lamina II consists of a dorsal or *outer zone* and a ventral or *inner zone*. In the outer zone, about one quarter of the thickness of the whole lamina, cells are slightly smaller and more tightly packed than in the inner zone. Neurons in both zones of the lamina are round or elongated with their long axis oriented radially to the surface of the lamina (Fig. 9-15). The spindle-shaped cell bodies are hardly larger than the nucleus and give rise to rich dendritic trees from one or both poles of the soma (2496). The main axes of the dendritic arborizations are radial (i.e., perpendicular to the curved lamina). At the ultrastructural level cells of lamina II show a striking paucity of granular endoplasmic reticulum which is correlated with the absence of discrete Nissl bodies in light microscopy (348, 2097). Thus, the cytoplasm of cells in lamina II is unusually pale in comparison with other spinal neurons. The most char-

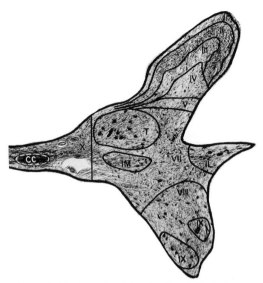

Figure 9-14. Structural lamination indicated on a thick section of human cord segment at T10. The central canal (*CC*), intermediomedial nucleus (*IM*) and nucleus dorsalis (*T*, of Clarke, nucleus thoracicus) are identified. Compare with Figure 9-13 (Thionin stain, photograph, ×14).

acteristic feature of the substantia gelatinosa is the presence of numerous small unmyelinated axons grouped in bundles running parallel to the long axis of the spinal cord, or perpendicular to that axis. Large myelinated axons representing primarily dorsal root fibers, pass through lamina II into deeper regions of the spinal gray. Myelinated fibers, frequently in bundles, are especially common in the medial half of lamina II.

As central processes of spinal ganglion cells approach the dorsal root entry zone small, fine fibers shift into lateral portions of the rootlets, while larger fibers, segregated medially, and enter the posterior white column medial to the posterior horn (348, 1297, 1300, 1490, 2106, 2107, 2373). Upon entering the spinal cord root fibers bifurcate into ascending and descending branches. Fibers of small caliber in the lateral division, unmyelinated and poorly myelinated, contribute to the dorsolateral fasciculus of Lissauer and occupy positions both medial and lateral to the entering rootlet. Larger fibers and their ascending and descending collaterals pass medial to, or through, the posterior horn; the bulk of these fibers project to deep laminae of the spinal gray.

Afferent fibers to lamina II are derived from collaterals in: (a) the dorsolateral fasciculus, (b) the dorsal funiculus and (c) parts of the lateral funiculus adjacent to the posterior horn (2496). Collateral fibers from these sources enter the substantia gelatinosa in a radial fashion and form flame-shaped terminal arborizations which establish synaptic contact with large numbers of neurons (Fig. 9-15). Fibers entering from the posterior funiculus traverse medial parts of laminae I and II, penetrate parts of laminae IV and V and recurve dorsally and laterally to enter lamina II from its ventral surface. Terminal arborizations within lamina II have a columnar arrangement with little overlap. Synaptic profiles with round synaptic vesicles were found to be the dominant type in lamina I and the outer zone of lamina II (2100).

Anterograde transport of HRP via spinal dorsal roots reveal that the outer zone of lamina II receives terminations from the very finest afferent fibers, while the inner zone of this lamina receives endings from some of the finest fibers as well as from small myelinated fibers (1490). Physiological observations on morphologically identified cells in laminae I and II suggest that thinly myelinated primary afferents from nociceptors end mainly in lamina I, while unmyelinated afferents from nociceptors, thermoreceptors and mechanoreceptors terminate predominantly in lamina II (1492). Soma location could not always be correlated with afferent input, but cell bodies of nociceptive and thermoreceptive neurons tended to be in lamina I, or the outer zone of lamina II, while innocuous mechanoreceptive neurons tended to be in the inner zone of lamina II (Fig. 9-15).

The majority of neurons in lamina II send axons into the dorsolateral fasciculus, or into the adjacent lateral fasciculus proprius, although some cells give rise to fine axonal plexuses retained within this lamina (669, 2496). Cells in medial parts of lamina II give rise to commissural fibers that can be followed into the contralateral substantia gelatinosa. Axons originating from cells of lamina II have always been traced back into this same lamina at different levels. None of these axons have been followed into other structures which might forward impulses to known sensory pathways. Thus, lamina II has been regarded as a "closed

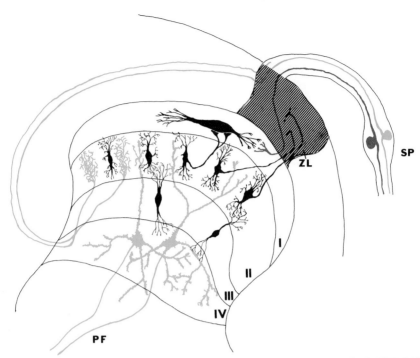

Figure 9-15. Schematic diagram of cutaneous input into the posterior gray horn. I, II, III and IV represent laminae of Rexed; *SP* is the spinal ganglion and *ZL* (shaded area) is the zone of Lissauer. Primary nociceptive afferents (*red*) enter lateral parts of the root entry zone, traverse the zone of Lissauer and synapse upon distal dendrites of larger cells in the posteromarginal nucleus (lamina I). Gelatinosa neurons in lamina II provide axons, or axon collaterals, that synapse on the soma of cells in lamina I and longer axons that ascend/or descend in the zone of Lissauer to ultimately return to lamina II at other levels. Non-nociceptive primary afferents (*blue*) enter as part of the medial division of root fibers by either passing medial to, or through the superficial gray laminae. These larger caliber fibers enter lamina II from its ventral aspect and end in terminal arbors near gelatinosa neurons and in relation to dendrites of large cells of the proper sensory nucleus in lamina IV. Large cells in lamina IV (*blue*) give rise to projection fibers (*PF*) some of which cross in the anterior white commissure and project to the thalamus.

system," although it can influence larger neurons in deeper laminae whose dendrites are embedded in lamina II (Fig. 9-15). Because neurons in lamina II appear organized to exert their main synaptic influences upon the larger cells in laminae III and IV, it has been postulated that the substantia gelatinosa may function as a controlling system modulating synaptic transmission from primary sensory neurons to secondary sensory systems (1298, 1300, 1492, 1665, 2496, 2662).

Emerging neurochemical and neuropharmacological data indicate that laminae I and II contain high concentrations of substance P, an undecapeptide, synthesized in spinal ganglia and transported via dorsal root fibers to terminals in these laminae (1122, 2005, 2507). Substance P is a polypeptide originally detected in equine brain and independently isolated from rat brain (440, 723). This peptide, widely and selectively distributed in the central nervous system, has especially high concentrations in areas receiving sensory afferents (Fig. 9-32). This distribution has led to speculations that it may have properties of a neurotransmitter in primary sensory systems. In axon terminals substance P appears to be associated with large round vesicles 60 to 80 nm in diameter (2005).

It has also been demonstrated that the spinal gray contains opiate receptors which are highly concentrated in laminae I and II (1125, 1418). Opiate receptors which mediate all pharmacological effects of opiates have been found to be concentrated on synaptic membranes (1978). Since opiates presumably cause analgesia by disrupting pain mechanisms, the distribution of opiate receptor sites in the central nervous system and the mechanism of opiate actions at

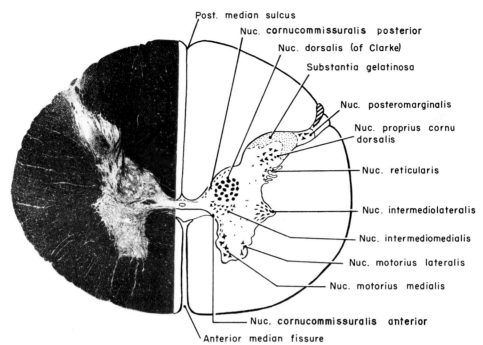

Post. median sulcus
Nuc. cornucommissuralis posterior
Nuc. dorsalis (of Clarke)
Substantia gelatinosa
Nuc. posteromarginalis
Nuc. proprius cornu dorsalis
Nuc. reticularis
Nuc. intermediolateralis
Nuc. intermediomedialis
Nuc. motorius lateralis
Nuc. motorius medialis
Nuc. cornucommissuralis anterior
Anterior median fissure

Figure 9-16. Section through the twelfth thoracic segment of the adult human spinal cord. Important cell groups are identified on the right (Weigert's myelin stain, photograph).

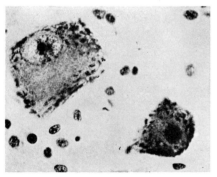

Figure 9-17. Photomicrograph of two cells in the dorsal nucleus of Clarke of human spinal cord (cresyl violet stain).

these sites seem essential to understanding nociceptive processes. The binding affinity of opiate receptors is closely correlated with the dose required to elicit pharmacological responses. A comparison of opiate receptor binding in the cervical spinal cord following multiple dorsal rhizotomies revealed a 50% loss of opiate receptors on the side of dorsal root sections (1418). The distribution of enkephalin, an endogenous opioid peptide, appears to parallel that of opiate receptor sites in the primate brain (2341). Thus, opiate receptors and their natural ligand

compose a "pain suppression system" present at every level of the neuraxis (1976). It also has been postulated that enkephalin may presynaptically inhibit the release of substance P considered to have an excitatory role in central transmission of impulses associated with pain (1220).

Lamina III forms a band across the posterior horn parallel with laminae I and II, except that the lateral bend is not so sharp (Figs. 9-12, 9-14, 9-19 and 9-21). The neurons of this lamina are not so closely packed as in lamina II, but are similarly round or spindle-shaped. Cells show more variations in size and in general are larger than those in lamina II; most of the cells are oriented transversely to the lamina and vertically to its surface (Fig. 9-15). Occasionally an exceptional large cell may be seen, but such cells properly belong to lamina IV. The border between lamina II and III is well-defined due to the presence of large numbers of medium-sized and small axons in lamina III which form a meshwork of fibers running longitudinally (2100). Neurons of lamina III have a large light-staining nucleus, relative scant cytoplasm and small amounts of Nissl substance (2097, 2135).

Golgi-stained reconstructions of neurons

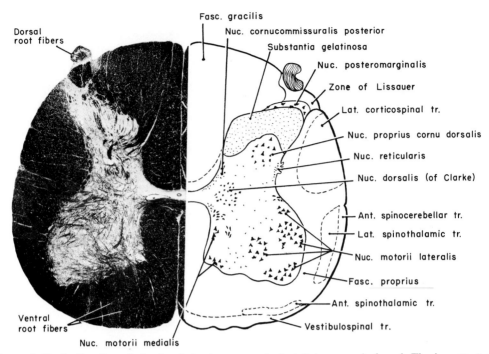

Fasc. gracilis
Dorsal root fibers
Nuc. cornucommissuralis posterior
Substantia gelatinosa
Nuc. posteromarginalis
Zone of Lissauer
Lat. corticospinal tr.
Nuc. proprius cornu dorsalis
Nuc. reticularis
Nuc. dorsalis (of Clarke)
Ant. spinocerebellar tr.
Lat. spinothalamic tr.
Nuc. motorii lateralis
Fasc. proprius
Ant. spinothalamic tr.
Ventral root fibers
Vestibulospinal tr.
Nuc. motorii medialis

Figure 9-18. Section through the fourth lumbar segment of adult human spinal cord. The important cell groups and fiber tracts are identified (Weigert's myelin stain, photograph).

in lamina III reveal that the dendritic ar-borizations of some cells extend dorsally into laminae I and II and ventrally into laminae IV and V (1598). The dorsally di-rected dendrites radiate into the substantia gelatinosa over a considerable rostrocaudal distance. Axons of these neurons emerge from the proximal part of one ventral den-drite, bifurcate a number of times, and the collaterals form a dense plexus in laminae III and IV. Although the length of these axons is great they appear to ramify en-tirely within the gray matter and have been regarded primarily as interneurons trans-mitting impulses from incoming afferent fibers to the cells of origin of sensory tracts. Most of the primary afferent fibers to cells in lamina III are intermediate to thick fi-bers that follow a recurring course to enter the ventral aspect of the lamina II (1490, 2101). Ultrastructural studies indicate di-verse synaptic populations in the posterior horn derived from difference sources. The round synaptic profiles, dominant in lami-nae I and II, decline in numbers in lamina III, where flattened synaptic vesicles pre-dominate (2100). Thus, most cells in lamina III appear anatomically organized to func-tion as interneurons. Although a few of the

larger neurons in this lamina may contrib-ute to ascending sensory pathways, most of the long ascending sensory fibers originate from cells of laminae I, IV and V (34, 2574, 2575, 2727).

Lamina IV, the thickest of the first four laminae of the posterior horn, extends straight across the gray column (Figs. 9-19 and 9-21). The borders of this lamina are sometimes diffuse and its cells, which vary greatly in size, give it a less compact ap-pearance than lamina III. Cells of this lam-ina are round, triangular or star-shaped; a few very large cells are especially conspic-uous. The cytoplasm of these cells is more abundant than in the cells of lamina III and the plentiful Nissl substance in the large cells appears as fine evenly distributed granules (2135). The dendrites of cells in lamina IV radiate upward into the substan-tia gelatinosa in a candelabra fashion par-allel to the primary afferent fibers (348, 2496). These dendrites have well-developed spines and it seems likely that a large part of the dendritic surface is covered with synaptic contacts of larger primary afferent fibers (Fig. 9-15); primary afferents termi-nating on the somata of these neurons are rare (1296, 1300). Neurons of lamina IV

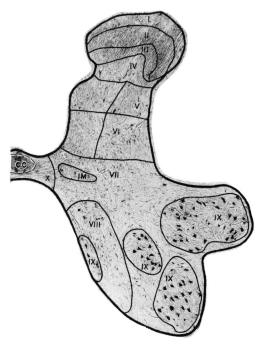

Figure 9-19. Structural lamination indicated on a thick section of human cord segment at L5. The central canal (*CC*) and intermediomedial nucleus (*IM*) are identified. Compare with Figure 9-18 (thionin stain, photograph, ×7.5).

sions, except in the thoracic region (Fig. 9-14). Many fiber bundles pass through the lateral zone, giving it a reticulated appearance. The lateral part of lamina V gives rise to a reticular process (i.e., reticular nucleus), prominent at cervical levels (Figs. 9-9–9-11). The dorsal boundary of this lamina is diffuse while the ventral border is well-defined. Neurons of lamina V are highly variable in size and shape and commonly are triangular or star-shaped, although spindle-shaped neurons are seen. Cells have large clear nuclei, relatively large amounts of cytoplasm and fine Nissl granules. Coarse Nissl granules occur only in the largest cells. Dendrites of some neurons in lamina V extend dorsally in lamina II in the same manner as the majority of cells in lamina IV (2496). Dorsal root fibers synapse upon dendrites of cells in lamina V in the substantia gelatinosa, and descending suprasegmental fiber systems (e.g., corticospinal and rubrospinal fibers) appear to establish synaptic contacts upon cells and their processes within lamina V. Neurons in lamina V, like those in lamina IV, contribute fibers that enter the spinothalamic tracts on the opposite side of the spinal cord (34, 2574, 2575).

Lamina VI is a broad layer at the base of the posterior horn and extends across its width. This lamina is present only in the cord enlargements (Figs. 9-1 and 9-5). There is no lamina VI between T4 and L2 (Figs. 9-14 and 9-21) where lamina V forms the dorsal boundary of lamina VII. Like lamina V, it is divided into medial and lateral regions (Figs. 9-12 and 9-19). The smaller, more compact, medial region contains numerous dark-staining medium and small-sized cells. The larger lateral region contains triangular or star-shaped neurons. Many dorsal root group I muscle afferents terminate in the medial zone of layer VI, while descending pathways are known to project to cells in the lateral zone. Physiological studies indicate functional differences between laminae in the dorsal horn (2661). Cutaneous afferents are distributed more dorsally than those concerned with proprioceptive sense or kinesthesis, but with few exceptions no lamina can be related to particular sensory modalities. There is some evidence that a group of cells in lamina VI in the cervical enlargement,

respond to low intensity stimuli, such as light touch, and their discharge frequency parallels the stimulus intensity (2072). Because of these properties they have been referred to as "wide dynamic range neurons." Cells in laminae III and IV correspond to the *proper sensory nucleus* (nucleus proprius cornu dorsalis) of the older terminology (Figs. 9-13, 9-16, 9-18 and 9-20).

In Golgi preparations and in degeneration studies there is no evidence that the axons of cells in lamina IV give rise to axons that cross in the anterior white commissure and enter the anterolateral funiculus (2496). Nevertheless studies using antidromic stimulation and the retrograde transport of HRP indicate that axons of some of these cells cross at spinal levels and ascend to thalamic levels (34, 2574, 2575). These cells and others in laminae I and V thus contribute fibers to the spinothalamic tracts (Figs 9-15 and 10-6).

Lamina V is a broad zone extending across the neck of the posterior horn, which is divided into medial and lateral subdivi-

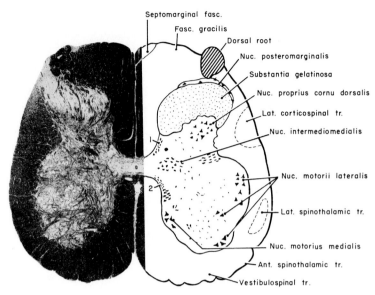

Figure 9-20. Section through the third sacral segment of adult human spinal cord. The important cell groups and fiber tracts are identified. *1*, Nucleus cornucommissuralis posterior; *2*, nucleus cornucommissuralis anterior (Weigert's myelin stain, photograph).

designated as the *centrobasal nucleus*, gives rise to an uncrossed tract projecting to the cerebellum (1638, 1995). These cells are considered as the origin of the rostral spinocerebellar tract. The centrobasal nucleus is a major terminus of dorsal root fibers (2333).

Lamina VII occupies a large heterogeneous region anterior to laminae V and VI, extending across the spinal gray on each side. This region, also known as the *zona intermedia* (intermediate gray), has boundaries which vary at different spinal levels (Fig. 9-7). In the cervical and lumbosacral enlargements lamina VII extends laterally and ventrally into the anterior horn and contains cell groups of lamina IX embedded in it (Fig. 9-23). In the thoracic region lamina VII occupies the zona intermedia and the base of the anterior horn; lamina VIII which forms its ventral border is arched dorsally (Figs. 9-7 and 9-14). Lamina VII gives a fairly homogenous appearance with evenly distributed light-staining nerve cells, a large number of which are internuncial. In particular regions well-defined cell columns are readily recognized. These well-defined cell columns are the dorsal nucleus, the intermediolateral nucleus and the intermediomedial nucleus.

The *dorsal nucleus of Clarke* forms a prominent round or oval cell column in the medial part of lamina VII that extends throughout thoracic and upper lumbar segments (Figs. 9-7, 9-13, 9-14 and 9-16). The large multipolar or oval cells of this nucleus have coarse Nissl granules and eccentric nuclei (Fig. 9-17). This nucleus achieves its greatest size in lower thoracic and upper lumbar segments. Collaterals of dorsal root afferents establish secure synapses upon cells of this nucleus at their levels of entrance and at adjoining levels which exhibit extensive overlap (941). The large cells of the dorsal nucleus give rise to the uncrossed fibers of the posterior spinocerebellar tract.

Lamina VII and adjacent parts of laminae V and VI also give rise to crossed fibers that ascend in the anterior spinocerebellar tract (1638, 1903). Many of these cells receive nonsynaptic excitation and disynaptic inhibition from ipsilateral group I*b* muscle afferents.

The *intermediolateral nucleus* consists of a cell column which occupies the apical region of the lateral horn in thoracic and upper lumbar segments (T1 through L2 or L3). Cells of this nucleus are spindle-shaped or ovoid with vesicular nuclei and fine Nissl granules (Figs. 9-13, 9-14 and 9-16). These cells, considerably smaller than somatic motor neurons, give rise to preganglionic sympathetic fibers that exit via the ventral root and reach various sympathetic ganglia

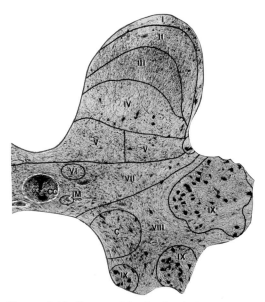

Figure 9-21. Structural lamination indicated on a thick section of human cord segment at S4. Structures identified are the commissural nucleus (*C*), central canal (*CC*), and the intermediomedial nucleus (*IM*). Compare with Figure 9-20 (thionin stain, photograph, ×15).

via the white rami communicantes. *Sacral autonomic nuclei* occupy a corresponding position in the lateral part of lamina VII of segments S2, S3 and S4 (2285), even though no lateral horn is present (Fig. 9-20). Cells of these nuclei resemble those of the intermediolateral cell column, but give rise to preganglionic parasympathetic fibers that exit via the sacral ventral roots to form the "pelvic nerves." The fibers synapse upon postganglionic neurons in, or near, the walls of pelvic viscera; postganglionic fibers in turn innervate the pelvic viscera (Fig. 8-10).

The *intermediomedial nucleus*, unlike other cell columns described in lamina VII, extends virtually the entire length of the spinal cord (Figs. 9-12, 9-14, 9-16, 9-19 and 9-21). This nucleus consists of a group of small and medium-sized cells with a triangular shape that lie in the most medial part of lamina VII, lateral to the central canal. The nucleus consistently receives a small number of fibers from the dorsal root at all levels (416, 2333). It has been suggested that the intermediomedial nucleus may receive visceral afferent fibers and serve as an intermediary relay in transmission of impulses to visceral motor neurons (1994).

Lamina VIII includes a zone at the base

of the anterior horn, but its size and shape differs at various cord levels. In the cord enlargements, this lamina occupies only the medial part of the anterior horn (Figs. 9-12, 9-19 and 9-23); at other levels it extends across the base of the anterior horn ventral to lamina VII (Fig. 9-14). Cells of this lamina vary greatly in size but are mostly triangular and stellate-shaped. The cells have relatively large amounts of cytoplasm and contain large Nissl granules. Axons of some medially located neurons are considered to cross the midline in the anterior white commissure. This lamina constitutes an entity of importance since specific descending fiber systems terminate upon cells in this region. Descending spinal tracts terminating, in part, within lamina VIII include the vestibulospinal, the medial longitudinal fasciculus, the pontine reticulospinal and the tectospinal (Figs. 9-8 and 10-24).

Lamina IX consists of several distinct groups of somatic motor neurons (Figs. 9-8, 9-11–9-14, 9-16 and 9-18–9-21). In thoracic regions of the cord several islands of motor neurons occupy the ventral part of the anterior gray horn, but in the cord enlargements greatly increased numbers of motor neurons form larger groups. Anterior horn cells of this lamina are large multipolar neurons (30 to 70 μm in diameter) regarded as the prototype of motor neurons. These cells have large central vesicular nuclei, coarse Nissl bodies, multiple dendrites and large axons which contribute to the ventral root. Somatic efferent neurons are largest in size and number in the cervical and lumbar enlargements where the cell groups spread both laterally and dorsally (Figs. 9-11 and 9-18).

The lateral nuclear masses are always sharply delimited. Within each nuclear group both large and small perikarya are rich in Nissl bodies. The smaller medial nuclear masses often are less sharply defined and share a diffuse border with lamina VIII (Figs. 9-14 and 9-19).

The large somatic motor cells of the anterior horn which innervate striate muscle are referred to as alpha (α) motor neurons. Scattered among these large motor cells are a number of smaller neurons (gamma (γ) neurons) which give rise to efferent fibers; these emerge via the ventral root and supply the contractile elements of the muscle spindle (i.e., intrafusal muscle fibers).

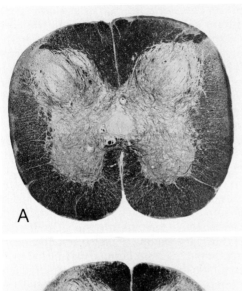

A

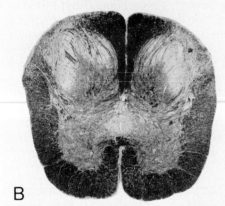

B

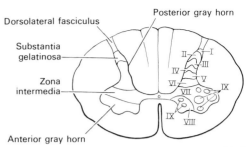

Figure 9-23. Schematic drawing through the eighth cervical spinal segment with the laminae of Rexed (2135, 2136) on the *right* and more general divisions of the spinal gray indicated on the left (Reproduced with permission from M. B. Carpenter: *Physiological Basis of Rehabilitation Medicine*, edited by J. A. Downey and R. C. Darling, W. B. Saunders, Philadelphia, 1971.)

Figure 9-22. Photomicrographs of transverse sections through the fifth sacral (*A*) and first coccygeal (*B*) spinal segments of the adult human spinal cord. Note the abundance of spinal gray in the anterior and posterior horns, the thickness of the gray commissures, the size of the gray surrounding the central canal and the configuration of fasciculus gracilis (Weigert's myelin stain).

Gamma efferent fibers play an essential role in the maintenance of muscle tone and bring the muscle spindle under control of spinal and supraspinal influences (Fig. 9-34). Studies of the retrograde transport of HRP from muscle to spinal neurons in the anterior horn indicate qualitative differences between α and γ motor neurons (2447). The γ motor neurons, most of which are less than 37 μm in average somal diameter, exhibited the heaviest and largest intracytoplasmic granules; cells in the α motor neuron range (i.e., somal diameters greater than 37 μm) showed less intensely stained, smaller HRP granules. While it is

suggested that γ neurons may take up and transport more HRP per unit cell volume than α motor neurons, this difference may be due to a variety of qualitative features that distinguish these cells. In addition to the α and γ motor neurons, the anterior gray horn contains a large population of internuncial neurons about which relatively little is known. Although physiological investigations have suggested that some small internuncial neurons (i.e., Renshaw cells) receive recurrent collaterals of α motor neurons and exert inhibitory influences upon adjacent motor neurons (673, 674, 2133, 2134), Golgi studies have failed to reveal short-axoned cells anywhere within the anterior horn that might correspond to these cells (2278). Most of the internuncial neurons of the anterior horn project fibers into propriospinal pathways.

Motor nuclei in the anterior horn have been subdivided and named on the basis of their location in the gray matter (Fig. 9-24). As shown in Figure 9-24, there is a topographical distribution of perikarya whose axons supply the different muscle groups of the extremity.

Somatic Efferent Neurons

These neurons, which contribute axons to the ventral roots of respective spinal nerves, are organized into named nuclear groups which may vary from segment to segment (Figs. 9-11, 9-13, 9-18 and 9-20). Large multipolar neurons have 3 to 20 dendrites with ramifications which extend into laminae VII and VIII; some longitudinally oriented dendrites may enter adjacent spinal segments (2278, 2414). Axons of α motor neurons arise primarily from the axon hillock, are quite thin in the initial unmyelinated segment (i.e., 3.5 μm), exhibit a variable course in the gray matter and increase in diameter as they enter the white matter (576). A large number of these axons give off multiple collaterals in the gray matter which become myelinated and ramify among α motor neurons (Fig. 9-25) upon which some terminals make direct synaptic contact (576, 577). Each cell has a large central vesicular nucleus and coarse Nissl bodies in the cytoplasm (Figs. 4-2E and 4-8A). These somatic efferent neurons are largest in the lumbar and cervical enlargements and smaller in the thoracic segments of the spinal cord (Fig. 9-14). Scattered among the large anterior horn cells are γ neurons which give rise to γ efferent fibers (Fig. 9-34).

In the ventral part of lamina VII, a collection of small internuncial neurons considered to have unique functional characteristics have been identified physiologically but not anatomically (2132–2134, 2278, 2730). These small neurons, commonly call "Renshaw cells," have been considered to receive recurrent collaterals of α motor neuron axons and to give rise to short axons terminating upon the same or adjacent motor neurons. This recurrent inhibitory pathway from motor axon collaterals via Renshaw cells back to α motor neurons has been regarded as a classic example of a negative feed-back mechanism (2729). Observations indicating that no short-axoned Golgi type II cells could be identified in the anterior horn (2278) and that collaterals of α motor neurons synapse directly on adjacent α motor neurons (576, 577) raises skepticism concerning the concept of the so-called "Renshaw cells." Recurrent collaterals of α motor neurons and their postulated relationships with "Renshaw cells" are schematically diagrammed in Figure 9-24.

The large anterior horn cells are organized into medial and lateral groups, and each group has several subdivisions.

Medial Nuclear Group. This cell group or column is divisible into a posteromedial and anteromedial group. The latter extends throughout the whole cord and is most prominent in C1, C2, C4, T1, T2, L3, L4, S2 and S3. The nucleus of the hypoglossal

nerve in the medulla appears to be a rostral continuation of this column. The posteromedial group is smaller and most distinct in the cervical and lumbar enlargements (Fig. 9-24). It may be missing in the sacral portions of the cord. The medial motor cell column innervates the short and long muscles attached to the axial skeleton.

Lateral Nuclear Group. This motor cell group innervates the rest of the body musculature. In the thoracic segments, it is small and undivided and innervates the intercostal and other anterolateral trunk muscles (Fig. 9-13). In the cervical and lumbar enlargements, it is enlarged and a number of subgroups may be distinguished. The group is especially prominent in those segments which participate in the innervation of the most distal portions of the extremities. Here may be distinguished anterolateral, posterolateral, anterior, central and retroposterolateral groups (Figs. 9-18 and 9-24). The exact innervation of individual muscles in the extremities by each of these groups has not been completely worked out, but in general the more distal muscles are supplied by the more lateral cell groups. Passing from the most mesial part of the anterior horn to its lateral periphery, α motor neurons successively innervate muscles of the trunk, shoulder and pelvic girdle, upper leg and arm, and lower leg and arm. The retroposterolateral group supplies the muscles of the hand and foot. Experimental denervation studies in animals have produced variable results. Section of specific peripheral motor nerves of the cat produced central chromatolysis in discrete anterior horn cells. Cell columns that supplied nerve fibers to the dorsal divisions of the ventral primary ramus were located anterolaterally; cell groups placed posteromedially contributed fibers to the ventral division of the ventral primary ramus (2201).

Multipolar neurons found along the lateral and medial borders of the anterior gray horn in the thoracic, lumbar and sacral segments of the spinal cord are known as spinal border cells (532). These border cells form the *nucleus pericornualis anterior*, considered to contribute fibers to the anterior spinocerebellar tracts. Similar neurons have been identified in the posterior and intermediate regions of the anterior gray horn of the monkey (2410).

Data based upon retrograde cell changes

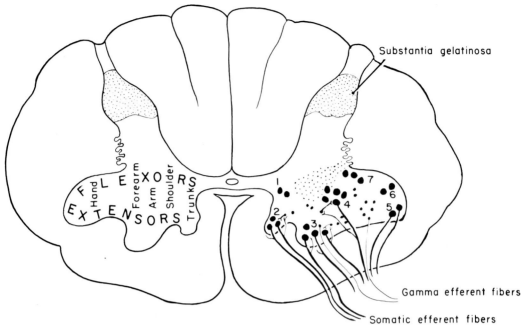

Figure 9-24. Diagram of motor nuclei in anterior gray horn of a lower cervical segment of spinal cord. On the *left* is shown the general location of anterior horn cells that send motor axons to specific muscle groups of the upper extremity. Motor nuclei indicated on the *right* are: *1*, posteromedial; *2*, anteromedial; *3*, anterior; *4*, central; *5*, anterolateral; *6*, posterolateral; *7*, retroposterolateral. Smaller anterior horn cells send axons (gamma efferents) to supply small muscle fibers of neuromuscular spindle (Fig. 9-33). Note the collaterals from somatic efferent axons that return to gray matter and synapse on small medially placed "Renshaw cells." Smaller cells appearing as the *dotted zone* in the intermediate gray indicate the area of the internuncial neuron pool.

following sectioning and crushing of peripheral nerves in various combinations indicate that motor neurons supplying flexor limb muscles are aligned longitudinally in dorsolateral regions of the lateral cell column, while extensor motor neurons lie ventral to flexor motor neurons (2435). A schematic representation of α motor neurons innervating the muscles of the upper extremity is depicted in Figure 9-24. Neurons in the most ventral portion of the anterior horn between the medial and lateral cell columns in cervical segments C3, C4 and C5 give rise to axons which form the phrenic nerve (2435). Dendrites of these neurons display a striking longitudinal orientation (Fig. 9-26).

Visceral Efferent Neurons

Axons of these neurons pass by way of the ventral roots and white rami communicantes to the various sympathetic ganglia. They are small ovoid or spindle-shaped cells with thin, short dendrites, vesicular nuclei and fine chromophilic bodies (Figs.

4-7E and 9-14). They range in size from 12 to 45 μm, and may be divided into two groups.

Intermediolateral Nucleus (Figs. 9-13 and 9-14). This nucleus consists of several adjacent cell columns. The most lateral apical cell group constitutes the lateral horn. The nucleus begins in the lower portion of C8 and extends caudally through L2 or L3. Axons of neurons in the intermediolateral nucleus leave the cord in the ventral roots of spinal nerves T1 and L3 (214, 2029) to terminate in the ganglionated sympathetic chain, or in more peripheral ganglia along the aorta (Figs. 8-1 and 9-28). Each preganglionic axon has synaptic endings upon the dendrites and cell bodies of many postganglionic neurons in outlying sympathetic ganglia.

Sacral Autonomic Nuclei. Scattered small neurons are found along the lateral surface at the base of the anterior gray horn in sacral segments S2, S3 and S4 (Fig. 9-20). Such cells bear a striking resemblance to those found in the intermediolateral nu-

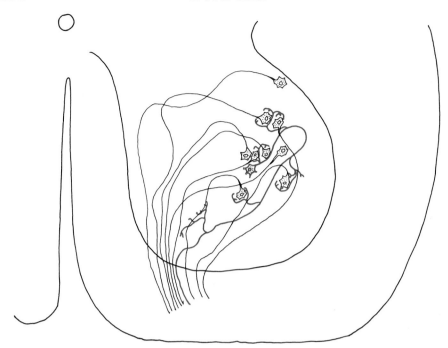

Figure 9-25. Diagram of transverse reconstructions of the trajectories of axons of motor neurons injected intracellularly with horseradish peroxidase (HRP). One α motor neuron (*red*) demonstrates recurrent collaterals that establish direct synaptic contacts with other α motor neurons. Axon collaterals of α motor neurons are not restricted to the ventromedial region of the anterior horn referred to as the "Renshaw cell area." (Based upon Cullheim et al. (577) and Cullheim and Kellerth (576).)

cleus. Axons of these scattered cells leave the cord in the corresponding ventral roots as preganglionic (sacral) parasympathetic fibers. These fibers in turn have multiple synapses with many postganglionic cells located in or near the wall of the pelvic viscera (Fig. 8-1).

Posterior Horn Neurons

These cells and their processes are confined entirely to the central nervous system. In the posterior and intermediate gray especially, they receive the collaterals or direct terminations of dorsal root fibers. In turn, they send their axons either directly to anterior horn cells of the same segments or to the white matter, where, by bifurcating, they become ascending and descending longitudinal fibers, forming intersegmental tracts of varying length (Fig. 9-29). The cells vary in size, form and internal structure. Some are organized into definite cell groups that are easily distinguished in transverse sections; others are scattered irregularly in the gray matter.

Posteromarginal Nucleus. This nucleus forms a thin layer of cells covering the tip of the posterior horn and situated in lamina I (Figs. 9-13–9-15 and 9-20). They are large, tangentially arranged stellate or spindle-shaped cells reaching a diameter of over 50 μm. Cells of the posteromarginal nucleus receive axons of primary afferent fibers conveying impulses related to nociceptive and thermal stimuli and axons from cells in the substantia gelatinosa (Fig. 9-15) (1491, 1803). Axons of cells in this nucleus contribute fibers to the contralateral spinothalamic tract (2727) and give rise to descending propriospinal projections that may influence motor neurons (332). Cells of this nucleus are found throughout the cord, and are most numerous in the lumbosacral segments.

Substantia Gelatinosa. This structure, forming the outer caplike portion of the head of the posterior horn, is present at all spinal levels and is best developed in the enlargements and in the first two cervical spinal segments (Figs. 9-8, 9-11, 9-15 and 9-18). The substantia gelatinosa corresponds to Rexed's lamina II. Variations in size and

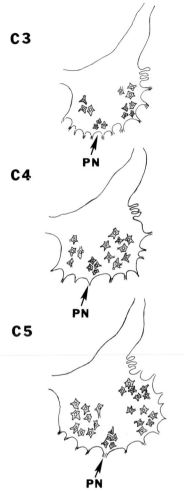

Figure 9-26. Schematic diagram of some cell groups in the anterior gray horn in cervical segments C3, C4 and C5. Phrenic nerve motor neurons (*PN*) lie ventrally between medial and lateral somatic cell columns. (Based upon Sterling and Kuypers (2435).)

configuration of the substantia gelatinosa are related to the size of the respective dorsal roots and the spinal level. The nucleus is composed of tightly packed spindle-shaped cells oriented radially that give rise to rich dendritic arborizations. Small unmyelinated axons course longitudinally in the substantia gelatinosa and bundles of myelinated dorsal root fibers pass through this lamina to deeper regions of the spinal gray. Afferent fibers project to the substantia gelatinosa in a radial fashion from the dorsolateral fasciculus, the dorsal funiculus and parts of the lateral funiculus (2496). Two distinct zones are recognized in the

substantia gelatinosa: (a) an outer zone which receives very fine afferent fibers related to nociceptive stimuli and (b) an inner zone receiving thinly myelinated fibers related to innocuous mechanoreceptive neurons (1491, 1492). Axons of cells in the substantia gelatinosa enter the dorsolateral fasciculus or the fasciculus proprius, but usually they are traced back to portions of lamina II at different levels (Fig. 9-15). Because none of the neurons in the substantia gelatinosa appear to relay impulses in rostrally projecting sensory pathways, this prominent structure has been regarded as a "closed system" which may modulate synaptic transmission of primary sensory neurons (1300, 1492, 2496, 2662).

Proper Sensory Nucleus. This nucleus occupies the head and neck of the posterior horn and corresponds to Rexed's laminae III and IV as seen in Figures 9-11, 9-13, 9-15, 9-16 and 9-18. Cells of this nucleus are of mixed types. Round or spindle-shaped cells which predominate dorsally are oriented vertically, while in deeper parts of the nucleus, round, triangular and polygonal cells with abundant Nissl substance are conspicuous. Dendrites of cells in the proper sensory nucleus radiate into the substantia gelatinosa where they make synaptic contact with primary afferent fibers (Fig. 9-15). Axons of larger cells in this nucleus cross in the anterior white commissure and contribute fibers to the spinothalamic tracts (Fig. 9-18) (34, 2574). Cells composing this poorly defined cell column are found at all spinal levels but are most numerous in lumbosacral segments. Lateral to the nucleus proprius the reticular process of the posterior horn protrudes finger-like extensions into the lateral funiculus (Figs. 9-9–9-11). Cells of this process are part of lamina V and have been called the *reticular nucleus*. The reticular process is most evident in cervical spinal segments.

Dorsal Nucleus of Clarke. This nucleus is a striking cell column in the medial portion of lamina VII at the base of the posterior horn. The nucleus begins to be well defined in C8 and extends through the thoracic and upper lumbar segments, being most prominent in T10, T12 and L1 (Figs. 9-14, 9-16 and 9-17). Below L3 it becomes indistinguishable, although occasional cells may be found.

Intermediomedial Nucleus. This nucleus is a rather diffusely organized cell group in the medial part of lamina VII lateral to the central canal. It is not as sharply outlined as the intermediolateral nucleus occupying the lateral horn (Figs. 9-14 and 9-16). Small- and medium-sized cells, 10 to 24 μm in size, are found in this location in varying numbers throughout the spinal cord (Fig. 9-16).

Central Cervical Nucleus. This nucleus is located in Rexed's lamina VII in upper four cervical spinal segments and forms an interrupted cell column consisting of a series of discrete cell groups (Fig. 9-31). Cells are fairly large, polygonal in shape, and resemble motor neurons. This group of cells lies lateral to the intermediomedial nucleus (579, 2136). Cells of the central cervical nucleus receive direct projections from dorsal root ganglion cells (1994, 2333) and give rise to a crossed spinocerebellar tract (579, 1637).

Two less definite cell columns extending the length of the cord are the *nuclei cornucommissurales posterior* and *anterior* (Fig. 9-20). The former, in section, is a thin cell strip occupying the medial margin of the posterior horn and extending along the border of the posterior gray commissure. It lies over the column of Clarke when the latter is present. The anterior is a similar cell group along the medial surface of the anterior horn and anterior gray commissure. These nuclei consist of small- and medium-sized spindle-shaped cells whose axons probably form intersegmental tracts in the posterior and anterior white funiculi, respectively.

ARRANGEMENT OF ENTERING AFFERENT FIBERS

Central processes of cells in the spinal ganglia enter the dorsolateral aspect of the spinal cord in small fascicles over a considerable distance (Fig. 9-2). The dorsal roots break up into a number of filaments, or rootlets, which enter the spinal cord in a linear manner. Peripheral processes of spinal ganglion cells convey impulses centrally from various somatic and visceral receptors. As central processes of spinal ganglion cells approach the dorsal root entry zone, small fine fibers become segregated in lateral portions of the rootlets and

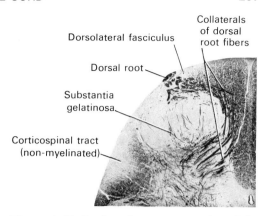

Figure 9-27. Portion of transverse section of the lumbar spinal cord in an infant showing entrance of dorsal root fibers and collaterals (Weigert's myelin stain, photograph).

enter lateral parts of the dorsal horn and the dorsolateral fasciculus directly (348, 1297, 1300, 1490, 2106, 2107, 2373). Larger fibers, shifting medially in the rootlets, enter the posterior columns directly or traverse medial parts of the posterior horn in passage to deeper laminae of the spinal gray (Figs. 9-27 and 9-28). Thick myelinated fibers of the *medial bundle* are described as representing the central processes of spinal ganglion cells conveying impulses from large encapsulated somatic receptors, such as neuromuscular spindles, neurotendinous organs, Pacinian corpuscles and Meissner's corpuscles (Fig. 9-28). The smaller, less conspicuous *lateral bundle*, composed of thinly myelinated fibers, is described as representing the central processes of smaller ganglion cells related to free nerve endings, tactile, thermal and other somatic and visceral receptors. Upon entering the spinal cord, central processes of each spinal ganglion cell divide into ascending and descending branches (2106), which in turn give rise to numerous collaterals (Fig. 9-29). Most of the collateral branches are given off in the segment of entry, where they either relay impulses to second order neurons, or participate in intrasegmental reflexes (Fig. 9-29). Primary ascending and descending branches extending into adjacent spinal cord segments, together with their collaterals, constitute the anatomical basis of intersegmental reflexes, and the relay of impulses to secondary sensory pathways (Figs. 9-28 and 9-29). The longer

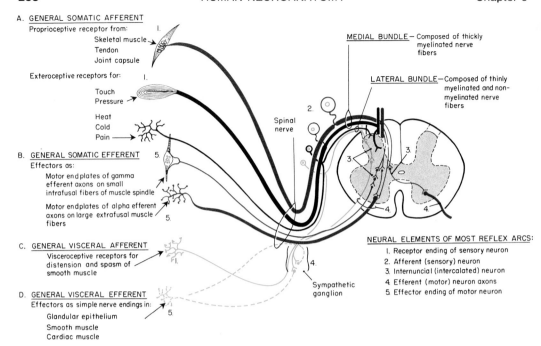

Figure 9-28. Diagram of functional components of a thoracic spinal nerve, and the arrangement of dorsal root fibers as they enter the spinal cord. Skeletal muscle afferent and efferent fibers are indicated in *red*. Visceral afferent and efferent fibers are shown in *blue*. An afferent fiber from a Pacinian corpuscle (*black*) and a thin pain fiber (*black*) also are shown. Numbers in the diagram correspond to neural elements that form reflex arcs.

ascending primary branches of the medial bundle enter the ipsilateral posterior funiculus, and many of these ascend without synapse as far as the medulla. Fine, thinly myelinated and unmyelinated fibers of the lateral bundle of the dorsal root, conveying impulses related to pain, thermal and light tactile sense, enter the medial part of the *zone of Lissauer (fasciculus dorsolateralis)* and terminate directly in portions of laminae I and II (1490, 1491) (Figs. 9-7, 9-15 and 9-18). Physiological data coupled with detailed anatomical studies indicate that lamina I and the outer zone of lamina II receive direct projections from cutaneous nociceptors, but have no direct input from cutaneous receptors responding to innocuous stimuli (1491). Primary afferent fibers terminating in the inner zone of lamina II are a mixture of fine and small myelinated fibers related physiologically to innocuous mechanoreceptive neurons (1492).

Zone of Lissauer. This zone (fasciculus dorsolateralis) is composed of: (a) fine myelinated and unmyelinated dorsal root fibers, which enter medial parts of the bundle, and (b) a large number of endogenous propriospinal fibers which interconnect dif-

ferent levels of the substantia gelatinosa (669, 2107, 2496). According to Chung and Coggeshall (458) 80% of the axons in the dorsolateral fasciculus are unmyelinated in the cat and approximately 50% of the axons represent primary afferent fibers, derived from the entering dorsal roots. In Golgi preparations axons of cells in laminae I, II and III have been followed into lateral parts of the zone of Lissauer and most of these fibers have been traced back to lamina II at other levels. Because few, if any, of the axons of cells in the substantia gelatinosa appear to relay impulses into known sensory pathways and the dendrites of larger sensory neurons in laminae III and IV extend radially into lamina II, this structure has been regarded as a modulator of synaptic transmission from primary to secondary sensory neurons (1298, 1300, 1665, 2496).

Most of the primary afferent fibers entering laminae III and IV are intermediate to thick fibers that pass through or around lamina II and after a recurring course in the gray matter, approach cells in the proper sensory nucleus from a ventral direction (Fig. 9-15). Primary afferent fibers

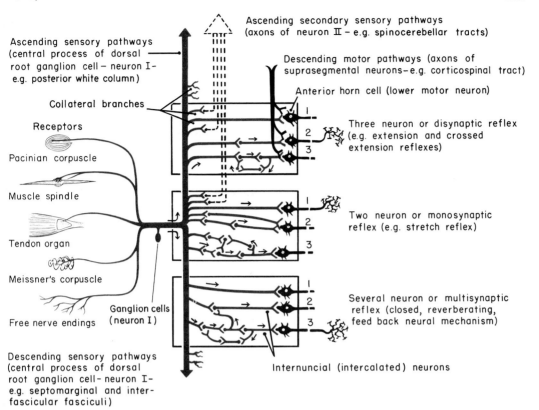

Ascending secondary sensory pathways
(axons of neuron II – e.g. spinocerebellar tracts)

Ascending sensory pathways
(central process of dorsal
root ganglion cell – neuron I–
e.g. posterior white column)

Descending motor pathways (axons of
suprasegmental neurons–e.g. corticospinal tract)

Anterior horn cell (lower motor neuron)

Collateral branches

Receptors

Three neuron or disynaptic reflex
(e.g. extension and crossed
extension reflexes)

Pacinian corpuscle

Muscle spindle

Two neuron or monosynaptic
reflex (e.g. stretch reflex)

Tendon organ

Meissner's corpuscle

Several neuron or multisynaptic
reflex (closed, reverberating,
feed back neural mechanism)

Ganglion cells
(neuron I)

Free nerve endings

Descending sensory pathways
(central process of dorsal
root ganglion cell– neuron I–
e.g. septomarginal and interfascicular fasciculi)

Internuncial (intercalated) neurons

Figure 9-29. Diagram of major branches and collaterals of dorsal root ganglion cells within three spinal cord segments. On the left are various receptors that generate impulses in response to different kinds of stimuli. Impulses from muscle spindles initiate the myotatic or stretch reflex involving two neurons (monosynaptic reflex). Impulses from the tendon organ initiate disynaptic reflex circuits involving inhibitory mechanisms. Other reflex circuits may involve many neurons (multisynaptic). Also indicated are ascending and descending branches of dorsal root fibers in the posterior white column (see Fig. 10-1) and collateral pathways that project fibers to the cerebellum (see Fig. 10-9).

largely terminate on dendrites of these neurons. Most of the neurons of lamina IV appear to respond to low intensity stimuli, such as light touch (2072). Cells in laminae I, IV and V have been identified as giving rise to fibers that form the crossed spinothalamic tracts (34, 2574, 2575).

One of the principal sites of termination of large myelinated dorsal root fibers is the dorsal nucleus of Clarke (Fig. 9-30). Clarke's nucleus receives fibers from all ipsilateral spinal roots except the upper cervical roots (941, 2333). Studies of dorsal root afferents to Clarke's nucleus (941, 1499) indicate: (a) the greatest number of fibers come from dorsal roots of the hindlimb, (b) there is considerable overlap of different dorsal root fibers distributed to the nucleus and (c) fibers enter the nucleus via both ascending and descending collat-

eral branches of the dorsal root. Synapses of dorsal root afferents upon the cells of Clarke's nucleus appear unique in that terminal fibers have long parallel contact with the dendrites of Clarke's neurons, and unusually large terminal boutons are partially buried in depressions on the cell surface (2500). These "giant synapses" between dorsal root fibers and cells of the dorsal nucleus are said to be larger than any other spinal cord synapses. Anatomical observations are in agreement with physiological studies (1505) which show that selective stimulation of group I afferent fibers establish secure synaptic relationships with the cells of Clarke's nucleus.

Collateral branches of dorsal root fibers also are distributed to parts of the anterior horn (Figs. 9-28 and 9-34). According to Sprague (2411) and Sprague and Ha (2414),

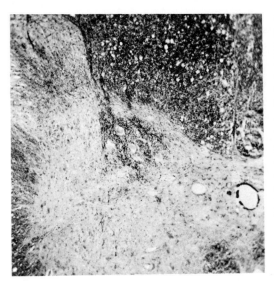

Figure 9-30. Photomicrograph of degenerated dorsal root fibers in the rhesus monkey projecting directly to the dorsal nucleus of Clarke at L2. Lumbar dorsal roots were sectioned proximal to the dorsal root ganglia (Nauta-Gygax stain, ×80).

dorsal root fibers become concentrated especially in the central part of lamina VI; from this region fibers pass in numerous small bundles into lamina IX where they arborize about the soma and dendrites of large motor neurons. Dorsal root fibers also give off collaterals which pass into lamina VIII. Since collaterals of dorsal root fibers passing to laminae VIII and IX traverse broad regions of lamina VII, it is likely that many fibers, or collaterals, end upon internuncial neurons in this lamina, as well as on dendrites of motor nuclei which extend beyond the limits of Rexed's lamina IX. Dorsal root fibers from group Ia afferent fibers projecting to lamina IX are involved in the monosynaptic myotatic reflex (Figs. 9-33 and 9-34). Group Ib and group II afferent fibers also generate synaptic potentials in central parts of laminae V, VI and VII (2414).

The central course of major branches and collaterals of dorsal root ganglion cells within three spinal segments are diagrammed schematically in Fig. 9-29. This simplified diagram summarizes information concerning sensory pathways and certain spinal reflexes.

Pain Mechanisms

Although pain of widely varying character, dimensions and intensity constitutes one of the most common complaints in medicine, the nature of pain is unresolved and is the subject of great controversy. Pain has been described as a sensory experience evoked by stimuli that injure or threaten to destroy tissue, which is defined introspectively by every man (1765). There are two opposing theories of pain: (a) the specific theory that regards pain as a specific sensory modality with unique peripheral and central apparatus and (b) the pattern theory which maintains that the nerve impulse pattern for pain is produced by intense stimulation of nonspecific receptors (1665). While there is convincing physiological evidence of specialization within the somesthetic system, the character, quality and amount of perceived pain are influenced by both psychological variables and sensory input. It has repeatedly been shown that stimulation of small diameter Aδ and C fibers evoke pain (15, 505, 2801), but this does not mean that impulses in these fibers always produce pain when they are stimulated. Cells in lamina I which receive thinly myelinated primary afferents respond to nociceptive stimuli and to no other stimuli (453, 1491, 1492). While some of these cells project to the contralateral thalamus (2575), these cells are not numerous and probably are not the main source of the spinothalamic tracts. In an attempt to explain the neural mechanism associated with pain Melzack and Wall (1665) proposed the *gate control theory of pain*. According to this theory: (a) the substantia gelatinosa functions as a gate control mechanism that modulates primary afferent input before these impulses impinge upon neurons that project to higher levels of the neuraxis, (b) primary afferent impulses in the posterior column system trigger central mechanisms that influence gate control and (c) transmission neurons which give rise to ascending sensory pathways are responsible for the perception and responses to pain. Recently this theory has been revised as a consequence of additional evidence (2662). The restated gate control theory is based upon three points: (a) while small diameter fibers (Aδ and C) respond only to nociceptive stimuli, other fibers with lower thresholds increase their discharge frequency in response to noxious stimuli, (b) cells in the spinal cord excited by nociceptive stimuli may be facilitated or inhibited by impulses conveyed by primary afferent fibers signal-

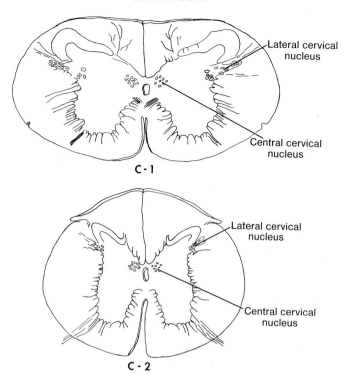

C - 1

C - 2

Figure 9-31. Drawings of the first two cervical spinal segments in a dog showing the locations of the central cervical nucleus and the lateral cervical nucleus. (Based on Cummings and Petras (579).)

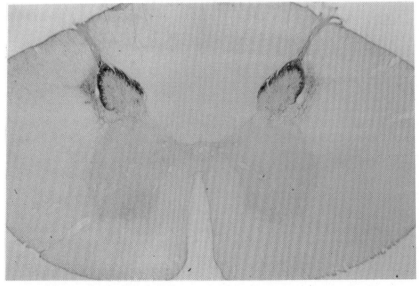

Figure 9-32. Photomicrograph of the monkey spinal cord revealing the localization of substance P. in lamina I and parts of lamina II. Tissue has been treated by immunocytochemical technics that stain substance P, which is present only in laminae of the dorsal horn that receive peripheral pain fibers. The morphine-like peptide enkephalin, also present in lamina I, may regulate the input of painful stimuli by modulating (i.e., inhibiting) the release of substance P. (Reproduced with permission from T. M. Jessell and L. L. Iversen: *Nature,* **268:** 549–551, 1977, and courtesy of Professor Stephen Hunt, Cambridge University.)

ing innocuous stimuli and (c) descending systems from higher levels of the neuraxis modulate the excitability of neurons that transmit signals initiated by noxious stim-uli. Clinical application of the gate control concept has demonstrated that transcutaneous stimulation of large caliber peripheral nerves raises the threshold of central neurons by increasing inhibition which may relieve pain in patients with peripheral nerve disease (1522, 1807, 2663).

The most important advance in the understanding of pain mechanisms has been the identification of opiate receptor binding sites which are concentrated upon synaptic membranes (1978). Because these binding sites mediate all pharmacological effects of opiates, universally regarded as the most powerful agents in disrupting pain mechanisms, opiate receptors must play a dominant role in the control of pain. While most regions of the central nervous system have some opiate receptors, their density varies greatly; only the white matter and the cerebellum appear totally devoid of opiate receptors (1379). In the spinal gray opiate receptors are especially concentrated in Rexed's laminae I and II which have been identified as containing neurons responding to nociceptive stimuli (1125, 1418, 1491, 1492). The central nervous system contains an endogenous opioid, enkephalin, which has been isolated and synthesized, whose distribution appears to parallel that of opiate receptors (1167, 2341). Met^5-enkephalin appears identical in peptide sequence with a fragment of a previously isolated pituitary protein, β-lipotropin. Other fragments of β-lipotropin have been identified from pituitary extracts and termed endorphins (978). Although enkephalin and β-endorphin exhibit similar opiate receptor binding activity, β-endorphin is more potent, has a longer period of action and produces behavioral disturbances as well as analgesia (1168). Thus the opiate receptors and endogenous opiates, such as enkephalin and β-endorphin, compose an intrinsic "pain suppression system" that modulates sensory processes at multiple levels of the neuraxis (1976). The opiate receptors concentrated in laminae I and II probably represent the first level at which these suppressor mechanism act to modulate pain. It has been suggested that enkephalin may also presynaptically inhibit the release of substance P (Fig. 9-32) which is regarded as having excitatory influences upon transmission of impulses associated nociceptive stimuli (1220).

Spinal Reflexes

The five essential elements required for most spinal reflexes are: (a) peripheral re-

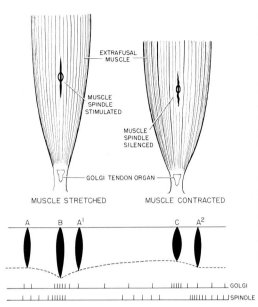

Figure 9-33. Diagram showing the anatomical and functional relationships of the muscle spindle and the Golgi tendon organ to extrafusal muscle fibers. The muscle spindles are arranged in "parallel" with the extrafusal muscle fibers, so that stretching the muscle causes the spindles to discharge. Contraction of the muscle tends to "unload" or "silence" the muscle spindles. The Golgi tendon organs are arranged in "series" with respect to the extrafusal muscle fibers. Thus the Golgi tendon organs can be discharged by either a stretch of the tendon or a contraction of the muscle. The threshold of the Golgi tendon organ is relatively higher than that of the muscle spindle. The *lower diagram* summarizes the functional characteristics of the muscle spindle and Golgi tendon in relation to changes in muscle length. At *A*, the muscle is shown at its resting length, and the slow spontaneous discharge of the tendon organ and muscle spindle is indicated. At *B*, the muscle is stretched and both receptors discharge, though the adaptation of the muscle spindle is more rapid. At A^1, the muscle resumes its original length and tension, and there is a temporary reduction in the frequency of spontaneous firing of the muscle spindle. At *C*, where the muscle is contracted and shortened, the muscle spindle is silenced, but the rate of discharge of the tendon organ is increased. At A^2, the muscle is stretched out to its resting length, and the muscle spindles are therefore discharged, while the tendon organs are silenced by the drop in tension (973).

ceptors, (b) sensory neurons, (c) internuncial neurons, (d) motor neurons and (e) terminal effectors. The *myotatic* or *stretch reflex* is a monosynaptic reflex dependent upon two neurons. Stretch-sensitive proprioceptive endings located in muscle (muscle spindle) and tendon (Golgi tendon organ)

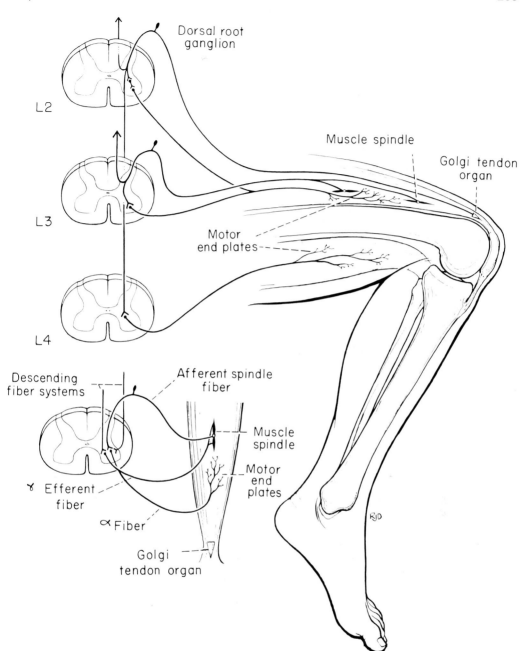

Figure 9-34. Schematic diagram of patellar tendon reflex. Motor and sensory fibers of the femoral nerve associated with spinal segments L2, L3 and L4 mediate this myotatic reflex. The principal receptors are the muscle spindles, which respond to a brisk stretching of the muscle effected usually by tapping the patellar tendon. Afferent fibers from muscle spindles are shown entering only the L3 spinal segment, while afferent fibers from the Golgi tendon organ are shown entering only the L2 spinal segment. In this monosynaptic reflex, afferent fibers entering spinal segments L2, L3 and L4 and efferent fibers issuing from the anterior horn cells of these levels complete the reflex arc. Motor fibers shown leaving the L4 spinal segment and passing to the hamstring muscles demonstrate the pathway by which inhibitory influences are exerted upon an antagonistic muscle group during the reflex. The *small diagram below* illustrates the γ loop. Gamma efferent fibers pass to the polar portions of the muscle spindle. Contractions of the intrafusal fibers in the polar parts of the spindle stretch the nuclear bag region and thus cause an afferent impulse to be conducted centrally. The afferent fibers from the spindle synapse upon an α motor neuron, whose peripheral processes pass to extrafusal muscle fibers, thus completing the loop. Both α and γ motor neurons can be influenced by descending fiber systems from supraspinal levels. These are indicated separately.

are the receptors stimulated by a sudden brisk stretch of muscle. The *muscle spindle*, consisting of bundles of specialized slender muscle fibers (intrafusal fibers) surrounded by a connective tissue capsule, is attached to the endomysium of extrafusal muscle fibers (Fig. 6-11). Stretching of the noncontractile nuclear bag region (equatorial region) of the muscle spindle constitutes the mechanical stimulus required to fire the annulospiral or primary afferent fiber (group Ia) of this receptor. The γ efferent fibers from the smaller anterior horn cells terminating in the polar (contractile) portions of the muscle spindle (intrafusal muscle fibers) bring this receptor under the control of spinal and supraspinal influences. *Golgi tendon organs* are found in tendons close to their muscular attachments (Figs. 6-15 and 6-16). As first pointed out by Fulton and Pi-Suñer (826), the muscle spindle is arranged in "parallel" with extrafusal fibers, so that stretching of a muscle causes the spindle to discharge, while contraction of the extrafusal fibers tends to "unload" the spindle. The Golgi tendon organ is in "series" with extrafusal muscle fibers and thus can be caused to discharge by either a stretch or a contraction of the muscle (Fig. 9-33). Current physiological belief, based largely upon indirect evidence, indicates that the low threshold muscle spindles are the prime receptors involved in the stretch reflex. However, γ efferent fibers to the muscle spindle can exert potent influences upon the activity of this receptor. The myotatic reflex can be elicited in almost any muscle by sharply tapping either the muscle, or its tendon, in such a way as to produce a brief sudden stretch of the muscle. Thus, striking the tendon of the quadriceps femoris muscle provokes a forceful contraction of the stretched muscle and a quick extension of the leg at the knee (Fig. 9-34). In this example, both the sensory and motor nerve fibers leave and enter the quadriceps muscle as constituents of the femoral nerve. It will be recalled that parts of two, three or more myotomes are incorporated in each muscle, and that two, three or more spinal nerves and cord segments provide sensory and motor fibers. The femoral nerve is composed of sensory and motor fibers from spinal nerves L2, L3 and L4. Thus, the synapses between these sensory and motor fibers must be within spinal cord segments L2, L3 and L4. The myotatic reflex is clinically useful in determining the levels of motor integrity of the nervous system, and also may reveal evidence of release of higher control.

Afferent fibers from Golgi tendon organs (group Ib) have disynaptic inhibitory influences upon α motor neurons (Fig. 9-34). Although Golgi tendon organs have a higher threshold than the muscle spindles, afferent discharge of Ib fibers can exert inhibitory influences upon α motor neurons which reduce muscle tone. Unlike the muscle spindle, the Golgi tendon organ does not receive efferent fibers from the central nervous system.

As shown in this schema, other spinal reflexes have one or more internuncial neurons interposed between sensory and motor neurons (*2* and *3* in Fig. 9-29), and some of these may form complex circuits. An anterior horn cell (lower motor neuron) thus may be facilitated, or inhibited, by the sum total of all the impulses that play upon it through literally thousands of synaptic terminals. Such synaptic endings may be terminals of incoming sensory fibers, internuncial neurons or several of the descending motor pathways arising from higher levels of the neuraxis. This is the basic organization of the spinal cord segment and its attached spinal nerves.

CHAPTER 10

Tracts of the Spinal Cord

The ascending and descending fibers of the spinal cord are organized into more or less distinct bundles which occupy particular areas in the white matter. Fiber bundles having the same origin, course and termination are known as tracts or fasciculi. It is customary to divide the white matter of the spinal cord into three funiculi: posterior, lateral and anterior (Figs. 9-2 and 9-6). Thus a funiculus may contain several fasciculi, but owing to the overlapping and intermingling of fibers, these may not be demarcated sharply. In general, long tracts tend to be located peripherally, while shorter tracts tend to be situated medially.

LONG ASCENDING SPINAL TRACTS

Although dorsal root afferent fibers entering the spinal cord convey impulses from all general types of somatic and visceral receptors, the impulses conveyed rostrally in the spinal cord are segregated so that impulses concerned with pain, thermal sense, touch and kinesthesis (sense of movement and joint position) from various body segments ascend together in more or less specific tracts, sometimes widely separated from each other. Ascending tracts not only convey impulses concerned with specific sensory modalities that reach consciousness, but they also transmit impulses from stretch receptors and tactile receptors that project directly, or via relay nuclei in the brain stem to the cerebellum. These impulses are not concerned with conscious sensory perception. Ascending impulses projected to the cerebellum are considered to be concerned largely, but not exclusively with the regulation of muscle tone and with the coordination of motor function.

Posterior White Columns (*fasciculus gracilis and fasciculus cuneatus*). Since the posterior funiculus is composed predominantly of dorsal root fibers, both the

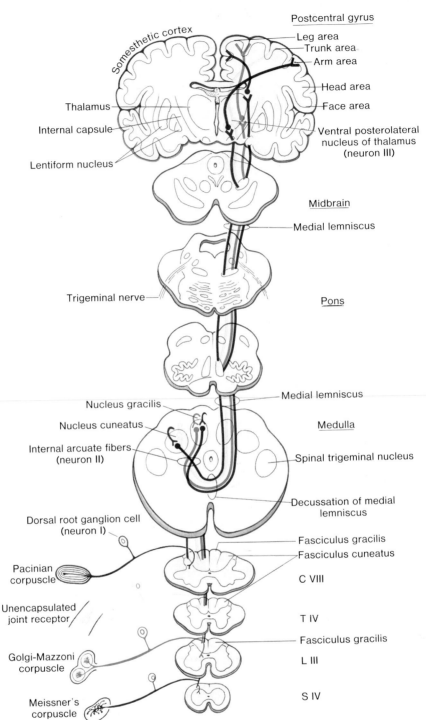

Figure 10-1. Schematic diagram of the formation and course of the posterior white columns in the spinal cord and the medial lemniscus in the brain stem. The posterior white columns are formed from uncrossed ascending branches of spinal ganglion cells; fibers forming the medial lemniscus arise from cells of the nuclei gracilis and cuneatus, cross in the lower medulla and ascend to the thalamus. Impulses mediated by this pathway largely concern discriminating tactile sense (touch and pressure) and kinesthetic sense (position and movement). Different receptors shown at various spinal levels on the left generate impulses conveyed centrally by this system. Spinal ganglia and afferent fibers entering the spinal cord at different levels (*red*, sacral; *blue*, lumbar; *yellow*, thoracic; *black*, cervical) are color coded. Letters and numbers indicate segmental levels of the spinal cord.

ascending and descending courses of these fibers will be described (Fig. 9-29).

A large proportion of heavily myelinated fibers of the dorsal root enter the posterior funiculus medial to the posterior horn, where they bifurcate into long ascending and short descending branches. Ascending fibers from lower levels gradually are shifted medially and posteriorly as they continue upward in the posterior funiculus of the spinal cord. Longer ascending fibers are displaced medially by shorter ascending dorsal root fibers entering the spinal cord at successively higher levels. This pattern of ascending fibers in the posterior columns results in an overlapping laminar arrangement in which the longer lumbosacral fibers are most medial, the shorter cervical fibers are most lateral, and the thoracic fibers occupy intermediate positions (Figs. 10-1 and 10-2). The number of ascending fibers derived from a particular dorsal root bears a relationship to the size of the root. Dorsal roots of the cervical and lumbar enlargements contribute the largest number of fibers.

In the cervical and upper thoracic regions of the spinal cord, the posterior funiculus is divided by a posterior intermediate sulcus into a medial *fasciculus gracilis* and a lateral fasciculus cuneatus (Fig. 9-11 and 10-1). The posterior intermediate septum which separates the fasciculus gracilis from the fasciculus cuneatus becomes discernible at about T6 (Fig. 9-5). Thus the fasciculus gracilis is present at all spinal levels and contains the long ascending branches of fibers from sacral, lumbar and the lower six thoracic dorsal roots. The fasciculus cuneatus, lateral to the septum, contains long ascending branches of the upper six thoracic and all cervical dorsal roots.

Since many ascending fibers in the posterior columns are relatively short and terminate in parts of the posterior gray column at various levels, only a portion of dorsal root fibers in the fasciculi gracilis and cuneatus ascend ipsilaterally to terminate upon the posterior column medullary relay nuclei, namely, the nucleus gracilis and the nucleus cuneatus. Fibers in the posterior columns which reach the medulla constitute the first relay in the largest spinal afferent pathway to the cerebral cortex.

The central processes of dorsal root ganglion cells constitute the first neuron (neuron I, uncrossed) of this ascending pathway. Ascending fibers that reach the medulla via the fasciculus gracilis terminate upon the cells of the *nucleus gracilis*, while the fibers of the fasciculus cuneatus end about cells of the *nucleus cuneatus* (Fig. 10-1). Dorsal root fibers projecting to the nuclei gracilis and cuneatus terminate somatotopically within these nuclei (416, 2333). The neurons of the nuclei gracilis and cuneatus constitute the second neuron (neuron II) in this afferent system. The axons of neuron II sweep ventromedially as *internal arcuate fibers*, cross the midline and turn upward as a single discrete bundle known as the *medial lemniscus*. This crossed tract ascends through the medulla, pons and midbrain levels to terminate somatotopically in the ventral posterolateral (VPL) nucleus of the thalamus. Relay neurons of this thalamic nucleus (neuron III) send their axons through the posterior limb of the internal capsule to terminate in the appropriate sensory areas of the cerebral cortex (Fig. 10-1). In this figure ascending sacral, lumbar, thoracic and cervical spinal root fibers can be followed from their level of entrance into the spinal cord to their termination in the posterior column medullary relay nuclei. Second order fibers arising from these nuclei decussate and form the medial lemniscus which projects to the contralateral thalamic sensory relay nucleus. The color coding in Figure 10-1 permits tracing the course of the impulse from the receptor to the somesthetic cortex.

The posterior white columns constitute one of the phylogenetically newer systems of the neuraxis concerned primarily with discriminating tactile and kinesthetic (i.e., sense of position and movement) sense. These fibers constitute part of a large highly specific sensory pathway in which single elements are responsive to one or the other of these forms of physiological stimuli, but not to both (2215). Fibers of this system are highly specific with respect to place, and endowed with an exquisite capacity for temporal and spatial discrimination. Thus these fibers conduct impulses from tactile receptors necessary for the proper discrimination of two points simultaneously applied (spatial discrimination) and for exact tactile localization. Rapid suc-

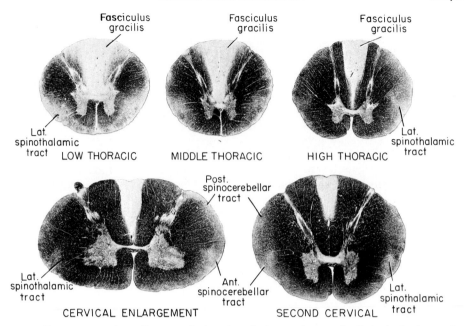

Figure 10-2. Transverse sections of human spinal cord crushed some time previously in the lumbosacral region. In the posterior white columns the progressive diminution of the degenerated area is due to passage into the gray matter of short and medium length ascending branches of lumbosacral dorsal root fibers. The progressive increase in normal fibers adjacent to the posterior horns is due to the addition of ascending branches of dorsal root fibers entering above the level of the injury (Weigert's myelin stain).

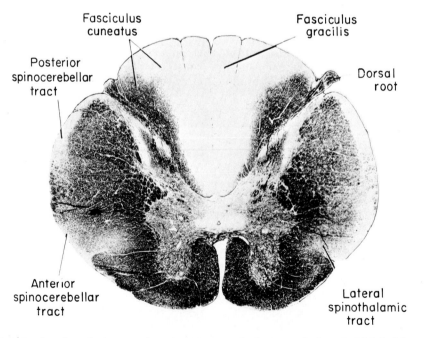

Figure 10-3. Section through the second cervical segment of a human spinal cord which had been crushed previously in the lower cervical region. Ascending branches of dorsal root fibers in the fasciculi gracilis and cuneatus are degenerated and demyelinated bilaterally, except for fibers in lateral parts of the fasciculi cuneatus which entered above the level of the lesion (about C6). This lesion also produced degeneration in most of the fibers of the spinocerebellar and spinothalamic tracts (Weigert's myelin stain, photograph).

cessive stimuli, produced by applying a tuning fork to a bony prominence or skin, result in a sense of vibration. "Vibratory sense" is not a specific sensory modality, but a temporal modulation of tactile sense (352). The end organs involved in perception of vibratory sense probably are Pacinian corpuscles found in subcutaneous connective tissue and in periosteum. Impulses conveying this form of temporally modulated tactile sense are considered to ascend in both the posterior and lateral columns of the spinal cord (352). The ascending fibers in the posterior columns conduct impulses from receptors on joint surfaces and in joint capsules, which are excited by movement, and are of great importance because they convey information concerning the position of different parts of the body (kinesthesis).

The posterior columns also contain group Ia and Ib muscle afferents. Most of these fibers ascend for variable distances, leave the posterior columns and terminate upon portions of the dorsal nucleus of Clarke. An important exception exists with respect to group Ia and Ib fibers from cervical and upper thoracic segments (2333). These fibers, ascending in the fasciculus cuneatus to low medullary levels, terminate somatotopically in different portions of the *accessory cuneate nucleus*. The accessory cuneate nucleus has cells which resemble those of Clarke's nucleus and, like that nucleus, projects fibers to the cerebellum (Fig. 10-9, 11-9 and 11-10).

The *descending branches of the dorsal root fibers* vary in length, and become displaced medially and posteriorly as they pass to lower segments of the spinal cord. They are relatively shorter fibers, but some may descend a distance of ten or more segments. In the cervical, and most of the thoracic, spinal cord they form a small plug-shaped bundle, the *fasciculus interfascicularis* or *comma tract of Schultze*, lying in the middle of the posterior funiculus (Fig. 9-11 and 10-24). In the lumbar region they descend near the middle of the posterior septum in the *septomarginal fasciculus* (*oval area of Flechsig*), while in the sacral cord these fibers occupy a small triangle near the posteromedian periphery (*triangle of Phillippe-Gombault*) (Fig. 9-20). Besides the descending root fibers, the above named fascicles also contain descending fibers from cells of the posterior gray horn.

Studies based upon horseradish perioxidase (HRP) and autoradiography indicate that cells in the nuclei gracilis and cuneatus give rise to descending axons which pass in the ipsilateral posterior columns (333). These cells, located largely in ventral regions of the posterior column nuclei, appear to project to all spinal levels but the terminal fields established for the cervical spinal segments are specific for Rexed's laminae IV, V and possibly lamina I. These descending pathways are regarded as part of a feedback mechanism which may regulate the flow of sensory information to higher levels of the neuraxis.

Lesions of the posterior columns naturally abolish or diminish discriminating tactile and kinesthetic sense and the symptoms appear on the same side as the lesion. Mere contact and pressure appear normal; but tactile localization is poor, and two-point discrimination and vibratory sense are lost or diminished. There is loss of appreciation of differences in weight and inability to identify objects placed in the hand by feeling them. These symptoms are most acute in the fingers and hand. Position and movement sense is severely affected, especially in the distal parts of the extremities. Small passive movements are not recognized as movements, but as touch or pressure. Even in long excursions the direction and extent of the movement may not be perceived. Loss of position sense greatly impairs the performance of voluntary motor function. This sensory loss causes movements to be clumsy, uncertain and poorly coordinated (posterior column ataxia).

Since a fiber severed from its cell of origin degenerates, injury to the ascending fibers of the posterior white column will produce microscopic evidences of fiber degeneration. These large myelinated fibers frequently are involved totally, or in part, by toxins, or by demyelinating or metabolic diseases. Sections prepared by the Weigert method yield a "negative picture of myelin degeneration" after injury, for only the normal intact fibers are stained (Figs. 10-2 and 10-3). A knowledge of tract formation (Fig. 10-1) enables one to distinguish which region of the spinal cord has been injured sometime prior to death. The series shown in Figure 10-2 was made following injury in the lumbosacral region, and the antemortem neurological signs and symptoms involved the lower extremities and pelvis. Note the decrease of ascending degeneration in the fasiculus gracilis at the second cervical segment. Also observe the progressive increase of normal fibers that have entered the spinal cord above the level of the injury. Contrast the appearance of the second cervical segments shown in Figures 10-2 and 10-3. The antemortem posterior column symptoms were far more extensive in the patient with a cervical cord crush (Fig. 10-3). Here all ascending posterior column fibers were interrupted bilaterally, including part of the sensory fibers from the brachial plexus. Note that only a few normal upper cervical root fibers have entered the fasiculus cuneatus above the level of injury.

Sections of the cord prepared by the Marchi method demonstrate a "positive picture of fiber degeneration" (Fig. 10-4). In such preparations the degenerated myelin sheaths stain as fine brown or black granules. A section of the cervical cord after lumbar injury (Fig. 10-4) shows that degeneration in the posterior columns is limited to the most medial fibers within the fasciculus gracilis. Fibers in the fasciculus cuneatus appear normal, but evidence of Marchi degeneration is seen in other ascending tracts.

The Marchi method yields important information concerning the course of large well myelinated tracts, but it does not provide information concerning the terminations of degenerated fibers. Great care must be used in interpreting Marchi preparations, for this method often produces deceiving artifacts (2359, 2360).

Evidence of degeneration in the posterior columns also can be detected in Nissl stained sections after a considerable period of time. Relatively dense gliosis is present in the areas of degenerated fibers (Fig. 10-5).

Anterior Spinothalamic Tract. For many years it has been assumed that the spinothalamic tracts arose primarily from the large cells of the proper sensory nucleus (i.e., nucleus centrodorsalis, laminae III and IV of Rexed (2135) of the dorsal horn (Figs. 9-16, 9-18 and 9-23); axons of these cells were considered to cross obliquely in the anterior white commissure and ascend contralaterally as part of the spinothalamic system. Studies of Golgi stained prepara-

tions have failed to reveal any fibers arising from cells of lamina III and IV that could be followed into the anterior white commissure (1955, 2496). Attempts to identify the locations of neurons giving rise to the spinothalamic tract by antidromic activation of specific sensory thalamic relay nuclei (i.e. the VPL nucleus) in the monkey indicated that most cells are located contralaterally in laminae IV and V (34, 2575). Subsequent studies in the monkey utilizing HRP identified neurons contralaterally mainly in laminae I, IV and V, though some labeled cells were found in medial lamina VII and dorsal lamina VIII (2574). Labeled cells in these laminae were more numerous in lumbar spinal segments than in cervical segments. Similar studies in the cat, based upon small HRP injections in the thalamus, failed to label spinal neurons; these observations support degeneration studies indicating that in this animal spinal neurons do not project directly to the VPL nucleus of the thalamus (211, 2574).

It is well established that spinothalamic fibers cross in the anterior white commissure, and that the decussation takes place through several spinal segments. Fibers ascending contralaterally in the anterior and anterolateral funiculi form the anterior spinothalamic tract (Figs. 10-4 and 10-6). Fibers of the anterior spinothalamic tract are somatotopically arranged so that those originating from the most caudal segments of the spinal cord are situated laterally with respect to those from more rostral spinal segments. A small number of uncrossed fibers may ascend in the anterior spinothalamic tract; these are not indicated in Figure 10-6.

Fibers of the anterior spinothalamic tract usually are described as ascending without interruption to thalamic levels. As this tract ascends in the brain stem a conspicuous reduction in the number of fibers is evident. In the medulla the tract is located dorsolaterally to the inferior olivary nucleus, where it appears to join the lateral spinothalamic tract. At medullary levels some fibers of this tract, or collaterals, project into the brain stem reticular formation, while others terminate about cells of the lateral reticular nucleus of the medulla, a cerebellar relay nucleus. Fibers projected to these locations explain the reduction in size of this tract in the lower brain stem. At levels through the

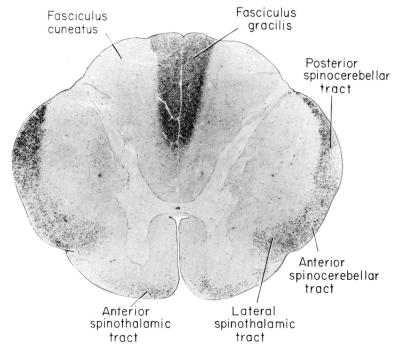

Figure 10-4. Section through second cervical segment of a human spinal cord which had been crushed several weeks previously in the upper lumbar region. The ascending degeneration appears as *black granules* in fibers of the fasciculi gracilis, the anterior and posterior spinocerebellar tracts and in the lateral and anterior spinothalamic tracts (Marchi stain, photograph).

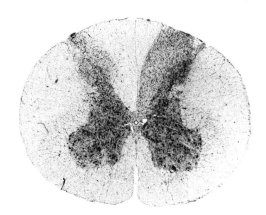

Figure 10-5. Photomicrograph of the fifth cervical spinal segment in a rhesus monkey following multiple cervical dorsal rhizotomies on the right and section of the C5 dorsal root on the left. Intense gliosis sharply outlines the fasciculus cuneatus on the right, while more restricted gliosis on the left occupies the area of degenerated C5 dorsal root fibers (Nissl stain; ×10).

upper pons and midbrain, the tract becomes closely associated with the medial lemniscus. At mesencephalic levels the anterior spinothalamic tract appears to divide into medial and lateral components (1299). The lateral component terminates in the posterior thalamic nucleus and in caudal parts of the VPL nucleus of the thalamus. A few fibers cross the midline and end in these same nuclei on the opposite side. The medial component of the tract projects into the periaqueductal gray and bilaterally into the paralaminar thalamic nuclei (i.e., nuclei near the internal medullary lamina of the thalamus). Axons reaching the VPL nucleus of the thalamus terminate somatotopically on neurons which in turn project to the postcentral gyrus.

The anterior spinothalamic tract transmits impulses associated with what is called "light touch" to higher levels of the neuraxis. Light touch is the sensation provoked by stroking an area of skin devoid of hair (glabrous skin) with a feather or wisp of cotton. This sensation supplements deep touch (pressure) and discriminative tactile sense conveyed in the posterior white columns. Because tactile sensation is transmitted centrally by both the posterior white columns and the anterior spinothalamic tracts, clinically this sensory modality is of

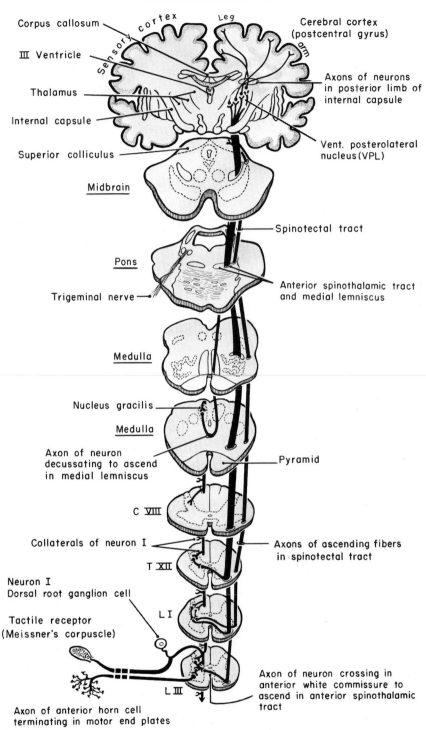

Figure 10-6. Schematic diagram of the anterior spinothalamic (*red*) and the spinotectal (*black*) tracts. These tracts arise from cells in multiple laminae of the spinal gray at all levels. The largest number of spinothalamic fibers appear to arise from cells in laminae I, IV and V contralaterally. The anterior spinothalamic tract conveys impulses associated with "light touch," the sensation produced by stroking glabrous skin with a wisp of cotton. The spinotectal tract ascends in close association with the anterior spinothalamic tract but terminates in deep layers of the contralateral superior colliculus and in parts of the periaqueductal gray; this tract conveys nociceptive impulses. Letters and numbers indicate segmental spinal levels.

limited value in localizing injuries of the spinal cord. Injury to the anterior spinothalamic tract in the spinal cord produces little, if any, disturbance in tactile sensibility. The pleasant or unpleasant character of certain sensations, however, is considered to be related to conduction in the anterolateral funiculi. Bilateral destruction of these columns may cause complete loss of such affective qualities as itching, tickling and libidinous feeling (766). According to Kerr (1299) the lateral component of the anterior spinothalamic tract which projects to VPL probably is associated with discriminatory functions, while fibers passing to the posterior thalamic nucleus and to the periaqueductal gray may be concerned with nociceptive stimuli.

Lateral spinothalamic Tract. Closely related to the anterior spinothalamic tract is the lateral spinothalamic tract. It is treated separately in view of its tremendous clinical importance. Its component fibers are more concentrated than those in the anterior spinothalamic tract, and it contains more long fibers that go directly to the thalamus (1297). The receptors of pain and thermal sense represent peripheral endings of the small- and medium-sized dorsal root ganglion cells, whose thin central processes enter the zone of Lissauer (Fig. 10-7). Statements made in regard to the cells of origin of the anterior spinothalamic tract apply also to the lateral spinothalamic tract. Thus it seems likely that cells largely in laminae I, IV and V and give rise to most of the axons that cross in the anterior white commissure and ascend in the opposite lateral funiculus, as the lateral spinothalamic tract (34, 2574). Fibers of this tract cross obliquely to the opposite side within the segment of entry, although some may ascend one segment before crossing. Fibers of this tract are medial to those of the anterior spinocerebellar tract (Figs. 10-4 and 10-24).

The fibers show an anteromedial segmental arrangement in the lateral spinothalamic tract. The most lateral and posterior fibers represent the lowest portion of the body, whereas the more medial and anterior fibers are related to the upper extremity and neck (Fig. 10-7). As shown on the left of level C8, there is also a lamination of the sensory modalities within this tract; fibers concerned with thermal sense are

posterior while fibers associated with pain are located more anteriorly. Injuries of this compact pathway ordinarily affect both pain and thermal sense. At higher levels this tract sends numerous collaterals into the brain stem reticular formation.

Detailed studies of anterolateral cordotomy in the monkey (229, 232, 1658) indicate that the thalamic projections of the spinothalamic system are more complex than classic studies suggest. Unilateral anterolateral cordotomy produces thalamic degeneration: (a) predominantly ipsilaterally in the VPL nucleus and (b) bilaterally in certain intralaminar nuclei and in a posterior thalamic nucleus (near the magnocellular part of the medial geniculate body). These anatomical observations, confirmed by physiological studies (1972, 2019, 2707), indicate that in the VPL nucleus: (a) the body surface is represented in a distorted, but orderly somatotopical manner, (b) cells of this nucleus are related to small specific receptive fields contralaterally and (c) most cells are not activated by noxious stimuli. In the posterior thalamic nucleus there is said to be a crude topographical representation; cells in this region are said to be activated from large receptive fields, both ipsilaterally and contralaterally, and respond to noxious stimuli.

Unilateral section of this tract produces a complete loss of pain and thermal sense (analgesia and thermoanesthesia) on the opposite side of the body. This contralateral sensory loss extends to a level one segment below that of the lesion, owing to the oblique crossing of fibers (Fig. 10-26). The anesthesia involves the superficial and deep portions of the body wall, but not the viscera, which appear to be represented bilaterally. The anogenital region is not markedly affected with unilateral lesions. After a variable period there is often some return of pain and thermal sensibility, due perhaps to the presence of uncrossed spinothalamic fibers. Such pain impulses also may ascend by shorter relays along spinospinal and spinoreticular pathways.

In certain instances bilateral surgical section of the lateral spinothalamic tracts (cordotomy) is performed at slightly different levels on selected patients to relieve pain and produce a complete and more enduring sensory loss. The spinothalamic and trigeminothalamic pathways both may be de-

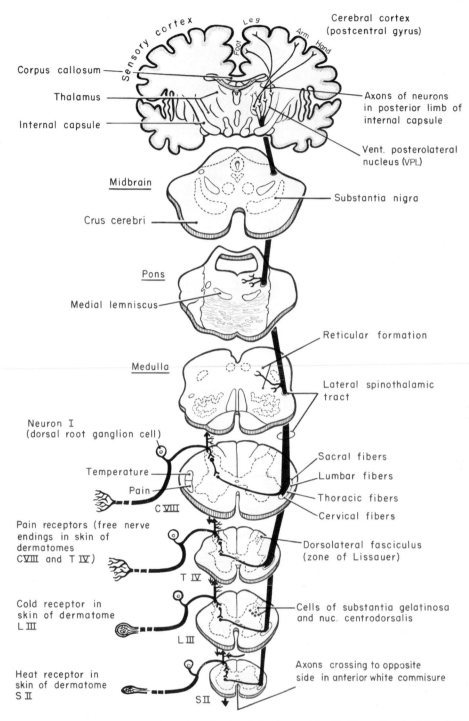

Figure 10-7. Schematic diagram of the lateral spinothalamic tract (*red*). The cells of origin of the lateral spinothalamic tract appear to be largely in laminae I, IV and V of Rexed. Fibers of this tract usually cross to the opposite side within one segment in the anterior white commissure. The lateral spinothalamic tract has a more complex termination in the thalamus than indicated here, conveys impulses associated with pain and thermal sense, and has a somatotopic lamination. Letters and numbers indicate segmental spinal levels.

stroyed by one laterally placed lesion in the medulla or midbrain, where these two tracts occupy a superficial position (Figs. 10-7 and 12-27). Interruption of both tracts at midbrain levels results in a loss of pain and thermal sense over the face, neck, trunk and extremities on the opposite side of the body.

Nathan and Smith (1804) presented evidence that in man the fibers subserving the sensation of bladder fullness and desire to micturate, and fibers associated with pain from the bladder, urethra and lower ureter, are all located in the lateral spinothalamic tract. They believe that fibers mediating touch, pressure or tension in the urethra ascend in the posterior white column.

It is evident from the above that the sensory impulses brought in by the dorsal roots are organized in the spinal cord into two main systems: discriminative (epicritic) and affective (vital, protopathic); the former are related to the long fibers of the posterior white columns and the latter to the shorter root fibers and the anterolateral white column. Discriminative sensibility carried by the longest fibers remains uncrossed in the spinal cord. Pain and thermal impulses, initially conveyed by the short fibers in the zone of Lissauer, may synapse one or more times before reaching cells that give rise to fibers crossing in the anterior white commissure that form the lateral spinothalamic tract.

This distribution of afferent impulses accounts for the curious sensory dissociation occurring in the hemisection of the spinal cord (Brown-Séquard syndrome), where there is loss of pain and thermal sense on the opposite half of the body below the level of the lesion, while the sense of position and movement, two-point discrimination and vibration are lost on the same side as the lesion (Fig. 10-26).

Spinocervical and Cervicothalamic Tracts. Experimental studies in the cat, which appears to lack an uninterrupted spinothalamic tract terminating in the VPL nucleus of the thalamus (34, 211, 335), suggest that spinocervical and cervicothalamic tracts may serve as its homologue (561, 562, 1748, 1749, 2517, 2518). Cells of origin of the spinocervical tract lie in lamina IV at all spinal levels and give rise to uncrossed fibers that ascend in the dorsolateral funiculus (561, 2517). These cells in the posterior

gray horn are monosynaptically activated by dorsal root afferents that respond chiefly to low threshold cutaneous stimuli (1421, 1539). Most of these units are activated by tactile stimuli from relatively restricted receptive fields, but additional activation results from pressure and pinching the skin. Axons of cells in lamina IV ascend ipsilaterally in the dorsolateral funiculus and synapse upon cells of the lateral cervical nucleus (Figs. 9-31 and 10-8). The *lateral cervical nucleus* is a longitudinal cell column, lateral to the posterior horn, in the lateral funiculus of the upper three cervical segments of the cat's spinal cord (2138). This nucleus is present in a variety of species, including man, although it is most prominent in carnivores (994, 2584). Cells of the lateral cervical nucleus are somatotopically organized (563). The lateral cervical nucleus gives rise to fibers that cross in the anterior white commissure at levels of the first and second cervical spinal segments, and ascend in association with the medial lemniscus to the thalamus, where they end in a restricted part of the VPL nucleus (210, 562, 1421, 1701). Retrograde transport studies based upon HRP indicate that virtually all of the cells of the lateral cervical nucleus project to the contralateral thalamus and terminate somatotopically (562). There also are indications that the dorsal column-medial lemniscal pathway and the spinocervicothalamic projection may be functionally linked, because some spinocervical collaterals end in the dorsal column nuclei and some cells of the dorsal column nuclei project to the lateral cervical nucleus (561).

Impulses transmitted via the spinocervicothalamic lemniscal pathway reach the cortex earlier than those mediated via the dorsal column-medial lemniscal pathway (1851). Its integrity is essential for the earliest portion of the cortical evoked potential in somatic sensory areas I and II (65), and according to Oscarsson and Rosén (1904), this pathway also activates the motor cortex. Single units of the spinocervical tract show spontaneous activity and respond to hair movement and thermal stimuli with a uniformly low threshold. The spinocervical tract, containing 2000 to 3000 fibers, 10 to 14 μm in diameter, is the most rapidly conducting pathway in the feline spinal cord. Anatomical studies suggest that the spinocervical tract may convey

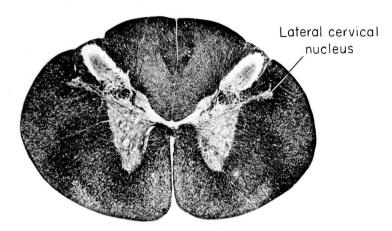

Figure 10-8. Photomicrograph of the first cervical segment of the cat spinal cord demonstrating the lateral cervical nucleus. Cells of the lateral cervical nucleus receive fibers of the spinocervical tract, considered the feline equivalent of the spinothalamic tract. Fibers arising from cells in the lateral cervical nucleus cross in the upper cervical spinal segments and ascend to the thalamus is association with the medial lemniscus (cresyl violet, ×100).

impulses related to painful stimuli and also plays a role in integration of motor functions.

Spinotectal Tract. The cells of origin of the small spinotectal tract are not known but they are presumed to arise from cells of the posterior horn. Fibers of this crossed tract, located in the anterolateral part of the spinal cord (Figs. 10-6 and 10-24), ascend in the spinal cord and brain stem in close association with the spinothalamic system (78, 2022). At midbrain levels fibers of the spinotectal tract project medially into the intermediate and deep layers of the superior colliculus. There is some evidence of more than one spinotectal tract; in addition to the classic pathway described above there are fibers that ascend ipsilaterally in the spinal cord and cross in the intertectal commissures (78). In the contralateral superior colliculus, crossed fibers terminate somatotopically in an orderly fashion in the caudal half of the colliculus. Some spinotectal fibers also terminate in lateral regions of the central gray substance. While the functional significance of the spinotectal tract is largely conjecture, evidence suggests that it is part of a multisynaptic pathway transmitting nociceptive impulses (1658). This view is supported by observations (1589, 2400) of behavioral reactions which suggest painful sensations as a consequence of stimulation of the superior colliculus and periaqueductal gray. The superior colliculus is a brain stem locus receiving multiple sensory inputs.

Posterior Spinocerebellar Tract. This prominent uncrossed ascending tract, situated along the posterolateral periphery of the spinal cord (Figs. 10-3, 10-4, 10-9 and 10-24), arises from the large cells of Clarke's column (dorsal nucleus) which extend from the third lumbar (L3) to the eight cervical (C8) segment. Afferent fibers reach the nuclei via the dorsal roots (Fig. 9-30). The cells of Clarke's nucleus give rise to large fibers which pass laterally in the ipsilateral white matter and ascend the entire length of the spinal cord. In the medulla fibers of this tract become incorporated in the inferior cerebellar peduncle (Figs. 2-25 and 2-31), enter the cerebellum and terminate in both rostral and caudal portions of the vermis. The tract first appears in the upper lumbar cord (L3) and increases in size until the upper limit of Clarke's nucleus is reached (C8). Since the column of Clarke is not present in lower lumbar and sacral spinal segments, impulses entering via these caudal dorsal roots, and destined for

Figure 10-9. Schematic diagram of the anterior (*red*) and posterior (*blue*) spinocerebellar tracts and the cuneocerebellar tract (*blue*). The posterior spinocerebellar tract arises from cells of the dorsal nucleus of Clarke and is uncrossed; it conveys impulses arising from muscle spindles and Golgi tendon organs. Fibers of the anterior spinocerebellar tract are crossed and arise from cells in parts of laminae V, VI and VII; fibers of this tract are activated by impulses from Golgi tendon organs. The cuneocerebellar tract, arising from cells of the

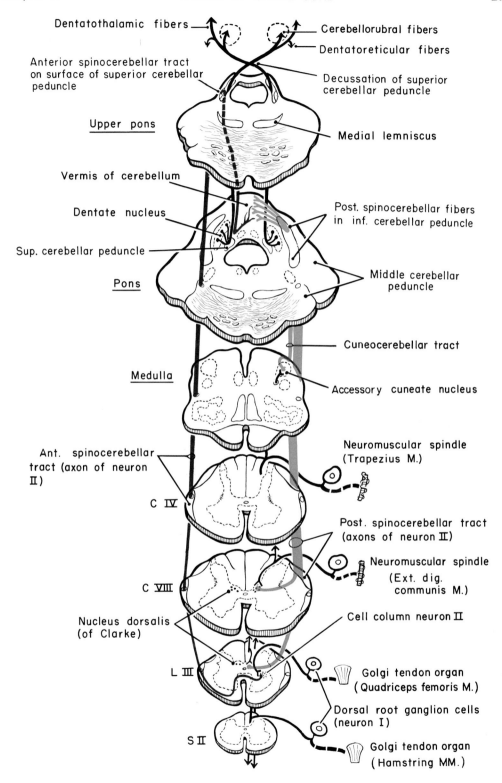

accessory cuneate nucleus in the medulla, is considered the upper limb equivalent of the posterior spinocerebellar tract; this tract is uncrossed. An uncrossed rostral spinocerebellar tract (not shown) is considered the upper limb equivalent of the anterior spinocerebellar tract in the cat. Letters and numbers indicate spinal levels.

the cerebellum, are first conveyed rostrally in the fasciculus gracilis by ascending branches of dorsal root fibers; at higher levels where Clarke's column is present, these fibers leave the fasciculus gracilis and enter the dorsal nucleus (Figs. 9-27 and 10-9).

Experimental evidence (416, 941, 1499, 2333) indicates that Clarke's nucleus receives both ascending and descending collaterals of dorsal root fibers, and a single dorsal root may supply afferent fibers to Clarke's nucleus in as many as six or seven spinal segments. Thus there is extensive overlapping of afferent fibers of certain dorsal roots in their termination in Clarke's nucleus. Clarke's nucleus receives afferent fibers via dorsal roots from all parts of the body except the head and neck (C1 to C4 dorsal roots), but functionally this nucleus appears related primarily to the hindlimb and caudal parts of the body.

Fibers of the posterior spinocerebellar tract have conduction velocities ranging from 30 to 110 m/sec (1505, 1900), and terminate ipsilaterally in the cerebellar vermal cortex (939). Areas of fiber termination in the anterior lobe of the cerebellum correspond to Larsell's lobules I to IV (Fig. 14-1), while those in posterior regions end mainly in parts of the pyramis and paramedian lobule. According to physiological studies (422, 511, 2371) these cerebellar cortical areas represent mainly the hindlimb.

The uncrossed pathway from periphery to cerebellum is composed of two neurons, the spinal ganglion cells and the cells of Clarke's column (dorsal nucleus) (Fig. 10-9). Degeneration studies in man have emphasized that the anterior and posterior spinocerebellar tracts are difficult to delimit as they form the margins of the lateral funiculus in the spinal cord. Many fibers of the anterior spinocerebellar tract move posteriorly as they ascend and become incorporated within the posterior spinocerebellar tract (2361).

Impulses relayed to the cerebellum via the posterior spinocerebellar tract arise from the muscle spindles and the Golgi tendon organs and from touch and pressure receptors. Neurons of Clarke's column receive monosynaptic excitation by group Ia and Ib afferent fibers via the dorsal root ganglion, and often there is additional ex-

citation from group II muscle spindle afferents (1900). There is no evidence that the posterior spinocerebellar tract is activated by stimulation of low threshold joint receptors. The synaptic linkage between group I afferents and the dorsal nucleus allows transmission of impulses at high frequencies, and little spatial summation is required for eliciting a discharge in the posterior spinocerebellar tract. The majority of neurons in Clarke's column are activated by either Ia or Ib afferents, but some neurons apparently receive excitation from both types of afferents. The occasional convergence of Ia and Ib excitation is said to be of little functional significance. Certain exteroceptive impulses are related to touch and pressure receptors in the skin, and slowly adapting pressure receptors in foot pads also are transmitted by the posterior spinocerebellar tract (1900).

Thus the posterior spinocerebellar tract relays impulses from stretch receptors, touch receptors and pressure receptors directly from spinal levels to particular parts of the cerebellum. The tract is somatotopically organized in its course and termination, and impulse transmission is little influenced by supraspinal mechanisms. Present information suggests that impulses conveyed by this tract are utilized in the fine coordination of posture and movement of individual limb muscles.

Anterior Spinocerebellar Tract. Situated along the lateral periphery of the spinal cord anterior to the posterior spinocerebellar tract, and posterior to the site of emergence of ventral root fibers (Figs. 10-3, 10-4 and 10-9), is the anterior spinocerebellar tract. Medial to this tract is the lateral spinothalamic tract. The tract makes its first appearance in the lower lumbar spinal cord. In upper cervical spinal segments some fibers of the tract become incorporated within the posterior spinocerebellar tract (2361). In the human brain stem the anterior spinocerebellar tract appears quite small.

Fibers of the anterior spinocerebellar tract were considered by Cooper and Sherington (532) to arise in lumbar spinal segments from cells in the periphery of the anterior horn, known as "spinal border cells" or the *nucleus pericornualis anterior*. Investigations by Hubbard and Oscarsson (1151) in the cat indicate that cells of origin of this tract occupy the lateral part of the base and neck of the posterior horn and the lateral part of the intermediate zone (i.e., parts of laminae V, VI and VII of Rexed). These cells form a column extending caudally as far as sacral (940), or coccygeal segments (993). The investigations of Ha and Liu (993) indicate that the cells of origin of the anterior spinocerebellar tract are widely distributed in the dorsolateral part of the anterior gray. Morphologically these neurons are almost impossible to distinguish from motor neurons in Nissl preparations of normal spinal cord. In the cat, cells of this scattered cell column extend rostrally to the L1 segment; there is no "forelimb" component. Fibers of the anterior spinocerebellar tract are less numerous than those of the posterior spinocerebellar tract, are composed uniformly large fibers (11 to 20 μm), have conduction velocities of 70 to 120 m/sec and are virtually all crossed.

This pathway to the cerebellum is composed of two neurons: neuron I in the dorsal root ganglia, and neuron II in the scattered cell groups at the base of the anterior and posterior horns in lumbar, sacral and coccygeal spinal segments. Fibers of neuron II cross in the spinal cord, and ascend through spinal cord, medulla and pons. At upper pontine levels the tract enters the cerebellum by coursing along the dorsal surface of the superior cerebellar peduncle (Fig. 10-9). Although physiological studies (422, 511) indicate that fibers of this ascending system cross initially at spinal levels and recross again within the cerebellum, anatomical studies in man suggest that only a small number of these fibers cross in the cerebellum (2362). Experimental studies show that the majority of fibers of this tract in the cat terminate contralaterally; about 10% end ipsilaterally and about 15%, after branching, end both ipsilaterally and contralaterally. Within the cerebellar cortex, fibers of this tract have a rostrocaudal distribution similar to that of the posterior spinocerebellar tract, except that the main area of termination is in the anterior lobe (lobules I to IV) (940, 1906).

Cells which give rise to the anterior spinocerebellar tract receive monosynaptic excitation from ipsilateral group Ib afferents, and polysynaptic excitation and inhibition from ipsilateral and contralateral flexor reflex afferents (1900). Fibers of this tract are activated by afferent impulses from Golgi tendon organs with receptive fields which often include one synergic muscle group at each joint of the ipsilateral limb. It is presumed that the fibers of this system convey information concerning movement or posture of the whole limb rather than information about movements in individual muscles. The significance of polysynaptic excitation and inhibition received via flexor reflex afferents remains obscure. Transmission of impulses in the anterior spinocerebellar tract is said to be controlled by supraspinal systems that might allow selection of information from either tendon organ afferents or flexor reflex afferents.

The effects of injury to these spinocerebellar tracts in the spinal cord are difficult to judge, since other tracts usually are involved simultaneously. Injury to the cerebellum itself results in a reduced muscle tone and in an incoordination of muscular activity (cerebellar ataxia or asynergia). There is no loss of kinesthetic sense as a consequence of these lesions since impulses projected to the cerebellum do not enter the conscious sphere.

Cuneocerebellar Tract. Since the column of Clarke is not present above C8, large fibers of cervical spinal nerves entering above this level ascend ipsilaterally in the fasciculus cuneatus. Fibers conveying impulses from group Ia and Ib muscle afferents and some cutaneous afferents pass to the *accessory cuneate nucleus*, a group of large cells in the dorsolateral part of the medulla with cytological features similar to those of the dorsal nucleus of Clarke (Figs. 10-9 and 11-9). The accessory cuneate nucleus in the monkey receives afferents via the dorsal roots from T7 to C1 (2333) which terminate in an overlapping systematic fashion (Fig. 11-10). Cells of the accessory cuneate nucleus give rise to the cuneocerebellar tract, the upper limb equivalent of the posterior spinocerebellar tract. Fibers of this tract known as posterior external arcuate fibers, enter the cerebellum as a component of the inferior cerebellar peduncle and terminate in the ipsilateral cerebellar cortex (lobule V). These cerebellar afferent fibers are distributed to the forelimb area of the intermediate zone in the anterior lobe and to forelimb areas of the pyramis and paramedian lobule (Fig. 14-1).

Rostral Spinocerebellar Tract. In carnivores another spinocerebellar pathway, the rostral spinocerebellar tract, has been described as the forelimb equivalent of the anterior spinocerebellar tract (1898, 1900, 1903, 1906). The cells of origin are rostral to the column of Clarke in the cervical spinal cord and they give rise to an uncrossed tract ascending in the anterior part of the lateral funiculus which enters the cerebellum via both inferior and superior cerebellar peduncles. Anatomical studies suggest that this tract may arise from the large neurons of the centrobasal nucleus located in lamina VI of the cervical enlargement (1636, 1995). This tract resembles the anterior spinocerebellar tract, except that it is uncrossed; fibers of the tract project ipsilaterally to lobules I to V of the anterior lobe of the cerebellum.

Another smaller crossed *cervicospinocerebellar* pathway arises from an interrupted column of cells in the upper cervical spinal cord (C1 to C4), known as the central cervical nucleus (Fig. 9-31) (579, 1636, 1637). This pathway conveys impulses from upper cervical spinal segments to cerebellum.

Thus in addition to the posterior and anterior spinocerebellar tracts, related primarily to the hindlimbs and caudal parts of the body, there are two equivalent tracts, the cuneocerebellar and the rostral spinocerebellar, that relay sensory information from the forelimbs and rostral parts of the body (1900). The posterior spinocerebellar and cuneocerebellar tracts are similar and convey information from muscle spindles, tendon organs and touch and pressure receptors in the skin. The anterior spinocerebellar and rostral spinocerebellar tracts are similar in that they convey impulses from tendon organ afferents and flexor reflex afferents, both with wide receptive fields.

Spino-olivary Pathways. These tracts appear to constitute another component of a spinocerebellar circuitry. Although physiological data indicate multiple spino-olivary tracts, the two best defined tracts have been designated as the posterior and anterior spino-olivary tracts (1901, 1903, 1905). Fibers of the posterior spino-olivary tract ascend in the posterior white columns to the nuclei gracilis and cuneatus; the posterior column nuclei relay impulses to parts of the accessory olivary nuclei. The multiple anterior spino-olivary tracts ascend contralaterally in the anterior funiculus and terminate upon portions of the dorsal and medial accessory olivary nuclei. Fibers contributing to the spino-olivary tracts arise from all levels of the spinal cord, are somatotopically organized and are activated by cutaneous afferents and group Ib afferents from Golgi tendon organs. Attempts to determine the cells of origin of anterior spino-olivary tracts using the retrograde transport of HRP in the cat have identified cells in lower lumbar segments in laminae IV and V and in medial regions of laminae VII and VIII (85). These studies confirm the crossed nature of these multiple tracts. The accessory olivary nuclei which receive the spino-olivary systems, give rise to crossed olivocerebellar fibers which project mainly to the anterior lobe of the cerebellum. Brodal (270) has referred to these spino-olivary-cerebellar linkages as the *indirect spinocerebellar pathways.*

Spinoreticular Fibers. Impulses from the spinal cord also project to widespread regions of the brain stem reticular formation. Spinoreticular fibers originate from all spinal levels, presumably from cells located in the posterior horn (263, 1657, 1751, 2229). These fibers ascend in the anterolateral funiculus, and those terminating in the medullary reticular formation are preponderantly uncrossed (Fig. 10-10). In the medulla these fibers terminate chiefly upon cells of the nucleus reticularis gigantocellularis and parts of the lateral reticular nucleus. The lateral reticular nucleus of the medulla (Fig. 11-8) is known to project to specific portions of the cerebellum, indicating that some fibers in this pathway are concerned with the transmission of exteroceptive impulses to the cerebellum. Large cells of the nucleus reticularis gigantocellularis project to spinal levels as well as to more rostral regions of the brain stem. Spinoreticular fibers passing to pontine levels are distributed bilaterally and are less numerous than those terminating in the medulla. Most of these fibers end in the nucleus reticularis pontis caudalis (266). A smaller number of spinoreticular fibers

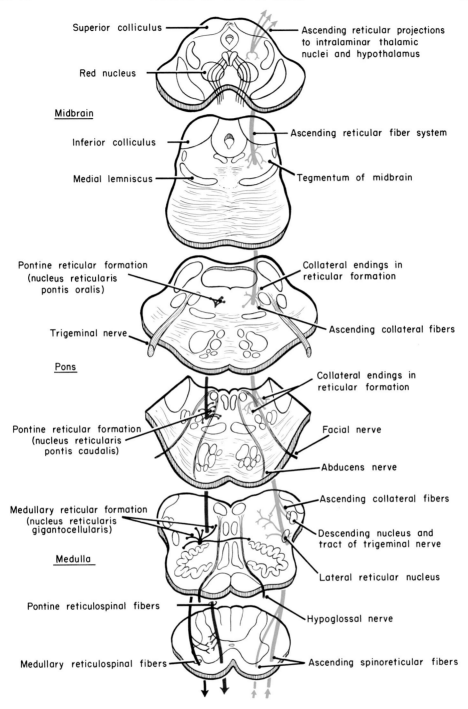

Figure 10-10. Schematic diagram of ascending and descending reticular fiber systems. Ascending spinoreticular projections and collaterals are shown on the *right* (*blue*). In this system collaterals are given off at various brain stem levels and the pathway is augmented by rostrally projecting reticular fibers. Pontine reticulospinal fibers (*red*) are uncrossed and originate largely from the nucleus reticularis pontis caudalis. Medullary reticulospinal fibers (*black*), predominantly uncrossed, arise from the nuclus reticularis gigantocellularis. Descending fibers from these sources are not topographically organized or sharply segregated in the spinal cord. (Based upon Olszewski and Baxter (1885), Brodal (266), and Nauta and Kuypers (1823).)

have been found in the reticular formation in the region of transition from pons to mesencephalon (1872). Functionally, the spinoreticular fibers represent part of a phylogenetically old, polysynaptic system which plays a significant role in the maintenance of the state of consciousness and awareness. This complex, referred to as the ascending reticular system (1756), is considered in more detail in Chapter 13.

Other Ascending Fiber Systems in the Spinal Cord. In addition to the ascending fiber systems mentioned in preceding sections, several other ascending pathways have been described. While the existence of these anatomical pathways seems certain, relatively little is known of their functional significance.

A *spinocortical tract* has been described in man and experimental animals (287, 1805). Fibers of this tract were said to arise from all levels of the spinal cord. Because axoplasmic transport studies have failed to identify any spinal neurons projecting directly to the cerebral cortex (288a), the existence of this tract appears doubtful. Other ascending fiber systems described include the spinovestibular, spinopontine and the already mentioned spino-olivary pathways.

Spinovestibular fibers project largely upon the dorsal part of the lateral vestibular nucleus and to parts of the inferior vestibular nucleus which do not receive primary fibers. These fibers ascend ipsilaterally in the spinal cord from levels as far caudally as lumbar segments (2040). Many fibers of this tract are partially intermingled with those of the posterior spinocerebellar tract.

Spinopontine fibers have been described as terminating upon pontine nuclei. It has been suggested that these fibers may transmit exteroceptive impulses to the cerebellum (2641).

LONG DESCENDING SPINAL TRACTS

The descending spinal tracts are concerned with somatic movement (motor function), visceral innervation, the modification of muscle tone, segmental reflexes and central transmission of sensory impulses. The largest and most important of these tracts arises from the cerebral cortex; all other descending spinal tracts arise from localized cell groups in the three lowest segments of the brain stem.

Corticospinal System. These tracts consist of all fibers which: (a) originate from cells within the cerebral cortex, (b) pass through the medullary pyramid and (c) enter the spinal cord. They constitute the largest and most important descending fiber system in the human neuraxis. In man each tract is composed of over 1,000,000 fibers of which some 700,000 are myelinated (1442, 1447, 1448). Approximately 90% of these myelinated fibers have a diameter of 1 to 4 μm; most of the remaining myelinated fibers range in caliber from 5 to 10 μm, but included among them are some 30,000 to 40,000 very large fibers having a thickness of 10 to 22 μm. Fibers of the corticospinal system arise from cells in the deeper part of lamina V in the precentral area (area 4), the premotor area (area 6), the postcentral gyrus (areas 3a, 3b, 1, 2) and adjacent parietal cortex (area 5) (540, 1245). Cells of origin of the corticospinal system, arranged in strips or clusters, vary greatly in size in different cortical areas (Fig. 10-11). The largest fibers arise mainly from the giant pyramidal cells of Betz in the precentral gyrus (area 4 of Brodmann; Fig. 19-5), but some may arise from adjacent cortical areas. These corticofugal fibers converge in the corona radiata and pass downward through the internal capsule, crus cerebri, pons and medulla (Figs. 2-11, 10-11 and 10-12). As this large tract descends in the brain stem, it passes close to the emerging root fibers of cranial nerves III, VI and XII. *Corticobulbar fibers* conveying impulses to motor nuclei of the brain stem are closely associated with corticospinal fibers in the internal capsule and brain stem. Cells of origin of corticobulbar fibers are found in the same cortical areas as corticospinal neurons but lie more superficially in lamina V and are quite uniform in size (1245). The corticospinal tract comes to the surface in the medullary pyramid. At the junction of medulla and cord, the fibers undergo an incomplete decussation giving rise to three tracts: (a) a large *lateral corticospinal tract* (crossed), (b) an *anterior corticospinal tract* (uncrossed) and (c) a small *anterolateral corticospinal tract* (uncrossed and illustrated in Fig. 10-12).

The majority of the fibers, 75 to 90%,

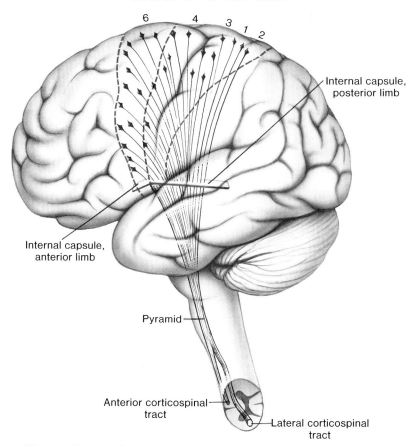

Figure 10-11. Schematic diagram of the lateral and anterior corticospinal tracts (*red*) showing their regions of origin and course. These tracts arise from cells of various sizes in the deep parts of lamina V.

cross in the pyramidal decussation and descend in the posterior part of the lateral funiculus as the lateral or crossed corticospinal tract, lying between the posterior spinocerebellar tract and the lateral fasciculus proprius (Figs. 10-12–10-15). In lower lumbar and sacral spinal segments, caudal to the posterior spinocerebellar tract fibers of the corticospinal tract reach the dorsolateral surface of the spinal cord (Fig. 10-16). In the uppermost cervical segments some fibers of that tract occupy, for a short distance, an aberrant position external to the posterior spinocerebellar fibers. The tract extends to the most caudal part of the cord and progressively diminishes in size as more and more fibers leave to terminate in the gray matter.

A smaller portion of the pyramidal fibers descend uncrossed as the anterior or direct corticospinal tract (bundle of Türck), oc-

cupying an oval area adjacent to the anterior median fissure (Figs. 10-11–10-15). It normally extends only to the upper thoracic cord, and innervates primarily the muscles of the upper extremities and neck. This tract is found only in man and the higher apes and shows considerable variation, because the proportion of decussating fibers is not constant. In extreme cases the tract may be absent. In rare cases, the pyramidal tract fibers of one or both sides may not cross at all and may form a huge anterior corticospinal tracts (2616).

Besides the two tracts discussed, there are other uncrossed corticospinal fibers which form the *anterolateral corticospinal tract* of Barnes (121) ("fibres pyramidales homolaterales superficelles" of Dejerine). This tract is composed of fine fibers which descend more anteriorly in the lateral funiculus (Fig. 10-12).

Corticospinal tract

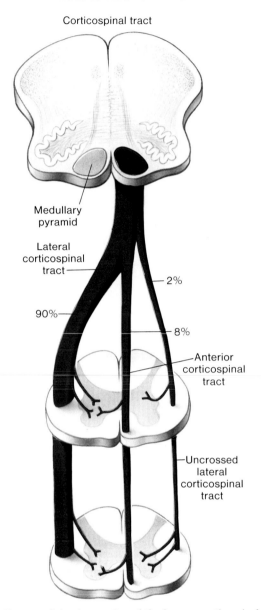

Medullary
pyramid

Lateral
corticospinal
tract

2%

90%

8%

Anterior
corticospinal
tract

Uncrossed
lateral
corticospinal
tract

Figure 10-12. Schematic diagram of the decussation of the human corticospinal tract (*red*). Approximately 90% of the corticospinal tract crosses in the lower medulla to form the *lateral corticospinal tract*. Of the fibers which do not decussate in the medulla approximately 8% form the *anterior corticospinal tract* which descends in the ventral funiculus; most of these fibers cross in cervical spinal segments. The small number of fibers in the *uncrossed lateral corticospinal tract* (121) remain uncrossed.

Figure 10-13. Schematic diagram of lateral and anterior corticospinal tracts—the principal descending motor pathways concerned with skilled, voluntary motor activity. The locations of the corticobulbar tracts at each level of the brain stem are indicated by *black areas* (*right side*). Letters and numbers indicate corresponding segments of the spinal cord.

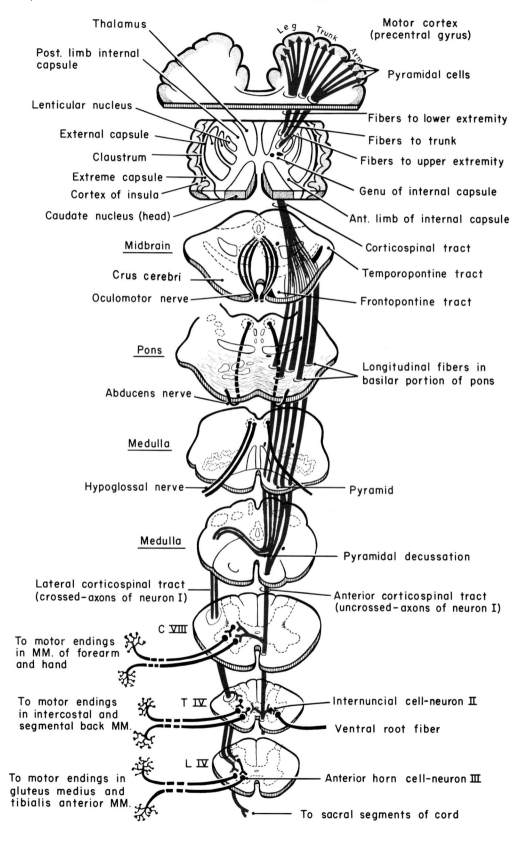

Thalamus

Post. limb internal capsule

Lenticular nucleus

External capsule

Claustrum

Extreme capsule

Cortex of insula

Caudate nucleus (head)

Motor cortex (precentral gyrus)

Leg Trunk Arm

Pyramidal cells

Fibers to lower extremity

Fibers to trunk

Fibers to upper extremity

Genu of internal capsule

Ant. limb of internal capsule

Midbrain

Crus cerebri

Oculomotor nerve

Corticospinal tract

Temporopontine tract

Frontopontine tract

Pons

Abducens nerve

Longitudinal fibers in basilar portion of pons

Medulla

Hypoglossal nerve

Pyramid

Medulla

Pyramidal decussation

Lateral corticospinal tract (crossed-axons of neuron I)

Anterior corticospinal tract (uncrossed-axons of neuron I)

C VIII

To motor endings in MM. of forearm and hand

T IV

To motor endings in intercostal and segmental back MM.

Internuncial cell-neuron II

Ventral root fiber

L IV

To motor endings in gluteus medius and tibialis anterior MM.

Anterior horn cell-neuron III

To sacral segments of cord

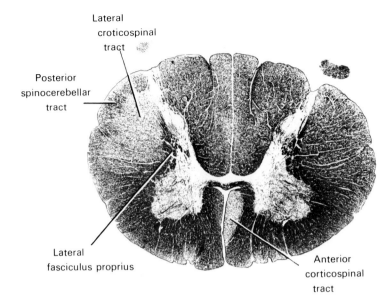

Figure 10-14. Transverse section through the cervical enlargement of an individual sustaining a vascular lesion of one medullary pyramid. The lateral corticospinal tract on the left and the anterior corticospinal tract on the side of the lesion are degenerated and demyelinated (Weigert's myelin stain, photograph).

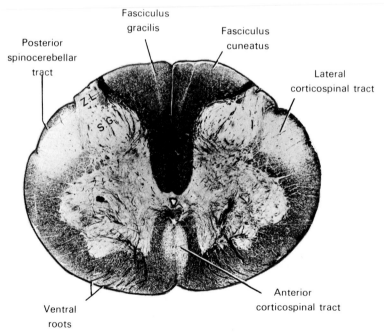

Figure 10-15. Section through the cervical enlargement of spinal cord of 7- to 8-month human fetus. The corticospinal tracts are unmyelinated at this stage and hence are unstained. *S.G.*, Substantia gelatinosa; *Z.L.*, zone of Lissauer (Weigert's myelin stain, photograph).

Fibers of the crossed lateral corticospinal tract enter the gray matter laterally in the region of the intermediate zone. Silver impregnation studies in the monkey indicate that fibers enter both dorsolateral and ventromedial parts of lamina VII; in the cervical and lumbosacral enlargements some fibers project beyond to motor neurons in

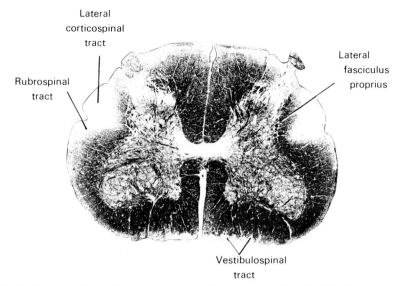

Lateral
corticospinal
tract

Rubrospinal
tract

Lateral
fasciculus
proprius

Vestibulospinal
tract

Figure 10-16. Section through fourth lumbar segment of a human spinal cord which had been crushed some time previously in the lower cervical region. The degenerated long descending tracts are unstained. Note that the lateral corticospinal tract reaches the lateral periphery of the spinal cord at this level and the vestibulospinal tract lies on the anterior surface of the cord (Weigert's myelin stain, photograph).

lamina IX (1409). In addition rostral parts of the precentral gyrus distributed fibers bilaterally to ventromedial parts of the intermediate zone (i.e. Rexed's lamina VIII). In the monkey Liu and Chambers (1500) describe corticospinal fibers passing into lamina VII and into the base of both the posterior and anterior horns. A few fibers of the lateral corticospinal tract have been described as crossing in the posterior and anterior gray commissures to end in the intermediate gray and the dorsomedial and central parts of the contralateral anterior horn.

The majority of axons in the anterior corticospinal tract have been found to cross in cervical spinal segments in the anterior white commissure and to terminate in the intermediate gray and the centromedial part of the anterior horn (Fig. 10-12). Fibers of the uncrossed lateral corticospinal tract remain uncrossed and terminate in the base of the posterior horn, the intermediate gray and central parts of the anterior horn. In an attempt to determine the differential distribution of corticospinal projections Coulter and Jones (541) injected ^{3}H-labeled amino acids into individual cortical areas. These studies demonstrated that fibers from the precentral motor cortex terminate

extensively in the intermediate zone (i.e., lamina VII) and in dorsolateral parts of the anterior horn (i.e., lamina IX), while areas of the somatic sensory cortex (areas 3b, 1, 2 and 5) each terminate in different though partially overlapping zones of the posterior horn. In the monkey it appears well established that some corticospinal fibers end in direct synaptic contact with anterior horn cells, although the majority of fibers are said to terminate on internuncial neurons in the intermediate zone. Some physiological and anatomical studies suggest a somatotopical organization in the monkey in which fibers from the precentral gyrus pass to epi-axial motor neurons, but not axial motor neurons (168, 1408, 1500, 2067, 2068). The contralateral projection is to neurons innervating distal (chiefly) and proximal limb muscles. The ipsilateral cortical projection is to motor neurons innervating proximal limb muscles.

It has been estimated that about 55% of all pyramidal fibers end in the cervical cord, 20% in the thoracic and 25% in the lumbosacral segments (2686). This would suggest that pyramidal control over the upper extremity is much greater than over the lower. Myelination of the corticospinal fibers begins near birth and is not completed until the end of the 2nd year.

The pyramidal tract conveys impulses to the spinal cord associated with volitional movements of the fingers and hand which form the basis for the acquisition of manual skills. Destruction of the tract produces a loss of voluntary movement that is most marked in the distal parts of the extremities. The proximal joints and grosser movement are less severely and permanently affected. At the onset of a vascular accident involving corticospinal fibers, there is a loss of tone in the affected muscles. But after a period of days, or sometimes weeks, the muscles gradually become resistant to passive movement (spasticity), and the deep tendon (myotatic) reflexes, especially in the leg, are increased in force and amplitude (hyperreflexia). On the other hand, the superficial reflexes, such as the abdominals, cremasteric and normal plantar, are lost or diminished.

In individuals of advanced age there is a tendency for the superficial abdominal reflexes to be absent. These reflexes are absent more often in females than in males (1580). Absence of the superficial abdominal reflexes is not in itself indicative of neurological disease. The abnormal plantar response, elicited by stroking the sole of the foot with a blunt instrument, is characterized by extension of the great toe and fanning of the other toes (*sign of Babinski*). The normal plantar response is a brisk flexion of all toes. The Babinski sign usually is indicative of injury to the corticospinal system, but it is not an infallible sign. The extensor toe response commonly can be elicited in the newborn infant, the sleeping or intoxicated adult or following a generalized seizure. It also may be absent in some patients with lesions of the corticospinal tract (1806).

The cause of the spasticity usually occurring in human hemiplegia is still a subject of considerable controversy. Lesions of the pyramidal tract in cats and monkeys produce a hypotonic paralysis, or paresis of discrete movements, although in the chimpanzee the hypotonia is more obscure (2565). Similarly, Fulton and Kennard (825) have reported that ablation of the motor area (area 4) in monkeys and chimpanzees produces a flaccid paralysis. When the motor area (area 4) and the premotor area (area 6) are both ablated, there is a slight increase in resistance to passive movements, but usually not of the degree that characterizes true clinical spasticity (see Chapter 19, page 690).

It must be remembered that the corticospinal tract is a complex fiber system arising from multiple cortical areas, and only a small part of it originates from the giant pyramidal cells of Betz in the precentral gyrus. These cells have been estimated to number between 34,000 and 40,000 in one hemisphere and probably account for the larger fibers (10 to 20 μm) in the corticospinal tract (1442, 1449). The more numerous finer fibers come in considerable part from other cortical regions. Thus there are at least two components in the pyramidal tract: a large and fine-fibered component from the motor area, and a fine-fibered one from all other areas that contribute fibers to the tract (Fig. 10-11). It is probable that fibers of the Betz cells are concerned with the finer isolated movements of the distal parts of the extremities, which are primarily affected in pyramidal lesions. The more numerous finer fibers may be related to grosser movement and tonic control, and injury to them may be the cause of the increase in muscle tone and the hyperactive deep tendon reflexes. These fibers which form an integral part of the pyramidal tract, its largest portion, descend uninterruptedly from the cerebral cortex through the medullary pyramids to the spinal cord.

The pyramidal cells and their axons constitute the "*upper motor neurons*" in contrast to the "*lower motor neurons*" (anterior horn cells), which directly innervate the skeletal muscle. The symptoms of a pyramidal tract lesion, loss of volitional movement, spasticity, increased deep tendon reflexes, loss of superficial reflexes and the sign of Babinski, therefore are designated as "upper motor neuron" type paralysis (spastic or supranuclear paralysis). In "lower motor neuron" paralysis, there is loss of all movement, reflex and voluntary, as well as loss of tone and atrophy of the affected muscles.

Paralysis of both arm and leg on one side is termed a *hemiplegia*, while paralysis of a single limb is called a *monoplegia*. *Diplegia* denotes the paralysis of two corresponding parts on opposite sides of the body, such as both arms. When both legs are paralyzed the term *paraplegia* is used.

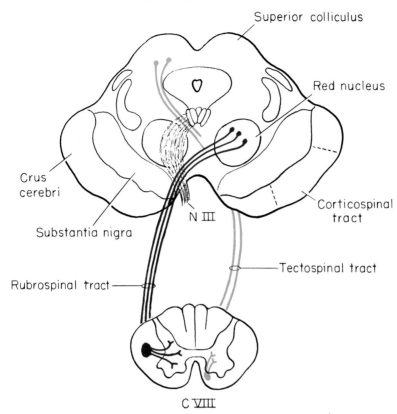

Superior colliculus

Red nucleus

Crus cerebri

N III

Substantia nigra

Corticospinal tract

Tectospinal tract

Rubrospinal tract

C VIII

Figure 10-17. Schematic diagram of the rubrospinal (*red*) and the tectospinal (*blue*) tracts. The rubrospinal tract arises somatotopically from cells of the red nucleus, crosses in the ventral tegmental decussation, and descends to spinal levels where fibers terminate in parts of laminae V, VI and VII. Tectospinal fibers arise from cells in deep layers of the superior colliculus, cross in the dorsal tegmental decussation, and descend in association with the medial longitudinal fasciculus. Fibers of the tectospinal tract are distributed to parts of laminae VIII, VII and VI only in cervical spinal segments.

Paralysis of all four extremities is known as *tetraplegia* or *quadriplegia.*

All descending spinal tracts, other than the corticospinal, arise from nuclear masses in the brain stem. Three descending tracts arise from the midbrain. These are the tectospinal, interstitiospinal and rubrospinal tracts.

Tectospinal Tract. Fibers of this tract arise from neurons in the deeper layers of the superior colliculus, a complex neural structure which serves primarily as an optic relay center (Figs. 10-17 and 10-18). The tract is formed by fibers that sweep anteromedially about the periaqueductal gray and cross the midline anterior to the medial longitudinal fasiculus in the *dorsal tegmental decussation.* In the upper brain stem this tract descends near the median raphe anterior to the medial longitudinal fasciculus; at medullary levels tectospinal fibers

become incorporated within the medial longitudinal fasciculus (Figs. 10-17 and 10-18). In the older literature tectospinal fibers are referred to as the predorsal bundle. In the spinal cord tectospinal fibers descend in the anterior part of the anterior funiculus near the anterior median fissure (Fig. 10-24). The majority of fibers terminate in the upper four cervical spinal segments, but a few reach lower cervical segments (51, 1855, 1991). Tectospinal fibers enter the ventromedial part of the anterior horn and radiate into laminae VIII, VII and parts of lamina VI (1855). None of these fibers terminates directly upon large motor neurons. The functional significance of the tectospinal tract is not known, but it is presumed to mediate reflex postural movements in response to visual and perhaps auditory stimuli.

The superior colliculus also gives rise to

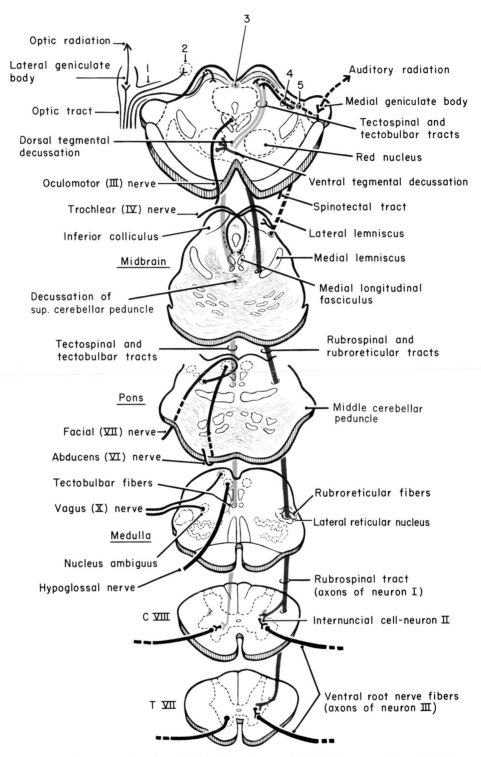

Figure 10-18. Diagram of the rubrospinal (*red*) and tectospinal (*blue*) tracts. Rubrospinal fibers arise somatotopically from the red nucleus, cross in the ventral tegmental decussation and descend to spinal levels where fibers terminate in parts of laminae V, VI and VII of Rexed. Crossed rubrobulbar fibers project to parts of the facial nucleus (not shown) and to the lateral reticular nucleus of the medulla (rubroreticular fibers). Uncrossed rubrobulbar fibers (not shown) descend in the central tegmental tract and terminate in the dorsal

fibers distributed bilaterally in the mesencephalic reticular formation and to medial regions of the contralateral pontine and medullary reticular formation (51). These fibers are referred to as *tectobulbar fibers*.

Rubrospinal Tract. Fibers of the rubrospinal tract arise from cells of the red nucleus, a well-defined structure in the central part of the mesencephalic tegmentum (Figs. 10-17, 10-18, 13-1 and 13-6). The red nucleus is a large, oval cell mass which in transverse sections has a circular appearance (Fig. 13-1). This nucleus is divided into a rostral parvocellular part and a caudal magnocellular part; the extent of these two divisions shows variations in size in different animals. In the monkey three distinctive types of neurons are found in the red nucleus: (a) large giant neurons with coarse, evenly distributed, Nissl granules which characterize the magnocellular part, (b) medium-sized triangular neurons with prominent nucleoli and a Nissl substance that does not form distinct granules, which characterize the parvocellular part and (c) small neurons, found in both magnocellular and parvocellular parts, which are achromatic and have scant cytoplasm (512, 1319, 1320, 2128, 2245). In the cat the rubrospinal tract arises from cells of all sizes in the caudal three-fourths of the nucleus (2039). In the monkey the rubrospinal tract arises largely from the magnocellular region which occupies the caudal third of the red nucleus (1275, 1411, 1632, 1893, 2023).

Rubrospinal fibers are given off from the medial border of the red nucleus, cross the median raphe immediately in the ventral tegmental decussation and descend to spinal levels, where fibers lie anterior to, and partially intermingled with, fibers of the lateral corticospinal tract (Figs. 10-17, 10-18 and 10-24). Fibers of the rubrospinal tract arise somatotopically from the red nucleus (2039). Projections to cervical spinal segments arise from dorsal and dorsomedial parts of the red nucleus, while fibers passing to lumbosacral regions of the spinal cord arise from ventral and ventrolateral parts of the nucleus. Thoracic spinal segments receive fibers that originate from intermediate regions of the nucleus. An example of retrograde transport of HRP from fibers and terminals of the rubrospinal tract to the contralateral red nucleus is shown in Figure 10–19. Somatotopic features are not evident here because uptake was mainly via injured fibers of the tract rather than terminals. While the rubrospinal tract extends the length of the spinal cord in most mammals, it has not been demonstrated below thoracic spinal segments in man (2437). Conclusions that the rubrospinal tract in man is rudimentary are based partially on the fact that cells of the human red nucleus are small and many of the rubrospinal fibers are thin and poorly myelinated. In the cat cervical spinal segments receive the greatest number of rubrospinal fibers and thoracic segments receive a smaller number of fibers than do lumbar segments (1104, 1856). Fibers of this tract enter the spinal gray laterally and radiate in fanshaped fashion into the lateral half of lamina V, lamina VI and dorsal and central parts of lamina VII (1855). These fibers terminate on somata and dendrites of large and small cells within these laminae (1856). Since rubrospinal fibers do not end directly upon anterior horn cells, impulses conveyed to spinal internuncial neurons in turn facilitate flexor α motor neurons.

In their descent through the brain stem, collateral fibers of the rubrospinal tract are given off which project to the cerebellum (547), the facial nucleus (542) and the lateral reticular nucleus of the medulla (542, 686, 1104, 1615, 1707, 2635). The parvocellular part of the red nucleus also gives rise to uncrossed rubral efferent fibers that project to dorsal parts of the principal inferior olivary nucleus (552, 686, 1707, 2023, 2635); these fibers are referred to as uncrossed rubrobulbar fibers (2632).

The red nucleus receives fibers from the cerebellum and the cerebral cortex. In the

lamella of the ipsilateral principal olivary nucleus. Tectospinal fibers arise from deep layers of the superior colliculus, cross in the dorsal tegmental decussation and descend initially ventral to the medial longitudinal fasciculus. At medullary levels these fibers become incorporated in the medial longitudinal fasciculus. Fibers of the tectospinal tract descend only to lower cervical spinal segments. Numbered midbrain structures include: *1*, the brachium of the superior colliculus; *2*, the pretectal area; *3*, commissure of the superior colliculus; *4*, spinotectal tract; and *5*, collicular fibers from the lateral lemniscus.

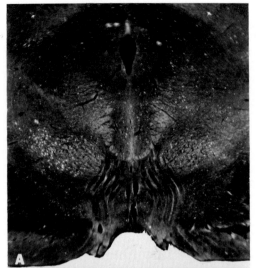

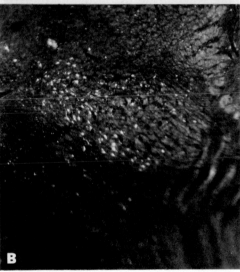

Figure 10-19. Photomicrographs of retrograde transport of horseradish peroxidase (HRP) to cells of the red nucleus from an injection into the contralateral lateral funiculus at the C2 spinal level in a squirrel monkey (dark field, *A*, ×12; *B*, ×26).

cat and monkey corticorubral fibers arise mainly from the "motor" cortex, descend ipsilaterally and terminate upon cells in all parts of the red nucleus (1411, 2163). Corticorubral fibers are somatotopically organized with respect to both origin and termination. The magnocellular part of the red nucleus receives cortical projections primarily from the precentral gyrus, while the parvocellular part receives fibers from the precentral gyrus, the adjacent premotor area, the supplementary motor area and

limited projections from parietal cortex (1411). Cortical projections to the red nucleus from the precentral and premotor areas have been confirmed by autoradiography in the monkey (1042). The parvocellular red nucleus receives a bilateral somatotopic projection from the precentral and premotor cortex; the most profuse contralateral projection arises from area 6 on the medial aspect of the hemisphere (partly within the supplementary motor area). Ipsilateral cortical projections from the precentral motor cortex end in the magnocellular part of the red nucleus. Thus the synaptic linkage of corticorubral and rubrospinal fibers, both of which are somatotopically organized, constitutes a two-neuronal pathway from the motor cortex to spinal levels. Cells of the red nucleus projecting to the spinal cord are excited monosynaptically by corticorubral projections (2588).

All parts of the red nucleus receive crossed cerebellar efferent fibers via the superior cerebellar peduncle. Fibers from the dentate nucleus project mainly to the rostral third of the red nucleus, while fibers from a part of the interposed nucleus (equivalent to the emboliform nucleus in man) pass to the caudal two-thirds of the nucleus (543, 755, 1632). Rubral afferent fibers from part of the interposed nucleus (anterior part) are somatotopically organized.

Stimulation of the red nucleus (2033, 2034) in the cat produces flexion in either the forelimb or hindlimb on the opposite side, depending upon which part of the nucleus is stimulated. Microelectrode studies (1138, 2257) have demonstrated that stimulation of cells in the red nucleus produces excitatory postsynaptic potentials in contralateral flexor α motor neurons, and inhibitory postsynaptic potentials in extensor α motor neurons. A convergence of rubrospinal fibers and primary afferents also provides for excitatory actions upon spinal interneurons involved in reflex pathways (1139). The most important function of the rubrospinal tract is the control of muscle tone in flexor muscle groups (1632). The rubrospinal tract excites flexor motor neurons via polysynaptic pathways, and stimulation of the red nucleus during locomotion enhances flexor muscle activity during the swing phase (1896). Modulation of activity in rubrospinal neurons according to locomotor rhythm occurs only when the cerebellum is intact. The spinocerebellar pathways participate in this modulation in that they provide the main inputs into regions of the cerebellar cortex which are somatotopically linked with the interposed nuclei (within the cerebellum), which in turn project to the red nuclei.

The *interstitiospinal tract* is uncrossed and forms a component of the descending medial longitudinal fasciculus (MLF); it will be discussed with that composite bundle.

Two major descending spinal tracts arise from the pons. These are the vestibulospinal and pontine reticulospinal tracts. The pontine and medullary reticulospinal tracts will be discussed together.

Vestibulospinal Tract. The vestibular nuclei constitute a cytological complex in the floor of the fourth ventricle in both the pons and medulla. The four major nuclei of this complex receive afferent fibers from the vestibular nerve and the cerebellum which are distributed differentially (Figs. 10-20, 10-21 and 12-17). The vestibulospinal tract, the principal descending spinal pathway from this complex, arises exclusively from the lateral vestibular nucleus. The *lateral vestibular nucleus* consists of a discrete collection of giant cells in the lateral part of the complex near the level of entry of the vestibular nerve root. Practically all cells of the lateral vestibular nucleus contribute fibers to the formation of this tract which descends the length of the spinal cord in the anterior part of the lateral funiculus (Figs. 10-20 and 10-21).

The vestibulospinal tract, like the rubrospinal tract, is somatotopically organized (2041). Cells in different portions of the lateral vestibular nucleus project fibers to specific levels of the spinal cord. The ventrorostral region of the nucleus projects fibers to cervical spinal segments, while cells in the dorsocaudal part of the nucleus pass to lumbosacral spinal segments. Fibers passing to thoracic spinal segments are derived from intermediate regions of the nucleus. While there is some overlap between regions sending fibers to particular spinal segments, there is a definite somatotopical arrangement. Fibers of the vestibulospinal tract descend the entire length of the spinal cord. Cervical and lumbar spinal segments

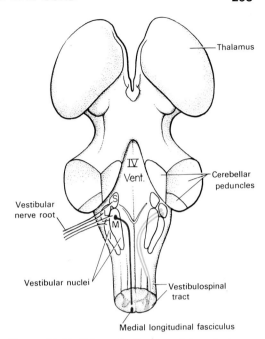

Figure 10-20. Schematic diagram of the spinal projections from the vestibular nuclei. The vestibulospinal tract (*blue*) arises only from cells of the lateral vestibular nucleus. This tract is uncrossed, somatotopically organized and concerned with the facilitation of extensor muscle tone. Vestibular fibers descending in the medial longitudinal fasciculus (*red*) arise largely from the medial vestibular nucleus and are mainly uncrossed. *S*, indicates superior vestibular nucleus, *L*, indicates the lateral vestibular nucleus and *I* and *M* indicate the inferior and medial vestibular nuclei.

receive the greatest number of vestibulospinal fibers. In cervical spinal segments fibers of the tract are located in the anterior part of the lateral funiculus, but in lumbosacral segments most of the fibers are found in the anterior funiculus (Figs. 9-11 and 10-16). Vestibulospinal fibers enter the gray matter and are distributed to all parts of lamina VIII and the medial and central parts of lamina VII (1857). These fibers form axodendritic and axosomatic synaptic contacts with all types of cells within these laminae, although axodendritic synapses are most numerous. Few vestibulospinal fibers appear to terminate directly on motor neurons, except in the thoracic spinal cord, where a few fibers may end upon cells of the anteromedial cell group. No cells of the inferior, medial or superior vestibular nuclei contribute fibers to the vestibulospinal tract and no fibers from the lateral vestib-

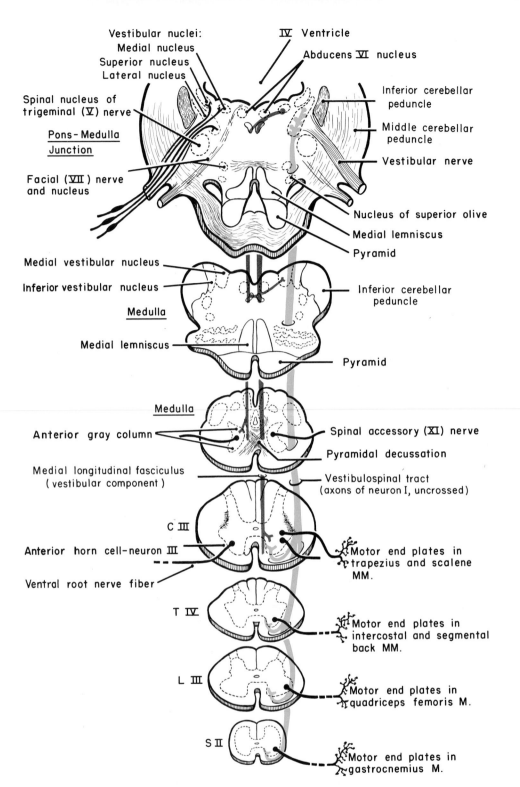

Figure 10-21. Schematic diagram of the vestibulospinal tract (*blue*) and descending vestibular fibers in the medial longitudinal fasciculus (*red*). Fibers of the vestibulospinal tract have a somatotopic origin in the lateral vestibular nucleus, descend the length of the spinal cord and terminate predominantly in lamina VIII of Rexed. Descending vestibular fibers in the medial longitudinal fasciculus arise from the medial vestibular nucleus. In the lower brain stem these fibers are bilateral, but in the cervical spinal cord they are ipsilateral. Letters and numbers indicate segmental spinal levels.

ular nucleus reach spinal levels via the medial longitudinal fasciculus (268, 382, 1857).

The vestibulospinal tract relays impulses to the spinal cord from the labyrinth and from specific portions of the cerebellum. Primary vestibular fibers terminate differentially and selectively upon cells in all four major divisions of the vestibular nuclear complex (2429, 2640). Projections to the lateral vestibular nucleus are restricted to its rostroventral part and represent predominantly input from the utricle. Electron microscopic findings indicate that primary vestibular fibers end upon perikarya and spines of proximal and distal dendrites of cells of all sizes in the lateral vestibular nucleus (1778). The cerebellum provides a large number of afferent projections to the vestibular nuclear complex. These fibers are derived from: (a) the "vestibular part" of the cerebellum (i.e., the nodulus, the uvula and the flocculus), (b) the fastigial nuclei and (c) the anterior lobe of the cerebellum (1776, 2637, 2643, 2646). "Vestibular parts" of the cerebellum project fibers to regions of all vestibular nuclei in a pattern similar to that of primary vestibular fibers, except that the projection to the lateral vestibular nucleus is scant (268). Fastigial projections to the vestibular nuclei are crossed and uncrossed, nearly symmetrical and end mainly in ventral portions of the lateral and inferior vestibular nuclei (135). Cerebellovestibular fibers from the anterior lobe of the cerebellum, representing Purkinje cell axons, are somatotopically arranged and terminate only in dorsal parts of the lateral and inferior vestibular nuclei (1776, 2637). It is apparent that vestibular influences upon the spinal cord are mediated largely by the vestibulospinal tract. The lateral vestibular nucleus, exerts facilitatory influences upon the reflex activity of the spinal cord and spinal mechanisms which control muscle tone. This perhaps is best exemplified in experimental decerebrate animals by the reduction of rigidity which follows lesions in the lateral vestibular nucleus or interruption of the vestibulospinal tract in the spinal cord. It also has been shown that electrical stimulation of points in the lateral vestibular nucleus produces increases in extensor muscle tone which may be localized to forelimb or hindlimb, depending upon the position of the electrode within the nucleus (2036). These

physiological findings confirm the anatomically described somatotopical origin of fibers in the lateral vestibular nucleus. Following stimulation of the lateral vestibular nucleus in the cat, excitatory postsynaptic potentials can be recorded intracellularly from extensor motor neurons, while the effects on flexor motor neurons are insignificant (2258, 2739). Excitatory vestibulospinal influences upon extensor muscles can be observed at rest and during locomotion (1895). Stimulation of the lateral vestibular nucleus during locomotion enhances the activity of extensor muscles during the stance phase of the step. Modulation of vestibulospinal neurons with locomotor rhythm occurs only when the cerebellum is intact. Anatomical data suggest that these facilitatory effects must be mediated via interneurons in laminae VII and VIII that influence extensor motor neurons, particularly those innervating limb muscles. The anterior lobe of the cerebellum inhibits neurons in the lateral vestibular nucleus and thus may exert a controlling influence upon labyrinthine activation.

Reticulospinal Tracts. Two relatively large regions of the brain stem reticular formation give rise to fibers that descend to spinal levels. One of these regions is in the pontine tegmentum, while the other lies in the medulla; hence it is proper to refer to these as the pontine and medullary reticulospinal tracts (Figs. 10-10 and 10-22).

The *pontine reticulospinal tract* arises from aggregations of cells in the medial pontine tegmentum referred to as the *nuclei reticularis pontis caudalis* and *oralis* (266, 1885, 2561). The caudal pontine reticular nucleus begins in the caudal pontine tegmentum and extends rostrally to the level of the motor trigeminal nucleus. This nucleus contains a number of giant cells in addition to various types of smaller cells. The oral pontine reticular nucleus, present in more rostral parts of the medial pontine tegmentum, extends into the caudal mesencephalon; giant cells are found only in the more caudal parts of this nucleus. Reticulospinal fibers arise from cells in all parts of the nucleus reticularis pontis caudalis but only from the caudal part of the nucleus reticularis pontis oralis. More than half of the large cells in the caudal pontine reticular nucleus project fibers to spinal levels (2561). The pontine reticulospinal

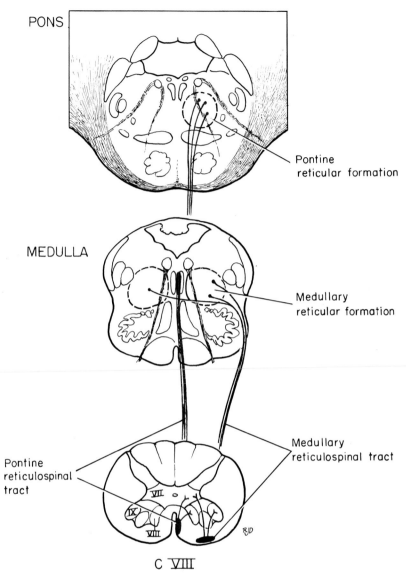

Figure 10-22. Schematic diagram of the reticulospinal tracts indicating their regions of origin, course and terminations. Pontine reticulospinal fibers (*red*) terminate in lamina VIII and adjacent parts of lamina VII. Medullary reticulospinal fibers (*black*) terminate chiefly in lamina VII, but some end in lamina IX.

tract is almost entirely ipsilateral and descends chiefly in the medial part of the anterior funiculus (Fig. 10-22). In the brain stem part of these fibers descend in close association with the medial longitudinal fasciculus. Pontine reticulospinal fibers are more numerous than those arising in the medulla, descend the entire length of the spinal cord and terminate in lamina VIII and adjacent parts of lamina VII (Fig. 10-22). A few pontine reticulospinal fibers cross at spinal levels in the anterior white commissure. The gray laminae that receive terminations of pontine reticulospinal fibers also contain terminals of vestibulospinal, tectospinal and interstitiospinal fibers. This spinal projection is not somatotopically organized.

The *medullary reticulospinal tract* arises from the medial two-thirds of the medullary reticular formation (266). The largest number of fibers arise from the *nucleus reticularis gigantocellularis,* lying dorsal to the inferior olivary complex and lateral to the paramedian region (Fig. 10-22). As the name of this nucleus implies, it is composed of characteristic large cells, but large cells are not as conspicuous in man as in lower animals. In addition, there are many medium-sized and small cells. Fibers of the medullary reticulospinal tract are mainly ipsilateral, but some fibers are crossed. The latter cross at medullary levels (129). The medullary reticulospinal tract descends the length of the spinal cord in the anterior part of the lateral funiculus (Figs. 10-10 and 10-22). Reticulospinal fibers from the pons and medulla are not sharply segregated in the spinal cord. Fibers entering the spinal gray radiate into all parts of lamina VII and terminate mainly in central parts of this lamina (Fig. 10-22). Other fibers are distributed in smaller quantities to laminae VIII and IX (129, 1854, 1855). Medullary reticulospinal fibers terminate in parts of the gray spinal laminae that also receive fibers from the rubrospinal and corticospinal tracts. Reticulospinal fibers from both the pons and medulla terminate upon cells of all sizes and on both the somata and dendrites. Impulses arising from the reticular formation which influence γ motor neurons probably are mediated largely by internuncial neurons in parts of laminae VII and VIII (695, 696).

Although information concerning the reticulospinal tracts in man is meager and incomplete, studies in animals indicate that these tracts descend the entire length of the spinal cord (129, 1854, 1855, 1991, 2417). Some of these fibers relay impulses from visceral nuclei while others are concerned with somatic activities.

The nuclei of the raphe which have serotonin (5-hydroxytryptamine, 5-HT) as their neurotransmitter give rise to projections distributed extensively in the reticular formation (202). Only the nucleus raphe magnus (medulla) and perhaps part of the nucleus raphe pontis appear to project to spinal levels. Cells of the nucleus raphe magnus give rise to bilateral spinal projections which descend in the dorsolateral funiculus (129). These fibers terminate most profusely in laminae I and II in the cervical and lumbar enlargements, but endings also are described in the intermediolateral cell columns of thoracic and lumbar spinal segments. Studies suggest that cells of the nucleus raphe magnus produce an analgesic effect by their inhibitory actions upon sensory neurons (128, 2075).

The brain stem reticular formation receives inputs from many sources, but direct corticoreticular projections seem especially important. Corticoreticular fibers arise from widespread areas of the cortex although the greatest number originate from the "motor area." While these fibers arise from different cortical areas, they mainly terminate in two fairly restricted regions of the reticular formation, one in the pons and one in the medulla (2227). In the pons these fibers end mainly in the nucleus reticularis pontis oralis and in the rostral part of the caudal pontine reticular nucleus. In the medulla such fibers terminate in the nucleus reticularis gigantocellularis. Corticoreticular fibers are distributed bilaterally with crossed preponderance. The regions of termination within the reticular formation correspond to those that give rise to the reticulospinal tracts. Thus the synaptic linkage of corticoreticular and reticulospinal fibers forms a pathway from the cortex to spinal levels. There is no evidence of a somatotopic arrangement within this system (266).

Experimental studies have demonstrated that stimulation of the brain stem reticular formation can: (a) facilitate or inhibit voluntary movement, cortically induced movement and reflex activity; (b) influence muscle tone; (c) affect inspiratory phases of respiration; (d) exert pressor or depressor effects on the circulatory system; and (e) exert depressant effects on the central transmission of sensory impulses. Areas of the medullary reticular formation from which medullary reticulospinal fibers arise appear to correspond closely with the regions from which inspiratory, inhibitory and depressor effects have been obtained (54, 2014, 2016, 2561). Areas of the brain stem reticular formation related to facilitatory influences, expiratory effects and pressor vasomotor phenomena are mainly rostral to the medulla and appear to extend beyond those regions which give rise to direct reticulospinal fibers (266). Thus some facilitatory influences from the upper brain stem reticular formation probably are not transmitted directly to spinal levels by reticulospinal pathways.

The reticular formation can influence muscle tone by acting upon γ motor neurons which innervate the contractile portions of the muscle spindle (696, 937). Inhibitory effects on the muscle spindle are obtained most easily from the medullary reticular formation, while facilitatory effects are elicited from more rostral regions. It is largely by this mechanism that the reticulospinal systems modify tendon reflex activity. The reticular formation and its great functional significance will be considered in more detail in Chapter 13.

Medial Longitudinal Fasciculus (MLF). The posterior part of the anterior funiculus contains a composite bundle of descending fibers that originates from different nuclei at various brain stem levels and is collectively referred to as the *medial longitudinal fasciculus* (abbreviated MLF). Such descending fibers represent only a portion of the brain stem tract that is designated by the same name, but is composed of both ascending and descending fibers (Figs. 10-20 and 10-21). In the brain stem and spinal cord, fibers of this tract are always near the median raphe and immediately ventral to the cerebral aqueduct, fourth ventricle or central canal (Figs. 10-20 and 10-21). Descending fibers of the medial longitudinal fasciculus in the spinal cord originate from the medial vestibular nucleus, the reticular formation, the superior colliculus (tectospinal fibers) and the interstitial nucleus of Cajal (interstitiospinal fibers). Fibers of this bundle form a well-defined tract only in the upper cervical segments of the spinal cord (Figs. 10-20, 10-21 and 10-24). Below that level most fibers are difficult to follow, although fibers have been traced to sacral levels. Most of these fibers are believed to terminate among internuncial neurons in the most medial part of the anterior horn.

Vestibular fibers descending in the medial longitudinal fasciculus arise only from the medial vestibular nucleus (Fig. 10-20), are predominantly ipsilateral in the spinal cord and terminate in the dorsal part of lamina VIII and adjacent parts of lamina VII (268, 391, 1573, 1853). Physiological studies suggest that fibers from the medial vestibular nucleus convey monosynaptic inhibitory influences directly to upper cervical motor neurons (28, 2742). This unusual direct pathway appears to play a role in the labyrinthine regulation of head positions. The largest component of descending fibers in the medial longitudinal fasciculus at spinal levels is the pontine reticulospinal tract; these fibers descend the length of the spinal cord and terminate mainly in lamina VIII and parts of VII (Fig. 10-22). Fibers of the interstitiospinal tract are uncrossed, descend in the most posterior part of the anterior funiculus near the anteromedian fissure and terminate in dorsal parts of lamina VIII and neighboring parts of lamina VII (1855, 2417). While most of the fibers of this tract are given off in upper portions of the spinal cord, some fibers project to sacral spinal levels.

Fastigiospinal Fibers. Although the cerebellum has been considered to exert its influences upon spinal activities solely via relay nuclei in the brain stem, recent evidence suggests that one of the deep cerebellar nuclei projects directly to cervical spinal levels (135, 821, 1635, 2541, 2741). Fastigiospinal fibers arise from cells in all parts of the fastigial nucleus, cross the midline within the cerebellum and emerge via the uncinate fasciculus. Fibers descend ventral to the spinal trigeminal tract where at some levels they are partially intermingled with fibers of the vestibulospinal tract. In the spinal cord fibers descending in the ventral part of the lateral funiculus, project into the anterior gray horn. In the cat these fibers were identified as far caudally as lower cervical spinal segments (2741). Fastigial neurons projecting contralaterally to cervical spinal segments can be activated by labyrinthine and somatic stimuli, but the significance of this pathway in motor control remains unknown.

Olivospinal Tract. This tract is considered to be composed of fine fibers, located on the anterior surface of the spinal cord at the zone of transition between the lateral and anterior funiculi. While this tract has been described as containing descending fibers from the inferior olivary nucleus, experimental studies indicate that this tract actually contains primarily spino-olivary fibers (289).

Descending Autonomic Pathways. The descending spinal tracts described in the preceding pages are parts of pathways by which impulses from the cerebral cortex and nuclei in various parts of the brain stem ultimately influence the activity of striated muscles through the somatic anterior horn cells. The spinal cord also contains descending fibers which arise from nuclear groups concerned with a variety of autonomic or visceral functions. These descending autonomic fibers terminate in relationship to spinal neurons that innervate visceral structures (i.e., smooth muscle, cardiac muscle and glandular epithelium) and influence their activity. Descending autonomic fibers originate from nuclei in the hypothalamus, visceral nuclei of the oculomotor complex, the locus ceruleus and certain cells of the solitary nuclear complex in the medulla. In addition, neurons in the reticular formation projecting fibers to spinal levels are concerned with a variety of visceral activities; some reticular neurons may merely relay impulses from more rostral visceral nuclei, while others possess intrinsic visceral properties. Although early studies (1585) suggested that neurons in the hypothalamus may descend to spinal levels, unquestioned anatomical evidence of a direct hypothalamic-spinal projection was dependent upon the retrograde transport of HRP (1412). Hypothalamic neurons projecting to spinal levels arise primarily from the: (a) paraventricular nucleus, (b) the dorsal part of the lateral hypothalamic area and (c) posterior hypothalamic regions dorsal to the mammillary body (2255). While the hypothalamic-spinal pathway is predominantly uncrossed, there are some crossed fibers. Descending hypothalamic efferent fibers studied by autoradiographic tracing technics, project to visceral nuclei in the medulla (i.e., dorsal motor nucleus of the vagus and the nucleus of the solitary fasciculus) as well as to spinal levels. Direct hypothalamic-spinal fibers descend in the lateral funiculus and terminate in relation to cells of the intermediolateral cell column in thoracic, lumbar and sacral levels. Thus these descending autonomic projections appear to directly influence preganglionic sympathetic and parasympathetic neurons at different levels (Fig. 10-23).

Although the visceral cell columns of the oculomotor complex have traditionally been considered to project preganglionic parasympathetic fibers only to the third nerve, recent evidence indicates certain visceral neurons project directly to spinal levels in the rat, cat and monkey (1520, 2255). Descending pathways from the Edinger-Westphal nucleus contribute fibers to the posterior column nuclei, pass caudally in the lateral funiculus and terminate in Rexed's lamina I and parts of lamina V (1520). Some of these fibers could be followed into lumbar spinal segments. It has been suggested these descending spinal projections may modulate sensory input, especially that related to nociceptive stimuli.

A small pigmented nucleus in the upper pons, known as the locus ceruleus (Figs. 12-30, 12-31 and 12-32) has been demonstrated to synthesize, store and release the neurotransmitter norepinephrine. This relatively small nucleus distributes fibers widely in the neuraxis and is regarded as a principal source of norepinephrine. Data are based upon the retrograde transport of HRP, fluorescence histochemistry and autoradiography. Fibers from this nucleus descend in the anterior and lateral funiculi, are largely uncrossed and appear to end in the anterior horn, the intermediate gray and the ventral half of the posterior horn (Fig. 10-23) (1859, 2006). The precise cellular regions of termination of these fibers in the spinal gray remain to be determined, but there is no doubt these fibers convey norepinephrine to their terminals.

Cells in the ventrolateral part of the solitary nucleus (Fig. 10-23) have been demonstrated to project to cervical and thoracic spinal segments by both retrograde (HRP) and anterograde (autoradiography) axoplasmic transport technics (1517). Fibers of this solitariospinal tract have been traced bilaterally, but predominantly contralaterally, to the region of the phrenic motor neurons at the C3–C5 level, to the thoracic anterior horns and the intermediolateral cell columns (Fig. 9-26). The largest number of fibers projecting to spinal levels from the solitary nuclear complex are found in cervical segments. It has been postulated that bifurcating axons distribute fibers bilaterally. The descending connections of cells in the solitary nuclear complex suggest that they provide excitatory inputs to phrenic and inspiratory interchondral motor neurons (660, 2435). Solitariospinal projections to the intermediolateral cell columns may be involved in cardiovascular reflexes of an orthostatic nature.

Other autonomic centers probably lie in the reticular formation of the midbrain, pons and medulla. These descending paths are diffuse and in the reticular formation they may be interrupted by relays. In the spinal cord these fibers descend mainly in the anterior and anterolateral portions of

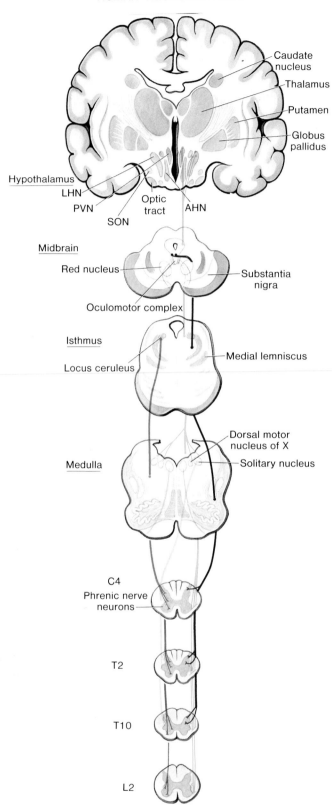

Caudate nucleus

Thalamus

Putamen

Globus pallidus

Hypothalamus
LHN
PVN
Optic tract
AHN
SON

Midbrain

Red nucleus

Substantia nigra

Oculomotor complex

Isthmus

Medial lemniscus

Locus ceruleus

Dorsal motor nucleus of X

Solitary nucleus

Medulla

C4
Phrenic nerve neurons

T2

T10

L2

the white matter, in close relation to the lateral fasciculus proprius system and the reticulospinal tracts. Lesions involving descending autonomic pathways in cervical spinal segments may produce an ipsilateral Horner's syndrome and other autonomic deficits. A descending excitatory pupillodilator pathway, situated near the spinothalamic tracts, has been identified in the cat (1516). This pathway is considered to terminate in the intermediolateral cell column of upper thoracic segments and to have norepinephrine as its transmitter (586).

ASCENDING AND DESCENDING SPINAL TRACTS

A series of schematic diagrams have represented the ascending and descending tracts of the spinal cord described in this chapter. It should be emphasized that at different levels of the spinal cord these tracts occupy slightly different positions, and that they show variations in size depending upon the particular level. Considerable intermingling and overlapping of fiber pathways are found at all spinal levels. Major ascending and descending spinal pathways are diagramed schematically in Figure 10-24.

Segmental Reflexes. In its simplest form a spinal reflex arc consists of only two neurons: an afferent peripheral neuron (spinal ganglion cell), and an efferent peripheral neuron (anterior horn cell) with a single synapse in the gray (Figs. 9-29 and 9-34). These monosynaptic reflexes are as a rule uncrossed and usually involve only one segment or closely adjacent ones. This same reflex arc, which is dependent upon impulses from the muscle spindles, plays a vital role in the unconscious neural control of muscular contraction during movement and the maintenance of posture. It was suggested (1671) that this reflex arc behaves as a servomechanism, or automatic control, which is activated by an "error signal" occurring in a closed loop and possessing power amplification. The closed loop consists of the muscle spindle, group Ia afferent fibers, the synapse with α motor neurons, and α fibers innervating extrafusal muscle (Fig. 9-34). The power amplification is provided by the contraction of extrafusal muscle. Thus contraction of the muscle opposes applied tension and tends to maintain the muscle at a constant length. The "error signal" may be considered to be the difference in the frequency of firing of the primary endings when the muscle is unloaded, and when it is loaded (1642).

Fasciculi Proprii. Only part of the collaterals of dorsal root fibers terminate directly upon anterior horn cells (767, 1113, 2414). Hence in most reflex arcs there is at least one central or internuncial neuron interposed between the afferent and efferent neurons. These central cells then send their axons to the motor cells of the same segment, or to higher and lower segments, for the completion of various intersegmental arcs. Many of the fibers are axons of internuncial cells which ascend or descend in the white columns of the same side. Others come from commissural cells and pass to the white matter of the opposite side. All these ascending and descending fibers, crossed and uncrossed, which begin and end in the spinal cord and connect its various levels, constitute the *spinospinal* or *fundamental* columns (*fasciculi proprii*)

Figure 10-23. Schematic diagram of descending autonomic projections to spinal cord from the hypothalamus, the Edinger-Westphal nucleus, the locus ceruleus and the nucleus of the solitary fasciculus. Direct fibers (*blue*) from the hypothalamus (i.e., paraventricular nucleus, PVN; dorsal part of the lateral hypothalamic nucleus (LHN) and the posterior hypothalamic area) project to the dorsal motor nucleus of the vagus nerve and the medial nucleus of the solitary fasciculus. This projection is mainly ipsilateral, but some fibers pass to contralateral nuclei. At spinal levels these fibers terminate largely in the ipsilateral intermediolateral cell column. Midline visceral neurons of the oculomotor complex (Edinger-Westphal nucleus) give rise to descending preganglionic parasympathetic fibers (*red*) distributed to Rexed's laminae I and V. Norepinephrine containing cells in the locus ceruleus and subceruleus project fibers (*purple*) to parts of the anterior horn, the intermediate gray and deep portions of the posterior horn. Cells mainly in the ventrolateral nucleus of the solitary fasciculus project fibers (*light blue*) predominantly contralaterally to phrenic motor neurons (C_3–C_5), to thoracic anterior horn cells and to the intermediolateral cell column. (AHN, anterior hypothalamic nucleus; SON, supraoptic nucleus). Based upon Saper et al. (2255), Loewy and Saper (1519), Nygren and Olson (1859 and Loewy and Burton (1517).

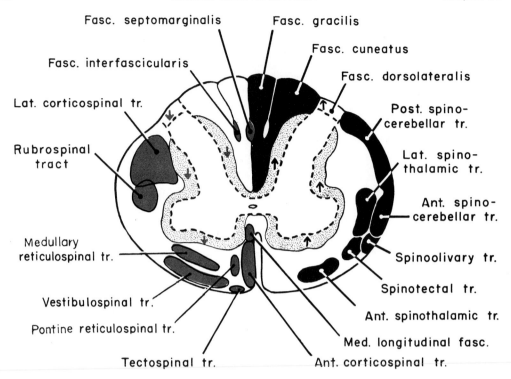

Figure 10-24. Diagram of ascending (*black*) and descending (*red*) pathways of the spinal cord. The fasciculus proprius system (*stippled*) and dorsolateral fasciculus contain both ascending and descending nerve fibers.

of the spinal cord (Figs. 9-7 and 10-24). A recent study of propriospinal neurons using HRP suggests that long descending axons arise ipsilaterally from lamina I and bilaterally from laminae V, VII and VIII (1639). The largest number of long descending fibers arise from cells in laminae VII and VIII; fibers crossing to the opposite side decussate at levels of cell origin. Descending branches of axons in lamina I may be implicated in modulation of sensory input, while neurons in laminae VII and VIII may influence motor neurons at more caudal levels of the spinal cord.

To this spinal reflex mechanism also belong the descending root fibers of the interfascicular and septomarginal bundles, previously described, and the collaterals and many terminals of ascending dorsal root fibers. Impulses entering the cord at any segment may travel along these fibers to higher or lower levels before synapsing directly or through internuncial neurons with the anterior horn cells (Fig. 9-29). These shorter fiber systems forming part of the

intrinsic reflex mechanism of the spinal cord are of major importance in a variety of reflexes.

The spinospinal fibers are found in all funiculi: posterior, anterior and lateral. They occupy the area adjacent to the gray matter and lie between the gray matter and the peripherally placed long tracts. They are most numerous in the anterolateral white columns. In the posterior funiculus they form a narrow zone along the posterior commissure and adjacent portions of the posterior horn. In general, the shortest fibers lie nearest the gray and connect adjacent segments while the longer fibers lie more peripherally.

There are no *isolated* reflexes and every neural reaction involving any given arc always influences, and is influenced by, other parts of the nervous system. The primitive nervous system is organized for the production of generalized muscle movements and total response. Studies of fetal behavior suggest that local reflexes appear later (496, 1085, 1140).

UPPER AND LOWER MOTOR NEURONS

One of the most important concepts in neurological diagnosis rests upon distinguishing the abnormalities of motor function which result from pathological involvement of, or injury to, the upper or lower motor neuron. This relatively simple, yet frequently puzzling, distinction forms one of the cornerstones of clinical neurology. The ability to distinguish upper and lower motor neuron lesions constitutes the first step in attempting to localize the site of a neural lesion that manifests itself by disturbances of normal motor function. Once the site of the neural lesion has been established, the clinician can begin to consider the pathological processes which might be responsible (386).

Lower Motor Neuron. Anterior horn cells (α motor neurons) and their axons, which innervate striated muscle, constitute anatomical and physiological units referred to as the final common motor pathway, or the lower motor neuron. The concept of the lower motor neuron is not limited to the spinal cord, even though it is most frequently used in that context. Cells of the motor cranial nerve nuclei (nerves III, IV, V, VI, VII, IX, X, XI and XII), which provide innervation for muscles of the head and neck, also must be classified as lower motor neurons, even though these nuclei form discontinuous cell columns in the brain stem. The anterior horn cells are regarded as the prototype for all motor neurons.

The segmental input to the lower motor neuron is profuse, both direct and indirect, and largely, but not exclusively, ipsilateral. Muscle spindle afferents (group Ia) project directly to the lower motor neuron (Figs. 9-28 and 9-34), while afferents from most other receptors, including the Golgi tendon organ (Fig. 9-34), influence the lower motor neuron indirectly via internuncial neurons. Afferent inputs from stretch receptors (i.e., muscle spindle and Golgi tendon organ) activate ipsilateral cell groups in the spinal cord, while afferent impulses from other sensory receptors are distributed by multisynaptic circuits to both sides of the spinal cord. The lower motor neuron also is under powerful indirect suprasegmental control provided by impulses transmitted via descending spinal systems (Fig. 10-24).

Lesions selectively involving the lower motor neuron result in weakness or paralysis, loss of muscle tone, loss of reflex activity and atrophy. All of these changes are confined to the affected muscles. *Weakness* or *paralysis*, occurring in affected muscles, bears a direct relationship to the extent and severity of the lesion. Since the anterior horn cells that innervate a single muscle extend longitudinally through several spinal segments, and since several such cell columns exist at each spinal level, a lesion confined to one spinal segment will cause weakness, but not complete paralysis, in all muscles innervated by this segment. Complete paralysis will occur only when the lesion involves the column of cells in several spinal segments that innervate a particular muscle, or the ventral root fibers that arise from these cells. Because most of the appendicular muscles are innervated by fibers arising from parts of three spinal segments, complete paralysis of a muscle resulting from a central lesion in the anterior horn indicates involvement of several spinal segments. Furthermore, because neighboring cell columns are likely to be affected at each level, such a lesion usually produces paralysis in muscle groups, rather than in individual muscles.

Since the lower motor neuron consists of the anterior horn cells and their axons, which innervate striated muscle, it becomes necessary to distinguish the motor deficits that occur as a consequence of lesions in spinal segments from those which occur in ventral roots, spinal nerves and peripheral nerves. A lesion in ventral root fibers usually produces motor deficits similar to those resulting from destruction of anterior horn cells. At certain levels (i.e., thoracolumbar and sacral) section of the ventral root fibers would produce additional autonomic deficits which might not accompany anterior horn cell lesions at the same level (Fig. 10-25). Lesions of mixed spinal nerves produce motor and sensory deficits that correspond to those of combined dorsal and ventral root lesions. While the motor deficit corresponds almost exactly to that seen with pure lesions of the ventral root, sensory disturbances and loss follow a dermatomal distribution and tend to be less extensive because of overlapping innervation characteristic of dermatomes (Figs. 7-10–7-12). With a peripheral nerve lesion, the muscle paralysis and sensory loss correspond to the distribution of the particular nerve (Figs. 7-11 and 7-12).

Loss of muscle tone, *hypotonia*, is a characteristic and constant finding in lower motor neuron lesions. Flaccidity of the affected muscles is evidenced by greatly diminished resistance to passive movement. This reduction in muscle tone results from the withdrawal of streams of impulses transmitted to muscles that normally maintain a state of variable, but sometimes sustained, contraction in some of the muscle units.

Reflexes in the affected muscles are diminished or lost (*areflexia*) in lower motor neuron lesions because the reflex arc is interrupted (Fig. 9-34). In this type of lesion the effector mechanism is destroyed.

Although paralysis, hypotonia and areflexia occur almost immediately following a lower motor neuron lesion, atrophy or muscle wasting does not become evident for 2 or 3 weeks. *Muscle atrophy* develops gradually and in time is obvious on inspection. Why muscles deprived of their innervation atrophy and degenerate is not adequately understood. It seems likely that the morphological and functional properties of muscle are dependent upon transmitter substances provided by the terminals of motor nerve fibers. Atrophy, of the type seen in lower motor neuron disease, does not result from depriving anterior horn cells of afferent impulses from either suprasegmental or segmental levels (2563).

In certain diseases of the lower motor neuron, the muscles exhibit small, localized spontaneous contractions known as *fasciculations*. These muscle twitches, visible through the skin, represent the discharge of squads of muscle fibers innervated by nerve fibers arising from a single lower motor neuron. Fasciculations occur asynchronously in different parts of various muscles and are thought to be due to a triggering of motor unit discharges that occur within the cell body of the motor neuron. Fasciculations of this type are interpreted as a disease process attacking the lower motor neurons in the anterior gray horn. Fasciculations commonly are seen in amyotrophic lateral sclerosis, occasionally in acute in-

flammatory lesions of peripheral nerves and rarely occur when anterior horn cells are rapidly injured or destroyed (i.e., in acute poliomyelitis).

The term *fibrillation*, frequently misused as the equivalent of the term fasciculation, refers to the small (10 to 200 μV) potentials of 1 to 2 msec duration that occur irregularly and asynchronously in electromyograms of denervated muscle. These spontaneous discharges cannot be observed through the skin and produce no detectable shortening of muscles.

Upper Motor Neuron. All of the descending fiber systems that can influence and modify the activity of the lower motor neuron constitute the upper motor neuron (Fig. 10-24). This is a more inclusive definition than that used by many clinicians who equate the upper motor neuron solely with the corticospinal system. The narrower concept has become a rule of thumb because of: (a) the overwhelming clinical importance of the corticospinal system and (b) the previously poorly defined functional influences of descending nonpyramidal fiber systems. Recent anatomical and physiological data concerning descending nonpyramidal fiber systems make it necessary to modify this venerable rule of thumb and to consider the concept of the upper motor neuron in its broadest sense. Descending impulses, transmitted to spinal levels by a group of heterogenous tracts, are concerned mainly with: (a) mediation of somatic motor activity, (b) control of muscle tone, (c) maintenance of posture and equilibrium, (d) suprasegmental control of reflex activity, (e) innervation of visceral and autonomic structures and (f) modification of sensory input.

Lesions involving the upper motor neuron, at a wide variety of locations and resulting from many different kinds of pathological processes, produce paralysis, alterations of muscle tone and alterations of reflex activity. Lesions destroying the upper motor neuron are rarely selective, usually incomplete and frequently involve adjacent pathways and nuclear structures. The degree of paresis or paralysis does not bear a direct relationship to the size of the lesion, or to the extent of involvement of the corticospinal tract (1447). Destruction of the upper motor neuron may result from vascular disease, trauma, neoplasm and infectious and degenerative diseases. Unilateral lesions in the cerebral hemisphere and brain stem produce contralateral paralysis, usually hemiplegia. Spinal lesions, most commonly the result of trauma, are usually bilateral and cause a paraplegia.

Immediately after an upper motor neuron lesion in the cerebral hemisphere, brain stem or spinal cord, the paralyzed limbs contralateral to the lesion usually are flaccid and the myotatic reflexes are depressed, or absent. After variable periods, the myotatic reflexes reappear in an exaggerated form in the paralyzed limbs. The superficial abdominal reflexes, elicited by stroking the skin over the abdomen, and the cremasteric reflexes in the male, disappear on the side of the paralysis. The plantar response, elicited by stroking the sole of the foot, becomes extensor. The latter response, known as the *sign of Babinski,* consists of extension of the great toe and fanning of the other toes. Although the sign of Babinski is of great clinical importance, the physiological mechanism underlying it is not understood.

After a variable period of time muscle tone in the affected limb gradually returns and ultimately exceeds that of the normal side. This exaggeration of muscle tone is referred to as *hypertonicity* or *spasticity.* The increase of tone is not exhibited by all muscles in the affected limbs. Spasticity selectively involves the antigravity muscles. In the affected upper extremity spasticity is present particularly in the adductors and internal rotators of the shoulder, in the flexors of the elbow, wrist and digits and in the pronators of the forearm. In the affected lower extremity spasticity develops in the adductors of the hip, the extensors of the hip and knee and in the plantar-flexors of foot and toes. *Spasticity* is relatively easy to describe but extremely difficult to define. Descriptively spasticity is characterized by: (a) increased resistance to passive movement, (b) extraordinarily hyperactive myotatic (deep tendon) reflexes that exhibit a low threshold, a large amplitude, an enlarged reflexogenous zone and have a briskness much greater than normal and (c) the presence of clonus (1594). *Clonus* is a manifestation of the exaggerated stretch reflex in which the contractions of one muscle group are sufficient to stretch antagonistic muscle groups and initiate myotatic responses in that muscle group. Clonus has a tendency to perpetuate itself in a synchronized manner. In some instances the threshold for this extreme exaggeration of the myotatic reflex is so low that passively moving a limb may initiate it.

The paralysis, which may appear complete at the onset of an upper motor neuron lesion, tends to become less severe in time. Even the weakness tends ultimately to involve one limb more than the other. The motor functions affected most are those associated with fine, skilled movements. Gross movements, and those which involve a whole limb, are least affected and show considerable restitution. Atrophy of the type seen with lower motor neuron lesions does not occur with upper motor neuron lesions. However, after a period of years some atrophy of disuse becomes evident.

Many hemiplegic patients recover considerable motor function in time. Those that become ambulatory have a characteristic gait. The paralyzed leg is circumducted at the hip *en bloc* and swung forward, because of the difficulty in flexing the knee. The foot is plantar-flexed and the toe of the shoe is dragged in a characteristic circular fashion. The arm on the affected side is flexed at the elbow and wrist, the forearm is pronated and the digits are flexed. The arm usually is held close to the body, but if the arm is swung at all in walking, it moves primarily at the shoulder. Upper motor neuron syndromes resulting from unilateral lesions in the brain stem or cerebral hemisphere produce contralateral disturbances of motor function. Unilateral brain stem lesions involving upper motor neurons frequently damage motor cranial nerves on the side of the lesion.

LESIONS OF THE SPINAL CORD AND NERVE ROOTS

The origin, course and terminations of ascending and descending spinal pathways are among the best documented pathways in the central nervous system (176, 266, 270, 280, 1632, 1806). However, considerable anatomical and physiological detail concerning these pathways continues to be developed from: (a) experimental anatomical studies in animals using silver impregnation technics and methods dependent upon anterograde and retrograde axoplasmic transport (554, 555, 1452, 1453), (b) neurophysiological stimulation and recording under controlled conditions and (c) detailed neuropathological studies in man.

The venerable study of secondary or Wallerian degeneration has been especially valuable in tracing fiber pathways (Fig. 10-25). When a nerve fiber is cut, not only does the part severed from the cell body undergo complete degeneration, but the cell body itself may exhibit pathological changes. Following transection of the axon, particularly close to the cell soma, the perikaryon undergoes swelling, there is apparent dissolution of Nissl substance, the cytoplasm acquires a "milky" appearance and the nucleus is displaced peripherally. These cell changes become fully developed after several days and are referred to as an *acute retrograde cell change or central chromatolysis*. Thus, if the spinal cord is transected, all the ascending fibers will degenerate above the level of injury ("ascending" degeneration). Their cell bodies, located below the injury, may show pathological changes (Figs. 4-2*E* and 4-33). Below the level of injury the descending fibers will degenerate ("descending" degeneration), since their cell bodies are above the cut. In the same way the central continuations of the dorsal root fibers may be determined by tracing secondary degeneration in the spinal cord after section of the dorsal roots proximal to the spinal ganglia (Fig. 10-25). Although chromatolysis of spinal ganglion cells might be expected following surgical section of the dorsal root in this location, only very minimal cell changes are seen (374, 1028). However, section of the mixed spinal nerve produces retrograde cell changes in the spinal ganglia (Fig. 7-5) and in some anterior horns (374). The location of the cell bodies whose axons form the ventral roots may be similarly determined by cutting the ventral root and ascertaining which cell bodies in the cord show retrograde changes (2201). The Marchi method (1601) which stains the degenerated myelin sheath has been useful in tracing the course of relatively large fiber bundles (Fig. 10-4). Silver impregnation technics (Figs. 4-2*F*, 9-30 and 9-25) provide more precise data concerning the course and termination of both myelinated and unmyelinated fibers (750, 896, 1068, 1819, 1821, 2721).

Axonal transport technics offer several important advantages over degeneration studies in tracing neural connections within the central nervous system. These methods depend upon essential physiological properties of nerve cells rather than upon destruction or injury. Small volumes of tritiated amino acids injected into localized collections of neurons are used to study anterograde transport of isotope via axons. Labeled precursors of protein and other macromolecules taken up by cell somata are synthesized, metabolized and transported into cell processes. Ultrastructural and biochemical evidence indicates that most protein synthesis occurs in ribosomes within cell perikarya and large dendrites (652). Axons passing through an area into which labeled amino acids have been injected do not incorporate the label into protein (555, 2482). Materials synthesized and transported via axoplasmic flow (2521) have various rates but two well-defined phases: (a) a "rapid phase" implicated in synaptic function which is in excess of 100 mm/day and (b) a "slow phase" of soluble material involved in the growth and maintenance of axons with rates of 1 to 5 mm/day (554). Labeled amino acids incorporated into a protein are not transported in a retrograde fashion, but in certain situations may be transported transneuronally (933, 2718). Isotope transported via axons to terminals can be traced in serial autoradiographs.

The enzyme HRP (molecular weight 40,000) transported in both anterograde and retrograde fashion, has been used mainly to study retrograde transport. The uptake of HRP at axon terminals and neuromuscular junctions appears to occur by pinocytosis into membrane-bound coated vesicles of different sizes (1452). As in other tissues most of the exogenous protein is seen in lysosomes or in multivesicular bodies that contribute to lysosomes. The intraaxonal transport of macromolecules within neurons involves many components which flow at different rates and in both directions. HRP is regarded as a sensitive marker because HRP organelles tend to fuse into larger membrane-bound vesicles and one molecule of enzyme can generate several molecules of visible reaction product (1451, 1814). The demonstration of HRP granules in neurons and their processes depends upon the ability of the enzyme to oxidize diaminobenzidine (DAB) or other chromagens (i.e., benzidine dihydrochloride or tetramethylbenzidine (TMB) in the presence of hydrogen peroxide to form an electron dense and light dense precipitate (936, 1027, 1678, 1680). TMB produces an intense blue reaction which can be identified readily under bright or dark field illumination. Reaction of tissue with chromagens and hydrogen peroxide results in a reaction product of fine, spherical granules within retrogradely labeled cells and within anterogradely labeled axons and axon terminals (Figs. 10-19 and 12-33). While there is no evidence that HRP is transported transneuronally, the enzyme may be taken up and transported by damaged axons. HRP injected into terminal axonal fields provides specific evidence of the location of the parent cell somata.

Certain fluorescent compounds also have been found to be transported in a retrograde fashion similar to HRP (158, 1345, 2425). Evans blue which fluoresces red and DAPI-primulin which fluoresces blue have been used in double labeling studies to identify populations of neurons in one locus that project divergent collaterals to different neural structures.

Dorsal Root Lesions. It should be obvious that cutting a dorsal root of a spinal nerve (i.e., dorsal rhizotomy) will abolish all of its incoming sensory impulses as well as interrupt the afferent arms of some segmental reflexes (Fig. 10-25). Due to the overlap of dermatomes in the periphery, destruction of one dorsal root does not result in diminished cutaneous innervation (hypesthesia); three consecutive dorsal roots must be destroyed before there is complete *anesthesia* in a dermatome (Fig. 7-10).

Muscle tone also is dependent upon the integrity of segmental reflexes, although two or more segments usually supply a single muscle. For example, total resection of dorsal root C5 will result in severe loss of muscle tone in the supraspinatus and rhomboid muscles (derived from cervical myotomes 4 and 5, mostly 5). Such a lesion also diminishes, but does not abolish, reflex tone in the deltoid, subscapularis, biceps brachii, brachialis and brachioradialis muscles (derived from cervical myotomes 5 and 6). However, if dorsal roots C5 and C6 are both destroyed, all sensory inputs via nerve fibers from these muscles are lost and there are no myotatic reflexes (*areflexia*). As a result the normal tone of these muscles is abolished completely (*atonia*). However, these muscles can still contract for their ventral root fibers remain intact.

The difference in the physiological deficits occurring with dorsal rhizotomies involving all roots to a limb and those sparing certain roots is impressive. Mott and Sherrington (1761) showed that complete deafferentation of an extremity resulted in virtual paralysis of the limb. Monkeys with such rhizotomies could not use the deafferented limb for walking, climbing or grasping. The motor deficits resulting from incomplete deafferentation of an extremity are quite different. If only one dorsal root distributing cutaneous afferents to any part of the hand or foot remained intact, little motor deficit resulted. These authors differentially sectioned certain dorsal roots and found that if cutaneous afferents alone were left intact, little impairment of function resulted. However, when muscle afferents were intact and cutaneous afferents were sectioned, the hand was virtually useless. From these studies, it was concluded that, "afferent impulses, both from the skin and from muscle, especially the former, as related to the palm or sole, are necessary for the carrying out of highest level movements." Subsequent investigations (1446) indicated that preservation of the C7 dorsal root appears to be of the greatest significance for use of the upper extremity. According to Twitchell (2593) monkeys with incomplete deafferentation of the arm direct movement of the limb by contact alone. These observations emphasize the important role that different sensory inputs play in the integration of motor function.

Ventral Root Lesions. Injury to the emerging ventral root of a spinal nerve produces deficits in segmental motor responses due to interruption of somatic efferent axons (Figs. 9-24, 9-28 and 10-25). If a thoracic or upper lumbar spinal nerve is injured, visceral efferent neurons (and reflexes) also would be involved (Figs. 8-1, 8-2, 9-28 and 10-25). Thus the destruction of the C8

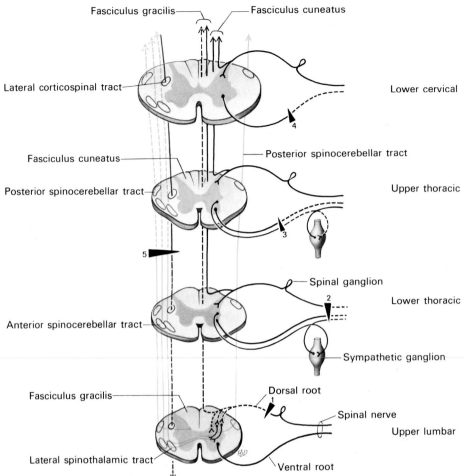

Figure 10-25. Simplified schematic diagram of degeneration resulting from certain lesions of the spinal nerves, spinal roots and spinal cord. Sites of lesions are indicated by small black wedges. Dorsal and ventral root fibers, peripheral nerve fibers, fibers in the posterior white columns and short relays are in *black*; ascending spinal tracts are *blue* and the corticospinal tract is *red*. A lesion of the dorsal root, *1*, at upper lumbar levels produces degeneration (*dashed lines*) in the posterior and anterior gray horns (not shown) and in parts of the fasciculus gracilis. No degeneration is present in other ascending spinal tracts because degeneration does not pass beyond the synapse. A lesion of a spinal nerve as at *2* produces peripheral degeneration (*dashed lines*) in somatic motor, sensory and postganglionic sympathetic fibers. A lesion of the ventral root at site *3* produces degeneration in somatic motor and preganglionic sympathetic fibers. A lesion at *4* produces degeneration only in somatic motor fibers distal to the lesion. The lesion at *5* destroys the lateral funiculus and produces ascending degeneration (*dashed lines*) in the posterior and anterior spinocerebellar tracts (*blue*) and in the spinothalamic tracts (only the lateral spinothalamic tract (*blue*) shown here) above the level of the lesion. This lesion also produces descending degeneration in the corticospinal tract (*red*) below the level of the lesion. Although other spinal tracts which would degenerate are not indicated, the same principle applies.

spinal ventral root would partly paralyze the small muscles of the hand (via median and ulnar nerves), whereas a lesion of both ventral roots C8 and T1 would produce a complete flaccid paralysis and atrophy of these muscles (Fig. 7-17). The inclusion of ventral root T1 in the injury would also interrupt most of the preganglionic visceral efferent fibers en route to the superior cer-

vical sympathetic ganglion (Figs. 9-28 and 10-29). Loss of these visceral motor fibers to the smooth muscle of the eye and levator palpebrae muscle results in a triad of clinical symptoms known as *Horner's syndrome* (page 228). This syndrome usually is accompanied by altered sweating on the face. Destruction of either the anterior horn cells (e.g., poliomyelitis), or their peripheral axons, results in a lower motor neuron lesion (Figs. 10-27 and 10-29), which deprives the appropriate muscles of the tonic influence of motor nerves.

If a mixed nerve is injured distal to the junction of the dorsal and ventral root (Fig. 10-25), the combined sensory and motor losses enumerated above will be present. It should be noted that if such combined nerve lesions are extensive, they may be followed by trophic changes in the skin (smoothness, dryness) and in capillary circulation (cyanosis). The trophic alterations presumably are due to the loss of peripheral vasomotor and afferent nerve fibers.

Spinal Cord Transection. Complete spinal cord transection immediately produces, below the level of the lesion, loss of all: (a) somatic sensation, (b) visceral sensation, (c) motor function, (d) muscle tone and (e) reflex activity. This state, referred to as *spinal shock*, is characterized by complete lack of neural function in the isolated spinal cord caudal to the lesion. Spinal shock occurs in all animals and man following complete transection of the spinal cord and is considered to be due to the sudden and abrupt interruption of descending excitatory influences. The period of spinal shock varies in different animals but in man ranges from 1 to 6 weeks and averages about 3 weeks. During this time there is no evidence of neural activity below the level of the lesion. The termination of the period of spinal shock is heralded by the appearance of the Babinski sign. A fairly orderly sequence of events follows which vary in duration. The various phases involved in the recovery of function in the isolated human spinal cord have been carefully analyzed by Kuhn (1388). These phases in recovery of neural function are: (a) minimal reflex activity (3 to 6 weeks), (b) flexor spasms (6 to 16 weeks), (c) alternate flexor and extensor spasms (after 4 months) and (d) predominant extensor spasms (after 6 months). The phase of minimal reflex activity is characterized by weak flexor responses to nociceptive stimuli, which begin distally and progressively involve proximal muscle groups in the extremities. During this period the Babinski sign can be obtained bilaterally, but the muscles are flaccid and the deep tendon reflexes cannot be elicited.

The phase of flexor muscle spasms is characterized by increasing tone in the flexor muscles and by stronger flexor responses to nociceptive stimuli, which progressively involve more proximal muscle groups. During this phase that the so-called *triple flexion response* is first seen. This involves flexion of the lower extremity at the hip, knee and ankle in response to a relatively mild nociceptive stimulus. The most exaggerated form of this reaction is the *mass reflex*, in which a relatively mild, and sometimes nonspecific, stimulus results in powerful bilateral triple flexion responses. These responses are characterized by repeated discharge of motor units throughout the caudal part of the spinal cord. The mass reflex appears to be due to the spread of afferent impulses from one segment to the next and dispersion of impulses in such a manner as to cause motor units to continue to fire after the exciting stimulus has been withdrawn. The mass reflex is distressing to the patient because it is almost impossible to control. This reflex becomes less severe about 4 months after spinal transection when extensor muscle tone gradually begins to increase. During this phase both flexor and extensor muscle spasms occur, but within a relatively short time extensor muscle tone predominates. It may be so great that the patient can momentarily support his weight in a standing position (1388).

Examination of the patient 1 year after complete spinal cord transection reveals the following: (a) complete paralysis below the level of the lesion, (b) loss of all sensation (somatic and visceral) below the lesion, (c) marked extensor muscle tone (spasticity) below the lesion (989, 990), (d) hyperactive deep tendon (myotatic) reflexes below the lesion, (e) clonus in both lower extremities and (f) bilateral Babinski signs. Paralysis of bowel and bladder, present from the time of spinal transection, constitutes one of the major problems, but with good nursing care, reflex emptying of bowel and bladder can be established. In many patients there is reflex spinal sweating in response to noxious stimuli. This type of sweating is not under thermoregulatory control. In the male there is also a disturbance of sexual functions.

Bladder and bowel functions are disturbed in all transections of the cord, for they are no longer under voluntary control. Interruption of descending autonomic fibers, particularly those *en route* to parasympathetic nuclei in the sacral cord (S2, S3, S4), leads to loss of rectal motility. There are reflex spasms of the external anal sphincters and fecal retention. Defecation occurs involuntarily after long intervals. If cord segments S2, S3 and S4 are destroyed (*conus medullaris syndrome*), there is a permanent paralysis of the external sphincter and fecal incontinence (Fig. 8-10). When these sacral segments are involved, there is in addition paralytic incontinence, and usually bladder distention, impotence and perianal, or saddle, anesthesia. However, normal sensory and motor function is retained in the lower extremities (conus medullaris syndrome).

Bladder disturbances usually occur in three phases after cord transection. At the outset there is always urinary *retention*, due to paralysis of the muscular bladder wall (detrusor muscle), and spasm of the vesicle sphincter. Two or 3 weeks later (range 2 days to 18 months) the second phase or *overflow incontinence* is observed. An intermittent dribbling of urine during this phase is due to gradual hypertrophy of the detrusor smooth muscle. The muscle overcomes the resistance of the external sphincter for short periods of time. Continued hypertrophy of the bladder wall eventually permits the bladder to expel small amounts of urine automatically, providing bladder infections have not intervened. This is the third phase, known as *automatic micturition*. Such automaticity of the bladder is poor if lumbar spinal cord segments are involved, and absent (paralytic incontinence) when the sacral segments are destroyed.

In partial or incomplete transection of the spinal cord, some ascending or descending fibers escape injury. The sensory deficits may not correspond to the level of motor loss, and some voluntary function may return within 1 or 2 weeks. Vasomotor and visceral disturbances usually are less pronounced, and irritative sensory phenomena are more common (e.g., pains, paresthesias, hyperesthesias). Marked priapism is more likely to accompany an incomplete transection of the cord. Haymaker

(1057) has stated that the only reliable criterion of total transection, in the early stages after spinal injury, is "a complete flaccid paraplegia with areflexia and complete sensory loss which lasts longer than 2 to 5 days."

Although complete transections of the spinal cord produce degeneration in ascending tracts above the level of the lesion (Fig. 10-2) and in descending tracts below the level of the lesion (Fig. 10-16), the lesion rarely is sharply localized, and considerable degeneration usually is present in nearly all systems in the immediate vicinity of the lesion.

Spinal Hemisection. Hemisection of the spinal cord is probably the most instructive spinal lesion for teaching purposes, in spite of the fact that precise lesions of this kind are encountered only rarely in clinical neurology. The signs and symptoms associated with hemisection of the spinal cord constitute the *Brown-Séquard* syndrome (Fig. 10-26). Neurological findings in the illustrated hemisection would include: (a) loss of sensory impulses transmitted by the posterior white columns from below the lesion on the same side, (b) an upper motor neuron lesion below the level of injury on the same side, (c) lower motor neuron symptoms and vasomotor paralysis in areas supplied by the injured segments on the side of the lesion, (d) bilateral loss of pain and thermal sense within the area of the lesion and (e) loss of pain and thermal sense below T12 on the opposite side of the body (i.e., lower extremity, genitals and perineum). With a lesion at the T12 spinal segment, sensory and upper motor neuron symptoms would be manifested through spinal nerves of the lumbar and sacral plexuses. The lower motor neuron damage at cord segment T12 would produce no atrophy in muscles of the lower extremity and the reflex arcs below the level of the lesion would remain intact.

Complete and incomplete transections of the human spinal cord may result from missile wounds or fracture-dislocation of vertebrae. Similar damage may follow ischemic necrosis due to occlusion or interruption of radicular arteries that supply the vulnerable upper thoracic segments (Fig. 20-1) of the spinal cord (215, 1688, 2802). Neoplasms also may compress the spinal

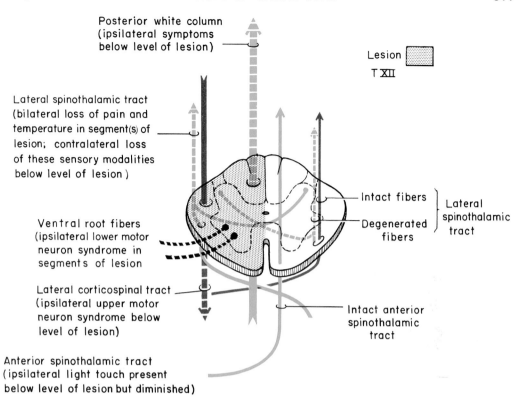

Posterior white column
(ipsilateral symptoms
below level of lesion)

Lesion
T XII

Lateral spinothalamic tract
(bilateral loss of pain and
temperature in segment(s) of
lesion; contralateral loss
of these sensory modalities
below level of lesion)

Intact fibers ⎫
Degenerated ⎬ Lateral spinothalamic tract
fibers ⎭

Ventral root fibers
(ipsilateral lower motor
neuron syndrome in
segments of lesion

Lateral corticospinal tract
(ipsilateral upper motor
neuron syndrome below
level of lesion)

Intact anterior
spinothalamic
tract

Anterior spinothalamic tract
(ipsilateral light touch present
below level of lesion but diminished)

Figure 10-26. Schematic diagram of degeneration associated with a spinal cord hemisection. Such a lesion produces the Brown-Séquard syndrome. The major degeneration occurs on the side of the lesion with ascending tracts degenerated above the lesion and descending tracts degenerated caudal to it. If the lesion involves only one spinal level contralateral degeneration would be minimal and confined to crossed fibers arising from the involved segment. *Arrows* indicate direction of impulse conduction, while *broken lines* indicated degenerated tracts.

cord and secondarily compromise the blood supply. In such spinal cord lesions, the symptoms are severe and the complications are numerous, regardless of the level of injury.

In spinal hemisection the basic principle with respect to degeneration pertains, in that virtually all degeneration is on the side of the lesion; ascending tracts will degenerate above the level of the lesion, and descending tracts will degenerate below the level of the lesion (Fig. 10-26). However, if the lesion involves several spinal segments, a small amount of degeneration may be detected in the contralateral spinothalamic tracts (and anterior spinocerebellar tract if the lesion involves lumbar spinal segments).

Amyotrophic Lateral Sclerosis. This spinal cord disease involves both upper and lower motor neurons. It is a progressive degenerative disease of unknown etiology, occurring with greatest frequency in the 5th and 6th decades of life, characterized by degeneration of the corticospinal tracts and the anterior horn cells. When degeneration of anterior horn cells begins in the cervical region (Fig. 10-27), the disease manifests itself by progressive muscular atrophy in the upper extremities, usually in the small intrinsic hand muscles, and spastic weakness of the muscles of the trunk and lower extremities. Muscular weakness usually is symmetrical and becomes generalized in the terminal phases of the disease. Fasciculations (i.e., involuntary twitching of muscle fascicles) in affected muscles can be observed and felt by the patient and the examiner. Myotatic irritability of affected muscles persists until atrophy is complete. Late in the course of this progressive disease, functional disturbances of the bladder

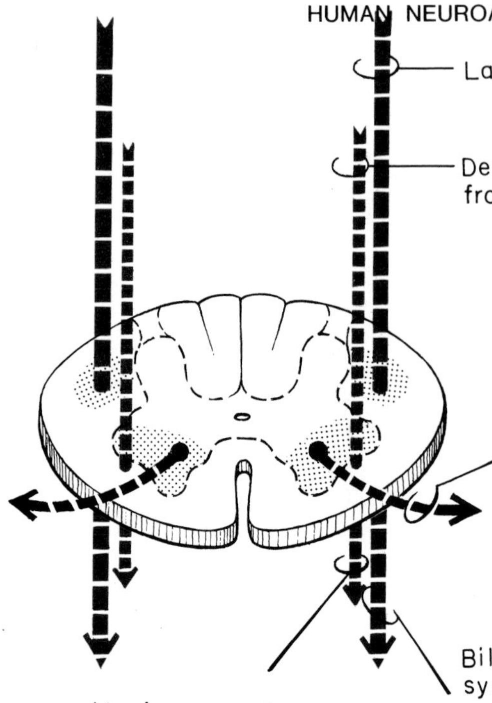

Lateral corticospinal tract

Descending autonomic fibers from higher levels

Bilateral lower motor neuron syndrome of all skeletal mm. supplied by anterior horn cells within segments of lesion.

(e.g. small mm. of hand)

Bilateral upper motor neuron syndrome of cord segments

May result in symptoms of visceral disturbance (e.g. bladder, rectum)

Lesion ▨

C VIII—TI

Figure 10-27. Schematic diagram of spinal cord pathology in amyotrophic lateral sclerosis, a syndrome which involves both upper and lower motor neurons. Although the upper motor neuron lesion may involve all spinal levels, lower motor neuron involvement initially may be localized at particular levels. *Arrows* indicate direction of impulse conduction and *broken lines* indicate degenerated nerve fibers.

and rectum may appear due to injury of descending autonomic fibers en route to lumbar and sacral segments of the cord.

Combined System Disease. The neurological manifestations of pernicious anemia result in degenerative changes in peripheral nerves and in the central nervous system. The anemia and the degenerative changes in the nervous system result from a deficiency of vitamin B_{12}. A defect in gastric secretion deprives these patients of an enzyme specifically required for absorption of vitamin B_{12}. Peripheral nerves and spinal tracts undergo varying degrees of degeneration. The degeneration in the spinal cord appears to affect especially the posterior white columns and the corticospinal tracts, but it is not confined to these systems (Fig. 10-28). Patients with this disease have both sensory and motor disturbances. The sensory disturbances include numbness and tingling, "pins and needles"

sensation, loss of position sense and loss of vibratory sense. These sensory disturbances are greatest in distal portions of the extremities and tend to be symmetrical. There is little impairment of tactile, thermal or pain sense. Weakness in the lower extremities is common and the gait may be spastic and ataxic. The myotatic reflexes in the lower extremities usually are reduced while those in the upper extremity are normal. The sign of Babinski can be elicited bilaterally. Moderate muscular wasting usually occurs in the late stages of the disease.

Syringomyelia. This is a chronic disease characterized pathologically by long cavities, surrounded by glial elements, that develop in relationship to the central canal of the spinal cord. These cavities may extend into the medulla (syringobulbia). Syringomyelia probably is related embryologically to an abnormal closure of the central

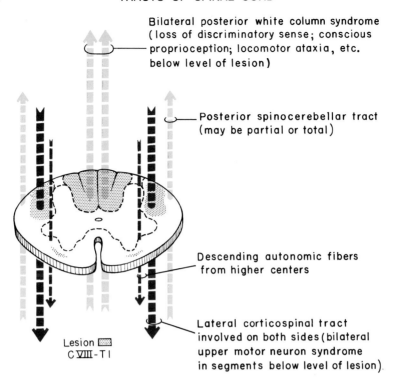

Bilateral posterior white column syndrome (loss of discriminatory sense; conscious proprioception; locomotor ataxia, etc. below level of lesion)

Posterior spinocerebellar tract (may be partial or total)

Descending autonomic fibers from higher centers

Lateral corticospinal tract involved on both sides (bilateral upper motor neuron syndrome in segments below level of lesion)

Lesion
C VIII-T I

Figure 10-28. Schematic diagram of the spinal degeneration seen in combined system disease, a neurological manifestation of pernicious anemia. Ascending fibers in the posterior columns and descending systems in the lateral funiculus are affected early, but other tracts and peripheral nerves may be involved. Spinal degeneration is fairly symmetrical. *Arrows* and *broken lines* indicate fiber systems which degenerate in the syndrome. The extent of degeneration in the posterior spinocerebellar tract is variable.

canal. Incomplete closure of the central canal may leave cavities around which a secondary gliosis develops. Characteristically syringomyelia involves the lower cervical and upper thoracic regions of the spinal cord. The affected region of the spinal cord is enlarged and transverse sections reveal a large irregular cavity containing a clear or yellow fluid.

The hallmark of this disease is an early impairment, or loss, of pain and thermal sense with preservation of tactile sense. This selective loss of pain and thermal sense, frequently noted first in the hands and forearms, results from interruption of decussating sensory fibers (i.e., spinothalamic tracts) in several consecutive segments. This kind of sensory loss is referred to as a "dissociated sensory" loss because other forms of sensation are preserved. Later the cavity may enlarge in a lateral, posterior, cranial or caudal direction, and it may destroy adjacent fiber tracts or gray matter. An example of such a case is illustrated schematically in Figure 10-29. Here

the lesion interrupts the crossing fibers of the lateral spinothalamic tract in cord segments C8 and T1. Axons distal to the lesion are separated from their cells or origin and undergo degeneration (*broken lines* in Fig. 10-29). Destruction of these crossing fibers from both sides of the cord results in a bilateral loss of pain and thermal sense in the distribution of spinal nerves and dermatomes of C8 to T1. All pain and temperature fibers of T1 are destroyed, but some of the C8 fibers are spared inasmuch as a few fibers ascend and cross in the C7 cord segment. This type of lesion results in a "dissociated sensory" loss as described above. The remainder of the lateral spinothalamic tract contains normal fibers that have crossed in spinal cord segments either above or below the area of the lesion. In this case, the lateral extension of the cavity also has destroyed the anterior gray horn and nerve fibers passing through it (Fig. 10-29). A patient with such a lesion would have symptoms and signs of a unilateral lower motor neuron lesion and a Horner's syn-

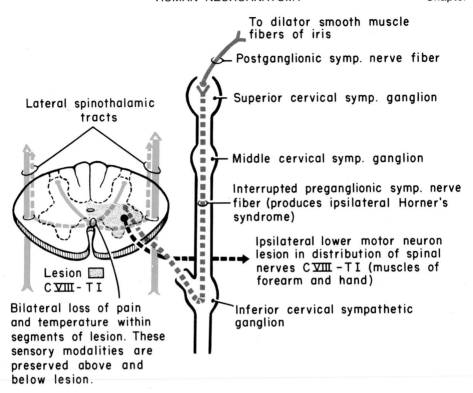

To dilator smooth muscle
fibers of iris

Postganglionic symp. nerve fiber

Superior cervical symp. ganglion

Lateral spinothalamic
tracts

Middle cervical symp. ganglion

Interrupted preganglionic symp. nerve
fiber (produces ipsilateral Horner's
syndrome)

Ipsilateral lower motor neuron
lesion in distribution of spinal
nerves C VIII – T I (muscles of
forearm and hand)

Lesion ▨
C VIII - T I

Inferior cervical sympathetic
ganglion

Bilateral loss of pain
and temperature within
segments of lesion. These
sensory modalities are
preserved above and
below lesion.

Figure 10-29. Schematic diagram of syringomyelia with lateral extension of the cavity into anterior gray horn of spinal cord. *Arrows* show direction of impulse conduction; *broken lines* indicate degenerated nerve fibers.

drome in addition to the classic sensory disturbances. These neurological findings aid in localizing the lesion to spinal segments C8 and T1.

Other Spinal Syndromes. There are many varieties of spinal cord lesions and syndromes in addition to those briefly described here. *Tabes dorsalis* (locomotor ataxia) is a central nervous system form of syphilis which produces degeneration in the central processes of dorsal root ganglion cells. This results in extensive demyelination and degeneration of fibers in the fasciculus gracilis. There is no unanimity of opinion as to why the degenerative lesions in tabes dorsalis have this selective character. The principal symptoms of tabes are attributable to degeneration and irritation of dorsal root fibers. Sensory loss, impairment of position and vibratory sense, radic-

ular pains and paresthesias all are related to dorsal root fibers. Ataxia and difficulty in walking are related to loss of position and kinesthetic sense. The patient compensates for these deficits by walking on a broad base with eyes directed to the ground. Muscle tone is greatly reduced and the myotatic reflexes in the lower extremities are greatly diminished or absent.

Multiple sclerosis is a demyelinating disease of unknown etiology characterized by widely disseminated lesions in the central nervous system. This disease which affects young adults frequently involves the white matter of the brain and spinal cord, but there is nothing selective about the location of the lesions. Early manifestations of the disease are followed by conspicuous improvement, but relapses are a striking and constant feature of the disorder.

CHAPTER 11

The Medulla

The medulla (myelencephalon), the most caudal segment of the brain stem, represents a conical, expanded continuation of the upper cervical spinal cord. Externally the transition from spinal cord to lower medulla is gradual, without sharp demarcation. The caudal limit of the medulla is rostral to the highest rootlets of the first cervical spinal nerve at about the level of the foramen magnum. Above the level of transition, the medulla increases in size and its external features become distinctive. Changes in the external appearance of the medulla are due chiefly to structural rearrangement and development of structures peculiar to the medulla. The development of the fourth ventricle causes structures previously located posteriorly to be shifted posterolaterally, while the appearance of the pyramids on the anterior surface partially obliterates the anterior median fissure. The oval eminences posterolateral to the pyramids, produced by the inferior olivary nuclei, give the medulla above the zone of transition a characteristic configuration. The gross features of the brain stem are shown in anterior and posterior views in Figures 11-1 and 11-2.

While the spinal cord throughout most of its length presents a relatively uniform internal organization, graded sections through the medulla disclose numerous important changes from level to level. Among the principal changes taking place in the medulla are the following: (a) the development of the fourth ventricle, representing the rostral continuation of the central canal of the spinal cord, (b) the replacement of the butterfly-shaped central gray of the spinal cord by large cellular aggregations and interlacing fibers constituting the reticular formation, (c) the decussation of the medullary pyramids, (d) the termination of ascending first order fibers contained in the fasciculi gracilis and cuneatus upon their respective nuclei, and the formation of a composite second order lemniscal pathway, (e) the gradual replacement of spinal fibers in the zone of Lissauer by fibers of the spinal trigeminal tract and (f) the appearance of groups of relay nuclei, most of which project fibers to the cerebellum.

In the floor of the fourth ventricle the sulcus limitans can be seen lateral to the median sulcus. This groove continues to demarcate afferent and efferent cell col-

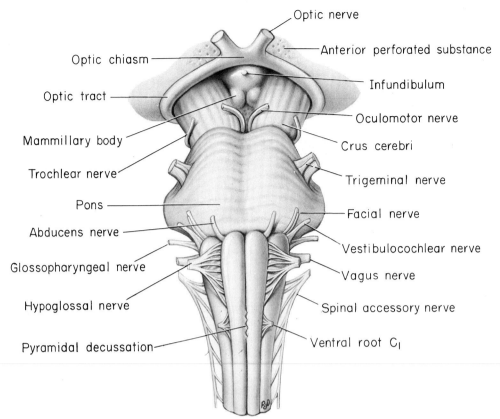

Figure 11-1. Drawing of the anterior aspect of the medulla, pons and midbrain.

umns (Fig. 11-17) as it did in the developing spinal cord (Fig. 3-4A). The reticular formation, phylogenetically one of the oldest portions of the neuraxis, represents the core of the brain stem. Structurally, it is composed of complex collections of cells of different sizes, types and shapes forming both diffuse cellular aggregations and circumscribed nuclei (Figs. 11-8 and 11-9). Fibers entering, leaving and traversing the reticular core seemingly pass haphazardly in all directions. However, studies of Golgi-stained preparations of this region (2274) indicate that fibers and cellular groups are organized in specific patterns. The reticular formation of the medulla is continuous with that of the pons and higher levels of the brain stem. Figure 11-3 indicates the level and plane of section of most of the brain stem photomicrographs described in this and succeeding chapters.

SPINOMEDULLARY TRANSITION

At the junction of the spinal cord and medulla (Figs. 11-4 and A-1) transverse sections resemble those of the upper cervical spinal cord with certain modifications. The substantia gelatinosa has increased in size, and larger descending myelinated fibers can be found in the zone of Lissauer. At this level the zone of Lissauer contains fine ascending root fibers from the uppermost cervical spinal nerves and coarser descending fibers of the trigeminal nerve (N. V) which enter at pontine levels and descend in the dorsolateral part of the brain stem. Some of these descending spinal trigeminal fibers can be found as low as the second cervical segment. The substantia gelatinosa becomes the spinal trigeminal nucleus at high cervical levels, and it retains the same relative position and size throughout the medulla. Descending trigeminal fibers terminate directly, or by collaterals, in parts of the spinal trigeminal nucleus.

A conspicuous increase in the gray surrounding the central canal is evident (Figs. 11-4 and 11-5). The lateral corticospinal tract has become clearly separated from the medial longitudinal fasciculus by its passage into the posterior part of the lateral funiculus. It is broken up into a number of

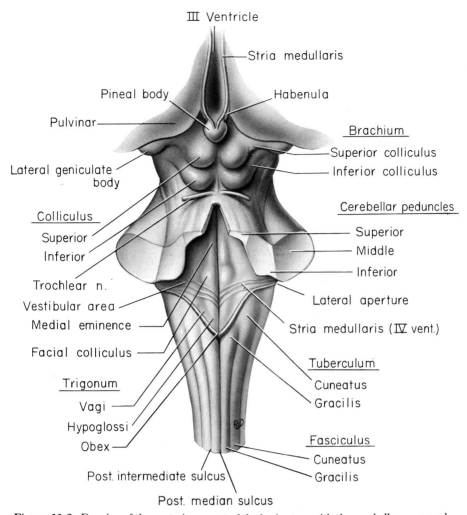

III Ventricle

Stria medullaris

Pineal body

Habenula

Pulvinar

Brachium
Superior colliculus
Inferior colliculus

Lateral geniculate
body

Colliculus
Superior
Inferior

Cerebellar peduncles
Superior
Middle
Inferior

Trochlear n.

Vestibular area

Lateral aperture

Medial eminence

Stria medullaris (IV vent.)

Facial colliculus

Tuberculum
Cuneatus
Gracilis

Trigonum
Vagi
Hypoglossi
Obex

Fasciculus
Cuneatus
Gracilis

Post. intermediate sulcus

Post. median sulcus

Figure 11-2. Drawing of the posterior aspect of the brain stem with the cerebellum removed.

obliquely or transversely cut bundles, between which are strands of gray matter. A few fibers of the spinal portion of the spinal accessory nerve can be seen arching posterolaterally to emerge from the lateral aspect of the spinal cord between the dorsal and ventral roots (Figs. 11-4 and A-1). Axons of somatic motor neurons in the anterior horn emerge as ventral root fibers of the first cervical spinal nerve. Rostrally these cells extend into the lower medulla (Fig. 11-7) where they are known as the *supraspinal nucleus* (1198). Fiber tracts in the white matter have the same arrangement as in cervical spinal segments.

Corticospinal Decussation. The most conspicuous features of sections through this level (Figs. 11-5, 11-6 and A-2) are the decussation of the corticospinal tracts, the first appearance of the nuclei of the poste-

rior columns and the development of the medullary reticular formation. The central gray has increased in size and lies mostly dorsal to the central canal.

Bundles of pyramidal fibers cross the midline ventral to the central gray and project dorsolaterally across the base of the anterior horn. These fibers cross in interdigitating bundles having a caudal, as well as transverse, direction; in transverse sections these bundles are cut obliquely, so that in some sections more pyramidal fibers may be present on one side. The corticospinal tract, which forms the pyramids, arises mainly from cells in the primary motor and somesthetic cortex, and undergoes an incomplete decussation in the lower medulla before entering the spinal cord. The largest number of fibers (nearly 90%) cross and descend in the posterior part of the lateral funiculus, as the lateral corticospinal tract (Figs. 10-11–10-13). Fibers of the anterior corticospinal tract retain their original position and project uncrossed into the anterior funiculus of the spinal cord (Figs.

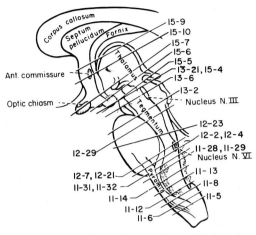

Figure 11-3. Outline of paramedian sagittal section of the brain stem indicating level and plane of transverse sections used to illustrate this and subsequent chapters. Figure numbers are opposite levels of section. Structures in this parasagittal outline are identified in Figure 15-2.

10-12 and 10-14). Some uncrossed fibers pass into the lateral funiculus on the same side. In a series of ascending sections the pyramidal decussation naturally is seen in reverse.

The corticospinal decussation forms the anatomical basis for the voluntary motor control of one half of the body by neurons in the opposite cerebral hemisphere. Injury of this tract anywhere above the decussation may cause paralysis of the contralateral extremities. For reasons that will be clear when the motor cortex is studied, the consequences of lesions confined to the corticospinal tract axons in the medullary pyramid have been of great interest. Due to the nature of the blood supply of the region, it is rare in man to encounter a lesion limited to the pyramid, and the motor deficit is usually a contralateral paresis sparing the face and tongue. In the case reported with the least damage beyond the pyramid, the paresis was accompanied by spasticity after an initial flaccidity (2203). In monkeys, it is possible surgically to interrupt the pyramid with minimal damage to the adjacent medulla (884, 2564, 2776). In these studies, there was a modest impairment of

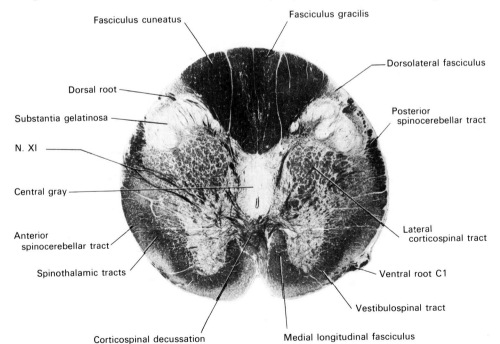

Figure 11-4. Transverse section through the junction of spinal cord and medulla. Some of the most caudal decussating fibers of the corticospinal tract can be seen passing into the posterior part of the lateral funiculus. The structure labeled substantia gelatinosa also contains cell groups of the spinal trigeminal nucleus (Weigert's myelin stain, photograph).

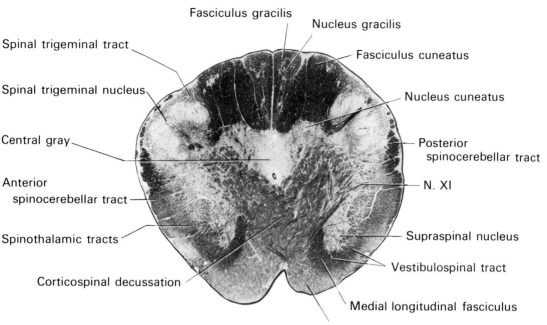

Fasciculus gracilis

Nucleus gracilis

Spinal trigeminal tract

Fasciculus cuneatus

Spinal trigeminal nucleus

Nucleus cuneatus

Central gray

Posterior spinocerebellar tract

Anterior spinocerebellar tract

N. XI

Spinothalamic tracts

Supraspinal nucleus

Vestibulospinal tract

Corticospinal decussation

Medial longitudinal fasciculus

Medullary pyramid

Figure 11-5. Transverse section of the medulla through the decussation of the corticospinal tract (Weigert's myelin stain, photograph).

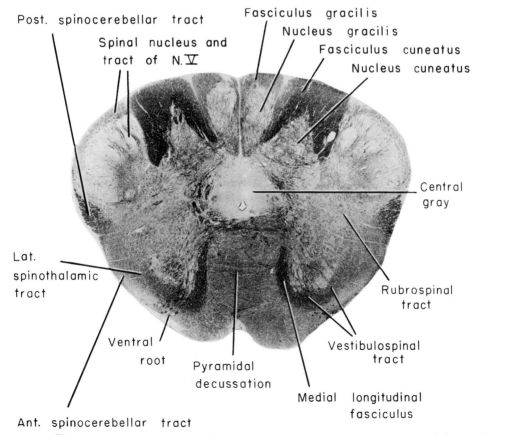

Post. spinocerebellar tract

Fasciculus gracilis

Spinal nucleus and tract of N. V

Nucleus gracilis

Fasciculus cuneatus

Nucleus cuneatus

Central gray

Lat. spinothalamic tract

Rubrospinal tract

Ventral root

Vestibulospinal tract

Pyramidal decussation

Medial longitudinal fasciculus

Ant. spinocerebellar tract

Figure 11-6. Transverse section of the medulla through the upper part of the corticospinal decussation (Weigert's myelin stain, photograph).

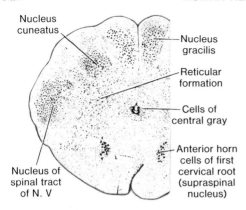

Nucleus cuneatus

Nucleus gracilis

Reticular formation

Cells of central gray

Anterior horn cells of first cervical root (supraspinal nucleus)

Nucleus of spinal tract of N. V

Figure 11-7. Section through medulla of 1-month infant at about same level as in Figure 11-5 (cresyl violet; photograph, with cell groups blocked in schematically).

contralateral limb movement, most noticeable in the distal limb joints, and hypotonia. The major deficit was inability to move individually the fingers of the contralateral upper limb to pick up small objects. However, if about 30% of the pyramidal tract fibers remain intact, it is possible with time and retraining to overcome the deficits of finger movement. The enduring deficit is loss of hand contact orienting responses and reflex sensory-motor adjustments (2295).

The substantia gelatinosa of the cervical spinal cord has now become the *spinal trigeminal nucleus* (Figs. 11-5–11-8). This nucleus is capped dorsolaterally by descending fibers of the *spinal trigeminal tract* which terminate in corresponding parts of this nucleus.

The anterior horn, still recognizable at this level, contains groups of motor neurons which contribute fibers to the first cervical and the spinal accessory nerves. On the medial border of the anterior horn is the medial longitudinal fasciculus which has been shifted laterally by the fibers of the corticospinal decussation (Figs. 11-5 and 11-6). On the ventral and lateral borders of the anterior horn are fibers of the vestibulospinal tract. The gray between the spinal trigeminal nucleus and the anterior horn has lost its definite continuity and is composed of scattered cells and fiber bundles. Fibers present in this area are corticospinal and short intersegmental fibers, comparable to those of the fasciculi proprii. This area of intermingled gray and white is the

most caudal part of the brain stem reticular formation.

Posterior Column Nuclei. In the posterior white columns nuclear masses have appeared in the fasciculi gracilis and cuneatus. These are the nuclei of the posterior funiculi, known respectively as the *nucleus gracilis* and *nucleus cuneatus*. The long ascending branches of the cells in the dorsal root ganglia, coursing in the posterior funiculus, terminate upon these nuclei (Figs. 9-29, 10-1 and 11-2). At these levels the fasciculus cuneatus is massive and only a small caudal part of the nucleus cuneatus protrudes into the ventral part of the fasciculus (Figs. 11-5 and 11-6). The nucleus gracilis is larger, occupies a more central position and is capped dorsally and laterally by fibers of the fasciculus gracilis. At progressively higher levels, increasing numbers of fibers terminate in these nuclei. The nuclei increase in size (Fig. 11-7) while the fasciculi correspondingly decrease (Fig. 11-8). At levels through the caudal part of the inferior olivary complex, the entire fasciculus gracilis and most of the fasciculus cuneatus have been replaced by their respective nuclei (Figs. 11-8 and 11-9).

In animals three cytologically distinct regions of the nucleus gracilis have been recognized (348, 1413, 2504): (a) a reticular region rostral to the obex characterized by a loose organization of cells, (b) a "cell nest" region caudal to the obex characterized by cell clusters and (c) a caudal region characterized by scattered cells occurring singly or in small clusters. Ascending dorsal root fibers project somatotopically to the nucleus gracilis (416, 746, 1024, 2660). According to Hand (1024) lumbosacral dorsal root fibers exhibit a somatotopic lamination chiefly in the "cell nest" region, while terminations in the reticular region are diffuse with intersegmental overlap. Certain physiological studies in the cat suggest that neurons in the nucleus gracilis exhibit rostrocaudal differences with respect to: (a) the size of the peripheral receptive fields which supply afferent input (923, 1557) and (b) segregation of sensory modality (921, 1387, 1973, 2752). Rostral portions of the nucleus (i.e., reticular region) are said to be related to deep pressure and joint movement, while the "cell nest" and caudal regions of the nucleus are related to hair and skin recep-

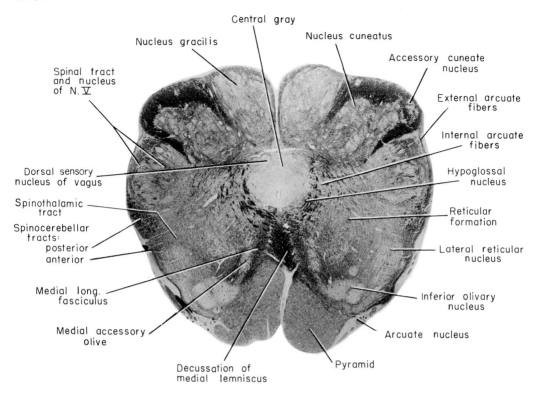

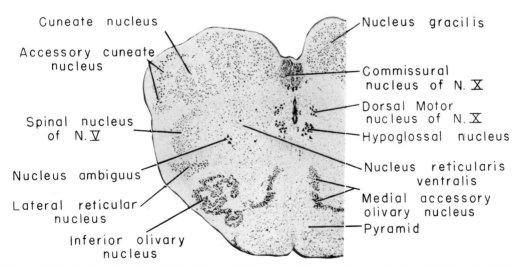

Figure 11-9. Section through medulla of 1-month infant about the same level as in Figure 11-8 (cresyl violet; photograph, with cell groups blocked in schematically).

tors. Other physiological data (1373), based upon single neuron analysis of posterior column nuclei, provide no evidence of rostrocaudal differentiation in terms of either somatotopy or modality segregation. The

latter finding supports experimental studies (1769, 2019) which indicate that: (a) the somatotopic organization of the posterior columns and the medial lemniscus is maintained at the level of the posterior column nuclei and (b) neural elements devoted to kinesthesis and tactile sense are intermingled in a single and mutual somatotopic pattern. Studies in the monkey indicate that lower thoracic, lumbar and sacrococcygeal dorsal roots project in overlapping somatotopic fashion throughout the rostrocaudal extent of the nucleus gracilis (416). Zones of the nucleus gracilis receiving terminal dorsal root fibers are organized so that: (a) roots of the lumbar enlargement project to irregular-shaped areas in the central core of the nucleus, (b) lower thoracic and upper lumbar roots project in serial fashion to narrow, oblique laminae lateral to the core region and (c) sacral and coc-cygeal dorsal roots project in serial fashion to crescent-shaped laminae in dorsomedial parts of the nucleus. The areas of the terminal projection zones in the nucleus gracilis are related to the size of the dorsal root and the number of ascending fibers they contribute to the fasciculus gracilis.

The nucleus cuneatus also exhibits regional differences in its cytoarchitecture (1649, 1885). According to Kuypers and Tuerk (1413) dorsal areas of the cuneate nucleus contain clusters of round cells with bushy dendrites, while basal areas contain triangular, multipolar and fusiform cells with long, sparse dendrites. These authors considered the round cell clusters to receive afferents principally from distal parts of the body and to be related to small cutaneous receptive fields. Triangular and multipolar cells were considered to receive afferents primarily from proximal parts of the limb and trunk, and were regarded as being related to larger cutaneous receptive fields. These studies suggested that dorsal root fibers have a dual termination with some fibers ending in cell clusters and others among basal triangular cells.

A systematic study of dorsal root projections to the cuneate nucleus in the monkey has shown that: (a) fibers from C1 through T1 terminate in both exclusive and overlapping zones, (b) fibers from C5 through C8 terminate in a central core region about which other dorsal root fibers terminate in oblique serial laminae, (c) rostral dorsal root fibers (C1 through C4) terminate in ventrolateral regions and (d) caudal dorsal root fibers (T1 through T7) terminate in dorsomedial regions (2333) (Fig. 11-10).

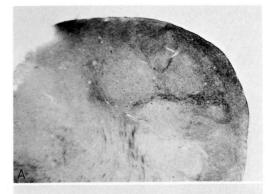

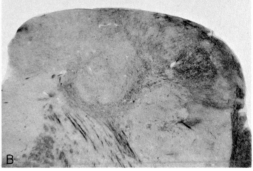

Figure 11-10. Photomicrograph of terminal degeneration in the cuneate and accessory cuneate nuclei in the monkey following section of the fifth (A) and sixth (B) cervical dorsal roots (Nauta-Gygax stain, ×16).

Comparisons of the patterns of dorsal root terminations in the nuclei gracilis and cuneatus in the monkey (416) suggest that in the nucleus gracilis: (a) overlapping terminations are more extensive and irregular than in the cuneate nucleus and (b) there is less autonomous terminal representation of individual dorsal root fibers in the nucleus gracilis.

Decussation of the Medial Lemniscus. In transverse sections of the medulla above the corticospinal decussation (Figs. 11-8, 11-9 and A-3), the nucleus gracilis reaches its greatest extent, and practically all fibers of the fasciculus gracilis have terminated in portions of the nucleus. Although the nucleus cuneatus is much larger than shown in Figures 11-6 or 11-7, a considerable number of fibers of the fasciculus cuneatus remain dorsal to the nuclei. From the nuclei gracilis and cuneatus, myelinated fibers arise which sweep ventromedially around the central gray. These fibers, known as *internal arcuate fibers*, cross the median raphe and contralaterally form a well-defined ascending bundle, the *medial lemniscus*. This large ascending fiber bundle can be readily followed through the brain stem to its termination in the ventral posterolateral nucleus (VPL) of the thalamus (Fig. 10-1). The medial lemniscus constitutes the second neuron of the posterior column pathway conveying kinesthetic sense and discriminative tactile sense to higher levels of the neuraxis. The decussation of the medial lemniscus provides part of the anatomical basis for sensory representation of half of the body in the contralateral cerebral cortex. Consequently, injury to the medial lemniscus causes characteristic kinesthetic and tactile deficits on the opposite side of the body.

Lateral to the cuneate nucleus is a group of large cells similar to those of the dorsal nucleus of Clarke, known as the *accessory cuneate* nucleus (Figs. 10-9, 11-8, 11-9, A-3 and A-4). This nucleus is considered to be the medullary equivalent of the dorsal nucleus (260, 1946, 2323). These nuclei share the following anatomical and functional features: (a) cells are morphologically similar with eccentric nuclei, (b) afferent fibers are derived from dorsal roots, (c) both nuclei give rise to uncrossed cerebellar afferent fibers and (d) both nuclei relay impulses from muscle spindles, Golgi tendon organs, type II muscle afferents and cutaneous afferents (1900, 1903). Ascending fibers conveyed by the fasciculus cuneatus and terminating in the accessory cuneate nucleus are derived from the same dorsal root ganglia as those projecting to the cuneate nucleus, namely those of cervical and upper thoracic spinal segments. Dorsal root fibers, projecting to the accessory cuneate nucleus, terminate somatotopically (1499, 2333), in overlapping laminae. In the monkey (2333) the pattern of termination of fibers from C1 through T1 dorsal roots in the accessory cuneate nucleus is similar to that of the cuneate nucleus in that fibers from: (a) C5 through C8 terminate in the central core region about which other dorsal root fibers terminate in oblique serial laminae; (b) rostral roots terminate in ventrolateral regions, while those from more caudal roots end in dorsomedial regions and (c) all of these roots, except C1 and C2, terminate throughout the rostrocaudal extent of the nucleus (Fig. 11-10). Fibers from the above-

mentioned dorsal roots terminating in the accessory cuneate nucleus end in both exclusive and overlapping zones; fibers from one dorsal root partially overlap the territory of the next highest root. Upper thoracic dorsal root fibers (other than T1) exhibit greater overlap and terminate in smaller zones in the lateral part of the nucleus.

Although fibers from parts of the fasciculus cuneatus terminate upon cells of the accessory cuneate nucleus, these cells do not contribute fibers to the formation of the medial lemniscus. Cells of the accessory cuneate nucleus give rise to uncrossed *cuneocerebellar fibers* that at higher levels enter the cerebellum via the inferior cerebellar peduncle (Fig. 10-9). Fibers of the cuneocerebellar tract, conveying impulses from receptors in muscles of the upper extremity and neck, represent the upper limb equivalent of the posterior spinocerebellar tract.

Spinal Trigeminal Tract. Afferent trigeminal root fibers, which enter the brain stem at upper pontine levels, descend in the dorsolateral part of the brain stem as the spinal trigeminal tract (Figs. 11-5, 11-6, 11-8, 11-12, 11-13 and 12-26). These fibers, originating from cells of the trigeminal ganglion, have a definite topographical organization within the tract. Central descending processes of cells are organized so that: (a) fibers of the mandibular division are most dorsal, (b) fibers of the ophthalmic division are most ventral and (c) fibers of the maxillary division occupy an intermediate position. Clinicopathological studies (734, 2366, 2522) suggest that fibers of the separate divisions extend caudally for different distances, with those of the mandibular division terminating at medullary levels and those of the ophthalmic division terminating in upper cervical spinal segments. Experimental studies (1294, 1370, 2141, 2558) indicate that there is little difference in the caudal extent of fibers in the different trigeminal divisions, and that some fibers from all divisions extend into upper cervical spinal segments. As this tract descends it becomes progressively smaller as fibers leave the tract and terminate in the adjacent spinal trigeminal nucleus. In the rostral medulla a surprisingly large number of trigeminal fibers in the dorsal part of the spinal trigeminal tract project medially to terminate in a restricted ventrolateral part of the nucleus solitarius (1292, 1294, 2141, 2558).

General somatic afferent fibers from the vagus, glossopharyngeal and facial nerves enter and descend in the spinal trigeminal tract. Vagal and glossopharyngeal fibers descend in the dorsomedial part of the tract for a considerable distance and terminate in the magnocellular division of the caudal part of the spinal trigeminal nucleus (1293, 1316, 2141, 2558). Only a modest number of facial nerve fibers enter the spinal trigeminal tract.

Spinal Trigeminal Nucleus. This nucleus, which lies along the medial border of the tract, extends from the level of entry of the trigeminal root in the pons to the second cervical spinal segment (Figs. 12-26–12-28). Fibers from the spinal trigeminal tract terminate upon cells of the nucleus at various levels throughout its extent. Cytoarchitecturally the spinal trigeminal nucleus has been subdivided into three parts (1882): (a) an *oral part* extending caudally to the level of the rostral pole of the hypoglossal nucleus, (b) an *interpolar part* extending caudally to the level of the obex and (c) a *caudal part* which begins at the level of the obex, closely resembles the posterior horn of the spinal cord and extends caudally as far as the second cervical spinal segment. The inner, medial part of the caudal subdivision, containing irregularly arranged medium-sized cells of triangular or multipolar shape, constitutes the magnocellular subnucleus (division). Fibers in different parts of the spinal trigeminal tract terminate within sharply circumscribed sectors of the spinal trigeminal nucleus. Fibers conveying impulses from the mandibular division terminate in dorsal parts of the nucleus, while fibers of the ophthalmic division terminate in ventral parts of the nucleus. A number of descending trigeminal fibers pass beyond the spinal trigeminal nucleus to terminate in dorsal parts of the reticular formation and portions of the solitary nucleus. Many neurons of the spinal trigeminal nucleus give rise to an extensive axonal plexus of small fiber bundles which lie adjacent to the nucleus. These so-called "deep bundles" emit collaterals which effectively link different levels of the spinal trigeminal nucleus (907).

In myelin stained sections, the spinal trigeminal nucleus has the same appearance as the translucent zone seen at the apex of the dorsal horn of the gray matter in the spinal cord, and the term *substantia gelatinosa* has been applied to both regions. More detailed cytological examination in both Nissl stained and Golgi impregnated material reveals several layers within both the dorsal horn of the cord and the spinal trigeminal nucleus. The former has been described on pages 244–247 where the laminar classification of Rexed is presented. The laminar configuration of the caudal part of the spinal trigeminal nucleus consists of four layers (903–905, 1368). Lamina I (marginal zone) contains many cells that are activated by nociceptive or thermal stimulation of the face and oral region (604, 640, 2071). Lamina II corresponds to the substantia gelatinosa and laminae III and IV constitute the magnocellular layers (1882).

Descending fibers in the spinal trigeminal tract convey impulses concerned with pain, thermal, and tactile sense from the face, forehead, and mucous membranes of the nose and mouth (Fig. 7-13). While other portions of the trigeminal complex are concerned with tactile sense, the spinal trigeminal tract and nucleus, pars caudalis, appear to be the only part of this complex uniquely concerned with the perception of pain and thermal sense. The most decisive evidence for this modality segregation is that medullary trigeminal tractotomy markedly reduces pain and thermal sense without impairing tactile sense (2346). Physiological studies (2071) indicate that the spinal trigeminal nucleus, pars caudalis, encodes nociceptive information in the same manner as the dorsal horn of the spinal cord. Cells are found which respond solely to oral and facial nociceptive stimulation as well as cells responding in a graded manner to a mechanical stimuli of increasing intensity. The cells responding to nociceptive stimulation are located within the nucleus and also in the subjacent reticular formation.

From the spinal nucleus fibers arise which form the secondary trigeminal tracts. These fibers arise, a few at each level, and cross through the reticular formation to the opposite side. Most of these fibers ascend to thalamic levels in association with the contralateral medial lemniscus (Fig. 12-27);

others appear to terminate upon cells of the reticular formation. These are trigemino-thalamic fibers which constitute the second neuron in the sensory pathway from face to cortex. Other uncrossed fibers ascend and descend on the same side, forming reflex connections with the motor nuclei of the hypoglossal, vagus, facial and other cranial nerves (Figs. 12-27 and 12-28). A considerable number of trigeminocerebellar fibers arise from the spinal trigeminal nucleus and enter the cerebellum via the inferior cerebellar peduncle (402).

Since the spinal trigeminal tract and nucleus are located close to the spinothalamic tract, injury to the dorsolateral region of the medulla produces the curious clinical picture of an alternating hemianalgesia and hemithermo-anesthesia of the face and body. There is loss or diminution of pain and thermal sense on the same side of the face, and on the opposite side of the body and neck (Fig. 12-27).

Groups of cells located lateral to spinal tract V and embedded in the fibers of the spinocerebellar tracts at the lateral edge of the medulla form the *paratrigeminal nucleus* (Fig. 11-11). Both cell bodies and fibers in the neuropile show substance P-like immunoactivity. In addition, the neuropile contains many serotonin (5-hydroxytryptamine, 5-HT)-containing afferent axons (443, 444). The function of the paratrigeminal nucleus is not known. Since it receives afferent axons from the intermediate nerve (142) and nucleus of the solitary tract (141) and sends efferent fibers to the gustatory region of the thalamus, it has been thought to represent a rostral extension of the portion of the nucleus of the solitary tract concerned with taste.

Reticular Formation. The reticular formation at the level of the decussation of the medial lemniscus occupies the region ventral to the posterior column nuclei and the spinal trigeminal complex and dorsolateral to the pyramid (Fig. 11-8). It contains numerous cells of various sizes arranged in more or less definite groups and is traversed by both longitudinal and transverse fiber bundles. At this level it is traversed by numerous internal arcuate fibers and smaller bundles of secondary trigeminal fibers. Cells in the above described region constitute the ventral reticular nucleus (Fig. 11-9). Peripheral to the reticular for-

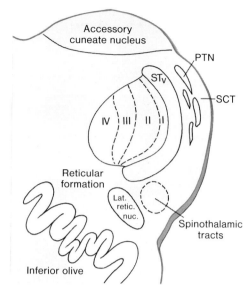

Figure 11-11. Schematic diagram of the laminar organization of the spinal trigeminal nucleus. Lamina I adjacent to the spinal trigeminal tract (ST_v) is called the marginal layer. Laminae II corresponds to the substantia gelatinosa and laminae III and IV form the magnocellular layers. *PTN* indicates the paratrigeminal nucleus and *SCT* the spinocerebellar tracts.

mation the long tracts retain their relative lateral and anterior positions. Fibers of the medial longitudinal fasciculus are dorsal to the pyramids and lateral to the decussation of the medial lemniscus.

The *lateral reticular nucleus of the medulla*, one of the distinctive reticular nuclei, is located ventrolaterally (Fig. 11-8). This nucleus begins caudal to the inferior olivary complex and extends rostrally to midolivary levels (Figs. 11-9 and 11-12). The nucleus consists of three cytoarchitectonic subdivisions: magnocellular, parvocellular and subtrigeminal. The large cell group is oriented ventromedially within the nucleus, dorsal to the inferior olive. The small cell group is situated dorsolateral to the large cell subdivision (1390, 2631). Neurons composing these subgroups project fibers to specific portions of the cerebellar cortex and deep cerebellar nuclei via the ipsilateral inferior cerebellar peduncle (1638), and receive a topographically arranged input from the spinal cord via spinoreticular pathways (1390). Electrophysiological studies show that the majority of cells in the lateral reticular nucleus respond to stimulation over large peripheral receptive fields involving both fore- and hindlimbs (2222). In

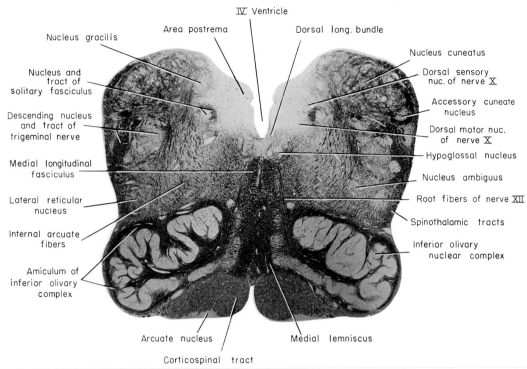

Figure 11-12. Transverse section of the medulla through the caudal part of the fourth ventricle, the area postrema and the lower part of the inferior olivary nucleus (Weigert's myelin stain, photograph).

view of the anatomical specificity of spinal projections to the lateral reticular nucleus, the physiological data suggest a substantial degree of convergence of afferent information at the spinal cord level (1390).

In addition to spinal input, the lateral reticular nucleus also receives crossed descending rubrobulbar axons (1104, 2635). While the lateral reticular nucleus can be considered to convey primarily exteroceptive information to the cerebellum, some cells of the nucleus also receive a vaginal input and are related to reproductive behavior (2205, 2206).

A description of chemically identified cell bodies and axon terminals in the lateral reticular nucleus is considered at the end of this section.

On the anterior aspect of the pyramid is the *arcuate nucleus*, whose position varies somewhat in different levels (Figs. 11-8 and 11-12–11-14). In rostral portions of the medulla the nucleus enlarges considerably (nucleus precursorius pontis) and appears to become continuous with the nuclei of the pons. Afferent fibers to this nucleus are derived from the cerebral cortex, and its

efferent fibers project as ventral external arcuate fibers to the cerebellum. Fibers from this small nucleus are thought to be crossed.

Area Postrema. Immediately rostral to the obex on each side of the fourth ventricle is the area postrema (Fig. 11-12), a slightly rounded eminence containing astroblast-like cells, arterioles, sinusoids and probably apolar or unipolar neurons (255, 353). The area postrema is one of several regions of the ependymal lining of the ventricular cavities which have a specialized structure (1342). Collectively these regions are referred to as *circumventricular organs* (Fig. 1-19). The area postrema is outside the blood-brain barrier, but axons or dendritic processes from nearby regions of the medulla enter the structure (480, 1746, 2620). The area postrema has been demonstrated to function as an emetic chemoreceptor trigger zone that responds to apomorphine and intravenous digitalis glycosides (218, 219). Electrical activity in the region of the area postrema is altered by intravenous administration of hypertonic solutions (481), and lesions result in altered Na^+/K^+

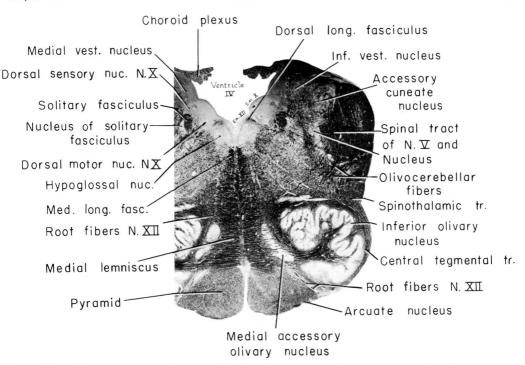

Figure 11-13. Transverse section of the medulla through the inferior olive complex rostral to that shown in Figure 11-12. *Em. X,* eminentia vagi; *Em. XII,* eminentia hypoglossi (Weigert's myelin stain, photograph).

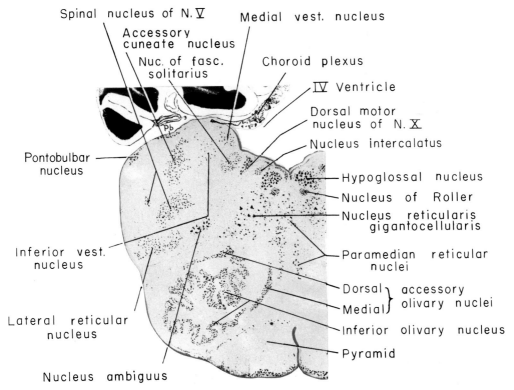

Figure 11-14. Section through midolivary region of the medulla (cresyl violet; photograph, with schematic representation of main cell groups).

excretion ratios in urine, which suggest a transient potassium retention by the kidney (2374). The chemical anatomy of the region is complex, and a number of putative transmitters have been identified.

Cranial Nerve Nuclei. At these levels, the cranial nerve nuclei, other than the spinal trigeminal nucleus, include the hypoglossal (N. XII) and those of the vagus (N. X) nerve (Figs. 11-9, 11-12 and 11-13). The latter nuclei are in the gray surrounding the central canal. Anterolateral to the central canal are small collections of typical large motor neurons which constitute the caudal portions of the hypoglossal nucleus. Lateral to the central canal collections of smaller spindle-shaped cells form the dorsal motor nucleus of the vagus nerve. These cells give rise to preganglionic parasympathetic fibers. Dorsal to the central canal on each side of the median raphe is the commissural nucleus of the vagus nerve. These cells represent the most caudal extension of the medial portion of the nucleus solitarius; they receive visceral afferent fibers. The nucleus ambiguus lies in the reticular formation dorsal to the inferior olivary complex and medial to the lateral reticular nucleus (Figs. 11-9 and 11-12).

CHEMICALLY IDENTIFIED NEURONS IN THE MEDULLA

When discussing the organization of a region of the brain it is not sufficient to consider only neuronal projections and arrangement of synapses; it is also necessary to know the neurotransmitters that are synthesized and released, and the density and distribution of postsynaptic receptor sites for that transmitter. The presence of transmitter synthetic enzymes and the relative affinities and kinetics of transmitter binding in relatively small regions of the central nervous system can be determined by biochemical methods, but details of topographic localization are not revealed. Recently developed immunohistochemical methods, together with refinements of earlier histochemical technics, make it possible to study the sites of synthesis and storage of known or suspected neurotransmitters and neuromodulators at the cellular and organelle levels of resolution. Autoradiographic techniques utilizing radioactive ligands can be used to study the distribution of transmitter binding sites in tissue slices. The information resulting from biochemical, histochemical and immunochemical studies has led to many new concepts of neuronal function. Initially these investigations emphasized the regional and topographical localization of transmitter related molecules. The functional significance of many of the putative transmitters identified is still obscure, but is a subject of active investigation.

In the medulla, the substances of greatest interest are: (a) acetylcholine; (b) the biogenic amines norepinephrine, epinephrine and serotonin; and (c) the peptides enkephalin, oxytocin, vasopressin and substance P. The location of neurons containing acetylcholine is determined indirectly by labeling the synthesizing enzyme choline acetyltransferase or visualizing the hydrolytic enzyme acetylcholinesterase. The latter may be found postsynaptically in neurons which are cholinoceptive, but not cholinergic, as well as in cells which synthesize acetylcholine. While there is a general correspondence between the localization of acetylcholinesterase and the presence of biochemically identified acetylcholine, there are regions where acetylcholinesterase is not associated with the presence of the transmitter. Cell bodies containing acetylcholinesterase are found in the cranial nerve motor nuclei, including the dorsal motor nucleus of X. Additionally, some cells of the sensory trigeminal nucleus and nuclei of the reticular formation contain the enzyme (2336).

When a radioactive ligand which binds to acetylcholine receptors with high specific activity is incubated with thin sections of brain tissue, the general distribution of binding sites can be observed in autoradiographs. The highest density of muscarinic acetylcholine receptors is found in the hypoglossal nucleus (cranial N. XII) and nucleus ambiguus (cranial nerves IX and X), with somewhat lower densities in the solitary nucleus and lateral reticular nucleus. Still lower density is observed in the dorsal motor nucleus of N. X (2669). Nicotinic acetylcholine receptors have their highest concentrations in the medulla in the dorsal motor nucleus of N. X (84).

The biogenic amines present in the medulla are norepinephrine, epinephrine and serotonin. Neurons containing the catecholamine dopamine are found only in the rostral brain stem at the level of the midbrain and diencephalon, and in some of the basal ganglia of the telencephalon. The enzyme phenylethanolamine-*n*-methyltransferase (PNMT) converts norepinephrine to epinephrine and is a convenient marker for cells synthesizing the latter amine. Immunohistochemically labeled PNMT is found in cell bodies of the lateral reticular nucleus of the medulla. This nucleus also contains noradrenergic neurons as well as acetylcholinesterase labeled cells. A second group of PNMT labeled cell bodies is located close to the midline in the dorsal reticular formation ventral and medial to the vestibular nuclei. Some of these cells are adjacent to the solitary nucleus (1119). PNMT labeled axons can be observed leaving the dorsal and the ventral groups of cell bodies to ascend through the reticular formation, and are probably the source of PNMT containing terminals in the tuberal region of the hypothalamus.

Most of the noradrenergic cell bodies of the medulla are scattered throughout the region of the lateral reticular nucleus and adjacent reticular formation (1482). Other noradrenergic cells occur near the midline, ventral to the hypoglossal nucleus (585, 2026).

The indole amine serotonin occurs largely in neurons whose cell bodies form the raphe nuclei of the brain stem (Fig. 11-15). These nuclei will be described later in this chapter (p. 335). Additional serotonin cells are found in the reticular formation (444).

Two pentapeptides, methionine-enkephalin (met-enkephalin) and leucine-enkephalin (leu-enkephalin), have been isolated from nervous tissue and appear to be endogenous ligands for opiate receptors (1169). Several lines of investigation suggest that these peptides may act as transmitters or modulators. The locations of cell bodies and terminals containing enkephalin have been determined by immunohistochemical methods (91, 752, 1117, 1126, 2596). In the medulla, enkephalin immunoreactive cell bodies occur in laminae II (substantia gelatinosa layer) and III of the caudal portion of the spinal nucleus of cranial N. V. Other enkephalin labeled cells are found in the solitary nucleus and a ventral cluster lying lateral to nucleus raphe magnus (Fig. 11-15). Axons and terminals containing enkephalin are generally seen in regions containing labeled cell bodies. In addition, moderately dense terminal plexuses occur in the motor nuclei of cranial nerves VII and XII and in parts of the reticular formation.

The study of the functional significance of neuronal pathways formed by enkephalin containing cells is still incomplete. The morphine agonist properties of enkephalin led to the analysis of the role of descending projections of enkephalin containing cells in mechanisms of nociception and analgesia (128, 129). Other studies have suggested that enkephalins and related peptides may have much broader functions, and it is now known that enkephalins and morphine bind to separate subclasses of opiate receptors. The organization of descending pain control systems is complex. Brain stem projections to the spinal cord other than those arising from enkephalin containing neurons in the medulla have been shown to affect spinal neurons which respond to noxious stimulation (995, 1111, 1626, 1876).

A surprising finding emerging from studies of biologically important peptides in the brain is the presence of posterior pituitary gland hormones in the brain stem. The nonapeptides oxytocin and vasopressin are synthesized by cells in discrete nuclei of the hypothalamus (see Chapter 16) and transported along axons to terminals in the posterior lobe of the pituitary. Double labeling experiments have demonstrated that the hypothalamic nuclei which innervate the posterior pituitary gland contain separate subpopulations of cells with descending projections (2483). The axons reaching the medulla contain mainly oxytocin and end in the solitary nucleus, dorsal vagal nucleus, lateral reticular nucleus and within lamina I (marginal layer) of the spinal nucleus of N. V (1754, 1842). When oxytocin is released into the circulation from the posterior lobe of the pituitary gland, it acts upon smooth muscle of the uterus during parturition and upon myoepithelial cells of the mammary gland during milk letdown. The function of this peptide in the medulla is unknown, but it is interesting to note that oxytocin containing axon terminals are found in or near regions rich in catechol-

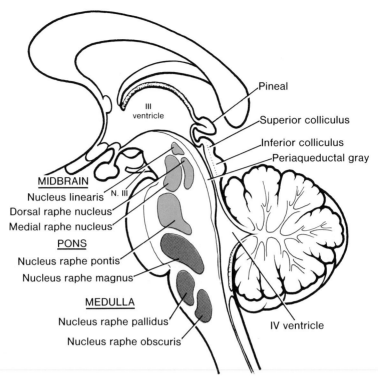

Figure 11-15. Schematic drawing of a midsagittal section of the brain stem indicating the positions of the raphe nuclei. Nuclei in *red* project to spinal levels, while those in *blue* have extensive projections to nuclei in the brain stem. Projections to diencephalic structures are most numerous from the dorsal and medial raphe nuclei and from the nucleus raphe pontis. The dorsal and medial raphe nuclei also project widely to telencephalic structures (130, 202).

amine and enkephalin containing terminals.

The final peptide considered is substance P, which was first isolated from the hypothalamus. It is found in some dorsal root ganglion cells and in terminals of spinal afferents which end in the superficial laminae of the gray matter of the posterior horn. The peptide is thought to be associated with the small spinal afferent fibers encoding nociceptive information. In the medulla, substance P containing terminals are prominent in superficial laminae of the caudal part of the spinal trigeminal nucleus and in the solitary nucleus. Less dense substance P labeled terminals are found in the nucleus raphe magnus (575).

OLIVARY LEVELS OF THE MEDULLA

The most characteristic features of the medulla are present in transverse sections through the inferior olivary complex (Figs. 11-9, 11-12, 11-13, A-4 and A-5). The central canal has opened into the fourth ventricle,

which widens progressively at higher levels. The tela choroidea and choroid plexus form a thin roof over the ventricle, while the floor of the fourth ventricle contains several rounded eminences formed by specific nuclear groups. The medial eminence, or *trigonum hypoglossi*, is produced by the nucleus of N. XII; the intermediate eminence, known as the *trigonum vagi*, overlies certain vagal nuclei; the lateral eminence in the fourth ventricle is the *area vestibularis*, which is occupied by the caudal poles of the medial and inferior vestibular nuclei (Figs. 11-2–11-14).

Although the nucleus gracilis has disappeared at this level and the nucleus cuneatus is greatly reduced in size, internal arcuate fibers can be seen sweeping ventromedially through the reticular formation to enter the contralateral medial lemniscus. At this level the medial lemnisci occupy triangular areas on each side of the median raphe, bounded ventrally by the pyramids and laterally by the inferior olivary nuclei.

Dorsal to the medial lemnisci on each side of the median raphe are the medial longitudinal fasciculi (Figs. 11-12 and 11-13). The spinal trigeminal nucleus and tract, somewhat inconspicuous in Weigert-stained sections, retain the same general position; the accessory cuneate nucleus is dorsal, and the fibers forming the inferior cerebellar peduncle are dorsolateral.

Inferior Olivary Nuclear Complex. The most characteristic and striking nuclear structure in the medulla is a convoluted gray band of cells known as the inferior olivary nuclear complex (Figs. 11-9, 11-12 and 11-13). This complex consists of: (a) the *principal inferior olivary nucleus*, appearing as a folded bag with the opening or hilus directed medially, (b) a *medial accessory olivary nucleus* along the lateral border of the medial lemniscus and (c) a *dorsal accessory olivary nucleus*, dorsal to the main nucleus (228). These nuclei are composed of relatively small, round or pear-shaped cells with numerous short branching dendrites. Fibers emerging from the inferior olivary nucleus fill the interior of the bag-shaped nucleus, pass through the hilus, traverse the medial lemnisci and course both through and around the opposite inferior olivary nuclei. These fibers traverse the reticular formation and parts of the spinal trigeminal complex to enter the contralateral inferior cerebellar peduncle. The accessory olivary nuclei and the most medial part of the main olivary nucleus are phylogenetically the oldest and project their fibers largely to the cerebellar vermis. The larger convoluted lateral portion of the main nucleus projects its fibers to the opposite cerebellar hemisphere (neocerebellum). The olivocerebellar projection is remarkably specific, and all parts of the cerebellar cortex, as well as the deep cerebellar nuclei, receive olivary projections (259). Olivocerebellar fibers end as climbing fibers (i.e., fibers which ascend Purkinje cell dendrites) in the cerebellar cortex (551, 675, 1018).

Climbing fibers produce a powerful excitatory action on Purkinje cells resulting in bursts of action potentials called complex spikes. Cells of the inferior olive have numerous gap junctions between dendrites (2385) and are electrotonically coupled (1503). This arrangement suggests that groups of cells in the inferior olive would tend to discharge synchronously.

As more and more olivocerebellar fibers are given off, the inferior cerebellar peduncle increases in size. While this peduncle is a composite bundle containing fibers from a large number of specific nuclei, olivocerebellar fibers constitute the largest component of this bundle (Figs. 11-28, 11-29 and 14-22).

The principal olivary nucleus is surrounded by a dense band of myelinated fibers, the *amiculum olivae*, composed largely of axons terminating in the nucleus. Descending fibers terminating upon cells of the inferior olivary complex arise from the cerebral cortex, the red nucleus and the periaqueductal gray of the mesencephalon (1683, 2632, 2638). Cortico-olivary fibers appear to arise from frontal, parietal, temporal and occipital cortex, descend in most of their course with corticospinal fibers and terminate bilaterally, primarily upon the ventral lamella of the principal olive. Rubro-olivary fibers and fibers arising from the periaqueductal gray of the mesencephalon enter a composite bundle known as the central tegmental tract and descend (Figs. 11-32, 12-1 and 12-4). These uncrossed fibers terminate in different portions of the principal olive. Noradrenergic axons from the pons also reach the inferior olive (2351). Rubro-olivary fibers end in the dorsal lamella while fibers from the periaqueductal gray, interstitial nucleus of Cajal, nucleus of Darkschewitsch and nearby regions terminate in the rostral parts of the principal and the medial and dorsal accessory nuclei (2249, 2638). Other brain stem projections to the olivary complex originate in the medial and inferior vestibular nuclei (2248), caudal part of the spinal nucleus of N. V, and the contralateral cerebellar cortex (164, 165). All parts of the dorsal column nuclei send axons to the contralateral olivary complex, especially the dorsal accessory nucleus (164, 165). Spino-olivary fibers, ascending in the anterior funiculus of the spinal cord, terminate largely on parts of the dorsal and medial accessory olivary nuclei; more than half of these fibers cross in the medulla. The inferior olivary nuclear complex is the largest of the medullary cerebellar relay nuclei.

The tracts ventrolateral to the reticular

formation have been pushed dorsally by the olivary nuclei. The anterior spinocerebellar, rubrospinal and spinothalamic tracts occupy the lateral periphery between the inferior cerebellar peduncle and the olivary complex. Fibers of the vestibulospinal tract are scattered along the posterior surface of the inferior olive. Posteriorly on each side of the medial raphe lie the medial longitudinal fasciculi, containing at this level predominately descending fiber bundles of mixed origin. Descending fibers in this tract are derived from certain vestibular nuclei, portions of the brain stem reticular formation and certain nuclei in the midbrain. The interstitial nucleus of Cajal (interstitiospinal tract) contributes a small number of fibers to the dorsomedial part of the medial longitudinal fasciculus. Tectospinal fibers from the superior colliculus form a loosely organized group of fibers in the ventral part of the bundle.

MEDULLARY RETICULAR FORMATION

The terms "brain stem" and "reticular formation" are used in varied ways by different authors (1384). In this text, brain stem refers to the supraspinal central nervous system exclusive of the cerebellum and cerebral hemispheres and would therefore include medulla, pons, midbrain and diencephalon.

We shall use the term reticular formation (formatio reticularis) to refer to a morphologically identified region extending throughout the lower brain stem (medulla through midbrain). The raphe nuclei constitute a part of the reticular formation, but will be described separately.

The term "reticular formation" describes portions of the brain stem core characterized structurally by a wealth of cells of various sizes and types, arranged in diverse aggregations, and enmeshed in a complicated fiber network. In a sense, the reticular formation constitutes a matrix within which "specific" nuclei and tracts are embedded. Cajal (348) considered reticular neurons to be composed largely of third order sensory neurons and, to a lesser extent, of second order motor neurons. Phylogenetically the reticular formation is very old. In primitive forms it may represent the largest part of the central nervous system. In higher vertebrates the reticular core of the brain stem constitutes a mass of considerable proportions, due in part to the process of encephalization. Although some authors have regarded the reticular formation as a diffusely organized brain stem component, anatomical studies (266) indicate that it is not diffusely organized, and that it can be subdivided into specific regions possessing distinctive cytoarchitecture, fiber connections and intrinsic organization. In spite of this, these regions cannot be considered as entirely independent entities, since complex fiber connections provide innumerable possibilities for interaction between the various subdivisions.

Golgi-stained sections of the reticular formation have yielded important information concerning its intrinsic organization. Such studies (2274) indicate that almost all reticular axons project for some distance in both rostral and caudal directions. A large number of these emit branching collaterals along their course which terminate in a variety of different types of endings. The majority of primary bifurcating axons are oriented in the longitudinal axis of the brain stem, but project collateral branches in all directions. Many of these collateral fibers arborize extensively about cranial nerve nuclei, and in some instances they may end upon both motor and sensory nuclei.

At one time the reticular formation was thought to consist mainly of neurons with short axons. However, Golgi impregnation studies do not reveal short axon (Golgi type II) cells (2274). Reticular neurons characteristically have many axon collaterals close to the parent cell body as well as long ascending or descending axons. Thus the organizational pattern of the reticular formation suggests that single reticular neurons may convey impulses both rostrally and caudally in addition to local synaptic actions (13, 2274).

The reticular formation proper begins in the medulla a little above the corticospinal decussation (Figs. 11-7 and 11-8). One of the particularly discrete nuclei of the reticular formation, the *lateral reticular nucleus* of the medulla, has been described (Figs. 11-8 and 11-9). In sections through the lower medulla, the area dorsal to the caudal half of the inferior olivary nucleus and medial to the lateral reticular nucleus is the location of the *nucleus reticularis ventralis* (Fig. 11-9). At higher levels the reticular area located medial and dorsal to the rostral half of the inferior olivary nucleus is occupied by the *nucleus reticularis gigantocellularis* (1885) (Figs. 11-14 and A-5). The latter nucleus is the rostral continuation of the nucleus reticularis ventralis. The nucleus reticularis gigantocellularis is a relatively large nuclear complex composed of characteristic large cells, as well as medium and small cells (Fig. 11-14). Giant cells in this nucleus are not as conspicuous in man as in lower forms. Descending fibers from this reticular nucleus form the medullary reticulospinal tract described earlier (Figs. 10-10 and 10-22) which has a largely inhibitory function.

At the mid-olivary levels of the medulla small groups of cells are situated near the midline, dorsal to the inferior olivary complex. These cells, which have been subdivided into a dorsal, a ventral and an accessory group, constitute the *paramedian reticular nuclei* (Fig. 11-14). Experimental studies (264) have shown that these reticular neurons project most of their fibers to the cerebellum.

The *nucleus reticularis parvicellularis* is a small-celled reticular nucleus situated dorsolaterally, medial to the spinal trigeminal nucleus and ventral to the vestibular area. This portion of the reticular formation has been referred to as the "sensory" part (266), since numerous studies have shown that collateral fibers from secondary sensory systems terminate in this region.

In essence the medullary reticular formation consists of three principal nuclear masses: (a) a *paramedian reticular nuclear group*, (b) a *central group* (i.e., the ventral reticular and gigantocellular reticular nuclei) and (c) a *lateral nuclear group* consisting of the lateral reticular and parvicellular reticular nuclei.

Afferent Fibers to the Medullary Reticular Formation. While the exact cells of origin of spinoreticular fibers have not been established, it is accepted generally that these fibers ascend almost exclusively in the anterolateral funiculus (1657, 2229). *Spinoreticular fibers* terminate largely in the caudal and lateral portions of the medullary reticular formation, including the caudal half of the nucleus reticularis gigantocellularis (Figs. 10-10 and 11-14). Al-though some fibers of this system project to more rostral regions of the brain stem reticular formation, fibers passing to the nucleus reticularis parvicellularis appear scanty.

A large number of spinothalamic fibers have been shown to terminate in a somatotopic fashion upon cells of the lateral reticular nucleus of the medulla (263). Since almost all cells of this nucleus give rise to fibers which pass to specific parts of the cerebellum, this nucleus is considered primarily a reticular relay nucleus in a spinocerebellar pathway. Physiological data support the thesis that exteroceptive impulses may be relayed to the cerebellum via this route (511).

Other important sources of afferents to the reticular formation are *collateral fibers* from second order sensory neurons, such as spinothalamic fibers, secondary auditory pathways, secondary fibers from the nucleus of the solitary fasciculus, secondary trigeminal pathways and secondary vestibular pathways. Collaterals from these diverse sources appear to terminate largely in the lateral region of the reticular formation, which has been referred to as the "sensory" part. It is notable that few, if any, collaterals from the medial lemniscus enter the brain stem reticular formation. Except for a modest number of trigeminal fibers (402, 2558), primary sensory fibers do not appear to terminate in the reticular formation.

Cerebelloreticular fibers in the medullary reticular formation terminate primarily in the region of the paramedian reticular nuclei. Fibers originating in the fastigial nuclei reach this region via the uncinate fasciculus (397, 2541), while fibers from the dentate nucleus pass via the descending division of the superior cerebellar peduncle (283, 411).

Corticoreticular fibers originate from widespread areas of the cerebral cortex, but the majority of these fibers arise from the sensorimotor areas (2227). These fibers for the most part terminate in areas of the reticular formation which give rise to reticulospinal fibers, the *nucleus reticularis pontis oralis*, the *nucleus reticularis pontis caudalis* and the *nucleus reticularis gigantocellularis* (Figs. 10-10, 10-22 and 11-14). Corticoreticular fibers are both crossed and uncrossed.

According to Golgi studies of afferents to the brain stem reticular formation, most of the long ascending and descending fiber systems, making connections in various regions, emit collateral or terminal fibers in planes perpendicular to the long axis of the brain stem. As a consequence of this arrangement, impulses from a wide variety of sources converge upon the reticular nuclei. The area of maximal overlap of afferent fields occurs in the medullary reticular formation, which gives rise to the largest number of long ascending and descending axons.

Efferent Fibers from the Medullary Reticular Formation. Ascending reticular fibers from the medulla arise from cells dorsal to the rostral half of the inferior olive and are localized in the medial two-thirds of the reticular formation. While most of these fibers originate from the nucleus reticularis gigantocellularis, some may arise from the nuclei reticularis ventralis and lateralis. These fibers ascend mainly in the area of the central tegmental fasciculus and are for the most part uncrossed (Fig. 12-4). Degeneration studies (1824) indicate that they terminate in parts of the intralaminar and reticular nuclei of the thalamus. This same area of the reticular formation also projects descending fibers to spinal levels (2561) (Figs. 10-10 and 10-22).

Efferent fibers from the paramedian reticular nuclei and the lateral reticular nuclei project to specific portions of the cerebellum. Fibers arising in the paramedian reticular nuclei, preponderantly uncrossed, terminate largely in the vermis of the anterior lobe (264). Cerebellar areas receiving fibers from the lateral reticular nucleus include the ipsilateral vermis, hemisphere and the flocculonodular lobule.

The medullary reticular formation, exclusive of the cerebellar projecting nuclei, may be divided into medial and lateral regions. The medial two-thirds of the reticular formation gives rise to most of the long ascending and descending fiber systems. Cells in the lateral third project axons medially and dendrites laterally.

The classical studies of Magoun and his collaborators (1593, 2140) demonstrated a powerful inhibition or facilitation of spinal and cranial motor activity upon stimulation of the brain stem reticular formation. Facilitation resulted from stimulation of the

dorsal and anterior pontomedullary and mesencephalic reticular formation, while inhibition followed activation of the ventral and posterior medial medullary reticular formation. Subsequently, it was found that low intensity stimulation produced excitation or inhibition limited to motor neurons innervating a single limb or body part (2413). Through the study of intracellular recordings in spinal motor neurons, it has been established that stimulation in nucleus reticularis pontis caudalis and the rostral dorsal part of nucleus reticularis gigantocellularis is capable of producing monosynaptic excitatory postsynaptic potentials in ipsilateral motor neurons supplying the neck, back and flexor and extensor muscles of the limbs (1985, 1986). Stimulation in the caudal and medial reticular formation produces disynaptic or multisynaptic inhibitory postsynaptic potentials in the same groups of ipsilateral motor neurons. Activation of the contralateral reticular formation also leads to weak inhibitory and excitatory postsynaptic potentials in spinal motor neurons. Thus, on the basis of physiological studies, the reticular formation can be divided into rostral facilitatory and caudal inhibitory zones.

Anatomical studies of the origin of reticulospinal axons reveals both a rostrocaudal and dorsoventral topographic arrangement (1336, 1985, 1986, 2549, 2795). In the spinal cord, reticulospinal axons from the pons form a medial tract in the ipsilateral ventromedial funiculus, and axons from the medulla form a lateral tract in ipsilateral ventrolateral funiculus. In addition, there is a crossed lateral tract. The pontine (medial) reticulospinal tract arises mainly from the region of the reticular formation in which electrical stimulation produces excitation of motor neurons. The organization of the medullary reticulospinal tract is more complex. Medullary (lateral) reticulospinal axons reaching the thoracic and lumbar levels of the cord arise from cells in the caudal and ventral medullary reticular formation, while axons destined for the cervical cord come from more rostrally situated cell bodies. The medullary reticulospinal tract consists of an admixture of excitatory and inhibitory axons (1985, 1986). Thus the pontine and medullary reticulospinal tracts of the spinal cord cannot be exclusively related to the functionally identified motor inhibitory and facilitatory zones of the pontomedullary reticular formation.

In addition to long ascending and descending connections, neurons within the reticular formation project to corresponding regions on the opposite side of the midline (2639).

Raphe Nuclei. Situated along the midline of the medulla, pons and midbrain are several groups of cells collectively called the raphe nuclei. The major nuclei that can be distinguished on the basis of cytoarchitectonics are shown in Figure 11-15. Many, but not all, of the raphe nuclei have neurons which synthesize serotonin. The midbrain and pontine serotonergic raphe cells send ascending axons to the diencephalon and cerebral cortex while the medullary serotonergic cells project to the spinal cord. (Fig 11-16). In the medulla, nuclei raphe magnus, raphe obscurus and raphe pallidus all contain serotonin cells (585, 2430). Much attention has been devoted to the physiological role of descending serotonergic neurons in the modulation of synaptic activity in pain related neurons of laminae I and V of the spinal cord (129) (also see Chapter 10, p. 297) (Fig. 11-16). Raphe stimulation also leads to inhibition of sympathetic preganglionic neurons (345).

In addition to the serotonin-containing cell bodies of the raphe nuclei, the medulla contains serotonin terminals (2430). Portions of the motor nucleus of N. VII, the caudal part of the spinal nucleus of N. V and the nucleus of the solitary tract receive a substantial serotonin innervation.

ASCENDING AND DESCENDING TRACTS

Ascending fibers of the medial lemniscus occupy an "L"-shaped area on each side of the median raphe posterior to the pyramid and medial to the inferior olivary complex (Figs. 11-12, 11-13 and 11-28). The spinothalamic tracts, which can no longer be designated as anterior and lateral, have merged and form essentially a single entity in the retro-olivary area. These tracts appear considerably smaller than at spinal levels, because an appreciable number of fibers terminate in the lateral reticular nucleus, and a number of spinoreticular fibers, which at spinal levels ascend in close asso-

ciation with these tracts, have passed medially into the gigantocellular reticular nucleus. The posterior spinocerebellar tract moves posteriorly at medullary levels and becomes incorporated into the inferior cerebellar peduncle (Fig. 11-28). The rostral spinocerebellar tract maintains a retro-olivary position and ultimately enters the cerebellum by coursing along the superior surface of the superior cerebellar peduncle. About one-third of the fibers of the rostral spinocerebellar tract enter the cerebellum via the inferior cerebellar peduncle; all other fibers of this uncrossed tract enter the cerebellum in association with the superior cerebellar peduncle (1900).

The medial longitudinal fasciculus (MLF) lies anterior to the hypoglossal nucleus adjacent to the median raphe (Figs. 11-12, 11-13 and 11-28). Rubrospinal fibers descend in a retro-olivary position close to the lateral reticular nucleus; some crossed descending rubral efferent fibers, terminating in this cerebellar relay nucleus, are properly called *rubrobulbar fibers*. Uncrossed rubrobulbar fibers, arising from rostral parts of the red nucleus, descend in the central tegmental tract and end upon cells in the dorsal lamella of the principal inferior olivary nucleus. At mid-medullary levels fibers of the vestibulospinal tract, which arise only from the lateral vestibular nucleus, are scattered in an area posterior to the inferior olivary complex. At more caudal levels, these fibers form a more compact bundle in the retro-olivary region. The medullary reticulospinal tract is not evident at these levels, but it cells of origin, the gigantocellular reticular nucleus, are present posteromedial to the inferior olivary complex (Fig. 11-12). The spinal trigeminal tract and nucleus occupy the same location as at more caudal levels.

INFERIOR CEREBELLAR PEDUNCLE

This peduncle is a composite group of tracts and fibers which assemble along the posterolateral border of the medulla and first form a distinct bundle at about mid-olivary levels (Fig. A-4). Throughout the upper medulla the addition of fibers increases the size of the structure until it forms a large, well-defined mass of myelinated fibers (Figs. 11-28, 11-29, 11-32 and A-5). Tracts and fibers forming this pedun-

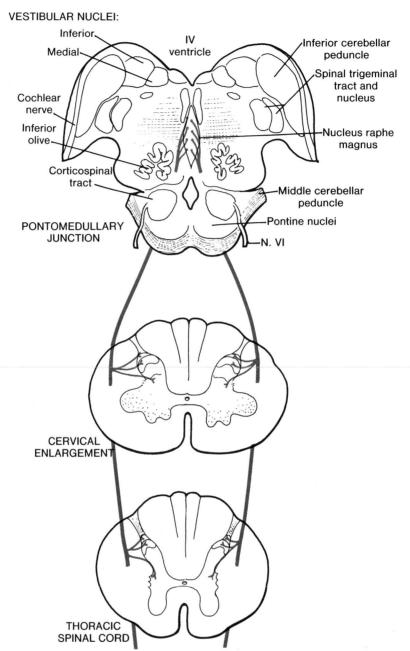

Figure 11-16. Schematic diagram of spinal serotoninergic projections from the nucleus raphe magnus. These projections are bilateral, descend in the dorsal part of the lateral funiculus and terminate upon cells in spinal cord laminae I, II and V, considered to receive nociceptive inputs. Large reticular neurons adjacent to the nucleus raphe magnus project fibers ipsilaterally to the same laminae in the posterior horn, but are not serotoninergic. Both of these pathways are considered links in an endogenous analgesia-producing system. Fibers from the nuclei raphe pallidus and obscuris (not shown) descend in the ventral quadrant of the spinal cord (129, 130).

cle originate in the medulla and spinal cord. The posterior spinocerebellar tract moves dorsally and enters the inferior cerebellar peduncle directly. Approximately one-third of the fibers of the rostral spinocerebellar tract enter this cerebellar peduncle. Crossed olivocerebellar fibers, originating from all parts of the inferior olivary com-

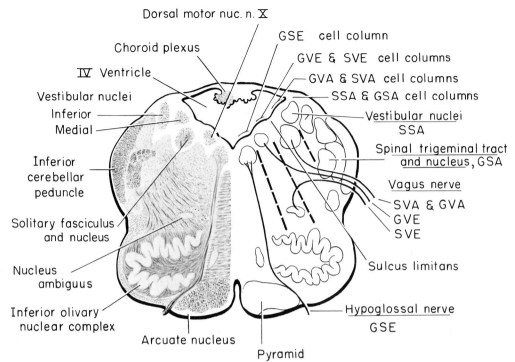

Figure 11-17. Schematic transverse section of the medulla showing its basic features. Cell columns related to functional components of the cranial nerve are indicated on the *right*. Functional components of cranial nerves are both general and special. The vestibular nuclei shown at this level (and auditory nuclei at higher levels) form the special somatic afferent (*SSA*) cell columns. The spinal trigeminal nucleus forms the general somatic afferent (*GSA*) cell column and receives fibers from cranial nerves with this functional component (i.e., N. V, N. VII, N. IX, N. X). Functional components of the vagus nerve (except GSA) are shown in relation to particular nuclei. The hypoglossal nucleus (and the nuclei of N. VI, N. IV and N. III at higher brain stem levels) gives rise to general somatic efferent (*GSE*) fibers. *Heavy dashes* separate the nuclei of the various cell columns on the *right* side.

plex, constitute quantitatively the largest group of fibers that enter the inferior cerebellar peduncle (Figs. 11-28, 11-32 and 14-22). A number of medullary nuclei contribute a relatively small number of fibers to the inferior cerebellar peduncle. These nuclei include: (a) the lateral reticular nucleus of the medulla, (b) the accessory cuneate nucleus, (c) the paramedian reticular nuclei, (d) the arcuate nucleus and (e) the perihypoglossal nuclei (i.e., the nucleus intercalatus, the nucleus of Roller and the nucleus prepositus) (Figs. 11-14 and 11-28). Fibers from the lateral reticular nucleus and the accessory cuneate nucleus are uncrossed, while those from the other nuclei are both crossed and uncrossed. At higher levels, the inferior cerebellar peduncle becomes covered laterally by fibers of the middle cerebellar peduncle (Figs. 11-32 and 12-2).

On the posterolateral aspect of the infe-

rior cerebellar peduncle a small group of closely packed, medium-sized cells can be seen (Fig. 11-14). These cells constitute the caudal portion of the *pontobulbar nucleus*. At more rostral levels this cell column assumes a progressively more ventral position, until at the junction of pons and medulla it forms a fairly large cell mass ventral to the inferior cerebellar peduncle (Figs. 11-29 and 11-31). The cells of this nucleus resemble those in the ventral portion of the pons and have been regarded as a caudal extension of the pontine nuclei.

CRANIAL NERVES OF THE MEDULLA

The schematic arrangement of the functional components of the cranial nerves of the medulla, and the cell columns to which they are related, is shown in Figure 11-17. This schema resembles that present in the spinal cord, although development of the fourth ventricle has shifted somatic and

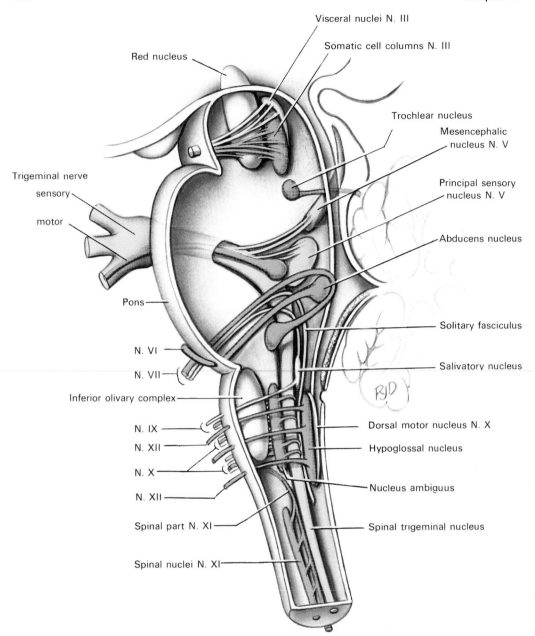

Figure 11-18. Schematic diagram of the intramedullary course of the cranial nerves in a midsagittal view. The brain stem is represented as a hollow shell except for cranial nerve components. General somatic (*GSE*) and special visceral (*SVE*) efferent components of cranial nerves innervating striated muscles are shown in *red*. General visceral efferent (*GVE*) components of cranial nerves III, VII, IX and X, representing preganglionic parasympathetic fibers, are shown in *yellow*. General somatic (*GSA*), general visceral (*GVA*) and special visceral (*SVA*) afferent components of the cranial nerves are in *blue*. (Modified from Elze (702).)

visceral afferent regions laterally. The functional components of a typical spinal nerve are four: (a) general somatic afferent (GSA), (b) general visceral afferent (GVA), (c) general somatic efferent (GSE) and (d) general visceral efferent (GVE). Functional

components of the cranial nerves include the four types found in spinal nerves, plus three additional special categories: (a) special somatic afferent (SSA), (b) special visceral afferent (SVA) and (c) special visceral efferent (SVE). Somatic efferent fibers in

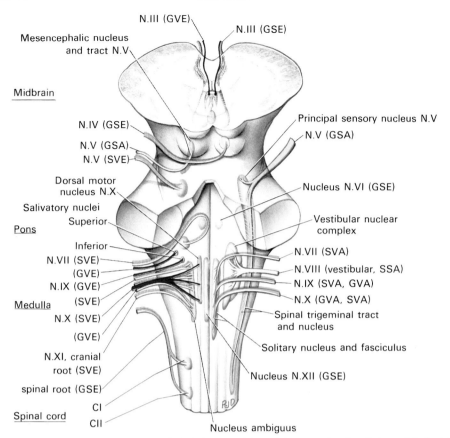

Figure 11-19. Schematic representation of the infratentorial cranial nerves showing their nuclei of origin and termination, their intramedullary course and their functional components. The cochlear nerve and nuclei are not shown (see Fig. 12-13). General somatic afferent (*GSA*) components of the trigeminal nerve (N. V) are shown in *light blue*. General and special visceral afferent (*GVA, SVA*) components of the facial (N. VII), glossopharyngeal (N. IX) and vagus (N. X) nerves are shown in *dark blue*. The vestibular nerve which differentially distributes special somatic afferent (*SSA*) fibers to the vestibular nuclear complex is *white*. Similarities in the intramedullary course of fibers in the spinal trigeminal tract, the vestibular nerve root and the solitary fasciculus are evident on the right. General somatic efferent (*GSE*) fibers from the oculomotor (N. III) and trochlear (N. IV) nuclei and those of the spinal root of the accessory nerve (N. XI) are *light red*. Only contributions from the first and second cervical segments to the spinal root of the accessory nerve are shown. Root fibers of the abducens (N. VI) and hypoglossal (N. XII) nuclei which exit ventrally and contain *GSE* fibers are not shown. Special visceral efferent (*SVE*) fibers from the branchiomeric cranial nerves (N. V, N. VII, N. IX, N. X and N. XI) are shown in *light red*. General visceral efferent (*GVE*) fibers, representing preganglionic parasympathetic components, of the oculomotor (N. III), facial (N. VII), glossopharyngeal (N. IX) and vagus (N. X) nerves are in *dark red*.

both spinal and cranial nerves are regarded as a general component.

In the medulla, as in the spinal cord, the sulcus limitans divides afferent and efferent cell columns. Special somatic afferent (SSA) cranial nerves in the medulla are represented by the auditory and vestibular components of the vestibulocochlear nerve (VIII). General somatic afferent (GSA) fiber components of cranial nerves V, VII, IX and X descend in the spinal trigeminal

tract. Fibers conveying taste (special visceral afferent, SVA) and general visceral afferent (GVA) impulses from components of cranial nerves VII, IX and X form a well-defined tract, the solitary fasciculus, which is embedded in the solitary nucleus (Figs. 11-12, 11-13, 11-18, 11-19 and 11-21). The above cell columns lie posterolateral to an extension of the sulcus limitans (Fig. 11-17). Ventromedial to this hypothetically projected line are the efferent cell columns.

The dorsal motor nucleus of the vagus nerve and the inferior salivatory nucleus of the glossopharyngeal nerve give rise to general visceral afferent (GVE) fibers. Cells of the nucleus ambiguus, located in the ventrolateral reticular formation posterior to the inferior olivary nuclear complex, give rise to special visceral efferent (SVE) fibers that pass peripherally as components of cranial nerves XI, X and IX (Figs. 11-18 and 11-19). These fibers innervate muscles of the pharynx and larynx derived from the third and fourth branchial arches (i.e., branchiomeric muscles). Other motor nuclei, having similar locations in the pons, supply special visceral efferent fibers to muscles derived from the first and second branchial arches via cranial nerves V and VII (Figs. 11-18 and 11-19). The general visceral efferent (GVE) components (parasympathetic) forming parts of cranial nerves III, VII, IX and X are indicated in Figures 11-18 and 11-19. The hypoglossal nucleus located in the floor of the fourth ventricle near the median raphe gives rise to general somatic efferent (GSE) fibers which innervate the muscles of the tongue. The general somatic efferent cranial nerve nuclei all lie near the median raphe and relatively close to the floor of the fourth ventricle or cerebral aqueduct. Other nuclei, at more rostral levels, belonging to this group are: the abducens, trochlear and oculomotor. Schematic diagrams showing these nuclei and their intramedullary course (Figs. 11-18 and 11-19) should help the student to understand the organization of the cranial nerves and their various components.

Hypoglossal Nerve. The hypoglossal nerve is a motor nerve (GSE) innervating the somatic skeletal musculature of the tongue. It also appears to contain some afferent fibers, since the muscle spindles of the tongue degenerate following section of the nerve. These afferent fibers may be derived in part from inconstant ganglion cells found on the hypoglossal roots (2514), but their principal source is still obscure. During fetal life the nerve apparently contains dorsal root fibers related to a small ganglion, but these disappear at a later period.

The nucleus of N. XII forms a column of typical multipolar motor cells about 18 mm long that occupies the central gray of the medial eminence. It begins caudal to the inferior olive and extends rostrally to the region of the striae medullares. Within the nucleus coarse myelinated fibers can be seen, which are the root fibers of the motor cells, and a network of finer fibers representing terminals of axons ending in the nucleus. The root fibers gather on the ventral surface of the nucleus, forming a series of rootlets which pass ventrally, lateral to the medial lemniscus, and emerge on the surface of the medulla between the pyramid and the inferior olivary complex (Figs. 11-1, 11-12, 11-13 and A-4).

The hypoglossal nuclei receive numerous fibers and collaterals from reticular neurons, which form delicate plexuses around the cells. Some of these fibers constitute the terminals of a "corticobulbar" fiber system effecting voluntary movements of the tongue. Fibers from the reticular formation are crossed and uncrossed. Other fibers to these nuclei probably are secondary glossopharyngeal, vagal and trigeminal fibers which mediate reflex tongue movements in a response to stimuli from lingual, oral and pharyngeal mucous membranes. Fibers from visceral centers also may terminate in the hypoglossal nuclei.

Immediately posterior to the hypoglossal nucleus is a small bundle of fibers in the periventricular gray known as the *dorsal longitudinal fasciculus* of Schütz (2291) (Figs. 11-12 and 11-13). This is a composite bundle of fibers consisting of ascending and descending components which are considered to be visceral in nature. While the prevailing conduction in this bundle appears to be in an ascending direction (329, 1820), descending fibers arising from medial and periventricular hypothalamic cell groups have been identified (1184, 1363, 1816), but these fibers do not extend caudally beyond the midbrain.

In the gray of the ventricular floor are several nuclear masses surrounding the hypoglossal nuclei whose functions and connections are not understood. The *nucleus intercalatus*, situated between the hypoglossal nucleus and dorsal motor nucleus of the vagus, is composed predominantly of small cells and a scattering of larger cells (Fig. 11-14). Rostral to the hypoglossal nucleus is the *nucleus prepositus* (Figs. 11-28

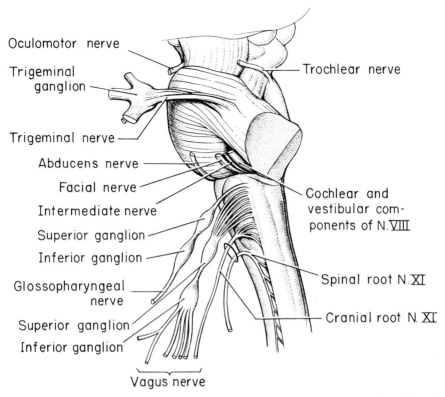

Oculomotor nerve

Trigeminal ganglion

Trochlear nerve

Trigeminal nerve

Abducens nerve

Facial nerve

Intermediate nerve

Superior ganglion

Inferior ganglion

Cochlear and vestibular components of N. VIII

Glossopharyngeal nerve

Superior ganglion

Inferior ganglion

Spinal root N. XI

Cranial root N. XI

Vagus nerve

Figure 11-20. Semidiagrammatic sketch of brain stem and cranial nerves showing their peripheral ganglia.

and 11-29), which extends from the oral pole of the hypoglossal nucleus almost to the abducens nucleus. It is composed of relatively large cells and a few smaller cells resembling those of the nucleus intercalatus, with which it is continuous at more caudal levels. The *nucleus of Roller*, composed of relatively large cells, lies ventral to the rostral pole of the hypoglossal nucleus and adjacent to its root fibers (Fig. 11-14). Collectively, the nucleus intercalatus, nucleus prepositus and nucleus of Roller constitute the so-called perihypoglossal nuclei.

Injury to the hypoglossal nerve produces a lower motor neuron paralysis of the ipsilateral half of the tongue with loss of movement, loss of tone and atrophy of the muscles. Since the genioglossus muscle effects protrusion of the tongue, the tongue, when protruded, will deviate to the side of the injury. The intrinsic muscles of the tongue alter the shape of the tongue; the extrinsic muscles alter its shape and position.

The juxtaposition of the emerging root fibers of N. XII and the corticospinal tract is the anatomical basis of the *inferior* or *hypoglossal alternating hemiplegia* resulting from ventral lesions of this area (Fig. 10-13). This syndrome consists of: (a) a lower motor neuron paralysis of the ipsilateral half of the tongue and (b) a contralateral hemiplegia.

Spinal Accessory Nerve. The accessory nerve usually is divided into cranial and spinal portions which form, respectively, the internal and external branches of the nerve (Fig. 11-20). The *cranial root* of the nerve arises from neurons in the caudal pole of the nucleus ambiguus (SVE). Axons of these cells emerge from the lateral surface of the medulla caudal to the lowest filaments of the vagus nerve. The cranial fibers of the accessory nerve join the vagus nerve and, as motor fibers of the inferior (recurrent) laryngeal nerve, innervate the intrinsic muscles of the larynx. The *spinal portion* of the accessory nerve originates from a cell column in the anterior horn extending from the fifth (or sixth) cervical segment to about the middle of the pyramidal decussation. Caudally cells of this column occupy a lateral process of the anterior horn, but at higher levels they tend to assume a more central position. Root fibers from these cells arch posterolaterally to emerge from the lateral aspect of the spinal cord between the dorsal and ventral roots (Fig. 11-4). Rootlets of the spinal part of the accessory nerve unite to form a common trunk (external branch) which ascends in the spinal canal posterior to the denticulate ligaments, enters the skull through the foramen magnum and ultimately exits from the skull via the jugular foramen, together with the vagus and glossopharyngeal nerves (Fig. 11-20). The spinal nucleus of N. XI, like all motor nuclei, receives direct and indirect fiber projections from a variety of sources which mediate reflex activity related to cephalogyric movements. The spinal portion of the accessory nerve supplies the sternocleidomastoid and upper parts of the trapezius muscles. Although contractions of the sternocleidomastoid muscle turn the head to the opposite side, unilateral lesions of N. XI usually do not produce any abnormality in the position of the head. Weakness in rotating the head to the opposite side can be detected on testing; when the neck is flexed, the chin tends to turn slightly to the paralyzed side. Paralysis of the upper part of the trapezius muscle is evidenced by: (a) downward and outward rotation of the upper part of the scapula and (b) a moderate sagging of the shoulder on the affected side. Weakness of the upper part of the trapezius muscle also can be tested by having the patient shrug his shoulders against resistance.

Vagus Nerve. This is a complex branchiomeric cranial nerve containing: (a) *general somatic afferent* (GSA) *fibers* distributed through the auricular branch of the vagus to the skin in back of the ear and the posterior wall of the external auditory meatus, (b) *general visceral afferent* (GVA) *fibers* from the pharynx, larynx, trachea, esophagus and thoracic and abdominal viscera, (c) *special visceral afferent* (SVA) *fibers* from scattered taste buds in the region of the epiglottis, (d) *general visceral efferent* (GVE; *preganglionic) fibers* to terminal parasympathetic ganglia innervating the thoracic and abdominal viscera and (e) *special visceral efferent* (SVE; *branchiomotor) fibers* to the voluntary striated muscles of the larynx and pharynx. General

somatic afferent fibers of the vagus nerve arise from cells of the superior ganglion of the vagus nerve, located in, or immediately beneath, the jugular foramen (Fig. 11-20). Both general and special visceral afferent fibers of the vagus nerve arise from the larger inferior vagal ganglion (nodosal ganglion). Afferent vagal fibers enter the lateral surface of the medulla ventral to the inferior cerebellar peduncle and usually traverse the spinal trigeminal tract and nucleus (Fig. 11-17). Cutaneous afferent fibers enter the dorsal part of the spinal trigeminal tract along with similar general somatic afferents from other branchiomeric cranial nerves. More numerous visceral afferent fibers of the vagus nerve pass dorsomedially into the nucleus and tractus solitarius (Figs. 11-17–11-19). Fibers entering the solitary fasciculus bifurcate into short ascending and longer descending components. Descending vagal components in the solitary fasciculus gradually diminish in number as collaterals and terminals are given off to the solitary nucleus. Some vagal visceral fibers descend caudal to the obex, where the solitary nuclei of the two sides merge to form the *commissural nucleus* of the vagus nerve (Fig. 11-9). A number of descending vagal fibers decussate and enter the contralateral half of the commissural nucleus (1256, 1257, 2141).

The *fasciculus solitarius* is formed by visceral afferent fibers contributed by the vagus, glossopharyngeal and facial (intermediate) nerves (Figs. 11-18 and 11-19). Fibers conveying taste from the anterior two-thirds of the tongue (chorda tympani) and from the posterior third of the tongue (glossopharyngeal nerve) enter rostral parts of the solitary fasciculus and mainly terminate in rostal parts of the solitary nucleus. Portions of the solitary fasciculus at the level of entry of the vagus nerve, and caudal to it, contain mainly general visceral afferent fibers, largely from the vagus nerve (142). The solitary fasciculus constitutes a composite descending bundle of visceral afferent fibers comparable to the spinal trigeminal tract which contains general somatic afferent fibers.

The *nucleus solitarius* can be divided on cytoarchitectonic criteria into several parts: (a) a medial part, dorsolateral to the dorsal motor nucleus of the vagus; (b) dorsome-

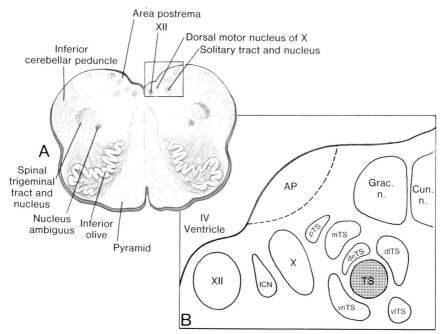

Figure 11-21. (*A*) Diagram of some of the major cell groups and tracts in the caudal medulla. The enclosed area in the dorsomedial portion of the diagram is shown in greater detail in *B*. (*B*) Schematic diagram of subnuclei forming the nucleus of the solitary tract which receive afferents from cranial nerves IX and X. Abbreviations used: *AP*, area postrema; *Cun. n.*, cuneate nucleus; *dlTS*, dorsolateral nucleus of solitary tract; *dnTS*, dorsal nucleus of solitary tract; *Grac. n.*, gracile nucleus; *ICN*, intercalated nucleus; *mTS*, medial nucleus of solitary tract; *pTS*, parvicellular nucleus of solitary tract; *TS*, solitary tract; *vlTS*, ventrolateral nucleus of solitary tract; *vnTS*, ventral nucleus of solitary tract; *X*, dorsal motor nucleus; *XII*, hypoglossal nucleus. (Based on Kalia and Mesulam (1256), Loewy and Burton (1517) and Beckstead and Norgren (142).

dial, dorsolateral, and ventrolateral subnuclei surrounding the *tractus solitarius*; and (c) a parvicellular subnucleus lying between the medial nucleus and the area postrema (Fig. 11-21). Although there is some variation, this general arrangement has been observed in both carnivores and primates (142, 1256, 1517). Cells of the medial part extend rostrally slightly beyond the dorsal motor nucleus of the vagus (Figs. 11-23 and 11-24); this part of the nucleus extends caudal to the fourth ventricle and merges with the corresponding cell column on the opposite side to form the commissural nucleus of the vagus nerve (Fig. 11-9) (2558).

The lateral subnuclei form a column of larger cells which partially or completely surrounds the solitary fasciculus (Figs. 11-13, 11-21 and 11-23). This part of the nucleus parallels the fasciculus throughout most of its length; rostrally it extends to the lower border of the pons while caudally its cells diminish in number and are difficult to distinguish from reticular neurons. The

enlarged rostral part of the solitary nucleus (i.e., the lateral part) receives mainly special visceral afferent (taste) fibers from the facial (intermediate) and glossopharyngeal nerves and is referred to as the *gustatory nucleus* (1792, 2141). The caudal and medial solitary nucleus receives mainly general visceral afferent fibers from the vagus nerve, along with some facial and glossopharyngeal fibers. Although visceral afferent axons to the solitary nuclear complex terminate over an extensive rostral-caudal portion of the structure, there is a viscerotopic pattern of endings within the subnuclei (1257). Alimentary tract afferents end in the parvicellular nucleus (991), pulmonary afferents synapse in the ventrolateral subnucleus (1517), and carotid sinus afferent endings are concentrated in the medial and dorsomedial subnuclei (1926) (Figs. 11-24 and 11-25).

In primates, the major secondary fiber systems originating from the solitary nucleus (NTS) project to structures in the

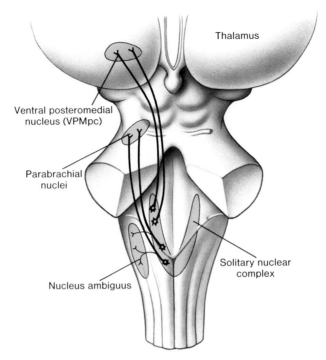

Figure 11-22. Schematic diagram of ascending projections of the solitary nuclear complex superimposed upon a posterior view of the brain stem. The solitary nuclear complex receives special visceral afferent fibers via the intermediate nerve and both special and general visceral afferent fibers via the glossopharyngeal and vagus nerves. Cells in rostral parts of the nucleus solitarius project ipsilaterally via the central tegmental tract to the small-celled part of the ventral posteromedial (*VPMpc*) nucleus of the thalamus. Caudal parts of the solitary nucleus which receive afferents largely from the glossopharyngeal and vagus nerves project fibers rostrally to the ipsilateral medial and lateral parabrachial nuclei, situated near the superior cerebellar peduncle. These caudal parts of the solitary nucleus also project collaterals to the nucleus ambiguus (141). The solitary nuclear complex, the nucleus ambiguus, the parabrachial nuclei and VPMpc are shown in *blue*. (Modified from R. M. Beckstead et al.: *Journal of Comparative Neurology*, **190**: 259–282, 1980.)

medulla, pons, and thalamus (141). At the level of the vagus nerve root entry zone, axons from cells in the caudal NTS pass ventrolaterally to reach the nucleus ambiguus and surrounding reticular formation. Rostrally directed axons from the medial NTS terminate in the parabrachial nuclei of the pons (Fig. 11-22). Lesions and single unit recordings suggest that these projections are part of the respiratory control mechanism. The prevagal part of the primate lateral NTS gives rise to a direct projection to a thalamic nucleus concerned with gustatory sensation (ventral posteromedial nucleus, pars parvicellularis (VPM$_{pc}$)) (Fig. 15-17). An additional ascending path between NTS and the hypothalamic paraventricular nucleus has been described in subprimate species (459, 460), which may play a role in cardiovascular

control of vasopressin (antidiuretic hormone) release from the neural lobe of the pituitary or activation of spinal sympathetic preganglionic neurons through axons of the paraventricular nucleus which reach the thoracic cord.

Other secondary fibers from the NTS go to various motor nuclei of the cranial and spinal nerves. As already stated, impulses pass to the hypoglossal and salivatory nuclei for lingual and secretory reflexes, either directly or through intercalated neurons. Impulses from the pharyngeal, respiratory and alimentary mucous membranes passing to the nucleus ambiguus probably are involved in pharyngeal and laryngeal reflexes. Additional impulses to the dorsal motor nucleus of N. X, the phrenic nucleus in the cervical spinal cord and the nuclei of the intercostal muscles in the thoracic cord are

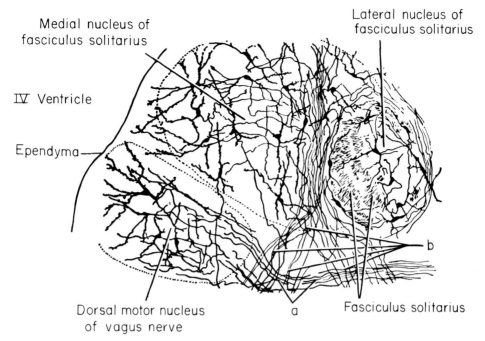

Figure 11-23. The vagal nuclei in the floor of the fourth ventricle based upon a drawing of a Golgi preparation of newborn cat (348). Efferent (preganglionic) fibers from the dorsal motor nucleus of the vagus nerve are indicated by *a*, while *b* indicates fibers from the medial and lateral (sensory) nuclei of the fasciculus solitarius forming secondary vagoglossopharyngeal pathways. The medial nucleus of the fasciculus solitarius extends caudally to the fourth ventricle and merges with the corresponding cell group on the opposite side, forming the commissural nucleus of the vagus nerve (Fig. 11-9). The lateral nucleus of the fasciculus solitarius extends rostrally, increases in size and parallels the fasciculus solitarius throughout most of its length.

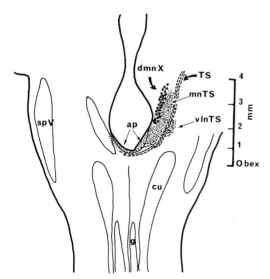

Figure 11-24. Line drawing of a horizontal section through the medulla showing the solitary tract (*TS*), medial and ventrolateral nuclei of the solitary tract (*mnTS, vlTS*), dorsal motor nucleus of vagus (*dmnX*), and the area postrema (*ap*) labeled with horseradish peroxidase (HRP) following an injection into the right inferior (nodose) ganglion of X. Survival time was 48 hr. The right side of the medulla is on the right side of the diagram and rostral is upward. Interrupted lines represent the position of sensory and motor fibers of X labeled with HRP reaction product. *Dots* indicate terminals of afferent projections and solid triangles show the location of retrogradely labeled cell bodies. Other abbreviations: *cu*, cuneate nucleus; *g*, gracile nucleus; *spV*, spinal trigeminal nucleus. (Reproduced with permission from M. Kalia and M. M. Mesulam: *Journal of Comparative Neurology*, **193:** 435–465, 1980.)

involved in coughing, vomiting and respiration. The connections with the spinal cord centers innervating the respiratory muscles probably are mediated by intercalated reticular neurons in the vicinity of the nucleus solitarius.

The region of the nucleus of the solitary tract is coextensive with the physiologically defined dorsal medullary respiratory "center" (1255). The ventral medullary respiratory "center" includes the nucleus ambiguus and surrounding reticular formation. Additional brain stem regions important for

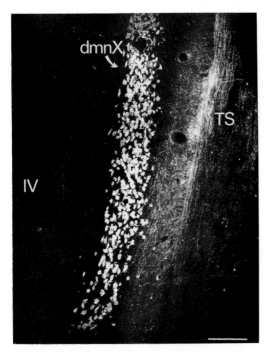

Figure 11-25. Darkfield photomicrograph from the medulla of a cat in which the inferior (nodose) ganglion of nerve X was injected with horseradish peroxidase. The medulla was sectioned in the horizontal plane. Rostral is toward the top, lateral is toward the readers right. In this section the right side of the medulla is on the right side of the plate. Survival time was 48 hr. Retrograde labeling is seen in perikarya of the dorsal motor nucleus of vagus and anterograde labeling occurs in the solitary nucleus and tract. Notice labeled fibers leaving the caudal half of the nucleus of the solitary tract which is situated between *TS* and *dmnX* in the lower half of the figure (calibration bar, 500 μm). (Reproduced with permission from M. Kalia and M. M. Mesulam: *Journal of Comparative Neurology*, **193:** 435–465, 1980.)

the regulation of respiration are found in the pons. The medial parabrachial nucleus and the adjacent nucleus of Kölliker-Fuse constitute the functionally defined "pneumotaxic center." An apneustic center has also been proposed, but has not been anatomically delineated. The parabrachial nuclei of the pons receive afferent connections from the solitary nucleus (1255) and in turn project to both the dorsal and ventral respiratory centers (344, 2508). An interesting feature of medullary cells projecting to the parabrachial nuclei is their orientation along the radial penetrating blood vessels (1318).

At the spinal segmental level, the reflex

organization of motor neurons innervating the diaphragm is similar to that for motor neurons innervating trunk and limb musculature (719).

The cells of the medullary "respiratory centers" not only are activated by vagal and other neural impulses, but also are affected directly by changes in their chemical environment (CO_2 accumulation, etc.). A loosely defined vasomotor "center" has been localized in the medulla with separate pressor and depressor zones. Recent studies have led to a revision of earlier concepts, placing greater emphasis on the distributed nature of neural networks in the brain stem concerned with cardiovascular control. A group of noradrenergic neurons (designated A5, see Table 16-1) located between the inferior olive and the emerging fibers of N. VII in the rostral medulla send axons to NTS, nucleus ambiguus, and sympathetic preganglionic neurons of the intermediolateral cell column in the thoracic cord. These anatomical features have led to the hypothesis that the A5 cell group is part of a network of cells acting upon smooth muscle and glands and importantly related to regulation of the cardiovascular system (1518). Some of the projections of the A5 cell group to other brain stem structures are illustrated in Figure 11-27.

The *dorsal motor nucleus of the vagus nerve* occupies the medial portion of the trigonum vagi in the floor of the fourth ventricle (Figs. 11-12, 11-14 and 11-17). It is a column of cells extending both cranially and caudally a little beyond the hypoglossal nucleus. The nucleus is composed of relatively small, spindle-shaped cells among which are larger cells with coarser chromophilic bodies and scattered melanin pigment. The functional significance of the several cell types is not clear. Cells of this nucleus give rise to preganglionic parasympathetic fibers (GVE) (Figs. 11-24 and 11-25). The axons of the cells from the dorsal motor nucleus pass ventrolaterally, traverse the spinal trigeminal nucleus and tract and emerge on the lateral surface of the medulla between the olive and the inferior cerebellar peduncle (Figs. A-4 and A-5).

The dorsal motor nucleus contains relatively few myelinated fibers, indicating that most of the terminals entering it are unmyelinated. These are principally secondary fibers from the sensory nuclei of the

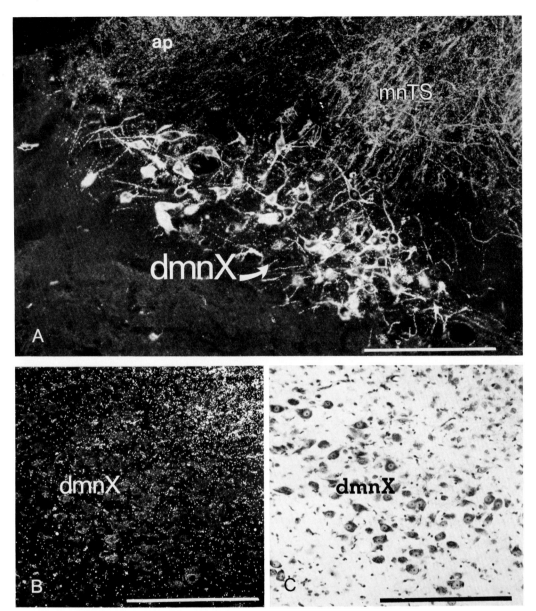

Figure 11-26. Photomicrograph of the medulla of cats in which the inferior (nodose) ganglion of nerve X was injected with either horseradish peroxidase or tritiated amino acid. The brain was sectioned coronally. Dorsal is toward the top and the midline to the readers left. In all photomicrographs, the rostral-caudal level is 1 mm rostral to the obex. (A) Darkfield photomicrograph. The inferior ganglion was injected with horseradish peroxidase 48 hr before the animal was prepared for histological examination. Retrograde labeling is seen in the dorsal motor nucleus of X (*dmnX*) and anterograde labeling is seen in the medial nucleus of the solitary tract (*mnts*) as well as dorsomedially in the area postrema (*ap*). Afferent fibers from the *mnts* are seen entering the *dmnX* and come into close contact with labeled perikarya (calibration bar, 250 μm). (B) Darkfield photomicrograph. The inferior vagal ganglion was injected with tritiated amino acid 5 days prior to preparation for examination. In the upper right hand corner, the *mnts* contains a high concentration of silver grains. The *dmnX* also contains a grain concentration that is above background level (calibration bar, 250 μm).) (C) Brightfield photomicrograph of exactly the same field as the one shown in B (calibration bar, 250 μm). (Reproduced with permission from M. Kalia and M. M. Mesulam: *Journal of Comparative Neurology*, **93**: 435–465, 1980.)

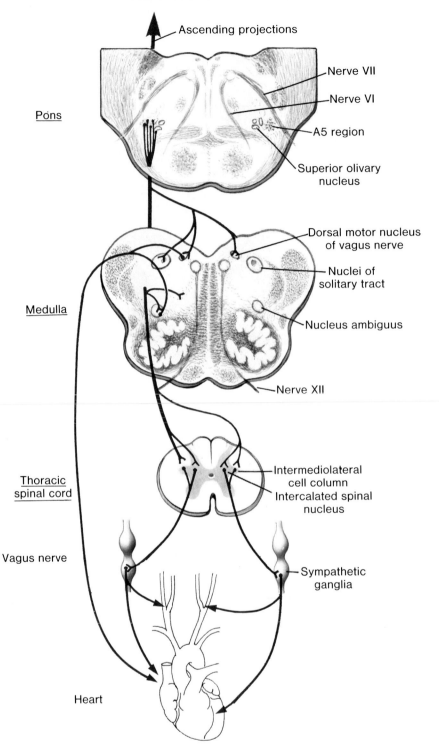

Figure 11-27. Schematic diagram of the descending projections of the A5 catecholamine cell group which lies lateral to the superior olivary nucleus and projects to: (a) medullary vasomotor areas, (b) preganglionic sympathetic neurons and (c) intercalated spinal neurons. Medullary nuclei receiving fibers from the A5 cell group include: (a) the nuclei of the solitary tract, (b) the dorsal motor nucleus of the vagus nerve, (c) the nucleus ambiguus, and (d) the paramedian and medial medullary reticular formation. Inputs reaching cells of the intermediolateral cell column and intercalated spinal neurons project to postganglionic sympathetic neurons which in turn project to the cardiovascular system. Electrical stimulation of the A5 cell group produces increases in systemic blood pressure and pulse pressure. Ascending projections from the A5 cell group have been described but not fully characterized. (Modified from Loewy and McKellar (1518).)

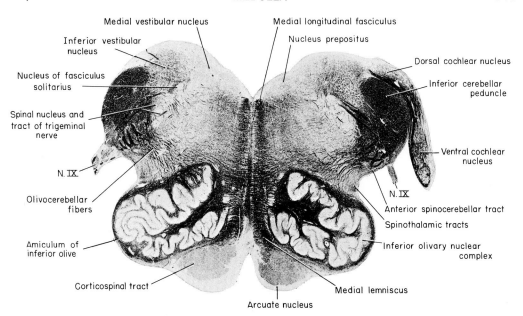

Figure 11-28. Transverse section of medulla of 1-month infant through the cochlear nuclei and ninth nerve (Weigert's myelin stain, photograph).

glossopharyngeal and vagus nerves, and from visceral centers (Figs. 11-24–11-26).

The *nucleus ambiguus* is a column of cells in the reticular formation about half way between the spinal trigeminal nucleus and the inferior olivary complex (Figs. 11-9, 11-12, 11-14, 11-17–11-19). This nucleus, extending from the level of the decussation of the medial lemniscus to levels through the rostral third of the inferior olivary complex, is composed of typical multipolar lower motor neurons. Fibers from the nucleus arch dorsally, join efferent fibers from the dorsal motor nucleus of the vagus nerve and emerge from the lateral surface of the medulla dorsal to the inferior olivary complex (Figs. 11-17–11-19). Caudal parts of the nucleus ambiguus give rise to the cranial part of the spinal accessory nerve, while rostral parts of this cell column give rise to glossopharyngeal special visceral efferent fibers (which innervate the stylopharyngeus muscle). Special visceral efferent fibers of the vagus nerve (and those from the cranial part of the accessory nerve which rejoin the vagus nerve) innervate the muscles of the pharynx and larynx (Figs. 11-17 and 11-19).

The nucleus receives various terminals, among which are both crossed and uncrossed corticobulbar fibers for the voluntary control of swallowing and phonation (Fig. 11-30). The nucleus also receives impulses from receptors in the pharyngeal and laryngeal muscles, and from secondary vagal, glossopharyngeal and trigeminal fibers. Fibers in these three nerves convey impulses from the oral, pharyngeal and respiratory mucosa that mediate various reflexes, such as coughing, vomiting, and pharyngeal and laryngeal reflexes.

A unilateral lesion of the vagus nerve is followed by ipsilateral paralysis of the soft palate, pharynx and larynx, which results in hoarseness, dyspnea and dysphagia. During phonation the soft palate is elevated on the normal side and the uvula deviates to the normal side. The palatal reflex is lost on the lesion side. Anesthesia of the pharynx and larynx results in an ipsilateral loss of the cough reflex. Destruction of visceral motor fibers of the vagus results in an ipsilateral loss of the carotid sinus reflex. As a rule visceral disturbances are not marked following a unilateral lesion of the vagus nerve. A unilateral lesion of the recurrent laryngeal nerve will result in hoarseness of the voice and coughing attacks which in time diminish and disappear. The abductor muscles of the larynx are affected first.

Bilateral lesions of the vagus nerves as a rule are fatal unless immediate precautions are instituted to prevent asphyxia, resulting from complete laryngeal paralysis. Paraly-

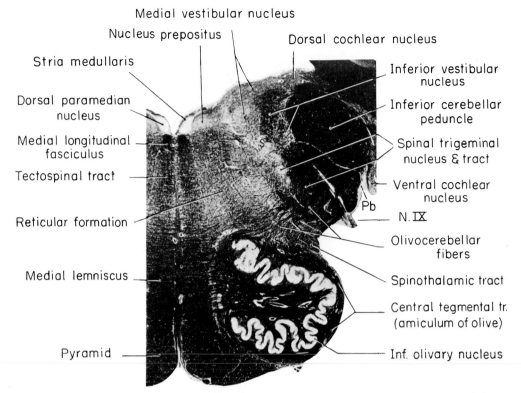

Medial vestibular nucleus

Nucleus prepositus

Dorsal cochlear nucleus

Stria medullaris

Inferior vestibular nucleus

Dorsal paramedian nucleus

Inferior cerebellar peduncle

Medial longitudinal fasciculus

Spinal trigeminal nucleus & tract

Tectospinal tract

Ventral cochlear nucleus

Pb

N. IX

Reticular formation

Olivocerebellar fibers

Medial lemniscus

Spinothalamic tract

Central tegmental tr. (amiculum of olive)

Pyramid

Inf. olivary nucleus

Figure 11-29. Transverse section through the upper medulla at the level of the cochlear nuclei and the root fibers of the glossopharyngeal nerve. *S* indicates the lateral nucleus of the fasciculus solitarius; *Pb* indicates pontobulbar nucleus (Weigert's myelin stain, photograph).

sis and atonia of the esophagus and stomach induce pain and vomiting with the hazards of aspiration. These lesions also result in loss of vagal respiratory reflexes, dyspnea and cardiac acceleration. Bilateral lesions most frequently are due to pathology within the medulla.

Glossopharyngeal Nerve. This nerve is related closely to the vagus nerve, having certain common intramedullary nuclei, and similar functional components. Fibers of this nerve enter and emerge from the medulla at levels rostral to the vagus nerve, but like the vagus nerve, they traverse the spinal trigeminal tract and nucleus (Figs. 11-17, 11-28 and 11-29). The glossopharyngeal is a mixed branchiomeric cranial nerve with the following functional components: (a) *general visceral afferent* (GVA) *fibers,* (b) *special visceral afferent* (SVA) *fibers* (taste), (c) a few *general somatic afferent* (GSA) *fibers,* (d) *general visceral efferent* (GVE) *fibers* and (e) a small number of *special visceral efferent* (SVE) *fibers.* Like the vagus nerve it has

two peripheral ganglia, a small *superior ganglion* in the jugular foramen and a larger extracranial *inferior (petrosal) ganglion* (Fig. 11-20).

Primary sensory neurons mediating general somatic sense (GSA) from cutaneous areas back of the ear lie in the superior ganglion; central processes of these cells enter the spinal trigeminal tract and nucleus. Cell bodies of visceral afferent fibers lie in the inferior ganglion. General visceral afferent fibers convey impulses concerned with tactile sense, thermal sense and pain from the mucous membranes of the posterior third of the tongue, the tonsil, the posterior wall of the upper pharynx and the Eustachian tube. Special visceral afferent fibers convey taste sensation from the posterior third of the tongue. Visceral afferent fibers enter the posterolateral part of the medulla and are distributed to rostral portions of the solitary fasciculus and its nucleus (Fig. 11-28). Rostral and lateral parts of the nucleus solitarius which receive fibers from the facial (intermediate) and glos-

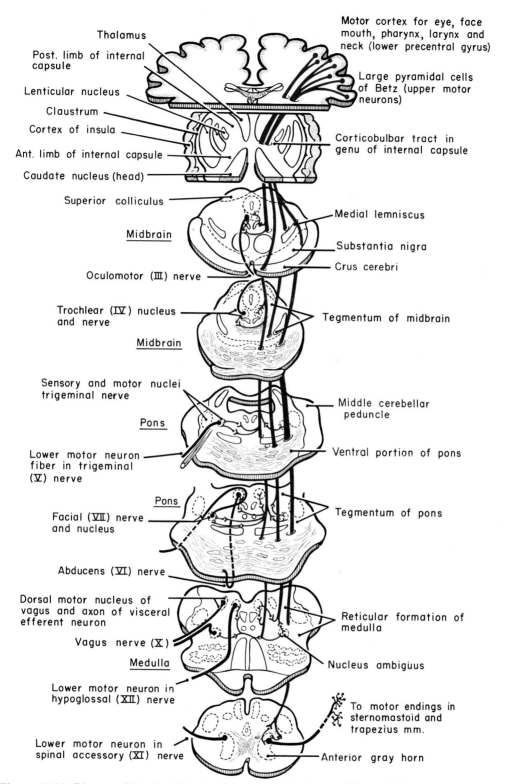

Figure 11-30. Diagram of "corticobulbar" pathways in the brain stem. Fibers of this upper motor neuron pathway to the motor cranial nerve nuclei arise in the cerebral cortex; pass caudally in the internal capsule, the crus cerebri and the ventral portion of the pons; and are distributed largely to neurons in the reticular formation bilaterally. Reticular neurons conveying the impulses to the motor cranial nerve correspond to the intercalated or internuncial neurons found at spinal levels. In man and primates this indirect system is paralleled by more recently developed direct corticobulbar fibers distributed to the motor nuclei of the trigeminal, facial and hypoglossal nerves. (Modified from H. G. J. M. Kuypers: *Brain*, **81**: 364–388, 1958.)

sopharyngeal nerves constitute what is called the *"gustatory nucleus."*

The *carotid sinus nerve* conveys impulses from the carotid sinus, a baroceptor located at the bifurcation of the common carotid artery. Increases in carotid arterial pressure excite carotid sinus baroceptors, and impulses are conveyed centrally by the glossopharyngeal nerve to the nucleus of the solitary tract (1926). Second order solitary neurons in turn excite cells of the dorsal motor nucleus of the vagus nerve and bring about reductions in heart rate and arterial pressure via cholinergic pre- and postganglionic vagal fibers that act upon the sinoatrial and atrioventricular nodes as well as the heart atrial muscle. The *carotid sinus reflex* involving glossopharyngeal visceral afferents and vagal general visceral efferents constitutes a mechanism for the regulation of arterial blood pressure.

General visceral efferent fibers, arising from the *inferior salivatory nucleus*, pass via the lesser petrosal nerve to the otic ganglion, situated below the foramen ovale and medial to the mandibular division of the trigeminal nerve. Postganglionic fibers originating from the cells of the otic ganglion convey parasympathetic secretory impulses to the parotid gland. Cells of the inferior salivatory nucleus are virtually impossible to distinguish from reticular neurons, but they are considered as a separate rostral cell group equivalent to the dorsal motor nucleus of the vagus.

Special visceral efferent fibers, as already described, arise from rostral portions of the nucleus ambiguus (Figs. 11-18 and 11-19). These fibers, small in number, innervate the stylopharyngeus muscle and perhaps portions of the superior pharyngeal constrictor muscle.

As the above description indicates, the glossopharyngeal nerve is predominantly a sensory nerve, and a nerve contributing preganglionic parasympathetic fibers to the otic ganglion. Isolated lesions of the glossopharyngeal nerve are rare. Disturbances associated with lesions of the nerve include: (a) loss of the pharyngeal (gag) reflex, (b) loss of the carotid sinus reflex and (c) loss of taste in the posterior third of the tongue. *Glossopharyngeal neuralgia* resembles trigeminal neuralgia in that the excruciating pain is paroxysmal and may be triggered by seemingly trivial stimuli such as coughing or swallowing. The pain associated with this syndrome radiates to regions behind the ear.

Swallowing, or deglutition, is a complex motor act which involves three identifiable neuro-regulatory systems: buccopharyngeal, esophageal and gastroesophageal (642). The effector neurons lie in the motor nuclei of cranial nerves V, VII, X (ambiguus) and XII. Unlike spinal motor neurons, those of the cranial motor nuclei have no recurrent collaterals which activate inhibitory interneurons. The neurons controlling the buccopharyngeal phase of deglutition are located in the medullary reticular formation close to the midline and dorsal to the inferior olive. These cells are found between the caudal border of the nucleus of N. VII and the rostral end of the inferior olive. The cells on each side of the midline can be considered "swallowing half-centers" which are coordinated through extensive interconnections.

Swallowing can be most readily initiated by stimulation of the endings of the internal branch of the superior laryngeal nerve (part of cranial N. X). Excitation of the maxillary division of cranial N. V and of cranial N. IX can also trigger deglutition. Afferent neurons convey information from oropharyngeal receptive fields to neurons in the lateral subnuclei of the solitary complex. Projections from the solitary nucleus to all the cranial motor nuclei involved have not been demonstrated anatomically, but it is likely that interneurons within the reticular formation are part of the reflex circuit.

CORTICOBULBAR FIBERS

Corticofugal fibers projecting into the lower brain stem are referred to as *corticobulbar fibers*. These fibers arise mainly from the precentral and postcentral gyri, and are distributed to: (a) sensory relay nuclei, (b) parts of the reticular formation and (c) certain motor cranial nerve nuclei in man and primates.

Sensory relay nuclei receiving corticobulbar fibers include the nuclei gracilis and cuneatus, the sensory trigeminal nuclei and the nucleus of the solitary fasciculus (282, 1404–1408, 1410, 1413, 2558, 2633, 2796). Corticobulbar fibers to the posterior column nuclei leave the corticospinal tract and enter these nuclei, by either passing among the fibers of the medial lemniscus, or by traversing the reticular formation. After unilateral cortical lesions degenerated terminal fibers are distributed bilaterally to the posterior column nuclei, but are most numerous contralaterally. There are suggestions of somatotopic projections between portions of the precentral and postcentral gyri and the nuclei gracilis and cuneatus, but considerable overlap also is evident (1406). According to Zimmerman et al. (2796), the projection from the primary somesthetic cortex in the rat is such that fibers from the forelimb cortical area pass to the nucleus cuneatus and those from the hindlimb area terminate in the nucleus gracilis. Studies of corticobulbar fibers projecting to the nuclei gracilis and cuneatus in the cat (1413) indicate that these fibers are distributed preferentially to portions of the nuclei containing loosely organized cells, and that few fibers from the cortex terminate in "cell nest" regions which receive ascending fibers from spinal dorsal roots. Fibers to all trigeminal sensory nuclei and the nucleus solitarius are derived from widespread cortical regions with the largest number arising from the frontoparietal region (282). Corticobulbar projections to trigeminal sensory nuclei appear to be nontopological (2796), although Kuypers (1406) suggests that in primates these fibers arise mainly from the postcentral gyrus. Corticofugal fibers to the nucleus solitarius terminate chiefly in its rostral part, near levels where facial and trigeminal afferents end.

Corticobulbar projections to the posterior column nuclei, and other sensory relay nuclei, constitute a mechanism by which descending cortical impulses can influence the transmission of ascending sensory impulses at the second neuron level. Both excitatory and inhibitory influences upon these sensory relay nuclei can be produced following stimulation of the cerebral cortex (922, 998, 1080, 1194, 1481). Experimental studies (921, 922) of descending cortical influences upon the nucleus gracilis suggest that excitatory and inhibitory actions are exerted differentially upon portions of the nucleus which are distinguishable on the basis of the size of the receptive field and sensory modality represented. Corticofugal

inhibitory influences were found mainly in middle portions of the nucleus where individual cells responded to movement of hair, light touch to foot pads, pressure at the base of a claw or subcutaneous pressure. These cells exhibited small receptive fields and were inhibited by stimuli applied outside the physiological receptive field (i.e., surround inhibition). Corticofugal excitatory effects were found mainly on the rostral, and the deep part of the middle region of the nucleus where individual cells responded mainly to touch and pressure. These cells with rather large receptive fields did not show the phenomenon of surround inhibition.

Corticoreticular fibers projecting to the lower brain stem arise from broad areas of the cerebral cortex, but the largest number originates from the motor, premotor and somesthetic areas (2228). These fibers descend with those of the corticospinal tract, but leave this bundle to enter the brain stem reticular formation. The largest number of these fibers terminate in two well circumscribed areas, one in the medulla and another in the pons. Terminations in the medulla are in the area of the nucleus reticularis gigantocellularis, while the pontine area of termination is mainly within the nucleus reticular pontis oralis. Corticoreticular fibers are distributed bilaterally, but with a slight contralateral predominance (2796). Some corticoreticular fibers also project to reticular cerebellar relay nuclei, such as the reticulotegmental nucleus in the pons, and the lateral reticular and paramedian reticular nuclei of the medulla. Regions of the reticular formation receiving corticofugal fibers give rise to: (a) long ascending and descending projections (281, 2561), (b) projections to the cerebellum (264, 511) and (c) abundant collateral fibers that project to cranial nerve nuclei (2274).

The *motor cranial nerve nuclei* innervating striated muscle receive impulses from the cerebral cortex via corticobulbar pathways. These fibers arise mainly from portions of the precentral gyrus, descend through the internal capsule and brain stem in association with the corticospinal tract (Figs. 2-11, 10-12 and 11-30) and constitute the upper motor neurons for the motor cranial nerve nuclei. Most fibers regarded as "corticobulbar" are distributed to neurons in the reticular formation which in turn relay impulses to the motor cranial nerve nuclei. In experimental studies (1404, 2634, 2796) in the cat and rat, it has not been possible to trace terminal degeneration directly into any motor cranial nerve nucleus. These findings present a parallel to that accepted for the spinal cord, in that relatively few corticospinal fibers terminate directly upon anterior horn cells (1999, 2503). This indirect system is supplemented in man and primates by corticobulbar fibers that project directly to certain motor nuclei, namely, the trigeminal, the facial, the hypoglossal and the supraspinal (1405). Fiber projections to the motor trigeminal and hypoglossal nuclei are bilateral and nearly equal (Fig. 11-30). Direct cortical projections to the facial nucleus are bilateral, but fibers passing to ventral cell groups, which innervate lower facial muscles, are most abundant contralaterally. These observations are in accord with clinical observations regarding one central type of facial palsy to be discussed fully in the next chapter. Many of the direct corticobulbar fibers correspond to what early authors referred to as aberrant pyramidal bundles. An example of these obliquely running fascicles, frequently seen in the medulla and lower pons, is shown coursing into the pontine tegmentum in Figure 12-24. The more numerous corticoreticular fibers represent part of the phylogenetically older indirect corticobulbar pathway in which neurons of the reticular core serve as internuncials. Direct corticobulbar fibers found in man and primates represent a more recently developed parallel system.

Thus the supranuclear innervation of the motor cranial nerve nuclei is largely bilateral and more complex than that present at spinal levels. Bilateral projections are most evident to those nuclei innervating muscle groups which as a rule cannot be contracted voluntarily on one side (Fig. 11-30). These include the laryngeal, pharyngeal, palatal and upper facial muscles. This same principle applies to the muscles of mastication and the extraocular muscles. Because unilateral stimulation of the motor cortex produces isolated contraction of contralateral lower facial muscles, certain cell groups of the facial nucleus are considered to receive predominantly crossed corticobulbar fibers.

The fact that unilateral stimulation of the motor cortex causes turning of the head to the opposite side has been interpreted as indicating that corticofugal fibers to nuclei innervating the sternocleidomastoid muscle probably are uncrossed, since contraction of this muscle turns the head to the opposite side. It seems likely that some uncrossed corticospinal fibers (Figs. 10-13 and 10-14) may project impulses to spinal accessory cell groups innervating this muscle and the upper part of the trapezius muscle, although direct fibers to these cells appear meager (1405). Eye movements elicited by electrical stimulation of the cerebral cortex are always conjugate, indicating that the supranuclear innervation of the nuclei of the extraocular muscles is bilateral.

Because cortical control of motor cranial nerve nuclei is largely bilateral, unilateral lesions interrupting corticobulbar fiber systems (upper motor neuron) produce comparatively mild forms of paresis. Slight weakness of tongue (genioglossus muscle) and jaw movements (pterygoid muscles) contralateral to the lesions usually can be detected. Weakness in these muscles is expressed by modest deviation of the tongue and jaw to the side opposite the lesion. However, marked weakness of lower facial muscles contralateral to the lesion is evident when the patient attempts to show the teeth, purse the lips or puff out the cheeks.

Bilateral lesions involving corticobulbar fiber systems produce a syndrome known as *pseudobulbar palsy*. This syndrome is characterized by paralysis or weakness of muscles which control swallowing, chewing, breathing and speaking, and may occur with little or no paralysis in the extremities, if lesions are localized. Loss of emotional control characterized by unrestrained and inappropriate outbursts of laughing and crying frequently form a part of the syndrome; these symptoms appear as the physiological expression of rather extensive bilateral lesions in the upper brain stem or at higher levels. Although there is marked paresis of the muscles of mastication and in the muscles of the face, tongue, pharynx and larynx, these muscles do not atrophy, since the lower motor neurons remain intact. After prolonged periods of time, contractures may appear in the muscles of the lips, tongue and palate (1057).

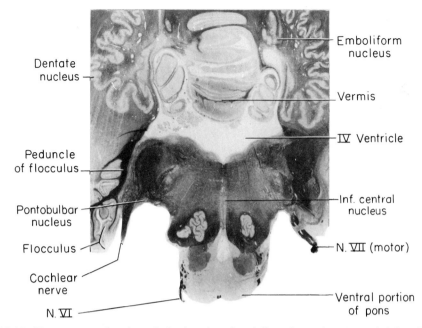

Dentate nucleus

Peduncle of flocculus

Pontobulbar nucleus

Flocculus

Cochlear nerve

N. VI

Emboliform nucleus

Vermis

IV Ventricle

Inf. central nucleus

N. VII (motor)

Ventral portion of pons

Figure 11-31. Transverse section through the junction of medulla and pons in a 1-month infant. Portions of the cerebellum containing large parts of the intracerebellar nuclei are attached. Structures in and around the tegmentum are identified in Figure 11-32 (Weigert's myelin stain, photograph).

Cranial nerves V, VII and IX through XII may be involved, together or in varying combinations, as a result of bilateral interruption of the corticobulbar tracts centrally (Fig. 11-30). Bilateral lesions involving "corticobulbar pathways" above pontine levels usually are the result of extensive demyelinating disease, vascular disease, thrombosis or neoplasms.

MEDULLARY-PONTINE JUNCTION

The fourth ventricle reaches its maximum width at the level of the lateral recesses (Figs. 11-2, 11-31 and A-6). These lateral extensions of the fourth ventricle pass external to the inferior cerebellar peduncle and the cochlear nuclei (Fig. A-5). The lateral wall of each recess is formed by the *peduncle of the flocculus*, a part of the floccular lobe of the cerebellum lying close to the lateral surface of the medulla (Fig. 11-31). The cochlear nerve, and the *dorsal* and *ventral cochlear nuclei* lie on the medial and ventral surfaces of the lateral recess. The *inferior cerebellar peduncle* has achieved its maximum size, and fibers of the cochlear nerve curve around its lateral and superior surfaces. At slightly more rostral levels, above the lateral recess, the

inferior cerebellar peduncle enters the cerebellum by passing posterolaterally. The fibers of this peduncle lie medial to the middle cerebellar peduncle (Fig. 11-32).

The hypoglossal and dorsal motor nucleus of the vagus are not present at these levels, although the rostral portion of the nucleus ambiguus is present and contributes special visceral efferent fibers to the glossopharyngeal nerve. Afferent fibers of N. IX enter the posterolateral aspect of the medulla ventral to the inferior cerebellar peduncle, traverse parts of the spinal trigeminal tract and nucleus, enter the fasciculus solitarius and in part terminate upon upper portions of the nucleus of that tract, the gustatory nucleus. Other fibers descend to lower levels. Above the level of entrance of N. IX the fasciculus solitarius cannot be distinguished readily, for it consists only of a small descending bundle of root fibers of N. VII.

Root fibers of the *cochlear* nerve, conveying impulses from the organ of Corti in the cochlea, enter the posterolateral margin of the upper medulla. Primary auditory fibers terminate upon two nuclear masses, the *ventral and dorsal cochlear nuclei*. The dorsal cochlear nucleus forms a prom-

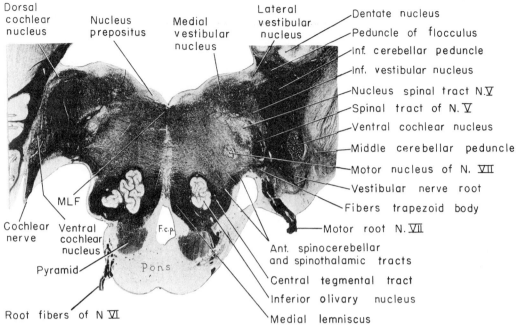

Dorsal cochlear nucleus
Nucleus prepositus
Medial vestibular nucleus
Lateral vestibular nucleus
Dentate nucleus
Peduncle of flocculus
Inf. cerebellar peduncle
Inf. vestibular nucleus
Nucleus spinal tract N.$\underline{V}$
Spinal tract of N. $\underline{V}$
Ventral cochlear nucleus
Middle cerebellar peduncle
Motor nucleus of N. $\underline{VII}$
Vestibular nerve root
Fibers trapezoid body
MLF
Cochlear nerve
Ventral cochlear nucleus
F.c.p.
Motor root N.$\underline{VII}$
Ant. spinocerebellar and spinothalamic tracts
Pyramid
Pons
Central tegmental tract
Inferior olivary nucleus
Root fibers of N $\underline{VI}$
Medial lemniscus

Figure 11-32. Transverse section of medulla of 1-month infant through caudal border of pons. *F.c.p.*, Foramen cecum posterior; *MLF*, medial longitudinal fasciculus (Weigert's myelin stain, photograph).

inence, the *tuberculum acusticum*, along the lateral border of the rhomboid fossa (Figs. 11-29, 11-32 and A-6). Cells of the dorsal cochlear nucleus are small, ovoid and fusiform, while those of the ventral nucleus are large, round cells with a dark-staining cytoplasm. Secondary auditory fibers arising from the dorsal and ventral cochlear nuclei become apparent at more rostral brain stem levels.

In the floor of the fourth ventricle the nucleus prepositus lies medially in the position previously occupied by the hypoglossal nucleus. Lateral to this nucleus are the vestibular nuclei (Figs. 11-28 and 11-32). At this level portions of the *medial* and *inferior vestibular nuclei* are seen. The inferior vestibular nucleus lies adjacent to the medial surface of the inferior cerebellar peduncle and is characterized by numerous, relatively coarse myelinated fiber bundles which course through it. These fibers, coursing in the longitudinal axis of the nucleus, are primary vestibular fibers and cerebellar efferent fibers which descend. The inferior vestibular nucleus has abundant reciprocal connections with vestibular portions of the cerebellum (391).

The inferior olivary complex is still present, but is reduced in size (Fig. 11-31). The accessory olivary nuclei have disappeared. Anterior to the olivary complex the fibers

of the pyramid are surrounded by pontine nuclei and some transverse fibers. The medial lemniscus and medial longitudinal fasciculus occupy the same positions as at more caudal levels, although they are slightly separated from the corresponding tract on the opposite side by more fully developed nuclei in the median raphe. Other ascending and descending tracts maintain the same relative positions as at lower medullary levels.

The junction of medulla and pons (Figs. 11-31 and 11-32) is characterized by: (a) passage of the inferior cerebellar peduncle into the cerebellum, (b) reduction in size and, ultimately, disappearance of the inferior olivary complex, (c) gradual incorporation of the corticospinal tract within the ventral part of the pons, (d) enlargement of the reticular formation and (e) appearance of cranial nerve nuclei and root fibers typical of this higher level.

Cranial nerves present at the junction of medulla and pons are the abducens, cochlear, vestibular and facial. The abducens nerve fibers emerge at the lower border of the pons lateral to the pyramids. All other cranial nerves at this level are grouped together at the *cerebellopontine angle*, formed by the junction of medulla, pons and cerebellum (Fig. 11-20). All of these nerves emerge from, or enter, the internal auditory meatus. The cochlear nerve is the most caudal and lateral, while the facial nerve is the most rostral and medial. The vestibular nerve lies between the cochlear and facial nerves. These cranial nerves will be described and discussed in the next chapter.

In the upper medulla the medial lemniscus reaches its full extent. It forms a vertical band of heavily myelinated fibers on either side of the raphe dorsal to the pyramids (Fig. 11-29). The formation and course of this tract are shown in Figure 10-1. The lateral and anterior spinothalamic tracts occupy a retro-olivary position (Fig. 11-29). Corticobulbar fibers leave the pyramids and pass dorsally into the reticular formation (Fig. 11-30); intercalated neurons lying in the reticular formation in turn project upon motor cranial nerve nuclei (2634).

The medial longitudinal fasciculus (MLF), tectospinal and tectobulbar tracts occupy an area dorsal to the medial lemniscus on each side of the median raphe. The tracts are partially separated by lighter-stained areas representing the raphe nuclei. At somewhat higher levels this position is occupied by the inferior central nucleus (Figs. 11-31 and 12-4). Other descending tracts, such as the rubrospinal and vestibulospinal, are difficult to distinguish in Weigert-stained material.

As the inferior cerebellar peduncle enters the medullary core of the cerebellum, it is covered externally by the fibers of the middle cerebellar peduncle, which arise from the ventral part of the pons. The development of the ventral portion of the pons envelops the medullary pyramids. The blind end of the anterior median fissure overhung by the pons is known as the *foramen cecum posterior* (Fig. 11-32). The attenuated rostral pole of the inferior olivary nucleus is flanked laterally by the fibers of the central tegmental tract and medially and ventrally by the medial lemniscus. The medial lemniscus gradually becomes flattened dorsoventrally and lies along the ventral border of the pontine tegmentum (Fig. 10-1). The light-staining area separating the medial lemnisci and the medial longitudinal fasciculi is occupied by raphe nuclei.

Experimentally, electrical stimulation of the lateral part of the medullary reticular formation and adjacent periventricular gray in lower animals (2670) produces elevation of arterial blood pressure and cardiac acceleration, probably as a consequence of activating sympathetic effectors. Descending pathways mediating these responses lie in the anterior and lateral funiculus of the spinal cord and are largely homolateral. Stimulations in the region of the obex, and in a wide area medial and ventral to the sympathetic area, produce a slowing of the heart rate. Part of this response appears to be vagal, but other evidence also suggests an inhibition of sympathetic neurons. Similar studies indicate that inspiratory and expiratory responses can be obtained from stimulations of circumscribed areas of the medulla (1833).

Multiple medullary structures may be simultaneously involved by vascular lesions, neoplasms or other disease processes. Symptoms and signs resulting from such lesions bear a close correlation to the specific neural structures involved, and their nature depends in part upon whether the lesions are irritative or destructive. Although vascular lesions are subject to considerable variation in location and extent, the distribution of the principal blood vessels within the medulla shows some constant features (Figs. 20-16 and 20-17). Lesions involving structures in the dorsolateral part of the medulla (lateral medullary syndrome) are probably the most common at this level and give rise to a constellation of symptoms and signs that are readily recognizable (580). While the classic feature of this syndrome is loss of pain and thermal sense in the ipsilateral half of the face and the contralateral half of the trunk and extremities, a variety of other severe symptoms occur. These include vertigo, nausea, vomiting, dysphonia, dysphagia, face and body pain, weakness of the face, disturbance of equilibrium and hiccup. This syndrome has been attributed largely to occlusion or disease of a single vessel, the posterior inferior cerebellar artery (Figs. 20-1, 20-5 and 20-7), but data (104) indicate that involvement of the vertebral artery and its smaller penetrating branches plays an equally important role in the production of the syndrome. Particular attention should be given to the neuronal structures which lie within the area of distribution of both the posterior inferior cerebellar and vertebral arteries (Figs. 20-16 and 20-17).

The Pons

The pons (metencephalon) representing the rostral part of the hindbrain, consists of two distinctive parts: (a) a *dorsal portion*, the pontine tegmentum and (b) a *ventral portion*, referred to as the pons proper (Fig. 12-1).

CAUDAL PONS

Dorsal Portion. The dorsal portion of the pons, known as the pontine tegmentum, is the rostral continuation of the medullary reticular formation. It contains cranial nerve nuclei, ascending and descending tracts and reticular nuclei (Fig. 12-1). Cranial nerve nuclei found in the pons are those of cranial nerves V, VI, VII and VIII. The ascending tracts in this part of the brain stem are similar to those found in the medulla. The medial lemniscus occupies a different position than in the medulla and its configuration is changed. This large, flattened, elliptical bundle, present on each side of the median raphe, lies anteriorly, just above the ventral portion of the pons (Figs. 12-1 and 12-2). Crossing fibers of the trapezoid body traverse ventral parts of the bundle on each side. The medial longitudinal fasciculi (MLF) are situated dorsally on each side of the median raphe as in the medulla. The spinothalamic and anterior spinocerebellar tracts are difficult to distinguish but occupy positions in the anterolateral tegmentum. The spinal trigeminal tract and nucleus lie medial to the inferior cerebellar peduncle. The vestibular nuclei are present in the floor of the fourth ventricle throughout the caudal pons (Fig. 12-2).

The pontine reticular formation is more extensive than the medullary reticular formation, but occupies a similar region. The medial two-thirds of the pontine reticular formation is represented by the pontine reticular nuclei (*nuclei reticularis pontis, pars caudalis* and *pars oralis*; Figs. 12-1 and 12-25) (266, 1884). The *pars caudalis* replaces the gigantocellular reticular nucleus of the medulla and extends rostrally to the level of the trigeminal motor nucleus (Fig. 12-3). The *pars oralis*, present in more rostral pontine levels, extends into the caudal mesencephalon (Fig. 12-25). The pontine reticular nuclei give rise to the pontine reticulospinal tract (Figs. 10-10 and 10-22). Lateral to the pars caudalis is a small-celled reticular nucleus (parvicellularis) similar to that described in the medulla. The median raphe contains the inferior central nucleus, and the subependymal area near the midline contains the nucleus of the *medial eminence* and the dorsal paramedian nucleus (Figs. 12-3 and 12-4).

The reticular formation posterolateral to the medial lemniscus contains a relatively large discrete bundle, the *central tegmental tract* (Figs. 12-1 and 12-4). This composite tract consists of descending fibers from midbrain nuclei that project mainly to the inferior olivary complex, and ascending fibers from the lower brain stem reticular formation that project to certain thalamic nuclei.

In addition to the structures described, the pontine tegmentum contains a number of cranial nerve nuclei and nuclei related to specific sensory systems. These include the cochlear and vestibular components of N. VIII, the motor and sensory components of the facial nerve, the abducens nerve and large portions of the trigeminal nuclear complex.

The *cerebellopontine angle*, formed laterally at the junction of pons, medulla and cerebellum, contains root fibers of the vestibulocochlear and facial nerves (Figs. 12-2 and 12-6). Fibers of the cochlear nerve root pass dorsally, lateral to the inferior cerebellar peduncle, to terminate upon cells in all divisions of both the dorsal and ventral cochlear nuclei (Fig. 11-32). Vestibular root fibers, slightly medial and rostral to those of the cochlear nerve, enter caudal portions of the pons by passing between the inferior cerebellar peduncle and the spinal trigeminal tract (Figs. 12-2 and 12-5). Primary vestibular fibers are distributed differentially within the vestibular nuclear complex in the floor of the fourth ventricle. A moderate number of vestibular fibers project to specific parts of the cerebellum via the juxtarestiform body, a structure medial to the inferior cerebellar peduncle (Fig. 12-7). Ventral to the vestibular nerve are the in-

termediate and facial nerves (Figs. 12-2 and 12-5). The intermediate nerve contains mainly special visceral afferent (taste; SVA) and general visceral efferent (parasympathetic; GVE) fibers. The larger motor root of the facial nerve is the most rostral and medial cranial nerve in the cerebellopontine angle.

The *motor nucleus of N. VII* appears as a pear-shaped gray mass in the lateral part of the reticular formation immediately dorsal to the superior olive (Figs. 12-1, 12-2 and 12-4). Within it may be seen the usual plexus of fine terminals and the coarser fibers which give origin to the facial nerve root. The root fibers form a complex intramedullary loop about the abducens nucleus whose continuity cannot be seen in any one section (Figs. 12-1, 12-5, 12-7 and 12-21). Fine bundles of fibers emerge from the dorsal surface of the facial nucleus, project dorsomedially toward the floor of the fourth ventricle and form a compact longitudinal bundle dorsal to the medial longitudinal fasciculus (Figs. 12-2 and 12-5). This bundle, medial to the abducens nucleus and dorsal to the medial longitudinal fasciculus, ascends for about 2 mm (Fig. 12-21). At the cranial border of the abducens nucleus the nerve makes a sharp lateral bend over the dorsal surface of the abducens nucleus, forming the *internal genu* of the facial nerve (Figs. 12-20 and 12-21). Fibers of the motor root of the facial nerve pass ventrolaterally, medial to the spinal trigeminal complex, and emerge from the brain stem at the cerebellopontine angle (Figs. 11-1 and 12-6).

The *abducens nucleus* (*N. VI*) is a rounded gray cellular mass in the lateral part of the medial eminence of the fourth ventricle. Together with the internal genu of the facial nerve, it forms the rounded prominence in the ventricular floor known as the *colliculus facialis* (Figs. 12-1–12-3 and 12-21). Its root fibers emerge from the medial surface of the abducens nucleus and descend to emerge at the caudal border of the pons (Figs. 11-1 and 12-1).

Ventral Portion. The ventral portion of the pons is a massive structure consisting of orderly arranged transverse and longitudinal fiber bundles between, and among, which are large collections of pontine nuclei (Figs. 12-1, 12-3 and 12-4). Longitudinal fiber bundles coursing through the ventral

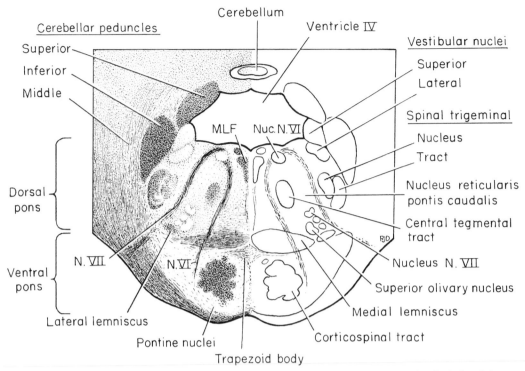

Figure 12-1. Semidiagrammatic drawing of a transverse section of the pons at the level of the abducens nucleus. The dorsal portion of the pons, constituting the tegmentum, contains the reticular formation, cranial nerve nuclei and ascending and descending tracts. The ventral portion of the pons contains the pontine nuclei, massive bundles of corticofugal fibers and the transverse fibers of the pons which form the middle cerebellar peduncle.

portion of the pons are: (a) corticospinal, (b) corticobulbar and (c) corticopontine (Figs. A-7–A-9). The largest groups of longitudinal fibers to traverse the ventral part of the pons are corticospinal; these fibers can be followed in continuity in sagittal section into the medullary pyramids (Figs. 2-23, 2-25, 10-13 and A-28). Corticobulbar fibers separate from the corticospinal tracts and enter the pontine reticular formation. Impulses pass to the motor cranial nerve nuclei directly and via intercalated neurons. While bundles of corticospinal fibers present a compact arrangement at rostral and caudal pontine levels, in the middle regions of the pons these bundles are broken up into a number of small fascicles by transversely oriented pontine fibers.

The most massive collection of longitudinally oriented fibers in the pons arise from broad regions of the cerebral cortex and terminate upon pontine nuclei. Corticopontine fibers arise from the cortex of the frontal (frontopontine), temporal (tempo-

ropontine), parietal (parietopontine) and occipital (occipitopontine) lobes, descend without crossing and end upon homolateral pontine nuclei. Corticopontine fibers from the primary sensorimotor cortex appear to be somatotopically organized and end upon circumscribed regions of the pontine nuclei (291). Each part of the cerebral cortex so far studied appears to give off fibers to several well defined areas within the pontine nuclei (292, 293). The corticopontocerebellar pathway is quantitatively the most important route by which the cerebral cortex can influence the cerebellar cortex. These projection systems appear to be somatotopically organized in a precise manner. The corticopontine fibers are most numerous in the rostral pons, where they form bundles difficult to distinguish from the pyramidal tracts (Fig. 12-29). Their number gradually diminishes as fibers terminate in the pontine nuclei. The corticopontine fibers and the transverse fibers to be described below do not become myelinated

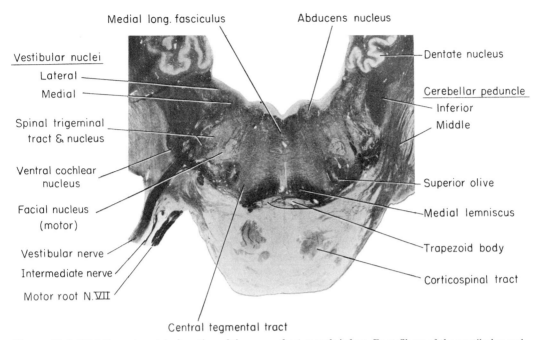

Medial long. fasciculus

Abducens nucleus

Vestibular nuclei

Lateral

Medial

Spinal trigeminal
tract & nucleus

Ventral cochlear
nucleus

Facial nucleus
(motor)

Vestibular nerve

Intermediate nerve

Motor root N.VII

Dentate nucleus

Cerebellar peduncle

Inferior

Middle

Superior olive

Medial lemniscus

Trapezoid body

Corticospinal tract

Central tegmental tract

Figure 12-2. Slightly asymmetrical section of the pons of a 1-month infant. Root fibers of the vestibular and facial nerves are present on the left (Weigert's myelin stain, photograph).

until some time after birth and are not distinguishable in brain sections of a 4-week infant stained by the Weigert technic (Fig. 12-2). They are shown in the adult pons in Figures 12-4, 12-21 and 12-29.

The transversely oriented fibers are axons of pontine nuclei (Fig. 12-3) which cross to the opposite side and form the massive *middle cerebellar peduncle*. In their transverse course these fibers pass dorsal, as well as ventral, to the corticospinal tract; the more dorsal fibers form the *deep layer*, while the more ventral ones constitute the *superficial layer* of the pons (Fig. A-26). Fibers of the middle cerebellar peduncle sweep dorsolaterally and somewhat caudally to enter the medullary core of the cerebellum superficial to the inferior cerebellar peduncle. The ventral portion of the pons thus may be considered as a relay station in an extensive, phylogenetically new, two neuronal pathway from the cerebral cortex to the cerebellar cortex. The first neuron in the cerebral cortex projects an uncrossed corticopontine fiber to the pontine nuclei. The second pontine neuron sends a crossed pontocerebellar fiber to the cortex of the opposite cerebellar hemisphere via the middle cerebellar peduncle. In addition a small number of fibers from

the superior colliculus (tectopontine fibers) descend ipsilaterally to terminate upon dorsolateral pontine nuclei (51). These fibers and fibers from the pontine nuclei are considered to transmit optic impulses to restricted regions of the cerebellum.

The pontine nuclei are large, closely packed cellular aggregations situated between the transverse and longitudinal fibers (Fig. 12-3). In caudal regions the cells form a ring around the compact pyramidal tract, which more rostrally is broken up into smaller bundles by islands of pontine cells. In a general way the cells may be grouped into lateral, medial, dorsal and ventral nuclear masses (Fig. 12-21). In the lateral groups the polygonal cells are relatively large- or medium-sized; in the paramedian region cells are smaller. Although the dendrites of these cells ramify around adjacent cell bodies, their axons, almost entirely crossed, form the middle cerebellar peduncle. Among these cells are found curiously shaped Golgi type II cells whose dendrites are beset with numerous hairlike processes, and whose short, branching axons terminate in the vicinity of the cell body.

Certain nuclei in the pontine tegmentum, like the reticulotegmental nucleus, project fibers into the ventral part of the pons

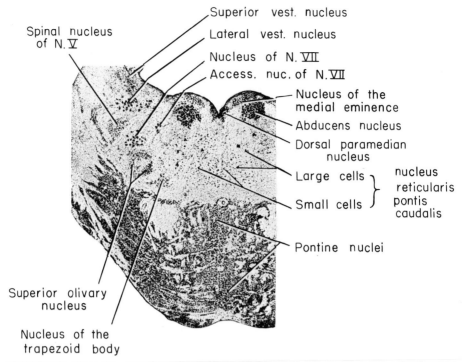

Figure 12-3. Section through pons and pontine tegmentum of 3-month infant at about same level as Figure 12-2 (Cresyl violet; photograph, with schematic representation of cell groups).

which enter the cerebellum via the contralateral middle cerebellar peduncle (Figs. 2-25, 12-25, 12-30, A-8 and A-9). The reticulotegmental nucleus is regarded by some as a tegmental extension of the pontine nuclei (1199).

VESTIBULOCOCHLEAR NERVE

The vestibulocochlear nerve (N. VIII) consists of two distinctive parts: (a) the cochlear part concerned with audition and (b) the vestibular part conveying impulses concerned with equilibrium and orientation in three-dimensional space. These two components of the vestibulocochlear nerve run together from the internal auditory meatus to the cerebellopontine angle, where they enter the brain stem (Figs. 11-1 and 12-6). Each of these nerves has distinctive central nuclei and connections.

Cochlea. The cochlear portion of the labyrinth consists of a fluid-filled tube, coiled in a spiral of about two and a half turns, that serves as the auditory transducer (Figs. 12-8 and 12-9). The cochlea is partitioned by two membranes, the basilar membrane and vestibular (Reissner's) membrane, to form the scala vestibuli, the scala tympani and the cochlear duct (scala media) (Figs. 12-9 and 12-10). Energy from sound waves is transmitted to the base of the scala vestibuli (oval window) by the foot plate of the stapes. The round window located at the base of the scala tympani is covered by a flexible membrane that accommodates to changes in hydrostatic pressure.

The *organ of Corti*, the auditory transducer, lies in the cochlear duct; the receptor organ consists of one row of inner hair cells and three rows of outer hair cells (Figs. 12-9–12-11). The tectorial membrane, attached at one end to the spiral limbus, overlies the hair cells (Fig. 12-10). The basilar membrane is not under tension, but has a stiffness that varies 100-fold from one end to the other. This membrane is narrowest and stiffest at the base of the cochlea and widest and most pliable near the helicotrema (910).

The energy of sound waves is transmitted in air to the tympanic membrane; in the middle ear the energy is transmitted by the ear ossicles. The piston-like action of the

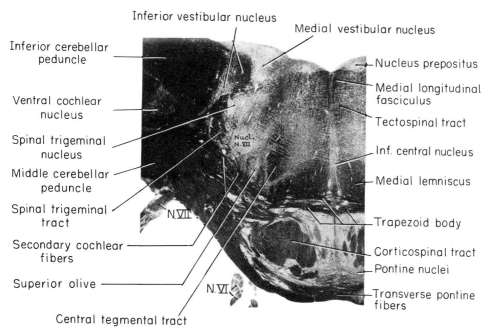

Figure 12-4. Transverse section of the adult pons at the level of emergence of the facial nerve root (Weigert's myelin stain, photograph).

stapes transmits the energy of sound waves to the perilymph in the scala vestibuli. Energy transmitted to the perilymph produces traveling waves in the basilar membrane that move from the base of the cochlea to the apex (146). Maximum displacement of the basilar membrane at different distances from the stapes can be correlated with specific sound frequencies. Displacement of the basilar membrane in response to an acoustic stimulus causes bending of hairs of the hair cells in contact with the tectorial membrane. The precise manner in which these forces produce excitation of primary auditory neurons is not known.

Cochlear Nerve and Nuclei. The larger cochlear division of N. VIII enters the brain stem lateral and somewhat caudal to the vestibular division (Fig. 11-32). Its fibers originate in the *spiral ganglion*, an aggregation of bipolar cells situated around the modiolus of the cochlea (Figs. 12-9, 12-10 and 12-13). The longer central processes of these cells form the cochlear nerve, while the short peripheral ones end in relation to the hair cells of the organ of Corti (Figs. 12-9 and 12-13). Fibers of the cochlear nerve terminate upon two nuclear masses, the *dorsal* and *ventral cochlear nuclei*, located on the lateral surface of the inferior cere-

bellar peduncle (Figs. 11-28, 11-32 and 12-12). Although the dorsal and ventral cochlear nuclei represent a more or less continuous cell mass dorsolateral and lateral to the inferior cerebellar peduncle, they have distinctive cell types, cytoarchitectural organization and divisions.

The *dorsal cochlear nucleus* forms an eminence on the most lateral part of the floor of the fourth ventricle, known as the *acoustic tubercle*. The acoustic tubercle lies dorsal to the inferior cerebellar peduncle and forms the floor of the lateral recess of the fourth ventricle (Figs. 12-5 and 12-12). In most mammals the dorsal cochlear nucleus has a distinct lamination evident in Nissl preparations (242, 1908, 2061, 2453). The *molecular layer*, beneath the ependyma of the lateral recess, contains small round neurons with scant cytoplasm which often are clustered in islands. The *fusiform layer* is composed of evenly distributed pyramidal cells oriented radially (i.e., with long axes perpendicular to the surface of the dorsal cochlear nucleus). This layer of conspicuous cells gives the dorsal cochlear nucleus its distinctive lamination. The *polymorphic layer*, the deepest and thickest, contains a diverse population of cells, including small granule cells, pyramidal cells,

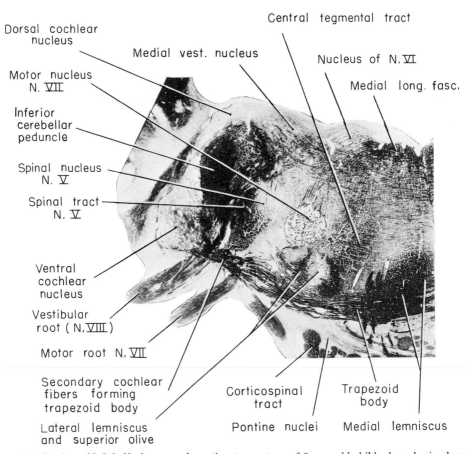

Dorsal cochlear nucleus

Medial vest. nucleus

Central tegmental tract

Nucleus of N. VI

Medial long. fasc.

Motor nucleus N. VII

Inferior cerebellar peduncle

Spinal nucleus N. V

Spinal tract N. V

Ventral cochlear nucleus

Vestibular root (N. VIII)

Motor root N. VII

Secondary cochlear fibers forming trapezoid body

Corticospinal tract

Trapezoid body

Lateral lemniscus and superior olive

Pontine nuclei

Medial lemniscus

Figure 12-5. Section of left half of pons and pontine tegmentum of 3-year old child whose brain showed a complete absence of the left cerebellar hemisphere and middle cerebellar peduncle. The origin of the trapezoid fibers from the ventral cochlear nucleus is clearly shown. Note fibers of the dorsal acoustic stria passing into the tegmentum from the dorsal cochlear nucleus (2458) (Weigert's myelin stain, photograph).

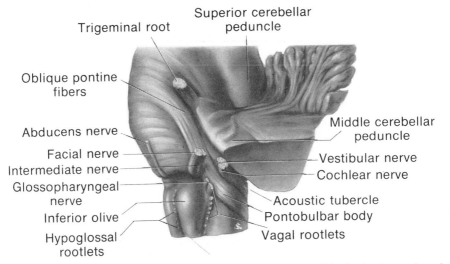

Trigeminal root

Superior cerebellar peduncle

Oblique pontine fibers

Abducens nerve

Facial nerve

Intermediate nerve

Glossopharyngeal nerve

Inferior olive

Hypoglossal rootlets

Middle cerebellar peduncle

Vestibular nerve

Cochlear nerve

Acoustic tubercle

Pontobulbar body

Vagal rootlets

Figure 12-6. Lateral view of the cerebellopontine angle from a dissection of the brain stem and cerebellum. (Reproduced with permission from F. A. Mettler: *Neuroanatomy.* C. V. Mosby Co., St. Louis, 1948.)

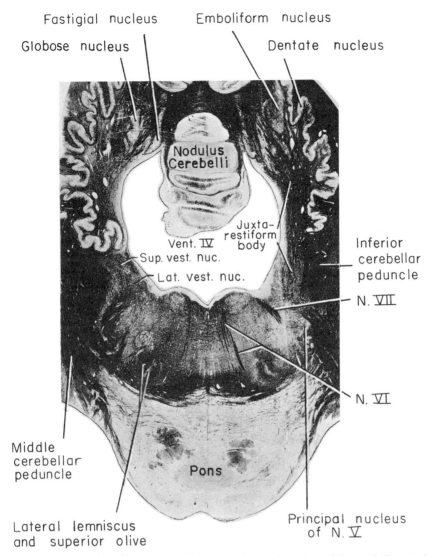

Fastigial nucleus

Globose nucleus

Emboliform nucleus

Dentate nucleus

Nodulus Cerebelli

Juxta-restiform body

Vent. IV

Sup. vest. nuc.

Lat. vest. nuc.

Inferior cerebellar peduncle

N. VII

N. VI

Middle cerebellar peduncle

Pons

Lateral lemniscus and superior olive

Principal nucleus of N. V

Figure 12-7. Transverse section of the pons, pontine tegmentum and portions of the cerebellum at the level of the abducens nuclei of 1-month infant (Weigert's myelin stain, photograph).

multipolar cells and occasional giant cells (1907). In man the above described lamination is indistinct.

The *ventral cochlear nucleus* has been subdivided into anteroventral and posteroventral cochlear nuclei on the basis of topography, cytology and functional characteristics (Fig. 12-12). Each of these subdivisions is tonotopically organized and has an orderly sequential representation of the auditory spectrum (2209, 2210). The *anteroventral cochlear nucleus* lies in the most rostral part of the cochlear nuclear complex between the vestibular nerve root and the peduncle of the flocculus. Cells of the an-

teroventral cochlear nucleus are predominantly ovoid or spherical in shape, and are densely packed in rostral parts of the nucleus. In the posterior part of this nucleus, near the entry zone of the cochlear root, cells are more widely spaced and larger. In addition to ovoid cells this region of the nucleus also contains globular cells with eccentric nuclei which bulge on the cell surface (95, 242, 1907).

The *posteroventral cochlear nucleus* begins at the level of entrance of the cochlear root into the brain stem and continues to the caudal tip of the cochlear complex where it is capped posteriorly by the dorsal

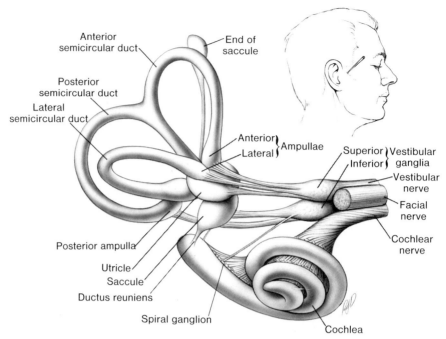

Figure 12-8. Drawing of the labyrinthine and cochlear apparatus, their ganglia and nerves with anatomical orientation. The cochlea has been rotated downward and laterally to expose the vestibular ganglia.

cochlear nucleus (242, 2453) (Fig. 12-12). Although the posteroventral cochlear nucleus contains several distinct types of neurons, multipolar cells of various sizes predominate, especially rostrally (1907). The caudal pole of this nuclear subdivision contains octopus cells, so-called because most of the dendrites are gathered together on one side of the cell body.

Primary Auditory Fibers. These fibers, representing the central processes of cells in the spiral ganglion, enter the cochlear nuclei, bifurcate in an orderly sequence and are distributed to both dorsal and ventral cochlear nuclei (1529). Experimental studies (1759, 2056) indicate that, after partial and complete lesions of the cochlea, degenerated fibers can be found in all parts of the cochlear nuclear complex. Ascending branches of the auditory nerve root terminate in a rostrolateral to caudomedial gradient in the anteroventral cochlear nucleus chiefly upon spherical and globular cells. Descending branches of the root terminate in a ventral to dorsal pattern in the posteroventral and dorsal cochlear nuclei. Fibers in the posteroventral nucleus end upon globular, multipolar and octopus cells. Fibers to the dorsal cochlear nucleus terminate about cells in the deep polymorphic layer and on the deep dendrites of the pyramidal cells.

One of the characteristic features of the auditory system is the pattern of *tonotopic localization* evident at various levels. In the cochlea it has been shown that high tones are received in the basal coils, while the apical portion is sensitive to low frequencies (573, 2516). Anatomical studies suggest that apical cochlear fibers terminate in ventral parts of the dorsal cochlear nucleus and in the ventral nucleus, while fibers from basal portions of the cochlea end in the dorsal part of the dorsal cochlear nucleus (1486). Physiological evidence (2208, 2209), based upon microelectrode studies of neuron frequency sensitivity in the cochlear nuclear complex, indicates that each major division possesses its own frequency sequence, and that each division seems to have a full tonal spectrum. In all three divisions of the cochlear complex in the cat (i.e., dorsal nucleus and anterior and posterior parts of the ventral nucleus) neurons responding to higher frequencies are dorsal, while those responding to lower frequencies are ventral. Thus there appears to be multiple tonotopic representation in the cochlear nuclear complex which suggests that primary cochlear fibers bifurcate and terminate in an orderly dorsoventral sequence throughout the nuclear complex.

Auditory Pathways. Secondary auditory pathways in the brain stem are complex and many details regarding their exact composition and course are uncertain. Most of the available information concerning these pathways is based upon studies in animals (Fig. 12-13). Secondary auditory fibers arising from the dorsal and ventral cochlear nuclei are grouped into three acoustic striae (10, 122). The three acoustic striae project to auditory relay nuclei on both sides of the brain stem (i.e., nuclei of the superior olivary complex and trapezoid body) and also contribute fibers to the lateral lemniscus, the principal ascending auditory pathway in the brain stem.

The *dorsal acoustic stria* arises from the dorsal cochlear nucleus, arches medially around the superior surface of the inferior cerebellar peduncle and projects across the midline of the dorsal pontine tegmentum (2452, 2453). A few fibers in this stria appear to terminate in the contralateral lateral superior olivary nucleus, but the main bundle enters the opposite lateral lemniscus directly (Fig. 12-13). Degeneration studies indicate that these fibers and their collaterals terminate in part upon the contralateral ventral and dorsal nuclei of the lateral lemniscus and project to major terminations in the central nucleus of the inferior colliculus on the opposite side (2452).

The *intermediate acoustic stria* arises from cells in the posteroventral cochlear nucleus, courses dorsally through parts of the dorsal cochlear nucleus and enters the tegmentum by passing around the inferior cerebellar peduncle (2452). In the ipsilateral tegmentum these fibers approach the dorsal aspect of the superior olivary complex where they are distributed to retro-olivary and periolivary nuclear groups. Fibers of the intermediate acoustic stria continue across the median raphe posterior to the trapezoid body to be distributed to retro-olivary and periolivary nuclei contralaterally (2452, 2453, 2674). None of these fibers appears to terminate in the principal nuclei of the superior olivary complex.

Other fibers in the intermediate acoustic stria contribute to the contralateral lateral lemniscus; these fibers pass to terminations in the ventral nucleus of the lateral lemniscus and inferior colliculus (2674). Because the retro-olivary and periolivary nuclei are known to give rise to fibers of the olivo-cochlear bundle that pass peripherally to make synaptic contact with outer hair cells, the posteroventral nucleus, which projects prominently to these nuclei, must play a significant role in this modulating system (2453, 2674).

The *ventral acoustic stria* arises from the ventral cochlear nucleus (2457, 2673), and courses medially along the ventral border of the pontine tegmentum to form the trapezoid body (Figs. 12-5 and 12-13). Many of these fibers pass through or ventral to the medial lemniscus, cross the raphe and reach the dorsolateral border of the opposite *superior olive*, where they turn upward to form a longitudinal ascending bundle known as the *lateral lemniscus*. Other trapezoid fibers terminate in the homolateral and contralateral nuclei of the superior olive and the trapezoid body, two nuclear masses interposed in the secondary cochlear pathway (Fig. 12-13). Fibers from these nuclei join the lateral lemniscus of the same or the opposite side.

The dorsal acoustic stria, is larger than the intermediate stria and the ventral stria is larger than the other two combined. In their passage through the tegmentum there is a diminution in the number of fibers in the various striae due to terminations in the reticular formation, the superior olivary nuclei and the trapezoid nuclei. The superior olivary and trapezoid nuclei (Fig. 12-5) give rise to a number of tertiary auditory fibers which ascend mainly in the lateral lemniscus of the same side (2444). Thus the lateral lemniscus consists primarily of crossed secondary fibers contributed by the three auditory striae and tertiary fibers from the superior olive and trapezoid nuclei. No direct fibers from the cochlear nuclei ascend in the ipsilateral lateral lemniscus (122). The number of ascending fibers in the lateral lemniscus is small compared with the total number of fibers arising from the dorsal and ventral cochlear nuclei.

The *superior olivary complex* is the most caudal level of the auditory pathway at

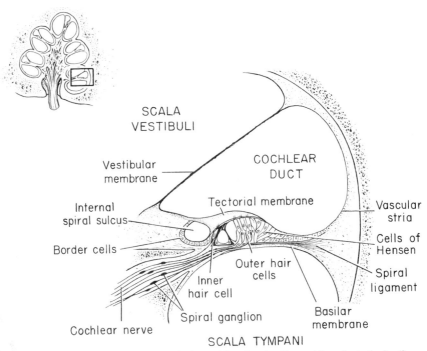

Figure 12-9. Drawing of a radial section through the cochlea showing the cochlear duct, the basilar membrane, the organ of Corti, and the tectorial membrane. The small *diagram in the upper left* is an axial section of the cochlea. The *area enclosed in the rectangle* is reproduced in detail in the large drawing.

which ascending fiber systems issuing from the two sides converge (2453). Binaural interaction in the superior olivary complex plays an important role in sound localization. The complex, located in the ventral part of the caudal pontine tegmentum, consists of several nuclei: (a) the lateral superior olivary nucleus, (b) the medial superior olivary nucleus, (c) the nuclei of the trapezoid body and (d) the preolivary and periolivary nuclei.

The *lateral superior olivary nucleus* has a conspicuous S-shaped configuration in carnivores, but in primates and man it is oval with dorsal and ventral indentations (Figs. 12-5 and 12-21). The lateral superior olive in man consists of about six clusters of cells which do not present a sharply circumscribed configuration (2455). The *medial superior olivary nucleus* forms a slender obliquely oriented cell column medial to the lateral superior olive; the dorsal tip of the cell column is closest to the midline. Spindle-shaped cells of the medial superior olivary nucleus emit dendrites from both poles of the neurons. In addition to the main nuclei described above, there are other smaller diffusely arranged cell groups

that belong to the superior olivary complex. Diffusely arranged cells ventral to the superior olivary complex are referred to as the *preolivary nuclei*, while cells dorsal to the main complex are designated as the *retro-olivary* cell group. The *periolivary nucleus* lies dorsal and medial to the medial superior olivary nucleus.

The *trapezoid body* forms a conspicuous bundle of transverse fibers in the ventral part of the pontine tegmentum (Figs. 12-4, 12-5 and 12-21). These fibers arise principally from the ventral cochlear nucleus and sweep medially in a gentle arc toward the median raphe. Most of these fibers cross to the opposite side, passing through or ventral to the medial lemniscus, and reach the ventrolateral portion of the tegmentum (Fig. 12-5). Here they turn sharply in a longitudinal direction to form the principal ascending auditory pathway, the lateral lemniscus (Fig. 12-13). The turn is made just dorsolateral to the *superior olivary complex* (Figs. 12-21 and A-29). This is a cellular column, about 4 mm long, extending from the level of the facial nucleus to the motor nucleus of the trigeminal nerve; it is in contact ventrally with the lateral

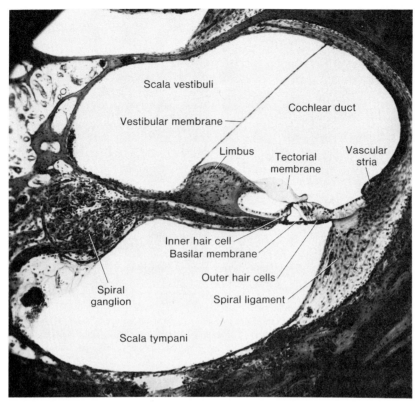

Figure 12-10. Photomicrograph of a radial section through the cochlea in man similar to the schematic drawing in Figure 12-9. Note the cells of the spiral ganglion.

portion of the trapezoid body (Figs. 12-3 and 12-5). The superior olive receives collaterals of secondary cochlear fibers and contributes fibers to the trapezoid body and lateral lemniscus. The medial accessory superior olivary nucleus receives afferents bilaterally from the anteroventral cochlear nuclei and gives rise to fibers that ascend in the ipsilateral lateral lemniscus (1907, 2444). From the region dorsal to the medial accessory olivary nucleus a bundle of fibers, the *peduncle of the superior olive*, passes dorsomedially toward the abducens nucleus (Figs. 12-2 and A-7).

Other smaller cellular aggregations related to the trapezoid body are difficult to see in Weigert preparations (Fig. 12-5). They include the *trapezoid nuclei*, which are scattered among the trapezoid fibers medial and lateral to the superior olive.

The *lateral lemniscus*, the principal ascending auditory pathway in the brain stem, courses rostrally in the lateral part of the tegmentum. Initially this bundle lies lateral to the superior olivary complex (Figs. 12-5 and 12-13), but at isthmus levels its position is more dorsal (Fig. 12-29).

The *nuclei of the lateral lemniscus*, located along the course of the principal ascending auditory bundle extend from the rostral pole of the superior olivary complex to levels through the caudal part of the inferior colliculus (Fig. 12-29). Two nuclei are distinguished: a ventral nucleus and a dorsal nucleus. The *ventral nucleus of the lateral lemniscus*, a compact aggregation of cells in the ventrolateral tegmentum, appears immediately rostral to the lateral preolivary nuclei and is surrounded ventrally and laterally by fibers of the lateral lemniscus. The *dorsal nucleus of the lateral lemniscus* appears at more rostral pontine levels and is composed of cell clusters located within fascicles of the lateral lemniscus (Fig. 12-29). The oral pole of the dorsal nucleus of the lateral lemniscus lies immediately ventral to the inferior colliculus. The dorsal and ventral nuclei of the lateral lemniscus of both sides receive inputs arising from the anteroventral cochlear nuclei

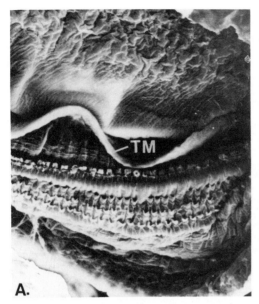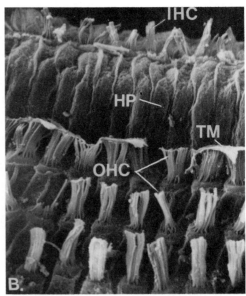

Figure 12-11. Scanning electron micrographs of the cochlea of the rhesus monkey. (*A*), View of the basal coil of the cochlea with the tectorial membrane (*TM*) reflected (×450). (*B*), Surface view of the hair cells of the cochlea after removal of the tectorial membrane (*TM*), except for fragments attached to outer hair cells (*OHC*). *IHC*, inner hair cells; *HP*, head plate of inner pillar (×2100). (Reproduced with permission from M. Rivera-Dominguez et al.: *Brain Research*, **65:** 159–164, 1973.)

(2673). Other fibers ascending in the lateral lemniscus probably contribute terminals or collaterals to these nuclei. The extent to which the nuclei of the lateral lemniscus contribute to the principal ascending auditory pathway is unknown, but it probably is substantial. When the lateral lemniscus reaches the midbrain, most of its fibers terminate directly in the central nucleus of the inferior colliculus (2456). Some fibers may reach the colliculus of the opposite side through the commissure of the inferior colliculi. The small number of remaining fibers in the lateral lemniscus may project directly to the medial geniculate body (2456, 2769). Thus fibers from the inferior colliculus, and possibly a few from the lateral lemniscus, constitute the *brachium of the inferior colliculus* (Fig. 12-13).

The nucleus of the lateral lemniscus gives rise to fibers which decussate and enter the inferior colliculus of the opposite side. The inferior colliculi are interconnected via commissural fibers and probably some fibers project to the superior colliculi. Physiological studies (2212) suggest that some neurons of the inferior colliculus are sensitive to interaural time relationships of binaurally applied stimuli, while others are

sensitive to small interaural intensity differences. These data indicate that certain neurons in the inferior coliculus may be concerned with the localization of a sound source.

It is evident from the above that the auditory pathway receives contributions from a number of intercalated nuclear masses and has a more complex composition than sensory systems considered heretofore. There is also a considerable ipsilateral ascending component consisting of ascending fibers arising mainly from the superior olivary complex. It is difficult to state the number of neurons involved in the auditory pathway from the periphery to the cortex, but the principal ones are: (a) cells of the spiral ganglion whose central processes form the cochlear nerve, (b) secondary fibers from the dorsal and ventral cochlear nuclei which form the three auditory striae and contribute primarily crossed fibers to the lateral lemniscus, (c) the nuclei of the superior olivary complex and the trapezoid body that contribute to the lateral lemnisci, (d) the nuclei of the lateral lemniscus which receive and contribute fibers to the bundle of the same name, (e) the inferior colliculus which receives fibers

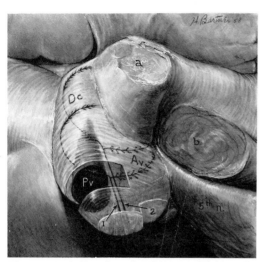

Figure 12-12. Drawing of cochlear nuclei from the lateral surface of the brain stem of a cat. Major divisions of the cochlear nuclei are indicated: *Dc*, dorsal cochlear nucleus; *Pv*, posteroventral nucleus; *Av*, anteroventral nucleus. Branches of central processes of the spiral ganglion cells are distributed to all divisions of cochlear nuclei and in each division neurons responding to higher frequencies are most dorsal. Fiber *1* is derived from the middle turn of the cochlea, while fiber *2* comes from the basal turn; *a* represents cut edges of the inferior and superior cerebellar peduncles; *b* is the cut edge of the middle cerebellar peduncle; *5th n* is the trigeminal nerve root. (Reproduced with permission from J. E. Rose et al.: In *Mechanisms of the Auditory and Vestibular Systems,* edited by G. Rasmussen and W. Windle. Charles C Thomas, Springfield, Ill., 1960.)

from the lateral lemniscus and projects via its brachium to the medial geniculate body and (f) the medial geniculate body, which gives rise to geniculocortical fibers (auditory radiation) that project to the transverse temporal gyri of Heschl (Figs. 2-10 and 12-13). Some crossed fibers in the dorsal and intermediate acoustic striae may pass via the lateral lemniscus directly to the medial geniculate body (2452), 2456, 2751). Most of the auditory impulses reaching the auditory cortex are conveyed by higher order neurons. Physiological studies indicate a definite tonotopic localization in the inferior colliculus (27, 1676, 2211). Units of the central nucleus of the inferior colliculus are characterized by sharp tuning and binaural responses, while those in the pericentral and external nuclei are very broadly tuned (Fig. 13-4). There is a systematic representation of the cochlea

within the pericentral nucleus and a highly ordered representation of the cochlea in the central nucleus of the inferior colliculus. Isofrequency contours in the central nucleus parallel cellular laminae with low frequencies represented dorsally and high frequencies represented ventrally. In the medial geniculate body low frequencies are perceived laterally and high frequencies are represented medially in the principal division (25, 26). Physiological data concerning the tonotopic representation of auditory impulses at the cortical level are discussed in Chapter 19.

Because of the large number of intercalated nuclei in the course of the auditory pathway (i.e., superior olive, trapezoid nucleus, nucleus of the lateral lemniscus, inferior colliculus), the cochlear reflex connections are exceedingly complex. It seems likely that all of the relay nuclei along the auditory pathway are involved to some degree in reflex circuits by which various motor phenomena occur in response to cochlear stimulation. Experimental evidence suggests that a descending conduction system, from the auditory cortex to the cochlea (2120), is associated with the classical ascending auditory system.

Efferent Cochlear Bundle. One of the most interesting cochlear reflex connections is the *olivocochlear bundle* or the *efferent cochlear bundle* described by Rasmussen (2118, 2119). Crossed and uncrossed components of the olivocochlear bundle project from the brain stem to the cochlea in a number of vertebrates, including man, and form a pathway by which the central nervous system may influence its own sensory input (833, 2120). Electrical stimulation of the crossed olivocochlear bundle in the cat results in a reduction of auditory nerve fiber responses to acoustic stimuli (839). Fibers of the crossed olivocochlear bundle in the cat arise from the region dorsal to the medial accessory superior olive (the medial periolivary nucleus), pass dorsally in the pontine tegmentum and cross the midline beneath the genu of the facial nerve (Fig. 12-14). Contralaterally these fibers emerge from the brain stem in association with the vestibular nerve. In the inner ear, fibers of this bundle pass via the vestibulocochlear anastomosis into the cochlear nerve and traverse the cochlear

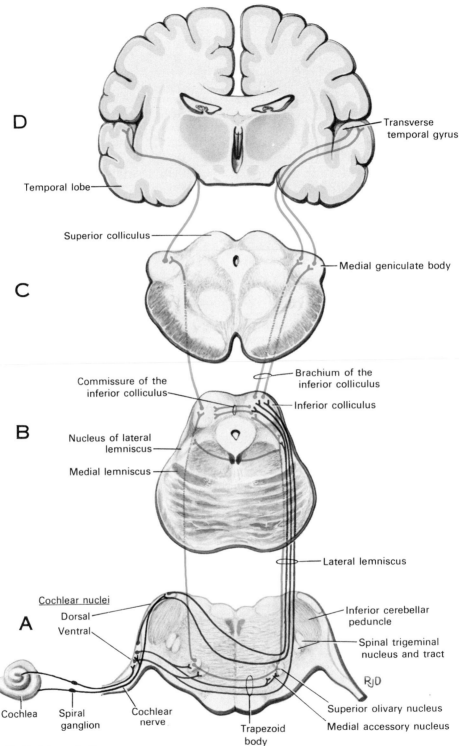

Figure 12-13. Schematic diagram of the auditory pathways. Primary auditory fibers arising from the spiral ganglion are in *black*. Secondary auditory fibers arising from the dorsal and ventral cochlear nuclei and forming the acoustic striae are in *red*. Auditory fibers arising from relay nuclei are in *blue*. *A*, Medulla; *B*, level of inferior colliculus; *C*, level of superior colliculus and medial geniculate body; *D*, transverse section through the cerebral hemisphere. (Reproduced with permission from M. B. Carpenter: *Core Text of Neuroanatomy.* Williams & Wilkins, Baltimore, 1978.)

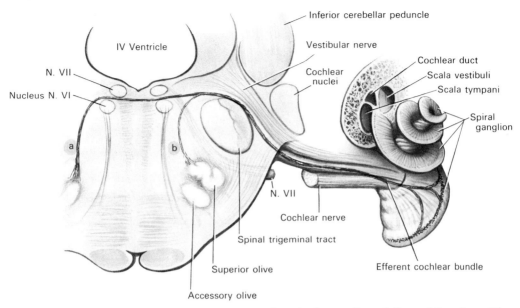

Figure 12-14. Schematic drawing of efferent cochlear fibers in the cat. Crossed fibers of the olivocochlear bundle (*red, a*) arise from cells dorsal to the accessory superior olivary nucleus, pass dorsomedially toward the floor of the fourth ventricle and cross to the opposite side. Uncrossed fibers of the olivocochlear bundle (*red, b*) arise from cells dorsal to the superior olivary nucleus, join the crossed fibers and pass peripherally in association with the vestibular nerve. Peripherally efferent cochlear fibers join the cochlear nerve via the vestibulocochlear anastomosis and are distributed to the hair cells of the cochlea. (Modified from Rasmussen (2120).)

spirals before projecting into the organ of Corti (2119). The uncrossed fibers of the olivocochlear bundle appear to arise from the region dorsal to the superior olive (the lateral periolivary nucleus) and join fibers of the crossed bundle in the ipsilateral vestibular nerve (1535). In the cat approximately 20% of the fibers in the olivocochlear bundle are uncrossed (2120). Peripherally crossed and uncrossed fibers of the olivocochlear bundle make synaptic contact with the outer hair cells (1317, 2357, 2358, 2409).

In the basal turn of the cochlea each outer hair cell receives 6 to 8 efferent nerve endings (2408), but this number is reduced gradually as the cochlear apex is approached. Certain efferent axons also enter the inner spiral bundle and appear to synapse with spiral ganglion fibers beneath the inner hair cells (2356, 2406). There are indications from electron micrographic studies that some fibers of the olivocochlear bundle are unmyelinated (2531). Studies of the origins of the crossed fibers of the olivocochlear bundle in the cat utilizing an acid phosphatase method suggest that these fibers arise from the dorsomedial periolivary nucleus, the ventral trapezoid nu-

cleus and portions of the medial trapezoid nucleus (1535).

In addition to the efferent cochlear bundle, which represents an inhibitory feedback system to the primary sensory receptor, the cochlear nuclei receive descending efferent fibers from various relay nuclei in the auditory pathway (2121). Structures giving rise to these fibers include the inferior colliculus, the nuclei of the lateral lemniscus and the principal superior olive. These descending pathways may inhibit impulses concerned with certain frequencies of the auditory spectrum and in this way result in a relative enhancement of those impulses not subject to inhibition. This phenomenon is referred to as auditory sharpening.

Other acoustic reflex mechanisms involve middle ear muscles, such as the stapedius and tensor tympani, which serve as regulators of auditory input to the cochlea. Both of these reflex pathways involve neurons of the ventral cochlear nucleus, the trapezoid body and the medial superior olive (217). In the reflex involving the stapedius muscle, fibers from the medial accessory superior olive project bilaterally to facial motor neurons. Contractions of the stapedius muscle serve to dampen the oscillations of the ear ossicles. In the reflex involving the tensor tympani muscle, fibers from the medial accessory superior olive project bilaterally to trigeminal motor neurons that innervate that muscle. The threshold for the tensor tympani reflex is relatively high and its significance in man is obscure. Acoustic reflexes which involve closing of the eyes and turning of the head in response to sudden loud noise are presumed to implicate auditory projections to the brain stem reticular formation.

Lesions of the Auditory System. Destruction of the cochlear nerve, or the cochlear nuclei, causes complete *deafness* on the same side. Among the more common disorders is the so-called acoustic neurinoma, a perineural fibroblastoma that arises from cells of the Schwann sheath. Although this benign tumor probably originates from the vestibular portion of the eighth nerve, loss of hearing with, or without, tinnitus usually is the first symptom. Unilateral loss of hearing usually is gradual and may not be noticed by the patient until it is severe. In time, other cranial nerves almost invariably are involved; these include the vestibular, trigeminal and facial nerves. Since the secondary cochlear pathways are both crossed and uncrossed, lesions of one lateral lemniscus or of the auditory cortex cause a bilateral diminution of hearing (partial deafness) that is most marked in the contralateral ear. Removal of one temporal lobe causes an impairment of sound localization on the opposite side, especially as regards judgment of the distance from which the sound is coming (1964).

Conduction deafness due to disease of the middle ear should be distinguished from nerve deafness. In conduction deafness the ossicular chain fails to transmit vibrations from the tympanum to the oval window and to the scala vestibuli and scala media (i.e., cochlear duct; Fig. 12-9). When the ossicular chain is broken, vibrations of the tympanum pass via the air of the middle ear to the round window; this is inefficient because it lacks the impedence matching of the ossicular chain and considerable sound energy is lost. Hearing loss due to interruption of the ossicular chain ranges from 30 decibels for low tones to 65 decibles in the middle range. Fixation of the ossicular chain resulting from middle ear infections, or otosclerosis, is more common than interruptions of the ossicular chain. In *otosclerosis* even air conduction is impaired because the membrane covering the round window is thickened. Early in the course of the disease patients with otosclerosis have either a loss of appreciation of low tones, or a mild loss in the entire auditory range. Later there is a marked perceptual deficit for high tones. Tinnitus, without vertigo, is common, and many patients hear better in the presence of loud noises (*paracusis*).

Labyrinth. The vestibular portion of the inner ear consists of three *semicircular ducts*, the *utricle* and the *saccule* (Figs. 12-8 and 12-15). Receptors in these structures are concerned with equilibrium and orientation in three-dimensional space. The semicircular ducts, concerned with kinetic equilibrium, are arranged at right angles to each other and represent approximately the three planes of space. One end of each duct has a dilatation, the ampulla, containing a ridge or crista oriented transversely to the duct. The columnar epithelium of the *crista ampullaris* is composed of neuroepithelial hair cells which constitute the vestibular receptor. Each crista is covered by a gelatinous cupula. Angular acceleration causes displacement of endolymphatic fluid and movement of the cupula which stimulates the hair cells. Corresponding ducts on opposite sides of the head function in pairs (i.e., the horizontal ducts are in the same plane and the anterior duct of one side is in the same plane as the posterior duct of the opposite side). The cristae of the semicircular ducts are stimulated by rotatory movement (i.e., angular acceleration) which causes movement of endolymphatic fluid and deflection of hairs of the sensory epithelium. Endolymphatic flow is greatest in the pair of ducts most nearly perpendicular to the axis of rotation.

The utricle and saccule each have a similar patch of sensory epithelium, the *macula utriculi* and *macula sacculi*, but here the hair cells are in contact with a gelatinous covering containing small calcareous concretions or particles, the *otoliths*. The utricle and saccule together constitute the so-called "otolith organ." The utricular macula, concerned primarily with static

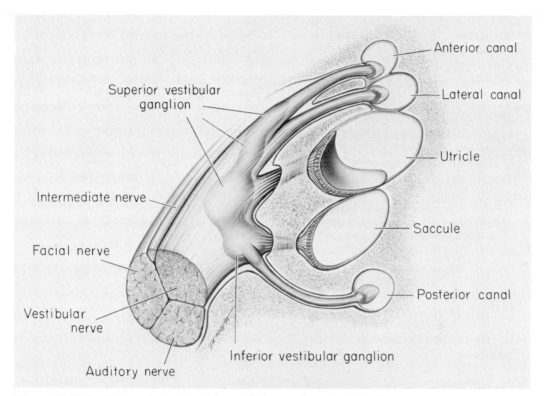

Figure 12-15. Semischematic drawing of the vestibular ganglia and peripheral branches innervating anatomically distinctive portions of the labyrinth. Cells in the superior vestibular ganglion are arranged in a spiral fashion. Cells in the superior and distal portion of this ganglion innervate the cristae of the anterior and lateral semicircular ducts. The broader proximal part of the superior vestibular ganglion contains cells which innervate the macula of the utricle. Cells of the inferior vestibular ganglion innervate the macula of the saccule and the crista of the posterior semicircular duct. The superior and inferior vestibular ganglia are joined by an isthmus of cells. The relationships between the facial, intermediate, vestibular and auditory nerves are shown on the left. (Reproduced with permission from B. M. Stein and M. B. Carpenter: *American Journal of Anatomy*, **120:** 281–318, 1967.)

equilibrium, responds to changes in gravitational forces, and to linear acceleration. Macular impulses convey information regarding the position of the head in space, the hair cells being stimulated by the otolithic particles, whose position varies under the influence of gravity. Physiological studies of peripheral otolithic neurons in the monkey suggest that the saccule has an equilibratory function (743). Saccular neurons appear sensitive to dorsoventral (i.e., anteroposterior axis of body) accelerations, while utricular neurons are most sensitive to vertical accelerations in the longitudinal axis of the body. Saccular afferents have a lower resting discharge and a lower sensitivity than utricular afferents.

Anatomical studies (1529, 2429) demonstrate that afferent nerve fibers from the saccular macula do not join the cochlear nerve and that they are distributed to the vestibular nuclei in a manner similar to that of nerve fibers from the utricular macula and the semicircular ducts.

Vestibular Nerve and Nuclei. The maculae and cristae are innervated by cells of the vestibular ganglion (ganglion of Scarpa), an aggregation of bipolar cells located in the internal auditory meatus. The vestibular ganglion can be divided into superior and inferior vestibular ganglia which are connected by a narrow isthmus (Figs. 12-8 and 12-15). The shorter peripheral processes of these cells go to the receptor cells of the maculae and cristae; the longer central processes form the vestibular nerve. Cells of the superior vestibular ganglion innervate the cristae of the anterior and lateral semicircular ducts and the macula of the utricle. Cells of the smaller inferior vestibular ganglion innervate the crista of the posterior semicircular duct and the macula of the saccule (415, 2429). The vestibular nerve enters the cerebellopontine angle medial to the cochlear nerve. Vestibular root fibers pass dorsally between the inferior cerebellar peduncle and the spinal trigeminal tract, and bifurcate into short ascending and long descending branches which are distributed to the vestibular nuclei (Figs. 11-19 and 12-16). Some primary vestibular fibers (i.e., root fibers) continue without interruption to particular parts of the cerebellum; these fibers reach the ipsilateral half of the cerebellum via the juxtarestiform body (Fig. 12-7) and project mainly to the cortex of the nodulus, uvula and flocculus (276, 415). The largest number of primary vestibular fibers terminate differentially in the four vestibular nuclei in the floor of the fourth ventricle (Figs. 12-17 and 12-18). The vestibular nuclei are the inferior, lateral, medial and superior. Because of the long rostrocaudal extent of the vestibular nuclei, usually only two nuclei can be seen in any one transverse section (Figs. 12-16, 12-17, A-4, A-5 and A-6).

The *inferior vestibular nucleus* begins caudally in the medulla medial to the accessory cuneate nucleus and extends rostrally medial to the inferior cerebellar peduncle to the point near the entrance of the vestibular nerve root (Fig. 12-4). Cytoarchitecturally the nucleus is composed of small- and medium-sized cells except in its most rostral part, where scattered large cells resemble those of the lateral vestibular nucleus. In the ventrolateral and caudal parts of the nucleus, a number of rather large cells form several densely packed groups. These cells (*group f* of Brodal and Pompeiano (278)) are of particular interest because they do not receive primary vestibular fibers and many of them project fibers to the cerebellum. In fiber-stained sections, the inferior vestibular nucleus is characterized by bundles of longitudinally oriented fibers, part of which are descending primary vestibular fibers. These descending fiber bundles facilitate the delineation of the inferior and medial vestibular nuclei (Figs. 11-29 and 12-4).

The *lateral vestibular nucleus* (Deiters'

nucleus), located laterally in the ventricular floor at the level of entrance of the vestibular nerve, extends rostrally to the level of the abducens nucleus. This nucleus is characterized by multipolar giant cells with coarse Nissl granules. Although most of the cells of this nucleus are regarded as giant cells, considerable variations in cell size are found (Fig. 12-3). The nucleus also contains varying types of smaller cells. Cells of all sizes are intermingled throughout the nucleus except in a small dorsolateral protrusion that consists only of medium-sized cells. There are some regional differences in the relative number and size of giant cells, which are most abundant in the caudal part of the nucleus. The giant cells in the lateral vestibular nucleus have numerous boutons on their soma, while small cells have relatively few boutons (1778).

The *medial vestibular nucleus* occupies the floor of the fourth ventricle medial to the inferior and lateral vestibular nuclei (Figs. 12-4 and 12-16). Its rostral and caudal boundaries are indistinct. Rostrally it fuses dorsolaterally with the superior vestibular nucleus.

Cells of the medial vestibular nucleus are small- and medium-sized, closely packed and fairly evenly distributed. Dorsolaterally some of the larger cells resemble those of the lateral vestibular nucleus, although none are true giant cells. The medial and inferior vestibular nuclei can be distinguished readily at all levels in myelin-stained preparations because bundles of longitudinally coursing fibers are not present in the medial vestibular nucleus (Fig. 12-4).

The *superior vestibular nucleus* lies dorsal and mostly rostral to the lateral vestibular nucleus in the angle formed by the floor and the lateral wall of the fourth ventricle (Figs. 12-1 and 12-7). The superior cerebellar peduncle forms the dorsolateral border of the nucleus throughout most of its rostrocaudal extent. The mesencephalic and principal sensory nuclei of the trigeminal nerve are adjacent to the nucleus medially and ventrally, in its rostral two-thirds. The rostral pole of the nucleus is difficult to delimit. Peripheral cells in this nucleus are loosely scattered, medium- and small-sized, and round or spindle-shaped. Cells in the central region of the nucleus

VESTIBULAR NUCLEI   VESTIBULAR GANGLIA

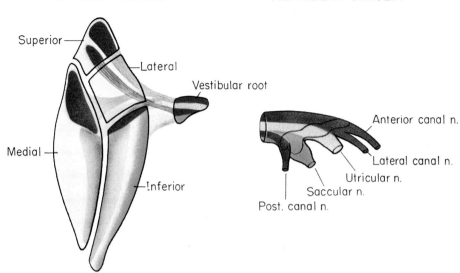

Figure 12-16. Diagrammatic representation of the relationship between portions of the vestibular ganglia and central fibers projecting to parts of the vestibular nuclear complex. The vestibular ganglia are shown in a modified transverse plane, while the vestibular nerve root and the vestibular nuclear complex are drawn in a stylized fashion, as they would appear in horizontal sections of the brain stem. Only the principal central projections of distinctive parts of the vestibular ganglia are shown. Portions of the vestibular ganglia innervating the cristae of the semicircular ducts (*red*) project primarily to the superior vestibular nucleus and rostral parts of the utricle project central fibers primarily to parts of the inferior and medial vestibular nuclei. Fibers from portions of the inferior vestibular ganglion innervating the macula of the saccule (*blue*), project mainly to dorsolateral parts of the inferior vestibular nucleus. Some cells in the vestibular ganglia project fibers to parts of all vestibular nuclei, so that each part of the labyrinth has a unique as well as common projection, within the vestibular nuclear complex. (Reproduced with permission from B. M. Stein and M. B. Carpenter: *American Journal of Anatomy,* **120:** 281–318, 1967.)

are large, stellate in shape and form clusters (268); this part of the nucleus receives most of the primary vestibular fibers.

Besides the main vestibular nuclei described above, there are several smaller accessory nuclei (268, 278), one of which consists of strands of cells between the root fibers of the vestibular nerve (interstitial nucleus of the vestibular nerve; Fig. 12-17).

Primary Vestibular Fibers. These fibers project to all four vestibular nuclei and the interstitial nucleus of the vestibular nerve, but their distribution has been considered to be differential (2640). Upon entering the brain stem, primary vestibular fibers bifurcate into ascending and descending branches. Ascending branches supply the superior vestibular nucleus, rostral parts of the medial vestibular nucleus, and give off collaterals to the ventral part of the lateral vestibular nucleus (Fig. 12-16). Descending branches form the so-called descending root of the vestibular nerve, which

provides fibers to the inferior vestibular nucleus and collaterals to the caudal parts of the medial vestibular nucleus (2429). Quantitatively the largest number of primary vestibular fibers pass to the inferior vestibular nucleus. Vestibular terminals are not distributed equally to all of the regions of the vestibular nuclei. Certain areas in each of the vestibular nuclei do not receive primary vestibular fibers (2640). In the superior vestibular nucleus, primary vestibular fibers terminate mainly in the central regions of the nucleus. In the lateral vestibular nucleus, primary vestibular fibers are found only in the ventral parts of the nucleus. Electron microscopic findings confirm that these fibers establish synaptic contact primarily with the soma and dendritic stems of small cells (1777). The large giant cells receive fewer synaptic endings from primary vestibular fibers. The dorsal half of the lateral vestibular nucleus is the largest regional area in this nuclear complex

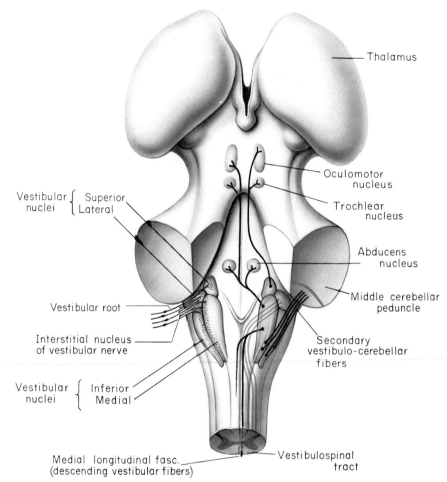

Figure 12-17. Schematic diagram of some of the principal fiber projections of the vestibular system. On the left the relationships and spatial disposition of the four main vestibular nuclei are indicated. Among the afferent root fibers are the cells of the interstitial nucleus of the vestibular nerve. Dotted areas in the vestibular nuclei represent the regions of the nuclear complex which receive the largest number of primary vestibular fibers. These areas are: (a) the ventral half of the lateral vestibular nucleus, (b) the lateral part of the medial vestibular nucleus, (c) the dorsomedial part of the inferior vestibular nucleus and (d) the central part of the superior vestibular nucleus. On the right, secondary projections from some of the individual vestibular nuclei are shown schematically. Fibers from the superior vestibular nucleus (*red*) ascend ipsilaterally in the medial longitudinal fasciculus (MLF) and terminate in parts of the trochlear and oculomotor nuclei. Ascending projections from the rostral part of the medial vestibular nucleus (*black*) to the nuclei of the extraocular muscles are predominantly crossed. A small number of uncrossed ascending fibers from lateral vestibular nucleus are not shown. Fibers from caudal parts of the medial vestibular nucleus descending in the MLF are shown in *black*. The somatotopically organized vestibulospinal tract (*blue*) arises only from the lateral vestibular nucleus. Secondary vestibulocerebellar fibers (*black*) arise from caudal parts of the inferior and medial vestibular nuclei.

devoid of primary vestibular fibers (1529, 2429, 2640). The medial vestibular nucleus receives primary vestibular fibers throughout large regions of its rostral part, but caudally terminations are mainly in lateral regions near the inferior vestibular nucleus (Fig. 12-16). Primary vestibular fibers are found throughout the rostrocaudal extent of the inferior vestibular nucleus, except in

its ventrolateral part (Figs. 12-16 and 12-17). A more recent silver degeneration study indicates that primary vestibular afferents are more widely distributed in the vestibular nuclei than previously recognized (1350). Following complete lesions of the vestibular ganglion, the terminal fields of vestibular nerve were found to extend to the cytoarchitectonic boundaries of all vestibular nuclei, except the lateral, where terminals were confined to a ventral region. Of the so-called accessory vestibular nuclei, only the interstitial nucleus of the vestibular nerve and cell group y (dorsal to the inferior cerebellar peduncle) receive primary vestibular fibers.

Studies of the central projections of cell groups of the vestibular ganglia that innervate distinctive parts of the labyrinth indicate a specific organization (2429). This organization in the monkey was determined by producing small lesions in specific parts of the vestibular ganglia and tracing degeneration: (a) distally to the receptor epithelium and (b) centrally into the vestibular nuclei (Fig. 12-16). Cells of the superior vestibular ganglion, innervating the cristae of the anterior and lateral ducts, give rise to central fibers which: (a) occupy rostral and lateral parts of the vestibular root and (b) project mainly to the superior vestibular nucleus and oral portions of the medial vestibular nucleus (Fig. 12-16). Cells of the superior vestibular ganglion, innervating the macula of the utricle, mainly descend in the dorsomedial part of the inferior vestibular nucleus. Collaterals of these fibers pass to dorsolateral parts of the medial vestibular nucleus caudally. Cells of the inferior vestibular ganglion, innervating the crista of the posterior duct, pass in caudal parts of the vestibular root and terminate mainly in portions of the superior and medial vestibular nuclei. Central fibers from cells of the inferior vestibular ganglion, innervating the saccular macula, mainly descend in dorsolateral parts of the inferior vestibular nucleus. Cell groups within the vestibular ganglia, innervating selectively individual receptor components of the labyrinth, have major unique central projections within the ipsilateral vestibular nuclei and less extensive projections to all parts of the complex. The interstitial nucleus of the vestibular nerve appears distinctive in that this nucleus receive fibers from all cell groups of the vestibular ganglia (Fig. 12-17).

Tritiated amino acids injected into the semicircular ducts in the monkey may be taken up by terminals in the sensory epithelium and transported to the vestibular ganglia and by the central processes of the bipolar cells (134). An autoradiograph of a sagittal section through the vestibular nu-

clei demonstrates the regions of termination of primary vestibular fibers (Fig. 12-18).

Primary vestibulocerebellar fibers traverse portions of the lateral and superior vestibular nuclei and enter the cerebellum via the juxtarestiform body. Most of these fibers are distributed to the cortex of the ipsilateral nodulus, uvula and flocculus (276). Studies in the monkey, based upon discrete lesions in specific parts of the vestibular ganglia, indicate that cells in all parts of these ganglia project fibers to the ipsilateral nodulus and uvula (415). These fibers appear to end as mossy fibers in the granular layer of cerebellar cortex. Cells of the vestibular ganglia innervating the cristae of the anterior and lateral ducts and the maculae of the utricle and saccule have distinctive regions of termination in the folia of the ipsilateral flocculus. While many of these fibers appear to end as mossy fi-

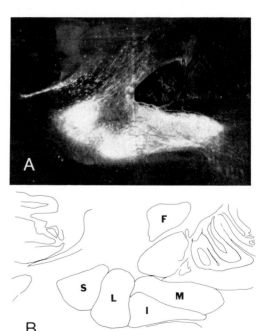

Figure 12-18. (*A*), Sagittal section through the brain stem in a rhesus monkey demonstrating transport of ^{3}H-labeled amino acids from the labyrinth to the vestibular nuclei in an autoradiograph (cresyl violet, dark field, × 20). (*B*), Outline drawings of the fastigial (*F*) and vestibular nuclei: S, superior vestibular nucleus; L, lateral vestibular nucleus; I, inferior vestibular nucleus; M, medial vestibular nucleus. Although primary vestibular afferents project to all ipsilateral vestibular nuclei, only the ventral half of the lateral vestibular receives terminals from this source.

bers, others enter the molecular layer of the cerebellar cortex as climbing fibers. Although a few primary vestibular fibers may end in the dentate nucleus, there is no conclusive evidence that such fibers terminate in the fastigial nucleus. At least one study suggests that primary vestibulocerebellar fibers are confined largely to the ipsilateral nodulus and flocculus and are relatively sparse (1351).

Afferent Projections to the Vestibular Nuclei. The vestibular nuclei receive a large number of afferent fibers from sources other than the vestibular ganglion. According to Brodal (268) vestibular afferents from the cerebellum outnumber those from any other source. Cerebellar projections to the vestibular nuclei arise from: (a) the "vestibular part," (b) the "spinal part" and (c) the fastigial nucleus. The "vestibular part" of the cerebellum, consisting of the flocculus, nodulus and ventral portion of the uvula, projects ipsilaterally chiefly to parts of the superior, medial and inferior vestibular nuclei (72). The lateral vestibular nucleus receives only a few afferents from this source. Projections from the "spinal part" of the cerebellum, represented mainly by the vermis of the anterior lobe, are ipsilateral to the dorsal part of the lateral vestibular nucleus and the dorsorostral part of the inferior vestibular nucleus (2643). The latter projection somatotopically links the forelimb region of the anterior lobe with the forelimb region of the lateral vestibular nucleus. These fibers, axons of Purkinje cells, are known to have a monosynaptic inhibitory influence upon neurons of the lateral vestibular nucleus mediated by γ-aminobutyric acid (GABA) (441, 781, 1189). Indirect projections from "spinal parts" of the cerebellum to the vestibular nuclei are relayed by the fastigial nuclei. The cortex of the cerebellar vermis projects upon the fastigial nucleus which in turn gives rise to vestibular projection. Fastigial efferent fibers follow a complex course, best described in relation to other efferent systems from the deep cerebellar nuclei (see p. 482, Chapter 14). Autoradiographic studies indicate that the fastigial nucleus projects bilaterally and nearly symmetrically upon ventral portions of the lateral and inferior vestibular nuclei (135). This pathway is regarded as excitatory in nature.

The vestibular nuclei do not receive descending fibers from the cerebral cortex, the corpus striatum, the superior colliculus or the nuclei of the posterior commissure (2043). Descending fibers from the interstitial nucleus of Cajal project via the medial longitudinal fasciculus to the medial vestibular nucleus. These fibers appear to be the only descending vestibular afferent fibers arising from cells within the brain stem.

Secondary Vestibular Fibers. The vestibular system and its projections constitute the most widely dispersed special sensory system in the neuraxis. The vestibular nuclei, which receive primary vestibular fibers, serve as a distributing center for secondary pathways. Secondary vestibular fibers project to specific portions of the cerebellum, certain motor cranial nerve nuclei and to all spinal levels. In addition to the primary vestibulocerebellar fibers described above, there are a number of secondary vestibulocerebellar fibers originating from specific portions of the inferior and medial vestibular nuclei (Fig. 12-17). These fibers arise from lateral and caudal parts of these nuclei, traverse the juxtarestiform body and project to the nodulus, uvula, flocculus and the fastigial nuclei. Within the cerebellum these fibers are distributed bilaterally, but with ipsilateral preponderance, except for fibers passing to the flocculus. The latter fibers are distributed ipsilaterally (286). The fastigial nuclei and certain portions of the cerebellar cortex give rise to fibers that project back to the vestibular nuclei to be distributed in a selective manner (135, 381, 2541, 2646). These cerebellar efferent fibers plus both primary and secondary vestibulocerebellar fibers mainly course medial to the inferior cerebellar peduncle in the *juxtarestiform body*. Thus the vestibular nuclei serve as an important relay station for the transmission of impulses to and from the cerebellum.

The cells of the lateral vestibular nucleus give rise to the uncrossed vestibulospinal tract, which descends throughout the length of the spinal cord in the anterior and lateral funiculi (Figs. 10-20, 10-21 and 12-17). These fibers, arising from cells of all sizes within the nucleus, are somatotopically organized (2041). In the brain stem, these fibers do not have a direct course. Upon leaving the lateral vestibular nucleus the fibers pass ventromedially and caudally, successively occupying positions dorsomedial to the motor nucleus of N. VII and the nucleus ambiguus; from a retro-olivary locus fibers pass into the spinal cord. The vestibulospinal tract has a more important functional relationship with the spinal cord than any other descending vestibular fiber system. The lateral vestibular nucleus also receives somatotopically organized afferent fibers from the fastigial nucleus and the cortex of the cerebellar vermis. Crossed and uncrossed fastigiovestibular fibers are distributed fairly symmetrically within the ventral half of the lateral vestibular nucleus (135). The modes of termination of fastigial fibers in the lateral vestibular nuclei are not conclusively established but few fibers appear to end on large neurons (2646). Cerebellovestibular fibers from the vermis, largely the anterior lobe, are distributed ipsilaterally mainly in the dorsal halves of the lateral and inferior vestibular nuclei. These fibers terminate upon cells of all sizes, but in the lateral vestibular nucleus the majority make synaptic contact with large cells (1776, 2643). Thus the lateral vestibular nucleus receives impulses from the vestibular nerve and various parts of the cerebellum, and conveys impulses to spinal levels that mediate responses in axial and appendicular musculature (280). Impulses relayed to spinal levels via the lateral vestibular nucleus have facilitating influences upon extensor muscle tone and spinal reflex activity.

Medial Longitudinal Fasciculus (MLF). Fibers from all of the vestibular nuclei pass medially in the region of the abducens nucleus and enter the MLF. Vestibular fibers in the MLF are both crossed and uncrossed and many bifurcate into ascending and descending branches (Figs. 10-20 and 12-17).

Descending vestibular fibers in the MLF projecting to spinal levels arise primarily, if not exclusively, in the medial vestibular nucleus. These fibers, both crossed and uncrossed, descend in the MLF until they reach the pyramidal decussation, where they shift ventrolaterally to enter the sulcomarginal region of the anterior funiculus. In their course they may project fibers into the lower brain stem reticular formation. Although these fibers are present bilat-

erally in the medulla, at spinal levels almost all fibers are ipsilateral. Some fibers may descend as far as upper thoracic segments, but most fibers end at cervical levels. Some vestibular fibers descending in the MLF synapse directly upon α motor neurons. Experimental evidence indicates that these fibers exert direct inhibitory influences upon cervical motor neurons (2742). The superior, lateral and inferior vestibular nuclei do not contribute descending fibers to the MLF that reach spinal levels (382, 1853, 2041).

The MLF also contains nonvestibular descending fibers from: (a) the interstitial nucleus of Cajal (interstitiospinal tract), (b) the superior colliculus (tectobulbar and tectospinal tracts, sometimes referred to as the predorsal bundle), (c) the pontine reticular formation (reticulospinal tract) and (d) more rostral brain stem nuclei projecting to particular portions of the inferior olivary complex. The largest group of descending fibers in the MLF are the pontine reticulospinal fibers (Figs. 10-10 and 10-22).

Ascending fibers in the MLF are mostly vestibular and arise from portions of all vestibular nuclei and the interstitial nucleus of the vestibular nerve (279). These ascending vestibular fibers project primarily to portions of the nuclei of the extraocular muscles (i.e., the abducens, trochlear and oculomotor) and bring the innervation of these muscles under the influence of vestibular, and possibly cerebellar, regulation. A small number of ascending fibers in the MLF bypass the oculomotor nucleus to terminate in the interstitial nucleus of Cajal (lateral to the MLF near the oculomotor nucleus) (Figs. 13-18, 13-19 and 13-20). Although it has been presumed that vestibular impulses projected rostrally to thalamic relay nuclei, identification of these nuclei has proved elusive. Physiological technics indicate that short latency vestibular responses are found in the monkey in the ventral posterior inferior (VPI) and the ventral posterolateral (VPL) thalamic nuclei (605–607, 1489). VPI is a distinctive cytoarchitectonic subdivision of the ventral posterior nucleus of the thalamus, located ventral to VPL and VPM. These authors suggest that VPI is closely associated with somesthetic areas of the cortex. Combined anatomical and physiological studies in the cat using horseradish peroxidase (HRP) suggest that most vestibular impulses project to the VPL nucleus of the thalamus contralaterally (199). Axoplasmic transport data suggest that ascending vestibular projection are bilateral and terminate in scattered regions of VPLo (pars oralis) and VPI (1423).

Ascending fibers in the MLF, arising from individual vestibular nuclei, have both differential and overlapping projections to the nuclei of the extraocular muscles (387, 1573). Fibers from the superior vestibular nucleus ascend exclusively (Fig. 12-17), enter the ipsilateral MLF rostral to the abducens nucleus and project primarily to the trochlear nucleus and the dorsal nucleus of the oculomotor complex (i.e., inferior rectus muscle) (Fig. 13-15). Ascending fibers from the medial vestibular nucleus enter the MLF at the level of the abducens nucleus, are both crossed and uncrossed, and project bilaterally, asymmetrically and differentially to the nuclei of the extraocular muscles. Projections of the medial vestibular nucleus are to: (a) the abducens nucleus (bilateral), (b) the contralateral trochlear nucleus, (c) the contralateral intermediate cell column (i.e., inferior oblique muscle) and (d) the ipsilateral ventral nucleus (i.e., medial rectus muscle) of the oculomotor complex (Fig. 13-15). Ascending fibers from the lateral vestibular nucleus arise only from ventral parts of the nucleus and are uncrossed. The inferior vestibular nucleus gives rise to relatively few fibers ascending in the MLF. Studies based upon the retrograde transport of HRP in the cat and monkey indicate that vestibular projections to the oculomotor nuclear complex are derived mainly from the superior and medial nuclei (951, 2426). The superior vestibular nucleus projects ipsilateral to the oculomotor complex, while projections from the medial vestibular nucleus and cell group y are bilateral.

In addition to the above ascending vestibular projections, the MLF contains ascending projections from abducens internuclear neurons that cross and terminate in specific portions of the oculomotor nuclear complex (107, 393, 951, 2394, 2425, 2426). This system of connections between the abducens nucleus of one side and that part of the oculomotor nucleus which innervates the contralateral medial rectus muscle

serves to mediate conjugate horizontal eye movements. In essence this coordinates lateral gaze which requires simultaneous contractions of the lateral rectus muscle on one side and the medial rectus muscle on the opposite side (Fig. 12-19).

The MLF, together with the tectospinal and tectobulbar tracts, represents a complex system of fibers which becomes myelinated very early in development. This bundle extends from the rostral part of the midbrain to the caudal medulla, where fibers pass into the sulcomarginal area of the anterior funiculus of the spinal cord. Below the level of the abducens nuclei most fibers of the bundle are descending; above these nuclei ascending fibers predominate.

The interaction between the vestibular nuclei of the two sides of the brain stem has been documented anatomically and physiologically (382, 1414, 2327). Studies based upon HRP indicate that commissural units are located mainly in the superior and medial vestibular nuclei (835). Since the superior and medial vestibular nuclei receive imputs largely from the semicircular ducts, commissural connections would appear to interrelate activities on the two sides resulting from stimulation of these portions of the labyrinth.

Efferent Vestibular System. The vestibular end organ receives an efferent innervation which arises bilaterally and symmetrically from cells located along the lateral border of the abducens nucleus and medial to the superior vestibular nucleus (837, 908, 2675). These neurons form a well-circumscribed cell column 500 μm in length containing about 200 cells in the squirrel monkey. Processes of these efferent neurons pass peripherally with the vestibular nerve to innervate the hair cells in the cristae of the semicircular ducts and the maculae of the utricle and saccule. Unlike the efferent cochlear bundle, vestibular efferent fibers appear to exert excitatory effects; these effects are bilateral upon neurons innervating each of the five end organs of the labyrinth (908). This excitatory activity cannot be converted to inhibition by changes in the parameters of stimulation or by variations in the afferent background discharge. Although the role of the vestibular efferent projection in vestibular function is unknown, it has been postulated that it may function to modulate the dynamic

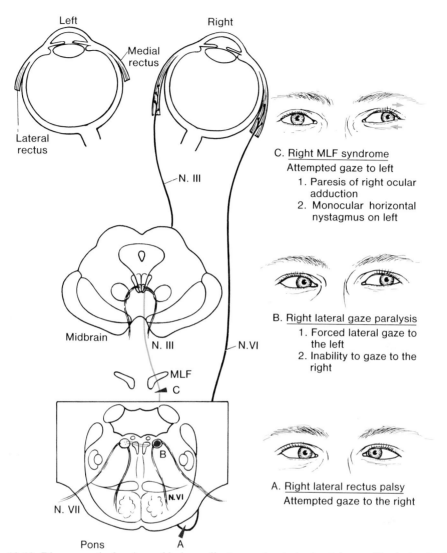

Figure 12-19. Diagrammatic drawings of lesions affecting conjugate horizontal gaze. The lesion (*red*) at *A*, involving the right abducens nerve as it leaves the brain stem, produces a paralysis of the right lateral rectus muscle. In the sketch of the eyes at *A* the patient is attempting to gaze to the right: the right eye is somewhat adducted and the left eye is fully adducted. This patient would experience diplopia on attempted right lateral gaze. The lesion (*red*) in the abducens nucleus (*B*) would destroy lower motor neurons and abducens internuclear neurons whose axons enter the opposite MLF and ascend to the ventral nucleus (which innervates the medial rectus muscle) of the oculomotor complex. A patient with such a lesion would have a right lateral gaze paralysis and both eyes would be forcefully directed to the left field of gaze. A unilateral lesion (*red*) in the right MLF (*blue*) at *C* would interrupt axons of abducens internuclear neurons arising from the left abducens nucleus. This lesion would produce dissociated horizontal eye movements. On attempted gaze to the left there would be a paresis of right ocular adduction (*C*) and monocular horizontal nystagmus in the left abducting eye, indicated by *arrows*.

range of afferents to match expected accelerations.

FUNCTIONAL CONSIDERATIONS

Physiological studies (497, 500, 756, 2494) indicate that secondary vestibular fibers and impulses transmitted via the MLF are essential for conjugate eye movements. The investigations cited have shown that selective stimulation of individual semicircular ducts, or of the nerves from the ducts, produces conjugate deviations of the eyes in specific directions. Primary responses obtained by this type of stimulation are abolished following section of the MLF rostral to the abducens nuclei. The observation that nystagmus produced by labyrinthine stimulation is not abolished by section of MLF (152, 1526, 1527, 2399) suggests that this vestibular phenomenon probably involves circuits within the reticular formation.

Clinically, lesions involving the MLF rostral to the abducens nuclei produce a disturbance of conjugate horizontal eye movements known as *anterior internuclear ophthalmoplegia* (454, 489, 2401, 2405). The salient features of this syndrome are: (a) a paresis or paralysis of ocular adduction on attempted lateral gaze to the opposite side, (b) horizontal nystagmus, either more pronounced or exclusively present in the abducting eye, and (c) preservation of ocular convergence. In most of the clinical cases examined pathologically, brain stem lesions have been so extensive as to preclude reliable anatomical correlations. Available data indicate that paresis of ocular adduction on attempted lateral gaze to the opposite side occurs ipsilateral to unilateral lesions of the MLF (Fig. 12-19). Thus, with a right unilateral lesion of the MLF, the patient could abduct the left eye on attempted gaze to the left, but the right eye could not be adducted. Monocular nystagmus would occur in the left abducting eye.

Bilateral lesions of the MLF rostral to the abducens nuclei, in patients with demyelinating disease, may result in dissociated horizontal eye movements on attempted lateral gaze to both the right and left sides. These findings have been confirmed experimentally in the monkey (152, 153, 2311). In the monkey the syndrome has been produced unilaterally and bilaterally by discrete lesions in the MLF rostral to the abducens nucleus (405, 418). Ascending degeneration resulting from unilateral lesions in the MLF rostral to the abducens nucleus is confined to the ipsilateral MLF and is distributed differentially to the ventral nucleus of the oculomotor complex, a cell group that innervates the ipsilateral medial rectus muscle. Such lesions produce no degeneration in any of the contralateral nuclei of the extraocular muscles. The paresis of ocular adduction on attempted lat-

eral gaze to the opposite side is due to interruption of ascending fibers from abducens internuclear neurons after they have crossed to the opposite MLF (393). An adequate explanation for the monocular horizontal nystagmus seen in this syndrome has eluded both clinicians and investigators. Large bilateral lesions of the MLF between the abducens nuclei in the monkey may produce bilateral paresis of all horizontal eye movements (both abducting and adducting eye movements), without impairment of vertical eye movements or ocular convergence. Unilateral lesions of individual vestibular nuclei in the monkey do not produce dissociated (i.e., disconjugate) eye movements (384, 1573, 2595).

Mechanisms governing equilibrium (i.e., maintenance of appropriate body position) and orientation in three-dimensional space are largely reflex in character and depend upon afferent inputs from several sources. The most important of these are: (a) kinesthetic sense conveyed by the posterior column-medial lemniscal system from receptors in joints and joint capsules, (b) impulses conveyed centrally by spinocerebellar systems from stretch receptors in muscles and tendons, (c) the suprasegmental kinesthetic sense provided by the vestibular end organ and (d) visual input from the retina. Among the sensory systems that contribute to the maintenance of equilibrium, the labyrinth constitutes a highly specialized receptor that is stimulated by the *position* or *changes in position* of the head. When the head is moved, either by contraction of the neck muscles or by shifting the body as a whole, the cristae are stimulated and effect compensatory reflex adjustments of the eyes and limb muscles needed for the particular movement (kinetostatic reflexes). As long as the position of the head remains unchanged the new attitude is sustained by impulses originating in the macula of the utricle. The sustaining (static) reflexes are initiated by the gravitational pull of the otolithic membrane on the macular hair cells.

The vestibulospinal tracts and descending fibers from the pontine reticular formation exert a strong excitatory influence upon muscle tone, particularly extensor tone. Descending vestibular impulses in the MLF exert inhibitory influences upon cervical motor neurons (2742). Normally muscle tone is maintained by a balance of inhibitory and facilitatory influences from higher centers, a large part of which are considered to be mediated by the brain stem reticular formation. If the influences of these higher centers are removed in an experimental animal, such as the cat, by transection of the brain stem at the intercollicular level (i.e., between the superior and inferior colliculi), a condition known as *decerebrate rigidity* develops. This condition is characterized by tremendously increased tone in the antigravity muscles. Increased muscle tone seen in this condition appears to be an expression of facilitation of γ motor neurons, which thereby increase the firing rate of muscle spindles; this in turn influences the firing of α motor neurons to maintain the tonic state (Fig. 9-34). In this experimental preparation, the facilitatory pathways of the reticular formation and the vestibulospinal tract remain active, while inhibitory elements of the reticular formation no longer function. Inhibitory regions of the reticular formation are considered to be dependent upon descending impulses from higher levels, while the facilitating regions of the reticular formation receive impulses from ascending afferent systems. This form of rigidity can be abolished, or reduced, by destruction of the labyrinth, the vestibular nuclei or the vestibulospinal tract. Surgical section of several successive dorsal or ventral spinal roots will abolish the phenomenon segmentally.

Labyrinthine stimulation, irritation or disease cause vertigo and objective signs such as unsteadiness, staggering, postural deviation, deviations of the eyes and nystagmus. In some instances nausea, vomiting, vasomotor changes and prostration occur. The term *vertigo* refers to a subjective sense of rotation, either of the individual or his environment; this term should not be regarded as a synonym for dizziness or giddiness. *Nystagmus*, one of the most prominent objective signs, is a rhythmic involuntary oscillation of the eyes characterized by alternate slow and rapid ocular excursions. Clinically, nystagmus is named for the direction of the rapid phase, but the slow phase is the primary physiological movement. The nausea and vomiting which occur with motion sickness are mainly the result of stimulation of the utricle. Since the labyrinths are antagonistic to each other, the elimination of one causes the other to be overactive until accommodation takes place.

Tests for vestibular function, based upon stimulation of the semicircular canals or vestibular nerve endings, include: (a) the rotating chair test (Bárány chair), (b) the caloric test (i.e., thermal stimulation which changes the temperature of the endolymph) and (c) the galvanic test which stimulates nerve endings directly. In the first of these testing procedures, the slow phase of the nystagmus, deviation of the eyes, postural deviation and pastpointing are all in the direction of the previous rotation, and can be correlated with the direction of endolymphatic flow. The sensation of vertigo is in the opposite direction (609). It is not possible to test the otoliths directly.

FACIAL NERVE

The facial nerve and the intermediate nerve usually are discussed together although they subserve separate functions (Figs. 12-1 and 12-2). Functional components of these nerves include: (a) *special visceral efferent* (SVE, branchiomotor) *fibers*, (b) *general visceral efferent* (GVE, parasympathetic) *fibers*, (c) *special visceral afferent* (SVA, taste) *fibers* and (d) a few *general somatic afferent* (GSA, sensory) *fibers*.

Special visceral efferent (SVE) *fibers* of the motor component innervate the muscles of facial expression, the platysma, the buccinator, the posterior belly of the digastric and the stapedius muscles. The motor nucleus of N. VII forms a column of multipolar neurons in the ventrolateral tegmentum dorsal to the superior olivary nucleus and ventromedial to the spinal trigeminal nucleus (Figs. 12-1, 12-2, 12-20 and 12-21).

The facial nucleus is composed of several distinct cell groups (544, 1927, 2629) which innervate specific facial muscles. Most authors recognize at least four cell groups, designated as dorsomedial, ventromedial, intermediate and lateral. The dorsomedial cell group give rise to the posterior auricular nerve which innervates auricular muscles and the occipital muscle. The ramus colli which innervates the platysma muscle arises from be ventromedial cell group.

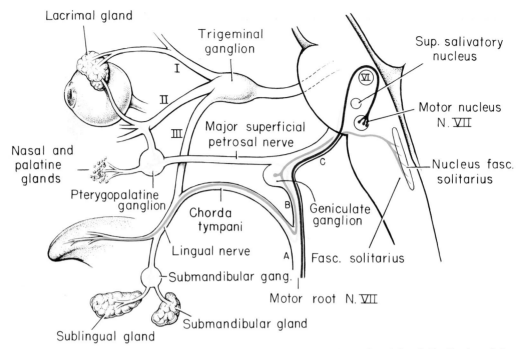

Figure 12-20. Diagram showing the functional components, organization and peripheral distribution of the facial nerve. Special visceral efferent fibers (motor) are shown in *red*. General visceral efferent fibers (parasympathetic) are in *yellow*, and special visceral afferent fibers (taste) are in *blue*. *A, B,* and *C* denote lesions of the facial nerve at the stylomastoid foramen, distal to the geniculate ganglion, and proximal to the geniculate ganglion. Disturbances resulting from lesions at these locations are described in the text (pp. 388–389).

Cells in the medial group are considered to innervate the stapedius muscle (217). The temporal and zygomatic branches of the facial nerve, related to the intermediate cell group, supply the frontalis, orbicularis oculi, the corrugator supercilli and the zygomaticus. The lateral cell group gives rise to the buccal branches which innervate the buccinator muscle and the buccolabial muscles. It is uncertain as to which cell groups innervate the stylohyoid and the posterior belly of the digastric muscle (544). Comparisons of the cell groups of the facial nucleus in animals and man (2629) reveal a close correspondence, except that in man the lateral cell group (buccolabial muscles) is especially prominent while the medial cell group is very small.

A few muscle spindles have been described in facial muscles (227, 2628). The presence of muscle spindles suggests the existence of γ efferent fibers, and leads to the assumption that γ neurons are mixed with α neurons in the facial nucleus.

Efferent fibers from the facial motor nucleus emerge from its dorsal surface and project dorsomedially into the floor of the fourth ventricle. These fibers pass medial toward the abducens nucleus and ascend for a short distance longitudinally in the floor of the fourth ventricle dorsal to the MLF (Fig. 12-21). Near the oral pole of the abducens nucleus, root fibers of the facial nerve make a sharp lateral bend around the rostral border of the abducens nucleus and pass ventrolaterally. In their course the fibers pass medial to the spinal trigeminal complex, lateral to the superior olivary nucleus and emerge from the brain stem near the caudal border of the pons, at the cerebellopontine angle (Figs. 11-32, 12-1, 12-4, 12-6 and 12-7). Root fibers looping around the abducens nucleus form the *internal genu* of the facial nerve.

The facial motor nucleus receives afferent fibers from a number of sources. Among these are: (a) secondary trigeminal fibers from the spinal trigeminal nucleus (348, 403) involved in corneal and other trigeminofacial reflexes, (b) direct corticobulbar fibers (Fig. 11-30) which project bilaterally, but with important regional differ-

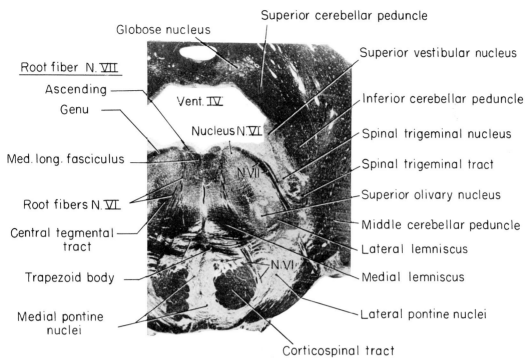

Superior cerebellar peduncle

Globose nucleus

Root fiber N. VII

Ascending

Genu

Vent. IV

Superior vestibular nucleus

Inferior cerebellar peduncle

Nucleus N. VI

Spinal trigeminal nucleus

Med. long. fasciculus

N VII

Spinal trigeminal tract

Root fibers N. VI

Superior olivary nucleus

Central tegmental
tract

Middle cerebellar peduncle

Lateral lemniscus

Trapezoid body

N VI

Medial lemniscus

Medial pontine
nuclei

Lateral pontine nuclei

Corticospinal tract

Figure 12-21. Transverse section of the adult pons through the abducens nucleus showing the root fibers of the abducens and facial nerves (Weigert's myelin stain, photograph).

ences (1404), (c) indirect corticobulbar fibers which convey impulses to the facial nucleus via relays in the reticular formation (1404, 1405, 2634) and (d) crossed rubrobulbar fibers (542) which project only to cell groups (i.e., dorsomedial and intermediate) innervating the upper facial muscles. In addition descending fibers from the mesencephalic reticular formation project ipsilaterally to portions of the facial nucleus (542). Secondary or tertiary auditory fibers, considered to reach the facial nucleus, are thought to mediate certain acousticofacial reflexes. These reflexes include closing of the eyes in response to a sudden loud noise, and contraction of the stapedius muscle to dampen the movements of the ear ossicles. Recent studies of the neuronal organization of acoustic middle ear reflexes indicate that pathways involved in the stapedius reflex involve three or four neurons: (a) primary auditory neurons, (b) processes of cells of the ventral cochlear nucleus which form the trapezoid body and (c) neurons in the ipsilateral and contralateral medial superior olivary nucleus which project to facial motor neurons that innervate the stapedius muscle (217). On clinical grounds it has

been suggested that impulses from the thalamus or globus pallidus may reach portions of the facial nucleus indirectly, since pathology involving these structures has been said to produce a *mimetic* or *emotional* type facial palsy (1725, 1726). The pathways which may be involved in this type of facial palsy are unknown.

The *intermediate nerve*, which emerges between the facial motor root and the vestibular nerve (Fig. 12-2), contains afferent and general visceral efferent fibers. Afferent fibers (SVA and GSA) arise from cells of the geniculate ganglion, located at the external genu of the facial nerve (Fig. 12-20). *Special visceral afferent* (SVA) *fibers* convey gustatory sense (taste) from the anterior two-thirds of the tongue via the chorda tympani nerve. Centrally these fibers enter the solitary fasciculus and terminate upon cells in the rostral part of the solitary nucleus, sometimes referred to as the gustatory nucleus. General somatic afferent (GSA) fibers convey cutaneous sensory impulses from the external auditory meatus and the region back of the ear; centrally these fibers enter the dorsal part of the spinal trigeminal tract (142).

There are observations which suggest that the facial nerve may carry impulses of deep pain and deep pressure from the face (1178). In some cases in which the trigeminal nerve has been sectioned for the relief of facial neuralgia, deep pain sense due to pressure has persisted. The question is not settled, but most investigations suggest that both deep and superficial pain probably are mediated by the trigeminal nerve (2366).

General visceral efferent (GVE) *fibers* in the intermediate nerve classically are described as arising from the *superior salivatory nucleus*. This poorly defined nucleus probably consists of scattered neurons in the dorsolateral reticular formation (Figs. 11-18, 11-19 and 12-20). Retrograde transport studies indicate that preganglionic parasympathetic neurons form an uninterrupted dorsal cell column extending from the medulla into the pons (516). Cells of the dorsal motor nucleus of the vagus form the caudal portion of this column; cells in more rostral regions are less compact and distributed over a wide region of the reticular formation. In the pons cells of this column lie between the nucleus of the solitary tract and the facial motor nucleus. The overlapping origins of neurons contributing to the glossopharyngeal and intermediate nerves raises a question concerning the appropriateness of a nomenclature that distinguishes separate salivatory nuclei as inferior and superior.

Preganglionic parasympathetic fibers from what is called the superior salivatory nucleus pass peripherally as a component of the intermediate nerve, but near the external genu of the facial nerve they divide into two groups: (a) one group that passes to the pterygopalatine ganglion via the major superficial petrosal nerve and (b) another group that projects via the chorda tympani nerve to the submandibular ganglion (Fig. 12-20). Synapses with postganglionic neurons occur in the pterygopalatine and submandibular ganglia. Postganglionic fibers from the pterygopalatine ganglion give rise to secretory and vasomotor fibers that innervate the lacrimal gland and the mucous membrane of the nose and mouth. Postganglionic parasympathetic fibers from the submandibular ganglion pass to the submandibular and sublingual salivary glands.

Lesions of the Facial Nerve (*Bell's palsy*). Lesions producing paralysis of facial movements, the sometimes disturbances of taste and secretory function, may involve fibers of the facial nerve within the brain stem or in their peripheral course. The particular deficits which result depend upon the location of the lesion and its extent. A complete lesion of the motor part of the facial nerve as it emerges from the stylomastoid foramen (*A*, Fig. 12-20) produces paralysis of all ipsilateral facial movements. The patient is unable to wrinkle the forehead, close the eye, show the teeth, purse the lips or whistle. On the side of the lesion the palpebral fissure is widened, the nasolabial fold is flattened and the corner of the mouth droops. Although corneal sensation is present, the corneal reflex is lost on the side of the lesion because motor fibers participating in this reflex are destroyed. A lesion of this nerve distal to the geniculate ganglion (*B*, Fig. 12-20) produces all of the deficits found with a lesion at *A*, plus impairment of secretions from the sublingual and submandibular salivary glands, hyperacusis and sometimes impairment of taste over the anterior two-thirds of the tongue. Impairment of salivary secretion results from interruption of preganglionic parasympathetic fibers from the superior salivatory nucleus. *Hyperacusis* is caused by paralysis of the stapedius muscle, which normally functions to dampen the oscillations of the ear ossicles. Taste may not always be impaired by such lesions since some fibers may take an aberrant course with the major superficial petrosal nerve. Lesions of the facial nerve proximal to the geniculate ganglion (*C*, Fig. 12-20) produce all of the deficits encountered with lesions at *A* and *B* and in addition, invariably result in complete loss of taste over the anterior two-thirds of the tongue. Lacrimation also is impaired on the side of the lesion as a consequence of destruction of parasympathetic fibers to the pterygopalatine (sphenopalatine) ganglion. With complete lesions in this location no regeneration of sensory fibers takes place. Aberrant regeneration of preganglionic parasympathetic fibers may occur, since the cell bodies lie within the central nervous system. In this aberrant regeneration, fibers previously synapsing upon postganglionic neurons of the submandibular ganglion established new relationships with cells of the pterygopalatine ganglion. Thus a stimulus which previously produced a salivary response may provoke lacrimation on the side of the lesion (syndrome of "crocodile tears"). The true etiology of Bell's palsy is poorly understood. It is tacitly presumed that most facial palsies of this type are due to compression of the nerve secondary to an unexplained swelling in the bony facial canal.

Central lesions involving corticobulbar and corticoreticular fibers projecting upon reticular neurons, which in turn discharge upon cells of the facial nucleus, produce a marked weakness of muscles in the lower half of the face contralaterally, especially in the perioral region. Muscles of the upper facial region concerned with wrinkling the forehead, frowning and closing the eyes are not affected. The accepted explanation of this upper motor neuron facial paralysis is that corticobulbar fibers projecting to the upper part of the facial nucleus (supplying muscles of the upper face and forehead) are distributed bilaterally, while corticobulbar projections to the lower part of the facial nucleus (supplying muscles of the lower face) are predominantly crossed. Although a completely satisfactory explanation is still lacking as to why a capsular hemiplegia in man is accompanied by paresis only in the lower facial muscles, the anatomical observations of Kuypers (1405) support the accepted thesis. This author found direct bilateral corticobulbar projections to the facial nucleus, but noted that ventral cell groups (regarded as innervating lower facial muscles) of the contralateral facial nucleus received more fibers than the same cell groups of the ipsilateral facial nucleus.

Even in the presence of a central type facial paralysis, as described above, mimetic or emotional innervation of the facial muscles may be preserved. In response to a genuine emotional stimulus, the muscles of the lower face will contract symmetrically while smiling or laughing. Actually, contractions of facial muscles on the paretic side may begin earlier and last longer than on the normal side (1726). Mimetic or emotional innervation of facial muscles is largely involuntary. Evidence suggests that impulses from higher levels of the neuraxis, other than those arising in the cerebral cortex, must reach the facial nuclei and bring about emotional facial expression. The neural mechanism for emotional facial innervation appears distinct and separate from that controlling voluntary facial movement. Thus two different types of central facial paresis are recognized, one concerned with voluntary facial movement, and another involving emotional facial expression. Each of these types of central facial paresis can occur alone, since the central pathways are different, but with certain lesions both voluntary and mimetic facial paralyses can occur together. The neuroanatomical pathways mediating emotional facial innervation are unknown.

ABDUCENS NERVE

The abducens is the motor nerve (GSE) innervating the lateral rectus muscle of the eye. The nucleus forms a column, about 3 mm in length, of typical somatic motor cells in the lateral part of the medial eminence (Figs. 12-3, 12-7, and 12-21). Fibers of the facial nerve form a complicated loop about the nucleus. Root fibers of the abducens nerve emerge from the medial aspect of the nucleus and pass ventrally through the pontine tegmentum and lateral to the corticospinal tract (Figs. 12-1, 12-7 and 12-21). They emerge from the brain stem at the caudal border of the pons (Figs. 11-1, 11-18 and A-7). This slender nerve in its long intracranial course traverses the cavernous sinus and the superior orbital fissure *en route* to the lateral rectus muscle.

Axonal transport and physiological studies indicate that the abducens nerve may be unique among all motor cranial nerves in that its nucleus appears to contain: (a) typical motor neurons giving rise to root fibers that innervate the lateral rectus muscle and (b) internuclear neurons whose axons cross the midline and ascend via the contralateral MLF to specific subdivisions of the oculomotor nuclear complex (107, 393, 834, 951, 1096, 2394, 2425, 2426). Retrograde labeling technics suggest that axons of about 50% of the cells in the abducens nucleus may be retained within the brain stem (2425). Abducens internuclear neurons are uniformly distributed throughout the nucleus and although neurons contributing fibers to the nerve root are slightly larger than internuclear neurons these two cell populations cannot be distinguished by simple morphological criteria (2394).

The abducens nucleus receives afferent inputs from the medial vestibular nuclei, the reticular formation and the superior vestibular ganglion (836, 948, 1578). Afferent fibers from the medial vestibular nucleus are predominantly ipsilateral and both populations of abducens neurons receive the same profile of disynaptic excitation and inhibition from the labyrinth (107). Abducens nucleus afferents from the *paramedian pontine reticular formation* (PPRF) are primarily uncrossed, while those from the vestibular ganglion are ipsilateral. The nucleus prepositus hypoglossi which receives a vestibular input is said to project bilaterally to the abducens nuclei (836). Corticobulbar fibers convey impulses to abducens nuclei bilaterally via intercalated neurons in the reticular formation (Fig. 11-30).

Lesions of the abducens nerve in the brain stem, or in its long intracranial course, cause ipsilateral paralysis of the lateral rectus muscle (Fig. 12-19). Because contraction of the medial rectus muscle on the affected side is unopposed, the eye is strongly adducted. The contralateral eye is unaffected and can move in all directions. The patient has diplopia (double vision) on attempting to gaze to the side of the lesion; two images are seen side by side. This is called horizontal diplopia. *Diplopia* results because light reflected by an object in the visual field does not fall upon corresponding points of the two retinae.

Lateral Gaze Paralysis. Unilateral lesions of the abducens nucleus produce a weakness, or paralysis, of lateral gaze toward the side of the lesion. The syndrome of *"lateral gaze paralysis"* differs from a simple paralysis of the lateral rectus muscle in that both eyes are forcefully and conjugately directed to the side opposite the lesion, and movement of both eyes toward the side of the lesion is severely limited, or impossible (Fig. 12-19). Ocular convergence usually is preserved. The abducens appears to be the only motor cranial nerve in which disturbances associated with lesions of root fibers and nucleus are not identical.

All ocular movements, whether horizontal, vertical or rotatory, require reciprocal activity in the extraocular muscles producing these movements. Conjugate lateral gaze requires simultaneous appropriate contractions of the lateral rectus muscle on one side and the medial rectus muscle of the opposite side. The central neural mechanisms underlying conjugate eye movements are just beginning to be understood. The observation that paralysis of vertical or horizontal eye movements can occur independently implies that there are separate anatomical sites at some distance from each other that generate vertical and horizontal eye movements. However many conjugate eye movements have both vertical and horizontal components so precisely synchronized that centers controlling vertical and horizontal eye movements must be functionally connected and coordinated. Considerable evidence suggests that the pontine "center for lateral gaze" and the abducens nucleus probably constitute a single entity (386, 393, 407, 951, 2394, 2425).

The localized region most concerned with vertical eye movements lies in the tegmental area rostral to the oculomotor complex in the zone of transition between diencephalon and mesencephalon (337). Large cells in this area lie among fibers of the MLF and have been referred to as the *rostral interstitial nucleus of the MLF*, an entity distinct from interstitial of Cajal which lies lateral to the oculomotor complex. The important question as to how horizontal and vertical components of conjugate eye movements are coordinated suggests that the PPRF which projects directly to the abducens nucleus and to the rostral interstitial nucleus of the MLF may be the encoding site (337). Bilateral lesions of the PPRF may cause paralysis of both horizontal and vertical gaze (151). Projections from the PPRF to the abducens nucleus are primarily uncrossed; those to the rostral interstitial nucleus of the MLF also are uncrossed and ascend outside of the MLF. The rostral interstitial nucleus of the MLF projects ipsilaterally to the oculomotor nuclear complex (2426).

Discrete lesions in the abducens nucleus in the monkey produce paralysis of ipsilateral lateral gaze that is enduring (407). Such lesions produce degeneration in the root fibers of the abducens nerve and ascending degeneration in the contralateral MLF. These ascending fibers are distributed differentially to the contralateral ventral nucleus of the oculomotor complex, a cell group innervating the medial rectus muscle on that side. Labeling of cells of the abducens nucleus with ³H-labeled amino acids results in transport of the isotope in the same manner as described for degeneration studies (393) (Figs. 12-22 and 13-17). Thus lateral gaze paralysis due to lesions of the abducens nucleus appears to be due to destruction of both populations of neurons that compose this nucleus, namely: (a) motor neurons that supply root fibers innervating the ipsilateral lateral rectus muscle and (b) abducens internuclear neurons that simultaneously excite oculomotor neurons that innervate the contralateral medial rectus muscle. Lesions involving the abducens nerve anywhere in its long course do not affect abducens internuclear neurons.

Lesions of the medial longitudinal fasciculus rostral to the abducens nucleus produce paresis of ipsilateral ocular adduction on attempted lateral gaze to the opposite side (i.e., anterior internuclear ophthalmoplegia). Such a lesion in the monkey produces ascending degeneration in the MLF selectively distributed to the ipsilateral ventral nucleus of oculomotor complex (418). These data have suggested that the paresis of ocular adduction which forms one of the principal features of anterior internuclear ophthalmoplegia is a consequence of interruption of the crossed ascending axons of abducens internuclear neurons in the MLF (Fig. 12-19). Experimental studies have shown that lesions limited to individual vestibular nuclei do not produce paresis of ocular adduction (1573).

Because of the proximity of emerging root fibers of the abducens nerve to the corticospinal tract, lesions in the caudal pons involving both of these structures produce the so-called *middle alternating hemiplegia* (Fig. 11-30). This syndrome is characterized by paralysis of the ipsilateral lateral rectus muscle and a contralateral hemiplegia. This condition resembles the *inferior alternating hemiplegia* seen with comparable medullary lesions which involve the hypoglossal nerve and the medullary pyramid.

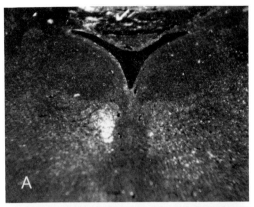
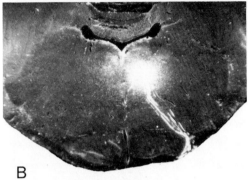

Figure 12-22. Dark field photomicrographs of transport of ³H-labeled amino acids injected into the right abducens nucleus in a rhesus monkey. In (*B*) anterograde transport from the injection site is seen ipsilaterally in the root fibers of the abducens nerve and crossing the midline to ascend in fibers in the medial longitudinal fasciculus (MLF). Ascending transport via the contralateral MLF seen in (*A*) is a consequence of labeling abducens internuclear neurons (*A*, ×18; *B*, ×6). (Reproduced with permission from M. B. Carpenter and R. R. Batton: *Journal of Comparative Neurology*, **189**: 191–209, 1980.)

ROSTRAL PONS

Transverse sections through the upper pons at the level of root fibers of the trigeminal nerve (Figs. 12-23, 12-24 and A-8) reveal important changes when compared with sections at lower pontine levels (Figs. 12-2, 12-4 and 12-21). The fourth ventricle is narrower, although its roof is still formed by the cerebellum. Within the cerebellum portions of all the deep cerebellar nuclei can be seen (Fig. 12-23), and fibers of the inferior and middle cerebellar peduncles enter the cerebellum close to each other (Fig. 12-23). At slightly higher levels fibers of the superior cerebellar peduncle form the dorsolateral wall of the fourth ventricle (Fig. 12-24).

The ventral portion of the pons is larger than at lower levels but still contains trans-

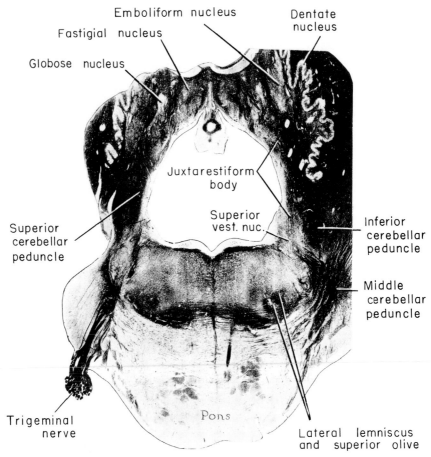

Emboliform nucleus

Dentate nucleus

Fastigial nucleus

Globose nucleus

Juxtarestiform body

Superior vest. nuc.

Superior cerebellar peduncle

Inferior cerebellar peduncle

Middle cerebellar peduncle

Trigeminal nerve

Pons

Lateral lemniscus and superior olive

Figure 12-23. Section of pons, pontine tegmentum, and part of cerebellum through the root of the trigeminal nerve of 1-month infant. (Weigert's myelin stain, photograph).

verse and longitudinal fibers, as well as large masses of pontine nuclei. Corticospinal and corticopontine tracts here consist of numerous fiber bundles less compactly arranged than in the caudal pons. Fibers within the raphe of the pons are probably reticulocerebellar fibers arising from cells in the pontine tegmentum (Fig. 12-24).

In the dorsal part of the pons the medial lemniscus is traversed by the transverse fibers of the trapezoid body. Lateral to the medial lemniscus and closely associated with fibers of the trapezoid body is the rostral pole of the superior olivary nucleus (Fig. 12-23). Ventrolaterally the lateral lemniscus is becoming a well-defined bundle (Fig. 12-24). The spinothalamic and anterior spinocerebellar tracts are located lateral to the medial lemniscus. The position

of the medial longitudinal fasciculus is unchanged from lower levels. Longitudinally cut fibers of the facial genu appear lateral to the medial longitudinal fasciculus (Fig. 12-24). Fibers of the central tegmental tract form a fairly discrete bundle in the reticular formation dorsal to the lateral part of the medial lemniscus (Fig. 12-24).

Pontine Reticular Formation. This cell group, occupying the central core of the tegmentum, is somewhat reduced in size. Dorsal to the facial genu the nucleus of the medial eminence remains. The central reticular area contains the *nucleus reticularis pontis oralis*, the rostral continuation of the more caudal pontine reticular nucleus (Fig. 12-25). This cell group extends rostrally into the caudal mesencephalon, where its oral boundaries become indistinct. The more caudal part of this nuclear mass contains scattered giant cells, like those which characterize the medial two-thirds of the medullary reticular formation. Some of the larger cells at this level give rise to the uncrossed reticulospinal fibers; others give rise to ascending fibers which pass rostrally in the central tegmental tract. A single cell with a dichotomizing axon may project fibers both rostrally and caudally. Ascending fibers from parts of the nuclei reticularis pontis oralis and caudalis pass to parts of the intralaminar nuclei of the thalamus. These ascending fibers and those originating more caudally in the brain stem participate in activation of broad regions of the cerebral cortex.

In the ventral part of the tegmentum immediately dorsal to the medial lemnisci is a moderately large group of multipolar cells known as the *nucleus reticularis tegmenti pontis*, or the reticulotegmental nucleus (Fig. 12-25). These cells have been considered as a medial tegmental extension of the pontine nuclei, which they resemble in certain respects. Portions of the reticulotegmental nucleus receive a bilateral and an ipsilateral projection from the frontal and parietal cortex (271). In addition, this nucleus receives a large bundle of cerebellar efferent fibers via the descending division of the superior cerebellar peduncle (283, 411). Since this nucleus projects virtually all its fibers to the cerebellum, it must play a role in integrating impulses from the cerebral cortex and from portions of the cerebellum, prior to their projection to the cerebellum. Projections of this nucleus to the cerebellar vermis are both crossed and uncrossed, while those to the hemisphere are entirely crossed (276a). In the raphe region dorsal to the reticulotegmental nucleus is the *superior central nucleus*, a closely packed aggregation of relatively small cells. This nucleus is more prominent at isthmus levels (Figs. 12-25, 12-29 and 12-30).

Afferent root fibers of the trigeminal nerve traverse the lateral portion of the pons, reach the dorsolateral pontine tegmentum and terminate in specific nuclei of the trigeminal nerve. Lateral to the entering root fibers is a large gray cellular mass, the *nucleus sensorius principalis* of the trigeminal nerve (Fig. 12-25). Small groups of root fibers can be seen entering this nucleus (Figs. 12-23 and 12-24). Medial to

the trigeminal root fibers and the principal sensory nucleus is a smaller oval collection of large cells whose efferent fibers emerge medial to the afferent fibers. This is the *motor nucleus* of the trigeminal nerve. A small bundle of afferent fibers coursing dorsally between the motor and sensory nuclei toward the ventricular surface constitutes the *mesencephalic tract of the trigeminal nerve* (Fig. 12-24). Although these are afferent fibers, they arise from large unipolar cells situated in the central gray matter along the lateral border of the ventricle (Figs. 12-24 and 12-25).

TRIGEMINAL NERVE

The trigeminal, the largest cranial nerve, contains both sensory and motor fibers (Figs. 11-1 and 12-23). *General somatic afferent* (GSA) *fibers* convey both exteroceptive and proprioceptive impulses. Exteroceptive impulses of touch, pain and thermal sense are transmitted from: (a) the skin of the face and forehead (Fig. 7-13), (b) the mucous membranes of the nose, the nasal sinuses and the oral cavity, (c) the teeth and (d) extensive portions of the cranial dura. Impulses concerned with deep pressure and kinesthesis sense are conveyed from the teeth, periodontium, the hard palate and temporomandibular joint. In addition, afferent fibers convey impulses arising from stretch receptors in the muscles of mastication. *Special visceral efferent fibers* (SVE; branchiomotor) innervate the muscles of mastication, the tensor tympani and the tensor veli palatini. Afferent fibers constitute the sensory root while efferent fibers form the smaller motor root.

Trigeminal Ganglion. The afferent fibers, except those associated with pressure and stretch receptors, have their cell bodies in the large, flattened, crescent-shaped *trigeminal ganglion* (Figs. 1-10 and 2-25). This semilunar-shaped ganglion, located in a dural cleft on the cerebral surface of the petrous bone in the middle cranial fossa, is composed of typical unipolar ganglion cells (2579) (Figs. 12-26 and 12-27). The peripheral processes of these cells form the three main divisions of the trigeminal nerve: ophthalmic, maxillary and mandibular. The first two are wholly sensory, but incorporated in the mandibular branch is the entire motor root supplying the muscles of mas-

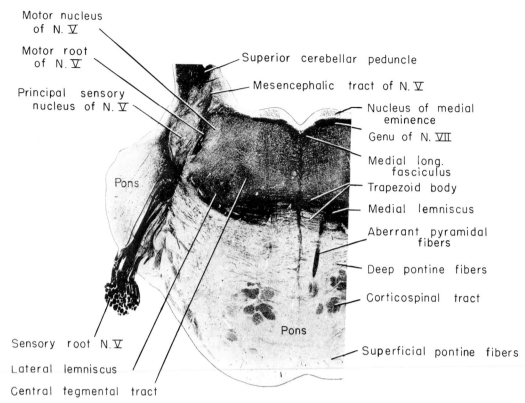

Motor nucleus of N. V

Motor root of N. V

Principal sensory nucleus of N. V

Superior cerebellar peduncle

Mesencephalic tract of N. V

Nucleus of medial eminence

Genu of N. VII

Medial long. fasciculus

Trapezoid body

Medial lemniscus

Aberrant pyramidal fibers

Deep pontine fibers

Corticospinal tract

Pons

Pons

Sensory root N. V

Lateral lemniscus

Central tegmental tract

Superficial pontine fibers

Figure 12-24. Section of pons and pontine tegmentum through entrance of trigeminal nerve of 1-month infant (Weigert's myelin stain, photograph).

tication. The ophthalmic branch innervates the forehead, upper eyelid, cornea, conjunctiva, dorsum of the nose, and mucous membranes of the nasal vestibule and the frontal sinus (Fig. 7-13). The maxillary division supplies the upper lip, lateral and posterior portions of the nose, upper cheek, anterior portion of the temple, and mucous membranes of the nose, upper jaw, upper teeth and roof of the mouth to the palatopharyngeal arch. Sensory fibers of the mandibular branch are distributed to the lower lip, chin, posterior portions of the cheek and the temple, external ear, and mucous membranes of the lower jaw, lower teeth, cheeks, anterior two-thirds of the tongue and floor of the mouth. All three divisions of the trigeminal nerve contribute sensory fibers to the dura. The dura of the posterior fossa also is innervated by fibers from the tenth cranial and the upper three spinal nerves (1315, 1966).

The central processes of cells in the trigeminal ganglion form the sensory root which passes through the lateral part of the

pons and enters the tegmentum, where many fibers divide into short ascending and long descending branches (Figs. 11-19 and 12-28). Other fibers descend or ascend without bifurcation (2744). The short ascending fibers and their collaterals terminate in the principal sensory nucleus lying dorsolateral to the entering fibers. The long descending branches form the spinal trigeminal tract, whose longest fibers reach the uppermost cervical segments of the spinal cord; terminals and collaterals to the spinal trigeminal nucleus are given off *en route* (Fig. 12-28).

Spinal Trigeminal Tract and Nucleus. Root fibers entering the spinal trigeminal tract have a definite topographical organization (1294, 1301, 2764). Fibers of the ophthalmic division are most ventral, fibers of the mandibular division are most dorsal and those of the maxillary division are intermediate (Fig. 12-26). This inverted laminar arrangement of fibers results from medial rotation of the trigeminal sensory root as it enters the brain stem and persists

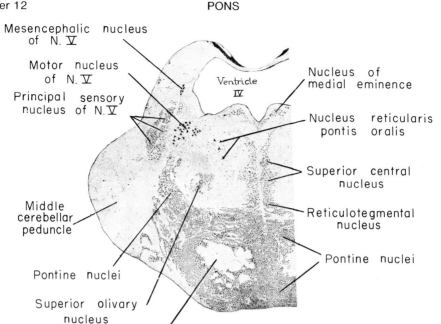

Figure 12-25. Section through pons and pontine tegmentum at about same level as Figure 12-24 of 1-month infant (cresyl violet; photograph, with cell groups schematically blocked in).

throughout the length of the tract. The tract extends from the level of the trigeminal root in the pons to the uppermost cervical spinal segments (Figs. 12-26 and 12-27). While it has been suggested that fibers in different divisions of the trigeminal nerve descend in the spinal trigeminal tract for different distances (1566, 2366), studies based upon better technics indicate that the laminar arrangement of fibers in the different divisions of the tract persists throughout its length with little intermingling of fibers (593, 1294, 1370). Fibers of the spinal trigeminal tract terminate upon cells of the spinal trigeminal nucleus, which forms a long cell column medial to the tract. Rostrally the nucleus merges with the principal sensory nucleus, while caudally it blends into the substantia gelatinosa of the first two cervical spinal segments. Fibers of the spinal trigeminal tract project into that part of the spinal trigeminal nucleus immediately adjacent to it (593). Thus, there is a sharp segregation of terminal fibers within parts of the nucleus and virtually no overlap of fibers from the different divisions of the nerve. The mandibular division of the spinal trigeminal tract also contains small groups of GVA fibers from the facial,

glossopharyngeal and vagus nerves which project dorsomedially into the nucleus solitarius (1292, 2141, 2558), a finding suggesting that some descending fibers in this tract may serve visceral functions. Autoradiographic studies based upon injections of ³H-labeled amino acids into the trigeminal ganglion indicate that central processes of cells in the ophthalamic and mandibular divisions also enter the ventrolateral part of the nucleus of the solitary tract (142).

In addition the spinal trigeminal tract contains some general somatic afferent (GSA) fibers from the facial, glossopharyngeal and vagus nerves, most of which occupy dorsomedial locations.

Cytoarchitecturally the spinal trigeminal nucleus has been subdivided into three parts (1882): (a) a *pars oralis* extending caudally to the rostral third of the inferior olivary nucleus, (b) a *pars interpolaris* extending from the pars oralis to the decussation of the pyramids and (c) a *pars caudalis* extending caudally as far as the second cervical spinal segment. Physiological studies in the cat reveal that a somatotopic map of the face exists at all levels within the spinal trigeminal nucleus (2664). Throughout the nucleus the face is repre-

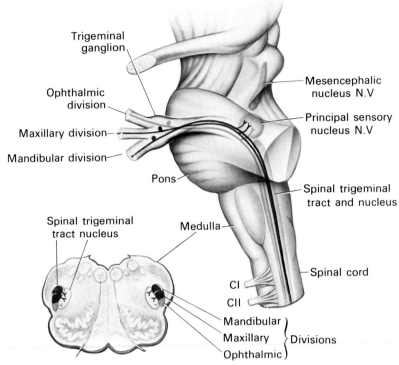

Figure 12-26. Diagram of the topographical arrangement of the fibers in the spinal trigeminal tract. The laminar arrangement of fibers from the different divisions of the trigeminal nerve persists throughout its length, although fibers leave the tract at all levels to terminate upon cells of the spinal trigeminal nucleus. (Reproduced with permission from M. B. Carpenter: *Core Text of Neuroanatomy.* Williams & Wilkins, Baltimore, 1978.)

sented in upside down fashion with the jaw dorsal and the forehead ventral. Cells of the pars oralis receive impulses from the head, mouth, nose and eyes, have small receptive fields, and the dominant representation is of internal structures. The pars interpolaris, with small receptive fields, is related mainly to cutaneous facial regions. The pars caudalis has large receptive fields and responds to light pressure over proximal parts of the face (i.e., forehead, cheeks and region of the jaw angle). Although neuronal receptive field size generally is related to peripheral innervation density, an extensive study of the trigeminal nuclear complex in the monkey failed to demonstrate any consistent variation of receptive field size throughout its rostrocaudal extent (1301).

In addition to fibers of the trigeminal nerve and general somatic afferent fibers from other branchiomeric cranial nerves, the spinal trigeminal nucleus receives corticobulbar fibers (282, 1404, 1413, 2796). These fibers arise mainly from the fronto-

Figure 12-27. Diagram of the secondary trigeminal tracts. The *ventral trigeminal tract (red)* conveys pain, thermal and tactile sense. These fibers originate from the spinal trigeminal nucleus, cross in the lower brain stem at various locations and ascend in association with the contralateral medial lemniscus. Secondary trigeminothalamic fibers from the principal sensory nucleus, conveying touch and pressure (*blue*) ascend by two separate pathways. Fibers from the ventral part of the principal sensory nucleus of N. V cross and ascend in association with the contralateral medial lemniscus. Fibers from the dorsomedial part of the same nucleus ascend uncrossed as the *dorsal trigeminal tract*. Both the ventral and dorsal trigeminal tracts project to the ventral posteromedial nucleus of the thalamus. The brain stem location of the ascending lateral spinothalamic tract is indicated in *black* on the *right side*. The ophthalmic (V^1), maxillary (V^2), and mandibular (V^3) divisions of the trigeminal nerve are identified. *1*, Free nerve ending; *2*, thermal receptor; *3*, Meissner's corpuscle; *4*, neuromuscular spindle; *5*, motor end plate in muscle of mastication.

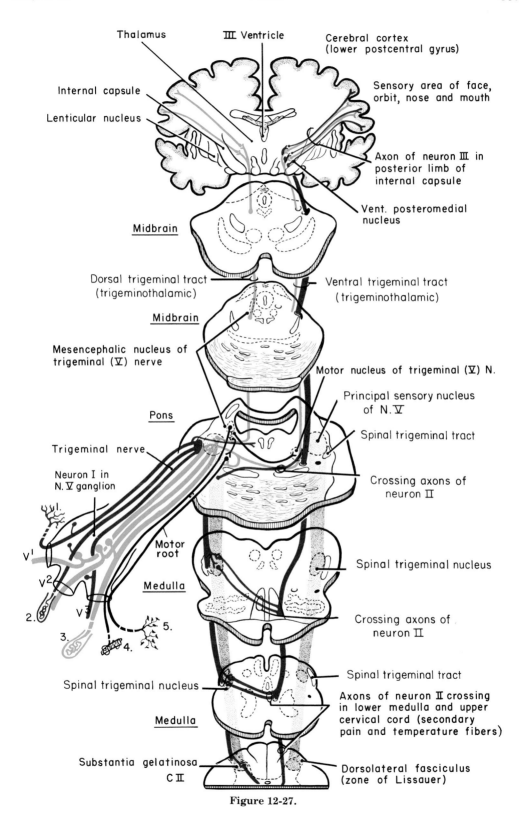

Figure 12-27.

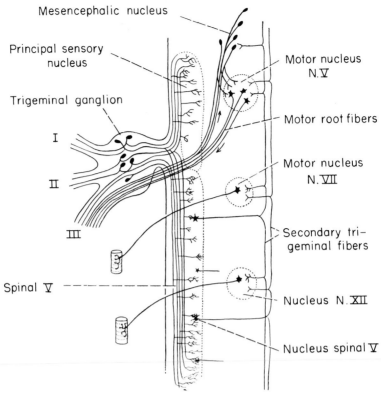

Figure 12-28. Diagram of the trigeminal nuclei and some of the trigeminal reflex arcs. *I*, Ophthalmic division; *II*, maxillary division; *III*, mandibular division. (Modified from Cajal (348).)

parietal cortex and are predominantly crossed. Physiological studies (594) indicate that corticobulbar fibers projecting to the pars oralis and pars caudalis mediate both inhibitory and excitatory effects. Observations suggest that inhibitory effects are presynaptic in nature.

There is considerable clinical evidence that lesions of the spinal trigeminal tract result chiefly in loss, or diminution, of pain and thermal sense in the area innervated by the trigeminal nerve, but do not affect tactile sensibility. It is probable that the nonbifurcating descending fibers mediate exclusively pain and thermal sense, while the bifurcating ones convey tactile sensibility. Hence in lesions of the spinal trigeminal tract many tactile fibers may be destroyed, but the ascending branches of these fibers still reach the principal sensory nucleus and touch sensibility remains intact. Clinically there is no doubt that pain and thermal sense are handled entirely by the spinal trigeminal tract and nucleus, while touch

and two-point discrimination are in large part related to the principal sensory nucleus (Figs. 12-27 and 12-28). However, physiological studies (1371, 2664) indicate that it is extremely difficult to isolate and identify neurons in the spinal trigeminal nucleus uniquely concerned with pain. Neurons at nearly all levels of the nucleus respond to tactile stimuli (1370).

The composition, location and relationships of the spinal trigeminal tract and nucleus are of considerable diagnostic and surgical importance. It should be noted that virtually no overlap exists between the cutaneous areas supplied by the three peripheral divisions of the trigeminal nerve, a finding in sharp contrast to the extensive overlap characteristic of spinal dermatomes (Fig. 7-13). Neurosurgical studies (2346) have demonstrated that trigeminal tractotomy can relieve various forms of facial pain including trigeminal neuralgia (tic douloureux). The importance of this procedure is that it selectively eliminates, or greatly reduces, pain and thermal sense without impairing tactile sense. Meticulous examination of such patients (2653, 2688) frequently reveals that tactile sense is mildly impaired and that there is not a complete loss of any sensory modality. One notable advantage of this procedure is that corneal sensation is not abolished, and the corneal reflex is not lost (although it may not be as brisk). The fact that section of this tract caudal to the level of the obex has produced complete facial analgesia is cited as supporting the thesis that the caudal part of the nucleus is concerned chiefly with pain.

Principal Sensory Nucleus. This nucleus lies lateral to the entering trigeminal root fibers in the upper pons (Figs. 12-24 and 12-28). Root fibers conveying impulses for tactile and pressure sense enter the principal sensory nucleus and are distributed in a manner similar to that described for the spinal trigeminal nucleus. Fibers of the ophthalmic division terminate ventrally, fibers of the maxillary division are intermediate and fibers of the mandibular division are most dorsal (1294, 1301). Cells of the principal sensory nucleus have an ovoid configuration in transverse sections, and consist of small- to medium-sized neurons with relative large nuclei (Fig. 12-25). Caudally this nucleus merges with the pars oralis of the spinal trigeminal nucleus and the level of transition is indistinct (Fig. 12-28). Cells of the principal sensory nucleus have large receptive fields, show high spontaneous activity and respond to a wide range of pressure stimuli with little adaptation (2664).

Mesencephalic Nucleus. This nucleus of the trigeminal nerve forms a slender cell column near the lateral margin of the central gray of the upper part of the fourth ventricle and cerebral aqueduct (Figs. 12-25, 12-26 and 12-28). The nucleus is composed of large unipolar neurons which extend from the level of the motor nucleus into the rostral midbrain. Studies of neurons in this nucleus have revealed many bipolar and multipolar cells as well, but most cells resemble those of the dorsal root ganglion (1953, 1954). However, unlike dorsal root ganglion cells, these cells lie within the central nervous system, are not encapsulated, and often have more than one process. The principal processes of these cells

form a slender sickle-shaped bundle, the *mesencephalic tract of the trigeminal nerve* (Figs. 12-24–12-29 and A-8), which descends to the level of the trigeminal motor nucleus, provides collaterals to motor cells and appears to emerge as part of the motor root. Cells of this nucleus commonly are regarded as afferent peripheral neurons which have been "retained" within the central nervous system, but proof that these cells arise from the neural crest in mammals is still lacking (1953, 1954).

Afferent fibers of the mesencephalic nucleus of the trigeminal nerve convey proprioceptive impulses (pressure and kinesthesis) from the teeth, periodontium, hard palate, muscles of mastication and joint capsules (38, 39, 535, 536, 1998). It appears likely that these fibers may be concerned with the mechanisms which control the force of the bite. The mesencephalic nucleus also receives afferent impulses from stretch receptors in the muscles of mastication. Action potentials can be recorded in the mesencephalic nucleus in response to stretching the masticatory muscles (530, 536). Scattered ganglion cells found along the motor root appear related to the mesencephalic nucleus and are considered to convey impulses from stretch receptors in the mylohyoid and diagastric muscles. Although most afferent fibers of the mesencephalic nucleus course peripherally with fibers of the motor root, experimental evidence (535) indicates that some fibers from this nucleus pass peripherally in all three divisions of the trigeminal nerve. One author (1960) considers cells of the mesencephalic nucleus to be homologous to cells of the dorsal nucleus of Clarke, but some impulses relayed by this nucleus reach consciousness and must be relayed to thalamic levels.

Connections of the mesencephalic nucleus are more extensive than previously believed (1953). Some fibers leave the mesencephalic tract and enter the white matter of the cerebellum, possibly connecting with the deep cerebellar nuclei. Other fibers have been traced to the roof of the cerebral aqueduct, the base of the cerebellum and to the region of the superior colliculi.

Some authorities have suggested that deep sensibility of the lingual, facial and extraocular muscles is mediated by fibers

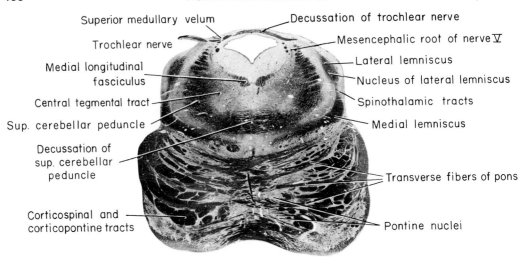

Figure 12-29. Section of the isthmus of an adult brain at the level of the decussation and exit of the trochlear nerve (Weigert's myelin stain, photograph).

of the fifth nerve (529, 530). Other studies indicate that a localized part of the trigeminal ganglion contains cells whose afferent fibers convey impulses from muscle spindles in the extraocular muscles (1599). Cells, in a part of the ganglion which forms the ophthalmic division, respond with a sustained increase in discharge rate when the extraocular muscles are stretched; the discharge ceases as soon as the stretched muscles are released. These short latency responses are abolished by section of the ophthalmic division of the trigeminal nerve. Deep sensibility from the face also is considered to be mediated by the trigeminal nerve, but the possibility remains that this may be supplemented by facial nerve afferents.

Motor Nucleus. The motor nucleus of the trigeminal nerve forms an ovoid column of typical multipolar motor cells that lies medial to the motor root and the principal sensory nucleus (Fig. 12-25). Its coarse efferent fibers emerge internal to the entering sensory root and pass underneath the trigeminal ganglion to become incorporated in the mandibular branch (Figs. 12-27 and 12-28). Among the terminals ending in the nucleus are collaterals from the mesencephalic root and other afferent trigeminal fibers. These fibers furnish a two-neuron arc for reflex control of the jaw muscles. Additional secondary trigeminal fibers, both crossed and uncrossed, provide reflex control of the jaw muscles to superficial stimuli,

especially from the lingual and oral mucous membranes. As in the case of other motor cranial nerve nuclei, many corticobulbar fibers do not terminate directly upon cells of the motor trigeminal nucleus but pass to reticular neurons, which in turn project to motor cells (Fig. 11-30).

Secondary Trigeminal Pathways. Secondary trigeminal pathways originate from cells in the principal sensory and spinal trigeminal nuclei and project to higher levels of the brain stem. Collaterals of these fibers provide numerous, largely uncrossed projections to motor nuclei of the brain stem involved in complex reflexes (Fig. 12-28).

Axons from cells within the spinal trigeminal nucleus pass ventromedially in the reticular formation, cross the median raphe and become associated with the contralateral medial lemniscus (402, 1824, 2366, 2652, 2654). These secondary trigeminal fibers retain their close association with the contralateral medial lemniscus as they ascend in the brain stem (Fig. 12-27). At thalamic levels these fibers leave the medial lemniscus and terminate in a selective manner about cells of the ventral posteromedial (VPM) nucleus of the thalamus. Crossed axons from cells of the spinal trigeminal nucleus which ascend in the brain stem with the medial lemniscus form the *ventral trigeminal tract* (ventral trigeminothalamic tract).

Some efferent fibers from the spinal tri-

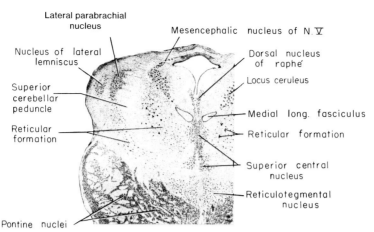

Figure 12-30. Section through isthmus of 3-month infant (cresyl violet; photograph, with cell groups schematically blocked in).

geminal nucleus pass into the parvicellular part of the reticular formation, and others arborize about cells of the nucleus reticularis gigantocellularis; a moderate number of fibers project to the cerebellum via the inferior cerebellar peduncle.

The relationship of the spinal trigeminal tract and nucleus to the spinothalamic tracts in the brain stem should be noted in Figure 12-27. The location of the latter tract is represented in *solid black dots* on the right side at each level. Vascular lesions in the lower medulla involving structures in this dorsolateral area frequently interrupt these pathways and produce a syndrome characterized by: (a) loss of pain and thermal sense over the face ipsilaterally and (b) loss of pain and thermal sense, and impairment of tactile sensation over the contralateral half of the body (Figs. 20-16 and 20-17). The involvement of other structures in this region produces additional neurological deficits.

Secondary trigeminal fibers originating from the principal sensory nucleus are both crossed and uncrossed. Cells in the dorsomedial part of the nucleus give rise to a small bundle of uncrossed fibers which ascends to ipsilateral thalamic nuclei (379, 2559). These uncrossed fibers, constituting the *dorsal trigeminal tract* (681, 1936, 2614, 2652, 2751), ascend in the dorsal pontine tegmentum; at mesencephalic levels they occupy a position near the periaqueductal gray (Fig. 12-27). At the level of the fasciculus retroflexus the fibers make a ventro-

lateral bend and enter the medial part of the ventral posteromedial (VPM) nucleus of the thalamus. Because afferent fibers terminating in the dorsal part of the principal sensory nucleus are associated primarily with the mandibular division (1294), it has been suggested that fibers of the dorsal trigeminal tract may subserve a unique function.

Neurons in the ventral part of the principal sensory nucleus of N. V give rise to a larger crossed bundle of trigeminothalamic fibers which ascends in association with the contralateral medial lemniscus, in a manner similar to that described for the ventral trigeminal tract (1936, 2238, 2559, 2652, 2665, 2751). These crossed secondary trigeminal fibers also terminate in the ventral posteromedial (VPM) nucleus of the thalamus.

As previously mentioned the mesencephalic nucleus of the trigeminal nerve is anomalous in that the primary sensory neurons are found in this brain stem nucleus rather than in the trigeminal ganglion. While there is convincing evidence that fibers from this nucleus convey impulses from pressure, joint and stretch receptors, the pathway by which these impulses are transmitted centrally remains obscure. It seems likely that processes of cells in the mesencephalic nucleus of the trigeminal nerve may project to the cerebellum (1953, 2764). Since a significant part of the input to this nucleus comes from stretch receptors, and impulses from most stretch receptors in other parts of the body are relayed to the cerebellum, this hypothesis seems reasonable.

Trigeminal Reflexes. The numerous secondary *reflex* fibers arising from the terminal nuclei of N. V ascend and descend in the dorsolateral part of the reticular formation, giving off terminals or collaterals to various motor nuclei (Fig. 12-28). These are largely uncrossed and provide connections for reflexes initiated by stimulation of the skin of the face, the oral and nasal mucous membranes, and muscles, tendons and bones of the jaw and face. Among the most important of these reflexes is the corneal reflex.

The *corneal reflex* is elicited by stimulation of the cornea with a wisp of cotton and produces bilateral blinking and closing of the eyes. The blinking and closing of the eyes is effected by impulses reaching the facial nuclei on both sides. Evidence suggests that secondary trigeminal fibers project bilaterally to the facial nuclei. Following an injury to the ophthalmic division of the trigeminal nerve, corneal sensation and the corneal reflex are lost on that side because the afferent limb of the reflex arc has been destroyed. However, corneal sensation remains on the opposite side and stimulation of that cornea will produce bilateral blinking and eye closure, indicating that the efferent limb (facial nucleus and nerve) of the reflex arc is intact. In patients with peripheral facial palsies, corneal sensation will be present on both sides, but no corneal reflex can be elicited on the side of the lesion because the efferent limb of the reflex arc has been destroyed. However, stimulation of the cornea on the side of the lesion will cause blinking and closure of the opposite eye (consensual response).

Other reflexes involving secondary trigeminal fibers which project impulses to cranial nerve nuclei include: (a) the *lacrimal* or *tearing reflex*, in which impulses pass to the superior salivatory nucleus of the intermediate nerve; (b) *sneezing*, in which impulses probably pass to the nucleus ambiguus, respiratory centers in the reticular formation and into the spinal cord (i.e., phrenic nerve nuclei and anterior horn cells innervating the intercostal muscles); and (c) *vomiting*, in which impulses pass predominantly to vagal nuclei (i.e., dorsal motor, ambiguus and solitary).

The *jaw jerk*, or masseter reflex, is a monosynaptic myotatic reflex. This reflex is elicited by placing the examiner's index finger over the middle of the patient's chin (mouth slightly open) and tapping gently with a reflex hammer. The response is a bilateral contraction of the masseter and temporal muscles. This reflex involves the mesencephalic nucleus and collaterals given off by it to the motor nucleus.

ISTHMUS OF THE HINDBRAIN

The narrow portion of the hindbrain, situated rostral to the cerebellum, which merges with the midbrain is known as the *isthmus rhombencephali*. The most rostral levels of this region, near the junction with the midbrain, demonstrate characteristic features (Figs. 12-29, 12-30 and A-9). As in more caudal brain stem sections three regions are distinguished, namely, a roof, the tegmentum and a ventral pontine portion. The roof consists of a thin membrane, the *superior medullary velum*, which covers the most superior portion of the fourth ventricle. The fourth ventricle, greatly reduced in size, resembles the *cerebral aqueduct* of the midbrain. The ventricle is bounded ventrally and laterally by the central gray matter. The root fibers of the *trochlear nerve* (N. IV) completely decussate in the superior medullary velum. They originate from nuclei which lie more rostrally in the ventral part of the central gray. The fibers arch dorsally and somewhat caudally around the fourth ventricle, decussate in the roof and emerge caudal to the inferior colliculus (Fig. 11-2). Only the decussation is seen at this level. The trochlear nerve innervates the superior oblique muscle of the eye.

The lateral lemniscus lies near the lateral surface of the tegmentum, forming the major part of the external structure known as the *trigonum lemnisci*. Groups of cells among its fibers constitute the *nucleus of the lateral lemniscus*, one of several intercalated nuclei in the auditory pathway (Figs. 12-13, 12-29 and 12-30).

The medial lemniscus is a flattened band extending transversely in the ventrolateral tegmentum, and the spinothalamic tract is in its usual position between the medial and lateral lemnisci. Included in the medial lemniscus are the secondary trigeminal fibers. The dorsal trigeminal tract ascends in the dorsal part of the reticular formation, lateral to the medial longitudinal fasciculus (Fig. 12-27). Thus at this level the principal ascending sensory pathways form a peripheral shell of fibers which enclose the pontine tegmentum. The ventral portion of the pons remains considerably larger than the tegmental portion (Figs. 12-29, A-26 and A-27). The pontine nuclei are extensive and lie in sheets between the numerous bundles of corticospinal and corticopontine fibers.

Superior Cerebellar Peduncle. Fibers of this large bundle ascend from the hilus of the deep cerebellar nuclei into the dorsolateral part of the rostral pontine tegmentum. It initially forms a crescent-shaped bundle dorsolateral to the fourth ventricle (Fig. 12-23), but at more rostral levels of the isthmus it lies medial to the lateral lemniscus (Fig. 12-29). The superior cerebellar peduncle arises from the dentate, emboliform and globose nuclei and forms the most important efferent fiber system of the cerebellum. Upon entering the brain stem, fibers of the superior cerebellar peduncle move ventrally and medially. In the caudal midbrain this major cerebellar efferent bundle decussates completely (Figs. 12-29, 13-2 and 14-16). Some of its fibers end in the red nucleus; others continue directly to the ventral lateral nucleus of the thalamus (Figs. 14-16 and 15-14*A*). A relatively small number of fibers of the superior cerebellar peduncle descend lateral to the superior central nucleus to terminate in the reticulotegmental nucleus in the upper pons, and the paramedian reticular nuclei in the medulla (283, 411). These cerebelloreticular fibers form part of a cerebelloreticular feedback pathway, since these reticular nuclei project fibers back to the cerebellum (Fig. 14-16).

Fibers of the anterior spinocerebellar tract which ascend in the lateral part of the reticular formation to levels of the upper pons become concentrated on the lateral surface of the superior cerebellar peduncle (Fig. 10-9). These fibers reverse their direction and enter the cerebellum by passing caudally along the dorsolateral border of the superior cerebellar peduncle. As these fibers descend in the superior medullary velum they terminate in the anterior lobe of the cerebellar vermis (Fig. 14-1). The majority of the fibers cross to the opposite side within the cerebellum. Part of the fi-

bers of the rostral spinocerebellar tract also enter the cerebellum in association with the superior cerebellar peduncle.

As fibers of the superior cerebellar peduncle move ventromedially toward their decussation they divide the reticular formation into medial and lateral parts (Fig. 12-29). In the lateral part is a fairly dense collection of cells known as the *pedunculopontine tegmental nucleus* (i.e., the pedunculopontine nucleus). Cells of this nucleus are partially traversed by fibers of the superior cerebellar peduncle (Figs. 13-3, 17-15 and 17-20). Compact and diffuse portions of this nucleus extend rostrally into the caudal midbrain (1885). This nucleus receives cortical projections from the precentral gyrus (1411), and descending fibers from the globus pallidus and substantia nigra (398, 419, 1438, 1825). The efferent projections of the pedunculopontine nucleus are mainly to the substantia nigra.

Locus Ceruleus. Near the periventricular gray of the upper part of the fourth ventricle is an irregular collection of medium-sized pigmented cells referred to as the *locus ceruleus* or *nucleus pigmentosus pontis* (Figs. 12-30–12-32). This nucleus appears at levels slightly rostral to the principal sensory nucleus of N. V where it lies ventromedial to the mesencephalic root and nucleus of the trigeminal nerve. The large globular neurons of the mesencephalic nucleus of N. V, partially intermingled with those of the locus ceruleus ventrally, extend further dorsally and rostrally in a linear fashion at the margin of the central gray (Figs. 12-26 and 12.31). Cells of the locus ceruleus are of at least two types: (a) medium-sized oval or round cells with eccentric nuclei and fairly large clumps of melanin pigment granules and (b) small oval cells with scant cytoplasm usually free of pigment (1885, 2239). Ventrolateral to the locus ceruleus is a more diffuse collection of similar cells which forms the *nucleus subceruleus* (1885).

Although the locus ceruleus is a relatively small structure, it can be identified readily in gross sections of the brain stem because of its pigmentation and location. The significance of this small pigmented nucleus remained unknown until it was demonstrated by a sensitive fluorescence technic that its cells contained catecholamines, nearly all of which are norepinephrine (Fig.

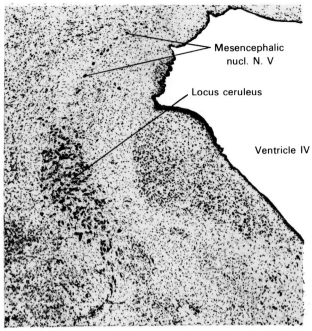

Figure 12-31. Photograph of the cell groups surrounding the periventricular gray at isthmus levels. Cells of the locus ceruleus contain melanin pigment granules and high concentrations of norepinephrine. Globular cells of the mesencephalic nucleus of N. V are present along the dorsal border of the locus ceruleus and extend dorsally and rostrally at the margin of the central gray.

12-32) (60, 585, 1380, 1879, 2598). Unlike other brain stem norepinephrine cells which are found largely as scattered neurons in the lateral tegmentum, the locus ceruleus is a compact nucleus that projects fibers to portions of the telencephalon, diencephalon, midbrain, cerebellum, pons, medulla and spinal cord (1225, 1482, 1555, 1582, 1859, 1879, 2006, 2598). Information concerning the widespread projections of locus ceruleus and the nucleus subceruleus have been developed through a variety of different anatomical, histochemical, biochemical and pharmacological methodologies applied in ingenious ways. The Falck-Hillarp (731) fluorescent technic permitted identification of the locus ceruleus as a norepinephrine cell group and provided an analysis of the pattern of brain innervation by central catecholamine-producing neurons (827). Although studies using a variety of technics have been employed to determine the projections of the locus ceruleus, none is without pitfalls. The most consistent, complete and reliable data appears to have been derived from anterograde and retrograde axoplasmic transport studies (225, 1223, 1225, 1555, 1630, 2006), but these studies were possible only because of information obtained by other methods.

The major ascending projection from the locus ceruleus passes rostrally through the mesencephalon lateral to the medial longitudinal fasciculus and ventrolateral to the central gray. In the caudal diencephalon the main ascending bundle of noradrenergic fibers enters the medial forebrain bundle via the mammillary peduncle (Fig. 16-7) and the ventral tegmental area. These fibers accompany the medial forebrain bundle to and through the lateral hypothalamus (Fig. 16-9). This ascending pathway continues rostrally to levels of the anterior commissure where it divides into bundles innervating the diencephalon and telencephalon. The stria medullaris component turns caudally to innervate midline portions of the thalamus, while the stria terminalis component supplies the amygdaloid nuclear complex. Other efferent fibers from the locus ceruleus pass via the fornix to the hippocampal formation and as a component of the cingulum bundle to the cingulate cortex, the subiculum and the hippocampal formation. The most rostrally projecting fibers from the locus ceruleus pass from the medial forebrain bundle into the external capsule which distributes fibers to rostral, dorsal and lateral cortex of the frontal lobe. Smaller groups of fibers separating

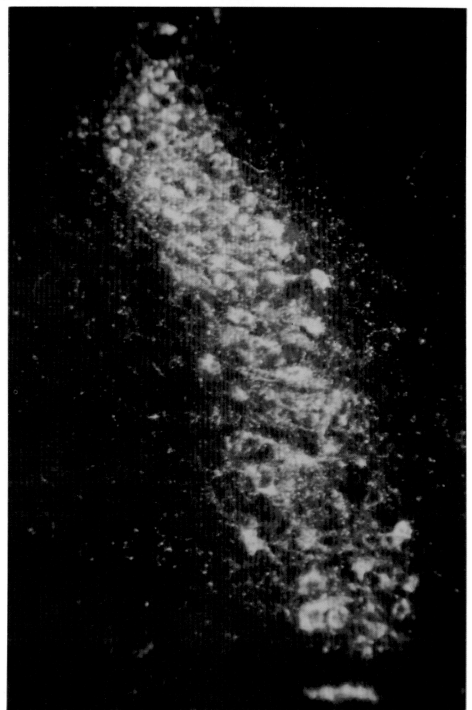

Figure 12-32. Photomicrograph of neurons containing norepinephrine in the locus ceruleus of the rat. The norepinephrine-containing cells were reacted with glyoxylic acid which converts norepinephrine into a fluorescent chemical derivative that can be viewed in the fluorescence microscope. (Courtesy of Drs. Jacqueline McGinty and Floyd Bloom, Salk Institute, La Jolla, Calif.)

from the main bundle, which is referred to as the dorsal catecholamine pathway, project into the periaqueductal gray and the periventricular gray of the third ventricle.

One of the most profuse projections is to the thalamus where terminals are found in the intralaminar thalamic nuclei, the anterior nuclear group and the lateral geniculate body. In addition to these ipsilateral pathways, smaller numbers of fibers cross to the opposite side via the tegmental decussation, the posterior commissure, the supraoptic commissures and the anterior commissure. After decussating these noradrenergic pathways have a distribution similar to those on the ipsilateral side.

Norepinephrine-containing fibers project to the cerebellar cortex via the superior cerebellar peduncle and terminate around Purkinje cell somata and in the lower third of the molecular layer (2006). Biochemical analysis of discrete nuclei of the brain stem and glyoxylic acid fluorescence histochemistry demonstrate the highest norepinephrine content in the trigeminal motor nucleus, the nucleus of the solitary tract, the dorsal motor nucleus of the vagus and the dorsal raphe nucleus (1482). Bilateral lesions of the locus ceruleus or subceruleus do not significantly alter the norepinephrine content of these nuclei, but such lesions decrease the norepinephrine content of the superior and inferior colliculi, the medial geniculate body, the interpeduncular nucleus, the pontine nuclei and the principal sensory nucleus of the trigeminal nerve. These observations suggest that the locus ceruleus complex innervates mainly primary sensory and association nuclei, while norepinephrine-containing neurons scattered in the lateral tegmentum probably innervate primary motor and visceral nuclei. Fluorescent histochemical and retrograde transport studies indicate that both the locus ceruleus and the subceruleus project fibers to spinal levels via the anterior funiculus and ventral parts of the lateral funiculus; some of these fibers reach lumbar spinal segments (1412, 1859).

The remarkable feature of the locus ceruleus projection is its wide distribution throughout the neuraxis. With the exception of the midbrain raphe serotonin projection system, no other cell group of the reticular formation has been shown to have such an extensive projection. The projection of the locus ceruleus directly to the neocortex is unique in that it does not involve synaptic relays in the thalamus (1225). Retrograde HRP studies based upon transport of the enzyme from a large number of sites within the neuraxis suggest a regional topography within the locus cer-

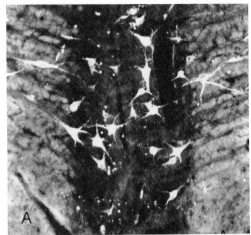
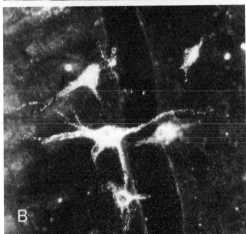

Figure 12-33. Photomicrographs of retrograde transport of horseradish peroxidase (HRP) from the C2 spinal segment to the nucleus raphe magnus in a squirrel monkey (dark field, *A*, ×80; *B*, ×200).

uleus (1630). These data imply that the locus ceruleus is composed of several distinct subdivisions.

The locus ceruleus and its efferent projections have been considered to play a role in paradoxical sleep, facilitation and inhibition of sensory neurons and control of cortical activation (456, 1222, 1249, 1487, 1793, 2256). In addition descending noradrenergic fibers from the locus ceruleus may supply preganglionic sympathetic neurons in the intermediolateral cell column at thoracic and upper lumbar levels (1859).

Raphe Nuclei. In addition to the cell groups of the pontine reticular formation previously described, the pons contains cell groups in the median raphe which properly

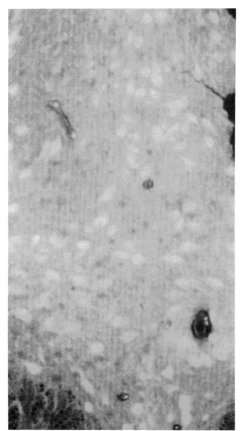

Figure 12-34. Fluorescent photomicrograph of serotonin-containing neurons in the dorsal nucleus of the raphe. (Courtesy of Dr. George K. Aghajanian, School of Medicine, Yale University.)

belong to the reticular formation, but appear to serve distinctive functions (284, 2505).

The raphe nuclei of the human brain have not been studied extensively, and the variations in nomenclature used are confusing. Detailed cytological descriptions of these nuclei in the cat (2505) suggest similarities to the raphe nuclei in man (1885). The raphe nuclei of the medulla (i.e., nucleus raphe obscurus, nucleus raphe pallidus and nucleus raphe magnus) are smaller and more restricted than similar nuclei in the pons (Figs. 11-15 and 11-16). The *inferior central nucleus* appears in the median raphe at the junction of pons and medulla (Fig. 11-31) and at caudal pontine levels (Fig. 12-4). This nucleus may represent the rostral part of the nucleus raphe magnus. The *nucleus raphe pontis* consists of several small cell groups, dorsal and rostral to

the inferior central nucleus. The rostral extension of the pontine raphe nuclei is the *superior central nucleus* (Figs. 12-25 and 12-30), a large aggregation of closely packed small- and medium-sized cells. Decussating fibers of the superior cerebellar peduncle pass through the superior central nucleus (Fig. 12-29). On each side of the midline, dorsal to the medial longitudinal fasciculus, is the *dorsal nucleus of the raphe* (Fig. 12-30). This nucleus extends rostrally in the ventral central gray into the caudal midbrain and merges with the *dorsal tegmental nucleus* (Fig. 13-3). Anatomical studies indicate that most of the pontine raphe nuclei give rise to long ascending projections (284). The superior central nucleus (median nucleus of the raphe) receives descending fibers from the medial forebrain bundle and some fibers from the fasciculus retroflexus (Fig. 18-7) (1816). The dorsal tegmental nucleus receives fibers from the mammillotegmental tract and projects impulses back to the mammillary bodies.

Histofluorescence technics demonstrate that the nuclei of the raphe region have a yellow fluorescence distinctive for serotonin (5-hydroxytryptamine, 5-HT) which can be demonstrated best by the use of monoamine oxidase inhibitors (Fig. 12-34) 585, 2010, 2598). These cells present a sharp contrast with the norepinephrine-containing neurons in lateral parts of the pontine reticular formation, particularly the locus ceruleus, which have a green fluorescence (Fig. 12-32).

The principal ascending fibers arise from serotonin cell bodies located in the dorsal nucleus of the raphe and in the superior central nucleus (201, 202, 515, 2598). The major ascending pathway from the rostral raphe nuclei passes through the ventral tegmental area (Tsai), medial parts of the fields of Forel and joins the medial forebrain bundle in the lateral hypothalamus. Fibers leaving this main ascending bundle enter the substantia nigra, the intralaminar thalamic nuclei, the stria terminalis, the septum and the internal capsule. The most rostral projections terminate mainly in the frontal lobe, although some fibers are distributed throughout the neocortex. The dorsal nucleus of the raphe selectively innervates the substantia nigra, the lateral geniculate body, the neostriatum, the pyriform lobe, the olfactory bulb and the amygdaloid nuclear complex (Fig. 12-34). The superior central nucleus is particularly associated with serotonergic fibers projecting to the interpeduncular nucleus, the mammillary bodies and the hippocampal formation. Other ascending fibers from these nuclei radiate into the mesencephalic reticular formation and the periventricular gray. Ascending projections from the caudal raphe nuclei are less numerous and distributed to the superior colliculus, the pretectum, and the nuclei of the posterior commissure. Histological and enzymatic studies of ascending serotonergic pathways suggest that the superior central nucleus projects mainly to mesolimbic structures, such as the hippocampus and the septal nuclei, while the dorsal nucleus of the raphe has a major projection to the mesostriatum (neostriatum) (873).

Descending projections of the dorsal nucleus of the raphe are modest, but they include fibers distributed to the locus ceruleus and the parabrachial nuclei (i.e., noradrenergic cells surrounding the superior cerebellar peduncle (Fig. 12-30) (202). The superior central nucleus gives rise to a significant descending bundle projecting fibers to: (a) the cerebellum via the middle cerebellar peduncle, (b) the locus ceruleus and (c) large regions of the pontine reticular formation (Fig. 12-30). Although the nuclei raphe pontis and raphe magnus have diffuse projections in the brain stem, they also project to spinal levels (Fig. 12-33). Autoradiographic studies of the nucleus raphe magnus suggest that descending fibers project primarily to structures concerned with nociceptive and/or visceral afferent input (129). Structures receiving efferents from the nucleus raphe magnus, largely via the dorsal longitudinal fasciculus, include the dorsal motor nucleus of the vagus, the solitary nucleus and the spinal trigeminal nucleus (pars caudalis). Projections of this nucleus to the spinal cord are bilateral and are distributed by fibers descending in the lateral funiculus (Figs. 10-23 and 11-16). These fibers terminate in the marginal zone (lamina I), the substantia gelatinosa (lamina II) and in parts of laminae V, VI and VII. Because electric stimulation of the nucleus raphe magnus inhibits the discharge of neurons associated with nociceptive sensory input, evidence suggests that this nucleus may be linked to endogenous analgesic mechanisms (127, 748, 2726). This thesis is strengthened by the close correspondence between the terminal projections of this nucleus and opiate receptor binding sites (1977).

Serotonin and the raphe nuclei have been implicated in the regulation of diverse physiological processes such as the regulation of sleep (1249), aggressive behavior (2313), and a variety of neuroendocrine functions (515, 2779).

Structurally, the serotonin molecule is similar to a portion of the larger *d*-lysergic acid diethylamide (LSD) molecule in that both contain an indole nucleus. LSD is a hallucinogenic drug considered to be the prototype of a psychotomimetic drug (i.e., a drug whose effects mimic psychosis (838, 2767). The argument was advanced that psychotic phenomenona might be due to either decreased amounts of brain serotonin or the synthesis of an endogenous compound that antagonized the action of serotonin in the brain. Microelectrode studies demonstrated that LSD produced a specific depression of activity in raphe neurons which contain serotonin (21, 1001). These observations led to the hypothesis that LSD acts to depress the activity of serotonin-containing neurons which through disinhibition, cause a release of activity in neurons in the visual system, the limbic system and in many other brain areas (22). Destruction of serotonin neurons, inhibition of its synthesis, or blockade of its receptors consistently produces an animal that is hypersensitive to virtually all environmental stimuli and hyperactive in virtually all situations. By a general inhibitory action in the central nervous system serotonin may serve to modulate and maintain behavior within specific limits. Studies indicate that as the overall level of motor activity or arousal increases, so does the activity of serotonin-containing cells. As an animal becomes quiescent and drowsy, the activity of these cells diminishes. Neurons of the raphe fire slowly as an animal enters sleep, and during rapid eye movement (REM) sleep the cells stop firing. These findings suggest that, under the influence of hallucinogenic drugs, the individual is fully awake but the brain serotonin system is depressed and behaving as it does during sleep (1196).

Recent investigations indicate that both serotonin and norepinephrine-containing neurons in the reticular formation play roles in the active mechanisms that control sleep states (1249). Sleep is not a single phenomenon. Sleep states can be quantitatively measured and correlated with biochemical, pharmacological and structural alterations. Inhibition of serotonin synthesis, or total destruction of serotonin-containing neurons, in the raphe system is described as producing to total insomnia. Serotonin appears to be involved in the mechanism of what is called *slow wave sleep*, a state characterized by the posture of sleep, myotic pupils and cortical electrical activity (electroencephalogram) which displays spindles and slow waves. In addition, serotonin-containing neurons appear to have a "priming" effect upon the cells of the locus ceruleus which serve as the "triggering" mechanism for what is called *paradoxical sleep* (456, 1249). Paradoxical sleep occurs intermittently after variable periods of slow wave sleep and is characterized by: (a) abolition of antigravity muscle tone; (b) reductions in blood pressure, bradycardia and irregular respiration; (c) bursts of REM (rapid eye movements) and (d) an electroencephalogram (EEG) which resembles that of the waking state. Lesions in caudal portions of the raphe nuclei suppress paradoxical sleep relative to slow wave sleep, while bilateral lesions of the locus ceruleus cause a selective suppression of paradoxical sleep. Data in the cat indicate that after bilateral lesions of the locus ceruleus paradoxical sleep returns nearly to the normal range in about 2 weeks in spite of extensive norepinephrine depletion in the cortex, thalamus and midbrain (1224).

At this point the student will find it instructive to review the blood supply of the medulla and pons (Chapter 20, p. 725). Familiarity with the internal organization of the hindbrain and the connections of the cranial nerves should give the reader an appreciation of the neurological syndromes which follow sudden occlusion of arteries of the vertebrobasilar system. Lower brain stem lesions associated with syringobulbia, demyelinating diseases and tumors frequently begin in localized regions and produce specific neurological signs and symptoms.

The Mesencephalon

The midbrain, or mesencephalon, is the smallest and least differentiated division of the brain stem. Like other parts of the infratentorial brain stem it can be divided into three parts: (a) the *tectum* or quadrigeminal plate, dorsal to the cerebral aqueduct, (b) the massive *crura cerebri* on the ventrolateral surfaces, and (c) the *tegmentum*, centrally, representing the rostral continuation of the pontine tegmentum. The cerebral aqueduct, surrounded by the central gray substance (i.e., periaqueductal gray), separates the tectum from the tegmentum (Fig. 13-1). The term *cerebral peduncle* denotes one-half of the midbrain, excluding the tectum, and consists of two parts: (a) a dorsal part, the tegmentum, and (b) a ventral part, the crus cerebri. These two parts of the cerebral peduncle are separated from each other by a large pigmented nuclear mass, the *substantia nigra* (Figs. 13-1, A-10 and A-27).

The midbrain contains the trochlear and oculomotor nuclei and neural structures concerned with ocular and visual reflexes.

Relay nuclei constituting important parts of the auditory and visual systems also are prominent, along with pathways interrelating higher and lower portions of the neuraxis. The principal nuclear masses and fiber pathways can be observed and studied at two typical levels, namely, the levels of the inferior and superior colliculi. The latter level is shown diagrammatically in Figure 13-1.

INFERIOR COLLICULAR LEVEL

The transition from isthmus to midbrain is associated with changes mainly in the tectum and tegmentum (Figs. 12-29, 12-30, 13-2, 13-3, A-9 and A-10). Comparison of these levels reveals that: (a) the fourth ventricle has become the cerebral aqueduct, (b) the superior medullary velum is replaced by two rounded eminences, the inferior colliculi, and (c) fibers of the superior cerebellar peduncles have begun to decussate. The ventral part of the pons is reduced in size and, at slightly more rostral levels, undergoes a reorganization as the massive

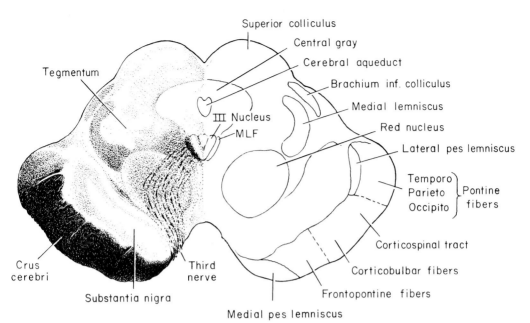

Figure 13-1. Schematic transverse section through the rostral midbrain. *MLF*, medial longitudinal fasciculus.

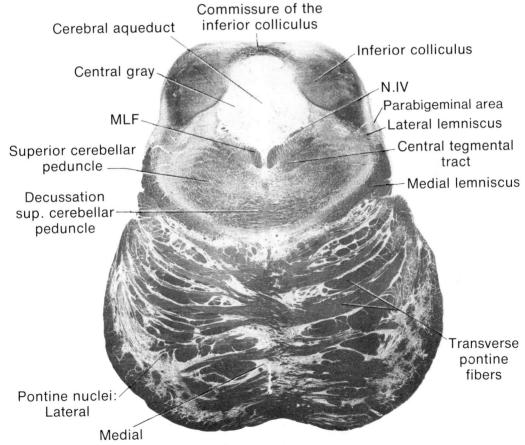

Figure 13-2. Transverse section of the adult midbrain through the inferior colliculus. Large fascicles of corticospinal and corticopontine fibers (unlabeled), cut in cross section, are located among the bundles of transverse pontine fibers. (Weigert's myelin stain, photograph.)

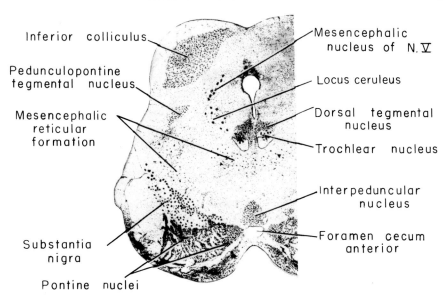

Figure 13-3. Section through inferior colliculi of midbrain. Three-month infant. (Cresyl violet, photograph with schematic representation of main cell groups.)

crura cerebri appear (Figs. 13-3 and 13-6). In some sections, portions of the heavily pigmented substantia nigra are evident dorsal to the most rostral pontine nuclei. Fibers of the lateral lemniscus, located near the lateral surface of the tegmentum, migrate dorsally and enter the inferior colliculus. These fibers envelop the inferior colliculus and form its capsule (Figs. 13-2 and 13-3).

Inferior Colliculi

These distinctive large cellular masses can be divided into three main subdivisions: (a) an ovoid central, cell mass called the central nucleus, (b) a thin dorsal cellular layer, the pericentral nucleus, often referred to as the cortex, and (c) an external nucleus which surrounds the central nucleus laterally, ventrally and rostrally (860, 2194, 2195). The *central nucleus* consists of densely packed small, medium and large cells which are to some extent segregated and arranged in parallel rows or laminae (2194). The central nucleus can be divided into a smaller dorsomedial division consisting mainly of large cells and a larger ventrolateral division composed mainly of medium and small cells with a pronounced laminar arrangement of cells, dendrites and axons (Fig. 13-4). In the ventrolateral division of the central nucleus, laminae form an overlapping onion-like series of concentric curved shells, most of which are incomplete

except for those closest to the center of curvature. The thickness of the laminae is determined by the dendritic ramifications of the principal cell types, referred to as fusiform and bitufted. It is probable that these laminae provide the basis for the tonotopic organization of neurons in the nucleus. Multipolar and large neurons have dendrites which cross one or more laminae and may form the basis for interactions between laminae. Each of these subdivisions contain complete and partial representations of the cochlea and have different afferent and efferent connections (1676, 2232).

The *pericentral nucleus* is a thin sheet of densely packed cells extending over the dorsal and posterior surfaces of the inferior colliculus (Fig. 13-4). This nucleus overlies both major divisions of the central nucleus, and its lateral border is continuous with the external nucleus (2195). Although the pericentral nucleus has been described as having a layered "cortical" structure, Golgi studies suggest only a predominance of certain cell types at different depths of the nucleus. This nucleus is composed of spiny and aspiny cells. Small spiny neurons are found at all depths in the pericentral nucleus, while large spiny neurons, overlying the large-celled division of the central nucleus, project axons into it. Large aspiny neurons are fusiform or multipolar; den-

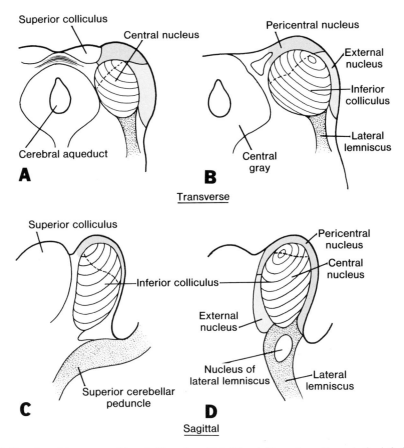

Figure 13-4. Drawing of transverse (*A* and *B*) and sagittal (*C* and *D*) sections through the inferior colliculus outlining the nuclear subdivisions. The pericentral nucleus is indicated in *red*, and the external nucleus in *blue*. The central nucleus in *white* shows contours of the laminae in the ventrolateral division. *Black dashes* indicate the division of the central nucleus into the large-celled dorsomedial part and the ventrolateral laminated part. Laminae in the central nucleus represent a given frequency band across the width of the nucleus and form the basis for the tonotopic organization of neurons. The disc-shaped laminae in dorsal regions are not as thick and represent the lower frequencies; high-frequency octaves are represented ventrally (27, 1676, 2194, 2195).

drites of multipolar neurons extend throughout the depth of the pericentral nucleus, and their axons project toward the brachium of the inferior colliculus. The largest cells are in deepest parts of the nucleus.

The *external nucleus* is composed of cells of various sizes, similar to those found in the central nucleus but less densely packed (2194). This nucleus appears almost continuous with the pericentral nucleus but is traversed by fibers of the lateral lemniscus and the brachium of the inferior colliculus (Fig. 13-4). Physiological studies indicate that the external nucleus is not an auditory relay nucleus like the central nucleus, but a nucleus related primarily to acousticomotor reflexes (27).

The inferior colliculus serves as a relay nucleus in transmitting auditory impulses to the medial geniculate body which in turn projects to the primary auditory cortex. Most cells respond to binaural stimulation and many cells may encode within spatio-temporal discharge patterns information about sound localization. Physiological studies in the cat indicate a definite tonotopic localization within the central and pericentral nuclei of the inferior colliculus (27, 1676, 2211). Neurons in the central nucleus of the inferior colliculus are arranged in a laminar pattern that represents a given frequency band of nearly constant thickness across the width of the nucleus. Isofrequency contours parallel the cellular laminae described in anatomical studies

(1676, 2194) and are tilted down rostrally. Advancement of an electrode from dorsal to ventral in the inferior colliculus consistently gives a sequence of frequencies from low to high in the central nucleus. The disc-shaped laminae representing the lowest frequencies (i.e., dorsal regions) are not as thick or as extensive as those representing middle and high frequency octaves (i.e., ventral region). The frequency representation in the central nucleus simply reflects the proportional representation of frequencies along the cochlear partition, in which low frequencies are perceived at the apex of the cochlea and high frequencies at the base. The central nucleus of the inferior colliculus is a tightly organized structure bearing specific relationships to the cochlea and with elements sharply tuned to different sound frequencies. These data suggest that small sections of the basilar membrane of approximately equal length are represented across individual anatomically defined cellular laminae within the nucleus (1676). This tonotopic organization applies only to the ventrolateral division of the central nucleus.

The pericentral nucleus demonstrates some evidence of a tonotopic organization in which high frequencies are located externally and low frequencies are found near the margins of the central nucleus (27). This nucleus contains units with such broad tuning characteristics that the concept of best frequency is difficult to apply. The majority of these units receive only a contralateral monaural input, and many units are labile and show habituation to repeated identical stimuli. Axons of neurons in the pericentral nucleus project to areas around the ventral division of the medial geniculate body which in turn project to nonprimary auditory cortex (2388). The overall behavior of units in the pericentral nucleus and their monaural input suggest that cells in this nucleus may subserve a role in directing auditory attention (1203).

Efferent fibers from the ventromedial division of the central nucleus of the inferior colliculus project via the brachium of the inferior colliculus to the small-celled ventral part of the medial geniculate body (1374, 1735, 2052, 2194). Anterograde and retrograde transport studies indicate that cells in the ventromedial division of the inferior colliculus distribute fibers in a distinct laminar pattern within the ventral part of the medial geniculate nucleus (Fig. 15-19) that suggests an orderly tonotopic organization (1374). Cells in the dorsal division of the central nucleus and in the pericentral nucleus send fibers to the dorsal part of the medial geniculate body. Thus, the dorsal division of the central nucleus and the pericentral nucleus of the inferior colliculus receive fibers from the auditory cortex but not from the lateral lemniscus. These nuclei ultimately send impulses back to the periauditory cortex via the dorsal part of the medial geniculate body (1374). Cells of the ventral part of the medial geniculate body project tonotopically upon the primary auditory cortex (331).

The inferior colliculus receives fibers from the lateral lemniscus, the opposite inferior colliculus and the auditory cortex (Fig. 12-13). The auditory cortex projects fibers bilaterally to the inferior colliculi; these fibers terminate in the pericentral nucleus and in the dorsomedial division of the central nucleus (631, 2194, 2195). Corticofugal fibers enter the ipsilateral inferior colliculus via the brachium of the inferior colliculus, and some fibers cross to the opposite side via the commissure of the inferior colliculus. The dorsomedial division of the central nucleus also receives direct commissural connections from the corresponding region of the opposite inferior colliculus. Both dorsomedial and ventrolateral divisions of the inferior colliculus receive ascending fibers from the lateral lemniscus. Lateral lemniscal fibers entering the ventromedial division of the inferior colliculus run along the full length of each lamina, follow its curves and are major determinants of the laminar organization. As these fibers traverse a lamina, axons establish synaptic contacts throughout its extent (2194). In addition to receiving fibers from the auditory cortex, the pericentral nucleus receives ascending fibers from the dorsal nucleus of the lateral lemniscus (2195). Cells in the pericentral nucleus project fibers into the central nucleus which course parallel to its laminae, but there is no evidence of a projection in the opposite direction. Detailed neuroanatomical and neurophysiological studies based upon the retrograde transport of horseradish peroxidase

(HRP) have identified specific auditory relay nuclei in the brain stem that project to the central nucleus of the inferior colliculus (7, 2232).

Other efferent fibers pass to the opposite inferior colliculus, to the superior colliculus and to lower relay nuclei in the auditory system (2120). Few, if any, tectospinal fibers arise from the inferior colliculus (2769).

Parabigeminal Area. Ventrolateral to the inferior colliculus is a fairly well-defined zone known as the *parabigeminal area*, lying between the lateral lemniscus and the periphery (Fig. 13-2). It is composed mainly of obliquely, or transversely, running fibers, among which are scattered cells or groups of cells constituting the *parabigeminal nucleus.* This small oval nucleus in the lateral midbrain receives a substantial projection from the superficial layers of the superior colliculus and has a visuotopic organization (935, 946, 2320). Cells of each parabigeminal nucleus project bilaterally upon superficial layers of the superior colliculi and show a regional organization; rostral parts of the nucleus project contralaterally and cells in caudal parts of the nucleus project to the ipsilateral superior colliculus (689, 950). Cells of the parabigeminal nucleus respond briskly and consistently to visual stimuli, can be activated by both moving and stationary spot stimuli and have receptive fields similar in size to those of the superficial layers of the superior colliculus (2320). The parabigeminal nucleus has a representation of the entire contralateral visual field and at least the central part of the ipsilateral field. Findings suggest that the parabigeminal nucleus functions with the superior colliculus in processing visual information.

The Trochlear Nerve. The nucleus of the trochlear nerve is a small compact cell group in the ventral part of the central gray that appears to indent the dorsal surface of the medial longitudinal fasciculus (Figs. 13-3 and 13-5). The nucleus consists of a column of typical somatic motor cells that in essence constitute a small caudal appendage of the oculomotor nuclear complex. Root fibers emerging from the nucleus curve dorsolaterally and caudally in the outer margin of the central gray, decussate completely in the superior medullary velum and exit from the dorsal surface of the brain stem caudal to the inferior colliculus (Figs. 2-24, 2-25, 11-2, 12-29, 13-2, 13-3 and A-9). Peripherally the slender nerve root curves around the lateral surface of the brain stem, passes between the superior cerebellar and posterior cerebral arteries and enters the cavernous sinus (Fig. 20-10). This cranial nerve innervates the superior oblique muscle that serves to: (a) intort the eye when abducted, and (b) depress the eye when adducted. Lesions involving the trochlear nerve alone are unusual, and detection of resulting disturbances of extraocular movement by inspection is difficult. Diplopia resulting from such a nerve lesion is vertical and maximal on attempted downward gaze to the opposite side. Patients with trochlear nerve lesions complain especially of difficulty in walking downstairs. Tilting of the head to the opposite side, seen in some patients with trochlear nerve lesions, is a posture which compensates for the weakness of ocular intortion on the lesion side (488).

Tegmental and Interpeduncular Nuclei. The narrow aqueduct, somewhat triangular in section, is surrounded by a broad layer of central gray substance that contains numerous diffuse cell groups. In the raphe region several nuclei are present at this level (Fig. 13-3). The *dorsal nucleus of the raphe* has expanded and is flanked laterally by the *dorsal tegmental nucleus* (Figs. 11-15, 12-30 and 13-3). This nucleus, composed mainly of small cells in the central gray dorsomedial to, and between the trochlear nuclei, has been called the *supratrochlear nucleus* (1885). Although the dorsal nucleus of the raphe and the dorsal tegmental nucleus are adjacent to each other, only the dorsal nucleus of the raphe synthesizes and transports serotonin. Immediately ventral to the medial longitudinal fasciculus, the cells near the raphe constitute the *ventral tegmental nucleus,* which appears to be a continuation of the superior central nucleus of the pons.; these nuclei usually are designated together as the *superior central nucleus.*

In histofluorescent studies, serotonin-containing neurons (5-HT cells) have been located in pontine and mesencephalic raphe nuclei (Fig. 12-34); these cell groups have been identified as the dorsal nucleus of the raphe (group B7), the median nucleus of

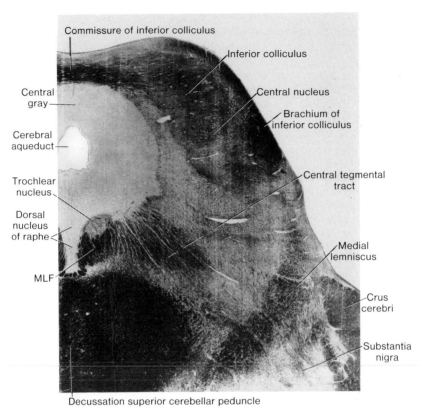

Commissure of inferior colliculus
Inferior colliculus
Central gray
Central nucleus
Brachium of inferior colliculus
Cerebral aqueduct
Trochlear nucleus
Central tegmental tract
Dorsal nucleus of raphe
MLF
Medial lemniscus
Crus cerebri
Substantia nigra
Decussation superior cerebellar peduncle

Figure 13-5. Photograph of the right dorsal quadrant of a section through the rostral part of the inferior colliculus. (Weigert's myelin stain.)

the raphe (superior central nucleus, group B8) and the lateral cell group (B9) (585). Detailed anatomical and biochemical studies reveal that cell groups B7 and B8 give rise to two distinct but overlapping ascending systems that have serotonin (5-HT) as their neurotransmitter (201, 202, 873, 1737, 1878, 2532). Although these ascending serotoninergic systems are overlapping, they each have distinctive features; the ascending pathways arising from the dorsal nucleus of the raphe (B7) have been called the *mesostriatal system*, while those arising from the median raphe nucleus (B8) have been referred to as the *mesolimbic system* (873). The dorsal nucleus of the raphe (B7) projects to the periaqueductal gray and gives rise to fibers that ascend in the medial forebrain bundle and that project to the substantia nigra, the hypothalamus, the intralaminar thalamic nuclei, the lateral geniculate body, the striatum, the amygdaloid nuclear complex and broad regions of the

frontal cortex. The median raphe nucleus (B8) projects fibers to the midbrain reticular formation, the hypothalamus, including the mammillary bodies, the septal area, the entorhinal cortex and the hippocampal formation. The median raphe nucleus, unlike the dorsal nucleus of the raphe, gives rise to descending fibers projecting to the cerebellum, the locus ceruleus, the reticular formation of the lower brain stem and the raphe nuclei of the pons and the medulla (202). Serotonin conveyed by these systems is believed to act as an inhibitory neurotransmitter (1001, 1878).

In the raphe region of the ventral tegmentum is the *interpeduncular nucleus*, a collection of medium-sized, multipolar, slightly pigmented cells (Fig. 13-3). This nucleus, situated immediately dorsal to the interpeduncular fossa, is prominent in most mammals but comparatively small in man. Fibers from the habenular nucleus project to the interpeduncular nucleus via the fasciculus retroflexus (Figs. 15-6 and 16-7); some fibers in this bundle bypass the interpeduncular nucleus and are distributed to the superior central nucleus, the dorsal tegmental nucleus and caudal regions of the central gray (1816). The dorsal tegmental nucleus also receives fibers from the interpeduncular nucleus and from the mammillary bodies (via the mammillotegmental tract). The dorsal tegmental nucleus appears related to the *dorsal longitudinal fasciculus* (of Schütz), a small but complex pathway in the ventromedial part of the central gray (Fig. 16-10). Although the prevailing direction of conduction in this bundle appears to be ascending, it contains some descending elements, but few of these reach pontine levels. The pathways described above contstitute part of the complex system by which impulses related to the limbic system are projected to midbrain levels. It is also apparent that ascending systems arising from the raphe nuclei at these levels convey serotonin to terminals in selective, but widely dispersed, loci within the diencephalon and forebrain. Impulses conducted via these pathways are thought to be concerned primarily with visceral and behavioral functions.

Corticofugal fibers (corticospinal, corticopontine and corticobulbar) on the ventral surface of the brain stem undergo a rearrangement and at higher levels begin to form the *crus cerebri* (Fig. 13-3). At slightly higher levels these fibers are separated from the tegmentum by a mass of gray matter, the *substantia nigra* (Figs. 13-6, A-10 and A-11).

SUPERIOR COLLICULAR LEVEL

Transverse sections of the rostral midbrain appear strikingly different from those through the inferior colliculus in that: (a) the flattened superior colliculi form the rostral part of the tectum (Figs. 13-6–13-8), (b) the oculomotor nuclei form a V-shaped complex ventral to the central gray and root fibers of the oculomotor nerve emerge from the interpeduncular fossa (Figs. 13-1, 13-6 and 13-18), (c) the red nuclei, surrounded by fibers of the superior cerebellar peduncle, occupy the central tegmental region (Figs. 13-1, 13-6 and 13-14), and (d) the substantiae nigrae achieve their maximum size ventral to the tegmentum and dorsal to

the crura cerebri (Fig. 13-6). Fibers of the brachium of the inferior colliculus lie on the lateral surface of the tegmentum (Fig. 13-6). The medial lemniscus appears as a curved bundle dorsal to the substantia nigra and lateral to the red nucleus. Fibers of the spinothalamic and spinotectal tracts lie medial to the most dorsal part of the medial lemniscus.

Superior Colliculi

The superior colliculi are two flattened eminences which form the rostral half of the tectum (Figs. 2-24, 2-25, 13-6 and A-11). In submammalian vertebrates the optic tectum, a structure homologous with the mammalian superior colliculus, has a complex laminated structure resembling that of the cerebral cortex and is the primary termination of the optic tract. Beginning with reptiles, the importance of the superior colliculus in visual discrimination progressively diminishes as an increasing number of optic fibers establish more extensive connections with the thalamus and cortex. In man the superior colliculi have become reduced in size and serve primarily as reflex centers, influencing the position of the head and eyes in response to visual, auditory and somatic stimuli (920). The superior colliculus is concerned primarily with the detection of the direction of movement of objects in the visual fields (2436), and in this way it facilitates visual orientation, searching and tracking. Cells in deeper layers of the superior colliculus appear to respond to auditory, somatic and visual stimuli, sometimes separately and sometimes in different combinations (920). The deep layers of the superior colliculus receive inputs not only from diverse relay nuclei of the somesthetic and auditory system but also from catecholamine-containing nuclei, the deep cerebellar nuclei, the zona incerta, the substantia nigra and various regions of the reticular formation (689). These deep layers have many anatomical and physiological characteristics of the brain stem reticular formation. In contrast, the superficial layers of the superior colliculus have features that characterize specific sensory structures. Most of the afferents to the superficial layers are derived from the retina and visual cortex. Physiologically the superficial lay-

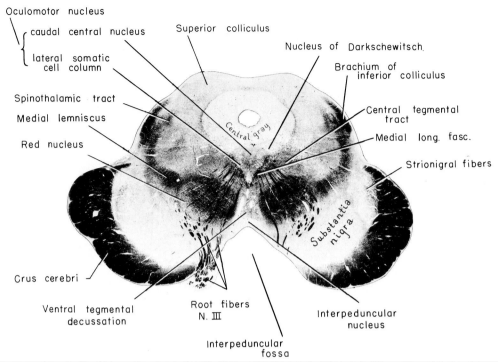

Figure 13-6. Transverse section of adult midbrain through the level of the oculomotor nerve. (Weigert's myelin stain, photograph.)

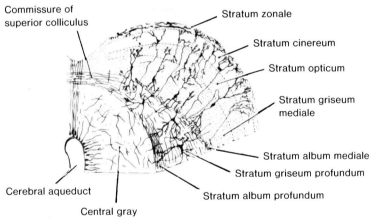

Figure 13-7. Drawing of the cellular lamination and organization of the superior colliculus based upon Golgi preparations from a human fetus.

ers respond only to visual stimuli and exhibit relatively small receptive fields.

Further efferent fibers arising in the superficial layers of the superior colliculus project to regions of the pulvinar and posterior thalamus that form parts of an extrageniculate visual pathway which parallels the geniculostriate system (51, 427, 946, 1039).

Each colliculus still shows in a rudimentary form the complex laminated structure found in lower forms and consists of several alternating layers of gray and white matter (Figs. 10-18, 13-7 and 13-8). From the surface inward these layers are: (a) the *stratum zonale* (mainly fibrous), (b) the *stratum cinereum* (outer gray layer), (c) the *stratum opticum* (superficial white layer), and (d)

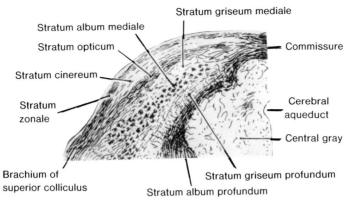

Figure 13-8. Drawing of the myelinated fiber structure of the superior colliculus based upon Weigert-stained sections.

the *stratum lemnisci* consisting of middle and deep, gray and white layers (Figs. 13-7 and 13-8). The stratum zonale is composed of fine nerve fibers arising mainly from the occipital cortex and entering through the brachium of the superior colliculus. Among the fibers are small, mostly horizontal cells with tangentially or centrally directed axons. The stratum cinereum consists of radially arranged cells whose dendrites pass peripherally and whose axons project inward. The larger cells lie deepest. The stratum opticum is composed mainly of fibers from the ganglion cells of the retina, and corticotectal fibers arising from the visual cortex. These fibers enter the stratum opticum via the brachium of the superior colliculus and pass into the superficial and middle gray layers. Corticotectal fibers from the frontal lobe (Brodmann's area 8) reach superficial and middle layers of the superior colliculus via a transtegmental approach and are thought to participate in mechanisms related to saccadic eye movements (1395, 1396). The stratum lemnisci, composed of medium-sized and large stellate cells, receives heterogenous inputs from diverse sources, most of which are somatosensory and auditory. These deep layers of the superior colliculus receive afferents from: (a) the spinal cord (i.e., spinotectal tract), (b) somatosensory relay nuclei (i.e., nucleus cuneatus, lateral cervical nucleus, and spinal trigeminal nucleus), (c) catecholamine-containing nuclei (i.e., locus ceruleus, dorsal nucleus of the raphe and parabrachial nuclei), (d) the inferior colliculus and a variety of auditory relay nuclei, (e) the deep cerebellar nuclei, (f) the substantia nigra (Fig. 13-10) and various parts of the brain stem reticular formation (689, 1212, 1658). Thus the superior colliculi are composed of two structurally and functionally distinct components, the superficial layers that receive most of their input from the retina and the visual cortex, and the deep layers that receive input from multiple sources, respond to a variety of different stimuli and appear to function in a manner similar to the reticular formation (427, 689, 1039).

The superior colliculus receives its principal input from: (a) the retina, (b) the cerebral cortex, (c) the inferior colliculus and (d) the spinal cord.

Retinotectal fibers arise from ganglion cells of the retina and pass via the optic nerve and optic tract to the superior colliculus via its brachium. These fibers leave the optic tract rostral to its principal termination in the lateral geniculate body. Fibers arise from all portions of the retina of each eye, but crossed fibers are most numerous. Impulses from the contralateral homonymous halves of the visual field project upon the superior colliculus in an orderly fashion (Fig. 13-9). Contrary to earlier studies, optic fibers project to all parts of the superior colliculus, including the anterolateral third of this structure, where the fovea is represented (582, 1153). Physiological and autoradiographic studies in the monkey indicate that upper quadrants of the contralateral visual field are represented in medial parts of the superior colliculus, while the lower quadrants project impulses to lateral regions of this structure. The contralateral peripheral visual field is

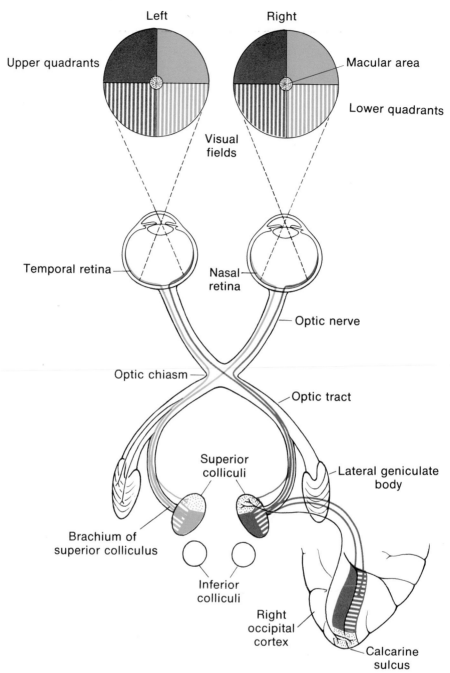

Figure 13-9. Diagrammatic representation of the projections of the retinae and striate cortex upon the superior colliculi in the monkey. Retinotectal fibers from the ipsilateral temporal and contralateral nasal halves of the retinae, which subserve the contralateral homonymous visual field, project to the superior colliculus. Cells in portions of the retinae concerned with the contralateral peripheral visual field project to the posterior two-thirds of the superior colliculus. Upper quadrants of the contralateral peripheral visual field (*solid blue* and *red*) are represented in medial region of caudal parts of the superior colliculus, while lower quadrants of the contralateral peripheral visual field (*blue* and *red stripes*) are represented in lateral regions. Portions of the retinae concerned with central vision (i.e., within 10° of the fovae centralis; *blue* and *red dots*) are represented in the rostral third of the superior colliculus. Although retinotectal fibers arise from portions of the retina of each eye, crossed fibers are most numerous. Corticotectal fibers from the striate cortex, shown on the *right*, project to all parts of the superior colliculus via its brachium. There is a correspondence in the superior colliculus of retinotectal and corticotectal terminations that represent both central and peripheral parts of the visual field.

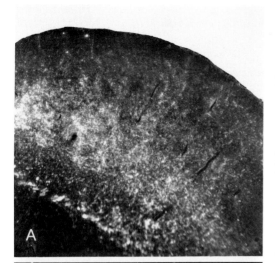

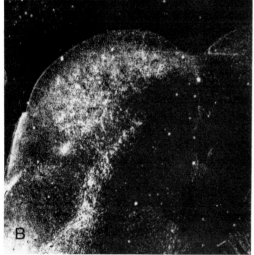

Figure 13-10. Dark field photomicrographs of autoradiographs, demonstrating the regions of termination of nigrotectal fibers in the monkey. Nigrotectal fibers arise from cells of the pars reticulata and project transtegmentally (*B*) to terminations mainly in the middle gray layers (*A*) of the superior colliculus. (Reproduced with permission from A. Jayaraman, R. R. Batton, and M. Carpenter: *Brain Research,* **135:** 147–152, 1977 (1212).)

surface of the superior colliculus (stratum cinereum) which becomes thinner in lateral regions and may show gaps or "holes" devoid of silver grains. Although less label is transported to the ipsilateral superior colliculus, silver grains appear as a series of "puffs" or clumps. The region corresponding to the optic disc of the opposite eye has been identified near the center of the superior colliculus; this area receives only an ipsilateral input (1153). In the superior colliculus the representation of the contralateral eye is dominant, a finding that contrasts with the equal representation of the two eyes in the lateral geniculate bodies and in the striate cortex. The temporal monocular crescent of the visual field is represented only posteromedially in the contralateral superior colliculus. In the cat and a variety of nonprimates a direct projection from the temporal retina to a small rostral region of the opposite superior colliculus has been demonstrated (1038).

Corticotectal fibers arise from portions of the frontal, temporal, parietal and occipital lobes. The most substantial and highly organized projection arises from the visual cortex (848, 1411, 2732). These fibers enter the stratum opticum and terminate in the superficial and middle gray layers of the superior colliculus, in the same manner as fibers from the retina. Corticotectal fibers from the visual cortex project ipsilaterally and are so organized that parts of striate cortex related to a particular part of the retina send fibers to that region of the superior colliculus. Thus there is a correspondence in the superior colliculus of retinotectal and corticotectal terminations that represent both central and peripheral parts of the retina (848, 2732). Superior portions of the retina (i.e., inferior half of the visual field) are represented superiorly in the visual cortex and laterally in the superior colliculus, while inferior portions of the retina (i.e., superior half of the visual field) are represented inferiorly in the visual cortex and medially in the superior colliculus. Thus many of the same cells of the superior colliculus receive distinct, but related, inputs from the ganglion cells of the retina and cells of the striate cortex. The macular representation in the superior colliculus receives inputs from both the striate cortex and the retina. Cells in the rostral part of the superior colliculus represent the

represented in the posterior two-thirds of the superior colliculus, while the central visual field (i.e., within 10° of the fovea) occupies the remaining rostral third.

Autoradiographic studies have brought out significant differences in the mode of termination and distribution of contralateral and ipsilateral retinotectal fibers (947, 1038, 1153). On the side contralateral to the eye injected with radioactive label, silver grains form a continuous layer beneath the macular area of the retina. At this brain stem level there is an interaction and integration of peripheral visual impulses with the more complex output of the visual cortex. Although retinal and visual cortical projections to the superior colliculus are similar, there are certain differences: (a) retinotectal projections are bilateral, (b) corticotectal fibers are unilateral, and (c) only corticotectal projections have some terminals in the stratum zonale.

Cortical projections from the frontal eye field (Brodmann's area 8), redetermined by autoradiographic technics, indicate terminations in the middle gray layer, the stratum opticum and the stratum zonale (1396). These fibers terminate largely in medial regions of the superior colliculus throughout its rostrocaudal extent. Cells in superficial layers respond to visual stimuli, while those in the middle gray layers discharge vigorously before the onset of saccadic eye movements. Fibers from the auditory cortex project mainly to deep layers in caudal parts of the superior colliculus that receive no input from the visual system (631).

Spinotectal fibers usually are cited as the principal somatosensory afferents to the deep layers of the superior colliculus, but recent retrograde transport studies suggest that these fibers are not numerous. While some somatosensory input to the superior colliculus arises from cells in the dorsal horn (lamina IV), the major sources of such afferents are the posterior column nuclei (particularly the nucleus cuneatus), the lateral cervical nucleus and parts of the spinal trigeminal nuclear complex (689). Regardless of the locations of the cells of origin, somatosensory input to the deep layers of the superior colliculus is topographically organized with the head represented rostrally, the forelimbs posterolaterally and the remainder of the body posteromedially (751, 2427). The somatotopic representation is distorted in that regions related to the head and forelimb are unusually large.

Brain stem afferents to the superior colliculus have been shown to arise from the inferior colliculus and a number of auditory relay nuclei (689, 2052, 2515). Projections to deep layers of caudal parts of the superior colliculus arise mainly from the external and pericentral nuclei of the inferior colliculus. Other auditory relay nuclei projecting fibers to the superior colliculus include the ventral nucleus of the lateral lemniscus and the nuclei of the trapezoid body.

The *commissure of the superior colliculus* (Figs. 13-7 and 13-8) interconnects primarily regions of the deep and intermediate gray layers in the rostral halves of the superior colliculi (688). In addition to commissural fibers interconnecting corresponding regions of the colliculi, this bundle contains some fibers projecting to noncorresponding areas of the colliculus and some decussating elements of both tectal and nontectal origin. It has been postulated that the commissural projection reciprocally connecting the deep gray layers may be related to motor functions, since all major brain stem efferents rise from the two deep layers. Commissural fibers may mediate mutually suppressive effects on the output of the colliculi to prevent competing responses in the opposite direction. While the commissure may function in relation to eye movements involved in visual tracking, the superior colliculi also functions to provide orientation to acoustic and somatic stimuli.

As the preceding discussion indicates, the superior colliculus can be partitioned into two zones: (a) the superficial layers which receive primarily visual afferents, and (b) a deep layer which receives a heterogeneous multimodal input. Although the superficial layers of the superior colliculus, the stratum zonale, the stratum cinereum and stratum opticum have projections distinct from that of all deeper layers, they also project to the deep layers (1036). In general the superficial layers give rise to ascending fibers and the deep layers project descending fibers to nuclei in the brain stem and spinal cord. The superficial layers of the superior colliculus project fibers to subdivisions of the ipsilateral pulvinar, the dorsal and ventral lateral geniculate nuclei and perhaps the pretectum (51, 154, 427, 946, 1039). The pulvinar receives the most extensive projection from the superficial layers of the colliculus and in turn projects upon extrastriate cortical areas (areas 18 and 19) (155, 897). Thus the superficial layers of the superior colliculus give rise to *tectothalamic fibers*, part of which convey visual information to the extrastriate cortex via the pulvinar. It also has been shown in the primate that cells in the most superficial layers of the superior colliculus project upon the dorsal lateral geniculate body (1037). These *tectogeniculate fibers* terminate in intralaminar geniculate regions adjacent to the magnocellular layers which are thought to contain interneurons. Thus, visual pathways to the cortex via the superior colliculus and the lateral geniculate body are not entirely separate. The deep layers of the superior colliculus also give rise to ascending fibers that project to the posterior and intralaminar thalamic nuclei (1039).

Descending tectofugal fibers largely arise from laminae of the superior colliculus ventral to the stratum opticum and can be grouped into uncrossed tectopontine and tectobulbar tracts, and crossed tectobulbar and tectospinal projections.

Uncrossed tectopontine and *tectobulbar fibers* project to the ipsilateral dorsolateral pontine nuclei, the lateral part of the reticulotegmental nucleus and to the nucleus reticularis pontis oralis (51, 1036, 1039, 1272). In addition, deep layers of the superior colliculus project fibers to the cuneiform nucleus and the external nucleus of the inferior colliculus. Superficial layers of superior colliculus give rise to a substantial ipsilateral projection to the parabigeminal nucleus, a structure that has bilateral regionally organized projections to the superior colliculus (950, 1036). The dorsolateral region of the pontine nuclei which receives fibers from the superior colliculus also receives inputs from the visual and auditory cortex (292, 848) and from the pretectum and ventral lateral geniculate body; this collection of pontine nuclei projects to lobules VI and VII of the cerebellar vermis (276a) and are responsive to visual, auditory and somatosensory stimuli (2369). Tectoreticular fibers distributed to the midbrain and pontine reticular formation play a role in the electroencephalogram (EEG) arousal response (1217). Some tectofugal fibers enter the accessory oculomotor nuclei (i.e., the nucleus of Darkschewitsch and the interstitial nucleus of Cajal), but none appear to enter the oculomotor complex (51, 1600, 1935, 2116, 2494).

Crossed tectobulbar and tectospinal fibers decussate in the dorsal tegmental decussation at midbrain levels and descend near the median raphe (Fig. 10-18); at medullary levels these fibers become incorporated within the medial longitudinal fasciculus. Tectospinal fibers continuing to cervical spinal segments descend in the medial part of the anterior funiculus (Fig. 10-24). In the brain stem this crossed projection is referred to as the *predorsal bundle*. Fibers from this bundle project to the reticulotegmental nucleus and to both rostral and caudal portions of the pontine reticular formation (1036). At medullary levels, crossed tectobulbar fibers terminate in parts of the medial accessory olivary nucleus (i.e., nucleus β). Tectospinal fibers descending only to cervical spinal segments terminate in laminae VIII, VII and VI (1855).

Functional Considerations. Each superior colliculus receives a visual input from the contralateral visual field. In addition, it receives an ipsilateral projection from the visual cortex supplying information concerning only the contralateral visual field. These two systems are precisely and topographically organized at all levels. Unilateral lesions of the superior colliculus in a variety of animals produce: (a) relative neglect of stimuli in the contralateral visual field, (b) deficits in perception involving spatial discriminations and tracking of moving objects, (c) heightened responses to stimuli in the ipsilateral visual field, and (d) no impairment of eye movements (2412, 2416). These disturbances undergo considerable attenuation in time, but they indicate that the superior colliculus contributes to the coordination of head and eye movements used to localize and follow visual stimuli.

Physiological studies in the cat indicate that the collicular receptive fields are two to four times larger than the receptive fields in the visual cortex. A receptive field in the visual system is defined as that region of the retina (or visual field) over which one can influence the firing of a particular ganglion cell (1375). The receptive field consists of a central circular region and a concentric surround. Most collicular cells respond only to moving stimuli and three-fourths of these cells show directional selectivity (582, 2436). These cells respond vigorously to movement in one direction, poorly, or not at all, to movement in the opposite direction, and are nonresponsive to stationary stimuli flashed on and off within the receptive field. In the superior colliculus the preferred directional selectivity is parallel to the horizontal meridian of the visual field and toward the periphery of the visual field. Thus most units in the right superior colliculus have receptive fields in the left visual field and responded best to stimuli moving from right to left. Cells in the superficial layers of the superior colliculus are most responsive to small moving objects.

In animals in which the visual cortex has been removed, cells of the superior colliculus lose their directional sensitivity to moving objects in the visual field (2714). While in the normal animal cells in the superior colliculus can be driven by stimuli to either eye, following ablations of the visual cortex, these cells respond only to stimuli in the contralateral eye. Thus, the superior colliculus cannot perform its normal function as a detector of specific movements within the visual field when deprived of input from the visual cortex.

It appears well established that stimulation of the superior colliculus results in contralateral conjugate deviations of the eyes (80, 2459), even though this structure has no projections to the nuclei of the extraocular muscles. Part of these responses may be mediated by colliuclar projections to the interstitial nucleus of Cajal which projects to specific subdivisions of the contralateral oculomotor complex (404, 2426). The superior colliculus also has projections to the pontine paramedian reticular formation (PPRF) which projects directly to the ipsilateral abducens nucleus (343). Although the PPRF has no direct connections with the oculomotor complex, impulses relayed via abducens internuclear neurons can influence subdivisions of the oculomotor nuclear complex (393).

Electrical stimulation of the superior colliculus in alert monkeys also elicits short-latency saccadic eye movements (2193, 2280). The amplitude and direction of these saccades are a function of the site stimulated within the superior colliculus; medial regions of the colliculus are associated with upward components, while lateral regions have downward components (2389). Chronic microelectrode recordings in the intermediate and deep layers of the superior colliculus have shown maximal discharges of neurons prior to eye movements

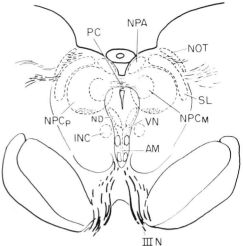

Figure 13-11. Outline drawing of a brain stem section through the most compact portion of the posterior commissure (*PC*). At this level, the nucleus of the optic tract (*NOT*), the sublentiform nucleus (*SL*), the nucleus of the pretectal area (*NPA*) and the nuclei of the posterior commissure (*NPC*) are well developed. The anterior median nucleus (*AM*) is present, but the dorsal visceral nuclei (*VN*) of the oculomotor complex have not separated into medial and lateral cell columns. Additional abbreviations: *INC*, interstitial nucleus of Cajal; *ND*, nucleus of Darkschewitsch; *NPC_M*, nucleus of posterior commissure, pars magnocellularis; *NPC_P*, nucleus of posterior commissure, pars principalis; *III N*, oculomotor nerve. (Reproduced with permission from M. B. Carpenter and R. J. Pierson: *Journal of Comparative Neurology,* **149:** 271–300, 1973 (414).)

in particular directions. These studies indicate that the superior colliculus is involved in coding the location of an object relative to the fovea and in eliciting saccadic eye movements that produce foveal acquisition of the object (2389).

The Pretectal Region

This region lies immediately rostral to the superior colliculus at levels of the posterior commissure (Figs. 13-11 and 15-5). Several distinct cell groups within this region are related to the visual system. The nuclei of the pretectal region include: (a) the nucleus of the optic tract, (b) the sublentiform nucleus, (c) the nucleus of the pretectal area, (d) the pretectal olivary nucleus, and (e) principal pretectal nucleus (87, 414, 1261, 1386). The nucleus of the optic tract consists of an irregular plate of large cells along the dorsolateral border of the pretectum at its junction with the pul-

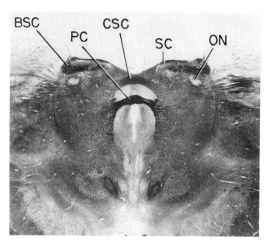

Figure 13-12. Photomicrograph of a myelin-stained section at junction of pretectum and superior colliculus in the rhesus monkey. Abbreviations: *BSC*, brachium of the superior colliculus; *CSC*, commissure of the superior colliculus; *ON*, pretectal olivary nucleus; *PC*, posterior commissure; *SC*, superior colliculus. (Weil stain.) (Reproduced with permission from: M. B. Carpenter and R. J. Pierson: *Journal of Comparative Neurology*, **149:** 271–300, 1973 (414).)

vinar (Fig. 13-11). The sublentiform nucleus forms a crescent-shaped group of small- and medium-sized cells medial to the nucleus of the optic tract. The nucleus of the pretectal area occupies a dorsomedial part of the pretectum throughout its extent. The pretectal olivary nucleus (or olivary nucleus of the superior colliculus) forms a sharply delimited cell group at levels through caudal parts of the posterior commissure and rostrolateral parts of the superior colliculus (Fig. 13-12). This nucleus and the nucleus of the optic tract are considered to be derived from a common ontogenetic matrix. The principal pretectal nucleus lies ventral to the sublentiform nucleus and its boundaries are difficult to distinguish. These nuclei receive fibers from the optic tract, the lateral geniculate body, certain areas of the cortex and probably from the posterior thalamic nuclei (848, 886, 887, 1074, 2009, 2263). The pretectal region is considered to be principal midbrain center involved in the *pupillary light reflex* (1590, 1591, 2111).

Degeneration studies in the monkey indicate that fibers from the pretectal olivary nucleus, which receives both crossed and uncrossed retinofugal fibers, cross in the posterior commissure and project to spe-

cific components of the visceral nuclei of the oculomotor complex (Fig. 13–18) (414). Retrograde transport studies using HRP confirm that the pretectal olivary nucleus is the main source of afferents to the visceral nuclei of the oculomotor complex (2426). Fibers from the nuclei of the posterior commissure, projecting bilaterally to other visceral nuclei, partially decussate ventral to the cerebral aqueduct (Fig. 13-18). Because of the complex crossed and uncrossed projections to the visceral nuclei of N. III, only relatively large lesions involving multiple structures in the pretectum impair the pupillary light reflex.

The Posterior Commissure

The region of transition from midbrain to diencephalon is marked dorsally by the *posterior commissure*. The posterior commissure lies immediately rostral to the superior colliculus at the place where the cerebral aqueduct becomes the third ventricle (Figs. 2-27, 13-11, 13-12, 13-13*A* and 13-16*B*). Fibers of the posterior commissure are surrounded rostrally, laterally and ventrally by cells known collectively as the nuclei of the posterior commissure (Fig. 13-11) (412). Although the posterior commissure is a fairly good sized bundle and appears to contain several different fiber components, its entire composition is unknown. The posterior commissure is considered to contain: (a) fibers from the pretectal nuclei, (b) fibers from the nuclei of the posterior commissure (Fig. 13-11), and (c) fibers from the interstitial nucleus and the nucleus of Darkschewitsch (Fig. 13-19). Fibers from the pretectal olivary nucleus (Fig. 13-12) cross in the commissure to the same nucleus on the opposite side and give collaterals to the visceral nuclei of the oculomotor complex (Fig. 13-18). Lesions in the posterior commissure are said to reduce, but not eliminate, the consensual pupillary light reflex in the cat (1592). In the monkey, interruption of fibers of the commissure in the midline produces no detectable change in the pupillary light reflex as measured in infrared pupillograms (414). Lesions in the nuclei of the posterior commissure, interrupting fibers from the interstitial nuclei of Cajal, produce bilateral eyelid retraction and impairment of vertical eye movements (404).

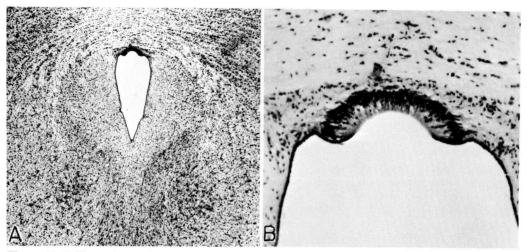

Figure 13-13. Photomicrographs of the subcommissural organ in the rhesus monkey. *A* shows the position of the structure in the roof of the aqueduct beneath the posterior commissure. *B* contrasts the tall columnar cells of the subcommissural organ with the cells of the ependyma. (Nissl stain, ×16; ×100.)

The *subcommissural organ* is a modified ependymal plate in the roof of the cerebral aqueduct immediately beneath the posterior commissure (Figs. 1-19 and 13-13). This periventricular organ consists of ciliated columnar cells which appear to have a secretory function (2755). The secretory product of these cells, in all species except man, is condensed to form a strand of proteinaceous material (Reissner's fiber) that extends through the aqueduct, the fourth ventricle and into the spinal canal. Cells of the subcommissural organ are different than the usual ependymal cells in that they have projections into the ventricular lumen covered with protruding microvilli, an abundance of rough endoplasmic reticulum and microtubules; these cells also show pinocytotic vesicles near the cell surface (506). These data, based upon scanning and transmission electron microscopy, suggest that cells of the subcommissural organ are active in secretion and possibly in absorbing substances from the cerebrospinal fluid. The function of the subcommissural organ in man is unknown, but it has been suggested that it may serve as a volume receptor (877), play an important role in control of salt and water balance (876, 1617), and be concerned with thirst and water intake.

The Oculomotor Nerve

The Oculomotor Nuclear Complex. The oculomotor nuclear complex is a collection of cell columns and discrete nuclei which: (a) innervate all the extraocular muscles except the lateral rectus and the superior oblique, (b) supply the levator palpebrae muscle, and (c) provide preganglionic parasympathetic fibers to the ciliary ganglion. Functional components of the nerve are categorized as *general somatic efferent* (GSE) and *general visceral efferent* (GVE). This complex lies ventral to the central gray in the midline in a "V"-shaped trough formed by the diverging fibers of the medial longitudinal fasciculus (MLF); it extends from the rostral pole of the trochlear nucleus to the upper limit of the midbrain (Figs. 13-6, 13-11, 13-12, 13-14 and 13-15). The nuclear complex consists of paired lateral somatic cell columns, midline and dorsal visceral nuclei and a discrete midline dorsal cell group called the caudal central nucleus.

The *lateral somatic cell columns*, composed of large motor-type neurons, innervate the extraocular muscles (2677). The dorsal cell column (or nucleus) innervates the inferior rectus muscle, the intermediate cell column innervates the inferior oblique muscle and the ventral cell column supplies fibers to the medial rectus muscle (Fig. 13-15). Root fibers arising from these cell columns are uncrossed. A cell column medial to both the dorsal and intermediate cell columns, referred to as the medial cell column, provides crossed fibers that innervate the superior rectus muscle.

The *caudal central nucleus* is a midline

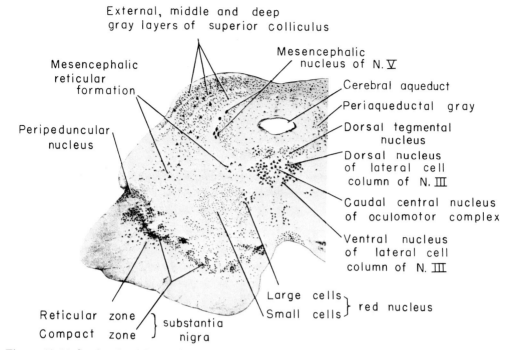

External, middle and deep
gray layers of superior colliculus

Mesencephalic
reticular
formation

Mesencephalic
nucleus of N. Ⅴ

Cerebral aqueduct

Periaqueductal gray

Peripeduncular
nucleus

Dorsal tegmental
nucleus

Dorsal nucleus
of lateral cell
column of N. Ⅲ

Caudal central nucleus
of oculomotor complex

Ventral nucleus
of lateral cell
column of N. Ⅲ

Large cells ⎤
Small cells ⎦ red nucleus

Reticular zone ⎫
Compact zone ⎭ substantia nigra

Figure 13-14. Section through superior colliculi of midbrain. Three-month infant. (Cresyl violet, photograph in which the main cell groups have been schematically blocked in.)

somatic cell group found only in the caudal third of the complex (2678). This nucleus gives rise to crossed and uncrossed fibers that innervate the levator palpebrae muscle (Figs. 13-14 and 13-15).

Visceral nuclei of the oculomotor nuclear complex consist of two distinct nuclear groups which are in continuity rostrally, and often are collectively referred to as the *Edinger-Westphal nucleus* (Figs. 13-11, 13-15 and 13-16A). The most rostral of these are the *anterior median nuclei*. The anterior median nuclei lie rostral to the somatic cell columns and consist of two slender, paired cell columns lying on each side of the median raphe (Figs. 13-11 and 13-18). Further caudally these nuclei elongate in a dorsoventral dimension and lie between rostral portions of the lateral somatic cell columns (principally the dorsal cell columns). Dorsally and rostrally cells of the anterior median nucleus merge with the dorsal visceral cell columns (Figs. 13-15 and 13-16A), which form the Edinger-Westphal nucleus in the strict sense (2679). The dorsal visceral cell columns lie dorsal to the rostral three-fifths of the somatic cell columns. Rostrally each nucleus is composed of two cell types: medium-sized round cells

which occupy a medial region, and smaller lightly staining cells in a lateral region (412). Further caudally the cell group divides into a medial cell column of medium-sized cells and a distinct small-celled lateral cell column that lies slightly more dorsal. The anterior median nuclei and the lateral visceral cell column receive fibers from the contralateral pretectal olivary nuclei which cross in the posterior commissure (2426) (Fig. 13-18). The anterior median and medial visceral cell columns receive bilateral projections from the nuclei of the posterior commissure which partially decussate ventral to the aqueduct (414). Both the anterior median nucleus and the medial dorsal visceral cell columns give rise to uncrossed preganglionic parasympathetic fibers that emerge with somatic root fibers (326). These fibers pass to the ciliary ganglion and synapse upon postganglionic neurons which give rise to the short ciliary nerves. Postganglionic nerve fibers innervate the ciliary body, concerned with the mechanism of accommodation, and the sphincter of the iris (pupillary light reflex). According to Warwick (2679), practically all of the cells of the ciliary ganglion (97%) innervate the intrinsic ocular musculature; only a small

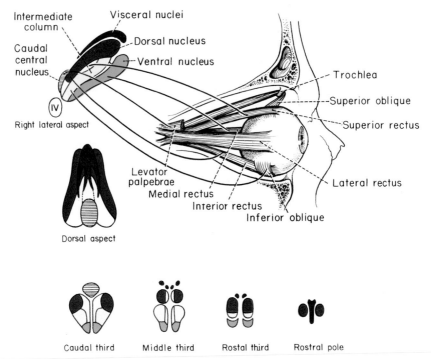

Figure 13-15. Schematic representation of the localization of the extraocular muscles within the oculomotor nuclear complex, based upon studies in the rhesus monkey (2677). Cell columns composing the complex are shown in lateral, dorsal and transverse views through various levels. The visceral motor (parasympathetic) cell columns are shown in *black*. The ventral nucleus (*blue*) innervates the medial rectus muscle. The dorsal nucleus (*red*) innervates the inferior rectus muscle. The intermediate cell column (*yellow*) innervates the inferior oblique muscle. The cell column (*white*) medial to the dorsal and intermediate cell columns innervates the superior rectus muscle. The caudal central nucleus (*lined*) supplies fibers to the levator palpebrae superioris. Fibers innervating the medial rectus, inferior rectus and inferior oblique muscles are uncrossed; fibers supplying the levator palpebrae muscle are both crossed and uncrossed, while those to the superior rectus muscle are crossed. The *drawing in the upper right* shows the positions of the extraocular muscles in relation to the globe and the bony orbit.

per cent of the cells supply axons to the sphincter pupillae. Small cells in the lateral visceral cell column have not been demonstrated to give rise to fibers emerging with the oculomotor nerve root (326, 414).

Although classically the visceral nuclei of the oculomotor nuclear complex (i.e., the Edinger-Westphal and anterior median nuclei) have been considered the sole source of preganglionic parasympathetic fibers passing to the ciliary ganglion, studies based upon the retrograde transport of HRP in the cat and monkey indicate that visceral neurons in this complex project to the lower brain stem (1519), the cerebellum (2465) and the spinal cord (430, 1412, 1519, 1520). Following HRP injections of the spinal cord in the monkey, cells in both medial and lateral cell columns of the Edinger-Westphal nucleus were retrogradely la-

beled, while no label was present in the anterior median nuclei or in the nucleus of Perlia (326). Descending fibers from distinctive visceral nuclei of the oculomotor complex project to the posterior column nuclei and the Rexed's laminae I and V as far caudally as lumbar spinal segments (Fig. 10-23).

The so-called central nucleus of Perlia, a midline cell group regarded as playing a role in ocular convergence, has been difficult to identify in the brains of man and monkey (462, 2680). While there is little evidence that it is associated with ocular convergence, some cells of the nucleus have been demonstrated to project to the ciliary ganglion (326).

Neuromuscular spindles identified in the extraocular muscles are thought to act as low threshold stretch receptors (528, 531).

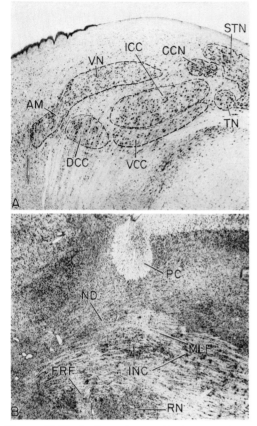

Figure 13-16. *A*, photomicrograph of a sagittal section through the oculomotor complex slightly removed from the midline in a rhesus monkey. The continuity of the anterior median (*AM*) and dorsal visceral cell columns (*VN*) is evident. Other nuclei identified are: *DCC*, dorsal (somatic) cell column; *VCC*, ventral (somatic) cell column; *ICC*, intermediate (somatic) cell column; *CCN*, caudal central nucleus; *TN*, trochlear nucleus; and *STN*, supratrochlear (dorsal raphe) nucleus. (Nissl stain, ×20.) *B*, parasagittal section through the posterior commissure (*PC*) and the medial longitudinal fasciculus (*MLF*), demonstrating the relationships between the nucleus of Darkschewitsch (*ND*), the interstitial nucleus of Cajal (*INC*) and the red nucleus (*RN*). *FRF* indicates fasciculus retroflexus. (Nissl stain, ×20.) (Reproduced with permission from M. B. Carpenter and P. Peter: *Journal fur Hirnforschung*, **12:** 405–408, 1970/71 (412).)

Evidence suggests that afferent impulses from eye muscle spindles are conveyed by cells in the trigeminal ganglion which form part of the ophthalmic division (1599).

The root fibers of the oculomotor nucleus pass ventrally in a number of bundles, some coursing medial to, and some traversing, the red nucleus. Ventrally the fibers con-

verge and emerge from the interpeduncular fossa on the anterior aspect of the midbrain (Figs. 2-8, 2-25 and 11-1). Visceral fibers emerge with rootlets in the rostral part of the oculomotor nerve. Spreading of the root fibers through and around the red nucleus is an expression of the intraradicular expansion of the red nucleus during embryological development (Fig. 13-6).

The Accessory Oculomotor Nuclei. Grouped under this designation are three nuclei closely associated with the oculomotor complex. These nuclei are the interstitial nucleus of Cajal, the nucleus of Darkschewitsch and the nuclei of the posterior commissure.

The *interstitial nucleus* is a small collection of multipolar neurons situated among, and lateral to, the fibers of the MLF in the rostral midbrain (Figs. 13-11, 13-13*A*, 13-16*B* and 13-20). This nucleus gives rise to fibers that cross in the ventral part of the posterior commissure and are distributed contralaterally to all somatic cell columns of the oculomotor complex except the ventral (404). In addition it projects fibers bilaterally to the trochlear nuclei and ipsilaterally to the medial vestibular nucleus (2043) and spinal cord (Fig. 13-19).

The *nucleus of Darkschewitsch* is formed by small cells which lie inside the ventrolateral border of the central gray dorsal and lateral to the somatic cell columns of the oculomotor complex (Figs. 13-11, 13-13*A*, 13-16*B* and 13-20). The nucleus projects fibers into the posterior commissure but does not send fibers into the oculomotor nuclear complex or the lower brain stem levels (2426). The *nuclei of the posterior commissure* have been previously described (page 425).

Afferent connections of the Oculomotor Complex. The oculomotor nuclear complex receives impulses from a variety of structures. Impulses are conveyed indirectly from cerebral cortex, the superior colliculus and certain regions of the reticular formation, while direct projections to the nuclear complex arise from specific parts of the vestibular nuclei, the interstitial nucleus of Cajal, the abducens nucleus, parts of the perihypoglossal nuclei, the rostral interstitial nucleus of the MLF, the pretectal olivary nucleus and regions of the brain stem reticular formation. Although

no direct corticobulbar fibers reach the oculomotor complex, impulses from the cerebral cortex are conveyed by corticoreticular
fibers to reticular neurons which relay these
impulses.

The superior colliculus does not give rise
to direct projections to the oculomotor
complex; it seems likely that impulses from
this structure reach the oculomotor complex via either the interstitial nucleus of
Cajal or the brain stem reticular formation
(51, 1036). The interstitial nucleus of Cajal
gives rise to fibers that cross in the ventral
part of the posterior commissure and pass
to all somatic cell columns, except the ventral, on the opposite side (Fig. 13-19) (387
and 404). Although discrete lesions in the
interstitial nucleus in monkeys do not produce detectable disturbances of oculomotor
function, physiological evidence indicates
that the nucleus plays a role in vertical and
rotatory eye movements (1606).

Secondary vestibular fibers arising from
parts of the medial and superior vestibular
nuclei and from cell group y project to the
oculomotor nuclear complex via the MLF
(2426). Cells in these nuclei, labeled after
unilateral HRP injections in the oculomotor complex in the monkey, were found
bilaterally in the medial vestibular nuclei
and cell group y (with contralateral preponderance) and ipsilaterally in the superior
vestibular nucleus. These fibers terminate
in a specific fashion upon cells in the lateral
somatic cell columns and the interstitial
nucleus of Cajal (1573). This vestibulo-
oculomotor pathway serves to integrate the
receptor activities of the labyrinth and visual systems which provide information concerning orientation in three-dimensional
space.

As indicated in Chapter 12, the abducens
nucleus contains two populations of neurons: (a) cells whose axons emerge via the
abducens nerve and innervate the lateral
rectus muscle, and (b) internuclear neurons
whose axons enter the contralateral MLF
and ascend to the oculomotor nuclear complex (2394, 2425). Ascending axons of abducens internuclear neurons project to terminations in the contralateral ventral cell
column whose neurons innervate the medial rectus muscle (341, 393). These internuclear projections from the abducens to
the oculomotor nucleus underlie the neural

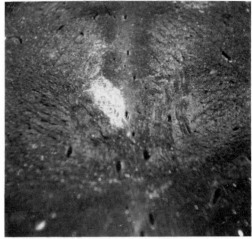

Figure 13-17. Dark field photomicrograph of an autoradiograph through the middle third of the oculomotor nuclear complex in a rhesus monkey, showing
a dense collection of silver grains over the ventral
nucleus. A small but less dense collection of silver
grains lies over cells located in part of the dorsal
nucleus. Silver grains are present in terminals of fibers
originating from contralateral abducens internuclear
neurons (see Fig. 12-22). (Reproduced with permission
from M. B. Carpenter and R. R. Batton: *Journal of
Comparative Neurology*, **189:** 191–209, 1980 (393).)

mechanism responsible for conjugate horizontal gaze (Fig. 13-17).

Several studies of afferent projections to
the oculomotor nuclear complex based
upon the retrograde transport of HRP indicate a distinct projection from cells of the
nucleus prepositus hypoglossi (834, 951,
2426). The nucleus prepositus receives an
input from the flocculus and also projects
to that structure (43, 106, 817). In addition,
the nucleus prepositus receives dysynaptic
vestibular projections. The suggestion that
the nucleus prepositus may project ipsilaterally in a monosynaptic excitatory fashion
upon neurons of the oculomotor complex
concerned with vertical eye movements
(106, 817) is supported by autoradiographic
evidence of a direct projection to the medial
nucleus, a cell group that provides crossed
innervation to the superior rectus muscle
(393). Physiologically the projection from
the nucleus prepositus appears related to
upward eye movements.

Because paralysis of vertical or horizontal eye movements can occur independently, it has been suggested that there are
separate anatomical sites for the generation

of vertical and horizontal eye movements. However, since many eye movements have both vertical and horizontal components, these anatomical sites must be functionally connected. The paramedian pontine reticular formation (PPRF) is regarded as the supranuclear structure responsible for conjugate horizontal eye movements (498, 499, 1277, 1542). Physiological recordings of unit activity related to vertical eye movements have identified a site at the transition between the mesencephalon and diencephalon as the supranuclear structure concerned with the generation of vertical eye movements (337). Cells concerned with vertical eye movements lie ventral to the nucleus of Darkschewitsch, rostral to the interstitial nucleus of Cajal and are situated among fibers of the MLF rostral to the oculomotor nuclear complex. This locus has been referred to as the rostral interstitial nucleus of the MLF (RiMLF) (337). Cells of the RiMLF are activated in short bursts before vertical eye movements in light, in darkness and in response to vestibular and optokinetic stimuli. Subsequent autoradiographic studies have demonstrated that the PPRF projects fibers to the RiMLF which ascend outside of the boundaries of the MLF (342). The RiMLF also receives inputs from the superior and lateral vestibular nuclei. The PPRF has projections to the abducens nucleus but no direct connections with the oculomotor nuclear complex. Unilateral HRP injections of the oculomotor nuclear complex result in labeling of cells in the ipsilateral RiMLF, indicating that these cells project directly to the oculomotor nucleus (2426). The above described oculomotor afferents terminate only upon somatic efferent cell columns.

Lesions of the Third Nerve. Lesions of the third nerve produce an ipsilateral lower motor neuron paralysis of the muscles supplied by the nerve. There is an external strabismus (squint) due to the unopposed action of the lateral rectus muscle, inability to move the eye vertically or inward, drooping of the eyelid (ptosis), dilatation of the pupil (mydriasis), loss of the pupillary light reflex and convergence, and loss of the accommodation reflex. The nearness of the emerging root fibers of N. III to the corticospinal tract in the crus cerebri may lead to the inclusion of both structures in a single lesion, which causes an alternating hemiplegia similar to those already described for the sixth and twelfth nerves (Fig. 10-13). In this case, there is an ipsilateral lower motor neuron paralysis of muscles innervated by N. III, combined with a contralateral hemiplegia. Since at this level the corticobulbar and corticospinal fibers are close to each other, there also may be contralateral paresis (weakness) of the muscles innervated by the cranial nerves, especially those of the lower face and tongue. This constitutes the *superior* or *oculomotor alternating hemiplegia* clinically known as *Weber's syndrome.*

PUPILLARY REFLEXES

Light shone on the retina of one eye causes both pupils to constrict. The response in the eye stimulated is called the *direct pupillary light reflex,* while that in the opposite eye is known as the *consensual pupillary light reflex.* Pathways involved in the pupillary light reflex are not entirely known but involve: (a) axons of retinal ganglion cells which pass via the optic nerve, optic tract and brachium of the superior colliculus to the pretectal area, (b) axons of pretectal neurons which partially cross in the posterior commissure and terminate bilaterally in visceral nuclei of the oculomotor complex (Fig. 13-18), (c) preganglionic parasympathetic fibers from the visceral nuclei which course with fibers of the third nerve and synapse on cells in the ciliary ganglion (Fig. 8-1), and (d) postganglionic fibers from the ciliary ganglion which project to the sphincter of the iris. Section of the posterior commissure reduces, but does not abolish, the consensual pupillary light reflex.

The term *anisocoria* is used to denote pupillary inequality. In man and monkey the direct and consensual pupillary light reflexes are exactly equal (1534). In the cat the direct pupillary light response is stronger than the indirect response because most retinofugal fibers are crossed. In man, anisocoria results only from lesions involving the efferent pathways from the oculomotor complex or pretectal fiber systems passing to it.

The *accommodation-convergence reaction* occurs when gaze is shifted from a distant object to a near one. This reaction

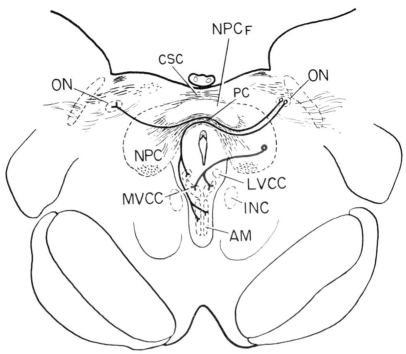

Figure 13-18. Schematic drawing of the brain stem through the caudal part of the posterior commissure, showing the course of fibers projecting to the visceral nuclei of the oculomotor complex. Fibers (*red*) from the nuclei of the posterior commissure (*NPC*) enter the ipsilateral central gray and project primarily to the medial visceral cell columns (*MVCC*); these fibers partially cross ventral to the cerebral aqueduct and some terminate in the anterior median nuclei. Fibers (*black*) from the pretectal olivary nucleus (*ON*) pass through the posterior commissure (*PC*), enter the central gray and project to the contralateral lateral visceral cell column (*LVCC*) and bilaterally to the anterior median nuclei (*AM*). There are some commissural projections from ON to the corresponding nucleus contralaterally. Additional abbreviations: *CSC*, commissure of superior colliculus; *INC*, interstitial nucleus of Cajal; *NPC_F*, nucleus of posterior commissure, pars infracommissuralis. (Reproduced with permission from M. B. Carpenter and R. J. Pierson: *Journal of Comparative Neurology*, **149**: 271–300, 1973 (414).)

involves: (a) simultaneous contractions of both medial recti muscles for convergence, (b) contractions of the ciliary muscles, which relax the suspensory ligament of the lens and cause the lens to assume a more convex shape, and (c) pupillary constriction. In this reflex, retinal impulses must first reach the visual cortex and be relayed via corticofugal fibers to brain stem centers. It is presumed that the corticofugal fibers involved in this response reach the superior colliculus and pretectal region where they are relayed, directly or indirectly, to the visceral nuclei oculomotor complex.

Under normal circumstances, accommodation always is accompanied by pupillary constriction, but certain central nervous system lesions can impair or abolish the pupillary light reflex without affecting accommodation. Such lesions occur with central nervous system syphilis (tabes dorsalis) in which the pupils are small (miosis) and do not react to light, but the accommodation reaction remains. This is the *Argyll Robertson pupil*. The precise location of the responsible lesion is unknown.

In intense illumination, contraction of the pupil may be accompanied by closure of the eyelids, lowering of the brow and general contractions of the face, designed to shut out the maximal amount of light. In so far as they are not volitional, these reflex movements probably are mediated through the superior colliculi and the tectobulbar tracts.

The central pathways for pupillary dilatation are incompletely known. Dilatation occurs reflexly on shading the eye or scratching the side of the neck with a pin, and it is a constant feature in severe pain and extreme emotional states. Experimental evidence points to a path from the frontal cortex to the region of the hypothalamus, one of the autonomic integrating centers of the brain stem. Descending fibers from the hypothalamus pass via the reticular formation (and periventricular region) and directly to spinal levels. Impulses conveyed by these fibers reach cells of the intermediolateral cell column in upper thoracic spinal (C8 to T1) segments (Fig. 10-23). The latter spinal segments send preganglionic fibers by way of the upper two or three rami communicantes and the sympathetic trunk to the superior cervical ganglion, from which postganglionic fibers go to the dilator muscle of the iris (Fig. 10-29). Interruption of these descending fibers, which course in the dorsolateral tegmentum, at all levels of the brain stem caudal to the hypothalamus will produce a *Horner's syndrome*. In a Horner's syndrome due to a brain stem lesion, the pupil shows relatively little dilatation to adrenalin. If the lesion producing this syndrome involves postganglionic sympathetic fibers, adrenalin causes mydriasis and lid retraction on the affected side but not on the normal side. This hypersensitivity of the pupil to adrenalin seen with lesions involving the postganglionic fibers is an example of denervation sensitivity (488).

NUCLEI OF THE MESENCEPHALIC TEGMENTUM

The midbrain tegmentum, the region ventral to the cerebral aqueduct and dorsal to the substantia nigra, contains the trochlear and oculomotor nuclei, the mesencephalic reticular formation, the red nuclei and many scattered collections of cells. The most conspicuous structure in the midbrain tegmentum at the level of the superior colliculus is the red nucleus.

The Red Nucleus

The red nucleus, a distinctive part of the mesencephalic reticular formation, has been distinguished as an entity because of its central position in the midbrain tegmentum, its particular vascularity (and color) and its capsule formed by fibers of the superior cerebellar peduncle. In transverse sections the red nucleus appears oval, but in sagittal sections it has an elliptical shape

with a blunt oral and a tapered caudal pole (Figs. 13-21, 15-1 and 17-17). The nucleus extends from the caudal diencephalon to the decussation of the superior cerebellar peduncle. The red nucleus is traversed in its oral part by fibers of the fasciculus retroflexus (Fig. 15-5), in its central part by rootlets of the oculomotor nerve and in its caudal and lateral regions by fibers of the superior cerebellar peduncle.

Since classic comparative studies of Hatschek (1050), it has been customary to recognize magnocellular and parvocellular portions of the red nucleus. The magnocellular part tends to occupy caudal parts of the structure; it is more extensive in lower mammals and has been considered as the cell group which gives rise to the rubrospinal tract. The small-celled, or parvocellular, portion forms the bulk of the nucleus (Fig. 13-14); its development parallels the growth of the deep cerebellar nuclei, particularly the dentate nucleus. Between the cells of the nucleus are numerous small bundles of myelinated fibers which give a punctate appearance to the nucleus in transverse sections. These are primarily fibers of the superior cerebellar peduncle which traverse the nucleus and terminate in parts of it.

Cytological studies of the red nucleus in the monkey reveal three distinctive types of neurons: (a) large multipolar neurons 50 to 70 μm in diameter with prominent nucleoli and a cytoplasm containing coarse Nissl granules (magnocellular part), (b) medium-sized cells, 20 to 30 μm in diameter, with a triangular or fusiform shape (parvocellular part), and (c) small achromatic neurons, 10 to 15 μm in diameter, found in all parts of the nucleus (1319, 1320). Golgi preparations in the monkey have provided details concerning these neurons. Giant neurons have star-shaped, ovoid or elongated cell bodies with prominent somatic spines; dendrites of these cells radiate in all directions and have a few isolated spines. Medium-sized neurons, largely representing cells of the parvocellular part of the nucleus, have shorter, less robust dendrites with branching collaterals. Small neurons have delicately branched dendrites and short axons.

Connections of the Red Nucleus. Afferent fibers projecting to the red nucleus are derived from two principal sources, the deep cerebellar nuclei and the cerebral cortex. Fibers from both of these sources appear to terminate somatotopically within the red nucleus. Fibers of the superior cerebellar peduncle, arising from the dentate, emboliform and globose nuclei, undergo a complete decussation in the caudal midbrain, and both enter and surround the contralateral red nucleus. Fibers from the dentate nucleus terminate mainly in the rostral third of the red nucleus (543, 755), while fibers from the emboliform nucleus (anterior interposed nucleus) project somatotopically to the caudal two-thirds of the nucleus (Figs. 14-16 and 14-17). There is a complex mediolateral and caudorostral correspondence between portions of the anterior interposed and the opposite red nucleus. The caudal portions of the red nucleus, which are linked somatotopically with the contralateral interposed nucleus (and paravermal cerebellar cortex), project somatotopically to spinal levels (Fig. 10-18). Thus indirect pathways are present by which impulses from the cerebellar cortex and the anterior interposed nucleus can be conveyed somatotopically to spinal levels via the red nucleus. This indirect pathway involves two midbrain decussations (i.e., the superior cerebellar peduncle and the rubrospinal tract). The terminal distribution of fibers from the globose nucleus (posterior interposed nucleus) is in the medial part of the magnocellular part of the red nucleus (69). Physiological interrelationships between the cerebellar cortex, the interposed nuclei and the red nucleus indicate that excitatory influences of the interposed nuclei upon the large cells of the red nucleus are suppressed by stimulation of the cerebellar cortex. Cortical inhibition, mediated by Purkinje cell axons, is followed by enhanced excitability of interposed neurons whose discharges result in depolarization of red nucleus neurons (2566).

Corticorubral fibers, mainly from the percentral gyrus (1411, 2163), originally were described as projecting ipsilaterally and somatotopically upon cells in all parts of the red nucleus. Thus corticorubral and rubrospinal fiber systems together constitute a somatotopically linked nonpyramidal pathway from the motor cortex to spinal levels. Autoradiographic tracing technics in the monkey have revealed projections to the parvicellular part of the red nucleus to be bilateral and somatotopic from both the precentral and premotor cortex (1042). Fibers from the face area end in medial vertical lamina in the parvicellular division of the red nucleus, while fibers from the arm and leg areas terminate in intermediate and lateral laminae, respectively, of the same subdivision. The most profuse contralateral projection is from the medial portion of area 6 which is coextensive with the supplementary motor area. Homolateral projections from the limb areas of the precentral motor cortex are to the magnocellular part of the red nucleus and correspond to the established origins of the rubrospinal tract (2039).

The efferent projections of the red nucleus are to the spinal cord, the brain stem and the cerebellum. Experimental data for the cat (2039) indicate that rubrospinal fibers arise chiefly, but not exclusively, from cells of all sizes in the caudal three-fourths of the red nucleus. Cells in dorsomedial parts of the nucleus project fibers to cervical spinal segments, while cells in ventral and ventrolateral locations project to lumbosacral spinal segments; fibers passing to thoracic regions of the spinal cord and arise from intermediate parts of the red nucleus. Cervical spinal segments receive the largest number of rubrospinal fibers. In the monkey, rubrospinal fibers arise almost exclusively from the caudal magnocellular part of the nucleus (1411).

Rubrospinal fibers issue from the medial margin of the red nucleus, cross the median raphe in the *ventral tegmental decussation (of Forel)* and descend in the brain stem in close association with the branchiomeric motor cranial nerve nuclei (Fig. 10-18). In the upper pons some crossed descending rubral collaterals separate from the rubrospinal tract, traverse portions of the trigeminal nuclei and enter the cerebellum in association with the superior cerebellar peduncle (273, 1104).

Rubrocerebellar fibers terminate in the anterior nucleus interpositus (547). This direct (and crossed) rubrocerebellar feedback is somatotopically organized.

Rubrobulbar projections are both crossed and uncrossed. Crossed rubrobulbar fibers project to the principal sensory nucleus of the trigeminal nerve, and some of these fibers extend caudally into the pars oralis of the spinal trigeminal nucleus (686, 1615, 1707). At more caudal levels, fibers separating from the rubrospinal tract enter the lateral aspect of the facial nucleus and terminate in dorsomedial and intermediate cell groups whose neurons innervate musculature of the upper part of the face (542, 544, 1707). Similar observations have been made in autoradiographic studies (686). Rubrobulbar fibers ending upon motor neurons of the facial nucleus probably are not involved in the neural mechanism of mimetic facial innervation, since this phenomenon involves predominantly perioral facial muscles. In the medulla, crossed rubrobulbar fibers end in the lateral reticular nucleus, the accessory cuneate nucleus and the nuclei gracilis and cuneatus (542, 686, 1615, 2635).

Uncrossed descending rubral efferents, from the parvocellular part of the nucleus, enter the central tegmental tract and project to the dorsal lamella of the principal inferior olivary nucleus (686, 1707, 2023, 2635). These fibers, referred to as *rubro-olivary fibers*, constitute the largest contingent of rubrobulbar fibers.

From the above discussion it is apparent that descending rubral efferent fibers, other than those in the rubrospinal tract, are organized to project impulses to the cerebellum via: (a) direct rubrocerebellar fibers, or (b) rubrobulbar fibers which pass to cerebellar relay nuclei.

Older studies suggested that cells in the red nucleus project fibers to thalamic nuclei in parallel with fibers of the superior cerebellar peduncle. Most of the supporting data was based upon lesions destroying portions of both of these structures. Doubts concerning ascending projections from the red nucleus were cast by Kuypers and Lawrence (1411) who described a lesion destroying most of the thalamus in a monkey that failed to produce cell loss or retrograde cell changes in any part of the red nucleus. In other studies it was shown that interruption of the central tegmental tract produced a complete cell loss in the parvocellular part of the red nucleus, suggesting that no part of this nucleus projected rostrally (2023). The most conclusive data, based upon autoradiographic tracing technics, revealed no

transport of isotope from cells of the red nucleus to the thalamus (686).

Functional Considerations. It is evident from the above that the red nucleus is a way station interposed in a variety of complex pathways. It is organized to relay impulses from the cerebral and cerebellar cortex to the spinal cord, as well as to participate in various neural mechanisms by which some impulses can be fed back to the cerebellum.

In lower mammals the midbrain contains a center for the integration of complex postural reflexes which enable an animal to change from an abnormal to a normal position (righting reactions). This center may be located in the magnocellular portion of the red nucleus or in the adjacent reticular formation. The rubrospinal tract excites flexor motor neurons via polysynaptic pathways, and stimulation of the red nucleus during locomotion enhances flexor muscle activity during the swing phase (1896). Vestibulospinal influences have a similarly enhancing effect upon extensor muscles during the stance phase of the step (1895). The cerebellum apparently modulates the activity of both rubrospinal and vestibulospinal neurons to provide appropriate locomotor rhythms.

Conflicting statements in the literature suggest that stimulation of the red nucleus in animals produces flexion of ipsilateral forelimb and extension of the contralateral forelimb. This reaction, generally known as "the tegmental response," frequently can be obtained from regions of the mesencephalic reticular formation dorsal and lateral to the red nucleus. The studies of Pompeiano (2033, 2034) indicate that stimulation of the red nucleus *per se* elicits flexion in the contralateral extremities, which is mediated by the rubrospinal tract (2039). It has been demonstrated that stimulation of the red nucleus in the decerebrate cat gives rise to: (a) excitatory postsynaptic potentials in the contralateral flexor α motor neurons, and (b) inhibitory postsynaptic potentials in contralateral extensor α motor neurons.

Because the red nucleus receives a large proportion of its afferents from the cerebellum by way of the superior cerebellar peduncle, it is possible to relate certain phenomena associated with cerebellar stimulation to the red nucleus. These observations concern mainly the anterior interposed nucleus which projects the majority of its fibers to the caudal two-thirds of the contralateral red nucleus. Reciprocal somatotopic relationships exist between the anterior interposed nucleus and the contralateral red nucleus (543, 547). Stimulation of specific parts of the nucleus interpositus (anterior part) in decerebrate preparations produces flexion in either the ipsilateral forelimb or hindlimb (1583, 2035, 2037). These flexor responses, mediated by the red nucleus, occur ipsilaterally because of the double crossing of the fiber systems involved (i.e., superior cerebellar peduncle and rubrospinal tract) (Fig. 14-17).

Lesions of the Red Nucleus. Clinically, unilateral lesions of the mesencephalic tegmentum involving the red nucleus are described as producing a syndrome characterized by contralateral motor disturbances that are variously designated as tremor, ataxia and choreiform activity, and an ipsilateral oculomotor palsy. The motor disturbances associated with this syndrome, known as the *syndrome of Benedikt,* have been attributed to destruction of the red nucleus. Experimentally produced lesions in the red nucleus in a variety of different animals (377, 684, 1186, 1790, 2088) have not produced disturbances equivalent to those reported in man. Isolated lesions of the red nucleus in the monkey (377) produce transient tremor and ataxia, enduring hypokinesis and ipsilateral oculomotor disturbances. It is of interest that unilateral lesions in the red nucleus in monkeys, with virtually complete degeneration of the contralateral superior cerebellar peduncle, produce no additional neurological disturbances (378). These findings suggest that the abnormal motor disturbances (i.e., dyskinesia) resulting from lesions of the mesencephalic tegmentum, including the red nucleus, are primarily a consequence of interruption of cerebellar efferent fibers in the superior cerebellar peduncle. In the monkey, neither lesions of the red nucleus nor section of the rubrospinal tract abolishes cerebellar disturbances produced by lesions of the deep cerebellar nuclei.

Mesencephalic Reticular Formation

The midbrain reticular formation is less extensive than the pontine reticular for-mation caudal to it. While the red nucleus is recognized as a distinctive part of the reticular formation, classically it is customary to reserve this term for structures lateral and dorsal to the red nucleus. According to detailed studies (1884, 1885), the principal reticular nuclei of the mesencephalon are: (a) the nucleus tegmenti pedunculopontinus (pedunculopontine nucleus), (b) the nucleus cuneiformis, and (c) the nucleus subcuneiformis.

The *pedunculopontine nucleus* lies in the lateral part of the midbrain tegmentum ventral to the inferior colliculus (Fig. 13-3). The nucleus consists of two parts, a compact part located dorsolaterally and a small-celled diffuse part located ventrally. Fibers of the superior cerebellar peduncle traverse portions of the nucleus as they shift ventromedially to decussate. The pedunculopontine nucleus appears to receive inputs from multiple sources. Afferent fibers to the pedunculopontine nucleus arise from the cerebral cortex (1042, 1411), the medial pallidal segment (419, 1313, 1825) and the substantia nigra (140, 398, 1729). Projections of the pedunculopontine nucleus appear to be ascending, with the largest number of fibers projecting to the pars compacta of the substantia nigra; a small number of fibers project to the medial pallidal segment (140, 398, 627). The known connections of this small nucleus appear to form a mesencephalic loop circuit that may modulate the activities of nigral and pallidal neurons (Figs. 17-19 and 17-20).

The *nuclei cuneiformis* and *subcuneiformis* lie between the tectum, dorsally, and the pedunculopontine nucleus. The nucleus cuneiformis extends throughout the rostrocaudal extent of the midbrain where it lies directly ventral to the superior and inferior colliculi (687). This nucleus increases in size at more rostral levels and merges with the pretectum. Most of the nucleus is composed of small- and medium-sized oval or fusiform cells. The nucleus subcuneiformis lies ventral to the nucleus cuneiformis. Descending fibers from the cuneiform nucleus cross in the ventral tegmental decussation and project to terminations in the reticulotegmental nucleus, the medial pontine and medullary reticular formation, the nucleus raphe magnus and in parts of the facial nucleus (687). Some fibers also end in parts of the medial accessory olivary nucleus. Ascend-

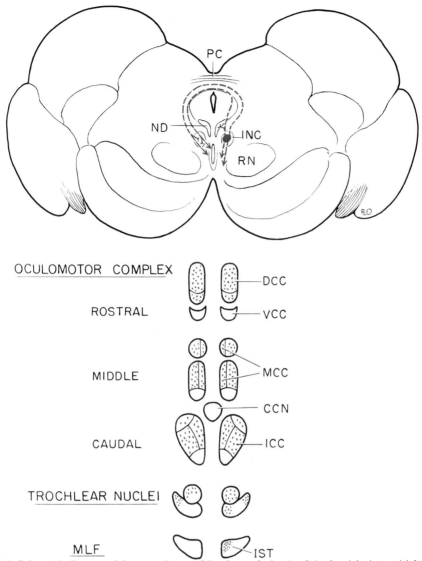

Figure 13-19. Schematic diagram of degeneration resulting from a lesion (*red*) in the right interstitial nucleus of Cajal (*INC*). The lesion destroyed: (a) cells which give rise to fibers that cross in the ventral part of the posterior commissure and fibers which descend in the ipsilateral *MLF*, and (b) fibers from the opposite interstitial nucleus which have crossed in the posterior commissure and traverse the lesion *en route* to the oculomotor complex. Fairly symmetrical differential degeneration (*red stippling*) in the oculomotor complex was greatest in the intermediate (*ICC*) and medial cell columns (*MCC*), somewhat less profuse in the dorsal cell columns (*DCC*) and absent in the ventral cell columns (*VCC*) and in the caudal central nucleus (*CCN*). Degeneration in the trochlear nuclei was bilateral but was greatest ipsilaterally. Fibers of the interstitiospinal tract (*IST*) were concentrated in the dorsomedial part of the MLF. *ND*, indicates the nucleus of Darkschewitsch, *PC*, indicates the posterior commissure and *RN* denotes the red nucleus. (Reproduced with permission from M. B. Carpenter, J. W. Harbison, and P. Peter: *Journal of Comparative Neurology*, **140**: 131–154, 1970 (404).)

ing projections of the cuneiform nucleus are to the pretectal nuclei, the nuclei of the posterior commissure, the posterior hypothalamus, the zona incerta and the paraventricular and the caudal intralaminar thalamic nuclei (690). The widespread connections of the midbrain reticular forma- tion are considered to mediate the varied somatic and visceral responses elicited by electrical stimulation of this region. These responses in the cat can be integrated into elaborate defense or attack behavior characterized by pupillary dilatation, widening of the palpebral fissures, flattening of the ears and aggressive and vicious behavior (1176, 2314).

The *interpeduncular nucleus* occupies a small triangular space dorsal to the interpeduncular fossa (Figs. 13-3 and 13-6). Cells of this nucleus are small, spindle-shaped, lightly staining and compactly arranged. The interpeduncular nucleus receives fibers from the habenular nuclei via the fasciculus retroflexus (Figs. 15-6 and 16-7).

The *central gray substance* (periaqueductal gray) surrounding the cerebral aqueduct is composed of small oval or spindle-shaped cells. The *nucleus of Darkschewitsch* is a rather indistinct cell group just inside the ventrolateral border of the central gray (Figs. 13-11, 13-16*B* and 13-20). The *dorsal tegmental nucleus* lies within the ventral central gray, mainly caudal to the trochlear nucleus and lateral to the raphe (Fig. 13-3). Fibers from this nucleus and from a collection of more caudally located cells known as the *ventral tegmental nucleus* ascend to the mammillary bodies, the lateral hypothalamic areas and the preoptic and septal areas (979, 1824). These fibers travel in the dorsal longitudinal fasciculus (of Schütz), the mammillary peduncle, and some continue rostrally in the medial forebrain bundle (Fig. 16-7).

FUNCTIONAL CONSIDERATIONS OF THE RETICULAR FORMATION

The anatomical organization of the medullary and pontine reticular formation has been described. It will be recalled that the medullary reticular formation consists essentially of four zones: (a) the nuclei of the raphe, (b) the paramedian reticular nuclei, (c) a medial region constituting roughly the medial two-thirds of the reticular formation regarded as an "effector" area, and (d) a smaller lateral region referred to as the "sensory" or "receptive" part because of the large number of collateral fibers projected to it from secondary sensory pathways. The pontine reticular formation has essentially the same divisions, except that the "sensory" portion is smaller and clearly evident only in the caudal pons.

Physiological investigations in animals have yielded important information concerning the functions of the reticular formation. Magoun and Rhines (1593, 1594) found that electrical stimulation of the ventromedial zone of the medullary reticular formation inhibited or reduced most forms of motor activity. Stimulation in this region produced inhibition of the patellar tendon reflex, the flexion reflex of the foreleg and the blink reflex. In addition, it inhibited extensor muscle tone in decerebrate animals and responses to stimulation of the motor cortex in intact animals. All inhibitory effects were bilateral, but ipsilateral inhibition sometimes could be obtained at a lower threshold. No inhibitory effects could be elicited from the most lateral part of the medullary reticular formation. Regions of the medullary reticular formation from which inhibitory responses are obtained correspond closely to the area occupied by the nucleus reticularis gigantocellularis (except for its most rostral part) and part of the nucleus reticularis ventralis. Since these nuclei give rise to medullary reticulospinal fibers, these inhibitory influences probably are mediated directly by this fiber system (2561). This thesis is further supported by the fact that medullary inhibition can still be obtained by electrical stimulation following chronic midbrain and pontine hemisection (1835). Nevertheless, there is evidence that higher centers projecting to medullary reticular units may produce inhibition of motor activity and of extensor muscle tone. Such higher centers include the anterior lobe of the cerebellum and certain cortical regions (1594).

A far greater region of the reticular formation facilitates reflexes at segmental levels, and movements in response to cortical stimulation. This facilitatory area extends rostrally uninterruptedly from the upper medulla through the pontine and mesencephalic tegmentum into caudal regions of the diencephalon. Bilateral facilitatory effects can be evoked at any level within this long stretch of the reticular formation. The facilitatory region of the reticular formation includes many areas from which no direct reticulospinal projections arise. Facilitatory effects produced by stimulation of the rostral and dorsal parts of the nucleus reticularis gigantocellularis, or of the nuclei reticularis pontis caudalis and oralis, presumably could reach spinal levels by direct reticulospinal fibers originating in these nuclei. Descending polysynaptic pathways would appear to mediate facilitatory effects obtained from regions of the

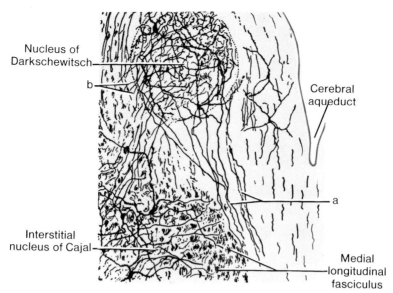

Figure 13-20. Relationships of the nucleus of Darkschewitsch and the interstitial nucleus of Cajal to the central gray (surrounding the cerebral aqueduct) and the medial longitudinal fasciculus. *b*, collateral fibers terminating in the nucleus of Darkschewitsch; *a*, fibers leaving this nucleus. Drawing based upon Golgi preparations from a newborn kitten (after Cajal (348)).

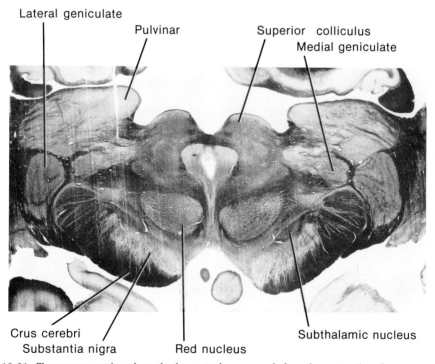

Figure 13-21. Transverse section through the rostral mesencephalon, demonstrating the manner in which diencephalic nuclei surround dorsal and lateral portions of the mesencephalon. (Weigert's myelin stain, photograph.)

midbrain and diencephalon, which have no direct reticulospinal projections.

The descending influences of the brain stem reticular formation are not limited to inhibition and facilitation of reflex and somatic motor activity. As commented upon earlier, respiratory responses can be obtained by electrical stimulation of the reticular formation. Maximal inspiratory responses can be obtained from stimulating points within the nucleus reticularis gigantocellularis (2561), while expiratory effects are evoked chiefly from the parvicellular reticular nucleus in the medulla. Vasomotor depressor effects generally are obtained from areas within the nucleus reticularis gigantocellularis and the most rostral part of the nucleus reticularis ventralis. Pressor effects usually are evoked by stimulations outside of the reticular regions which project fibers to spinal levels.

Although nearly all parts of the central nervous system are capable of exerting detectable influences upon the heart and blood vessels, the primary vasomotor control center is located in the reticular formation of the medulla. Transections of the brain stem as far caudal as the lower third of the pons have no significant effect upon arterial blood pressure or on the tonic discharge of the inferior cardiac nerve. Successively more caudal transections produce: (a) an increasing drop in blood pressure, and (b) a reduction in the discharge of cardiac accelerator impulses (112). The bulbar pressor and depressor areas constitute a central cardiovascular mechanism which reflexly regulates blood pressure and the parameters of the heart rate. In the intact animal a normal arterial pressure is dependent upon the bulbar pressor area. Activity in the pressor area is independent of afferent influx. Vagal cardiac centers, assumed to lie in the dorsal motor nucleus of N. X, must be intimately integrated with neurons in pressor areas; activity of vagal units are subject to reflex excitation and inhibition.

While it is well known that α motor neurons can be influenced by stimulation of the reticular formation, the investigations of Granit (937) indicate that these effects are not necessarily due to reticulospinal volleys impinging directly upon these neurons, since activity of γ motor neurons can influence α motor neurons through the γ loop (Fig. 9-34). Granit and Kaada (938) demonstrated that repetitive electrical stimulation of the facilitating regions of the brain stem tegmentum increased the efferent discharge of γ motor neurons, and increased the rate of discharge from the muscle spindle. On the other hand, inhibition of the γ discharge was produced by stimulating the medullary inhibitory region. These data suggest that a large part of the excitation of α motor neurons results from firing of the γ efferents, which are actively controlled by the reticular formation. The inhibition of extensor muscle tone in a decerebrate animal by stimulation of the medullary reticular formation (2536) is a dramatic example of this potent influence.

The discovery that the activity of the muscle spindle could be modified by descending reticular projections suggested that the reticular formation might affect the initiation and transmission of other sensory impulses. Hagbarth and Kerr (998) demonstrated that synaptic transmission of sensory impulses in the spinal cord could be depressed by stimulation of the reticular formation. Likewise, potentials evoked in the posterior column nuclei following stimulation of the posterior columns could be depressed or abolished by stimulation of the reticular formation.

Recent studies indicate that neurons in the raphe and medullary reticular formation, and possible fibers originating elsewhere and passing through the reticular formation, are critical for analgesia produced by opiates and brain stem stimulation (129, 130, 995). The nucleus raphe magnus, located ventrally in the rostral medulla, projects bilaterally to spinal levels via the dorsolateral funiculus; terminals of these fibers are found in laminae I and II, which receive fibers conveying nociceptive inputs (Figs. 9-15, 11-15 and 11-16). Electrical stimulation of the serotoninergic neurons of the nucleus raphe magnus has an analgesic effect produced by inhibitory actions upon sensory neurons (128, 129, 2075). In the primate spinothalamic tract, neurons with nociceptive inputs also are inhibited by stimulation of the nucleus raphe magnus (136, 2726). Neurons in the nucleus reticularis gigantocellularis have ipsilateral spinal projections which partially overlap those from the nucleus raphe magnus (129) but descend in the ventral quadrant of the spinal cord. Observations in the monkey show that stimulation of the medullary reticular formation can both inhibit and excite neurons of the spinothalamic tract (995). These studies imply that the nucleus reticularis gigantocellularis can determine the effectiveness of cutaneous stimuli in evoking activity in ascending pathways mediating sensory experience, such as pain.

Moruzzi and Magoun (1756) have demonstrated that the facilitatory region of the brain stem reticular formation also acts in an ascending direction to influence the electrical activity of the cerebral cortex. The pioneer investigations of Berger (160, 161) indicated that in man and lower mammals wakefulness, sleep, alertness and relaxation were characterized by strikingly different electroencephalographic patterns. Wakefulness and alertness are characterized by fast low-voltage activity, while at least one form of sleep is associated with the appearance of slow high-voltage waves.

Fundamental insight into the underlying brain mechanisms was provided by Bremer (246) who compared the electroencephalograms (EEG) of animals following high spinal transections (*encéphale isolé*) and decerebration (i.e., transection of the midbrain at the intercollicular level, *cerveau isolé*). In the encéphale isolé preparation the EEG displayed the waking pattern, while in the cerveau isolé preparation the EEG exhibited a pattern characteristic of the sleeping state. These experiments pointed to a potent ascending electrotonic influence generated in the lower brain stem. While it was well known that a variety of different stimuli could change the EEG from a synchronized pattern (i.e., sleep state), to a desynchronized one (i.e., alert state), the puzzling feature was how impulses channeled in the classic ascending pathways could exert such broad and diffuse electrotonic changes in the cerebral cortex. The observations that stimulation of the brain stem reticular formation could activate and desynchronize the EEG and produce behavioral arousal without discharging the classic lemniscal pathways suggested the concept of a second ascending system (1756). This second ascending system, exerting powerful influences upon broad regions of the cerebral cortex has become known as the ascending reticular activating system (ARAS).

The *ascending reticular activating system* has been shown to respond to peripheral, splanchnic, trigeminal and vagal nerve stimulation, as well as to auditory, vestibular, visual and olfactory stimuli (170, 245,

613, 808, 809, 863, 1566, 1756, 2423). Interruption of the long ascending specific sensory pathways in the brain stem does not prevent impulses from reaching the reticular activating system and evoking the characteristic EEG arousal response (808, 1756, 2424). Lesions in the rostromedial midbrain tegmentum abolish the EEG arousal reaction elicited by sensory stimulation (807, 1586), even though the long ascending sensory pathways are intact. Thus, two functionally distinct, but inter-related, pathways must project to diencephalic levels. The long ascending sensory pathways, located peripheral to the reticular core, constitute the *lemniscal system*. This system is concerned largely with the transmission of specific sensory impulses to particular thalamic relay nuclei. The lemniscal systems (i.e., the medial lemniscus, lateral lemniscus, spinothalamic tracts and secondary trigeminal projections) are oligosynaptic specific sensory pathways. Although electrical stimulation of the lemniscal systems produces arousal (809, 1588, 2422), this is not considered a direct effect. The second pathway, the *ascending reticular activating system* occupies central regions within the brain stem reticular formation that receive collateral fibers from surrounding specific sensory systems. Physiologically this system is regarded as a multineuronal, polysynaptic system within which collaterals conveying impulses from various sensory systems lose their identification with specific sensory modalities. The continuous subliminal facilitating effect of these nonspecific afferents upon the reticular activating system play an important role in wakefulness, alerting and arousal.

Anatomical and physiological data are in agreement concerning the distribution of collaterals from secondary sensory systems within the reticular formation. Collaterals are given off by secondary fibers in the auditory and vestibular systems, as well as from the nuclei of the solitary tract, the trigeminal nuclei, the vagal nuclei and the spinothalamic tracts. Visual impulses reach the reticular formation via tectoreticular fibers (51, 1036). Anatomically it is significant that direct spinoreticular fibers are more numerous than collaterals from the spinothalamic tracts and have a wider distribution within the reticular formation.

The medial lemniscus, unlike other long ascending sensory systems, does not contribute collaterals to the reticular activating system. Experimental studies (2198, 2231) indicate that the secondary trigeminal collaterals given off at pontine levels are a particularly potent source of tonic influence to the reticular activating system, exceeding in importance the contributions by other sensory cranial nerves.

The cerebral cortex also plays a role in altering the state of consciousness and alertness by influencing reticular neurons that mediate the arousal responses (247, 806, 1210). Such a role has been suggested by the well known arousal effect of psychic stimuli. Areas of the cerebral cortex from which the arousal responses can be obtained by nonconvulsive electrical stimulation include loci on the orbitofrontal surface, the frontal convexity, the sensorimotor cortex, the posterior parieto-occipital cortex, the superior temporal gyrus and the cingulate gyrus. Corticoreticular fibers, which originate from all parts of the cerebral cortex, convey excitatory impulses to the reticular neurons, whose ascending discharges participate in the arousal response. Corticoreticular fibers project most abundantly to two regions of the brain stem reticular formation: (a) the nucleus reticularis pontis oralis, and (b) the nucleus reticularis gigantocellularis (2227).

As noted earlier lateral regions of the brain stem reticular formation are regarded as the "sensory" part, while the larger, more medial region, which projects both long ascending and descending fibers, is considered the "effector" portion. Although physiological studies of ascending transmission in the reticular formation suggest chains of neurons which fire successively, it has not been possible to demonstrate short-axoned, Golgi type II cells in the reticular formation (2274). Since approximately one-third of the cells in the "effector" reticular regions give rise to long ascending fibers in the reticular core, it appears likely that these fibers form the structural basis of the ascending reticular activating system (281). Rapidly conducted impulses in the reticular core are transmitted by the main long ascending axons, while slowly conducted impulses are conveyed by collaterals or by circuitous pathways involving laterally dispersed collaterals. The main long ascending pathway of the brain stem reticular formation appears to be the *central tegmental fasciculus* (Figs. 12-4, 12-21 and 12-29), a large composite bundle that also contains descending fiber systems (266, 1824). This bundle occupies a large part of the bulbar tegmentum, but at mesencephalic levels it is displaced dorsally so that its fibers occupy a position adjacent to the central gray and dorsal to the red nucleus (Fig. 13-6). At diencephalic levels the central tegmental tract projects into the subthalamic region and to the intralaminar nuclei of the thalamus. Although the precise regions of origin of ascending fibers within this system have not been delineated, most evidence indicates that ascending fibers originate throughout the longitudinal extent of the medulla and pons (281); reticular pathways ascending beyond the midbrain appear to arise largely from levels rostral to the inferior olivary nuclei. The central tegmental tract also contains abundant short ascending fibers which form a multineuronal system for intrareticular conduction (1824).

Ascending reticular projections to the hypothalamus arise from medial regions of the caudal midbrain and are distinct from those contained in the central tegmental tract (1824). These projections are represented largely by three bundles: (a) the dorsal longitudinal fasciculus (Schütz) situated ventrally in the central gray, (b) fibers of the mammillary peduncle which originate in the medial tegmental region (Fig. 16-7) and terminate in the mammillary body and lateral hypothalamus (1816), and (c) the medial forebrain bundle, which contains certain ascending components from several sources.

Anatomical and physiological data are in agreement concerning the diencephalic projections (hypothalamus, subthalamic region and intralaminar nuclei of the thalamus) of the ascending reticular activating system, but the means by which these structures influenced the activity of the cerebral cortex took longer to establish (231, 809, 2230). While the EEG arousal response is mediated in part by the intralaminar nuclei (1756), projections from these nuclei to the cerebral cortex could not be followed by degeneration technics. Recent evidence indicates that the intralaminar thalamic nuclei project profusely upon the neostriatum and give rise to an extensive collateral system that projects diffusely upon the cerebral cortex (1234).

It is significant that bilateral interruption of lemniscal systems in the brain stem leaves the animal with an electrocorticogram characteristic of the wakeful state. After lesions in the upper reticular core which spare the lemniscal system, the EEG changes to that of the sleeping state. After lesions in the rostral midbrain interrupting somatic and auditory pathways (without destroying the ascending reticular system), tactile and auditory stimuli produce an EEG arousal, although no tactile or auditory impulses reach the thalamus by the specific sensory pathways. The central reticular core may be regarded as a common system of neurons with multiple relays which are discharged equivalently by all sensory systems projecting collaterals to it. Such a common system is not involved in the conscious perception of any sensory modality, but is concerned with afferent functions common to all types of sensory experience, namely, alerting and attracting attention. The nonspecific sensory impulses ascending in the reticular activating system appear to sharpen the attentive state of cortex and create optimal conditions for the conscious perception of sensory impulses mediated by the classical pathways.

A differential susceptibility of these two systems to the action of depressant drugs contributes to the production of the anesthetic state (81, 243, 808, 1311). The undiminished persistence of impulses in the lemniscal systems, and the blocking of impulses in the ascending reticular core, in anesthetic states (e.g., ether and certain barbiturates) suggest that many effects may be due to the blockage of synaptic transmission in the multineuronal activating system.

Long-term studies (2415) of cats with extensive rostral midbrain lesions interrupting the specific lemniscal pathways bilaterally produce consistent alterations of behavior. Such animals exhibit: (a) a marked reduction of somatic and autonomic signs of affective behavior, (b) inattention to, and poor localization of, visual, auditory, tactile and nociceptive stimuli, (c) stereotyped hyperexploratory behavior,

largely independent of stimuli in the external environment, and (d) changes in eating, grooming, excretory and sexual habits. In spite of these changes, these animals show essentially normal behavioral and EEG arousal.

In man, lesions of the brain stem often produce disturbances of consciousness which range from fleeting unconsciousness to deep and sustained coma (347). As Magoun (1586) has stated, "It is not easy for the physiologist to put his finger upon consciousness, though it is present abundantly and for long periods of time." One of the accepted working definitions of consciousness is, "an awareness of environment and of self" (485). In all forms of disturbed consciousness due to brain stem lesions, there is a loss of crude awareness. With lesions of the lower brain stem, unconsciousness usually is accompanied by respiratory and cardiovascular disturbances and, often, increased muscle tone. The loss of consciousness frequently is sudden in onset, and depression of vital functions leads to extreme states which may be fatal. Lesions of the upper brain stem most commonly produce hypersomnia characterized by muscular relaxation, slow respiration and an EEG pattern showing large amplitude slow waves. The level of unconsciousness usually is not deep, and some patients can be aroused briefly. If the patient develops decerebrate rigidity, there is usually coma, but these phenomena are not always correlated. A variant of hypersomnia seen with upper brain stem lesions is referred to as *akinetic mutism* (coma vigil). In this variant the EEG pattern resembles that associated with slow sleep, but eye movements remain normal. Many patients with such lesions survive for months in this state. With lesions at all levels of the brain stem, liability to unconsciousness is related to the rapidity with which the lesions develop. Lesions associated with hemorrhage produce sudden unconsciousness and coma; slowly developing lesions, such as tumors, may not disturb consciousness for a considerable period of time. This subject has been reviewed extensively by Plum and Posner (2018). Although there is probably no center uniquely concerned with consciousness, there are indications that the functional integrity of the brain stem reticular formation is essential for its maintenance. This further suggests that a healthy cerebral cortex cannot by itself maintain the conscious state.

As described in Chapter 12, the principal ascending fibers from serotoninergic neurons lie in the dorsal (supratrochlear) and median (superior central nucleus) raphe nuclei of the midbrain (Fig. 11-15). The major ascending pathway of serotoninergic fibers from these nuclei is through the ventral tegmental area (Fig. 16-7) where fibers join the medial forebrain bundle (202, 1737, 2598). A number of these fibers pass dorsally to enter the habenular nuclei, while others project rostrally in the internal medullary lamina of the thalamus. Fibers in the medial forebrain bundle project medially into the hypothalamus and laterally through the internal capsule to the striatum and amygdaloid nuclear complex. Ascending fibers continuing in the medial forebrain bundle divide into several components that pass via: (a) the stria medullaris to the thalamus, (b) the stria terminalis to the amygdala, (c) the fornix to the hippocampus, (d) cingulum bundle to the cortex on the dorsomedial aspect of the hemisphere and (e) the medial olfactory stria to the olfactory bulb (1737). The raphe nuclei of the midbrain and their extensive ascending fiber systems have close functional relationships with both the ascending reticular activating system and the limbic system. There is considerable evidence that the general inhibitory action of serotonin in the central nervous system serves to modulate and maintain behavior within certain limits. Hallucinogenic drugs, such as LSD, depress the serotoninergic system and the release of inhibition results in a hypersensitivity to environmental stimuli and hyperactivity in a brain otherwise behaving as if it were asleep (1196).

SUBSTANTIA NIGRA

The substantia nigra is the most voluminous nuclear mass of the human mesencephalon, extending throughout its length and into the caudal diencephalon (Figs. 13-1, 13-3, 13-6, 13-14 and 13-20). It is rudimentary in lower vertebrates, makes its definite appearance in mammals, and reaches its greatest development in man. For descriptive purposes the substantia ni-

gra commonly is divided into two parts: (a) the pars compacta, a cell-rich region composed in man of pigmented neurons containing melanin, and (b) the pars reticulata, a cell-poor region adjacent to the crus cerebri. Some ultrastructural studies do not support the division of the substantia into two parts, even though cells vary in size and regional distribution, and the specific orientation of dendrites and the connections of each division are different (100, 1105, 2159). The compact zone appears as an irregular band of closely packed, polygonal or pyramidal cells containing melanin granules. Pigmented cells are found in the substantia nigra of a wide variety of mammals (1609); the intensity of the pigmentation in primates is greater than in any other order and reaches maximum intensity in man. In man, pigmented cells do not appear in the substantia nigra until the fourth or fifth year of life. The compact zone extends to the most caudal part of the midbrain, where it is covered ventrally by the pontine nuclei (Fig. 13-3). The pars reticulata, also known as the stratum intermedium, lies close to the crus cerebri and is composed of scattered cells of irregular size and shape.

The division of neurons of the substantia nigra into "large" and "small" cells is not so apparent at the electron microscopic level (101). Neurons rich in cytoplasmic organelles probably represent the large neurons, while pale cells with a paucity of organelles appear to be the small neurons, but there are numerous intermediary forms. Most of the larger neurons, characterized by a deeply lobulated nucleus and a well-developed eccentric nucleolus, have been considered to be dopaminergic (Fig. 13-22). Three types of nigral neurons have been described in the rat: (a) large neurons distributed exclusively in the pars reticulata, (b) medium-sized neurons in the pars compacta (Fig. 13-23), and (c) small, short-axoned cells found in both the pars compacta and the pars reticulata (986). Large neurons, found throughout the pars reticulata, appear most prevalent in rostrolateral regions, are enveloped by a thin astrocytic sheath and are embedded in a neuropil of small unmyelinated fibers. Medium-sized neurons, closely grouped in the pars compacta, are invariably separated by thin astrocytic sheaths and contain inclusions

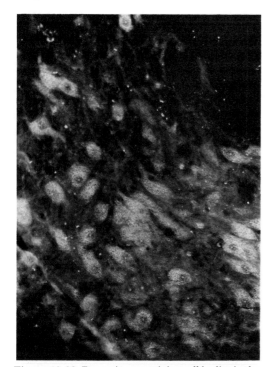

Figure 13-22. Dopamine-containing cell bodies in the pars compacta of the substantia nigra of the squirrel monkey. Green fluorescence in the cell bodies extends into some of the large processes which contribute to the background fluorescence. (Fluorescence photomicrograph, ×400.) (Courtesy of Dr. David L. Felton, School of Medicine, Indiana University.)

composed of whorls of concentric cisternae. Small neurons (10 to 12 μm), comprising roughly 10% of the pars compacta and 40% of the pars reticulata, have a paucity of cytoplasmic organelles, lack an organized Nissl substance and have short axons. The small nigral neurons with short axons may function as interneurons (2298).

Golgi studies demonstrate that nigral neurons give rise to long radiating dendrites with few branches. Relatively smooth dendrites are oriented in two main directions. Dendrites of cells in the pars reticulata and in the caudal pars compacta are oriented primarily in rostrocaudal directions. Dendrites of most cells in the pars compacta have a dorsoventral orientation. Thus the dendritic fields of cells in the pars compacta and pars reticulata overlap extensively in the pars reticulata (2159). The surface of nigral dendrites is covered with boutons whose numbers increase with the distance from the soma and are separated from

the neighboring neuropil by protoplasmic sheets of astroglia. Although axons of nigral neurons are difficult to impregnate by the Golgi technic, a prominent feature of the substantia nigra is the enormous number of thin unmyelinated axons coursing in a rostrocaudal direction.

Dorsomedial to the substantia nigra and ventral to the red nucleus is a region containing scattered cells of various sizes and shapes, among which are some large cells with melanin pigment. It is not certain whether some of these belong to the substantia nigra or to the tegmentum, but this region is regarded as a diffusely organized extension of the compact zone. This region is referred to as the *ventral tegmental area* (Tsai). Lateral to the substantia nigra, a layer of small cells, the *peripeduncular nucleus*, caps the dorsal surface of the crus cerebri (Fig. 13-14).

Neurotransmitters. Cells of the pars compacta contain high concentrations of dopamine (Fig. 13-22) and are recognized as the principal source of striatal dopamine (59, 585, 1127, 1734, 2298). This thesis is supported by evidence that: (a) lesions in the substantia nigra produce marked decreases in striatal dopamine (2024, 2025), and (b) the normally high concentrations of striatal dopamine are greatly reduced in the brains of Parkinsonian patients (692, 1144, 1145). The substantia nigra also contains the highest concentrations of glutamic acid decarboxylase (GAD), the enzyme that synthesizes γ-aminobutyric acid (GABA) (728, 1865). A study of the topographical distribution of GAD in the substantia nigra indicates that the highest concentration is in the medial part of the pars reticulata; GAD is lowest in the medial part of the pars compacta which contains the highest concentration of cell bodies (778). Subcellular fractionations show that about 85% of the GAD in the substantia nigra is present in particles, probably synaptosomes. The observation that lesions of the striatum produce large reductions in GAD suggests that only a small number of the GABA-ergic fibers in the substantia nigra could be derived from other sources.

The substantia nigra also contains serotonin (5-HT) and its synthesizing enzyme, tryptophan hydroxylase (308, 1005, 1923); 5-HT is taken up by dense core vesicles in fiber terminals mainly within the pars reticulata (827, 1005, 1940). The dorsal nucleus of the raphe appears to be the principal source of this serotoninergic pathway (324, 398, 515, 648, 1263). Stimulation of the dorsal nucleus of the raphe produces predominantly inhibition of spontaneous activity in single neurons of the substantia nigra (648).

The substantia nigra also contains a highly biologically active principle known as substance P which has been characterized as an undecapeptide (723). Substance P (SP) has been synthesized and used to produce antibodies for radioimmunological determinations of the regional distribution of SP in the brain (2571). Neurophysiological studies have demonstrated that SP has an excitatory action on neurons in many areas of the central nervous system (1121). The highest concentration of SP in any brain region is found in the substantia nigra where the substance is concentrated in nerve ending particles (596, 657, 2051). Neurons containing SP project from the striatum to the nigra and presumably synapse upon dendrites of dopaminergic neurons (841, 1137, 1262). It has been shown that strionigral fibers containing GABA and SP have a similar course, but that the cell bodies have distinct anatomical locations within the striatum (841). Neurons containing SP are concentrated in rostral portions of the striatum, while GABA-containing neurons projecting to the substantia nigra are distributed throughout the striatum. These data suggest that strionigral fibers containing GABA and SP are independent and that striatal neurons containing SP have a distinct localization.

The substantia nigra is implicated primarily in the metabolic disturbances considered to underlie parkinsonism (59, 143, 585, 828, 1127, 1145, 1734, 2025). Data based upon a histochemical fluorescence method (730, 731) indicated that dopamine, stored in varicosities in nerve terminals, is mainly concentrated in three areas of the telencephalon: (a) the striatum (i.e., caudate nucleus and putamen), (b) the nucleus accumbens septi, and (c) the olfactory tubercle (828). These terminal varicosities are fine, densely packed, and exhibit a diffuse green fluorescence. Dopamine is believed to be synthesized in the large pigmented cells in

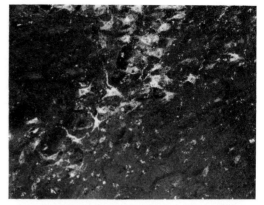

Figure 13-23. Dark field photomicrograph of horseradish peroxidase (HRP) transported from striatum to cells of the pars compacta of the substantia nigra in the monkey. (×200.)

the pars compacta. In contrast to the nerve terminals in the striatum, the concentrations of monoamines in large cells of the substantia nigra seem low, and monoamines occur mainly in the perinuclear cytoplasm (Figs. 13–22 and 13–23). Dopamine, synthesized in the substantia nigra, is continuously transported via axoplasmic flow to terminal varicosities in the striatum. Lesions in the substantia nigra cause conspicuous reductions in ipsilateral striatal dopamine as measured by fluorescent chemical and electron microscopic technics (59, 828, 1127, 2598). Large striatal lesions produce a distinct increase of monoamines (dopamine) in the large cells of the pars compacta which ultimately decreases as the cells undergo chromatolysis (59, 828, 2598). Following interruption of nigrostriatal axons, fluorescent material builds up in the axon proximal to the lesion. Ordinarily the levels of monoamines in the axons are too low to be demonstrated by the fluorescent technic. These observations appear significant in view of the fact that the brains of patients with parkinsonism show a virtual absence of dopamine in the striatum and substantia nigra (1144, 1145). Other complex interrelationships between dopamine and γ-aminobutyric acid (GABA) suggest that both the striatum and the substantia nigra may be involved in the neural mechanisms responsible for choreoid dyskinesia in Huntington's disease (181).

Cells in the *ventral tegmental area* (Tsai), medial to the substantia nigra and

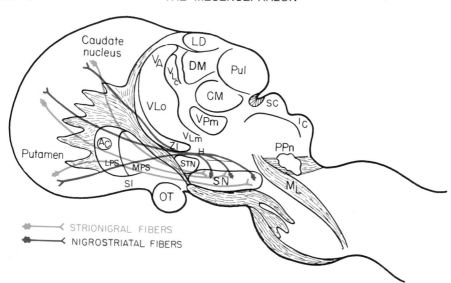

Figure 13-24.   Schematic diagram of the strionigral feedback system in a sagittal plane. Strionigral fibers (*blue*) project topographically upon cells of the pars reticulata of the nigra and have γ-aminobutyric acid (GABA) as their neurotransmitter. Cells of the pars compacta of the nigra give rise to reciprocally arranged nigrostriatal fibers (*red*) which convey dopamine to specific loci within the striatum (413). Abbreviations: *AC,* anterior commissure; *CM,* centromedian nucleus; *DM,* dorsomedial nucleus; *H,* Forel's field, *IC,* inferior colliculus; *LD,* lateral dorsal nucleus; *LPS,* lateral segment of globus pallidus; *ML,* medial lemniscus; *MPS,* medial segment of globus pallidus; *OT,* optic tract; *PPn,* pedunculopontine nucleus; *Pul,* pulvinar; *SC,* superior colliculus; *SI,* substantia innominata; *SN,* substantia nigra; *STN,* subthalamic nucleus; *VA,* ventral anterior nucleus; *VLc, VLo* and *VLm,* ventral lateral nucleus, pars caudalis, pars oralis and pars medialis; *VPM,* ventral posterior medial nucleus; *ZI,* zona incerta.

dorsal to the interpeduncular nucleus, also contain dopamine. Fibers from these cells ascend to enter the medial forebrain bundle (2598). At levels of the anterior commissure, fibers of this bundle enter the nucleus accumbens and the nucleus of the stria terminalis, while other laterally projecting fibers enter the olfactory tubercle.

Nigral Afferent Fibers. Afferent fibers to the substantia nigra arise mainly from the caudate nucleus and the putamen (1747, 2237, 2613). *Strionigral fibers* are topographically organized (Fig. 13–24), but their extensive nature, organization and regions of termination were not appreciated until the investigations of Voneida (2626) and Szabo (2489–2491). These studies indicated that fibers from the head of the caudate nucleus project to the rostral third of the substantia nigra and have a mediolateral correspondence. Fibers from the putamen project to the caudal two-thirds of substantia nigra, with dorsal regions of the putamen related to lateral parts of the nigra, and ventral regions related to medial parts

of the nigra. While most of the strionigral fibers are regarded as terminating in the pars reticulata, this distinction appears less significant in view of the electron microscopic evidence that almost all afferents terminate in the pars reticulata (970, 1283, 2298). The majority of strionigral fibers establish symmetrical types of synapses on the soma, dendritic trunks or dendrites of nigral cells in the pars reticulata.

Studies of afferent projections to the substantia nigra based upon the retrograde transport of HRP also indicate that the caudatonigral projection system is arranged topographically (324). All portions of the caudate-putamen except the medial core were found to contain HRP-positive cells. In the positive areas a large percentage of cells (i.e., 30 to 50%) were found to participate in this projection, but only medium-sized cells (12 to 20 μm) contained the enzyme (324, 969).

Strionigral fibers are of two types, those that convey GABA to terminals in the pars reticulata (728, 1865) and fibers that contain substance P. Rostral portions of the striatum give rise to an independent parallel strionigral projection that conveys substance P to particles in nerve endings (596, 841). The concentration of substance P is highest in the pars reticulata (1773).

Pallidonigral projections have been identified largely on the basis of retrograde transport of horseradish peroxidase; labeled terminals in the pars reticulata have transported the enzyme to cells in the lateral pallidal segment (324, 969, 1263). In the monkey the only part of the pallidum clearly demonstrated to project to the substantia nigra was the medial segment (1313). These fibers observed in sagittal autoradiographs descended in lateral parts of the substantia nigra to terminations in two locations: (a) in the pars lateralis immediately caudal to the subthalamic nucleus, and (b) near cells of the pars compacta in caudal parts of the nigra. Data concerning these fibers, considered to convey GABA to their nigral terminations, are incomplete but substantiated by a variety of different methods (1051, 1262, 1563).

Subthalamonigral fibers have long been postulated, but their polarity has remained in doubt. The application of axonal transport technics indicates that cells in the subthalamic nucleus project to the substantia nigra (1263). HRP injected into various parts of the substantia nigra was transported retrograde to cells in the subthalamic nucleus in the cat. Studies in the rat based upon a fluorescent double-labeling technic suggest that virtually all cells in the subthalamic nucleus project axons to both the substantia nigra and the globus pallidus (1344). An autoradiographic study of subthalamic efferent fibers indicated that labeled fibers from the nucleus entered the substantia nigra directly or via a fiber stratum interposed between the crus cerebri and substantia nigra (1812). Terminal fibers appeared in patchy areas, but were not present around clusters of pigmented cells. The impression from this study was that the major subthalamonigral projection is to the pars reticulata.

Projections from the raphe nuclei of the midbrain to the substantia nigra have serotonin (5-HT) as their neurotransmitter. The bulk of the serotonin neurons projecting to the forebrain are located in the dorsal and median raphe nuclei of the midbrain (60, 586, 2598). The dorsal nucleus of the raphe appears to be the principal source of serotoninergic projections to the substantia nigra which have an inhibitory action on single neurons, particularly those in the pars reticulata (324, 398, 515, 648, 1263). Even though many anatomical details are unresolved, the raphe nuclei of the midbrain appear to modulate the activities of the substantia nigra.

Although corticonigral fibers have been described by a number of investigators (2156), electron microscopic studies indicate that such fibers are absent in the cat (2164). According to Bunney and Aghajanian (324), HRP injections in the substantia nigra consistently label a few neurons in prefrontal cortex. This observation has received some support from autoradiographic studies indicating a few corticonigral fibers arising from areas 6 and 9. These fibers are described as ending in patches within the pars compacta (1395).

Nigral Efferent Projections. Nigral efferent fibers arising from the pars compacta and the pars reticulata are distinctive. Nigrostriatal fibers arise from the pars compacta and project topographically upon all parts of the striatum (i.e., caudate nucleus and putamen). Nigrothalamic and nigrotectal fibers arise from the cells of the pars reticulata.

Nigrostriatal fibers were first demonstrated by retrograde cellular degeneration in the substantia nigra following cerebral ablations that included portions of the striatum (1720). Subsequent studies showed that the retrograde cell changes in the substantia nigra could be correlated with the extent of striatal injury (744, 1682). Attempts to trace nigrostriatal fibers in Marchi preparations indicated that nigral efferent fibers ascended and entered both segments of the globus pallidus, but none could be followed into the caudate nucleus or putamen (1681a, 1682, 2113, 2220). These data suggest that nigrostriatal fibers become poorly myelinated in the globus pallidus. In spite of difficulty in identifying "classic" terminations of dopamine fibers on caudate neurons, evidence indicates asymmetrical synapses on spiny processes with postsynaptic thickenings. Nerve terminals containing dopamine have small granular vesicles about 500 Å in diameter (1127). The preponderance of data suggests that these fibers exert inhibitory influences upon striatal neurons (196, 1086, 1571, 2340).

Even though the fluorescent histochemical technic clearly demonstrated nigrostriatal projections, the Nauta silver impregnation method failed to provide evidence of a substantial projection (20, 406, 419). Investigations of nigral efferent projections using relatively short survival times and modified silver impregnation technics demonstrated nigrostriatal projections in both the cat and monkey (413, 1734). Discrete lesions involving primarily the caudal two-thirds of the nigra produce degeneration which ascended in the pars compacta, and the region immediately dorsal to it, to Forel's field H. Laterally projecting fibers from this locus traversed the internal capsule and the globus pallidus to enter the putamen. Anterograde silver degeneration studies suggest that strionigral and nigrostriatal fibers are topographically and reciprocally organized and may form a closed feedback loop (413, 2489, 2490, 2626). The reciprocal nature of strionigral and nigrostriatal fiber systems (Fig. 13–24) is substantiated by axoplasmic transport studies (1813). Horseradish peroxidase (HRP) injected into the striatum is transported: (a) in retrograde fashion from axon terminals to cells in the pars compacta (Fig. 13–23), and (b) in anterograde fashion by striatal neurons to terminals in the pars reticulata of substantia nigra. All studies using HRP are in agreement that the enzyme is transported in a retrograde fashion from the striatum to the cells of the pars compacta of the substantia nigra (1814, 2187). This is regarded as the heaviest retrograde label transported from the striatum. It is significant that no striatal label is transported to cells of the pars reticulata.

Retrograde transport studies of HRP in the cat and monkey provide data concerning the topographical organization of nigrostriatal projections (2492, 2493). The projections of the pars compacta to the striatum are organized in all principal planes. The rostral two-thirds of the substantia nigra is related to the head of the caudate nucleus, while neurons projecting to the putamen are located posteriorly. An inverse relationship exists dorsoventrally between the substantia nigra and the caudate nucleus, so that ventral parts of the pars compacta project to dorsal regions of the caudate nucleus and dorsally situated neurons in the nigra pass to ventral regions of the caudate nucleus. Lateral and posterior regions of the nigra are related to dorsal and lateral parts of the putamen. There is also a mediolateral correspondence between the cells of the substantia nigra and regions of fiber termination in the striatum.

Strionigral and nigrostriatal fibers appear to form a closed feedback loop in which strionigral fibers form the afferent limb and nigrostriatal fibers constitute the efferent limb that conveys dopamine to terminal varicosities in the striatum (Fig. 13–24).

In patients with paralysis agitans, there is a virtual absence of dopamine in the striatum and the substantia nigra (1145, 2011). An effective treatment for this metabolic disorder is large doses of L-dihydroxyphenylalanine (L-dopa), a precursor of dopamine, which passes the blood-brain barrier. The effectiveness of this drug can be enhanced by the use of a peripheral decarboxylase inhibitor (1608) which prevents systemic decarboxylation of L-dopa to dopamine. Thus, adequate L-dopa will be left unmetabolized systemically to enter the brain where the desired decarboxylation to dopamine can occur (Fig. 1-17).

Nigrothalamic fibers arise from the cells of the pars reticulata of the nigra and project rostrally to the large-celled part of the ventral anterior nucleus (VAmc), the medial part of the ventral lateral nucleus (VLm) and to the paralaminar part of the dorsomedial nucleus (DMpl) (Figs. 13–25 and 13–26). In their course these fibers closely parallel the mammillothalamic tract (409, 413, 419). Nigral lesions in the monkey which selectively destroyed portions of the pars reticulata are associated with terminal degeneration in thalamic nuclei and little or no degeneration in the striatum (409). This observation supported the conclusion that nigrothalamic fibers (nondopaminergic) arise exclusively from cells in the pars reticulata. Confirmation of the origin of nigrothalamic fibers has come from axonal transport studies (2158). Horseradish peroxidase (HRP) injected into medial thalamic nuclei and into VL in the cat resulted in retrograde transport of the label exclusively to cells in the pars reticulata. This study indicated that nigrothalamic fibers in the cat arise particularly from lateral parts of pars reticulata, as demonstrated in earlier degeneration studies in the monkey (419). Autoradiographic tracing studies of nigral efferent fibers in the monkey demonstrated that neurons in rostrolateral parts of the nigra projected preferentially and abundantly to thalamic nuclei (413). Isotope transported from nigral neurons was found in parts of three thalamic nuclei (Figs. 13–25 and 13–26), the medial part of the ventral lateral nucleus (VLm), the magnocellular part of the ventral anterior nucleus (VAmc) and the paralaminar part of the dorsomedial nucleus (DMpl). Since DMpl has been shown to have a specific connection with the frontal eye field, this nigral projection may be involved in mechanisms that control or modulate ocular movements (2299). Recent studies indicate that the connections of DMpl with area 8 are reciprocal; area 8 also projects to the contralateral frontal eye field and to the ipsilateral superior colliculus and pretectum (1395).

Nigrotectal fibers have been described in almost all degeneration studies, but initially this finding was interpreted to be a consequence of interruption of corticotectal projections (406, 419, 504, 1411). Uncertainty concerning nigrotectal fibers has been resolved by retrograde transport studies using HRP, which indicate that such fibers arise only from the pars reticulata of the substantia nigra (952, 1141, 2162). An autoradiographic study of nigrotectal projections in the monkey indicated that nigrotectal fibers: (a) arise only from the pars reticulata and project to the middle gray layers of the caudal two-thirds of the ipsilateral superior colliculus and to lateral regions of the central gray and (b) may be topographically arranged so that lateral parts of the substantia nigra project to lateral parts of the superior colliculus and medial regions of the substantia nigra project to medial parts of the superior colliculus. Some nigral neurons project bilaterally to the superior colliculus (1212). Projections of nigrotectal fibers are to portions of the superior colliculus which receive multimodal inputs not relayed to the visual system.

The use of a fluorescent retrograde double-labeling technic using Evans blue (fluoresces red) and a mixture of DAPI-primuline (fluoresces blue) has demonstrated that most cells in the pars reticulata of the substantia nigra project individually to either the thalamus or the superior colliculus (158). In addition, there are some cells with divergent axon collaterals that project to both the thalamus and the superior colliculus (double-labeled cells). Electrophysiological studies in the cat also indicate that some nigral axons innervate both thalamic nuclei and the superior colliculus (61, 62). Stimulation of the caudate nucleus produced inhibition of both collicular and thalamic neurons.

Nigrotegmental fibers arise from the pars reticulata and project to the pedunculopontine nucleus (140, 398, 1066, 1729). These fibers are nondopaminergic. It is of interest that the pedunculopontine nucleus receives its subcortical inputs from structures that receive striatal afferents (i.e., the medial pallidal segment and the substantia nigra) and that efferent from this nucleus largely project back to these nuclei (Figs. 17-19 and 17-20). The pars compacta of the substantia nigra also gives rise to a descending tegmental projection which terminates in the dorsal and median raphe nuclei (140).

The substantia nigra is the brain stem nucleus most intimately related to the largest part of the basal ganglia, namely, the neostriatum. The pars reticulata receives its major input from the caudate nucleus and putamen; these strionigral fibers have either γ-aminobutyric acid (GABA) or substance P as their neurotransmitter. Cells of the pars compacta are reciprocally arranged and convey dopamine to terminals within the striatum. Cells of the pars reticulata constitute an important and distinctive output component of the corpus striatal complex, which is different from that arising from the medial pallidal segment. The pars reticulata of the substantia nigra projects to different rostral ventral tier thalamic nuclei (i.e., the ventral anterior, pars magnocellularis, VAmc, and the ventral lateral nucleus, pars medialis, VLm) than the medial pallidal segment and also has a distinctive projection to the dorsomedial nucleus of the thalamus (DMpl). Nigrothalamic fibers and pallidothalamic projections collectively constitute the major out-

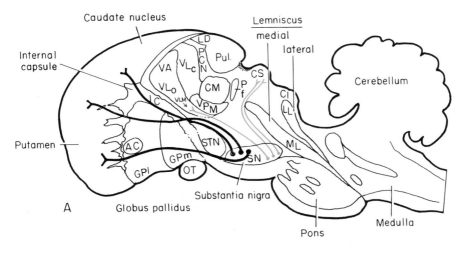

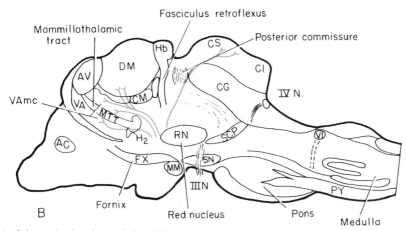

Figure 13-25. Schematic drawings of the efferent projections of the substantia nigra in sagittal sections. Ascending *nigrostriatal fibers* (*red*) arise from cells in the pars compacta and project through the internal capsule (*IC*) to terminations in the putamen and caudate nucleus (*A*). *Nigrothalamic* and *nigrotectal fibers* (*blue*) arise from cells in the pars reticulata (*A* and *B*). Nigrothalamic fibers (*blue*) project to medial parts of the ventral lateral nucleus (*VLm*), the magnocellular part of the ventral anterior nucleus (*VAmc*) and to the paralaminar part of the dorsomedial nucleus (*DM*). In part of their course these fibers parallel the mammillothalamic tract (*MTT*). Nigrotectal projections (*blue*) pass to middle gray layers in the caudal two-thirds of the superior colliculus (*A* and *B*). Not shown in this diagram are projections from the substantia nigra to the pedunculopontine nucleus (see Fig. 17-20). Drawing *A* is lateral to drawing *B*. Abbreviations: *AC*, anterior commissure; *AV*, anterior ventral thalamic nucleus; *CG*, central gray; *CI*, inferior coliculus; *CM*, centromedian thalamic nucleus; *CS*, superior colliculus; *DM*, dorsomedial thalamic nucleus; *FX*, fornix; *GPl* and *GPm*, lateral and medial segments of the globus pallidus, respectively; *H₂*, lenticular fasciculus; *Hb*, habenular nucleus; *LD*, lateral dorsal thalamic nucleus; *LL*, lateral lemniscus; *ML*, medial lemniscus; *MM*, mammillary body; *OT*, optic tract; *PCN*, paracentral thalamic nucleus; *Pf*, parafascicular nucleus; *Pul*, pulvinar; *PY*, medullary pyramid; *RN*, red nucleus; *SCP*, superior cerebellar peduncle; *STN*, subthalamic nucleus; *VA*, ventral anterior thalamic nucleus; *VLc* and *VLo*, ventral lateral thalamic nucleus (caudal and oral parts); *VPM*, ventral posteromedial thalamic nucleus; *VI*, abducens nucleus.

put system of the corpus striatum complex (390).

The substantia nigra is the principal site of the pathological process which underlies the metabolic disturbances associated with paralysis agitans (768, 1048, 1064, 2572). It is of interest that discrete lesions of the substantia nigra in the monkey, destroying

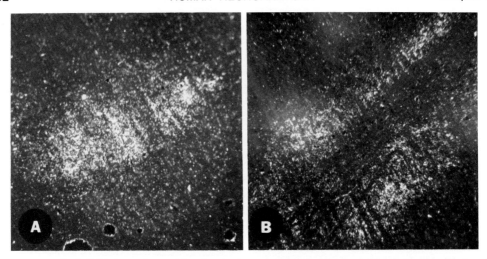

Figure 13-26. Dark field photomicrographs of sagittal autoradiographs, demonstrating transport of isotope from injections in the substantia nigra to thalamic nuclei. *A* shows transport to the paralaminar part of the dorsomedial nucleus (*DMpl*), while *B* shows isotope in terminals in the magnocellular part of the ventral anterior nucleus. The mammillothalamic tract passes obliquely through the ventral anterior nucleus in *B* (409).

up to 40% of the nucleus, do not produce alterations of muscle tone, impairment of associative movements, tremor or any detectable form of dyskinesia (406). Although these lesions interfere with a variety of neurotransmitters, they do not mimic the metabolic disturbances associated with paralysis agitans.

CRUS CEREBRI

The most ventral part of the midbrain contains a massive band of descending corticofugal fibers, the *crus cerebri*. According to Déjerine (608), the medial three-fifths of the crus cerebri contain somatotopically arranged corticospinal and corticobulbar fibers. Other authors (753, 1721, 2084) indicate that much smaller portions of the central part of the crus cerebri contain these fibers. In the classic view, fibers in the most lateral part of the central region are concerned with the lower extremity; the larger middle region contains fibers concerned with the upper extremity; and the most medial fibers of the central region are associated with the musculature of the face, pharynx and larynx. The extreme medial and lateral portions of the crus cerebri contain *corticopontine fibers*. Frontopontine fibers are medial, while corticopontine fibers from the temporal, parietal and occipital cortices are located laterally (Fig. 13-1).

More recent data indicate that corticospinal fibers in the internal capsule are largely confined to a compact region in the caudal part of the posterior limb of the internal capsule (174, 711, 880, 1023, 2363). Somatotopical organization of fibers destined for particular segmental levels appears relatively crude. These data suggest that the somatotopic arrangement of corticospinal fibers in the crus cerebri probably is much less precise than commonly depicted. In man, corticospinal fibers probably account for only 1 million of the 20 million fibers in the crus cerebri; the remaining fibers are largely corticopontine (2556).

Besides the above named tracts, there often are two fiber bundles which descend partly within the crus cerebri and partly in the region of the medial lemniscus, known as *pes lemnisci* (Fig. 13-1). The *medial* or *superficial pes lemniscus* detaches itself from the lateral portion of the crus cerebri, winds ventrally around the crus and forms a semilunar fiber bundle medial to the frontal corticopontine tract (Fig. 13-1). At lower levels the fibers leave the crus cerebri, pass dorsally through the substantia nigra and descend in or near the ventromedial portion of the medial lemniscus. The *lateral* or *deep pes lemniscus* detaches itself from the dorsal surface of the crus, runs for some distance in the lateral portion of the substantia nigra, then turns dorsally and descends in the region of the medial lemniscus (Fig. 13-1). Certain authors (608, 2612) regarded these bundles as aberrant corticospinal fibers which during phylogenesis became separated from the main tract by the increasing development of the dorsal pontine nuclei. According to Kuypers (1405), fibers of the pes lemnisci can be traced caudally through the pons to the level of the pyramidal decussation. A number of these fibers are distributed to the tegmentum of the pons and medulla. These fibers, undoubtedly corticobulbar, appear to project mainly into the reticular formation; few, if any, of these fibers pass directly to motor cranial nerve nuclei (Fig. 11-30).

At this juncture it is recommended that the blood supply of the midbrain be reviewed (Chapter 20). A more complete understanding of the structural organization of the midbrain should emphasize the importance of the vessels that supply this part of the brain stem. The principal vessels supplying parts of the midbrain include the posterior cerebral, the superior cerebellar, the posterior communicating and the anterior choroidal arteries (Figs. 20-14, 20-16 and 20-18). The numerous veins draining large portions of the diencephalon and basal regions enter the great cerebral vein in regions dorsal to the midbrain (Fig. 20-23). These veins and their tributaries are of major importance.

CHAPTER 14

The Cerebellum

The cerebellum is concerned with the coordination of somatic motor activity, the regulation of muscle tone and mechanisms that influence and maintain equilibrium. It is derived embryologically from ectodermal thickenings about the cephalic borders of the fourth ventricle, known as the rhombic lip (Figs. 3-12 and 3-14). Although this portion of the brain is derived from portions of the embryonic neural tube which lie dorsal to the sulcus limitans and receive sensory inputs from virtually all receptors, it is not concerned with sensory perception. No sensory information transmitted to the cerebellum enters the conscious sphere. Sensory information transmitted to the cerebellum is utilized primarily in the automatic regulation and control of motor functions. The cerebellum serves as an example of the important role sensory integrating mechanisms play in motor function. This metencephalic derivative functions in a supraseg-mental manner in that its integrative influences affect activities at all levels of the neuraxis. Although the cerebellum gives rise to one small tract (fastigiospinal) that projects directly to spinal levels, its major influences upon segmental levels of the neuraxis are mediated indirectly by brain stem nuclei that relay impulses to spinal levels.

GROSS ANATOMY

The gross anatomy of the cerebellum has been described in Chapter 2. From this discussion, it will be recalled that the cerebellum consists of: (a) a superficial gray mantle, the *cerebellar cortex*; (b) an internal white mass, the *medullary substance*; and (c) four pairs of *intrinsic nuclei* (Figs. 12-7, 12-23 and 14-14). Grossly the cerebellum may be divided into a median portion, the *vermis*, and two expanded lateral lobes or *hemispheres*. The cerebellar cortex is composed of numerous narrow *laminae* or

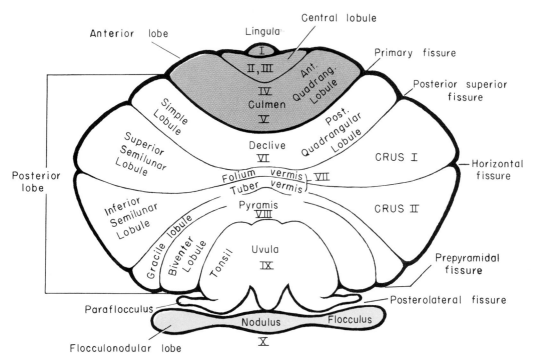

Figure 14-1. Schematic diagram of the fissures and lobules of the cerebellum (76, 1207, 1435). Portions of the cerebellum caudal to the posterolateral fissure (*blue*) represent the flocculonodular lobule (archicerebellum), while portions of the cerebellum rostral to the primary fissure (*red*) constitute the anterior lobe (paleocerebellum). The neocerebellum lies between the primary and posterolateral fissure. Roman numerals refer to portions of the cerebellar vermis only.

cerebellar *folia*, which in turn possess secondary and tertiary infoldings. Five deeper fissures divide the cerebellar vermis and hemispheres into lobes and lobules which can be identified in gross specimens as well as in midsagittal section (Figs. 2-29–2-32). These fissures are (a) the *primary*, (b) the *posterior superior*, (c) the *horizontal*, (d) the *prepyramidal* and (e) the *posterolateral* (prenodular). They form the basis for all subdivisions of the cerebellum (Fig. 14-1). In spite of a wealth of histological detail concerning the structural organization of the cerebellum, precise anatomical localization within various lobules is difficult, except in gross specimens. Precise identification of cerebellar lobules, laminae and folia in microscopic sections is difficult even in serial sections. Detailed atlases of the human (76) and monkey (1579) cerebella facilitate the microscopic study of cerebellar sections.

On developmental and functional bases, the cerebellum can be divided into three parts, archicerebellum, paleocerebellum and neocerebellum.

The *archicerebellum*, represented largely by the *nodulus*, the *two flocculi* and their peduncular connections (i.e., *flocculonodular lobe*), is the oldest part of the cerebellum and is the subdivision most closely related to the vestibular nerve and nuclei (*blue* in Fig. 14-1). The flocculonodular lobe is separated from the corpus cerebelli by the posterolateral fissure, the first fissure to develop in the cerebellum.

The *paleocerebellum*, consisting of all parts of the cerebellum rostral to the primary fissure, is referred to as the *anterior lobe* of the cerebellum (*red* in Fig. 14-1). In lower forms, the paleocerebellum forms the largest part of the cerebellum, while in man it constitutes a small subdivision which receives impulses primarily from stretch receptors. It is the part of the cerebellum considered to be most concerned with the regulation of muscle tone. Influences upon muscle tone mediated via the fastigial nuclei and cerebellovestibular projections reach spinal levels via the vestibulospinal, reticulospinal and fastigiospinal tracts. Impulses from the emboliform nucleus modify

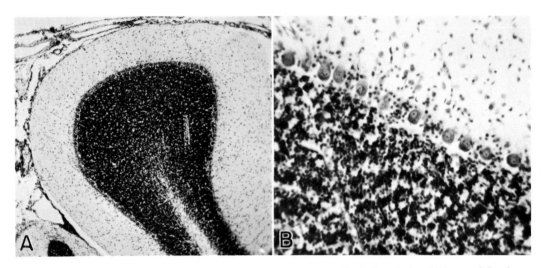

Figure 14-2. Sections through a folium of monkey cerebellar cortex. In *A* the relative thickness of the three cerebellar layers can be seen. Light spaces in the dark staining granular layer are the "cerebellar islands" containing the glomeruli. A single row of Purkinje cells above the granula layer is shown in *B* (photograph, Nissl stain, ×20, ×50).

muscle tone by projecting upon cells of the red nucleus which in turn project to spinal levels (1632). These fibers are shown in Figure 14-17.

The *neocerebellum*, phylogenetically the newest and the largest portion, includes all parts of the cerebellum between the primary and posterolateral fissures in both the vermis and lateral lobes and comprises the posterior lobe (Fig. 14-1). Lateral parts of the cerebellum, between the primary and the posterior superior fissures, are known as the *simple lobule*. The portions of the lateral lobe between the posterior superior fissure and the gracile lobule constitute the *ansiform lobule*. The horizontal fissure divides the ansiform lobule into major parts commonly known as *crus I* (superior semilunar lobule) and *crus II* (inferior semilunar lobule). Between the prepyramidal and posterolateral fissures are the biventer lobule and the cerebellar tonsil in the hemisphere, and the pyramis and uvula in the vermis. The neocerebellum is the portion of the cerebellum considered to be related primarily to coordination of skilled voluntary movements initiated at cortical levels. The major input to the neocerebellum is derived from broad regions of the cerebral cortex of the opposite hemisphere which project to pontine nuclei, that in turn give rise to crossed projections that collectively form the middle cerebellar peduncle.

The cerebellum is attached to the medulla, the pons and the midbrain by three paired cerebellar peduncles (Figs. 2–24, 2–25 and 2–31). These compact fiber bundles interconnect the archicerebellum, paleocerebellum and neocerebellum with the spinal cord, brain stem and higher levels of the neuraxis. The extensive nature of these connections suggests that the cerebellum serves as a great integrative center for the coordination of muscular activity. Before examining the afferent and efferent fiber systems of the cerebellum, the structure of the cerebellar cortex will be considered.

CEREBELLAR CORTEX

The cerebellar cortex is uniformly structured in all parts and extends across the midline without evidence of a median raphe. The cortex is composed of three well-defined layers containing five different types of neurons. These layers from the surface are: (a) the molecular layer, (b) the Purkinje cell layer and (c) the granular layer (Figs. 14-2–14-4).

The Molecular Layer. This consists principally of dendritic arborizations, densely packed thin axons coursing parallel to the long axis of the folia and two types of neurons (Figs. 14-2, 14-4 and 14-5). The cell density of this layer is low. The two types of cell bodies in the molecular layer are the basket cell and the outer (superfi-

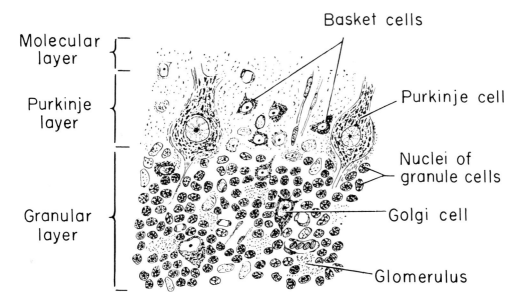

Figure 14-3. Drawing of portions of the three layers of the human cerebellar cortex (Nissl stain) (after Cajal (348)).

cial) stellate cell (Figs. 14-4 and 14-5). The dendritic ramifications of both types of these neurons are confined to the molecular layer, as are the axons of the outer stellate cells. The axons of the basket cells lie mainly in the molecular and Purkinje cell layers, but penetrate short distances into the granular layer. The cell processes of both cells are oriented transversely to the long axis of the folia. The *outer stellate cells*, located in the outer two-thirds of the molecular layer, have small cell bodies, short thin dendrites and fine unmyelinated axons (Figs. 14-4 and 14-5). The short thin dendrites ramify near the cell body, and fine unmyelinated short axons extend transversely to the folia to establish synaptic contacts with Purkinje cell dendrites.

The *basket cells* are situated in the vicinity of the Purkinje cell bodies (Figs. 14-3–14-5). These cells give rise to numerous branching dendrites that ascend in the molecular layer to produce a fan-shaped field in a sagittal plane. The unique feature of the basket cells are elaborate unmyelinated axons arising from one side of the cell body that course transversely to the folia. The axons of the basket cells, passing in the same plane as the dendritic arborizations of the Purkinje cells, give off one or more descending collaterals which form intricate terminal arborizations about the somata of

about 10 Purkinje cells. A single descending axon collateral may furnish terminal arborizations for more than one Purkinje cell, and Purkinje cells may receive axonal collaterals from several different basket cells. Basket cell axons divide and form a dense plexus about the Purkinje cell axon hillock (147). Thus a single basket cell may come in synaptic relationship with many Purkinje cells situated in a sagittal plane, its axon even extending to a neighboring folium (Fig. 14-4). It is evident from the above that besides the relatively few cells, the molecular layer is composed primarily of unmyelinated dendritic and axonal processes. These processes include the dendrites of the Purkinje cells, the transversely running axons of the granule cells, the axons of the outer stellate cells, the sagittally oriented axons of the basket cells, and the dendrites of basket and Golgi type II cells. Section of all these processes gives to the molecular layer its finely punctate appearance. Only in its deepest portion is there a narrow horizontal plexus of myelinated fibers composed of axonal collaterals of Purkinje cells (Fig. 14-4).

The Purkinje Cell Layer. This layer consists of a sheet of large flask-shaped cells relatively uniformly arranged along the upper margin of the granular layer (Figs. 14-2–14-6). Purkinje cells have a clear vesicular

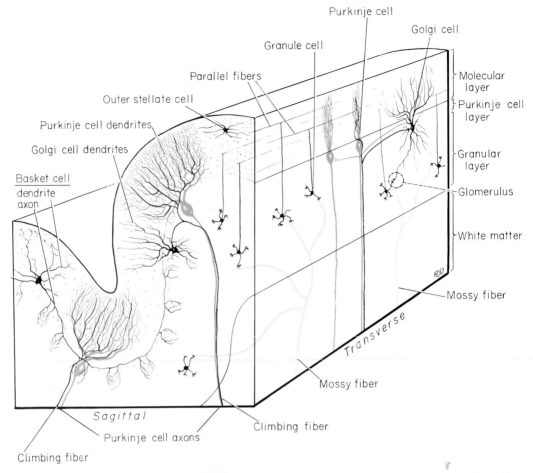

Figure 14-4. Schematic diagram of the cerebellar cortex in sagittal and transverse planes showing cell and fiber arrangements. Purkinje cells and cell processes (i.e., axons and dendrites) are shown in *blue*. Mossy fibers are in *yellow*; climbing fibers are shown in *red*. Golgi cells, basket cells, and outer stellate cells are in *black*. While the dendritic arborizations of Purkinje cells are oriented in a sagittal plane, dendrites of the Golgi cells show no similar arrangement. Layers of the cerebellar cortex are indicated.

nucleus with a deeply staining nucleolus and irregular Nissl granules usually arranged concentrically (Fig. 14-3). They are among the largest neurons in the central nervous system. Although the nucleus appears smooth and round in Nissl-stained sections, in electron micrographs the nuclear membrane is wrinkled or puckered on the side facing the dendritic tree (Fig. 4–11) (1920). Each cell gives rise to an elaborate dendritic tree which arborizes in a flattened fanlike fashion in a plane at right angles to the long axis of the folium (Figs. 14-4–14-7). The dendritic tree arises from the neck of the cell as two or three large primary dendrites which branch repeatedly. In the depth of a furrow the dendritic branches form a broad angle approximating 180°,

while near the crest of a folium dendritic branches form more acute angles (675). The full extent of the dendritic arborization can be appreciated only in sagittal sections of the cerebellum. Primary and secondary dendritic branches have a smooth surface, but tertiary branches are characterized by short rather thick spines, densely and regularly distributed over all surfaces. These thick dendritic spines are referred to as "*spiny branchlets*" (790) or "*gemmules*" (Figs. 4-6 and 14-6). Larger dendritic processes bear stubbier thorns known as *smooth branchlets*. The axon arises from the part of the Purkinje cell opposite to the dendrites, acquires a myelin sheath and passes through the granular layer to enter the underlying white matter (Figs. 14-4 and

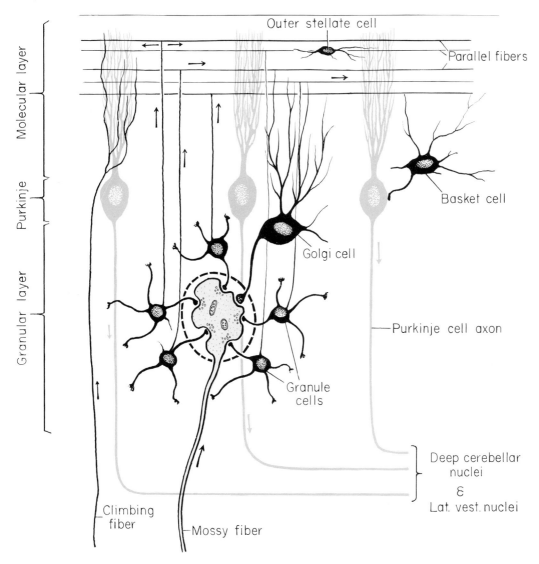

Figure 14-5. Schematic diagram of the cellular and fiber elements of the cerebellar cortex in the longitudinal axis of a folium. Excitatory inputs to the cerebellar cortex are conveyed by the mossy fibers (*yellow*) and the climbing fibers (*red*). The *broken line* represents a glia lamella ensheathing a glomerulus, containing: (a) a mossy fiber rosette, (b) several granule cell dendrites and (c) one Golgi cell axon. Axons of granule cells ascend to the molecular layer, bifurcate, and form an extensive system of parallel fibers which synapse on the spiny processes of the Purkinje cells. Purkinje cells and their processes are shown in *blue*. Climbing fibers traverse the granular layer and ascend the dendrites of the Purkinje cells where they synapse on smooth branchlets. *Arrows* indicate the directions of impulse conduction. Outer stellate and basket cells are shown in the molecular layer, but the axons of the basket cells which ramify about Purkinje cell somata are not shown. (Based on Gray (942) and Eccles et al. (675).)

14-5); most, but not all, of these axons pass to the deep cerebellar nuclei. Purkinje cell axons give rise to recurrent Purkinje collaterals (Fig. 14-4) which establish axo-somatic contacts with Golgi type II cells in the granular layer (1018). Some Purkinje cell collaterals may make synaptic contact with basket cells. Occasionally somewhat smaller, aberrantly placed Purkinje cells may be found in the granular or molecular layers. Since the axons of the Purkinje cells are the only ones to emerge from the cerebellar cortex and enter the white matter, all impulses entering the cerebellar cortex

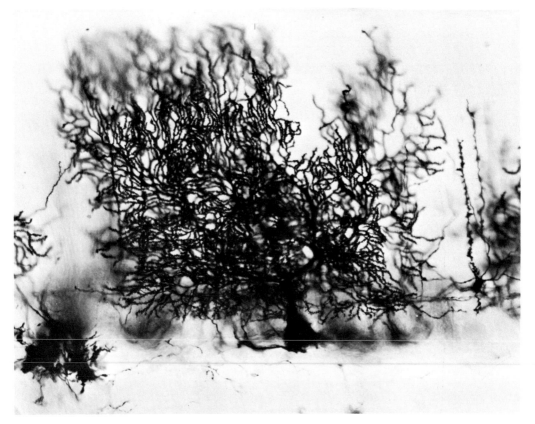

Figure 14-6. Photomicrograph of a single Purkinje cell and its rich dendritic arborizations in the molecular layer (×300). (Courtesy of the late Dr. C. A. Fox, School of Medicine, Wayne State University.)

must ultimately converge on these cells to reach the efferent cerebellar paths. Purkinje cell axons project to the deep cerebellar nuclei and to the dorsal half of the lateral vestibular nuclei; the projection of individual Purkinje cells depends upon their location in the cerebellar cortex. Histochemical studies indicate that γ-aminobutyric acid (GABA) is the neurotransmitter released at the synapse (780, 781). Electron microscopic studies indicate that the majority of terminal boutons are elliptical in shape (2642). Intracellular iontophoresis of horseradish peroxidase (HRP) into single Purkinje cells results in transport of the enzyme into both the dendritic tree and the axon (Fig. 14-7) (182, 1558).

The Granular Layer. In ordinary stains the granular layer presents the appearance of closely packed chromatic nuclei, not unlike those of lymphocytes; irregular light spaces here and there constitute the so-called "cerebellar islands" or "glomeruli" (Figs. 14-2–14-5). The *granule cells* are so

prodigious in number (3 million to 7 million granule cells/mm^3 of granular layer, (240)) that the residual space seems insufficient to accommodate their processes, fibers of passage and other intrinsic cells. Granule cell nuclei are round or oval in shape, and range in diameter from 5 to 8 μm; chromatin granules are aggregated against their nuclear membrane as well as clustered centrally. In light microscopic preparations it is unusual to distinguish the nucleolus of a granule cell. The nakedness of granule cell nuclei is said to be due to: (a) the complete absence of discrete Nissl granules and (b) the thinness of the rimming cytoplasm (792). In silver preparations these cells give rise to four or five short dendrites, which arborize in clawlike endings within the "glomeruli" (Fig. 14-5).

The scattered relatively clear areas in the granular layer, known as "cerebellar islands," contain glomeruli which are complex synaptic structures (Fig. 14-9). The unmyelinated axons of granule cells ascend

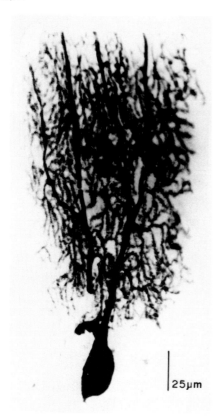

25µm

Figure 14-7. Photomicrograph of a single Purkinje cell labeled iontophoretically with horseradish peroxidase (HRP). This technic labels the dendritic arborization, the axon and axonal collaterals. (Courtesy of Dr. S. T. Kitai, School of Medicine, Michigan State University.)

vertically into the molecular layer, where each bifurcates into two branches which run parallel to the long axis of the folium. These parallel fibers practically fill the whole depth of the molecular layer and run transversely to the dendritic expansions of the Purkinje cells. In general parallel fibers are thicker in the lower third of the molecular layer. Granule cells in deep parts of the granular layer give rise to parallel fibers in deeper parts of the molecular layer, while cells in the more superficial parts of the granular layer provide parallel fibers in the upper part of the molecular layer (1920). Parallel fibers traverse layer after layer of Purkinje cell dendrites, like telegraph wires strung along the branches of a tree, and extend laterally in a folium (Fig. 14-4). Electron microscopic observations (797, 942, 1018) have shown that each dendritic spine of the Purkinje cell dendritic tree receives

a synaptic connection from a parallel fiber in the so-called "crossing-over" synapse. Fox and Barnard (790) estimated that each Purkinje cell in the cerebellar cortex of the monkey had a total of 60,000 dendritic spines and that from 200,000 to 300,000 parallel fibers projected through the territory of its dendritic tree. Other studies in cat, monkey and man (792) indicate that the estimate of 60,000 spines on a single Purkinje cell should be doubled. Each parallel fiber, extending about 1.5 mm from its bifurcation, has been estimated to traverse the dendritic trees of up to 500 Purkinje cells. The parallel fibers of the granule cells also make "crossing-over" synaptic contacts with the dendrites of outer stellate, basket and Golgi type II cells in the molecular layer (Fig. 14-5).

The *Golgi type* II cell usually is found in the upper part of the granular layer, but it may be seen in any part of this layer. These cells have vesicular nuclei and definite chromophilic bodies (Fig. 14-3). Dendritic branches of the Golgi cell extend throughout all layers of the cerebellar cortex, but are most extensive in the molecular layer. Unlike the dendrites of the Purkinje cell, arborizations are not restricted to a single plane (Figs. 14-4 and 14-5). In the molecular layer Golgi cell dendrites have sparse spines of different configurations irregularly distributed that are contacted by parallel fibers; the cell body is in contact with collaterals of climbing fibers and recurrent collaterals of Purkinje cells (1018, 2273). Many of the deep Golgi cells have dendrites that arborize almost entirely within the granular layer (675). The axonal arborization of the Golgi cell is extremely dense; it extends throughout the width of the granular layer but is restricted laterally to a region immediately beneath the cell body. The axons and dendrites of Golgi type II cells have complex relationships with the terminals of mossy fibers and the dendrites of granule cells.

In addition to the large Golgi cells described above, there is a small Golgi cell whose dendritic tree arises from several trunks which radiate outward from the cell body (1920). Groups of two or three small Golgi cells often are clustered together.

Cortical Afferent Input. Afferent fibers to the cerebellar cortex are supplied by tracts entering the cerebellum mainly

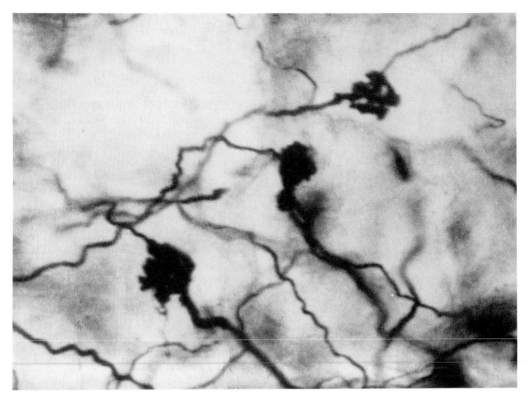

Figure 14-8. Mossy fiber rosettes in the granular layer of the monkey cerebellum as seen in a Golgi preparation. Although mossy fiber rosettes appear as solid structures under low magnifications, under oil immersion the rosettes appear as coiled convoluted fibers (×850). (Courtesy of the late Dr. C. A. Fox, School of Medicine, Wayne State University.)

via the inferior and middle cerebellar peduncles. These include the spinocerebellar, the cuneocerebellar, the olivocerebellar, the vestibulocerebellar and the pontocerebellar tracts as well as numerous smaller bundles. In addition there are cerebellar association fibers (666, 667) that pass from one folium to adjacent folia, and longer association fibers that connect different cortical regions on the same side. Structurally two types of afferent terminals are found in the cerebellar cortex, mossy fibers and climbing fibers.

The *mossy fibers*, so-called because of the appearance of their terminations in the embryo, are the coarsest fibers in the white matter. In the white matter these fibers bifurcate into numerous branches, before entering the granular layer, where the branches of a single fiber often go to adjacent folia. They pass into the granular layer, lose their myelin sheath and give off many fine collaterals. The mossy fiber retains its myelin sheath up to its point of continuity with a synaptic terminal known

as a rosette (942). Rosettes are the sites of synapses between mossy fibers and the clawlike terminals of granule cell dendrites. Mossy fiber rosettes are fine lobulated enlargements that occur along the course of branches and at terminals (Figs. 14-4, 14-5 and 14-8) (1920). A single mossy fiber and its branches may have as many as 44 rosettes (792). Under low magnification rosettes appear as solid structures in Golgi preparations, but under oil immersion they appear to be coiled, convoluted fibers (Fig. 14-8) (792). This view is confirmed by electron micrographs (Fig. 14-10) which also reveal synaptic vesicles, a concentration of mitochondria and a conspicuous core of neurofilaments and neurotubules (1774, 1920). A single mossy fiber rosette forms the center of each cerebellar glomerulus (Figs. 14-5 and 14-9). In the glomerulus it comes into synaptic relationship with granule cell dendrites and Golgi cell axons and dendrites. The spatial arrangement of the rosettes belonging to a single mossy fiber

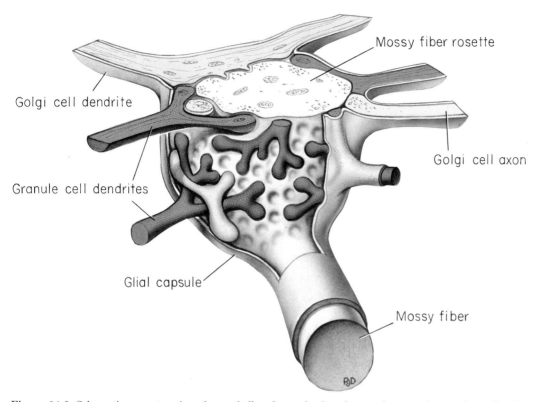

Golgi cell dendrite

Granule cell dendrites

Glial capsule

Mossy fiber rosette

Golgi cell axon

Mossy fiber

Figure 14-9. Schematic reconstruction of a cerebellar glomerulus based upon electron microscopic studies. A cerebellar glomerulus is formed by one mossy fiber rosette, the dendritic terminals of numerous granule cells (*red*), and terminals of Golgi cell axons (*yellow*). Proximal parts of Golgi dendrites (*blue*) also enter the glomerulus and establish broad synaptic contacts with the mossy fiber rosette. The entire nodular structure is ensheathed in a glial capsule. In this reconstruction the glomerulus is shown in horizontal section, and in a schematic three-dimensional view. (Based on Eccles et al. (675).)

makes it unlikely that two or more dendrites of the same granule cell establish synaptic contact with the same mossy fiber (675).

A *glomerulus* is a complex synaptic structure contained within the "cerebellar islands" of the granular layer (Figs. 14-4, 14-5 and 14-9). A cerebellar glomerulus is a nodular structure formed by: (a) one mossy fiber rosette, (b) the dendritic terminals of numerous granule cells, (c) the terminals of Golgi cell axons and (d) proximal parts of Golgi cell dendrites. The center of the glomerulus contains a single mossy fiber rosette with which the dendrites of about 20 different granule cells interdigitate (Figs. 14-8–14-10). The axonal ramifications of a Golgi cell form a plexus on the outer surface of the granule cell dendrites. The whole structure is encased by a single glial lamella (147, 675). Physiological evidence (677) indicates that in the glomerulus, the mossy

fiber-granule cell synapse is excitatory, while the Golgi axon-granule cell junction is inhibitory. Thus a glomerulus is basically a cluster in which two types of presynaptic fibers enter into a complex relationship with one postsynaptic element. The granule cell dendrites constitute the postsynaptic element. The Golgi cell functions as a negative feedback to the mossy fiber-granule cell relay; the main excitatory input to the Golgi cell is derived from the parallel fibers (Fig. 14-5).

Mossy fiber rosettes also establish wrinkled axosomatic synapses (*en marron*) on Golgi type II cell bodies. In the region of contact the mossy fiber terminal appears pressed into the fingerlike ridges of the Golgi II cell soma (446). Dendritic claws of granule cells make contact with the surface of the mossy fiber rosette not in contact with the Golgi II cell soma.

Climbing fibers, according to classic de-

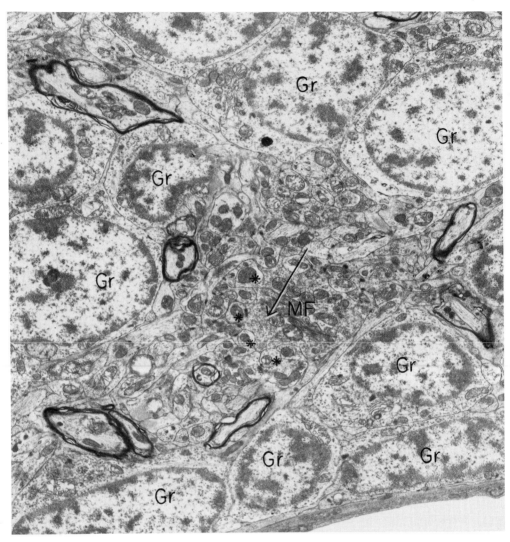

Figure 14-10. Electron micrograph of cerebellar glomerulus in the monkey. A mossy fiber rosette (*MF*) with dispersed synaptic vesicles (*arrow*) is surrounded by granule cells (*Gr*). Granule cell dendrites are indicated by asterisks. (×5600). (Courtesy of Dr. R. C. Henrikson, Albany Medical College.)

scriptions (348), arise from extracerebellar sources, ascend undivided through the white matter of the cerebellum and the medullary lamina of the folia, traverse the granular layer and project beyond the Purkinje cell somata to reach the dendrites of the Purkinje cells. In the molecular layer climbing fibers lose their myelin sheaths and split into a number of small fibers which climb ivy-like along the dendritic arborization of the Purkinje cell, whose branchings they closely imitate (Figs. 14-4 and 14-5). Climbing fibers contact only the smooth branchlets of Purkinje cell den-

drites; they do not contact the spiny branchlets on which parallel fibers synapse (792). Many climbing fibers have intracortical courses that change abruptly in the infraganglionic plexus (i.e., beneath the Purkinje cell layer). Some fibers may course transversely near the somata of five or six Purkinje cells before turning toward the surface to be deployed over the dendritic arbor of a Purkinje cell. Although a climbing fiber begins to divide and ramify at the level of the Purkinje cell body, its arborization is closely attached to the dendritic arbor of a single Purkinje cell. Golgi studies in a variety of species indicate that fine collaterals of climbing fibers may establish synaptic contact with adjacent Purkinje cells (2273), but these appear insignificant when compared with the repeated and abundant synaptic contacts that a climbing fiber makes with the dendrites of its own Purkinje cell (675). Light and electron microscopic studies indicate that climbing fiber collaterals also make contact with stellate, basket and Golgi cells (1018, 2273). Electron microscopic evidence indicates that although climbing fibers and basket cell axons partially overlap in their contact with portions of the Purkinje cell dendritic tree, there are no synaptic junctions between these fibers (445). Climbing fibers articulate primarily with the smooth branchlets of the dendritic tree, while basket cell axons are restricted to dendritic shafts. Additional electron microscopic data establish that collaterals of climbing fibers given off in the granular layer synapse directly upon the shafts of granule cell dendrites and the somata of Golgi II cells (447).

Physiologically the climbing fiber system is remarkably specific. Each climbing fiber possesses an extensive all-or-none excitatory connection with the Purkinje cell dendrites. Whenever the climbing fiber discharges, the Purkinje cell also discharges (676, 677). Morphological information suggests that stimulation of a climbing fiber not only excites a single Purkinje cell, but also a number of granule cells whose axons (parallel fibers) in turn excite Purkinje cells in the long axis of the folium. Thus excitation carried by parallel fibers will influence Purkinje cells surrounding a particular Purkinje cell which is excited directly by a climbing fiber. The potential inhibitory influence that climbing fibers may exert via Golgi II cells is more difficult to understand, but it is possible that their output may inhibit granule cells not strongly excited by mossy or climbing fibers (675).

The respective sources of the mossy and climbing fibers have been difficult to determine. Experimental evidence indicates that the mossy fibers degenerate following interruption of spinocerebellar and pontocerebellar tracts and lesions involving primary and secondary vestibulocerebellar fibers (265, 276, 1694, 1716, 1717, 2367). Mossy fibers are considered to constitute the principal afferent system to the cerebellar cortex and are the mode of termination of most cerebellar afferent systems.

The climbing fibers have been the center of great interest since their discovery by Cajal in 1888 because of their remarkable one-to-one relationship with dendritic branches of the Purkinje cell. These fibers have been thought to be recurrent axonal collaterals of Purkinje cells (1525), or recurrent axons of the deep cerebellar nuclei (424). There is now general agreement that climbing fibers, like mossy fibers, have exogenous origins (i.e., from nuclei outside of the cerebellum). Silver impregnation technics originally suggested that most climbing fibers originated from the inferior olivary complex (2502). This view was strengthened by electrophysiological results which concluded that climbing fibers originated only from the inferior olivary complex (425, 675, 2537). While some autoradiographic studies suggest that climbing fibers originate from the pontine nuclei, the medial reticular formation and the inferior olivary nuclear complex (1783), other studies indicate that nearly all climbing fibers arise from the inferior olive and are crossed (132, 551). Olivocerebellar fibers terminate in a pattern of thin sagittal strips that interdigitate with unlabeled strips (545). Because it has been shown that olivary neurons distribute fibers to different regions of the cerebellar cortex, it has been postulated that the empty strips receive climbing fibers from other unlabeled regions of the inferior olivary nucleus, rather than from extraolivary sources. This concept has been strengthened by data demonstrating that injections of ^{3}H-labeled amino acids into the pons, reticulotegmental nucleus, the lateral reticular nucleus, the spinal trigeminal nucleus, the inferior vestibular nucleus and the accessory cuneate nucleus labeled only mossy fibers (551).

Fluorescence microscopy has revealed a hitherto unrecognized fiber system in the cerebellar cortex which contains norepinephrine (1118). These fibers, detectable by their green fluorescence (Fig. 12-32), extend from the white matter into all layers of the cortex, are not restricted to any particular plane and are moderately concentrated in the Purkinje cell layer. This fiber system is considered to arise from the locus ceruleus (Figs. 12-30–12-32) and 13-3) and establish synaptic contacts with Purkinje cell somata (197, 1879, 2006). The number of fibers in this system is small, and without their fluorescent marker they cannot be recognized (1920). It is not clear how widely the fibers of the locus ceruleus are distributed in the cerebellum. An HRP study in the cat indicates that cells in the caudal half of the locus ceruleus project to the entire cerebellar vermis, the flocculus and the ventral paraflocculus (2379). These authors found no evidence of a projection to the cerebellar cortex of the hemisphere.

The raphe nuclei which synthesize and transmit serotonin (5-hydroxytryptamine, 5-HT) to various parts of the central nervous system project fibers to the cerebellum, presumably via periventricular routes (441). The largest number of serotonergic fibers appear to arise from the raphe nuclei of the pons and medulla (930, 2506), although nearly all raphe nuclei make some contribution. All parts of the cerebellar cortex receive afferents from the raphe nuclei, with the most profuse projections passing to lobules VII and X of the vermis and to crus I and II (930). Axons of raphe neurons: (a) terminate as mossy fiber rosettes in the granular layer, (b) terminate diffusely throughout all cortical layers without specialized junctions and (c) pass directly to the molecular layer where they bifurcate like parallel fibers and establish synaptic contacts with cerebellar interneurons (441). Serotonergic fibers differ from noradrenergic afferents in the molecular layer in that they do not synapse upon Purkinje cells.

Structural Mechanisms. The intricate geometric relationships of the structural elements in the cerebellar cortex have furnished many hypotheses concerning intracortical impulse transmission and the possible functions of individual neurons. Studies of the microphysiology of cerebellar neurons have yielded spectacular findings. There are several important initial considerations in understanding the neural mechanisms underlying cerebellar cortical function: (a) the output from the cerebellar cortex is mediated solely by discharges from Purkinje cells and (b) every Purkinje cell is subject to two distinct inputs. Excitation of Purkinje cells, via climbing fibers is direct,

while that via mossy fibers is indirect and involves relays in cerebellar glomeruli which are subject to inhibition. Mossy fiber impulses exert their synaptic excitatory action solely within the cerebellar glomerulus, where they excite granule cells whose axons (the parallel fibers) excite all cells with dendrites in the molecular layer (i.e., Purkinje, basket, stellate and Golgi cells). Impulses conveyed to dendrites in the molecular layer by parallel fibers result in excitation of: (a) a narrow band of Purkinje and Golgi cells in the longitudinal axis of the folia and (b) basket and outer stellate cells whose axons extend sagittally (transverse to the folia) on each side of the excited band of parallel fibers. This geometric configuration results in excitation of a narrow band of Purkinje cells, flanked on each side by Purkinje cells inhibited by basket and stellate cells (675). Although mossy fiber excitation of granule cells can be powerful, this excitation in the cerebellar cortex is all transformed into inhibition. Mossy fiber input is transformed into inhibition: (a) at the first synaptic relay by Golgi cell axons in the glomeruli and (b) at the second synaptic relays between parallel fibers and Purkinje, Golgi, basket and stellate cells. There is no excitatory action of any kind beyond the second synaptic relay in the cerebellar cortex. Outer stellate cells, basket cells and Golgi type II cells are inhibitory interneurons within the cerebellar cortex (679). The outer stellate cells synapse upon Purkinje cell dendrites in the molecular layer where their inhibitory influence is relatively localized. Basket cell inhibition is effected by axosomatic synapses upon Purkinje cell somata and involves 10 to 12 Purkinje cells in a sagittal plane (Fig. 14-4). Golgi cells intermittently inhibit afferent input to the cerebellar cortex at the mossy fiber-granule cell relay in the glomeruli (678). Because Golgi cell axons reach glomeruli throughout the depth of the granular layer, they could inhibit input via mossy fibers to parallel fibers for a distance of about 3 mm longitudinally, and over a distance of 5 or 6 Purkinje cells transverse to the folium (Figs. 14-4, 14-5 and 14-9). Although Purkinje cell axons represent the principal discharge pathway from the cerebellar cortex, recurrent axonal collaterals exert important influences upon Golgi cells and basket cells (Fig. 14-4). These axonal collaterals have a disinhibitory influence upon these cells (1018).

Climbing fibers have powerful, all-or-none, direct excitatory action upon the primary and secondary dendrites of a single Purkinje cell (676, 677). In addition the same climbing fiber has synaptic articulations with inhibitory interneurons, the Golgi type II, stellate and basket cells. On the basis that collaterals of the same neuron mediate the same effects, climbing fibers appear to excite interneurons within the cerebellar cortex. The excitation of basket cells results in inhibition of Purkinje cells on both sides of the single Purkinje cell receiving the main branches of a climbing fiber. A single basket cell theoretically could inhibit 7 rows of about 10 Purkinje cells. The excitation of Golgi cells via climbing fibers results in the inhibition of impulses through all glomeruli reached by the ramifications of the Golgi cell axon. This mechanism results in a depression of activity in Purkinje cells on both sides of the single Purkinje cell excited by the climbing fiber. The widespread inhibitory influence exerted by a single climbing fiber appears to be a device to silence the background for the Purkinje cell activated by the climbing fiber volley (675).

The cerebellar cortex thus has an exceedingly elaborate structural and functional organization in which multiple interactions influence input, conduction, synaptic articulations and the output which ultimately must pass via Purkinje cell axons to the deep cerebellar nuclei. The unique feature of the cerebellar cortex is that all excitatory activity, whether transmitted by mossy or climbing fibers, is transformed to inhibition at either the first (i.e., glomeruli, or climbing fiber) or second (i.e., parallel fiber) synaptic relay. This observation distinguishes the cerebellar cortex from all other regions of the central nervous system.

It has been estimated that the human cerebellar cortex contains 15 million Purkinje cells (240). The combined surface area of the dendritic branchlets and spines of one Purkinje cell in the monkey is said to be about 200,000 μm^2 (790). A synaptic area of such magnitude on each of 15 million cells provides an index of the elaborate activity of the cerebellar cortex. The fact that all parts of the cerebellar cortex have a similar structure has been interpreted to mean that specific functions are not precisely localized.

Purkinje cell axons represent the efferent pathway from the cerebellar cortex. These axons project mainly to the deep cerebellar nuclei, although some fibers from certain cortical areas bypass the deep cerebellar nuclei and project to portions of the vestibular nuclear complex. Direct cerebellovestibular fibers arise from the flocculonodular lobe (643, 644) and from portions of the vermis both anteriorly and posteriorly (665, 2643). Physiological studies indicate that the entire output of the cerebellar cortex is inhibitory (675, 1188–1191). Thus the axons of the Purkinje cells inhibit the cells with which they synapse, namely those of the deep cerebellar nuclei and portions of the vestibular nuclei. Biochemical and physiological studies indicate that the neurotransmitter responsible for Purkinje cell inhibition is GABA (780, 781, 1400, 1860). Purkinje cell collaterals taking origin from proximal portions of the axon (Fig. 14-4) exert inhibitory influences upon Golgi cells that in turn inhibit granule cells; this disinhibition tends to release granule cells whose axons excite Purkinje cells.

The majority of cerebellar cortical association fibers are short interconnections extending no more than two or three folia. Long association pathways have been traced only from the paravermal cortex, the lateral culmen and the lateral cortex of crus II (666). Anatomically the cortex of the vermis appears independent of that of the lateral hemispheres, in that association fibers in vermal cortex pass only to adjacent vermal folia, and the cortex of the lateral hemispheres does not project to the vermis (479, 666, 1204). Paravermal and lateral cortical areas of the anterior lobe give rise to long association fibers passing to the posterior folia of crus II on the same side. Long association fibers, crossing the midline, arise from lateral crus II, and terminate in folia of the contralateral crus II, the paramedian lobule and parts of the paraflocculus (665). Long and short association fibers in the cerebellar cortex are regarded as myelinated axonal collaterals of Purkinje cells (792).

Neuroglia. While most of the neuroglial

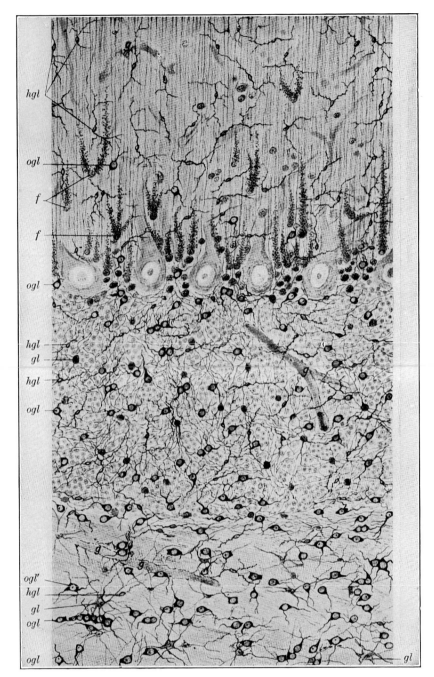

Figure 14-11. Arrangement of neuroglia cells in human cerebellar cortex; *f*, cells of Fañanas; *gl*, astroglia; *hgl*, microglia; *ogl*, *ogl'*, oligodendrocytes. (From Jakob (1202), after Schröder.)

elements in the cerebellar cortex are similar to those in other parts of the central nervous system, the architectonics of the neuroglia bear definite relationships to the three-layered neuronal structure (Fig. 14-11). Each cortical layer has a different population of neuroglial cell types, and one type, the Golgi epithelial cell, is unique to the cerebellar cortex (Fig. 14-12). The cerebellar cortex contains both astrocytes and oligodendrocytes. Astrocytes are primarily protoplasmic and have been divided into

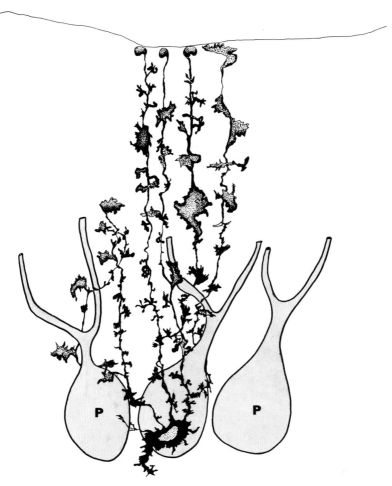

Figure 14.12. Drawing of a Golgi epithelial cells in the rat cerebral cortex. Purkinje cells are surrounded by Golgi epithelial cells whose somata bear ragged irregular appendages. Multiple processes of these glial cells extending upwards to the pial surface in candelabra-fashion bear irregular leaf-like appendages which project horizontally. These cells cannot be distinguished from Fañanas cells. (Based on Palay and Chan-Palay (1920).)

three classes: (a) the Golgi epithelial cell, (b) the lamellar or velate astrocyte and (c) the smooth astrocyte (1920). The Purkinje cell layer contains modified astrocytes known as the *Golgi epithelial cells* (348), or *Bergmann cells*. These neuroglial cells are true satellites of Purkinje cells in that they lie directly against the surface of Purkinje cells and form a nearly complete sheath around them (Fig. 14-12). Purkinje cells also are surrounded by Fañanas cells (Fig. 14-11), which in thin sections do not appear different in the electron microscope (1920, 2384). Each Bergmann cell gives rise to two or more processes which bifurcate and ascend in almost parallel lines to the pial surface. The upward prolongations of these processes course perpendicularly in the molecular layer and terminate at the surface of the cortex (i.e., limiting glial membrane) in conical expansions. These cells resemble miniature candelabra with their branches either clustered or spread out in parasagittal planes. The neuroglial processes of these cells lie between the dendritic arborizations of consecutive Purkinje cells (348). Electron micrographs indicate that the ascending processes of neighboring Bergmann cells are interdigitated to form a dense forest, rather than alternating palisades. Processes of Bergmann cells insulate the smooth branchlets of Purkinje cell dendrites from passing parallel fibers (792). This insulation appears absent only where climbing fibers come into synaptic relationship with the smooth branchlets. These specialized glial processes also may serve to confine transmitter substances to a particular synaptic site and in this way promote neuronal specificity (1982). The Golgi epithelial cell is characteristic of the Purkinje and molecular layers and is not found elsewhere. Golgi epithelial cells, Fañanas cells and protoplasmic astrocytes of the cerebellar cortex probably are all variants of a single cell type (1920).

The lamellar astrocyte is found chiefly in the granular layer, while the smooth astrocyte may be found in any layer, but is most common in the granular layer. Lamellar astrocytes are about the same size as granule cells, have a bean-shaped nucleus and may contain one or two nucleoli. The distribution and form of the glial processes of these cells are unusual. Numerous lamellar neuroglial processes pass between adjacent granule cells, dendrites and axons, forming open and confluent compartments. The number and extent of these processes is greater than might be expected. The lamellar processes separate one glomerulus from another in the cerebellar islands, and interweave with the dendrites and Golgi cell axons on the periphery of the glomeruli (1920).

Smooth astrocytes with long radiating processes, found in the molecular and granular layers, resemble stellate neuroglial cells, but are much smaller. Processes of these cells are kinky, contorted and branch repeatedly. Oligodendrocytes, seen throughout the cerebellar cortex, are most numerous in the granular layer and in the depths of the molecular layer where myelinated fibers are found.

THE DEEP CEREBELLAR NUCLEI

The corpus medullare is a compact mass of white matter, continuous from hemisphere to hemisphere, that is covered everywhere by the cerebellar cortex. It consists of afferent projections to the cerebellar cortex, efferent fibers from the cerebellar cortex and, to a lesser extent, association fibers connecting the various portions of the cerebellum. Some of these fibers cross to the other side in two cerebellar commissures: (a) a posterior commissure in the region of the fastigial nuclei and (b) an anterior commissure rostral to the dentate nuclei.

The corpus medullare is continuous with the three peduncles which connect the cerebellum with the brain stem: (a) the *inferior cerebellar peduncle*, which connects with the medulla; (b) the *middle cerebellar peduncle*, which connects with the pons; and (c) the *superior cerebellar peduncle*, which connects with the midbrain (Figs. 2-25 and 2-31). Medially and ventrally, near the roof of the ventricle, the corpus medullare splits into two white laminae, inferior and superior, which separate at an acute angle to form a tentlike recess (i.e., fastigium) in the roof of the fourth ventricle (Figs. 2-26, 2-27 and 2-32). The inferior medullary lamina passes caudally over the nodulus and becomes continuous with the tela choroidea and the choroid plexus of the fourth ventricle (Fig. 2-26). Laterally the inferior medullary velum extends to the flocculi, forming a narrow bridge connecting these structures with the nodulus (Fig. 2-31). The largest part of the medullary substance is continued rostrally, forming the superior medullary velum (Figs. 2-27 and 2-31). The latter is a thin white plate joining the two superior cerebellar peduncles; together these structures form the roof and lateral walls of the upper part of the fourth ventricle.

Imbedded in the white matter of each half of the cerebellum are four nuclear masses, the deep cerebellar nuclei (Figs. 12-7, 12-23 and 14-14). All deep cerebellar nuclei originate from condensations of cells that migrate outward from the germinal neuroepithelium of the fourth ventricle (1347). The four deep cerebellar nuclei start to differentiate simultaneously at early developmental stages and there is no evidence that individual cerebellar nuclei differ with respect to ontogenetic origin or age. Although four distinct deep cerebellar nuclei are recognized in most mammals, prior to the investigations of Snider (2368) most authors described these nuclei as a capriciously indented cell mass divisible into three nuclei: (a) the medial (fastigial), (b) the interposed and (c) the lateral (dentate). Studies in the monkey distinguish four cerebellar nuclei on the basis of fiber patterns, cellular morphology and the size, shape and orientation of cells (548). The strongest arguments supporting the existence of four individual deep cerebellar nuclei are obser-

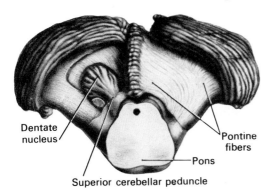

Dentate
nucleus

Pontine
fibers

Pons

Superior cerebellar peduncle

Figure 14-13. Drawing of a dissection of the superior surface of the cerebellum exposing the dentate nucleus. (Reproduced with permission from F. A. Mettler: *Neuroanatomy.* C. V. Mosby Co., St. Louis, 1948.)

vations indicating that each nucleus has unique connections. The four deep cerebellar nuclei in man, from medial to lateral, are the fastigial, globose (posterior interposed), emboliform (anterior interposed) and the dentate.

The Dentate Nucleus. This nucleus, the largest of the deep cerebellar nuclei, lies in the white matter of the cerebellar hemisphere close to the vermis (Fig. 14-13). It is a convoluted band of gray having the shape of a folded bag with the opening or hilus directed medially and dorsally (Fig. 14-14). In transverse section it has an appearance similar to that of the inferior olivary nucleus. It is found as a definite nucleus only in mammals, and it becomes greatly enlarged in man and the anthropoid apes. In anthropoid apes and man the dentate nucleus can be divided into an older dorsomedial portion (paleodentate) and a larger, newer ventrolateral portion (neodentate). Cells in the ventrolateral region of the dentate nucleus are smaller than those located dorsomedially (1437, 2553). The nucleus is composed mainly of large multipolar cells with branching dendrites. Axons of these cells acquire a myelin sheath while still in the nucleus and emerge from the cerebellum in the superior cerebellar peduncle (1437). Between these large cells are small stellate cells whose axons arborize within the nucleus. Golgi studies of the dentate nucleus in the rat and monkey reveal several varieties of large and small neurons and a segmentation of the nucleus into zones (441). Large dentate nucleus neurons

have radiating tortuous dendrites bearing occasional thorns. Large columnar neurons have elliptical cell bodies with long twisting dendritic branches which arise from a primary trunk; these cells occur only in two major zones of the nucleus. Afferent fibers from the Purkinje cells enter laterally and form a dense fiber plexus, the amiculum, around the nucleus.

The Emboliform Nucleus. This nucleus is a wedge-shaped gray mass close to the hilus of the dentate nucleus and often is difficult to delimit from the latter. It is composed of clumps of cells resembling those of the dentate nucleus (Figs. 12-23 and 14-14). In lower mammals the globose and emboliform nuclei form a continuous nuclear mass referred to as the *nucleus interpositus.* Two parts of the nucleus interpositus have been distinguished: (a) an anterior nucleus interpositus located rostrally close to the dentate nucleus that is homologous to the emboliform nucleus in man and (b) a posterior nucleus interpositus located more medially and caudally that is the homologue of the globose nucleus (548).

The Globose Nucleus. This nucleus consists of one or more rounded gray masses lying between the fastigial and emboliform nuclei (Fig. 14-14). It likewise contains large and small multipolar cells. Neurons in both the globose and emboliform nucleus give rise to axons projecting into the superior cerebellar peduncle.

The Fastigial Nucleus. This nucleus, the most medial of the deep cerebellar nuclei, lies near the midline in the roof of the fourth ventricle and in man is second in size to the dentate nucleus (Figs. 12-23 and 14-14). This nucleus is characterized by a population of densely packed cells of varying sizes. Large, medium and small cells are intermingled in dorsal parts of the nucleus, while small cells predominate ventrally (548). Cell strands emerging from the lateral border of the nucleus extend ventrolaterally towards the vestibular nuclei. Golgi studies indicate that both large and small cells have dendrites radiating in all directions which bear spines on distal branches (1640). Dendritic fields of neurons within the nucleus show extensive overlap, but there is no evidence of Golgi type II cells. Unlike the other deep cerebellar nuclei,

Emboliform nucleus   Dentate nucleus

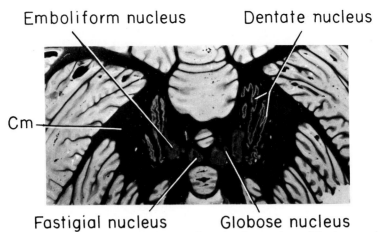

Cm

Fastigial nucleus   Globose nucleus

Figure 14-14. Horizontal section through adult cerebellum showing portions of the deep cerebellar nuclei and the corpus medullare (*Cm*) (Weigert's myelin stain, photograph).

cells of the fastigial nucleus give rise to both crossed and uncrossed axons; axons crossing to the opposite side are most numerous in rostral regions of the nucleus (394).

Connections of the Deep Cerebellar Nuclei

Corticonuclear Projections. The largest number of afferent fibers to deep cerebellar nuclei arise from Purkinje cells in the cerebellar cortex and have GABA as their neurotransmitter. All parts of the cerebellar cortex project upon the intrinsic nuclei. On the basis of cerebellar cortical projections to the deep cerebellar nuclei, the cerebellum has been divided into three rostrocaudal longitudinal zones: (a) a medial or vermal zone projecting to the fastigial nucleus, (b) a paravermal zone projecting to the interposed nuclei and (c) a lateral or hemispheric zone projecting to the dentate nucleus (665, 1205, 1206, 1348, 2627). These longitudinal corticonuclear zones are in addition to the classic division of the cerebellum into lobes and lobules. Physiological studies appear consistent with the longitudinal zonal division of the cerebellum, particularly with respect to afferent inputs (1903). Afferent fibers ending in a particular zone may not be distributed throughout its extent because of somatotopic features. The medial cortical zone, constituting the vermis proper, projects to the fastigial nucleus and is strictly unilateral (549, 1002). Fibers from the cortical lobules of the vermis project to the nearest region of the fastigial nucleus. This arrangement results

in a sequential representation of the cerebellar vermis in the fastigial nucleus. HRP injections of one fastigial nucleus result in retrograde transport of the enzyme to Purkinje cells in a narrow longitudinal zone of the ipsilateral vermis in folia of lobules I through X (394, 2236). While information concerning the paravermal and lateral longitudinal cerebellar zones is less precise, the same principle appears to apply. Studies of the projections of crus II and the paramedian lobule indicate that lesions in these parts of the cerebellum produce degeneration in portions of the three lateral deep cerebellar nuclei which vary with the location of the lesion (272, 550). Because the longitudinal zonal pattern, recognized during cerebellar corticogenesis, becomes distorted during later development, even small cortical lesions may involve more than one zone. The paraflocculus has been demonstrated to supply fibers to caudal and ventral parts of the dentate and the posterior interposed nuclei (1004). Studies based upon anterograde transport of HRP and ^{3}H-labeled amino acids appear to provide more precise data concerning the longitudinal zonal cortical projections to the deep cerebellar nuclei (182, 632, 2550). These data support the concept of three rostrocaudal zones projecting, respectively, to the fastigial, interposed and dentate nuclei, and other data indicate that nucleocortical fibers from the deep cerebellar nuclei project collaterals back to their specific cortical zones (931, 2551, 2552). Corticonuclear and nucleocortical fibers appear to have reciprocal relationships. Purkinje cell axons branch profusely upon entering the deep cerebellar nuclei and their terminal arborizations have a conical-shaped configuration (441). Purkinje cell axons have a powerful monosynaptic inhibitory action upon cells of the deep cerebellar nuclei (675).

Nucleocortical Projections. The conceptional division of the cerebellum into three sagittal zones, each consisting of a longitudinal strip of cerebellar cortex and the deep cerebellar nucleus to which its Purkinje cells project, has been strengthened by the observation that cells in the deep cerebellar nuclei project collaterals to the cortex in a specific manner. While it has long been suspected that the deep cerebellar nuclei provided collaterals to the cerebellar cortex (348, 424), axoplasmic transport technics provided conclusive evidence of this intrinsic cerebellar pathway (441, 929, 931, 2552). HRP injected into a localized region of the cerebellar cortex resulted in retrograde transport of the enzyme to cells of a single deep cerebellar nucleus, and injections of ^{3}H-labeled amino acids into the deep cerebellar nuclei could be traced autoradiographical into the cerebellar cortex. Studies in the cat indicate that cells in: (a) the fastigial nucleus project to the vermal cortex, (b) the interposed nuclei project to the paravermal cortex and (c) the dentate nucleus project to the cortex of the cerebellar hemisphere (441, 632, 929, 931, 2551, 2554). Present evidence suggests that nucleocortical and corticonuclear projections are reciprocally organized. Neurons in the deep cerebellar nuclei project back to the cerebellar cortical regions from which they receive input. These reciprocal projections do not appear to be organized in a strict one-to-one fashion in that projections from the cortex may not terminate on cells that give rise to return cortical projections (2550). In the primate the nucleocortical projections from the distinctive parts of the dentate nucleus are more complex than in lower forms in that the neodentate (ventrolateral) projects to the lateral hemisphere while the older (dorsomedial) paleodentate has projections to the vermis (2554). Axons of the deep cerebellar nuclei projecting to the cerebellar cortex arise from a heterogenous population of cells, similar to those that project fibers to the

thalamus and brain stem (2553). Electrophysiological studies indicate that some cells in the dentate and interposed nuclei have collateral axons which project via the superior cerebellar peduncle to the thalamus and inferior olive as well as to the cerebellar cortex (2553). Nucleocortical collaterals terminate in the granular layer of the cerebellar cortex (2552). Since the nucleocortical projection arises, at least in part, from axon collaterals of cerebellar efferent neurons, some of the same signals projected to brain stem nuclei by the deep cerebellar nuclei are fed back to the cerebellar cortical neurons. While the nature of this corticonuclear and nucleocortical loop is not understood at present, it seems that it must modulate cerebellar efferent activity in an important way. These projections from the deep cerebellar nuclei represent a major afferent system to the cerebellar cortex which has not previously been recognized.

Extracerebellar Inputs. Although the Purkinje cells exert inhibitory influences upon the deep cerebellar nuclei, these nuclei maintain a high frequency excitatory discharge (1191, 1192). This observation implies that unless the deep cerebellar nuclei are spontaneously active, they must receive excitatory inputs from extracerebellar sources. It is presumed that excitatory inputs from extracerebellar sources must overcome the tonic inhibitory output from the cerebellar cortex. The current thesis is that extracerebellar inputs to the deep cerebellar nuclei provide the tonic facilitation which predominates over the cortical inhibition and thus maintains the discharge of impulses directed towards brain stem nuclei (675).

Retrograde transport studies indicate that the dentate nucleus receives afferents from: (a) the pontine nuclei, (b) the principal inferior olivary nucleus, (c) the trigeminal sensory nuclei, (d) the reticulotegmental nucleus, (e) the locus ceruleus and (f) the raphe nuclei (441, 699). The largest number of afferent fibers appear to arise from the pontine nuclei, the inferior olivary nucleus and the reticulotegmental nucleus. Both ipsilateral and contralateral pontine nuclei project to the dentate nucleus, but the largest number of fibers arise from the opposite side (699). Olivocerebellar fibers, comprising one of the largest cerebellar afferent systems, pass to all parts of the cerebellar cortex and to the deep cerebellar nuclei (259). Afferent projections to the dentate nucleus are crossed and arise from cells of the principal inferior olivary nucleus (546). The interposed nuclei receive crossed fibers from the medial and dorsal accessory olivary nuclei, and the fastigial nucleus receives fibers from the dorsomedial cell column and nucleus β, caudal subdivisions of the medial accessory olive (269). It seems likely that these projections to the deep cerebellar nuclei are collaterals of climbing fibers. According to Eller and Chan-Palay (699) the dentate nucleus and the interposed nuclei receive bilateral projections from the reticulotegmental nucleus. The anterior interposed nucleus (i.e., the emboliform nucleus) receives a projection from the red nucleus which is crossed (546), and is reciprocal to the major projection from the anterior interposed nucleus.

The fastigial nucleus receives an input from caudal and dorsal regions of the medial and inferior vestibular nuclei and from cells of group x, located along the lateral borders of the inferior vestibular nucleus; these afferents are bilateral and fairly symmetrical in origin (2236). The fastigial nucleus also receives small inputs from the nucleus prepositus, the dorsal paramedian reticular nuclei, the reticulotegmental nucleus and the locus ceruleus (394, 2379, 2380). Although no primary vestibular afferents have been found to terminate in the fastigial nucleus, these fibers have been shown to end in the small-celled ventrolateral part of the dentate nucleus (276, 415).

The above findings suggest that practically all information transmitted to the cerebellar cortex also is conveyed to one or more of the deep cerebellar nuclei.

SOMATOTOPIC LOCALIZATION

The afferent fiber systems which convey sensory information to the cerebellum from receptors of various kinds in different parts of the body have been shown to be related to particular parts of the cerebellum. Electrophysiological studies have demonstrated in animals that exteroceptive impulses, such as tactile sense, audition and vision, give rise to action potentials in specific regions of the cerebellum (19, 2369, 2371).

The projection of exteroceptive impulses to the cerebellar cortex is somatotopically organized in a precise manner (Fig. 14–15). Tactile stimulation evokes potentials ipsilaterally in the anterior lobe and simple lobule, and bilaterally in the paramedian lobules. The leg area is represented in the central lobule, the arm in the culmen and the head and face in the simple lobule. The orientation was found to be reversed in the paramedian lobules with the leg representation most caudal and the head represented rostrally. Responses in this pattern were most easily obtained from skin receptors or cutaneous nerves. The head area was found partially to overlap the middle region of the vermis (i.e., simple lobule, folium and tuber and adjacent areas) where action potentials were recorded following auditory and visual stimuli. It has further been shown that the same somatotopic regions of the cerebellum could be activated by stimulating corresponding areas of the sensorimotor cortex contralaterally (2370). Stimulation of the auditory and visual cortex in cerebrum likewise produced potentials in the audiovisual representation in the cerebellum (1020). Many additional studies support in detail the somatotopic organization outlined above (1903).

CEREBELLAR CONNECTIONS

Afferent Fibers

The cerebellum receives afferent impulses from virtually all kinds of receptors located in all parts of the body. These impulses are relayed to the cerebellum by nuclei within the spinal cord and brain stem. The input includes impulses generated in cutaneous, stretch, vestibular, visual, and other receptors conveyed by both spinal and cranial nerves. Afferents from the vestibular apparatus appear unique in that these fibers pass directly into the cerebellum. The number of cerebellar afferent fibers exceeds the number of efferent fibers by an estimated ratio of 40:1 (1067). Most of the afferent fibers enter the cerebellum through the inferior and middle cerebellar peduncles, although a small number enter in association with the superior cerebellar peduncle.

The inferior peduncle consists of a larger, entirely afferent portion, the restiform body, and a smaller, medial, juxtarestiform

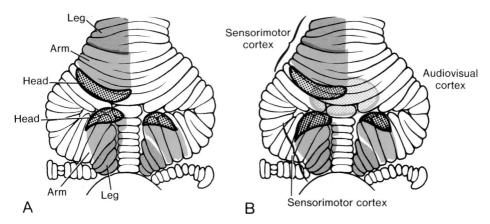

Figure 14-15. Schematic diagrams of somatotopic localization in the cerebellar cortex of the monkey. (*A*) Diagram of the tactile receiving areas of the cerebellum mapped by potentials recorded in response to movement of hairs on the left side of the body. (*B*) Diagram of cerebellar cortical areas responding to stimulation of the sensorimotor, auditory and visual cortex in the right hemisphere. The leg (*red*), arm (*blue*) and head (*black stipple*) are represented ipsilaterally in the anterior lobe and bilaterally in reversed fashion in the paramedian lobules. The auditory and visual cortex (*blue stipple*) are represented in the simple lobule, folium, tuber and adjacent cortex. (Based on Snider (2369).)

portion that contains both afferent and efferent fibers. The juxtarestiform body contains primarily vestibulocerebellar and cerebellovestibular fibers (Fig. 12–23). Although a number of brain stem nuclei project fibers directly to the deep cerebellar nuclei, quantitatively the largest number of cerebellar afferents terminate in the cerebellar cortex as climbing or mossy fibers. Most of the afferent input to the cerebellar cortex is relayed by brain stem nuclei such as the pontine nuclei, the inferior olivary nuclei and a number of smaller nuclei located in the medulla and pons. Nuclei of the brain stem which project most of their fibers to the cerebellum are referred to as *precerebellar nuclei*. The precerebellar nuclei receive afferents from a variety of sources and differ greatly with respect to size, cytoarchitecture and cerebellar connections.

Vestibulocerebellar Fibers. These fibers enter the cerebellum largely through the juxtarestiform body and can be classified as both primary and secondary. *Primary vestibulocerebellar fibers* arise from the vestibular ganglion and project to the ipsilateral nodulus, uvula and flocculus (276). In the monkey, fibers from all parts of the ganglion project to parts of the nodulus and uvula, while fibers from ganglion cells innervating the cristae of the semicircular ducts and the maculae of the

utricle and saccule project to different folia of the flocculus (415). Some primary vestibulocerebellar fibers end as climbing fibers in the flocculus. Retrograde transport studies using HRP suggest that nearly the entire vermis may receive afferents from the vestibular ganglion (1357).

Secondary vestibular fibers originate from the inferior vestibular nucleus and, to a lesser extent, from parts of the medial vestibular nucleus. Although primary and secondary vestibulocerebellar fibers have similar distributions, the number of secondary fibers is much greater. In addition secondary vestibular fibers pass bilaterally to the nodulus, uvula and the fastigial nuclei (286, 392). These observations have been confirmed in retrograde transport studies with the suggestion that secondary vestibulocerebellar fibers may have a more extensive distribution in the cerebellar vermis (1358).

Spinocerebellar Tracts. The spinocerebellar tracts arise from cell groups within the spinal cord and pass directly to the cerebellum. Their cells of origin receive primary dorsal root afferents. Included in this group are the posterior, anterior and rostral spinocerebellar tracts, as well as the cuneocerebellar tract which arises from the accessory cuneate nucleus.

The *posterior spinocerebellar tract* enters the inferior cerebellar peduncle and projects upon the rostromedial part of the anterior lobe (lobules I to IV, Fig. 14-1) and the lateral part of the pyramis and the paramedian lobule (940, 1437, 1900, 1903). Most of these fibers terminate ipsilaterally in longitudinally arranged zones in what corresponds to hindlimb regions. The posterior spinocerebellar tract conveys impulses from stretch receptors via group Ia and Ib muscle afferents, exteroceptive impulses from touch and pressure receptors in the skin and slow adapting pressure receptors (1900). Fibers of this tract do not convey impulses from low threshold joint receptors.

The *anterior spinocerebellar tract* ascends in the brain stem to rostral pontine levels and enters the cerebellum in association with the superior cerebellar peduncle (Figs. 10–9, 12–21). Fibers initially located dorsolateral to the superior cerebellar peduncle arch medially over this largely efferent bundle to enter the cerebellum. These fibers pass to essentially the same cortical areas as those of the posterior spinocerebellar tract. However, the main area of termination is in the anterior lobe; only a few fibers reach the pyramis and paramedian lobule (940). The majority of the fibers of this tract terminate in the cerebellum contralaterally with respect to the tract in the spinal cord (and ipsilateral to the cells of origin); about 15% of the fibers terminate bilaterally (940, 1437, 1900, 2362). The anterior spinocerebellar tract conveys impulses from group Ib and flexor reflex afferent fibers from the hindlimb and lower trunk.

Cuneocerebellar fibers arise from the accessory cuneate nucleus in the lower medulla, enter the inferior cerebellar peduncle and pass to the posterior part of the anterior lobe (lobule V, Fig. 14-1), the anterior folia of the simple lobule, the paramedian lobule and the depths of the prepyramidal fissure in the posterior vermis (939). Fibers of this afferent system are ipsilateral. The accessory cuneate nucleus is regarded as the medullary equivalent of the dorsal nucleus of Clarke, and the cuneocerebellar tract is regarded as the forelimb equivalent of the posterior spinocerebellar tract. This tract conveys impulses from group Ia and Ib muscle afferents and exteroceptive impulses from cutaneous afferents (Fig. 10–9).

Receptive fields for cutaneous impulses are smaller than those associated with the posterior spinocerebellar tract (1900).

Studies based upon the retrograde transport of HRP confirm observations concerning the origin and termination of cuneocerebellar fibers and indicate that some cells in the cuneate nucleus also project to lobule V of the anterior lobe and to the paramedian lobule (2165, 2382).

The *rostral spinocerebellar tract*, identified in the cat (1899, 1900), is the forelimb functional equivalent of the anterior spinocerebellar tract, but is uncrossed. This tract arises from cells rostral to the dorsal nucleus of Clarke (See p. 280), ascends in the anterior part of the spinal cord and enters the cerebellum via both the inferior and superior cerebellar peduncles. Fibers of this tract are distributed almost exclusively to the anterior lobe of the cerebellum in lobules I to V (Fig. 14-1). Fiber terminations are predominantly ipsilateral (1900, 1902). This tract is activated monosynaptically by group Ib muscle afferents and polysynaptically by flexor reflex afferents.

Pontocerebellar Projections. The pontine nuclei represent the largest collection of precerebellar nuclei and they constitute the most important relay in the conduction of impulses from the cerebral cortex to the cerebellum. Corticopontine fibers arise from all of the four major lobes of the cerebrum, descend in the internal capsule and crus cerebri and terminate on the ipsilateral pontine nuclei. The most massive cortical projections arise from the sensorimotor cortex and project in a somatotopical fashion onto two longitudinally oriented cell columns within the pontine nuclei (291). Each part of the cerebral cortex in the cat appears to project to several well-defined areas within the pontine nuclei (292, 293). Fibers from the temporal cortex terminate in the caudal pons and those from the frontal cortex end in the rostral pons. Studies in the monkey indicate that the motor area (area 4), the primary somatosensory area (areas 3, 1, 2), area 5 and portions of the visual cortex give rise to the major corticopontine fibers (296). Fibers from particular regions of the cortex end within longitudinally oriented columns. Although projections from the motor and somatosensory areas are somatotopically organized, they are separated from each other.

All cells of the pontine nuclei project their axons to the cerebellum via the middle cerebellar peduncle and most, but not all, of these fibers are crossed. Fibers projecting to the cerebellar hemisphere are mainly crossed, while projections to the vermis are bilateral (270). The nodulus appears to be the only part of the cerebellum that does not receive a pontine projection. Most of the pontocerebellar fibers terminate as mossy fibers (1694, 2367). The pontocerebellar projection appears to be precisely organized and recent HRP studies indicate that most cerebellar lobules receive afferents from two or more different sites within the pontine nuclei (275, 288, 1109). This pattern of termination suggests that impulses from different regions of the pontine nuclei may converge onto a particular cerebellar lobule.

The pontine nuclei also receive afferents from the superior and inferior colliculi (51, 1271) and from the deep cerebellar nuclei (135, 2627). The dorsolateral pontine nuclei, which receive fibers from the tectum project to regions of the cerebellum where visual and auditory impulses have been recorded.

Olivocerebellar Fibers. These fibers form the largest component of the inferior cerebellar peduncle. They arise from the contralateral inferior olivary nucleus and are distributed to all parts of the cerebellar cortex in an orderly pattern (Fig. 14–22A). In man, fibers from the medial portion of the principal olive and the accessory olives go to all portions of the vermis. A much larger component from the lateral portion of the principal olivary nucleus is distributed to the cerebellar hemisphere. The dorsal part of the olive projects to the superior surface of the cerebellum, while the ventral part projects to its inferior surface (1134). The olivocerebellar projection in young cats and rabbits has been worked out in detail by Brodal (259). The intracerebellar nuclei, as well as all parts of the cortex, receive olivary fibers, and the distribution is localized exquisitely, each portion of the olive projecting to a specific cerebellar area. Anterograde and retrograde axonal transport technics have demonstrated that the olivocerebellar projection is more complex than revealed by degeneration studies (259). These studies indicate that cerebellar lobules receive afferents from more than one region of the inferior olivary complex (269, 288, 290, 2644). It has further been shown that olivocerebellar fibers terminate in a pattern of thin sagittal strips that alternate with unlabeled strips which are supplied by fibers from another region of the inferior olive (545, 551). The inferior olive also sends fibers to the deep cerebellar nuclei which are crossed and are believed to be collaterals of fibers projecting to the cortex (269, 546).

The inferior olivary nucleus, a highly developed complex in man, is the major source of climbing fibers that have potent excitatory synapses on Purkinje cell dendrites (545, 551, 676, 677, 1018, 2502). The principal olivary nucleus receives descending fibers from the central tegmental tract, a composite bundle originating from multiple brain stem nuclei. Descending fibers in this tract passing to the principal part of the inferior olivary nucleus arise from the red nucleus, the central gray substance and the midbrain tegmentum. Fibers from the sensorimotor cortex pass to the ventral lamella of the principal olive via the crus cerebri and the pyramid (2632).

The most important afferents to the inferior olivary complex arise from the spinal cord. Spino-olivary fibers project to specific parts of the medial and dorsal accessory olivary nuclei. Spinal pathways belonging to the olivary system have been identified physiologically by their climbing fiber responses in the anterior lobe of the cerebellum (1709). Fibers arising in the spinal cord and ascending in the anterior funiculus form the anterior spino-olivary tract which terminates upon cells of the medial and dorsal accessory olivary nuclei (209). Fibers ascending in the posterior columns synapse upon the posterior column nuclei and project impulses contralaterally to the same olivary nuclei (670, 1259). These fibers form a dorsal (funicular) spino-olivary pathway. Additional spino-olivocerebellar pathways have been described, all of which project to sagittal zones in the anterior lobe. These sagittal projection zones display a somatotopic pattern in lobules IV and V of the vermis (1905). Spino-olivocerebellar pathways resemble the spinocerebellar tracts

(289). Responses in these systems are evoked by stimuli activating group II and III muscle afferents, cutaneous afferents and high threshold joint afferents with wide receptive fields. These impulses, referred to as *flexor reflex afferents*, also have actions upon segmental reflexes and are transmitted by several other ascending tracts. There is difficulty in interpreting the information transmitted by these pathways because it lacks modality specificity and permits only crude spatial discrimination. Certain evidence suggests that olivary neurons may convey specific information related to interneuronal activities at spinal and brain stem levels (1709). The spino-olivary systems may be activated by either flexor reflex afferents or by the corticospinal tract through a common set of interneurons, which are assumed to influence motor neurons and to be part of the segmental reflex arc. Thus, the spino-olivocerebellar system may monitor the activity of interneurons at spinal levels and transmit such signals to the cerebellum.

The inferior olivary nucleus also receives afferent fibers from the contralateral deep cerebellar nuclei which are topographically organized (2555). The dentate nucleus projects to the principal olivary nucleus and the interposed nuclei project to the medial and dorsal accessory olivary nuclei. Projections from the deep cerebellar nuclei to the inferior olive appear reciprocal to olivonuclear fibers, except that no fibers from the fastigial nucleus terminate in the inferior olive. These observations suggest that the activities of the inferior olivary nucleus may be modulated by feedback from the cerebellar nuclei.

Reticulocerebellar Fibers. Three nuclei of the reticular formation project fibers to the cerebellum and can be regarded as precerebellar nuclei: (a) the reticulotegmental nucleus, (b) the lateral reticular nucleus of the medulla and (c) the paramedian reticular nucleus.

The *reticulotegmental nucleus* (Figs. 12-25 and 12-30) receives afferents from the cerebral cortex and from the deep cerebellar nuclei (283, 411, 1411, 2227). Projections from the frontal and parietal cortex are bilateral but mainly ipsilateral and end in ventral parts of the nucleus (271). A larger and more important group of afferent fibers arise from the dentate and anterior interposed nuclei, enter the superior cerebellar peduncle, cross in its decussation and descend as the crossed descending limb of the superior cerebellar peduncle (277). Cerebellar projections from this nucleus pass via the middle cerebellar peduncle to vermal regions, particularly lobules VI and VII, and to the flocculus, but all parts of the cortex receive some fibers (1110). Projections of the reticulotegmental nucleus are bilateral and they end as mossy fibers in the granular layer. This nucleus participates in a cerebellar-reticular feedback system, but its efferent fibers do not project back to the deep cerebellar nuclei that supply it.

The *lateral reticular nucleus* of the medulla (Figs. 11-9 and 11-14), consisting of three cytologically distinct subdivisions, receives inputs from a variety of sources including the spinal cord (263, 1390), the cerebral cortex (298), the red nucleus (2635) and the fastigial nucleus (2645). Spinal afferents contained in the anterolateral funiculus terminate in a specific manner upon the small-celled part of the nucleus and appear to transmit exteroceptive impulses somatotopically (511).

Cerebellar projections of the lateral reticular nucleus arise from cells in all subdivisions, and enter the cerebellum via the inferior cerebellar peduncle. Degeneration and autoradiographic studies indicate that projections of the lateral reticular nucleus terminate as mossy fibers in the anterior lobe, in both vermal and intermediate parts, in the paramedian lobule and in lobule VII of the vermis (1391, 1638). The projection is bilateral with ipsilateral predominance. Horseradish peroxidase studies appear to demonstrate a topographical projection from the nucleus to the anterior lobe and the paramedian lobule, but these studies also suggest the entire cerebellar cortex may receive some fibers (295, 633, 930).

The *paramedian reticular nuclei* of the medulla (Figs. 11-14 and 14–16) receives afferent fibers from the spinal cord (274), the fastigial nucleus (135), the cerebral cortex (274, 2388) and the vestibular nuclei (1414). Projections from these nuclei are mostly uncrossed and terminate mainly in the vermis of the anterior lobe and in the pyramis and uvula (285). In addition some

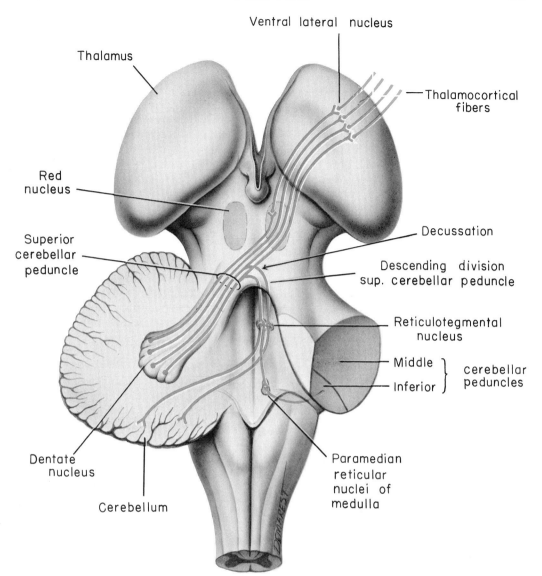

Figure 14-16. Diagram of the efferent fibers of the dentate nucleus. These fibers, contained in the superior cerebellar peduncle (*blue*) all decussate in the caudal mesencephalon. Ascending fibers project to the rostral part of the red nucleus and to the ventral lateral (VL) nucleus of the thalamus. Fibers of the descending division of the superior cerebellar peduncle project to the reticulotegmental nucleus, the paramedian reticular nuclei of the medulla, and to the inferior olivary nucleus (not shown). Descending fibers of the superior cerebellar peduncle constitute part of a cerebelloreticular system that conveys impulses back to the cerebellum.

fibers terminate in the fastigial nucleus (2236). HRP studies confirm that the majority of the efferent fibers of these nuclei project to the anterior lobe and to the vermis of the posterior lobe (2379). The dorsal paramedian reticular nucleus appears to be connected with a somewhat wider region of the cerebellar cortex than other nuclei of

this group. These nuclei, like others in the reticular formation projecting to the cerebellum, are involved in feedback systems.

Other Precerebellar Efferents. A number of other brain stem nuclei project smaller numbers of fibers to the cerebellar cortex. These precerebellar nuclei include the perihypoglossal nuclei, the trigeminal sensory nuclei, the nucleus of the solitary tract, the locus ceruleus and the raphe nuclei.

The *perihypoglossal nuclei* (Figs. 11-14 and 11-28) have been shown to project mainly to the vermis and fastigial nucleus in degeneration studies (2560). Studies based upon HRP transport indicate that these fibers have a wider distribution which includes the flocculus, paraflocculus and nodulus (43, 1354), as well as the fastigial nucleus and the anterior interposed nucleus (1559, 2236). The nucleus prepositus, the largest of the perihypoglossal nuclei, also gives rise to ascending fibers that terminate in the oculomotor nuclei.

Trigeminocerebellar fibers, both primary and secondary, from different subdivisions of the trigeminal nuclear complex have been described. Although primary trigeminocerebellar fibers have been observed in lower vertebrates (1084, 1432, 1433, 2764), their areas of termination in the cerebellum have not been established. Trigeminocerebellar fibers from the mesencephalic nucleus of N. V, studied in human fetal material (1953, 1954), enter the cerebellum in association with the superior cerebellar peduncle and are distributed to the dentate and the emboliform nuclei. These fibers are believed to conduct impulses from stretch receptors in the muscles of mastication and possibly also from the facial muscles. Secondary trigeminocerebellar fibers from the principal sensory and spinal trigeminal nuclei (402, 1434, 2764) enter the cerebellum via the inferior cerebellar peduncle and terminate in the upper culmen and declive (402, 1437, 2371, 2704).

Studies based upon retrograde transport technics indicate trigeminocerebellar fibers arising from the spinal and principal trigeminal nuclei are exclusively ipsilateral and project mainly to the simple lobule and the dorsal part of the paramedian lobule (1180, 2378). Most of the efferent fibers originate from the nuclei interpolaris and oralis of the spinal trigeminal complex and terminate as mossy fibers. According to some studies the motor trigeminal nucleus projects some fibers to the dentate nucleus (699, 1356). A small number of the cells in the nucleus of the solitary tract and a number of motor cranial nerve nuclei also project to the cerebellum (1356, 2247, 2378, 2381).

Projections from the raphe nuclei, which contain serotonergic neurons, have been traced to all parts of the cerebellar cortex, except lobule VI, by retrograde transport technics (2506). The most profuse projection is to vermal lobules VII and X and to crus I and II (930). According to Chan-Palay (441) axons of serotonergic neurons: (a) terminate as mossy fiber rosettes and (b) traverse the molecular layer like parallel fibers, but terminate on cortical interneurons, rather than on Purkinje cells.

Projections from the locus ceruleus, convey noradrenergic input to the cerebellum via the middle and superior cerebellar peduncles (1581, 2006). In the cerebellar cortex noradrenergic fibers terminate around Purkinje cell somata (457). The extent of the distribution of these fibers in the cerebellum is unclear; according to Somana and Walberg (2379) most fibers project to the cerebellar vermis, although a few project to the fastigial nucleus.

Efferent Fibers

Cerebellar efferent fibers arise from all of the deep cerebellar nuclei and from certain parts of the cerebellar cortex. Direct projections from the anterior and posterior vermis and from the so-called vestibulocerebellum (i.e., the flocculonodular lobule and adjoining parts of the uvula) pass to the ipsilateral vestibular nuclear complex and collectively constitute the cerebellovestibular projection. The largest and most widely distributed cerebellar efferent fibers arise from the deep cerebellar nuclei and are organized into two major systems contained in three separate bundles. The major efferent systems are the superior cerebellar peduncle and the fastigial efferent projection.

Superior Cerebellar Peduncle. The largest cerebellar efferent bundle, the superior cerebellar peduncle, is formed by fibers from the dentate, emboliform and globose nuclei. (Figs. 2-25, 12-23, 12-29 and 14-16). This composite group of fibers emerges from the hilus of the dentate nucleus and passes rostrally into the upper pons where it forms a compact bundle along the dorsolateral wall of the fourth ventricle (Figs. 2-24 and 2-25). At isthmus levels fibers of the superior cerebellar peduncle sweep ventromedially into the tegmentum (Fig. 12-29). All fibers of the superior cerebellar peduncle decussate at levels through the inferior colliculus (Fig. 13-2). Most of these crossed fibers ascend to enter and surround the contralateral red nucleus. A relatively small part of the fibers from the dentate nucleus terminate in the rostral third of the red nucleus (70, 543); the bulk of these fibers project to the thalamus and end in the ventral lateral (VL) nucleus (Fig. 14-16) (385, 441, 1207, 1659, 1708, 2160). Some of the fibers extend into caudal parts of the ventral anterior (VApc) and the rostral parts of the adjoining ventral posterolateral (VPL) thalamic nuclei (2538). A small number of fibers from the dentate nucleus project beyond VL to the rostral intralaminar thalamic nucleus, the central lateral nucleus (1660, 2110, 2538).

The ventral lateral nucleus of the thalamus projects in a topical fashion upon the primary motor area of the cerebral cortex (2650, 2655, 2657). Thus impulses from the dentate nucleus are conveyed via contralateral thalamic nuclei to the motor cortex (2599). In this manner, impulses from the dentate nucleus can influence activity of motor neurons in the cerebral cortex; impulses from the motor cortex are transmitted to spinal levels via the corticospinal tract. This system appears to be concerned primarily with the coordination of somatic motor function.

A relatively small number of cerebellar efferent fibers from the ventrocaudal dentate nucleus decussate in the caudal mesencephalon, pass dorsally and are distributed differentially within the lateral somatic cell columns of the contralateral oculomotor nuclear complex (417). Most of these fibers terminate about cells which innervate the superior rectus muscle on the opposite side (Fig. 13-15). The part of the dentate nucleus from which these fibers arise receives primary vestibular fibers (276, 415). Thus, this dentato-oculomotor projection may constitute a link in a vestibulo-oculomotor pathway (1003). This connection has been confirmed by autoradiographic tracing methods (441, 1616, 1708).

Another small group of fibers in the superior cerebellar peduncle decussate with the main bundle and descend in the ventromedial tegmentum of the brain stem near the median raphe. These fibers, constituting the descending division of the superior cerebellar peduncle, project to the reticulotegmental, the paramedian reticular nuclei and portions of the inferior olivary nucleus (283, 411, 1616, 2555). Because these nuclei are known to project to the cerebellum, this component of the superior cerebellar peduncle is a part of both a cerebelloreticular and a cerebello-olivary feedback system (Fig. 14-16).

Fibers from the emboliform and globose nuclei enter the superior cerebellar peduncle, undergo a complete decussation and surround caudal portions of the contralateral red nucleus, where many of these fibers terminate. According to Courville (543) fibers from the anterior interposed nucleus in the cat (which corresponds to the emboliform nucleus in man (754)) project somatotopically upon cells of the red nucleus. Two patterns of fiber organization have been recognized between these nuclei: (a) fibers distributed in a mediolateral sequence in the red nucleus have a caudorostral pattern of origin in the nucleus interpositus and (b) fibers terminating in a rostrocaudal arrangement in the red nucleus have a corresponding lateromedial origin in the nucleus interpositus. However, only fibers from the interposed nucleus terminating in a mediolateral arrangement in the red nucleus are regarded as having a somatotopic distribution (543, 1632, 2039). Thus rostral parts of the interposed nucleus project to hindlimb regions of the red nucleus (ventral and ventrolateral areas), while caudal parts of the nucleus project to forelimb regions of the red nucleus (dorsal and dorsomedial areas; Fig. 14-17). Because of the topographical projections of cerebellar cortex upon the deep cerebellar nuclei (549, 665, 1207) which are organized as three longitudinal zones, connections exist between: (a) the paravermal cortex and the red nucleus through the anterior interposed nucleus and (b) cerebellar cortex of the hemisphere and the red nucleus through the dentate nucleus (1632).

The pathway from the paravermal cortex to the contralateral red nucleus via the anterior interposed nucleus forms part of a somatotopic linkage that extends to spinal levels. Somatotopically organized rubrospinal fibers cross in the midbrain and descend to spinal levels. This small system involves two decussations, that of the superior cerebellar peduncle and that of the rubrospinal tract (Fig. 14-17). Thus im-

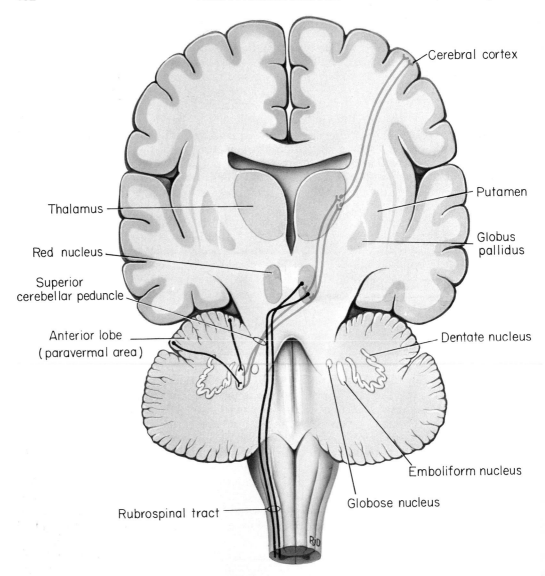

Figure 14-17. Schematic diagram of connections between the emboliform nucleus (anterior interposed nucleus) and the red nucleus. Axons of Purkinje cells (*black*) in the paravermal cortex of the anterior lobe of the cerebellum project somatotopically upon the emboliform nucleus. The most rostral cortical regions, concerned with the lower extremity (Figs. 14-15 and 14-20), project to the rostral part of the emboliform nucleus, while caudal regions, concerned with the upper extremity, project to caudal parts of this nucleus. Fibers from the emboliform nucleus (*blue*) project via the superior cerebellar peduncle to caudal portions of the contralateral red nucleus, and to the ventral lateral nucleus of the thalamus. Projections from the emboliform nucleus to the red nucleus terminate somatotopically. Rubrospinal fibers (*red*) arising from dorsomedial regions of the red nucleus project to cervical spinal segments, while fibers from ventrolateral parts of this nucleus project to lumbosacral spinal segments. Thus the somatotopic linkage is maintained from cerebellar cortex to spinal levels (after Courville (543) and Massion (1632)).

pulses conveyed from paravermal cortex to the spinal cord end on the same side. This system is concerned with mechanisms that can facilitate ipsilateral flexor muscle tone.

A number of studies indicate that axons from cells of the interposed nuclei also project to the ventral lateral nucleus of the thalamus after giving off collaterals to the red nucleus (69, 79, 675, 2553).

Fastigial Efferent Projections. The

efferent projections of the fastigial nucleus are unique in that: (a) they do not emerge via the superior cerebellar peduncle, (b) a large part of the efferent fibers cross within the cerebellum and (c) they project to nuclei at all levels of the brain stem (394). Crossed fibers from the fastigial nucleus emerge from the cerebellum via the *uncinate fasciculus* (*Russell*) which arches around the superior cerebellar peduncle (Figs. 14-18 and 14-19). Uncrossed fastigial efferent fibers project to the brain stem in the *juxtarestiform body* (Figs. 12-7 and 14-19). Crossed efferent fibers contained in the uncinate fasciculus arise from cells in all parts of the fastigial nucleus and outnumber uncrossed efferents in the juxtarestiform body. Although data from degeneration studies suggested that fastigial efferent projections to vestibular nuclei are bilateral and differentially distributed (381, 2541, 2646), autoradiographic data indicate that these projections are bilateral and symmetrical only to ventrolateral portions of the lateral and inferior vestibular nuclei (135). Fastigial projections to cell group f of the inferior vestibular nucleus and cell group x are entirely crossed. Some crossed fastigial efferents terminate in the nucleus parasolitarius. Fastigioreticular fibers arise predominantly from rostral parts of the nucleus, are mainly crossed and project to: (a) medial regions of the nucleus reticularis gigantocellularis, (b) parts of the caudal pontine reticular formation, (c) the dorsal paramedian reticular nucleus and (d) portions of the lateral reticular nucleus (2644a). Crossed fastigiopontine fibers separate from the uncinate fasciculus and pass ventrally to terminations in the dorsolateral pontine nuclei. A small number of crossed fastigiospinal fibers descend ventral to the spinal trigeminal tract and enter the ventral part of the lateral funiculus of the spinal cord. Following HRP injections into the spinal gray at various levels, it was determined that the largest number of contralateral fastigial axons probably terminated in the C2–C3 segments (821, 1635). Physiological evidence based upon antidromic stimulation of the upper cervical spinal cord and direct stimulation of the fastigial nucleus indicate that axons of fastigial neurons make monosynaptic contacts with motoneurons at the C2–C3 level (2740, 2741).

A small portion of the fibers in the uncinate fasciculus ascend in the dorsolateral part of the brain stem and project fibers to thalamic nuclei (397, 2541). Ascending fibers in the uncinate fasciculus arise from cells in the caudal part of the fastigial nucleus, decussate within the cerebellum and ascend contralaterally (71). These fibers project bilaterally to rostral parts of the superior colliculus and the nuclei of the posterior commissure (68). Most of the fibers in the ascending limb of the uncinate fasciculus project to contralateral diencephalic nuclei in a loosely organized bundle close to the medial geniculate body. These fibers project rostrally and dorsally directly into the ventral posterolateral (VPL) and ventral lateral (VL) thalamic nuclei (71, 135, 1308). A smaller number of fibers ascending near the central gray turn abruptly ventrolaterally and enter parts of VPL and VL. These fibers tend to terminate in prominent clusters in thalamic nuclei. These thalamic terminations suggest that ascending impulses from the fastigial nucleus probably are relayed to the primary motor cortex.

Cerebellovestibular Projections. Certain regions of the cerebellar cortex give rise to direct projections which pass to the vestibular nuclei. These fibers, representing axons of Purkinje cells, arise from the: (a) anterior and posterior cerebellar vermis and (b) from the vestibulocerebellum (i.e., the flocculonodular lobule). Thus the vestibular nuclei receive cerebellar afferents bilaterally from the fastigial nucleus and ipsilaterally from specific cortical regions. Direct projections from lateral parts of the cerebellar vermis terminate in dorsal regions of the ipsilateral lateral and inferior vestibular nucleus and are somatotopically organized (1002, 2637, 2643). Efferent fibers from the anterior lobe establish synaptic contacts on somata and dendrites of cells of all sizes in the lateral vestibular nucleus (1776). Fibers from the posterior part of the vermis also project to the lateral vestibular nucleus, but not in a somatotopical pattern. Because these fibers partially traverse the fastigial nucleus, they were a source of interpretative error in degeneration studies of fastigiovestibular projections (2646). Physiological studies demonstrate that stimulation of the anterior lobe of the cerebellum produces a monosynaptic inhibi-

longitudinal (sagittal) zones referred to as vermal, paravermal and lateral.

The *vermal zone* is the midline, unpaired portion of the cerebellum related to fastigial nuclei, and is concerned primarily with mechanisms that modify extensor muscle tone. Direct projections from the anterior and posterior vermis exert inhibitory influences upon the vestibular nuclei which could result in a reduction of extensor muscle tone. The projections of the fastigial nucleus which receive strictly ipsilateral afferents from the vermis (549) are to some extent bilateral, although crossed fibers are more numerous (394). These fibers pass to terminations in the vestibular nuclei where they are excitatory, and to broad regions of the reticular formation of the pons and medulla. A small number of crossed fastigiospinal fibers descending directly to the upper cervical spinal cord have excitatory influences upon motoneurons (2740). Finally, some crossed fastigial efferents projecting to thalamic nuclei probably make a contribution to coordinated somatic motor activity. According to Chambers and Sprague (438, 439) the vermal zone of the cerebellum is particularly concerned with control of posture, muscle tone, locomotion and equilibrium for the entire body.

The *paravermal zone* relates the paravermal cortex with the emboliform and globose nuclei. The emboliform nucleus (anterior interposed nucleus) projects somatotopically upon the caudal two-thirds of the contralateral red nucleus (543, 755). This somatotopically organized system is concerned with mechanisms that can facilitate ipsilateral flexor muscle tone via the rubrospinal tract (Fig. 14-17). The opposite red nucleus also receives some fibers from the globose nucleus (posterior interposed nucleus) which terminate in the most medial part of the nucleus (69). Both of the interposed nuclei have modest projections to the contralateral ventral lateral (VL) nucleus of the thalamus.

The *lateral zone* relates the cortex of the cerebellar hemisphere with the dentate nucleus which has projections primarily to the ventral lateral nucleus of the thalamus on the opposite side (Fig. 14-16). This, the largest cerebellar efferent system, appears to be concerned with the coordination of ipsilateral somatic motor activity. Impulses conveyed to the ventral lateral nucleus of

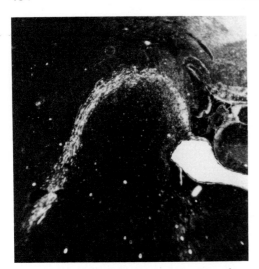

Figure 14-18. Dark field photomicrograph of ³H-labeled amino acids transported by fibers of the uncinate fasciculus as seen in an autoradiograph. (Reproduced with permission from R. R. Batton III et al.: *Journal of Comparative Neurology*, **174**: 281–306, 1977.)

tion of neurons of the lateral vestibular nucleus (1190).

Although the flocculonodular lobe is classically regarded as the "vestibulocerebellum," primary vestibulocerebellar fibers have a more extensive distribution in that they also project to ventral parts of the uvula and to the ventral paraflocculus (276). All of these parts of the "vestibulocerebellum," considered in its broadest sense, project fibers to the vestibular nuclear complex, except the paraflocculus (72). The flocculus and nodulus project fibers to portions of the four main vestibular nuclei; the uvula gives rise to fibers passing to portions of the superior, lateral and inferior vestibular nuclei. These fibers have an ipsilateral distribution.

CEREBELLAR ORGANIZATION

On the basis of cortical projections to the deep cerebellar nuclei and projections from the deep nuclei to the cerebellar cortex, the cerebellum has been divided into three sagittal zones of cortex and their connecting deep nuclei (182, 549, 632, 665, 929, 931, 1002, 1205, 1206, 1348, 2550–2552, 2627). This concept provides an elementary view of the functional organization of the cerebellum. In this simplified scheme the cerebellar efferent systems are related to three

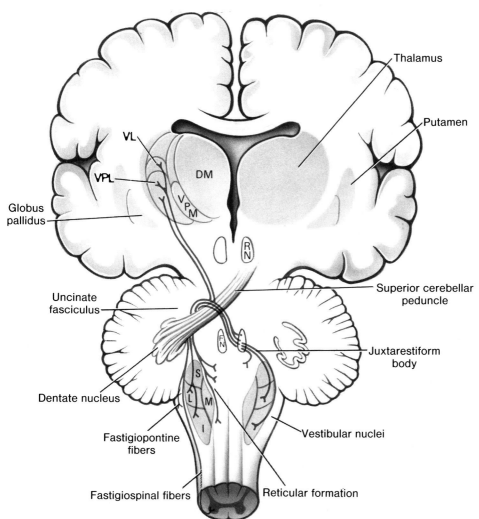

Figure 14-19. Schematic diagram of fastigial efferent projections. Crossed fastigial efferent fibers contained in the uncinate fasciculus arise from cells in all parts of the fastigial nucleus (*FN*) and outnumber uncrossed efferent fibers that emerge in the juxtarestiform body. Fastigiovestibular fibers project bilaterally and symmetrically upon ventral portions of the lateral (*L*) and inferior (*I*) vestibular nuclei. Fastigioreticular fibers arise predominantly from rostral parts of the fastigial nucleus. Crossed fastigiopontine fibers separate from the uncinate fasiculus and pass to the dorsolateral pontine nuclei. Crossed fastigiospinal fibers pass to upper cervical spinal segments and exert excitatory effects upon motoneurons. Ascending fastigial projections arise from caudal parts of the nucleus, are entirely crossed and ascending in dorsolateral parts of the midbrain tegmentum. These fibers project to parts of the superior colliculus, the nuclei of the posterior commissure and to the ventral posterolateral (*VPL*) and ventral lateral (*VL*) thalamic nuclei (135, 394). Abbreviations: *DM*, dorsomedial nucleus; *FN*, fastigial nucleus; *RN*, red nucleus; *VL*, *VPL* and *VPM*, ventral lateral, ventral posterolateral and ventral posteromedial thalamic nuclei; vestibular nuclei: *I*, inferior, *L*, lateral, *M*, medial and *S*, superior.

the thalamus are relayed to the motor cortex where they modify the activity of neurons projecting to spinal levels and to pontine nuclei.

Some relay nuclei at all brain stem levels, receiving part of the cerebellar output, project fibers back to the cerebellum. These pathways, referred to as feedback systems, appear similar to those found in electronic systems which provide controlling and regulating effects. The motor cortex in turn gives rise to frontopontine fibers, which convey impulses back to the contralateral cerebellar hemisphere via the pontine nu-

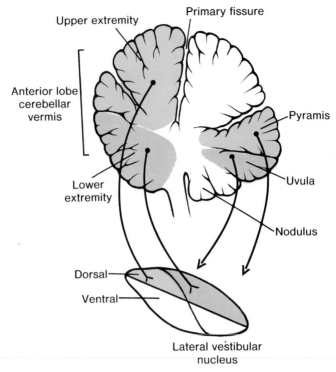

Figure 14-20. Schematic diagram of cerebellovestibular projections from the anterior and posterior vermis. Purkinje cell axons from the anterior vermis project somatotopically upon dorsal regions of the lateral vestibular nucleus and exert inhibitory influences. Similar direct projections from the pyramis and parts of the uvula which are not somatotopically arranged are shown by *arrows*. (Modified from Brodal et al. (280).)

clei and the middle cerebellar peduncle (Fig. 14-21). Other areas of the cerebral cortex also influence the activity of the cerebellum via corticopontine and ponto-cerebellar pathways. The central tegmental tract conveys impulses from the red nucleus and the midbrain tegmentum which reach the contralateral cerebellar hemisphere by way of parts of the inferior olivary nuclear complex. Certain fibers of the superior cerebellar peduncle that descend in the brain stem terminate upon reticular and olivary nuclei, which project fibers back to the cerebellum (Fig. 14-16). Efferent fibers from the red nucleus also project directly to the interposed nucleus (547).

Some of the neocerebellar connections in man are especially evident in Figure 14-22, which shows sections through the medulla, pons and isthmus from an individual in whom the left cerebellar hemisphere failed to develop (2458). There was also a correlated agenesis of all the afferent and efferent pathways to and from the the left cer-

ebellar hemisphere. The left dentate nucleus was represented by a minute structure, the right inferior olive was greatly reduced and the right red nucleus (not shown) and pontine nuclei were practically absent. All of the cerebellar peduncles on the left were greatly reduced in size. These preparations emphasize that in man the middle cerebellar peduncle and the olivo-cerebellar fibers are practically all crossed.

FUNCTIONAL CONSIDERATIONS

The cerebellum is concerned with the coordination of somatic motor activity, the regulation of muscle tone and mechanisms that influence and maintain equilibrium. Afferent cerebellar pathways convey impulses from a variety of different receptors, including the organs of special sense. Special attention has been directed to cerebellar afferent systems that convey impulses from stretch receptors in muscles and tendons. Although Sherrington referred to the cerebellum as "the head ganglion of the

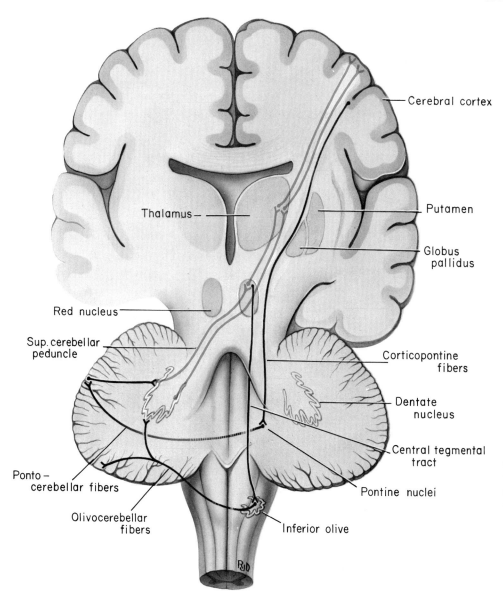

Cerebral cortex

Thalamus

Putamen

Globus pallidus

Red nucleus

Sup. cerebellar peduncle

Corticopontine fibers

Dentate nucleus

Central tegmental tract

Ponto-cerebellar fibers

Pontine nuclei

Olivocerebellar fibers

Inferior olive

Figure 14-21. Diagram of some of the principal afferent and efferent cerebellar connections. Cerebellar efferent fibers from the dentate nucleus are shown in *blue*. Corticopontine and pontocerebellar fibers (*black*) represent the most massive cerebellar afferent system. The principle inferior olivary nucleus receives uncrossed descending fibers from the red nucleus and periaqueductal gray via the central tegmental tract. Cortico-olivary fibers to the principal inferior olivary nucleus (not shown) pass via the medullary pyramids. Olivocerebellar fibers (*black*) cross, enter the inferior cerebellar peduncle, and are distributed to: (a) the cerebellar cortex as climbing fibers and (b) the deep cerebellar nuclei.

proprioceptive system," the cerebellum is not concerned with the conscious appreciation of muscle, joint, and tendon sense, or any specific sensory modality. The cerebellum receives a massive input from the stretch receptors (i.e., the muscle spindle and Golgi tendon organ) via the spinocerebellar and cuneocerebellar tracts; few impulses from these receptors are projected to the cerebral cortex (1642). The major afferent input from stretch receptors provides part of the neural mechanism that:

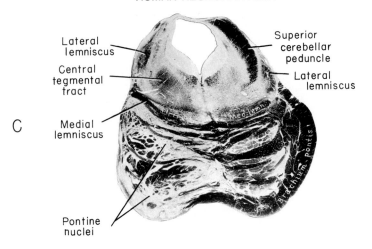

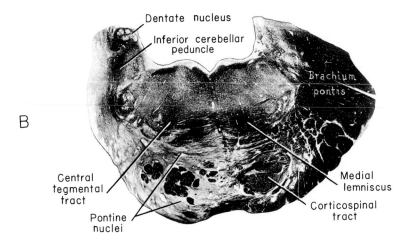

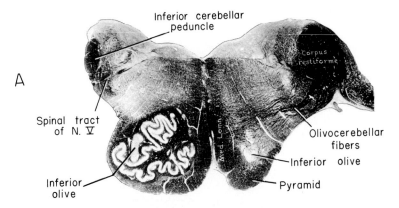

Figure 14-22. Transverse sections of the medulla (*A*), pons (*B*), and isthmus (*C*) from a case of left cerebellar agenesis (2458). These sections clearly demonstrate the crossed nature of olivocerebellar and pontocerebellar fibers (Weigert's myelin stain, photograph).

(a) effects gradual alterations of muscle tone for proper maintenance of equilibrium and posture and (b) assures the smooth and orderly sequence of muscular contractions that characterize skilled voluntary movement (1900).

Each movement requires the coordinated action (synergy) of a group of muscles. The agonist is the muscle which provides the actual movement of the part, while the antagonist is the opposing muscle which must relax to permit movement. Associated with these are other synergic or fixating muscles, which fix neighboring or even distant joints to the extent needed for the desired movement. Such synergistic motor activity requires not only complex reciprocal innervation but coordinated control of muscle tone and movement. The cerebellum provides this control for the somatic motor system in an efficient, automatic manner without our being aware of it.

There are certain general principles concerning disturbances resulting from cerebellar lesions. These principles are: (a) cerebellar lesions produce ipsilateral disturbances, (b) cerebellar disturbances usually occur as a constellation of intimately related phenomena, (c) cerebellar disturbances due to nonprogressive pathological changes show a gradual but definite attenuation with time and (d) cerebellar disturbances resulting from cerebellar lesions probably are the physiological expression of intact neural structures deprived of the controlling and regulating influences of the cerebellum. To a degree the severity of the disturbances reflects the magnitude of the lesion, but it is known from experimental studies that extensive lesions confined to the neocerebellar cortex may cause only transient or minimal disturbances (423, 1276). Lesions involving the deep cerebellar nuclei, particularly the dentate nuclei, or the superior cerebellar peduncle, produce severe and enduring disturbances.

Neocerebellar Lesions. Lesions involving the cerebellar hemispheres and the dentate nucleus affect primarily skilled voluntary and associated movements (i.e., movements related to the corticospinal system). The muscles become *hypotonic* (flabby) and tire easily. The deep tendon reflexes tend to be sluggish and often have a pendular quality. There are severe disturbances of coordinated movement referred to as *asynergia* in which the range, direction, amplitude and force of muscle contractions are inappropriate. Cerebellar asynergia can be demonstrated by many tests. Among these are tests of precise movements to a point; distances frequently are improperly gauged (*dysmetria*) and fall short of the mark or exceed it (*pastpointing*). Rapid successive movements, such as alternately supinating and pronating the hands and forearms, are poorly performed (*dysdiadochokinesis*). The patient is unable to adjust to changes of muscle tension. When the forearm is flexed at the elbow and held flexed against resistance, a sudden release of resistance causes the forearm to strike the chest. This is an example of the *rebound phenomenon*. These patients also demonstrate a *decomposition of movement* in which phases of complex movements are performed as a series of successive single simple movements.

The *tremor* seen in association with neocerebellar lesions occurs primarily during voluntary and associated movements (1132). This tremor is referred to as "intention tremor" because it is not present at rest. It involves especially the proximal appendicular musculature, but is transmitted mechanically to distal parts of the extremities. Tremor is most evident in the upper extremities because weight-bearing masks the disturbance in the lower extremities. Cerebellar tremor frequently is contrasted with the tremor seen in paralysis agitans, which is referred to as a "rest tremor," meaning that the tremor is present in the absence of voluntary and associated movement. Each of these types of tremor has unmistakable features and occurs in different syndromes. Nevertheless, "rest tremor" may occur in association with certain cerebellar lesions (1131). There are certain indications that the basic mechanisms involved in cerebellar tremor may underlie other kinds of tremor (383).

Ataxia is an asynergic disturbance associated with neocerebellar lesions which results in a bizarre distortion of voluntary and associated movements. It involves particularly the axial muscles, and groups of muscles around the shoulder and pelvic girdles. This disturbance is evident during walking and is characterized by muscle contractions which are highly irregular in force, amplitude and direction, and which occur asynchronously in different parts of the body. There frequently is unsteadiness in standing, especially if the feet are close together. The gait is broad-based and the patient reels, lurches and stumbles.

Nystagmus commonly is seen in association with cerebellar disease; it is most pronounced when the patient directs the eyes laterally toward the side of the lesion. This disturbance consists of an oscillatory pattern in which the eyes slowly drift in one direction and then rapidly move in the opposite direction to correct the drift. Although nystagmus seen in association with cerebellar disease has been considered as an expression of asynergic phenomena in the extraocular muscles, many pathological processes which affect the cerebellum also involve the underlying brain stem and the vestibular nuclei located in the floor of the fourth ventricle.

Speech disturbances are common in association with cerebellar lesions of long standing. Speech often is slow and monotonous, and some syllables are unnaturally separated. There is a slurring of speech and some words are uttered in an explosive manner. These disturbances appear to be due to loss of control over the coordination of laryngeal and respiratory muscles involved in speech.

Archicerebellar Lesions. Lesions involving portions of the posterior cerebellar vermis (i.e., nodulus and uvula) and probably portions of the flocculus produce what has been called the *archicerebellar syndrome*. Such lesions affect the axial musculature and the bilateral movements used for locomotion and maintenance of equilibrium. The patient sways and is generally unsteady when standing; when walking he staggers and has a tendency to fall backward or to either side. The gait resembles that of a drunken individual in that it is broad-based, jerky and highly incoordinate. If the muscles involved in speech are affected, articulation is jerky and words are slurred; the words are often shot out with unnecessary force. Nystagmus and abnormal attitudes, if present, are usually ascribed to injury of the vestibular structures. Muscle tone is little affected, there is usually no tremor and there is no incoordina-

tion of arm or leg movements when the patient is resting in bed. This particular syndrome most commonly occurs in children as a consequence of a midline cerebellar tumor (medulloblastoma) that probably arises from cell-rests in the inferior medullary velum at the base of the nodulus.

Experimental studies (2594) indicate that ablations of the nodulus in dogs, demonstrated to be susceptible to motion sickness, render these animals immune to the emetic effects of motion. These findings suggest that the emetic responses of motion sickness involve neural mechanisms independent of the forebrain.

Anterior Lobe of the Cerebellum. Lesions of the anterior lobe of the cerebellum (paleocerebellum) in the dog and cat produce severe disturbances of posture and increased extensor muscle tone. These animals exhibit an extreme opisthotonus, tight closure of the jaw, hyperactive deep tendon reflexes, increased positive supporting mechanisms and periodic tonic seizures. Animals surviving these lesions regain the ability to walk without swaying of the head or trunk, and can perform voluntary movements without evident tremor (822). Conclusive information concerning ablations of the anterior lobe of the cerebellum in primates does not appear to be available. A clinical syndrome in man corresponding to that described in experimental animals has not been defined. The closest related phenomenon would appear to be the so-called "tonic seizure," which usually is related to compression of the brain stem. Other experimental studies (244) have shown that ablations of the anterior lobe of the cerebellum produce an exaggeration of decerebrate rigidity in the cat.

In what is now a classical experiment, Sherrington (2324) demonstrated that electrical stimulation of the anterior lobe of the cerebellum could inhibit the extensor muscle tone in a decerebrate animal. This experiment, confirming the early work of Loewenthal and Horsley (1512), indicated an important inhibitory action of the paleocerebellum upon muscle tone. Studies summarized by Dow and Moruzzi (645) indicate that facilitating effects also can be obtained by stimulation of the anterior lobe of the cerebellum, and that the rate of stimulation is critical in determining whether inhibition or facilitation occurs. With square wave stimulation, it was found that low repetitive rates (2 to 10 cycles/sec) caused a slow increase in ipsilateral extensor muscle tone, while rapid stimulation (30 to 300 cycles/sec) produced a relaxation of the muscles in the ipsilateral limbs. These opposite effects originally were interpreted as indicating that inhibitory and facilitatory neurons were intermingled in the cortex of the anterior lobe of the cerebellum. Further studies of these interesting phenomena (summarized by Brodal et al. (280)) indicate that these inhibitory and facilitatory influences must involve different parts of the fastigial nuclei and their fiber projections, as well as cerebellovestibular fiber projections (Figs. 14-19 and 14-20). Following lesions near the rostrolateral part of the fastigial nucleus, stimulation of the ipsilateral vermis of the anterior lobe with high frequency square waves (300 cycles/sec) produced a clear-cut increase in extensor rigidity on the side stimulated. This finding suggested that most of the inhibitory pathways had been interrupted by the lesion, while the facilitatory pathways remained intact. Following lesions near the rostromedial part of the fastigial nucleus, stimulation of the vermis of the anterior lobe with low frequency square waves (2 to 10 cycles/sec) caused inhibitory effects upon ipsilateral decerebrate rigidity, indicating that facilitatory fiber systems were interrupted by the fastigial lesion. After a unilateral total lesion of the fastigial nucleus, stimulation of the surface of the ipsilateral vermis of the anterior lobe yielded no responses (2412a, 2413), and the same effect was seen when the lesion was limited to the rostral part of the ipsilateral fastigial nucleus (1756a). Although a complete anatomical basis for these physiological observations cannot be provided, it seems likely that: (a) inhibitory influences obtained from stimulating the vermis of the anterior lobe of the cerebellum are mediated via the fastigial nucleus and act in part upon the ipsilateral reticular formation and (b) facilitatory influences obtained from stimulation of the vermis of the anterior lobe are mediated by parts of the fastigial nucleus that act upon the lateral vestibular nucleus (280). Cerebellovestibular fibers which pass through regions near the rostrolateral part of the fastigial nucleus

(2643) have been demonstrated to exert an inhibitory influence upon cells of the lateral vestibular nucleus (675, 1188, 1190). This is an example of direct cerebellar cortical inhibition upon cells of the lateral vestibular nucleus. There is no direct fiber projection from the cerebellar cortex to the reticular formation.

Other cerebellar mechanisms which can influence muscle tone involve the paravermal cortex, the nucleus interpositus and the contralateral red nucleus (1632); all of these structures are connected by somatotopically organized fibers. Stimulation of the rostral part of the interposed nucleus (anterior part) produces flexion in the ipsilateral hindlimb of the cat, while stimulation of the caudal part of this nucleus produces flexion in the ipsilateral forelimb (1583, 2035). These responses occur ipsilaterally because fibers of both the superior cerebellar peduncle and the rubrospinal tract are crossed (Fig. 14-17). Intracellular recordings in the red nucleus demonstrate that stimulation of the nucleus interpositus produces excitatory postsynaptic potentials with a monosynaptic latency (1632, 2587). The pathway between the interposed nucleus and the red nucleus is regarded as purely excitatory and impulses conveyed by this system have an important facilitatory influence upon flexor muscle tone; these impulses are conveyed to spinal levels by the rubrospinal tract. Although the Purkinje cell output from the cerebellar cortex is inhibitory, variations in the activity of those cells are responsible for the inhibition, or activation, of cells in the interposed nucleus which directly affects cells of the contralateral red nucleus.

Modification of Cerebellar Disturbances. Experimental studies in the monkey demonstrate that cerebellar dyskinesia, produced by lesions in the deep cerebellar nuclei, can be abolished by surgical section of the dorsal half of the lateral funiculus of the spinal cord at high cervical levels (400). Selective section of the anterior half of the lateral funiculus and the anterior funiculus of the spinal cord in these animals has no appreciable effect on the dyskinesia. Bilateral selective destruction of the posterior funiculi tends to exaggerate ataxia and asynergic disturbances, including tremor. These data suggest that impulses essential to the neural mechanism of experimental cerebellar dyskinesia in the monkey are transmitted to segmental levels via the lateral corticospinal tract. Since no fibers of the corticospinal tract are infrapallial in origin, and most are crossed, this implies that the neocerebellum must exert its regulating and controlling influences upon the contralateral motor cortex through the mediation of certain thalamic relay nuclei. This hypothesis is in accord with the well established finding that neocerebellar disturbances occur ipsilateral to cerebellar lesions.

Clinical experiences indicate that lesions in the contralateral thalamic nuclei can significantly modify and ameliorate cerebellar dyskinesia in man (522, 525, 1620). Experimental studies (403) in the monkey have demonstrated that lesions destroying significant parts of the ventral lateral nucleus of the thalamus can reduce the tremor associated with cerebellar lesions without destroying fibers of the corticospinal tract and without producing paresis. Thus this thalamic nucleus must be concerned with the mediation of certain cerebellar disturbances (Fig. 14-21). Physiological evidence also suggests that the cerebellothalamic cortical relay system may play an important role in the unconscious regulation of muscle tone. Following decerebellation in monkeys there is a decrease in the tonic sensitivity of muscle spindle afferents, presumably because fusimotor neurons are activated via the output of the cerebellum to the motor cortex which in turn influences corticospinal activity (881). It also has been shown that lesions in the motor cortex of the monkey decrease the muscle spindle response to stretch (883).

Localized cooling of the dentate nucleus in monkeys trained to perform various types of movement or movement sequences results in disturbances of movement that resemble those associated with lesions (302, 514). Cooling of the dentate nucleus affects the range, rate and force of skilled voluntary movement.

Computer Functions. Advances concerning the structural and functional components of the cerebellar cortex (675, 1920) suggest that in some way the cerebellum functions as a type of computer particularly concerned with smooth and effective control of movement. Present evidence suggests that the cerebellum integrates and organizes information flowing into it via numerous neural pathways, and that cerebellar output participates in the control of motor function by the transmission of impulses to: (a) brain stem nuclei (i.e., lateral vestibular and red nuclei) that project to spinal levels and (b) thalamic nuclei which can modify the activity of cortical regions concerned with motor function.

Every part of the cerebellar cortex receives directly, or indirectly, two different inputs, that of the mossy fibers and that of the climbing fibers. Although these inputs differ in their structural and functional characteristics, they appear to convey similar "sensory" information to particular areas of the cerebellar cortex. The only output of the cerebellar cortex, conveyed by Purkinje cell axons, is inhibitory. This inhibition is exerted upon the deep cerebellar nuclei and the lateral vestibular nucleus. The output of the deep cerebellar nuclei is excitatory, a fact which implies that excitatory, as well as inhibitory, impulses must reach these nuclei. Excitatory impulses passing to the deep cerebellar nuclei are considered to be derived from extracerebellar sources. Impulses are conveyed to these nuclei via collaterals of both climbing and mossy fibers (1323, 1559). The fact that the cerebellar cortex transforms all input into inhibition precludes the possibility of dynamic storage of information by impulses circulating in complex neuronal pathways, as in the cerebral cortex. The absence of reverberatory chains of neurons in the cerebellar cortex enhances its performance as a special kind of computer, in that it can provide a quick and clear response to the input of any particular set of information. Thus the cerebellum processes its input information rapidly, conveys its output indirectly to other parts of the nervous system, and has virtually no short-term dynamic memory.

CHAPTER 15

The Diencephalon

The rostral end of the brain stem, the diencephalon, is a nuclear complex composed of several major subdivisions (Figs. 15-1, 15-2 and 15-7). Although the diencephalon is relatively small, constituting less than 2% of the neuraxis (1218), it has long been regarded as the key to the understanding of the organization of the central nervous system. The diencephalon extends from the region of the posterior commissure rostrally to the region of the interventricular foramen. Laterally it is bounded by the posterior limb of the internal capsule, the tail of the caudate nucleus and the stria terminalis (Figs. 15-5, 15-7, 15-8). The third ventricle separates the diencephalon into two symmetrical halves, except in the region of the interthalamic adhesion where the medial surfaces of the thalami may be in continuity. The diencephalon is divisible into four major parts: the epithalamus, the thalamus, the hypothalamus and the subthalamus, or ventral thalamus. The medial and lateral geniculate bodies constitute distinctive subdivisions of the thalamus, referred to as the *metathalamus*. Adjacent to the diencephalon, but separated from it by the fibers of the internal capsule, are the corpa striata.

The region can be approached best through a graded series of photomicrographs of transverse sections. The level and plane of each section are indicated in Figures 15-2 and 15-3.

MIDBRAIN-DIENCEPHALIC JUNCTION

Rostral transverse sections of the midbrain reveal the addition of several discrete nuclear masses of the caudal thalamus closely surrounding the posterior and lat-

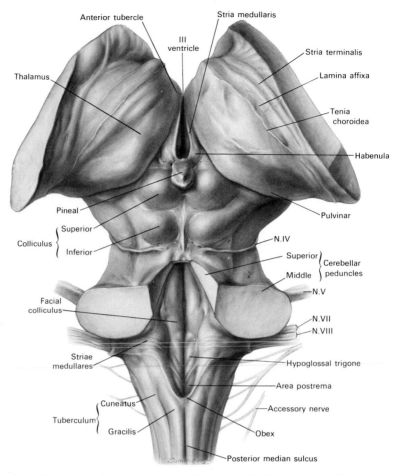

Figure 15-1. Posterior aspect of the brain stem with the cerebellum removed. This drawing shows the epithalamus and the pulvinar. (Reproduced with permission from F. A. Mettler: *Neuroanatomy*. The C. V. Mosby Co., St. Louis, 1948.)

eral surfaces of the mesencephalon. These structures include the *medial* and *lateral geniculate bodies* and the *pulvinar*. External to all of these is the *retrolenticular* portion of the internal capsule (Figs. 15-4, 15-5 and A-12). The pineal body lies dorsally between the superior colliculi, while portions of the mammillary bodies can be seen in the interpeduncular fossa (Fig. 15-4). Fibers from thalamic nuclei pass laterally into the internal capsule, through which they are distributed to various parts of the cerebral cortex. The internal capsule also contains corticofugal fibers projecting to thalamic nuclei. *Thalamocortical* and *corticothalamic fibers* constitute a large part of the internal capsule referred to as the *thalamic radiations.*

The pulvinar is a large nuclear mass dorsal to the medial and lateral geniculate bodies. Its dorsal surface is covered by a thin plate of fibers, the *stratum zonale* (Figs. 15-4–15-6). Fibers passing laterally from this nucleus contribute to the retrolenticular portion of the internal capsule (Figs. 15-4 and 15-28) and are distributed to the posterior parietal and occipitotemporal cortex. The innermost portion of the internal capsule, wedged between the pulvinar and lateral geniculate body, forms a triangular area known as the *zone of Wernicke*. This zone, composed of a mixture of transverse and longitudinal fibers (Fig. 15-4), contains the optic radiations. Intermingled with these are fibers from the pulvinar and the medial geniculate body.

Sections through more rostral levels (Figs. 15-5, and A-12) reveal a great expansion of the diencephalic nuclei, as well as significant, although less marked, changes in the midbrain. The pulvinar is much larger, the medial geniculate body is smaller, and some fibers of the optic tract can be seen entering the lateral geniculate body. Lateral to the pulvinar is the body of the caudate nucleus, separated from the pulvinar by fibers of the *stria terminalis* (Figs. 15-4–15-6). The cerebral aqueduct expands into the deeper third ventricle; the posterior commissure marks the midline dorsal boundary between midbrain and diencephalon. Superior to the posterior commissure is the stalk of the pineal body, enclosing the pineal recess of the third ventricle (Fig. 15-5). The superior colliculi are replaced by the pretectal region, considered to be a center for the pupillary light reflex (Fig. 15-5). The connections of the pretectal area and posterior commissure have been discussed in Chapter 13.

The oculomotor nuclei and their root fibers have largely disappeared, although portions of the most rostral visceral nuclei of the oculomotor complex are present in the midline area below the ventricle. Lateral to the rostral part of the oculomotor complex is a collection of relatively large cells, the *interstitial nucleus of Cajal* (Figs. 13-16*B*, 13-19, 13-20 and 15-5). The area lateral to the posterior commissure and ventral to the pretectum contains the *nuclei of the posterior commissure* (Fig. 13-11).

The medial portion of the red nucleus is transversed by a vertical fiber bundle, the *fasciculus retroflexus* or *habenulo-interpeduncular tract*. These fibers arise from the *habenular nucleus*, situated at a somewhat more rostral level (Figs. 15-6 and A-13). The capsular fibers of the red nucleus change from a longitudinal to a transverse direction and form a radiating bundle that extends from the dorsolateral surface of the red nucleus toward the ventral portion of the thalamus. This is the beginning of the *tegmental field H of Forel* or *prerubral field* (Fig. 15-6). Cells scattered among the fibers of Forel's field H and along its dorsal border constitute the *nucleus of the tegmental field of Forel* (nucleus of the prerubral field; Figs. 15-11 and 15-12).

CAUDAL DIENCEPHALON

Transverse sections through the habenular nuclei and the mammillary bodies (Fig. 15-6) reveal the structural organization of the caudal diencephalon. The *habenular nuclei* are two small gray masses forming triangular eminences on the dorsomedial surfaces of the thalami. These nuclei receive fibers mainly from the septal nuclei and the preoptic area via the striae medullares (Figs. 2-28, 15-1, 15-2 and 16-7). Some fibers crossing to the opposite side in the *habenular commissure* are not illustrated in Figure 15-6, but can be seen in Figures 2-28 and 15-1. Axons from the habenular nuclei form a well-defined bundle, the *fasciculus retroflexus*, which passes ventrally and caudally to terminate in the interpeduncular nuclei.

The third ventricle appears enlarged, and parts of it are seen in two locations (Figs. 15-6 and A-13). The main part of the third ventricle is present dorsally, where it is covered by a thin roof extending between the habenular nuclei and the striae medullares. The margins of this attachment (not shown in Fig. 15-6) on each side constitute the *tenia thalami*. A small part of the third ventricle, referred to as the *infundibular recess*, is present ventral to the mammillary bodies and dorsal to the infundibulum. The mammillary bodies, tuber cinereum and infundibulum are parts of the hypothalamus.

A progressive increase in the size of the thalamus is evident (Figs. 15-6 and A-13). The pulvinar has reached its greatest extent, and part of the lateral thalamic nuclear group, with which the pulvinar is continuous rostrally, also may be present. Ventral to the pulvinar are the ventral tier thalamic nuclei and the *centromedian nucleus*; the latter nucleus is delimited by a thin fibrous capsule. The medial geniculate body has disappeared and the lateral geniculate is greatly reduced.

EPITHALAMUS

The epithalamus comprises the pineal body, the habenular trigones, the striae medullares and the epithelial roof of the third ventricle (Figs. 2-28 and 15-8).

The Habenula. In man, the habenula consists of a small medial and a large lateral nucleus (Figs. 15-6 and 16-7). The medial nucleus consists of small, closely packed, deeply staining round cells; in the lateral nucleus, the cells are larger, paler and more loosely arranged. These nuclei receive the

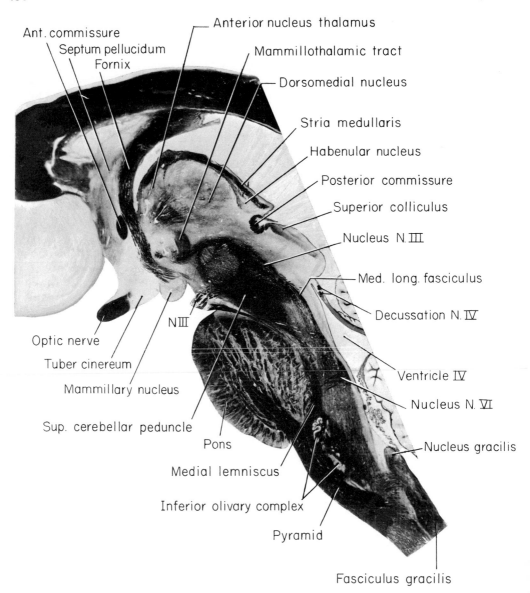

Figure 15-2. Sagittal section of brain stem through the pillar of fornix and root of the third nerve (Weigert's myelin stain, photograph).

terminals of the stria medullaris (Figs. 15-2 and 15-8) and gives origin to the habenulo-interpeduncular tract or fasciculus retroflexus, which terminates in the interpeduncular nucleus and certain midline reticular nuclei (Figs. 13-3, 15-6 and 16-7). The *stria medullaris* is a complex bundle composed of fibers arising from: (a) the septal nuclei, (b) lateral preoptic region (1816), (c) the anterior thalamic nuclei and (d) the globus pallidus (1079, 1438, 1811, 1825). The septal nuclei which receive fibers from both the

hippocampal formation and the amygdaloid nuclear complex project profusely to the medial habenular nucleus. Fibers from the lateral preoptic nucleus and the medial pallidal segment pass to the lateral habenular nucleus (Fig. 16-7). Some of the strial fibers cross to the opposite side in the habenular commissure.

Retrograde transport studies in the rat indicate that the lateral habenular nucleus receives afferents from the globus pallidus, the lateral hypothalamus, the substantia

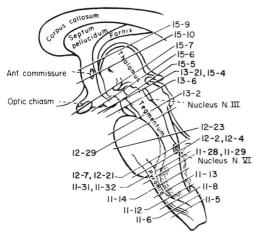

Figure 15-3. Outline of a paramedian sagittal section of brain stem, showing level and plane of the transverse sections of the figures indicated. For identification of structures, see Figure 15-2.

innominata and the lateral preoptic area, as well as from the ventral tegmental area and the midbrain raphe nuclei (1079). The smaller medial habenular nucleus receives afferents from posterior parts of the septal nuclei and the midbrain raphe nuclei. The medial habenular nucleus receives serotonergic projections from the raphe nuclei and adrenergic innervation from the superior cervical ganglion (186). Although the habenular nuclei are adjacent to each other they do not appear to have interconnections. These nuclei appear to be the sites of convergence of limbic pathways that convey impulses to rostral portions of the midbrain.

The Pineal Gland. The pineal body, or *epiphysis*, is a small, coned-shaped body attached to the roof of the third ventricle in the region of the posterior commissure (Figs. 15-1 and 15-5). It appears to be a rudimentary gland whose function in the adult is not fully known. It consists of a network of richly vascular connective tissue trabeculae in the meshes of which are found glial cells and cells of a peculiar type, the *pinealocyte*. These are cells of variable size with a pale nucleus, granular argentophilic cytoplasm and relatively few branching processes. Histofluorescence studies reveal that pinealocytes in the rhesus monkey have an intense yellow fluorescence characteristic of serotonin (2319). Mammalian pinealocytes are phylogenetically related to the neurosensory photoreceptor elements

present in the pineal body in fish and amphibia. During evolution these cells lose their outer photoreceptive segments and their synaptic processes disappear, so that the pineal can no longer convey photic stimuli directly to the brain (83). The pinealocytes become predominantly secretory cells but they remain indirectly photosensitive. The loss of central neural connections of the pineal is compensated for by the peripheral sympathetic system which provides innervation via the superior cervical ganglion. The mammalian pineal gland is regarded as an indirectly photosensitive neuroendocrine organ derived from embryonic neuroepithelium. The pinealocyte has one or more processes of variable length which from ultrastructural studies appear adapted for secretory function (1617). The club-shaped endings of these processes terminate close to the perivascular space surrounding capillaries that have fenestrations. Pinealocytes receive a direct innervation from sympathetic neurons which form recognizable synapses. True nerve cells do not appear to be present, although occasional cells with typical Nissl bodies have been observed by some investigators (1719).

The best known pineal secretions are the biogenic amines serotonin, norepinephrine and melatonin, but the gland also contains significant concentrations of identified hypothalamic peptides such as thyrotropin-releasing hormone (TRH), luteinizing hormone-releasing hormone (LHRH) and somatostatin (1617). The synthesis of serotonin from tryptophan involves two enzymes, tryptophan hydroxylase and aromatic amino acid decarboxylase, both of which are found in pinealocytes (1325). Only the raphe nuclei of the brain stem have higher levels of tryptophan hydroxylase. Serotonin is synthesized in pinealocytes and released into the extracellular space. Nerve endings in the pineal gland do not contain serotonin. Norepinephrine is synthesized in sympathetic neurons which terminate on pineal parenchymal cells and in the perivascular space (2083).

The pineal gland synthesizes melatonin from serotonin by the action of two enzymes sensitive to variations of diurnal light, *N*-acetyltransferase and hydroxyindole-*o*-methyltransferase (93, 1327). Daily fluctuations in melatonin synthesis are

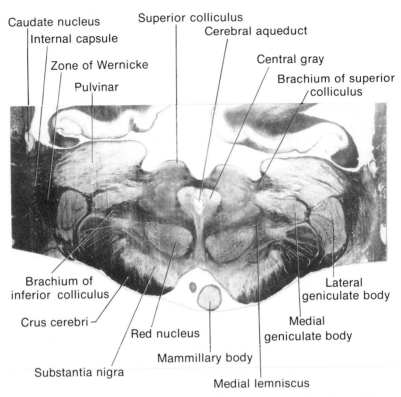

Figure 15-4. Transverse section through the rostral midbrain demonstrating relationship of midbrain and caudal portions of the thalamus (Weigert's myelin stain, photograph).

rhythmic and in direct response to the daily cycle of photic input. Light entrains the circadian clock mechanism to the environmental lighting cycle (1327, 1738) and also acts by an unidentified pathway to rapidly block the transmission of neural signals to the pineal gland (1328). N-Acetyltransferase activity is elevated during the night, but exposure to light results in the rapid "turn-off" of enzyme activity (1326). Exposure of a rat to constant light for 30 days results in a reduction of hydroxyindole-o-methyltransferase and the disappearance of the rhythm in N-acetyltransferase activity. If animals are blinded, the suppressive effects of light on hydroxyindole-o-methyltransferase are abolished, but the rhythm of N-acetyltransferase activity persists (93, 1327, 1733). Bilateral lesions of the suprachiasmatic nucleus of the hypothalamus (Fig. 16-1), which receives the retinohypothalamic tract, abolish the rhythm in pineal N-acetyltransferase activity and result in low levels of hydroxyindole-o-methyltransferase activity (1326). Such lesions abolish the circadian rhythms of spontaneous lo-

comotor activity and of both feeding and drinking (1758, 2027). Lesions of the suprachiasmatic nuclei also eliminate the circadian rhythm of the sleep-wakefulness cycle although ultradian rhythms with a 2- to 4-hr periodicity may show slight enhancement (1179). In female rats the normal estrous cycle is abolished by lesions of the suprachiasmatic nuclei (1758). These studies indicate that photo regulation of pineal N-acetyltransferase and hydroxyindole-o-methyltransferase is via the retinohypothalamic tract and suggest that the suprachiasmatic nuclei are the endogenous sources of signals which generate the circadian rhythms in pineal N-acetyltransferase activity and tonically elevate hydroxyindole-o-methyltransferase activity (1326). Failure to find a discrete area of the brain to which the suprachiasmatic nucleus projects efferent fibers (2479) supports the thesis that no other locus in the hypothalamus has primary importance for circadian pacemaker activity (1179). It seems likely that the retinohypothalamic projection alters pineal function by directly interacting with struc-

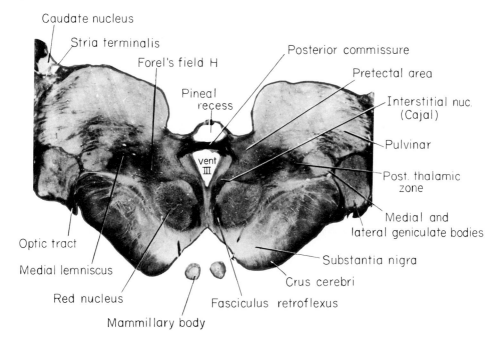

Caudate nucleus
Stria terminalis
Forel's field H
Pineal recess
Posterior commissure
Pretectal area
Interstitial nuc. (Cajal)
Pulvinar
vent III
Post. thalamic zone
Medial and lateral geniculate bodies
Optic tract
Medial lemniscus
Substantia nigra
Crus cerebri
Red nucleus
Fasciculus retroflexus
Mammillary body

Figure 15-5. Transverse section of the brain stem at the junction of mesencephalon and diencephalon. The posterior thalamic zone (nucleus), which receives collaterals from the spinothalamic tract, lies medial to the medial geniculate body (Fig. 15-18). This cell group lies caudal to the ventral posterior thalamic nucleus (Fig. 15-6) (Weigert's myelin stain, photograph).

tures in the suprachiasmatic nucleus. Environmental light can be regarded as having an entraining function and a transmission function. The effect of light in entraining the endogenous oscillator to the light cycle is slow, but the effect of light on signal transmission is rapid and probably accounts for the rapid "turn off" of *N*-acetyl-transfarese by light and the blocking of circadian rhythm by constant light.

Although a single neural pathway from the suprachiasmatic nucleus regulates both enzymes involved in the formation of melatonin by the pineal gland, details concerning these connections are not known. Localized injections of ^{3}H-labeled amino acids in the suprachiasmatic nucleus in the rat have not revealed a projection to any well-defined cell mass in the hypothalamus (2479). It is presumed on the basis of indirect evidence that the pathway from the suprachiasmatic nucleus to the pineal involves relays to the tuberal region of the hypothalamus, the medial forebrain bundle and spinal pathways that reach the intermediolateral cell column and cells of the superior cervical ganglion. Lesions in the superior cervical ganglion, the medial fore-

brain bundle and the retrochiasmatic region of the hypothalamus block the stimulatory effects of the suprachiasmatic nucleus upon pineal enzymes (1329, 1738, 1740). Thus the pineal gland appears to be a neurendocrine transducer that converts neural signals received via sympathetic neurons into an endocrine output, melatonin.

Pineal secretions which alter hypothalamic functions do so after they enter the general circulation or the cerebrospinal fluid (799, 1617). Daily fluctuations in pineal serotonin and melatonin are rhythmic in response to the cycle of photic input. Because of these rhythmic changes in pineal activity, it has been suggested that this gland functions as a biological clock that delivers signals that regulate both physiological and behavioral processes. These fluctations, called *circadian rhythms*, have a period of exactly 24 hr in the presence of environmental cues, while in the absence of such cues they only approximate the 24-hr cycle (180).

Early observations suggested that parenchymatous pinealomas were associated with depression of gonadal function and

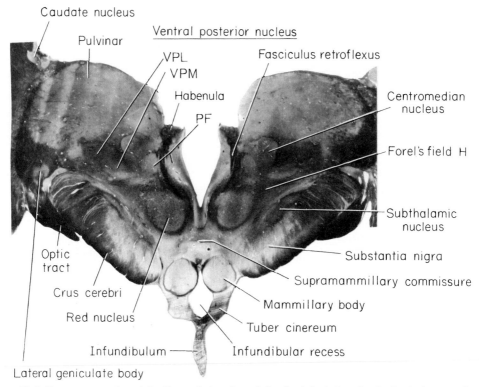

Figure 15-6. Transverse section of the diencephalon through levels of the habenula, the fasciculus retroflexus, the mammillary bodies, and the infundibulum. *VPL* and *VPM* indicate the ventral posterolateral and ventral posteromedial nuclei of the thalamus. *PF* indicates the parafascicular nucleus which surrounds the fasciculus retroflexus (Weigert's myelin stain, photograph).

delayed pubescence, while lesions which destroyed the pineal frequently were associated with precocious puberty (2130). These observations are consistent with experimental studies indicating that the pineal gland exerts an inhibitory influence on the gonads and the reproductive system (799). Experimental data suggest indoles and methoxyindoles synthesized in the pineal inhibit the secretions of pituitary gonadotropins. The inhibitory effects of these pineal principles are thought to act upon receptors sensitive to methoxyindoles located in the hypothalamus and in the midbrain.

Melatonin, which is a potent skin-lightening agent in amphibians, has no effect upon human skin, possibly because in man most melanin pigment is stored outside the melanocytes. The human pineal gland obtained at autopsy is capable of forming melatonin, and melatonin has been identified in the plasma of males during darkness (1617).

After the age of 16 calcareous bodies frequently are present in the pineal body. These calcareous bodies, consisting of calcium and magnesium phosphates and carbonates, form large conglomerations which often are visible in skull roentgenographs. Identification and measurements of the position of the pineal body in skull films can provide useful information, especially in the diagnosis of space occupying intracranial lesions.

THE THALAMUS

Transverse sections through the central part of the diencephalon demonstrate three major divisions of the diencephalon: (a) the thalamus, (b) the hypothalamus and (c) the subthalamic region (Figs. 2-15, 2-28, 15-6 and 15-7).

The narrow third ventricle, extending from the region immediately ventral to the striae medullares to the optic chiasm, completely separates the thalami. A shallow groove on the ventricular surface, the hy-

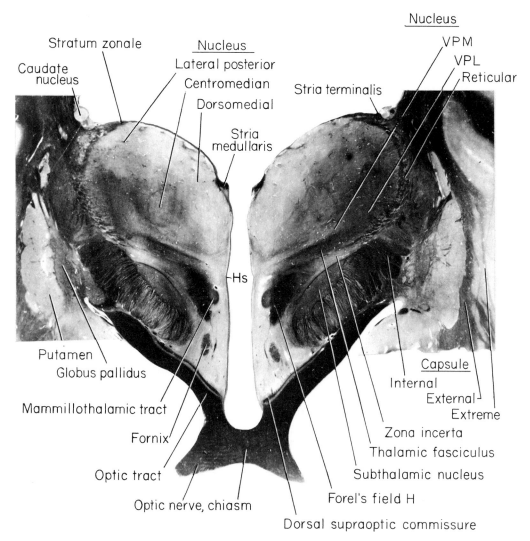

Figure 15-7. Transverse section through the diencephalon and corpus striatum at the level of the optic chiasm. *Hs* indicates the hypothalamic sulcus in the wall of the third ventricle. *VPM* and *VPL* refer to the ventral posteromedial and ventral posterolateral nuclei of the thalamus (Weigert's myelin stain, photograph).

pothalamic sulcus (Fig. 15-7), separates the dorsal thalamus from the hypothalamus. The dorsal surface of the thalamus is covered by the stratum zonale. At the junction of the dorsal and medial thalamic surfaces, fibers of the striae medullares are cut transversely and appear as small bundles of myelinated fibers.

The dorsal thalamus is divided into anterior, medial and lateral nuclear groups by a band of myelinated fibers, the internal medullary lamina of the thalamus (Fig. 2-28). The *anterior nuclear group* of the thalamus forms a rostromedial swelling known

as the anterior tubercle and is separated from other thalamic nuclei by a myelinated capsule (Figs. 15-1, 15-2 and 15-9). At slightly more caudal levels a curved band of myelinated fibers, the *internal medullary lamina*, separates the thalamus into medial and lateral nuclear groups. In the *lateral nuclear group*, ventral and lateral (dorsal) nuclear masses can be distinguished (Figs. 15-7 and 15-14). The ventral nuclear mass, extending nearly the entire length of the thalamus, is divisible into three separate nuclei: (a) a caudal, *ventral posterior nucleus*, (b) an intermediate, *ven-*

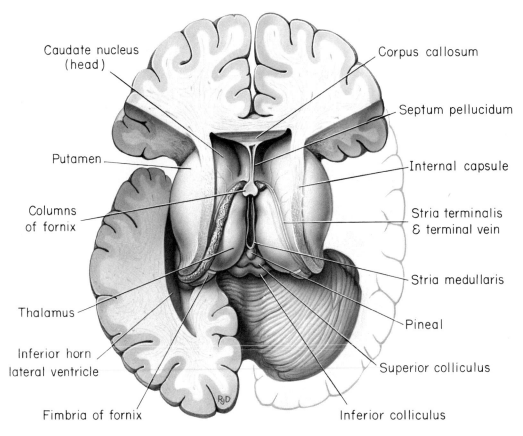

Figure 15-8. Drawing of a brain dissection showing gross relationships of the thalamus, internal capsule, corpus striatum and the ventricular system.

tral lateral nucleus and (c) a rostral, *ventral anterior nucleus.* The ventral posterior nucleus is subdivided into a ventral posterolateral nucleus, located laterally, and a ventral posteromedial nucleus, located medially (Figs. 15-11, 15-12 and 15-14). These are the ventral tier thalamic nuclei.

The lateral nuclear mass of the thalamus, located dorsal to the ventral nuclear mass discussed above, also is divided into three separate nuclei: (a) a greatly expanded caudal part, the *pulvinar,* (b) an intermediate part, the *lateral posterior nucleus* and (c) a more rostral part, the *lateral dorsal nucleus* (Figs. 15-13 and 15-14). These are the dorsal tier thalamic nuclei.

The medial nuclear group of the thalamus, located medial to the internal medullary lamina, contains the *dorsomedial nucleus,* a nuclear mass intimately related to the cortex of the frontal lobe (Fig. 15-7). Wedged between the dorsomedial nucleus and the ventral nuclei caudally is the *cen-*

tromedian nucleus, the largest of the intralaminar nuclei (Figs. 15-6, 15-7, and 15-12–15-14). The internal medullary lamina partially splits to surround this nucleus.

Along the lateral border of the thalamus, near the internal capsule, is a narrow band of myelinated fibers, the *external medullary lamina* of the thalamus. Cells located external to these fibers form a thin outer envelope, the *reticular nucleus* of the thalamus (Figs. 15-7, 15-11, 15-12 and 15-14). Ventrally the reticular nucleus becomes continuous with the zona incerta (Fig. 15-7).

The thalamic nuclei are particularly difficult to visualize in three dimensions (Fig. 15-14). In addition, the nomenclature is complex, and the fiber connections and the significance of the smaller thalamic nuclei remain unknown. In a general way, depending upon their connections, most of the major thalamic nuclei can be classified either as specific relay nuclei (R), or as

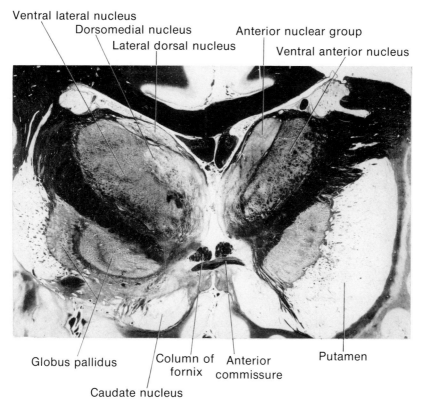

Ventral lateral nucleus
Dorsomedial nucleus
Lateral dorsal nucleus
Anterior nuclear group
Ventral anterior nucleus

Globus pallidus
Column of fornix
Anterior commissure
Putamen
Caudate nucleus

Figure 15-9. Photograph of an asymmetrical transverse section through rostral portions of the thalamus and corpus striatum. The right side reveals the most rostral level (Weigert's myelin stain). (Reproduced with permission from M. B. Carpenter: *Core Text of Neuroanatomy.* Williams & Wilkins, Baltimore, 1978).

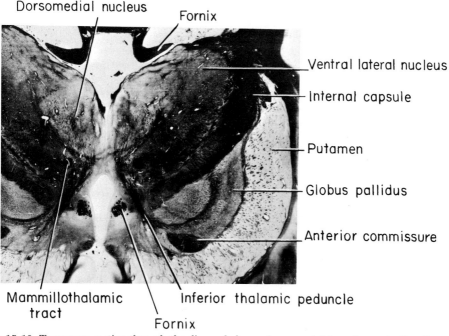

Dorsomedial nucleus
Fornix
Ventral lateral nucleus
Internal capsule
Putamen
Globus pallidus
Anterior commissure
Mammillothalamic tract
Inferior thalamic peduncle
Fornix

Figure 15-10. Transverse section through the diencephalon and corpus striatum demonstrating fibers of the inferior thalamic peduncle. The inferior thalamic peduncle consists of fibers from the amygdaloid complex, temporal neocortex, and possibly the substantia innominata which project to the dorsomedial nucleus of the thalamus. The inferior thalamic peduncle plus amygdaloid projections to the hypothalamus and preoptic regions constitute the *ansa peduncularis* (Weigert's myelin stain, photograph).

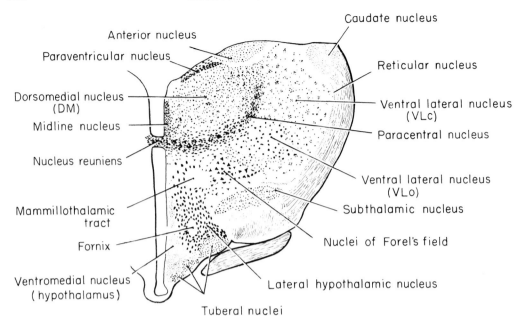

Figure 15-11. Drawing of a transverse Nissl section through the diencephalon at the level of the tuber cinereum showing nuclei of the thalamus and hypothalamus. (Modified from Malone (1596).)

association nuclei (*A*). The specific relay nuclei project to, and receive fibers from, well defined cortical areas related to specific functions. The association nuclei of the thalamus do not receive direct fibers from ascending systems, but project to association areas of the cortex. Other thalamic nuclei have predominantly, or exclusively, subcortical (*SC*) connections. Physiological and anatomical studies suggest that certain thalamic nuclei may have diffuse cortical (*DC*) connections. The following classification of thalamic nuclei is based upon functional and morphological data drawn from many sources, but especially from the works of Clark (463), Walker (2650, 2651, 2657), Olszewski (1883), Russell (2240), and van Buren and Borke (327). The major nuclear groups of the thalamus and the most important nuclei are in bold faced type. The abbreviations most frequently used to designate these nuclear subdivisions are in parentheses. Letters in italics indicate specific relay nuclei (*R*), association nuclei (*A*) and nuclei with subcortical (*SC*) or diffuse cortical (*DC*) projections.

A. **Anterior Nuclear Group**
 1. **Anteroventral nucleus** (AV) *R*
 2. Anterodorsal nucleus (AD) *R*
 3. Anteromedial nucleus (AM) *R*

B. **Medial Nuclear Group**
 1. **Dorsomedial nucleus** (DM)
  a. parvicellular part (DMpc) *A*
  b. magnocellular part (DMmc) *SC*
  c. paralaminar part (DMpl) *R*
C. **Midline Nuclear Group**
 1. Paratenial nucleus
 2. Paraventricular nucleus
 3. Reuniens nucleus
 4. Rhomboidal nucleus
D. **Intralaminar Nuclear Group**
 1. **Centromedian nucleus** (CM) *SC, DC*
 2. **Parafascicular nucleus** (PF) *SC, DC*
 3. Paracentral nucleus *SC, DC*
 4. Central lateral nucleus *SC, DC*
 5. Central medial nucleus *SC*
E. **Lateral Nuclear Group**
 1. **Lateral dorsal nucleus** (LD) *A*
 2. **Lateral posterior nucleus** (LP) *A*
 3. **Pulvinar** (P) *A*
  a. medial part
  b. lateral part
  c. inferior part *R*
F. **Ventral Nuclear Group**
 1. **Ventral anterior nucleus** (VA)
  a. parvicellular part (VApc) *R, SC, DC*
  b. magnocellular part (VAmc) *R, SC*
 2. **Ventral lateral nucleus** (VL)
  a. **oral part** (VLo) *R*
  b. **caudal part** (VLc) *R*
  c. medial part (VLm) *R*

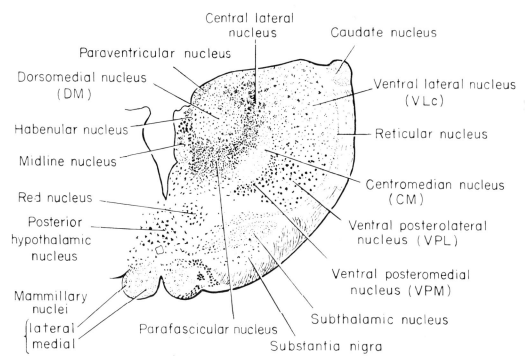

Figure 15-12. Drawing of a transverse Nissl section through the diencephalon at the level of the habenular nuclei and the mammillary bodies showing the nuclei of the thalamus and hypothalamus. (Modified from Malone (1596).)

3. **Ventral posterior nucleus** (VP) *R*
   a. **ventral posterolateral** (VPL) *R*
      aa. oral part (VPLo) *R*
      bb. caudal part (VPLc) *R*
   b. **ventral posteromedial** (VPM) *R*
      aa. parvicellular part (VPMpc) *R*
   c. ventral posterior inferior (VPI) *R*
G. **Metathalamus**
   1. **Medial geniculate body** (MGB) *R*
      a. parvicellular part (MGpc) *R*
      b. magnocellular part (MGmc) *R*
      c. dorsal part *R*
   2. **Lateral geniculate body** (LGB) *R*
      a. dorsal part *R*
      b. ventral part, *SC*
H. **Unclassified Thalamic Nuclei**
   1. Submedial nucleus
   2. Suprageniculate nucleus
   3. Limitans nucleus
I. **Thalamic Reticular Nucleus** (RN) *SC*

The gross appearance of the dorsal surface of the diencephalon exposed by dissection is shown in Figures 15-1 and 15-8. These illustrations demonstrate the relationships of the thalamus and epithalamus to surrounding structures. Figures 15-11 and 15-12 show portions of many major

thalamic nuclei at two important levels. The major subdivisions of the thalamus together with the established afferent and efferent thalamic projections are diagrammed in Figure 15-14. The cortical projection areas of the thalamic nuclei are diagrammatically represented in Figure 15-15. Examples of ascending thalamic afferent systems have been provided in diagrams for spinal pathways (Figs. 10-1, 10-6 and 10-7), for certain pathways originating in the brain stem (Figs. 12-13 and 12-27) and for the cerebellum (Figs. 14-16, 14-17 and 14-21). Review of these schematic diagrams will contribute to your understanding of thalamic organization. The illustrations in the atlas section provide additional material worthy of reference.

The Anterior Nuclear Group

The anterior nuclear group lies beneath the dorsal surface of the most rostral part of the thalamus, where it forms a distinct swelling, the anterior tubercle (Figs. 2-25, 15-1, 15-2, 15-9, 15-11, 15-14, A-16 and A-17). It consists of a large principal nucleus, the anteroventral (AV), and accessory nu-

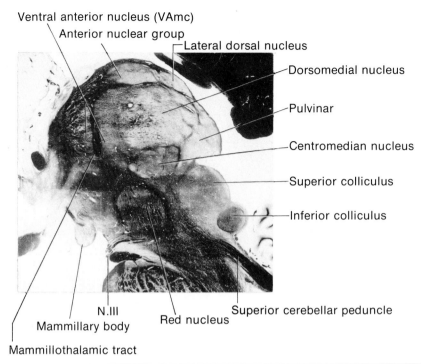

Ventral anterior nucleus (VAmc)
Anterior nuclear group
Lateral dorsal nucleus
Dorsomedial nucleus
Pulvinar
Centromedian nucleus
Superior colliculus
Inferior colliculus
N.III
Mammillary body
Red nucleus
Superior cerebellar peduncle
Mammillothalamic tract

Figure 15-13. Photograph of a sagittal section of the diencephalon through the mammillothalamic tract. Note the relationship between the dorsomedial nucleus, the centromedian nucleus and the pulvinar (Weigert's myelin stain).

clei, the anterodorsal (AD) and anteromedial (AM). The round or polygonal cells composing these nuclei are of medium or small size; they have little chromophilic substance, moderate amounts of yellow pigment and are separated from other thalamic nuclei by a capsule of myelinated fibers. The anterior nuclei receive the mammillothalamic tract and may send some fibers to the mammillary body (471) (Fig. 15-14B). Fibers from the medial mammillary nucleus project to the ipsilateral anteroventral and anteromedial nuclei, while the lateral mammillary nucleus projects bilaterally to the anterodorsal nucleus, but not to other subdivisions of the nuclear group (816). These observations have been confirmed by fluorescent retrograde double labeling technics which also indicate that cells of the lateral mammillary nucleus project fibers to both the thalamus and the midbrain tegmentum (1345). In addition, the anterior nuclei of the thalamus receive as many direct fibers from the fornix as from the mammillothalamic tract (2062). The cortical projections of the anterior nu-

clei are to the cingulate gyrus (areas 23, 24 and 32) via the anterior limb of the internal capsule (Fig. 15-15). The anterodorsal nucleus sends fibers to the posterior cingulate gyrus including the retrosplenial area, while the anteroventral nucleus projects to the middle and posterior cingulate cortex (1841). The anteromedial nucleus projects largely to the anterior cingulate cortex, but its diffuse projections extend into the entire limbic cortex and the orbitofrontal region. Although there is considerable overlap, the cingulate cortex receives most of its input from the anteroventral and anteromedial nuclei (1839). These cortical areas have been considered to project back to the anterior thalamic nuclei (804, 1697), but the bulk of the projections are via the cingulum to the entorhinal cortex (Fig. 18-13) (2090, 2094). Because the entorhinal cortex projects to the hippocampal formation, impulses following this course can affect hypothalamic activities. Fibers passing from the anterior nuclei to the habenular nuclei via the stria medullaris also have been described by some investigators.

The Dorsomedial Nucleus

The dorsomedial nucleus (DM) occupies most of the area between the internal medullary lamina and the periventricular gray (Figs. 15-2, 15-7, 15-10–15-14A and A-16). Three cytologically distinct regions of the nucleus are recognized: (a) a magnocellular portion, located rostrally and dorsomedially, consisting of fairly large, polygonal, deeply staining cells, (b) a larger dorsolateral and caudal parvicellular portion made up of small, pale-staining cells which tend to occur in clusters and (c) a paralaminar portion (pars multiformis) characterized by very large cells occupying a narrow band adjacent to the internal medullary lamina (610, 1395, 1467, 1883, 2318). The nucleus has connections with the centromedian and other intralaminar nuclei and with the lateral nuclear groups. The medial magnocellular division of the dorsomedial nucleus receives fibers from the amygdaloid complex, temporal neocortex and possibly the substantia innominata via the inferior thalamic peduncle (Fig. 15-10) (1817, 2059, 2060, 2705). Autoradiographic studies in the rat indicate that the basolateral amygdaloid nuclei project to the medial part of the dorsomedial nucleus and directly to portions of the anterior limbic cortex (1360). The medial subdivision of the dorsomedial nucleus also receives projections from the pyriform cortex and the olfactory tubercle, which suggests that portions of this nucleus may receive an olfactory input (1360, 1467). The caudal orbitofrontal cortex also has connections with the medial division of the dorsomedial nucleus (1818). Most of these fibers constitute components of the so-called *ansa peduncularis*. The ansa peduncularis consists of fibers of the inferior thalamic peduncle, plus fibers interconnecting the amygdaloid complex and the preoptico-hypothalamic region (1825).

The much larger parvicellular portion of the dorsomedial nucleus is connected by a massive projection with practically the entire frontal cortex rostral to areas 6 and 32 (Figs. 15-14 and 15-15). After extensive prefrontal cortical lesions, or lesions interrupting fibers to this region, nearly all small cells of the dorsomedial nucleus degenerate (804, 1568, 1697, 2318, 2649). Fibers projected by the parvicellular part of this nucleus are organized in such a way that cells in the rostral and caudal parts of the nucleus project to corresponding parts of the prefrontal cortex (1686). Anterograde axoplasmic transport studies indicate that cells of the dorsomedial nucleus project to all parts of the prefrontal cortex (i.e., rostral to the premotor area, area 6) including the cortex on the medial aspect of the hemisphere and the orbitofrontal cortex (2548). Retrograde transport of horseradish peroxidase (HRP) suggests that no cells of the dorsomedial nucleus project to the precentral motor cortex and that only the paralaminar part of the nucleus projects to the premotor area (1310). There are reciprocal connections between the dorsomedial nucleus and the granular frontal cortex (i.e., prefrontal cortex) and between the paralaminar subdivision and the premotor cortex (31). Particularly profuse reciprocal connections exist between area 8 (frontal eye field) and the paralaminar part of the dorsomedial nucleus (1395, 2299). The paralaminar part of the dorsomedial nucleus also receives a substantial projection from the pars reticulata of the substantia nigra (409, 413). It is of interest that although the magnocellular division of the dorsomedial nucleus receives projections from the amygdala, this connection is not reciprocal (1656).

The dorsomedial nucleus is thought to be concerned with integration of certain somatic and visceral impulses (2656). Some impulses relayed to the prefrontal cortex may enter consciousness and may thus influence or produce various feeling tones. Psychosurgical studies (i.e., prefrontal lobotomy) suggest that the dorsomedial nucleus may mediate impulses of an affective nature, and although these vary greatly among individuals, they may constitute part of the emotional experience that contributes to the formation of personality. Prefrontal lobotomy and lesions in the dorsomedial nucleus of the thalamus modify the patient's reaction to chronic pain, but it is doubtful if they eliminate pain.

The Midline Nuclei

The midline nuclei are more or less distinct cell clusters which lie in the periventricular gray matter of the dorsal half of the

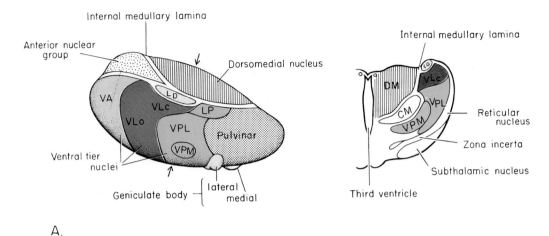

A.

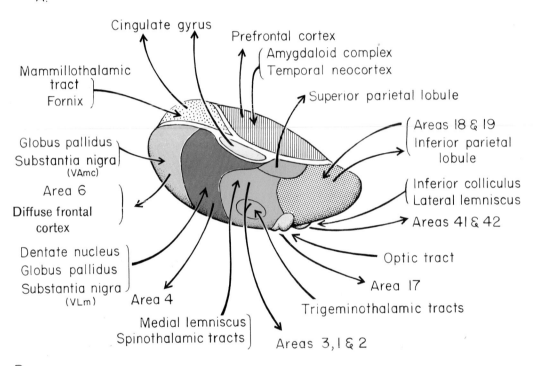

B.

Figure 15-14. Schematic diagrams of the major thalamic nuclei. An oblique dorsolateral view of the thalamus and its major subdivisions is shown in *A*. A transverse section of the thalamus at level of arrows, shown on the right in *A*, indicates: (a) the relationships between VPM and VPL and (b) the location of CM with respect to the internal medullary lamina of the thalamus. In *B*, the principal afferent and efferent projections of particular thalamic subdivisions are indicated. While most cortical areas project fibers back to the thalamic nuclei from which fibers are received, not all of these are shown.

ventricular wall and in the interthalamic adhesion (Figs. 15-11 and 15-12). They are small and difficult to delimit in man, but in the lower vertebrates they, together with some of the intralaminar nuclei, form the largest part of the thalamus (paleothala-

mus). They consist of small, fusiform, rather darkly staining cells resembling preganglionic autonomic neurons (1596), and are believed to be concerned with visceral activities. Efferent fibers from the midline thalamic nuclei have been demonstrated to

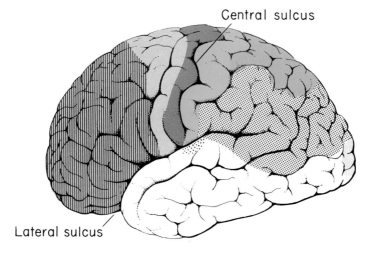

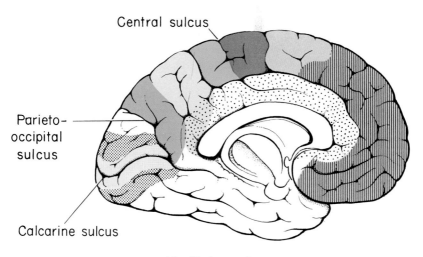

Medial surface

Figure 15-15. Diagram of the left cerebral hemisphere showing the cortical projection areas of thalamic nuclei. The color code is the same as in Figure 15-14. The diffuse projection of the ventral anterior nucleus (VApc) to the frontal lobe appears to largely overlap the projection of the dorsomedial nucleus (DM). Information concerning the cortical projection areas of some thalamic nuclei is incomplete.

project to the amygdaloid nuclear complex (1656). These fibers arise from the paraventricular nucleus, the central nuclear complex and the nucleus reuniens. Other evidence suggests that midline thalamic nuclei may also project to the anterior cingulate cortex (2624). Fine myelinated and unmyelinated fibers coursing in the periventricular gray are thought to relate these nuclei to the hypothalamus.

The more distinct midline cell groups include the *paratenial nucleus*, near the stria medullaris, and the *paraventricular nucleus*, in the dorsal ventricular wall (Fig. 15-11). In an attempt to homologize these ill-defined nuclei with the more developed nuclei of lower mammals, some authorities recognize several cell groups in this periventricular gray: the *nucleus reuniens*, the *rhomboidal nucleus* and the *median cen-*

tral nucleus. The reuniens, rhomboidal and median central nuclei all bear close relationships with the interthalamic adhesion (massa intermedia), when present. The latter structure is reported to be absent in about 30% of human brains (1741).

The Intralaminar Nuclei

The intralaminar nuclei (Figs. 15-6, 15-7, 15-11 and 15-14) are cell groups of variable extent infiltrating the internal medullary lamina, which separates the medial from the lateral thalamic mass. Their cells, although varying in size in the different nuclei, are usually fusiform and dark staining, and they resemble those of the midline nuclei. Their fiber connections are intricate and incompletely understood (Fig. 15-14*B*).

The Centromedian Nucleus (CM). This is the largest and most easily defined of the intralaminar thalamic nuclei (Figs. 15-6, 15-7 and 15-14); other intralaminar nuclei are smaller and some of their boundaries are indistinct. This prominent nucleus is located in the caudal third of the thalamus between the dorsomedial nucleus above and the ventral posterior nucleus below (Figs. 15-6, 15-7, 15-12 and 15-13). It is surrounded by fibers of the internal medullary lamina, except along its medial border, where it merges by interdigitations with the parafascicular nucleus (Figs. 15-6, 15-12 and 15-16). It is composed of small, loosely arranged, ovoid or round cells containing a considerable amount of yellow pigment. Cells in the lateral portion of the nucleus are small, while those in more medial regions bordering the dorsomedial nucleus are larger and more densely arranged. There has been considerable controversy concerning precise delimitation of the centromedian nucleus, particularly with respect to the border separating it from the parafascicular nucleus. According to Mehler (1651) only the ventrolateral small-celled region should be identified as the centromedian nucleus.

The Parafascicular Nucleus (PF). This nucleus lies medial to the centromedian nucleus and ventral to the caudal part of the dorsomedial nucleus (Figs. 15-6, 15-12 and 15-16). Caudally the boundary between the parafascicular nucleus and the centromedian nucleus is indistinct and somewhat arbitrary. The most distinguishing feature of the parafascicular nucleus is that its larger, more deeply stained cells surround the dorsomedial part of the fasciculus retroflexus; portions of the nucleus medial and lateral to this tract show no cytological differences (2651).

The Rostral Intralaminar Nuclei. The paracentral, central lateral and central medial nuclei are all associated with the internal medullary lamina of the thalamus rostral and dorsal to the centromedian nucleus. The paracentral nucleus (PCN) lies in the internal medullary lamina adjacent to the rostral part of the dorsomedial nucleus. Cells are large, dark-staining and multipolar and grouped into clusters between myelinated fiber bundles. Caudally the paracentral nucleus appears to fuse with the central lateral nucleus (CL) which lies dorsal to the centromedian nucleus and lateral to the dorsomedial nucleus (Figs. 15-11, 15-12 and 15-16). The central lateral nucleus is broader than the paracentral nucleus and composed of similar cells. The central medial nucleus lies adjacent to the medial part of the paracentral nucleus (1883, 2557).

Although it is widely recognized that the brain stem reticular formation probably is one of the principal sources of afferent impulses to the intralaminar nuclei of the thalamus, considerable controversy has developed concerning the manner in which these impulses are transmitted rostrally. According to physiological findings (1756, 2422), transmission of ascending impulses in the reticular formation is polysynaptic. Golgi studies of the intrinsic organization of the reticular core do not reveal neurons with short axons (Golgi type II cells), although such neurons might be expected on the basis of physiological evidence (2274). Anatomical studies indicate that "effector" regions of the reticular formation give rise to long ascending fibers which enter the area of the central tegmental tract (266, 281, 1824, 1932, 1933, 2274). Areas of the reticular formation from which the largest number of ascending fibers in this system originate correspond to parts of the nucleus reticularis gigantocellularis and nucleus reticularis ventralis (medulla) and to the nucleus reticularis pontis caudalis (pons) (Figs. 10-10, 11-9, 11-14 and 12-3). The most complete study of the diencephalic projec-

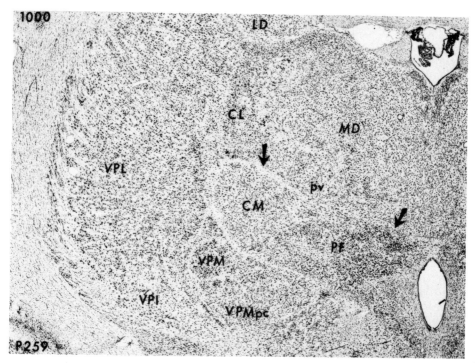

Figure 15-16. Photomicrograph of a transverse section of the thalamus through the ventrobasal complex and the intralaminar nuclei in the monkey. Abbreviations used: *CL*, central lateral nucleus; *CM*, centromedian nucleus; *LD*, lateral dorsal nucleus; *MD*, dorsomedial nucleus; *PF*, parafascicular nucleus, *pv*, ventral paralaminar part of dorsomedial nucleus; *VPI*, ventral posterior inferior nucleus; *VPL*, ventral posterolateral nucleus; *VPM*, ventral posteromedial nucleus; *VPMpc*, parvicellular part of *VPM*. *Arrows* on superior border of the internal medullary lamina define limits of *pv*. Numbers refer to animal and sequential section (cresyl violet, ×22). (Reproduced with permission from T. S. Roberts and K. Akert: *Schweizer Archiv für Neurologie, Neurochirurgie und Psychiatrie,* **92:** 1–43, 1963.)

tion of this system is that of Nauta and Kuypers (1824) based upon silver staining methods. These authors traced fibers from the central tegmental fasciculus into: (a) the centromedian-parafascicular nuclear complex, as well as the paracentral and central lateral nuclei, and (b) the subthalamic region. These ascending reticular projections are chiefly ipsilateral. The above findings have been confirmed in detail by Golgi studies (2274). Because action potentials in the brain stem reticular formation have been recorded with stimulation of almost every type of receptor, it has been presumed that activation of the ascending reticular system is due to "collateral" excitation derived from specific sensory pathways (Chapter 13).

As mentioned earlier (Chapter 10) with respect to the spinothalamic tract, anterolateral cordotomy (232, 1658) produces as-

cending degeneration which passes not only to the ventral posterolateral nucleus and the posterior thalamic nucleus, but also to the intralaminar thalamic nuclei. Unilateral anterolateral cordotomy produces bilateral degeneration in these nuclei which is greatest ipsilaterally, except in the intralaminar nuclei where nearly equal bilateral degeneration is distributed to parts of the paracentral and the central lateral nuclei (Fig. 15-12). These spinal afferents to parts of the intralaminar nuclei follow pathways in the brain stem that are independent of the classic spinothalamic trajectory (1658) and probably are related to a phylogenetically older system.

Other afferent fibers to the intralaminar nuclei originate from the dentate nucleus (501, 1049). Although fibers of the superior cerebellar peduncle have been described as passing to the centromedian nuclei, most of these fibers merely pass through this nucleus to the more rostral intralaminar nuclei. Most of these fibers terminate in the central lateral nucleus (385, 1075, 1654, 1660, 1971, 2419, 2538).

The centromedian (CM) and parafascicular (PF) nuclei receive afferent fibers mainly from forebrain derivatives. Area 4 projects fibers which are distributed throughout the centromedian nucleus, while area 6 projects to the lateral part of the parafascicular nucleus (1651, 1988, 1992). Some fibers to the centromedian-parafascicular complex (CM-PF) reach these nuclei by a circuitous route described by Rinvik (2157). These fibers descend in the internal capsule as far caudally as the junction of midbrain and diencephalon; they separate from the crus cerebri and project rostrally and dorsally to terminate in the CM-PF complex.

Autoradiographic studies confirm that cortical projections to the intralaminar thalamic nuclei arise from broad regions of the frontal lobe and are substantial (31, 1393, 1394). The precentral motor cortex (area 4) projects terminals to the paracentral, central lateral and centromedian thalamic nuclei. The cortical projection to the centromedian nucleus is massive, but greatest in ventral regions of the nucleus; some of these fibers cross the midline to corresponding parts of the same nucleus on the opposite side. The premotor area (area 6) sends afferents to parts of the central lateral nucleus and to the parafascicular nucleus. In the prefrontal cortex, only areas 8 and 9 project to the intralaminar nuclei and these fibers end in the parafascicular nucleus. Although most corticothalamic and thalamocortical projection systems are reciprocal, this generalization does not pertain to the intralaminar thalamic nuclei which have diffuse cortical projections that are in no sense reciprocal.

The centromedian nucleus also receives a large number of pallidal efferent fibers that separate from the thalamic fasciculus at nearly right angles (1313, 1398, 1438, 1825). A considerable part of these fibers are collaterals of pallidofugal fibers passing to the ventral anterior and ventral lateral thalamic nuclei (Figs. 15-14, 15-16, 17-11 and 17-14).

Retrograde transport studies using HRP in the cat confirm the projection of the motor cortex and the medial pallidal segment to the centromedian nucleus and also suggest that afferent fibers to this nucleus may arise from the pars reticulata of the substantia nigra, deep layers of the superior colliculus and the medial and lateral vestibular nuclei (1565). These authors consider it unlikely that the pallidal projection to the centromedian nucleus consists entirely of collaterals of fibers passing to the rostral ventral tier thalamic nuclei. A bilateral projection from the vestibular nuclei to the centromedian nuclei was prominent while that from the brain stem reticular formation was sparse and scattered.

While all of the efferent projections of the intralaminar nuclei are not known, the principal projection of the CM-PF nuclear complex is to the putamen (651, 803, 1234, 1340, 1397, 1567, 1651, 1685, 1814, 1827, 2055, 2115). The smaller and most rostral intralaminar nuclei project fibers to the caudate nucleus. These thalamostriatal fibers follow a wide curved path through the ventral anterior and rostral reticular nuclei of the thalamus, but do not appear to establish terminal connections within the ventral anterior nucleus (1651). Some of these fibers, however, may terminate in portions of the thalamic reticular nucleus (1227). The majority of the afferent projections to the striatum course dorsal to the globus pallidus. Although data are incomplete concerning the patterns of termination of thalamostriate fibers, these fibers end upon spiny striate neurons and some cells in the CM-PF complex project to portions of both the caudate nucleus and the putamen (1340, 1651). These data suggest that the striatum, like the cerebral cortex, is dependent upon thalamic input.

The intralaminar nuclei of the thalamus have long been regarded as having no cortical projections. This conclusion is based upon the absence of retrograde cell changes in these nuclei following virtually complete decortication (510, 2054, 2318, 2650, 2651) and the absence of degeneration traceable from lesions in the centromedian nucleus to any part of the cortex (471, 472, 1827). These observations have been difficult to reconcile with physiological studies indicating that the intralaminar nuclei are of extreme importance in the control and regulation of electrocortical activity over broad regions of the cerebral cortex. The view has been widely held that the intralaminar thalamic nuclei give rise to the so-called non-specific cortical afferents (1531), but this concept was not based on solid anatomical evidence. The introduction of retrograde transport technics utilizing HRP provided a means to further explore the projections of the intralaminar thalamic nuclei. Injections of HRP into the putamen produced intense labeling of the cells in the CM-PF complex and some labeling of cells in posterior parts of the central lateral nucleus, while HRP injections in various cortical areas produced intense labeling of cells in corresponding thalamic relay nuclei and relatively light labeling of cells in portions of the intralaminar nuclei (1234). These results have been interpreted to mean that the intralaminar thalamic nuclei project profusely to the striatum (i.e., thalamostriatal fibers) and sparsely and diffusely upon broad regions of the cerebral cortex. Cortical projections from the intralaminar thalamic nuclei are regarded as collaterals of thalamostriate fibers. These collateral fibers have overlapping cortical terminations with fibers of at least one cortical thalamic relay nucleus. Autoradiographic studies of projections of the intralaminar thalamic nuclei stress the dorsoventral and rostrocaudal organization of thalamostriate fibers and indicate that these fibers end in mosaic patterns similar to corticostriate projections (1078). Collaterals of the thalamostriate fibers, projecting to broad cortical areas, end in layers V and VI of the cerebral cortex.

The intralaminar thalamic nuclei show a striking development in primates and man, in relation to thalamic relay nuclei, suggesting that they may constitute a complex intrathalamic regulating mechanism concerned with diverse functions (463, 500a, 2079). A wide range of different functions have been ascribed to these nuclei. The intralaminar thalamic nuclei have been considered to serve as: (a) the thalamic pacemaker controlling electrocortical activities (618, 619, 1208, 2080), (b) part of a nonspecific sensory system (35, 2233), (c) a component of a central pain mechanism (33, 709, 1494) and (d) a modulator of striatal activities (1565). Most anatomical evidence indicates the spinal, trigeminal, reticular and cerebellar projections to the intralaminar thalamic nuclei end in the central lateral nucleus (213, 1230, 1565, 1651, 1824). This nucleus may be particularly concerned with pain mechanisms and sensory integration. The larger CM-PF nuclear complex appears more closely related to motor functions in that it receives major projections from the motor and premotor cortex and from the globus pallidus; this nuclear complex projects mainly to the striatum. The extent to which CM-PF may funnel sensory information into the striatum remains to be determined but it is suggested that impulses from the vestibular nuclei and deep layers of the superior colliculus may follow this route (1565). In any case there are suggestions that the different functions may be related to particular nuclei of the intralaminar thalamic group.

The Lateral Nuclear Group

The lateral nuclear group begins as a narrow strip some distance from the anterior limit of the thalamus, enlarges posteriorly and merges caudally with the pulvinar. This group consists of three nuclear masses arranged in rostrocaudal sequence, the lateral dorsal nucleus, the lateral posterior nucleus and the pulvinar (Fig. 15-14).

The Lateral Dorsal Nucleus (LD). This nucleus begins near the caudal part of the anterior nuclear group and extends caudally along the dorsal surface of the thalamus (Fig. 15-13). A well-defined myelin capsule surrounds the nucleus which in myelin-sheath-stained sections has light staining properties similar to that of the anterior nuclear group. The nucleus achieves its largest dimensions dorsal to the portion of the internal medullary lamina which contains the central lateral nucleus (Figs. 15-9 and 15-16). Topographically this nucleus has been considered as a posterior extension of the anterior nuclear group (1506, 2657). While many authors accept that this nucleus projects to the posterior parietal cortex (Fig. 15-15), recent data indicate that its fibers pass mainly to the cingulate gyrus, although some pass to the supralimbic cortex of the parietal lobe (1507, 1836). Retrograde transport studies indicate that HRP injected into all parts of the limbic cortex, except for the rostral region, labels

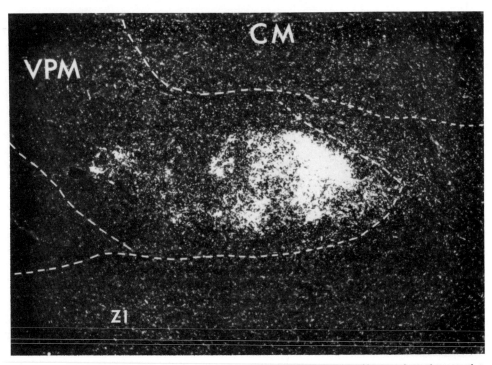

Figure 15-17. Photomicrograph of an autoradiograph demonstrating transport of isotope from the rostrolateral nucleus of the solitary fasciculus to the ipsilateral ventral posteromedial nucleus (pars parvicellularis). Abbreviations used: *CM*, centromedian nucleus; *VPM*, somatic part of the ventral posteromedial nucleus; *ZI*, zona incerta. (Reproduced with permission from R. M. Beckstead et al.: *Journal of Comparative Neurology*, **190:** 259–282, 1980.) (See Fig. 11-22.)

cells in the lateral dorsal nucleus (1839). The lateral dorsal nucleus also sends and receives fibers from the precuneal cortex. Afferent fibers to this nucleus are poorly understood.

The Lateral Posterior Nucleus (LP). This nucleus lies caudal, lateral and ventral to the lateral dorsal nucleus, and is composed of medium-sized cells evenly distributed (Figs. 15-14 and 15-18). The nucleus is irregular in shape and lies dorsal to the ventral posterolateral nucleus and adjacent to the lateral medullary lamina. Caudally the nucleus merges with the oral and medial parts of the pulvinar, from which it is not easily distinguished (1883). Unlike the lateral dorsal nucleus it has no myelin capsule. The input to this thalamic nucleus is poorly understood but it may receive inputs from adjacent primary relay nuclei, especially the ventral posterior nucleus (2657). Degeneration studies in the monkey and cat indicate that the superior and inferior parietal lobules project upon the lateral posterior nucleus; some fibers from the inferior parietal lobule also project to the lateral dorsal nucleus (1993, 2186). Area 5 of the parietal cortex, constituting part of the superior parietal lobe, has been demonstrated to transport isotope to laminar arrays of terminals distributed throughout the lateral posterior nucleus (1246). Some of these thalamic neurons appear to have reciprocal cortical connections. Retrograde transport studies indicate that the lateral posterior nucleus projects upon areas 5 and 7 (1957). Electrophysiological studies demonstrate that cortical areas 5 and 7 in monkey respond to stimulation of peripheral receptors and that both of these areas receive association fibers from the primary somesthetic cortex (1242, 1768). Area 7 in the monkey, considered the equivalent of the greatly expanded inferior parietal lobule in man, is concerned with the integration of sensory modalities that serve important cognitive and symbolic functions, and appears to have a heterogeneous afferent input (635).

The Pulvinar (P). This large nuclear mass, forming the most caudal portion of

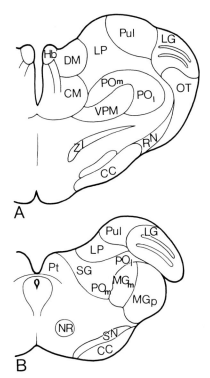

Figure 15-18. Outline drawings through two levels of the caudal thalamus in the cat showing relationships of the nuclei of the posterior thalamic complex to other thalamic nuclei. Two divisions of the posterior thalamic nuclei are recognized, a medial (*PO$_m$*) and a lateral (*PO$_l$*). In *B*, the posterior thalamic nuclei lie medial and dorsal to the magnocellular part of the medial geniculate nucleus (*MGm*); the medial nucleus, *PO$_m$*, appears continuous with the suprageniculate nucleus (*SG*). In *A*, PO$_m$ and PO$_l$ lie dorsal and lateral to the ventral posterior medial nucleus (*VPM*) and immediately caudal to the ventral posterolateral nucleus (*VPL*). Abbreviations used: *CC*, crus cerebri; *CM*, centromedian nucleus; *DM*, dorsomedial nucleus; *Hb*, habenular nucleus; *LG*, lateral geniculate body; *LP*, lateral posterior nucleus; *MG$_p$*, medial geniculate, parvicellular part; *NR*, red nucleus; *OT*, optic tract; *Pt*, pretectum; *Pul*, pulvinar; *RN*, reticular nucleus of thalamus; *SN*, substantia nigra; *ZI*, zone incerta. (Modified from Jones and Powell (1243).)

the thalamus, overhangs the geniculate bodies and the dorsolateral surface of the midbrain (Figs. 15-4–15-6 and 15-14). Because the pulvinar exhibits considerable cytological uniformity it is subdivided on a topographic basis into four parts: (a) a pars oralis, located between the ventral posterolateral and centromedian nuclei, (b) a pars inferior, located ventrally between the medial and lateral geniculate bodies, (c) a pars

medialis forming the medial half of the pulvinar and (d) a pars lateralis extending along the external medullary lamina which is traversed by fibers (1883). The basic element of the pulvinar is a lightly stained, medium-sized, multipolar cell, whose density and pattern of arrangement varies in the different subdivisions. Cells in the oral division of the pulvinar are small, light-staining and less dense than in any other part. The pars inferior, separated from the main body of the pulvinar by fibers of the brachium of the superior colliculus, is composed of large dark cells scattered among medium-sized elements. Small cells in the lateral pulvinar are arranged in oblique stripes separated by fiber bundles extending from the external medullary lamina. The medial nucleus contains evenly distributed medium-sized cells and very few fibers.

The nuclei of the pulvinar do not appear to receive inputs from long ascending sensory pathways, but the inferior division receives a projection from the superficial layers of the superior colliculus (154, 1039, 1941). This projection has been shown to represent topographically the contralateral visual field, with the lower visual field represented dorsomedially and the upper field ventrolaterally. Both the inferior pulvinar and the adjacent portion of the lateral pulvinar have reciprocal connections with occipital cortex, including striate cortex (1864). The inferior pulvinar and the adjacent lateral pulvinar each contain a representation of the contralateral visual hemifield and project retinotopically upon: (a) cortical areas 18 and 19 where fibers end in layers IV, III and I (155) and (b) the striate cortex (area 17) where fibers terminate upon the supragranular layers (2139). In contrast the dorsal lateral geniculate nucleus projects retinotopically largely upon the striate cortex (area 17) where fibers end upon cells in layer IV. These findings indicate three visuotopically organized inputs from the thalamus (lateral geniculate body, inferior pulvinar and adjacent lateral pulvinar) to the primary visual cortex which terminate upon different layers. Fibers from the inferior pulvinar and the adjacent lateral pulvinar passing to the supragranular layers of area 17 may be involved in visual association pathways (2139). Projections from the inferior pulvinar to cortical areas 17, 18 and 19 constitute the final link in an extrageniculate visual pathway. The lateral pulvinar does not receive a visual input from the superior colliculus, but parts of this nucleus have reciprocal connections with all recognized areas of the visual cortex.

The lateral nucleus of the pulvinar (other than that portion adjacent to the inferior pulvinar) projects to temporal cortex and receives reciprocal projections from the same region (2342, 2345, 2577). The medial pulvinar appears to have more distant projections than most divisions of the pulvinar in that fibers project to part of the frontal eye field (area 8) and to a small region of the lateral orbital cortex (222, 2576). These cortical areas have reciprocal projections with the medial pulvinar.

The Ventral Nuclear Mass

The ventral nuclear mass of the thalamus usually is divided into three separate nuclei: the *ventral anterior*, the *ventral lateral* and the *ventral posterior*. The ventral anterior nucleus is the most rostral and smallest of this group. The ventral posterior nucleus, the largest and most posterior of the group, is further subdivided into the ventral posterolateral and ventral posteromedial nuclei (Figs. 15-12, 15-14, 15-16 and 15-17). Although the *medial* and *lateral geniculate bodies* together constitute the *metathalamus*, these well defined nuclear masses may be considered as a caudal continuation of the ventral nuclear mass (Figs. 15-4, 15-5 and 15-14). The ventral nuclear group and the metathalamus constitute the largest division of the thalamus concerned with relaying impulses from other portions of the neuraxis to specific parts of the cerebral cortex. The most caudal parts of this complex are concerned with relaying impulses of specific sensory systems to cortical regions, while more rostral nuclei (ventral anterior and ventral lateral nuclei) relay impulses from the corpus striatum and cerebellum.

The Ventral Anterior Nucleus (VA). This subdivision of the thalamus lies in the extreme rostral part of the ventral nuclear mass where it is bounded anteriorly and ventrolaterally by the thalamic reticular nucleus (Fig. 15-14). Rostrally this nucleus occupies the entire thalamic region lateral to the anterior nuclear group (Fig. 15-9),

but caudally it becomes restricted to a more medial region. The mammillothalamic tract passes through the ventral anterior nucleus but does not form its medial border. The nucleus is composed of large and medium-sized multipolar cells arranged in clusters. The clustering of cells is particularly evident in rostrolateral parts of the nucleus due to thick myelinated fiber bundles coursing longitudinally within the nucleus.

A distinctive part of the nucleus adjacent to the mammillothalamic tract and along the ventral border of the nucleus is composed of large, dark, densely arranged cells (Fig. 13-26*B*). This subdivision, called the magnocellular part (VAmc) (1883), extends further caudal than the principal part of the ventral anterior nucleus (VApc). Thus there are two distinctive cytological subdivisions of the ventral anterior nucleus. Each of these subdivisions receives fibers from different sources. Afferent fibers to the ventral anterior nucleus (VApc) arise from the medial segment of the globus pallidus (Fig. 17-14) and reach the nucleus via the lenticular fasciculus and ansa lenticularis (1313, 1438, 1825, 1931, 2112, 2277). These fibers enter the thalamic fasciculus, turn dorsolaterally and are distributed in a rostrolateral direction within the ventral anterior nucleus. Pallidothalamic fibers projecting to the rostral ventral tier thalamic nuclei (i.e., VApc and VLo) appear organized in a specific manner (1398). Rostral parts of the medial pallidal segment project most profusely to VApc. More caudal parts of the medial pallidal segment project fibers to parts of the ventral lateral nucleus (VLo).

Some projections from the contralateral deep cerebellar nuclei also project to the ventral anterior nucleus (VApc) which appear to terminate largely in caudal and lateral portions of the nucleus. These projections are more prominent in the cat than in the monkey (1075, 1260, 1971, 2419). Projections to VApc from the deep cerebellar nuclei appear to represent a rostral extension of the principal termination in the ventral lateral nucleus. This is an example of an ascending fiber system that does not terminate entirely within a commonly recognized cytoarchitectonic subdivision of the thalamus (1075).

The magnocellular part of the ventral anterior nucleus (VAmc) receives a significant fiber projection from the substantia nigra (20, 409, 419, 504, 736). Nigrothalamic fibers arise from the pars reticularis, pass medially and rostrally through Forel's field H and follow a course that parallels that of the mammillothalamic tract (Figs. 13-25, 13-26, 15-2 and 15-9) (413). Terminals of nigrothalamic fibers form a dense felt-work about groups of cells in VAmc.

Cortical projections to the VA have been described in autoradiographic studies. Cortical area 6, projects primarily to VApc while fibers from area 8 terminate in VAmc (1394, 1395); fibers from the primary motor area do not reach any part of the nucleus (1393). Other afferent fibers, arising from the intralaminar and midline nuclei, may account for some of the characteristics of the nonspecific thalamic system exhibited by this nucleus (2277).

Information concerning the efferent projections of the VA is conflicting and incomplete. Some studies indicate that nearly all cells of the VA degenerate following hemidecortication (114, 1930), while others indicate virtually no cell changes in this nucleus (2651). In man over 50% of the cells in this nucleus remain following hemispherectomy (2054). A systematic investigation indicates that no significant cell changes in VA follow ablations limited to single cortical areas, including area 6, frequently cited as receiving a projection from this nucleus (373, 803). Cell loss and morphological alterations of remaining cells in VA were noted after large cortical ablations. This evidence suggested that the VA may have unusually widespread frontal cortical projections, probably on the basis of collateral systems.

Although it has been suggested that VAmc does not project to the cerebral cortex (2783), both Golgi and degeneration studies revealed projections from VAmc to the caudal and medial orbital cortex (373, 2277). Retrograde transport studies based upon HRP indicate a limited number of labeled neurons in VAmc after injections of rostral parts of the frontal lobe (1310). A systematic study of the thalmocortical projections to the frontal lobe using HRP indicates that obliquely oriented bands of cells in VApc project to frontal cortex rostral to the precentral gyrus; cells in medial bands project to the most rostral regions of

the prefrontal cortex while lateral bands of cells pass to more caudal regions, including portions of the premotor cortex (1310). In this study longitudinal bands of thalamic neurons were related to transverse strips of frontal cortex.

Subcortical projections from VA have been alluded to by many authors (1686, 2651), but their determination has been difficult because this nucleus is traversed by fibers from many sources. In spite of these difficulties it appears established that: (a) VAmc projects fibers to VApc, although this connection is not reciprocal, and (b) portions of VApc project to the intralaminar nuclei and the dorsomedial nucleus (373, 2277). Fibers from VA do not cross the midline to contralateral thalamic nuclei and none of the fibers from this nucleus project to the caudate nucleus.

Physiological data (1209, 1210, 2421) indicate that the ventral anterior nucleus may be functionally related to the intralaminar nuclei of the thalamus in that responses in widespread cortical areas can be evoked by repeated low frequency stimulation of the nucleus. Other authors have demonstrated that VA is essential for the recruiting response and that lesions in this nucleus block the responses elicited by stimulating the nonspecific thalamic nuclei (2350). The *recruiting response* is a surface negative response evoked by repetitive stimulation of the midline and intralaminar nuclei that waxes and wanes and can be recorded over broad areas of the cerebral cortex. The ventral anterior nucleus appears to be the pre-eminent site among thalamic nuclei for production of the recruiting response. Efferent projections from VA seems to form an anatomical substrate well suited for diffuse synchronous discharge to large regions of the frontal cortex and thalamus. Anatomical and physiological data are in agreement concerning the special role of the orbitofrontal cortex in "triggering" the recruiting response. This cortical response is abolished by ablations of the orbitofrontal cortex (2610) and reversibly diminished by cryogenic blockade of this cortical region (2350). Although VAmc has been considered to project preferentially to the orbitofrontal cortex, retrograde HRP studies (1310) suggest that the rostral midline thalamic nuclei may be the major thalamic source of afferents to this cortical region. The ventral anterior thalamic nucleus appears to exhibit characteristics of both the specific and nonspecific thalamic nuclei.

The Ventral Lateral Nucleus (VL). This nucleus, caudal to the ventral anterior nucleus, is composed of small and large neurons that show considerable differences in various parts of the nucleus (Figs. 15-10 and 15-11). This nucleus has been subdivided into three main parts (1883): (a) pars oralis (VLo), (b) pars caudalis (VLc) and (c) pars medialis (VLm). The largest subdivision (VLo) consists of numerous deep staining cells arranged in clusters. The pars caudalis (VLc) is less cellular but formed of scattered large cells. The pars medialis (VLm) begins ventral to VA and extends caudally toward the subthalamic region. A crescent-shaped thalamic area in the monkey caudal to VAmc and medial to VLo, designated as "area x" (1883), appears on the basis of connectivity to be an integral part of the ventral lateral nuclear complex (373, 1654, 1971).

Cerebellar efferent fibers contained in the superior cerebellar peduncle decussate in the mesencephalon and project profusely to the contralateral ventral lateral nucleus. While there is general agreement that cerebellar efferents to the thalamus terminate in regions rostral to those of the medial lemniscus, there have been discrepancies concerning the precise nuclear subdivisions which receive these fibers (1971, 2567). Cerebellar efferent fibers have been described as terminating in all subdivisions of the VL, except for the medial part of VLm, in portions of the VA and in portions of the ventral posterolateral nucleus (VPLo) (441, 1260, 1654, 1708, 2419). In addition cerebellar efferent fibers project to "area x" and the central lateral nucleus. In the monkey cerebellar projections to VA appear to be very modest (1260, 2419), but in the cat these fibers terminate in extensive regions of the nucleus (1075). Both degeneration and autoradiographic studies indicate that efferents from the deep cerebellar nuclei terminate in VLo, VLc, "area x," the central lateral nucleus (CL), the paralaminar part of the dorsomedial nucleus (DMpl) and the oral part of the VPL (441, 1260, 1654, 1708, 2419). Other investigators support most of these observations, but suggest that few, if any, cerebellar efferent fibers terminate in VLo which has long been regarded as a major thalamic terminus of this system (1402, 1403, 1971, 2538). This view is supported by retrograde transport studies which indicate that HRP injections confined to VLo in the thalamus retrogradely label only cells in the medial pallidal segment (2567). This same study has shown that HRP injections in VLc and VPLo retrogradely label cells in the contralateral deep cerebellar nuclei. The unresolved question is whether cerebellar and pallidal efferent terminations overlap in VLo (1075).

Pallidofugal fibers arising from the medial pallidal segment project to the ventral lateral nucleus of the thalamus via the thalamic fasciculus. The major projection from the globus pallidus is to the pars oralis, VLo, and the lateral part of the pars medialis (VLm) (1313, 1398, 1825). Pallidofugal fibers also project rostrally to ventral anterior nucleus (VApc) and give off collateral fibers to the centromedian nucleus (CM) (Figs. 17-11 and 17-14). Pallidothalamic projections are topographically organized and the most profuse projections to VLo arise from caudal regions of the medial pallidal segment (1398). These observations have been confirmed by retrograde transport studies (2567). The pars medialis of the ventral lateral nucleus (VLm) receives efferent projections from the medial pallidal segment and the pars reticulata of the substantia nigra but these are not overlapping. The medial part of the VLm receives nigral efferents while the lateral part of this nucleus receives pallidal efferents (409, 413, 1313, 1398).

It has long been presumed that the cerebellar and pallidal efferent fibers converged and terminated in VLo (and perhaps parts of VA) in overlapping fashion (1654). This view has been challenged by new data which suggest that cerebellar, pallidal and nigral efferents to VA and VL do not overlap but end in distinctive regions of the rostral ventral tier thalamic nuclei (409, 1075, 1313, 1398, 1971, 2567). This hypothesis presumes that integration of cerebellar and striopallidal activities takes place in the motor cortex since there is no anatomical evidence of internuclear connections at the thalamic level. Physiological studies offer some support for two separate systems regulating motor activity in that: (a) the cerebellum provides control for fast movements and (b) the striopallidum provides modulating influences over slower "ramp" movements (614, 615).

The ventral lateral nucleus of the thalamus receives a considerable number of fibers from the precentral cortex (463, 1478, 1479, 1686, 2615). These corticofugal fibers pass to both the pars oralis and the pars caudalis of VL (1883). Both areas 4 and 6 project profusely upon the ventral lateral nucleus, the thalamic reticular nucleus and the centromedian-parafascicular (CM-PF) complex (92, 971, 1988, 1990, 1992, 2157). Autoradiographic studies in the monkey demonstrate that area 4 projects to VLo, VLm, VLc and VPLo as well as to CM, the paracentral nucleus (PCN) and the central lateral nucleus (CL) (1393). The projection to VLc from area 4 is not as impressive as that from area 6, which also projects to "area x" (1394). The cortical projections of area 4 upon VLo and VPLo are topographically arranged.

Connections of the VL with the precentral cortex are reciprocal and topically arranged. Medial parts of the nucleus send fibers to the face area, lateral parts send fibers to the leg area and fibers from intermediate portions of the nucleus pass to cortical regions representing the arm and trunk (2650, 2655). Most of these fibers pass to area 4, but some may reach area 6 (Fig. 15-15). This topical arrangement of thalamocortical fibers passing to the precentral cortex is considered as the anatomical expression of the functional independence of different body parts in the primary motor area.

Retrograde transport studies based upon multiple injections of HRP into the precentral cortex result in labeling of cells in VLo, VLc and VPLo, indicating that these nuclei have reciprocal connections with the motor cortex (1310, 2445). Similar HRP injections of the postcentral gyrus do not label cells in any of the ventral lateral nucleus or in VPLo. It had been postulated that VPLo might receive sensory information from group I muscle afferents and convey this information to cortical area 3a in the depths of the central sulcus. These fibers were

thought to reach VPLo via the posterior column nuclei, but neither anterograde or retrograde transport studies support this thesis (2567). Physiological data indicate that the motor cortex is topographically organized in such a way that the caudal motor cortex, adjacent to the central sulcus, influences control of distal musculature, while more rostral motor cortex has control of proximal and axial musculature (2445). Both physiological and anatomical studies have shown that neurons in the ventral lateral nucleus of the thalamus have monosynaptic connections with corticospinal tract neurons and can exert potent influences upon the output of the motor cortex (2450, 2784). Through its inputs which arise from the deep cerebellar nucleus, the globus pallidus and the substantia nigra, the ventral lateral nucleus of the thalamus makes important contributions to the initiation of movement, the control of muscle tone and the regulation of cortical reflexes (882, 1211, 2355).

The Ventral Posterior Nucleus (VP). This nucleus, whose cells are among the largest in the thalamus, is composed of two main portions, the *ventral posteromedial* and the *ventral posterolateral* (Figs. 15-7, 15-12 and 15-14. The smallest subdivision of the VP is the *ventral posterior inferior nucleus* which lies ventrally adjacent to the thalamic reticular nucleus beneath parts of both the ventral posteromedial and posterolateral nuclei (Fig. 15-16). The VP is the largest primary somatic sensory relay nucleus of the thalamus and is referred to as the ventrobasal complex.

The Ventral Posterolateral Nucleus (VPL). This nucleus has been subdivided into a pars oralis (VPLo), characterized by very large, relatively uniform cells sparsely distributed, and a pars caudalis (VPLc) characterized by a wide range of cell size and a high cellular density. Both divisions of the nucleus contain medium-sized fiber bundles radiating in an oblique dorsal direction.

Three pathways convey somesthetic impulses from the spinal cord and somatosensory relay nuclei in the medulla: (a) the medial lemniscus, (b) the spinothalamic tract and (c) the cervicothalamic tract. In the cat the spinothalamic tract does not project to VPL of the thalamus but terminations are seen in other locations (213, 1230). The spinocervicothalamic system is particularly well developed in carnivores but also exists in primates (992, 2573, 2575). The two principal long ascending somesthetic pathways projecting to the thalamus in primates and man are the medial lemniscus (230, 232, 464, 1643, 2117, 2651) and the spinothalamic tracts (172, 229, 232, 464, 1658, 2651).

Fibers of the medial lemniscus course through the brain stem without supplying collateral or terminal fibers to the reticular formation, and enter the VPL (Fig. 15-14). Although older studies suggested that fibers of the medial lemniscus terminated profusely in all parts of VPL, more recent data indicate terminations almost entirely within VPLc (212, 1260, 2567). Degeneration and autoradiographic studies demonstrate a mediolateral topographical organization in the contralateral VPLc in which fibers originating from the cuneate nucleus terminate medially while those arising from the gracile nucleus end in the lateral part of VPLc (464, 1260, 2651). Small injections of HRP made into VPLo result in retrograde transport of the enzyme to cells of the deep cerebellar nuclei, but not to cells in posterior column nuclei (2567). Injections of HRP into VPLc result in retrograde labeling of cells in nuclei gracilis and cuneatus. Fibers of the medial lemniscus establish predominantly axodendritic contacts with cells in VPLc. In autoradiographs labeled terminals of medial lemniscus fibers, represented by silver grains, appear uniformly distributed and do not form patchy aggregations of silver grains, as commonly found in thalamic nuclei receiving cerebellar efferent fibers. With degeneration methods a small number of terminals were found in the medial part of the posterior thalamic nucleus, near the magnocellular medial geniculate nucleus (212) but terminations in this region were not found in autoradiographic studies (1260, 2567).

The spinothalamic tracts form a far less discrete ascending sensory pathway than the medial lemniscus and in the spinal cord they are intermingled with fibers destined for multiple sites in the brain stem. Much of our information concerning the ccurse and terminations of the spinothalamic tracts has been based upon the study of

degeneration following anterolateral cordotomy or hemisection of the spinal cord (229, 232, 1658). The spinothalamic tract, and fiber systems ascending with it, contribute a large number of projections and collaterals to various portions of the brain stem reticular formation at all levels. Fibers of the spinothalamic tract occupy a distinctive retro-olivary position in the medulla but become closely associated with the medial lemniscus in the pons. In the rostral midbrain spinothalamic fibers lie dorsal to the medial lemniscus and form a fairly discrete tract (Fig. 13-6). At the midbrain-diencephalic junction fibers of the spinothalamic tract enter the thalamus at the dorsomedial border of the medial geniculate nucleus. Fibers of the spinothalamic tract terminate mainly in three thalamic nuclei: (a) the medial part of the posterior thalamic nucleus, located medial and rostral to the magnocellular part of the medial geniculate nucleus (Fig. 15-5), (b) the ventral posterolateral nucleus (Fig. 15-6) and (c) the central lateral nucleus (CL) of the intralaminar group (Fig. 15-12) (213, 229, 232, 1297, 1302, 1650, 1653, 1655, 1658). Terminals in the posterior thalamic nucleus were most numerous ventromedially, while those in VPL were distributed unevenly over the entire nucleus (213). In the central lateral nucleus terminals were distributed about clusters of neurons. In addition to the above major terminations some spinothalamic fibers end in the transitional zone between VPL and VL (213, 1230). Ascending spinothalamic fibers are distributed bilaterally in VPLc, CL and the medial part of the posterior thalamic nucleus, but contralateral terminations are less numerous (213, 229, 232, 1658). It is not entirely clear where these fibers cross to the opposite side, but some fibers appear to cross in the posterior commissure, while others cross at lower brain stem levels. Anatomical data provide no evidence that fibers of the lateral and ventral spinothalamic tracts have distinctive thalamic terminations (1297) and the concept of separating this system into two tracts at spinal levels has been questioned.

The cervicothalamic tract, arising from the lateral cervical nucleus in the upper cervical spinal cord is particularly well developed in carnivores, which lack a typical spinothalamic tract terminating in VPL. Cells in the posterior horn of the spinal gray give rise to fibers of the spinocervical tract which ascend uncrossed in the lateral funiculus and end upon cells of the lateral cervical nucleus (1748, 1749, 2517). The lateral cervical nucleus gives rise to fibers that cross in the first and second cervical segments in the anterior white commissure and ascend in the brain stem in association with the medial lemniscus (210). Fibers of the cervicothalamic tract enter the thalamus via the medial lemniscus and terminate upon cells in the medial and lateral parts of VPL (210, 335, 1421). Some fibers of this tract are described as terminating in the medial part of the posterior thalamic nucleus (210). Thalamic projections of the cervicothalamic tract are entirely contralateral and no appreciable difference in thalamic terminations could be correlated with lesions in rostral or caudal parts of the lateral cervical nucleus. Comparisons of the pattern of thalamic terminations of the spinothalamic tract in the monkey with that of the cervicothalamic tract in the cat reveal striking similarities with respect to VPL. The combined thalamic terminations of the cervicothalamic and spinothalamic tracts in the cat closely resemble the total spinothalamic tract projection in the monkey (213).

Physiological studies (1766, 1767, 2019, 2020, 2214, 2215) indicate the precise and orderly fashion in which the contralateral body surface is represented in the VPL (external portion of the ventrobasal complex). There is a complete, although distorted, image of the body form; volume representation of a given part of the body is related to its effectiveness as a tactile organ (i.e., to its innervation density). Cervical segments are represented most medially and sacral segments most laterally. The thoracic and lumbar regions are represented only dorsally, while the regions concerned with the distal parts of the limbs extend ventrally. Each neuron of this complex is related to a restricted, specific and unchanging receptive field on the contralateral side of the body. Each neuron of the ventrobasal complex can be activated by either tactile stimulation of the skin, or mechanical alteration of deep structures (especially joint rotation), but by only one

of these. These neurons are regarded as place specific, modality specific, and concerned, almost exclusively, with the perception of tactile sense and position sense (kinesthesis). The functional properties of these thalamic neurons depends upon synaptic connections so secure that they are virtually unaffected by anesthesia (2020). Rostral parts of the ventrobasal complex which correspond to VPLo appear to have functional properties different from more caudal regions (VPLc) which receive fibers of the medial lemniscus (2020). Neurons in VPLo were described as having very large, and sometimes bilateral, receptive fields activated only by prolonged manipulation of deep tissue. Few cells of the ventrobasal complex appear to be activated by noxious stimuli (2019).

Although the terminology used by these authors differs from that used here, it is generally accepted that these superbly defined principles apply to man. The inner portion of the ventrobasal complex, known as the ventral posteromedial nucleus, contains the representation of the contralateral head, face and intraoral structures.

The Ventral Posteromedial Nucleus (VPM). This crescent-shaped nucleus with a relatively light-staining neuropil lies medial to the ventral posterolateral nucleus and lateral to the curved boundary of the centromedian nucleus (Figs. 15-6, 15-7, 15-12, 15-14 and 15-16). The VPM consists of two distinct parts: (a) a principal part composed of both small and large cells, designated simply as VPM, and (b) a small celled, light-staining part which occupies the medial apex of this arcuate-shaped nucleus, referred to as the pars parvicellularis (VPMpc). The principal part of VPM receives somatic afferent fibers from receptors in the head, face and intraoral structures, while VPMpc is concerned with taste (Fig. 15-17).

The precise boundaries of VPM are best defined on the basis of its fiber connections. The VPM receives ascending secondary trigeminal fibers which include: (a) crossed fibers from the spinal and principal sensory trigeminal nuclei, which ascend in association with the medial lemniscus (402), and (b) uncrossed fibers of the dorsal trigeminal tract (379, 2559), originating from the dorsal part of the principal sensory nucleus of N.

V. Retrograde transport of HRP from VPM in the cat and monkey labels, cells in the contralateral spinal trigeminal nucleus, particularly in the caudal half of the interpolar subdivision, and in ventral portions of the principal trigeminal nucleus (330). Ipsilaterally labeled cells are largely confined to the dorsomedial division of the principal nucleus which gives rise to the dorsal trigeminal tract. Some impulses from stretch receptors in the facial musculature may reach the VPM, but the pathways are not known. Experimental evidence (171, 1767) indicates that tactile impulses from the face and intraoral structures are transmitted bilaterally to parts of the VPM.

Although the central pathways conveying gustatory sense have been poorly understood, there is good reason to believe that sensory impulses concerned with taste are represented in the medial small-celled portion of the ventral posteromedial nucleus (VPMpc). Electrical stimulation of the chorda tympanic and glossopharyngeal nerves has been shown to evoke potentials in VPMpc with relatively short latencies (156, 193, 707) and VPMpc does not appear to respond to tactile stimuli from body surfaces (1767, 2214). Gustatory representation in the rat is said to be bilateral, while in the cat and monkey it is predominantly ipsilateral. Benjamin and Akert (157) have shown that ablations of the cortical taste area in the rat produce retrograde degeneration of thalamic neurons confined to VPMpc. Lesions in medial parts of the VPM in experimental animals impair taste (64, 198, 1951).

Gustatory impulses received by primary afferents in cranial nerves in the rat pass to the rostral part of the nucleus of the solitary fasciculus which relays impulses ipsilaterally to a secondary "pontine taste area" (1847, 1848). The "pontine taste area" in the rat is a wedged-shaped area of small cells situated between the mesencephalic root of the trigeminal tract and the superior cerebellar peduncle. Cells in this area lie on both sides of the superior cerebellar peduncle and are commonly referred to as the parabrachial nuclei (Fig. 12-30). Degeneration from lesions in these nuclei has been traced bilaterally via the dorsomedial tegmentum to VPMpc. Collaterals of fibers from this pontine taste area, described as passing to ventral forebrain regions, are considered as direct links to neural regions that may influence ingestive behavior. In the monkey isotope deposited in the nucleus of the solitary fasciculus, rostral to the entrance of vagal fibers, labels an ipsilateral bundle of fibers ascending directly to VPMpc via the central tegmental tract (Figs. 11-22 and 15-17) (141). Tritiated amino acids labeling intermediate parts of the nuclei of the solitary fasciculus were traced in ipsilateral fibers to both the parabrachial nuclei and VPMpc. HPR injections in VPMpc retrogradely labeled cells only in the lateral subdivision of the rostral part of the nucleus solitarius. These observations provide an understanding of the pathways by which gustatory sense is transmitted to the thalamus.

The Ventral Posterior Inferior Nucleus (VPI). This smallest subdivision of the ventral posterior nucleus lies ventrally between VPL and VPM (Fig. 15-16). The ventral border of the nucleus is adjacent to the reticular nucleus and the thalamic fasciculus. Cells of the nucleus are medium-sized and light-staining. Ascending afferents to VPI are incompletely known, but physiological evidence indicates that isolated stimulation of the vestibular nerve in the monkey evokes short latency responses in the nucleus (605, 606). These evoked responses are unchanged following total cerebellectomy, but are abolished by vestibular nerve section. Antidromic stimulation of parietal cortex suggests that neurons in VPI may project to caudal portions of the postcentral gyrus, near the junction of Brodmann's areas 2 and 5 (Fig. 19-5). In subsequent studies vestibular stimulation has evoked potentials in VPLo as well as VPI (607, 1489). Anatomical data based on axoplasmic transport in the monkey suggest ascending vestibular projections terminate bilaterally in small scattered regions of VPLo and to a lesser extent in VPI (1423). Most of the vestibular fibers ascend outside the limits of the medial longitudinal fasciculus and none were found to terminate in the posterior thalamic nuclei. Other data suggest that the vestibular nuclei have a direct projection to the centromedian nucleus (1565).

Cortical Connections of the Ventral Posterior Nucleus. The VP has a precise topical projection to the cortex (473, 477, 1372, 2651). Fibers project to the postcentral gyrus so that superior portions of the gyrus receive fibers from the lateral part of VPL; inferior portions of the gyrus near the lateral sulcus are supplied by fibers from VPM. Intermediate parts of VP project to intermediate parts of the postcentral gyrus (Fig. 15-15). This thalamocortical projection correlates precisely with the termination of ascending somatosensory systems in the ventral posterior nuclear complex. Cortical areas 3, 1 and 2 receive the specific projections of VPL and VPM.

Anterograde degeneration and physiological studies have shown that cells of VPL and VPM, which constitute the ventrobasal complex, project ipsilaterally to both the primary (S I) and secondary (SS II) somatosensory areas (984, 1240). The SS II lies along the superior bank of the lateral sulcus and in the monkey the greater part of SS II lies buried in the lateral sulcus (1239, 1241). Projections of the ventrobasal complex upon these cortical areas is topographic. It has been estimated that only about half of the neurons of the ventrobasal complex project to both cortical areas. Corticothalamic fibers arising in both S I and SS II project back to the ventrobasal complex in a topographical and reciprocal manner (1237). Retrograde labeling technics demonstrate that thalamocortical relay neurons projecting to S I are arranged in curved lamellae which extend throughout the rostrocaudal extent of the ventrobasal complex (1246). Aggregations of cells within the lamellae projecting to areas 3, 1 and 2 are intermingled and it seems unlikely that collaterals of one cell project to more than one cortical area. Tritiated amino acids injected into S I were transported to terminals in VPLc and VPM; no label was detected in cells of VPLo, VPI or the posterior thalamic nuclei.

The Posterior Thalamic Nuclear Complex. Caudal to the VPL there is a transitional diencephalic zone with a complex and varied cellular morphology referred to as the posterior thalamic nuclear complex (2218). The posterior nuclear complex (zone) lies caudal to VPLc, medial to the rostral part of the pulvinar and dorsal to the medial geniculate body (Fig. 15-5). The nuclear complex consists of the *supra-geniculate nucleus*, the *nucleus limitans* and an ill-defined region of heterogeneous cell types which extends rostrally toward the caudal pole of VPLc, referred to as the *posterior nucleus* (331). The suprageniculate nucleus is a pyramid-shaped cell mass that extends dorsomedially from the dorsal part of the principal division of the medial geniculate body (Fig. 15-18). The nucleus limitans is a narrow band of oval or spindle-shaped cells that separates the pretectum and medial nucleus of the pulvinar (1883); these cells merge laterally with those of the suprageniculate nucleus. The posterior nucleus, composed of small and medium-sized cells which lie rostral to the suprageniculate nucleus, extends rostrally toward VPLc and becomes continuous with VPI. The dorsal part of the posterior nucleus is difficult to distinguish from overlying regions of the pulvinar and the small-celled part of the suprageniculate nucleus. The magnocellular part of the medial geniculate nucleus lies ventral to the rostral part of the suprageniculate nucleus and ventral to the posterior nucleus (Fig. 15-18).

The posterior nucleus is of particular interest because it receives spinothalamic fibers and has been considered to be concerned with the perception of painful and noxious stimuli (213, 229, 232, 1297, 1302, 1650, 1653, 1655, 1658). Some studies also suggest that fibers of the medial lemniscus and cervicothalamic tract may terminate in this nucleus (210, 212). The medial part of the posterior nucleus also receives projections from the primary (S I) and the secondary (SS II) somatosensory cortex (1237, 1238), as well as from the auditory cortex (1063).

Physiological studies have suggested that cells in the posterior thalamic nucleus are activated by somatic sensory stimuli, but that mechano-receptive cells are not place specific and there is only a vague representation of the body image within this region (706, 2019). Cells of this region are not modality specific in that many cells may respond to tactile, vibratory or auditory stimuli. None of the cells in this thalamic region has been observed to be activated by gentle rotation of joints. The majority of cells in this region were described as responding to noxious stimuli. Neurons responding to nociceptive stimuli appeared related to large, and usually bilateral, receptive fields.

Neurons in the region of the posterior thalamic nucleus were originally considered to project in a sustaining fashion to the second somatic area (SS II), a cortical sensory representation on the superior bank of the lateral sulcus (2218) (see p. 664). More detailed physiological studies of a cortical area considered to represent the SS II in the monkey described two parts: (a) a rostral part which responded to low threshold tactile stimuli in an organized topographic fashion and (b) a caudal part with large receptive fields and poorly organized topographic features that responded to nociceptive stimuli (2708). Because the response properties of the caudal part of SS II appeared similar to those of the medial region of the posterior thalamic nucleus (1972, 2019, 2706), it was presumed that this nucleus projected to parts of SS II. Detailed studies in the cat and monkey (Fig. 15-18) indicate that cells in medial division of the posterior thalamic nucleus project to the retroinsular cortex and cells in the lateral division of this nucleus project to postauditory cortex (331). Neither of these cortical projections overlap recognized somatosensory or auditory areas. The retroinsular cortex, which receives projections from the medial part of the posterior thalamic nucleus, appears to respond to cutaneous stimuli from well-defined contralateral receptive fields located in the hand and foot (2190). These findings raise questions concerning the notion that cells of the posterior thalamic nucleus and SS II are concerned with perception of pain and noxious stimuli and are related. Although SS II is difficult to define physiologically (2190–2192, 2708, 2771), it can be identified anatomically on the basis of its connections with VPLc and the primary somesthetic cortex (331, 812, 1238, 1239, 1241, 1244). Cells in SS II respond to non-nociceptive stimuli and have a unique somatotopic organization (812, 2190–2192). For a further discussion of SS II, see page 664.

The Medial Geniculate Body

The medial geniculate body (MGB) lies on the caudal ventral aspect of the thalamus, medial to the lateral geniculate body (LGB) and dorsal to the crus cerebri (Figs. 15-4, 15-5 and 15-14). This large nuclear mass is the thalamic auditory relay nucleus, receiving fibers from the inferior colliculus via its brachium and giving rise to the auditory radiation (Figs. 2-9 and 12-13). Unlike auditory relay nuclei at lower brain stem levels, there are no commissural connections between the medial geniculate bodies. The medial geniculate nucleus consists of several subdivisions with distinctive cytoarchitecture and connections to which different designations have been given (1035, 1743, 1874). According to Morest (1743) the MGB consists of three main divisions referred to as medial, dorsal and ventral (Fig. 15-19). Several nuclei are described in each of the main subdivisions (1874). These subdivisions of the medial geniculate nucleus are not easily distinguished in ordinary histological preparations, but become apparent in Golgi preparations (1743–1745).

The ventral nucleus extends throughout most of the rostrocaudal length of the MGB and is bounded medially by the brachium of the inferior colliculus and ventrally by the surface of the MGB. Unlike all other major subdivisions of the MGB the ventral nucleus has a distinct laminar organization reminiscent of that seen in the lateral geniculate body. Cells of the ventral division are fairly constant in size and shape and have tufted dendrites, considered to be typical of neuronal populations having a homogeneous input. The lamination, produced by the dendritic pattern of tufted cells and fibers of the brachium of the inferior colliculus, is in the form of spirals or curved vertical sheets (Fig. 15-19). Data suggest that afferent fibers from the inferior colliculus enter particular laminae and remain continuously associated with the same, or contiguous dendritic layers. The lamination in the ventral division of the MGB is analogous to that in the lateral geniculate body (LGB), except the cellular laminae are not separated by bands of myelinated fibers. This laminar organization of the ventral division is considered to form the basis for the tonotopic localization (i.e., frequency discrimination) within the MGB (1744). The laminar organization of the ventral division of the MGB also resembles that of the ventrolateral division of the central nucleus of the inferior colliculus

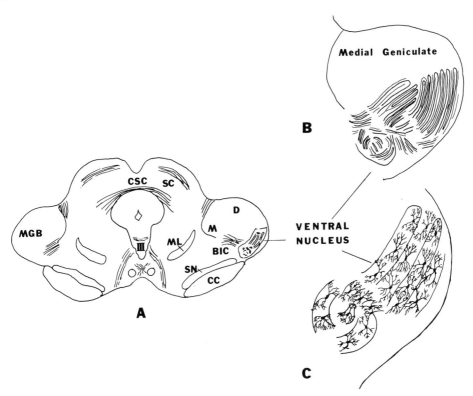

Figure 15-19. Transverse reconstructions of the fibrodendritic laminations in the ventral nucleus of the medial geniculate body in the cat based on Golgi preparations. (*A*) Transverse section of midbrain through the superior colliculus (*SC*) and medial geniculate body (*MGB*); *M* and *D* indicate the magnocellular and dorsal nuclei of the MGB. The laminated ventral nucleus of MGB is shown in *A*, *B*, and *C*. The lamination in the ventral nucleus, produced by the arrangement of dendrites of geniculate neurons and fibers in the brachium of the inferior colliculus, occurs in spirals and vertical sheets (*B*, *C*). (Based upon Morest (1744).) Abbreviation used: *BIC*, brachium of the inferior colliculus; *CC*, crus cerebri; *CSC*, commissure of the superior colliculus; *SN*, substantia nigra; *III*, oculomotor nucleus.

from which it receives its major input (429, 1374, 1735, 1743, 1874, 2194). Physiological mapping of ventral division of the MGB reveals that the lamination is related to the tonotopic organization, in which high frequencies are represented medially and low frequencies laterally (26, 840, 974). Neurons in the ventral division of the MGB give rise to the auditory radiation which terminates in the primary auditory cortex (Figs. 12-13, 19-23 and 19-24), where there is a spatial representation of tonal frequencies (429, 1838, 1875, 2087, 2750). The primary auditory cortex gives rise to reciprocal corticothalamic fibers that terminate in the ventral division of the MGB (631, 782, 1875). Both geniculocortical and corticogeniculate fibers are ipsilateral.

In man the principal cortical projection of the MGB is to the superior temporal convolution (transverse gyrus of Heschl) via the geniculotemporal or auditory radiations (Figs. 12-13, 15-14, 15-15 and 15-28). This cortical projection area (area 41) is presumed to have a tonotopic localization in which high tones are appreciated in medial regions and low tones in anterior and lateral regions (Fig. 19-5). The tonotopic localization at the cortical level is neither simple nor easily defined, but present evidence suggests it is similar to that in the monkey (Fig. 19-24) (1182, 1672).

The dorsal division of the MGB contains several nuclei, among which are the suprageniculate and the dorsal nuclei (1874). The dorsal nucleus is prominent at caudal levels of the MGB, where it is located dorsolaterally to the ventral division (Fig. 15-19). This nucleus receives projections from the lateral tegmental area, broadly defined as a region extending from the deep layers of the superior colliculus to the area adjacent to the lateral lemniscus (1374, 1874). The suprageniculate nucleus (Fig. 15-18) appears to receive projections from deep layers of the superior colliculus and the dorsal midbrain tegmentum (331, 1874).

The medial division, containing the largest cells in the MGB and lying dorsomedial to the ventral division, is known as the magnocellular part (Figs. 15-18 and 15-19). Rostrally the magnocellular part of the MGB borders the suprageniculate nucleus and the posterior thalamic nucleus. This division of the MGB receives an input from the inferior colliculus, the lateral tegmentum and spinal cord (211, 429, 1243, 1651, 1735, 1736, 1745, 1874). All nonlaminated portions of the medial geniculate body (i.e., the dorsal and medial divisions) send fibers ipsilaterally to at least five cytoarchitectonically distinct areas which form a cortical belt surrounding the primary auditory area (1875, 2087, 2750). There appears to be very little overlap in the cortical projections of these MGB subdivisions. One exception to the above concerns the caudal magnocellular part of the medial division which appears to project to most, if not all, of the cortical target areas of the medial geniculate body. Thus the cortical projection of the magnocellular MGB overlaps terminations of the ventral laminated part of the MGB in the primary auditory area and the terminations of all nuclei in other subdivisions projecting to the secondary auditory cortex. However, there is a difference in the cortical terminations of these fibers in that fibers from the magnocellular division terminate mainly in layer VI of the cortex while all other parts of the MGB send fibers primarily to cortical layer IV.

Although ascending pathways in the auditory system are paralleled by descending fiber linkages which can facilitate or inhibit transmission of impulses at numerous relay nuclei, or in the hair cells of the cochlea, the MGB does not participate in this descending system. Cortical projections from the primary and secondary auditory areas are back to the subdivisions of the MGB from which they receive afferents (429, 1875). Corticocollicular fibers arise largely from the primary auditory cortex and terminate mainly in the pericentral nucleus of the inferior colliculus (429, 631, 1875, 2195).

Dorsolateral

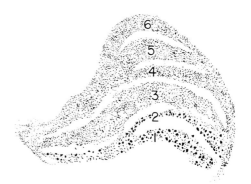

Ventromedial

Figure 15-20. Drawing of the cellular lamination of the lateral geniculate body with laminae numbered from the hilus. The magnocellular laminae (*1* and *2*) constitute the ventral nucleus. Parvicellular laminae *3* through *6* are referred to as the dorsal nucleus. Crossed fibers of the optic tract terminate in laminae *1*, *4*, and *6*; uncrossed optic fibers terminate on other laminae. Only cells in the dorsal nucleus project fibers to the visual cortex.

In addition the auditory cortex gives rise to corticopontine fibers that terminate in the dorsolateral pontine nuclei and in deep layers of the superior colliculus (294, 2388). The inferior colliculus, the second link in the descending system of auditory pathways, projects fibers via the lateral lemniscus to the olivary and cochlear nuclei (429, 1874).

The Lateral Geniculate Body

The lateral geniculate body (LGB), the thalamic relay nucleus for the visual system, lies rostral and lateral to the medial geniculate body (MGB), lateral to the posterior part of the crus cerebri and ventral to the pulvinar (Figs. 2-25, 15-4, 15-5, 15-14 and 15-20). This thalamic nucleus has an impressive laminated cellular structure which in transverse sections has a horseshoe-shaped configuration with the hilus directed ventromedially. Crossed and uncrossed fibers of the optic tract enter via the hilus and are distributed in a precise pattern. In man and most primates the LGB consists of six cellular layers or laminae arranged in two major subdivisions (465, 476, 1095). The six concentric cell layers, separated by intervening fiber bands, customarily are numbered from 1 to

6, beginning from the ventromedial hilar region (Fig. 15-20). Subdivisions of the LGB are the ventral nucleus (layers 1 and 2) consisting of large cells (magnocellular laminae) and the dorsal nucleus (layers 3 to 6) composed of small cells (parvicellular laminae) (1596). Both divisions of the lateral geniculate nucleus receive afferents from the ganglion cells of the retina (2252), but cells of the ventral nucleus do not project to the striate (visual) cortex (Fig. 15-21). The ventral magnocellular part of the LGB projects to the pretectum, the superior colliculus, the suprachiasmatic nucleus of the hypothalamus and the zona incerta (691, 2482). Direct projections from the retina have been shown to terminate in overlapping fashion in all of the structures receiving inputs from the ventral nucleus, except the superior colliculus; in the latter structure inputs from the retina and the ventral nucleus of LGB end in adjacent layers. The ventral nucleus, a derivative of the ventral thalamus, receives an input from the striate cortex (848) and has been considered to play a role in visuomotor integration because its efferent connections are entirely subcortical (338, 2482). Phylogenetically, the LGB first differentiates into three cell layers. It becomes six-layered in forms where the optic tracts show a partial decussation, the uncrossed and crossed portions each terminating upon three different laminae (463, 1712).

Layer 1 of the magnocellular division is present through all levels of the nucleus and extends laterally into the monocular segment, while layer 2 does not reach as far rostrally or laterally (1095). Occasionally small groups of large cells, extending into medial and caudal parts of the dorsal nucleus, can be traced into continuity with layer 1. The parvicellular layers of LGB, consisting of layers 3, 4, 5 and 6 in ventrodorsal sequence, are most easily distinguished in the caudal half of the nucleus in man (Fig. 15-22). As these layers are traced laterally they fuse in pairs: layer 4 with layer 6, and layer 3 with layer 5 (1095). In rostral parts of the dorsal nucleus the individual layers are more difficult to identify because layer 3 does not extend as far rostrally as layer 5, and layers 4 and 6 fuse medially as well as laterally.

The projection from the retina onto the LGB is very precise and crossed and un-

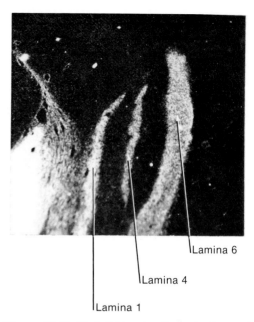

Figure 15-21. Dark field autoradiograph of part of the right lateral geniculate body in a monkey whose left eye was injected with [³H]leucine. Isotope conveyed by axoplasmic transport to terminals in laminae *1*, *4*, and *6* is evident (photograph, ×45).

crossed fibers in the optic tract end upon separate layers. Crossed fibers of the optic tract end upon layers 1, 4 and 6 while uncrossed fibers terminate in layers 2, 3 and 5 (Fig. 15-21). This pattern of laminar termination in the LGB has been established by the studies of anterograde degeneration following enucleation or section of the optic nerve (894, 983, 1074, 1416, 2546) and by study of transneuronal cell changes following similar lesions (892, 1095, 1221, 1641, 1713). These findings have been confirmed in studies in which one eye has been injected with tritiated amino acids and the retinofugal fibers have been traced in serial autoradiographs (1074, 1253, 2545). Two unique features related to crossed retinogeniculate fibers are reflected in structure. The monocular crescent of the visual field is subserved by receptor elements in the most medial part of the nasal retina (Fig. 15-23). Ganglion cells in this part of the retina project crossed fibers to the bilaminar segment of opposite LGB, located laterally where parts of layers 4 and 6 fuse (1095, 1252). The bilaminar segment produces a small reverse curve on the ventrolateral aspect of the LGB (Fig. 15-22). The optic disc, located in the nasal half of the

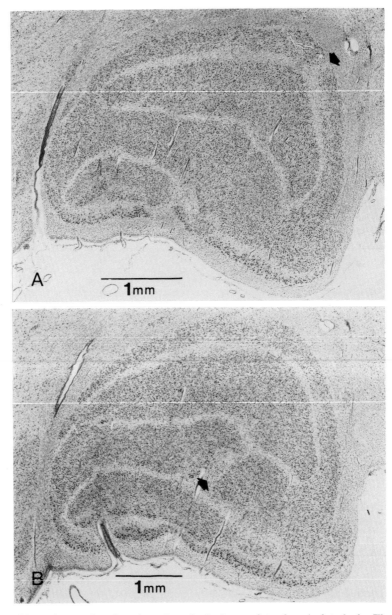

Figure 15-22. Photomicrographs of sections through the human lateral geniculate body. The blind spot is represented by discontinuities in layers 6 (*A, arrow*) and 4 (*B, arrow*). Layers 4 and 6 fuse laterally (*right*) in both *A* and *B* producing the bilaminar segment ventrally. The bilaminar segment receive an input from the most medial contralateral nasal retina that subserves the monocular visual field (i.e., the monocular crescent). (Reproduced with permission from T. L. Hickey and R. W. Guillery: *Journal of Comparative Neurology,* **183:** 221–246, 1979.)

retina, representing optic nerve fibers, has no photoreceptors and is responsible for the blind spot detectable on perimetry. The optic disc is represented in the contralateral LGB by cellular discontinuities in layers 4 and 6 which are found medial and caudal to the bilaminar segment (Fig. 15-22).

These cellular discontinuities in the mentioned laminae have been detected in the same parts of LGB in a large series of human brains and are regarded as a constant feature (1095).

Nissl preparations through the human lateral geniculate nucleus reveal a linear cellular organization in which the long axis of the cells tend to run perpendicular to the laminae. This linear cellular orientation corresponds to the orientation of small blood vessels running through the nucleus from its ventral surface (1095). Perikarya of the parvicellular layers are oriented perpendicular to laminae so that the long axis of the cells parallel "lines of projection" which indicate isorepresentation of points in the visual field (183, 1252).

The topographic representation of the retinal surface within the LGB is highly organized and precisely defined. In all mammals the contralateral half of the total visual field is represented in each lateral geniculate nucleus. The contralateral half of the binocular visual field is represented in all layers of the LGB, even though crossed and uncrossed fibers end in different layers. The projection locales in the six layers lie in perfect register so that any small area in the contralateral binocular visual field can be shown to correspond to a dorsoventral column of cells extending radially through all six layers parallel to the "lines of projection" (Fig. 15-23) (1252). The LGB consists of six sheets of cells bent in a horseshoe configuration, but in exact registration, so that columns of cells in the "lines of projection" receive inputs from corresponding points in the retina of each eye related to the contralateral binocular visual field. It should be stressed that binocular fusion does not occur in the LGB because retinogeniculate fibers end on different layers. Following section of the optic nerve anterograde degeneration or transneuronal degeneration (after long survivals) will occur in three layers of the LGB on each side. The layers in which degeneration of fibers or cells occur differs in accordance with the disposition of crossed (layers 1, 4 and 6) and uncrossed (layers 2, 3 and 5) retinal fibers (894, 983, 1095, 1641, 2031). Small lesions of the retina produce transneuronal degeneration in localized clusters of cells in three different layers on each side aligned according to the "lines of projection" (476, 850, 2031). The contralateral monocular visual field (monocular crescent) is related to receptor elements in the most medial nasal retina which are regarded as projecting only crossed fibers to the bilaminar segment located on the lateral surface of the LGB where parts of layers 4 and 6 fuse (Figs. 15-22 and 15-23). This appears to be the only region to which these fibers project (1095, 1252).

The "lines of projection" in the LGB also can be demonstrated by the study of retrograde cell degeneration in the LGB following small lesions in the striate cortex (849, 1095, 1252, 2213). Since one half of the visual field is represented topographically in the striate cortex of each hemisphere, the zone of retrograde cell degeneration in the LGB is bounded on each side by lines of projections. If a striate cortical lesion were small, the zone of degenerated cells in the LGB would form a narrow column of cells in the orientation of the projection lines. Large lesions of the striate cortex produce a larger zone of degeneration in the LGB bounded by sets of projection lines, referred to a geniculate segment (985). Cortical projection zones in geniculate segments involve cells of the dorsal nucleus in all layers. These observations indicate that neurons in the LGB with identical receptive fields form a column of cells extending through all laminae and that cells in the dorsal nucleus of LGB of this column project to the same region of the striate cortex.

Information concerning the retinotopic organization of retinofugal fibers in the optic nerve, chiasm, tract and lateral geniculate body in man and monkey is based upon considerable data (303, 476, 1095, 1149, 1150, 1252, 1597, 2031). In the optic nerve fibers from the four quadrants correspond approximately to their mutual positions in the retina in that fibers from upper quadrants remain superiorly while those from lower quadrants are found inferiorly. Retinal fibers from the macula occupy a central position. In the optic chiasm upper retinal fibers cross dorsally while lower retinal fibers cross ventrally. The partial decussation of fibers in the chiasm results in an intermingling of crossed and uncrossed fibers and a rearrangement of fibers in the optic tract in a pattern similar to that of their terminations in the LGB. Crossed and uncrossed fibers from superior retinal quadrants occupy medial regions of the optic tract and fibers from inferior retinal quadrants shift to lateral positions (Fig. 15-24). Fibers from the macula pass through central and peripheral regions of the optic

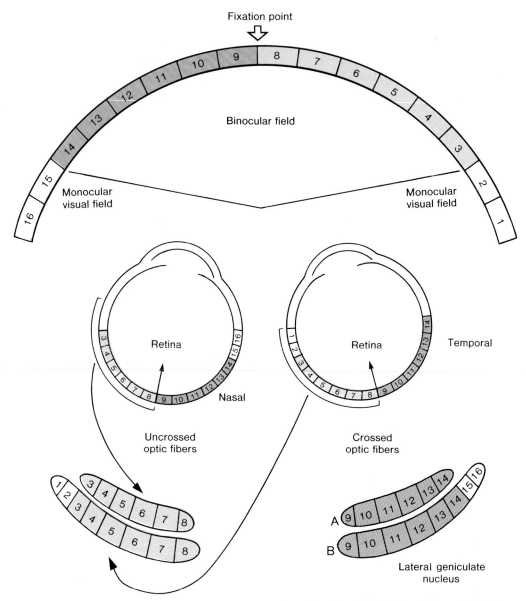

Figure 15-23. Schematic diagram showing the representation of the visual field in the retinae and in the layers of the lateral geniculate nucleus. Portions of the binocular visual field are shown in *red (left)* and *blue (right)*, while the monocular visual fields are *white*. Light from numbered sectors of both the binocular and monocular visual fields falls upon corresponding numbered sectors of the retinae. Crossed and uncrossed retinofugal fibers project upon columns of cells in different laminae of the lateral geniculate nucleus which are in exact registration, represented here by corresponding numbers. *A* represents laminae receiving uncrossed fibers (i.e., laminae 2, 3 and 5). *B* represents laminae receiving crossed fibers (i.e., laminae 1, 4 and 6). Light from the right monocular visual field (sectors 1 and 2) falls upon retinal receptors of the corresponding number in the most medial ipsilateral nasal retina. Crossed retinofugal fibers project to cell columns of the left lateral geniculate nucleus (1, 2). Cell columns 1 and 2 are best developed in laminae 4 and 6 which fuse to form the bilaminar segment. (Modified from Kaas, et al. (1252).)

nerve, but after decussating both crossed and uncrossed fibers lie in superior parts of the optic tract. The macular projection from the retina is extensively mixed with that from peripheral retinal areas in all but the most distal parts of the optic nerve (1149). Axons from the macular region of the retina are of fine caliber while those

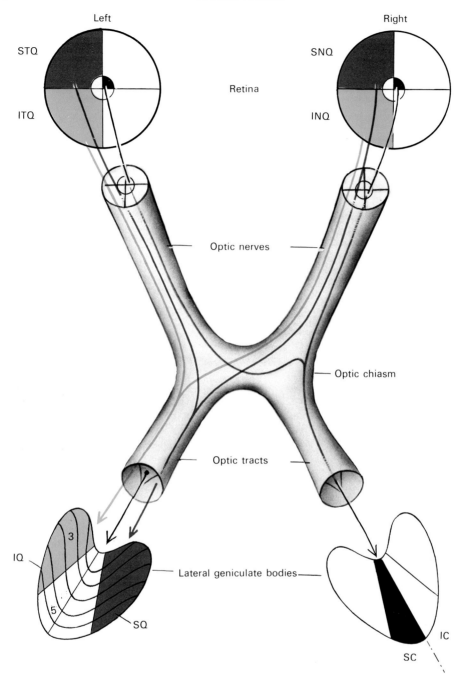

Figure 15-24. Schematic diagram of retinal ganglion cell projections through the optic nerves, optic chiasm and optic tracts to terminations within the lateral geniculate bodies. Superior peripheral quadrants of the retina on both sides (*SNQ*, superior nasal quadrant and *STQ*, superior temporal quadrant) shown in *red* project to the medial part (*SQ*) of the left lateral geniculate body (*red*). Inferior peripheral quadrants of the retina (*INQ*, inferior nasal quadrant and *ITQ*, inferior temporal quadrant) shown in *blue* project to the lateral part (*IQ*) of the left lateral geniculate body (*blue*). Superior central regions of the retina on nasal and temporal sides (*black*) on the opposite side project to the region of the right lateral geniculate body indicated by *SC*. Inferior central regions of the retina (*white*) project in the same fashion to the region of the right lateral geniculate body indicated by *IC*. The macular projection to the lateral geniculate is in the caudal region of the nucleus. Numbers in the left lateral geniculate body indicate two of the six laminae. (Based on Hoyt and Luis (1149) and Noback and Laemle (1843).)

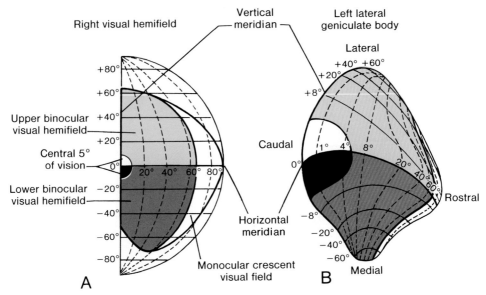

Figure 15-25. Schematic drawing of the right visual hemifield of the monkey (*A*) and its projection onto the dorsal surface of the unfolded left lateral geniculate body (LGB) (*B*). The vertical meridian is represented by the heavy *black* line on the left in both *A* and B; visual field zones of increasing eccentricity are represented serially in degrees by dashed lines. In the left lateral geniculate body visual field zones (dashed lines) are represented serially among the caudorostral axis of the nucleus in degrees. The horizontal meridian of the hemifield at 0 degrees is represented by a curved line in the caudorostral axis of the LGB (*B*); thin lines above and below the horizontal meridian indicate positive or negative elevations in degrees. Upper (*blue*) and lower (*red*) portions of the binocular visual hemifield indicated in *A* are represented by the same colors in *B*. The central 5° of vision, a generous estimate of the angle subtended by the fovea centralis, are shown in *black* and *white* at the intersection of the vertical and horizontal meridians. The monocular crescent (*white*) in *A* is represented along the rostral border of the LGB. (Based on Malpeli and Baker (1597).)

from nonmacular regions are large fibers. In the LGB the horizontal meridian of the visual field corresponds to an oblique dorsoventral plane that divides the nucleus into medial and lateral segments. Fibers from superior retinal quadrants of both eyes project to the medial half of the LGB; the inferior retinal quadrants send fibers to the lateral half of the nucleus (Fig. 15-24). The retinal projection from the macula is represented in a broad wedge-shaped sector in the caudal part of the LGB on both sides of the plane representing the horizontal meridian. Early studies suggested that macular fibers projected to central regions of the caudal two-thirds of the LGB (303, 476, 1399, 2031), but physiological data reveal that its projection is strictly limited to the caudal pole of the nucleus (1252, 1597). The macular representation accounts for about 12% of the total volume of the LGB and the caudal third of the nucleus represents the central 20% of vision. Retinal zones subserving the contralateral peripheral visual

field are represented serially along the caudorostral axis of the LGB (Fig. 15-25) with retinal fibers related to the most peripheral part of the visual field, the monocular crescent, projecting to the oral pole; other peripheral zones project to rostral regions of the nucleus caudal to its oral pole (1597). In rostral regions of the LGB there is no representation of central vision and mapping of the visual field is continuous across the horizontal meridian. The vertical meridian of the visual field, corresponding to the line separating temporal and nasal parts of the retina, is represented along the caudal margin of the nucleus from its medial to lateral borders (Fig. 15-25) where the edges of all layers are aligned (1252, 1597).

Physiological and anatomical evidence indicate at least three distinct classes of retinal ganglion cells and it is well known that retinofugal fibers provide inputs to several neural regions in addition to the LGB (233, 820, 2440). Retrograde transport studies in the monkey demonstrate that retinal ganglion cells of all sizes project to the parvicellular layers of the LGB, but only the largest ganglion cells of the peripheral retina have axons terminating in the magnocellular layers (325). Scattered ganglion cells of all sizes appear to project fibers to the superior colliculus. Retinofugal fibers entering various laminae of the LGB establish synaptic contact with the dendrites of geniculate neurons which are distributed within their particular lamina (361, 509, 981, 2498). Cells within this nucleus exhibit both convergence and divergence. Retinal afferent fibers may synapse with several neurons in the LGB (divergence), and each neuron of the LGB may receive inputs from several retinofugal fibers (convergence).

Laminae of the dorsal division of the LGB also contain substantial numbers of Golgi type II neurons which are regarded as playing an important role in processing visual information (981, 1017, 1415, 1944, 1945, 2498). Electron microscopic observations of the dorsal LGB in the monkey reveal the consistent occurrence of a synaptic arrangement in which retinal axon terminals establish synaptic contact with both relay neurons and Golgi type II cells (1017, 1944). This pattern of synaptic articulation appears to be a fundamental ultra-architectonic feature of the geniculate body as well as of other thalamic sensory nuclei and the authors refer to it as "the triadic synaptic arrangement." In this synaptic arrangement a retinal axon terminates upon dendrites of both a LGB relay neuron and a Golgi type II interneuron; the Golgi type II neuron is presynaptic to the same relay neuron that received a direct retinal ending. These "triads" are found throughout the LGB and in glial encapsulated synaptic complexes known as glomeruli. One interesting feature of the geniculate interneurons is that their dendrites are longer than their axon. This triadic synaptic arrangement is considered to serve as a mechanism for phasic inhibition of geniculate relay neurons. In this action it is assumed that the retinal axon excites both the geniculate relay neuron and the interneuron; the discharge of the interneuron in turn inhibits the same relay neuron excited by the retina afferent.

Glomeruli in the LGB constitute a synaptic complex of interlocking nerve processes of various origins which are arranged in a specific manner and separated from the environment by a capsule of glial processes (Fig. 15-26) (2497). The axon terminals of retinal afferents occupy the central position in these glomeruli. Unlike the cerebellar glomeruli which contain only one mossy fiber rosette, several club-shaped retinal afferents may occur in a LGB glomerulus. Other contributions to the glomeruli arise from Golgi type II cells and corticofugal fibers (Fig. 15-26). Glomeruli often are located at the bifurcation of stem dendrites of a LGB neuron. Axons of Golgi type II cells enter the glomeruli and establish synapses with relay cell (LGB neuron) dendrites; these cells are considered to be inhibitory in nature. The LGB glomerular complex contains: (a) axodendritic synapses on stem, secondary and peripheral dendrites and (b) axoaxonic synapses in which the presynaptic portion is contributed by terminals of the retinofugal fibers. The most remarkable feature of these glomeruli is the frequent occurrence of axoaxonic synapses. Some glomeruli of the LGB contain the triadic synaptic arrangement previously described. In the triadic arrangement the participating neural elements remain the same, but the receptive surfaces on geniculate relay neurons or Golgi type II cell may be either the soma or a dendrite (1017).

It is assumed that the synaptic arrangements within the LGB glomeruli are effective in the versatile processing of visual information. The interpretation of the structural arrangement within the LGB glomeruli suggests that optic afferents depolarizing Golgi cell terminals would presynaptically inhibit the inhibitory influence exerted by these cells upon geniculate body neurons (2497). This concept of presynaptic disinhibition by retinal afferents appears attractive because LGB neurons exhibit less activity if the visual field is uniformly illuminated than if there is a sharp contrast of light and dark projected upon the retina.

The lateral geniculate nucleus is the main end station of the optic tract. It projects to the calcarine cortex (area 17) by the geniculocalcarine tract or visual radiations (Fig. 15-31). Although both dorsal and ventral divisions of the LGB receive projec-

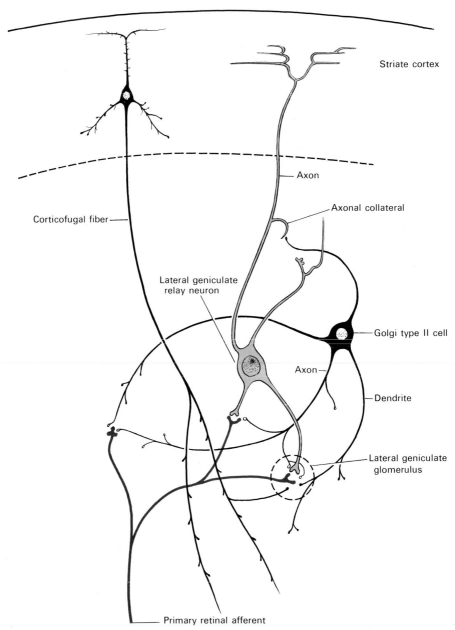

Figure 15-26. Schematic diagram of the neuronal arrangements in a glomerulus of the lateral geniculate body (LGB). A primary retinal afferent is indicated in *red*, while the LGB relay neuron is in *blue*. A corticofugal fiber and a Golgi type II cell are shown in *black*. The glomerulus contains a terminal of a primary retinal afferent, several club-shaped terminals of a LGB relay neuron, and contributions from both Golgi type II neurons and corticofugal fibers. This synaptic complex is enclosed in a capsule of glial processes, indicated by the dashed line. (Modified from Szentágothai (2497).)

tions of the optic tract, only the cells of dorsal division of the nucleus give rise to cortical projections (691, 1840, 2196, 2252, 2482). Cells of the dorsal division of the LGB project retinotopically primarily upon the striate cortex (area 17), but also upon the parastriate (area 18) and peristriate (area 19) cortex (691, 851, 875, 898, 1130, 1840, 2592, 2731, 2762). Quantitative data indicate that larger cells of the dorsal nucleus project to area 18, while cells of all sizes project to area 17 (875, 1130), and it has been suggested that the largest genic-ulate neurons may send collaterals to both areas 17 and 18. Geniculocortical fibers ter-minate largely in lamina IV of the striate cortex (851, 1163, 1536, 2731). The striate cortex has reciprocal connections with the LGB and also projects to the superior col-liculus and the pretectum. Retrograde HRP studies indicate that cells in lamina VI of the striate cortex project to both parvicel-lular and magnocellular divisions of the LGB, while cells in lamina V project to the superior colliculus and inferior pulvinar (875, 1537). Autoradiographic findings con-firm that fibers from area 17 project to all cell layers of the LGB (1129). These obser-vations point out that the relationships of the LGB with the striate cortex are not reciprocal in the strict sense because geni-culocortical fibers terminate upon lamina IV and corticogeniculate fibers arise from cells in lamina VI.

The great majority of LGB neurons in the parvicellular division project to the pri-mary visual cortex and have receptive field properties similar to those of retinal gan-glion cells, but there is essentially no mixing of excitatory signals at this level. The LGB is not a simple cortical relay nucleus, but a nucleus in which important transforma-tions of visual information occur through physiological processes involving the inhi-bition from a variety of sources that change the pattern and strength of neuronal re-sponses (810).

The Thalamic Reticular Nucleus

The thalamic reticular nucleus (RN) is a thin neuronal shell which surrounds the lateral, anterosuperior and anteroinferior aspects of the dorsal thalamus (Figs. 15-7, 15-11, 15-12 and 15-14). This thalamic nu-clear envelope develops embryologically from the mantle layer of the subthalamus and migrates dorsally between the external medullary lamina of the thalamus and the internal capsule (611, 1381). Morphologi-cally this nucleus is closely related to the zona incerta and the ventral division of the LGB. Although the reticular nucleus of the thalamus is a derivative of the ventral thal-amus, it surrounds the lateral aspect of the dorsal thalamus. Cells in this nucleus are heterogeneous in type, ranging from very small cells in dorsal regions to quite large cells in ventral and caudal regions (1227). Golgi studies of the reticular nucleus indi-cate that its neurons are similar to those of the brain stem reticular formation in that they are multipolar, vary in size from me-dium to large and lie immersed in a complex neuropil (2276). Dendrites of cells are long, relatively unramified and without specific orientation. The main axons of the majority of cells penetrate deeply into the thalamus, although some axons appear to run exclu-sively within the reticular nucleus. Auto-radiographic studies in the cat and monkey have shown that inputs to the reticular nucleus are derived from nuclei of the dor-sal thalamus and from the cerebral cortex (370, 1227). Fibers emanating from a partic-ular nucleus of the dorsal thalamus and destined for a specific cortical area give rise to collateral branches, or specific axons, that terminate in a particular part of the reticular nucleus that are constant for that nucleus. Corticothalamic fibers passing to-ward a particular nucleus of the dorsal thal-amus give collaterals to the same portions of the reticular nucleus as the target nu-cleus of the thalamus (1227). Cells of this same part of the reticular nucleus project back to the thalamic nucleus from which it receives an input. Both the intralaminar and the so-called relay nuclei of the dorsal thalamus project to the reticular nucleus and both receive fibers from it. Fibers pass-ing to the reticular nucleus from the intra-laminar thalamic nuclei are those that trav-erse the reticular nucleus en route to the striatum. The reticular nucleus is strategi-cally situated to sample neural activity passing between the cerebral cortex and nuclei of the dorsal thalamus, but it has no projection to the cerebral cortex (370, 1227, 2276). Cortical projections to the various parts of the reticular nucleus arise from the entire cerebral cortex and are topographi-cally organized (370). Although cells in the reticular nucleus are said to undergo degen-eration following cortical ablations (2207, 2216), degeneration occurs late and is less severe than in cortically dependent tha-lamic nuclei. It has been suggested that cell changes and cell loss in the reticular nuclei under these conditions might be transneu-ronal, but this is disputed. Injections of ^{3}H-labeled amino acids into the reticular nu-cleus and injections of HRP into various parts of the brain indicate that efferent

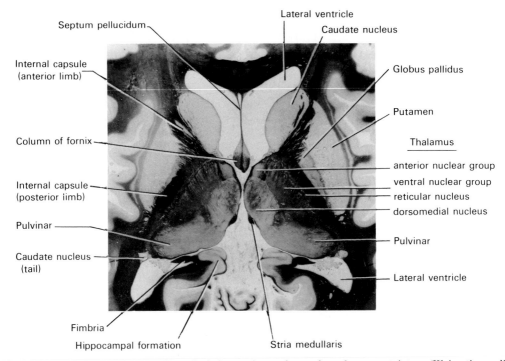

Figure 15-27. Horizontal section through thalamus, internal capsule and corpus striatum (Weigert's myelin stain, photograph).

fibers from this nucleus terminate only in dorsal thalamic nuclei; no fibers from the nucleus project to the ventral thalamus or to the cerebral cortex (1227). Suggestions that neurons in the reticular nucleus might have projections to the brain stem and striatum (2276) have not been substantiated. Descending fibers from the reticular nucleus have been found to terminate in parts of the medial geniculate body and caudal regions of the thalamus. Thus the reticular nucleus of the thalamus does not appear to be part of the so-called nonspecific thalamic pathway to the cerebral cortex. Since the major projections of this nucleus are to specific and nonspecific thalamic nuclei, it may serve to integrate intrathalamic activities. Physiological evidence supports the thesis that the reticular nucleus may act as a source of inhibitory neurons which act upon the major thalamic nuclei to "gate" the activity of thalamocortical relay neurons (815, 2078, 2281).

THE THALAMIC RADIATIONS AND INTERNAL CAPSULE

Fibers which reciprocally connect the thalamus and the cortex constitute the thalamic radiations. These thalamocortical and corticothalamic fibers form a continuous fan that emerges along the whole lateral extent of the caudate nucleus. Fiber bundles, radiating forward, backward, upward and downward, form large portions of various parts of the internal capsule (Figs. 2-11–2-13, 15-27 and 15-28). Although the radiations connect with practically all parts of the cortex, the richness of connections varies considerably for specific cortical areas. Most abundant are the projections to the frontal granular cortex, the precentral and postcentral gyri, the calcarine area and the gyrus of Heschl. The posterior parietal region and adjacent portions of the temporal lobe also have rich thalamic connections, but relatively scanty radiations go to other cortical areas (2650) (Fig. 15-15).

The thalamic radiations are grouped into four subradiations designated as the thalamic peduncles (Fig. 15-28). The *anterior* or *frontal peduncle* connects the frontal lobe with the medial and anterior thalamic nuclei. The *superior* or *centroparietal peduncle* connects the Rolandic area and adjacent portions of the frontal and parietal lobes with the ventral tier thalamic nuclei.

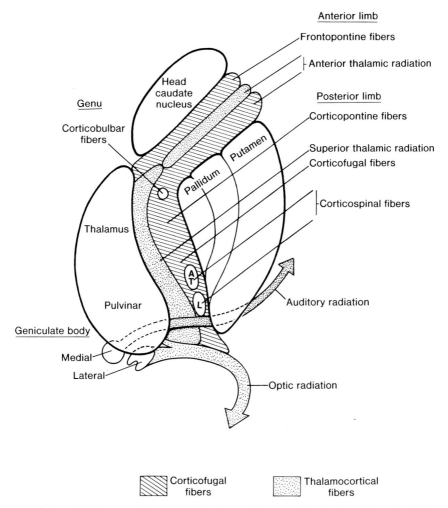

Figure 15-28. Schematic diagram of the right internal capsule as seen in a horizontal section similar to that shown in Figure 15-27. Corticospinal fibers in man occupy the caudal third of the posterior limb of the internal capsule.

The fibers, carrying general sensory impulses from the body and head, form part of this radiation and terminate in the postcentral gyrus (Figs. 15-14, 15-15 and 15-28). The *posterior* or *occipital peduncle* connects the occipital and posterior parietal convolutions with the caudal portions of the thalamus. It includes the optic radiations (geniculocalcarine) from the lateral geniculate body to the calcarine cortex (striate area). The *inferior* or *temporal peduncle* is small and includes the scanty connections of the thalamus with the temporal lobe and the insula. Included in this are the auditory radiations (geniculotemporal) from the medial geniculate body to the transverse temporal gyrus of Heschl (Fig. 15-28).

The cerebral hemisphere is connected with the brain stem and spinal cord by an extensive projection system. These fibers arise from the whole extent of the cortex, enter the white substance of the hemisphere and appear as a radiating mass of fibers, the *corona radiata*, which converges toward the brain stem (Figs. 2-11 and 2-13). On reaching the latter they form a broad, compact fiber band, the *internal capsule*, flanked medially by the thalamus and caudate nucleus and laterally by the lentiform nucleus (Figs. 15-27 and 15-28). Thus the internal capsule is composed of all the fibers, afferent and efferent, which go to, or come from, the cerebral cortex. A large part of the capsule is obviously composed of the thalamic radiations described above. The rest is composed mainly of corticofugal fiber systems (efferent cortical fibers) which descend to lower portions of the brain stem and to the spinal cord. These include the corticospinal, corticobulbar, corticoreticular and corticopontine tracts, as well as a number of smaller bundles.

The internal capsule, as seen in a horizontal section, is composed of a shorter *anterior* and a longer *posterior limb*, which meet at an obtuse angle, forming a junctional zone known as the *genu* (Figs. 2-12, 2-13, 15-27 and 15-28). The anterior limb lies between the lentiform and caudate nuclei. The posterior limb of the internal capsule (*lenticulothalamic portion*) lies between the lentiform nucleus and the thalamus. A *retrolenticular* part of the internal capsule extends caudally for a short distance behind the lentiform nucleus. In this caudal region a number of fibers passing beneath the lentiform nucleus to reach the temporal lobe collectively form the *sublenticular* portion of the internal capsule.

The *anterior limb* of the internal capsule contains the anterior thalamic radiation or peduncle, and the prefrontal corticopontine tract. The *genu*, and regions posterior to it, contains corticobulbar and corticoreticular fibers.

The *posterior limb* of the internal capsule contains: (a) corticospinal fibers, (b) frontopontine fibers, (c) the superior thalamic radiation and (d) relatively smaller numbers of corticotectal, corticorubral and corticoreticular fibers. Corticospinal fibers in man have classically been considered to lie in the posterior limb of the internal capsule relatively close to the genu (608). This traditional localization of corticospinal fibers in the internal capsule has been challenged by explorations using electrical stimulation and by careful pathological studies. More recent data suggest that corticospinal fibers are largely confined to a compact region in the posterior half of the posterior limb of the internal capsule (174, 711, 880, 1023, 2363). Evidence that fibers of the corticospinal tract are somatotopically arranged in this part of the internal capsule, with those destined for cervical, thoracic, lumbar and sacral spinal arranged in a rostrocaudal sequence, seems relatively crude. The classic view that corticospinal fibers

occupy the medial three-fifths of the crus cerebri and are somatotopically organized appears unreasonable on the basis of the number of fibers in the crus cerebri; corticospinal fibers in man probably account for only 1 million of the 20 million fibers in this massive bundle (2556). The somatotopic arrangement of corticospinal fibers in the crus cerebri probably is much less precise than commonly depicted.

The *retrolenticular portion* of the posterior limb contains the posterior thalamic radiations, including the optic radiations, parietal and occipital corticopontine fibers and fibers from the occipital cortex to the superior colliculi and pretectal region (Figs. 15-4 and 15-31). The *sublenticular portion*, difficult to separate from the retrolenticular, contains the *inferior thalamic peduncle* (Fig. 15-10), the auditory radiations (Figs. 2-10 and 15-28) and corticopontine fibers from the temporal and the parieto-occipital areas.

Thalamocortical and corticofugal fibers within the internal capsule occupy a comparatively small, compact area (Fig. 15-28). Lesions in this area produce more widespread disability than lesions of comparable size in any other region of the nervous system. Thrombosis or hemorrhage of the anterior choroidal, striate or capsular branches of the middle cerebral arteries (Fig. 20-13) are responsible for most lesions in the internal capsule. Vascular lesions in the posterior limb of the internal capsule may result in contralateral hemianesthesia of the head, trunk and limbs due to injury of thalamocortical fibers *en route* to the sensory cortex. There is also a contralateral hemiplegia due to injury of the corticospinal tract. Lesions of the internal capsule may also injure corticobulbar fibers which result in an upper motor neuron type weakness of certain cranial nerves; these disturbances are manifest particularly by contralateral facial weakness. Lesions in the posterior regions of the posterior limb may include the optic and auditory radiations. In such instances there may be a contralateral triad consisting of hemianesthesia, hemianopsia and hemihypacusis (Figs. 2-10, 15-28 and 15-31). More extensive vascular lesions may include the thalamus or corpus striatum, so that affective changes

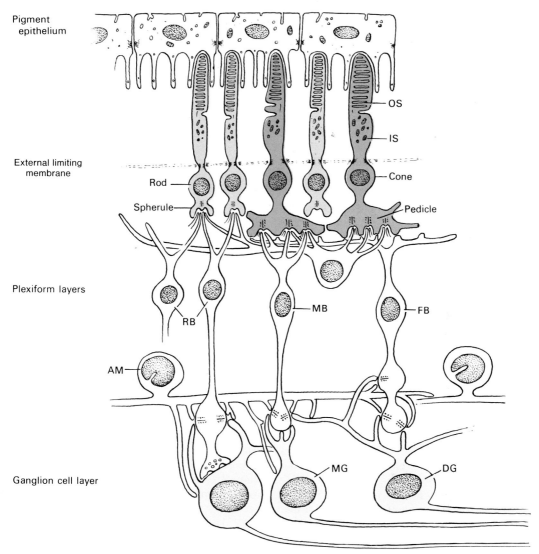

Figure 15-29. Schematic diagram of the ultrastructural organization of the retina. Rods (*blue*) and cones (*red*) are composed of an outer segment (*OS*), an inner segment (*IS*), a cell body and a synaptic base. Photopigments are present in the outer segments (OS) which are composed of laminated discs. The synaptic base of the rod is called a spherule, while the synaptic base of the cone is called a pedicle. In the plexiform layers *RB* indicates rod bipolar cells, *MB* a midget bipolar cell and, *FB* a flat bipolar cell. *AM* indicates an amacrine cell. Ganglion cells (*MG*, midget ganglion cell; *DG*, diffuse ganglion cell) and retinal afferents are in *yellow*. (Modified from Dowling and Boycott (646) and Noback and Laemle (1843).)

and symptoms due to injury of the basal ganglia may be added to those characteristic of injury to the internal capsule.

THE VISUAL PATHWAYS

The Retina. The retina arises as an evaginated portion of the brain, the optic pouch, which secondarily is invaginated to form the two-layered optic cup. The outer layer gives rise to pigmented epithelium. The inner layer forms the neural portion of the retina, from which are differentiated the bipolar rod and cone cells, the bipolar and horizontal neurons (confined within the retina itself) and the multipolar ganglionic neurons whose axons form the optic nerve (Fig. 15-29). The inner layer thus constitutes a fiber tract connecting two parts of the brain. Its fibers possess no Schwann sheaths, and its connective tissue investments represent continuations of the meningeal sheaths of the brain (i.e., pia, arachnoid and dura).

The rod and cone cells are visual receptors which react specifically to physical light. The cones, numbering some 7 million in the human eye, have a higher threshold of excitability and are stimulated by light of relatively high intensity. They are responsible for sharp visual definition and for color discrimination in adequate illumination. The rods, whose number has been estimated at more than 100 million, react to low intensities of illumination and subserve twilight and night vision. Close to the posterior pole of the eye, the retina shows a small, circular, yellowish area, the *macula lutea*, in direct line with the visual axis. The macula represents the retinal area for central vision, and the eyes are fixed in such a manner that the retinal image of any object is always focused on the macula. The rest of the retina is concerned with paracentral and peripheral vision. In the macular region the inner layers of the retina are pushed apart, forming a small central pit, the *fovea centralis*, which constitutes the point of sharpest vision and most acute color discrimination. Here the retina is composed entirely of closely packed slender cones.

The rods and cones are composed of an outer segment, a narrow neck, an inner segment, a cell body and a synaptic base (Fig. 15-29). Photopigments are present in the outer segments, where the photochemical reactions to light take place that give rise to the generator potential. The outer segment is composed of a series of laminated discs derived from the infolding of the plasma membrane. The photopigments, bound to the membranes of the discs, are constantly renewed. Rhodopsin is the photopigment of the rods in primates, and three pigments with maximum absorptions for blue, green and red are present in the cones (2647). The synaptic base of the cone is called a pedicle, while that of the rod is referred to as a spherule. Each cone pedicle has several invaginations which contain terminals of horizontal, midget bipolar and flat bipolar cells in a specific arrangement. Rod spherules have a single invagination containing multiple processes of horizontal and rod bipolar cells (Fig. 15-29) (1843). Each midget ganglion cell makes several synaptic contacts with a single midget bipolar cell. Diffuse ganglion cells establish synaptic contacts with all types of bipolar cells (646). Horizontal cells and amacrine cells constitute retinal interneurons. It is difficult to determine whether processes of horizontal cells are axons or dendrites, and it is possible that each process may be capable of both receiving and transmitting signals. Amacrine cells in the inner plexiform layer have no axon, but make synaptic contacts with all types of bipolar cells, other amacrine cells and the dendrites and somata of ganglion cells. The axons of ganglion cells, at first unmyelinated, are arranged in fine radiating bundles which run parallel to the retinal surface and converge at the optic disc to form the optic nerve. On emerging from the eyeball the fibers immediately acquire a myelin sheath, and there is a consequent increase in the size of the optic nerve.

Retinal ganglion cells are of different sizes, project to different sites and appear functionally to form at least three distinct classes (233, 325, 820, 1279, 2440). The physiologically distinct classes of ganglion cells are referred to as X, Y and W cells. The X class cells have slower conduction velocities than Y cells, exhibit sustained or tonic responses and project to the dorsal nucleus of the LGB and the pretectum. The Y cells have rapidly conducting axons, exhibit transient or phasic responses and project to both the dorsal nucleus of the LGB and the superior colliculus. The W ganglion cells have either tonic or phasic responses, very slow axonal conduction velocities and project to the superior colliculus and the pretectum. It has been suggested that: (a) the largest ganglion cells correspond to the Y cells, (b) medium-sized cells with narrow dendritic arborizations correspond to the X cells and (c) the smallest ganglion cells with the widest dendritic trees correspond to the W cells. Because the central projections of these classes of retinal ganglion cells differ, it is presumed that their functional roles also differ. The Y cells are present in much smaller numbers than either X or W cells. The retinal density of X and W cells is maximal in the area centralis and falls off

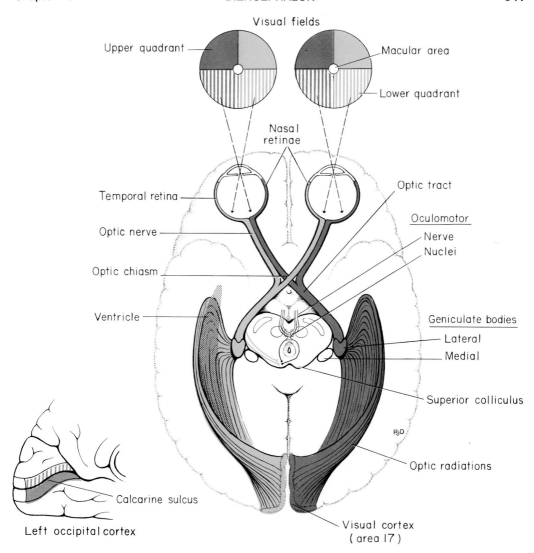

Figure 15-30. Diagram of the visual pathways viewed from the ventral surface of the brain. Light from the upper half of the visual field falls on the inferior half of the retina. Light from the temporal half of the visual field falls on the nasal half of the retina, while light from the nasal half of the visual field falls on the temporal half of the retina. The visual pathways from the retina to the striate cortex are shown. The plane of the visual fields has been rotated 90 degrees toward the reader. The insert shows the projection of the quadrants of the visual field upon the left calcarine (striate) cortex. The macular area of the retina is represented nearest the occipital pole. Fibers mediating the pupillary light reflex leave the optic tract and project to the pretectal region; other fibers relay impulses indirectly to the visceral nuclei of the oculomotor complex.

rapidly with eccentricity. Since W cells do not project to the dorsal nucleus of the LGB, it is presumed that X type ganglion cells must be concerned with central vision (820).

The Optic Nerves. These nerves enter the cranial cavity through the optic foramina and unite to form the optic chiasm, beyond which they are continued as the optic tracts. Within the chiasm a partial decussation occurs, the fibers from the nasal halves of the retina crossing to the opposite side, and those from the temporal halves of the retina remaining uncrossed (Fig. 15-30). In binocular vision each visual field, right and left, is projected upon portions of both retinae. Thus the images of objects in the right field of vision (*red* in

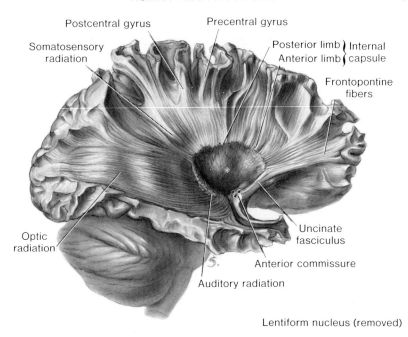

Figure 15-31. Drawing of a brain dissection showing the corona radiata. The lentiform nucleus has been removed and its position marked by an asterisk (*). The visual, auditory and somatosensory radiations are identified. (Reproduced with permission from F. A. Mettler: *Neuroanatomy*. C. V. Mosby Co., St. Louis, 1948.)

Fig. 15-30) are projected on the right nasal and the left temporal half of the retina. The right monocular crescent of the visual field projects upon retinal receptors only in the most medial part of the right nasal retina (Fig. 15-23). In the chiasm the fibers from these two retinal portions are combined to form the left optic tract, which represents the complete right field of vision. By this arrangement the whole right field of vision is projected upon the left hemisphere, and the left visual field upon the right hemisphere.

The Optic Tract. On each side the optic tract sweeps outward and backward, encircling the hypothalamus and the rostral portions of the crus cerebri. Most of its fibers terminate in the lateral geniculate body, although small portions continue as the brachium of the superior colliculus to the superior colliculi and pretectal area (Fig. 15-30). Although the existence of retinohypothalamic fibers has been suggested by many authors, only recently have these assumptions been confirmed. Using autoradiographic technics it has been established that retinal fibers terminate bilaterally in the suprachiasmatic nucleus of the hypothalamus in a variety of mammals, includ-

ing the monkey (1731, 1739, 2009, 2545). This direct projection from the retina has functional relevance to mechanisms of neuroendocrine regulation (see p. 497).

The lateral geniculate body gives rise to the geniculocalcarine tract which forms the last relay to the visual cortex. The superior colliculus is concerned with detection of movement with the visual fields and with the coordination of eye and head movements. The pretectal region is concerned with the pupillary light reflex.

The Geniculocalcarine Tract. This tract arises from the lateral geniculate body, passes through the retrolenticular portion of the internal capsule and forms the optic radiations, which end in the striate cortex (area 17), located on the medial surface of the occipital lobe. These fibers terminate on both banks of the calcarine sulcus (Figs. 2-5, 15-15, 15-30 and 15-31). All fibers of this radiation do not reach the cortex by the shortest route (Figs. 15-30 and 15-31). The most dorsal fibers pass almost directly backward to the striate area. Those placed more ventrally first turn forward and downward into the temporal lobe, and spread out over the rostral part of the inferior horn of the lateral ventricle;

these fibers then loop backward and run close to the outer wall of the lateral ventricle (external sagittal stratum) to reach the occipital cortex (Fig. 2-21). The most ventral fibers make the longest loop; some of these extend into the uncal region of the temporal lobe before turning backwards (Figs. 15-30 and 15-31).

Retinal areas have a precise point-to-point relationship with the lateral geniculate body, each portion of the retina projecting on a specific and topographically limited portion of the geniculate body (Figs. 15-23, 15-24 and 15-25). The fibers from the upper retinal quadrants (representing the lower visual field) terminate in the medial part, those from the lower quadrants in the lateral part of the geniculate body. The macula is represented by a wedge-shaped sector in the caudal part of the LGB on both sides of the plane representing the horizontal meridian (1597). The peripheral field, including the monocular crescent, is represented rostrally in the LGB and is continuous across the horizontal meridian (Fig. 15-25). A similar point-to-point relation exists between the geniculate body and the striate cortex. The medial half of the lateral geniculate body, representing the upper retinal quadrants (lower visual fields), projects to the superior lip of the calcarine sulcus via the superior portion of the optic radiation (Fig. 15-30). The lateral half of the lateral geniculate body, representing the lower retinal quadrants (upper visual field), projects to the inferior lip of the calcarine sulcus. These fibers occupy the inferior portion of the optic radiation. The macular fibers, which constitute the intermediate part of the optic radiation, terminate in the caudal third of the calcarine cortex. Those from the paracentral and peripheral retinal areas end in respectively more rostral portions.

Experimental studies (1375) with stationary spots of light indicate that the receptive fields of ganglion cells in the retina are organized in concentric zones with either an "on" or "off" type of discharge in the center and the reverse in the periphery or surround (Fig. 19-16). The concept of receptive fields in the visual system has been critically reviewed by Jacobs (1197). In the retina the receptive field consists of those receptors, rods and cones, and retinal neurons, which influence the excitability of a single ganglion cell. The retina is a composite of as many receptive fields as there are ganglion cells. Each receptive field is organized into two zones: (a) a small circular central zone and (b) a surrounding concentric zone referred to as the periphery or surround. These two zones are functionally antagonistic. Two general types of receptive fields have been described: (a) those with an "on" center and an "off" surround and (b) those with an "off" center and an "on" surround. If a light stimulus illuminates an "on" center, or an "on" surround, the ganglion cell will fire vigorously. If a spot of light strikes an "off" center, or an "off" surround, the ganglion cell is inhibited until the light is turned off; when the light is withdrawn, the ganglion cell will fire (Fig. 19-16). If the light stimulus illuminates both "on" and "off" zones, which exhibit mutual inhibition, the stimuli cancel each other. According to Dowling and Boycott (646), retinal connections account for the concentric circular receptive fields at the ganglion cell level. Impulses from the central zone are said to be mediated by direct connections between receptor cells, bipolar cells and ganglion cells, while the antagonistic annular surround zone has interposed connections with amacrine cells (i.e., between bipolar and ganglion cells).

The receptive fields of neurons in the lateral geniculate body appear similar with stationary spots of light (1155). The major difference between the receptive fields for ganglion cells and lateral geniculate cells is that cells of the LGB show a greater suppression of the receptive field periphery (1197). This suggests that LGB neurons receive multiple inputs from the optic tract. Single geniculate relay neurons receive inputs from more than one optic tract fiber (convergence), as well as inhibitory inputs from the visual cortex, cells within the geniculate body, and the brain stem reticular formation (810). These observations indicate no rearrangement of the organization of the receptive fields of the visual system occurs at the geniculate level. However, studies of single units in the striate cortex reveal that receptive fields at this level are not concentric and are particularly sensitive to "slits" of light or moving visual patterns oriented in specific directions (Fig. 19-17) (1156, 1157).

Clinical Considerations. Injury to any

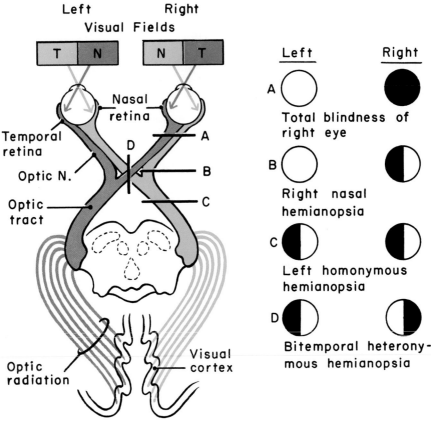

Figure 15-32. Diagram of common lesions within the visual pathway. On the *left*, *A* through *D* indicate lesions. Corresponding visual field defects are shown on the *right*. (Modified from Haymaker (1057).)

part of the optic pathway produces visual defects whose nature depends on the location and extent of the injury. During examination each eye is covered in turn as the retinal quadrants of the opposite eye are tested. Visual defects are said to be *homonymous* when restricted to a single visual field, right or left, and *heteronymous* when parts of both fields are involved. It is evident that homonymous defects are caused by lesions on one side anywhere behind the chiasm (i.e., optic tract, lateral geniculate body, optic radiations and visual cortex). Complete destruction of any of these structures results in a loss of the whole opposite field of vision (*homonymous hemianopsia*) (Fig. 15-32*C*); partial injury may produce *quadrantic homonymous* defects. Lesions of the temporal lobe, by compressing or destroying the looping fibers in the lower portion of the optic radiations, are likely to produce such quadrantic defects in the upper visual field. In-

jury to the parietal lobe may involve the more superiorly placed fibers of the radiations and cause similar defects in the lower field of vision.

Lesions of the chiasm may cause several kinds of heteronymous defects. Most commonly the crossing fibers from the nasal portions of the retina are involved, with consequent loss of the two temporal fields of vision (*bitemporal hemianopsia*) (Fig. 15-32*D*). Rarely, both lateral angles of the chiasm may be compressed; in such cases the nondecussating fibers from the temporal retinae are affected, and the result is loss of the nasal visual fields (*binasal hemianopsia*). Injury of one optic nerve naturally produces blindness in the corresponding eye with loss of the pupillary light reflex (Fig. 15-32*A*). The pupil will, however, contract consensually to light entering the other eye, since the pretectal reflex center is related bilaterally to visceral nuclei of the oculomotor complex. The pupillary light reflex will not be affected by lesions of the visual pathway above the brachium of the superior colliculus (Fig. 15-30).

FUNCTIONAL CONSIDERATIONS OF THE THALAMUS

All sensory impulses, with the sole exception of the olfactory ones, terminate in the gray masses of the thalamus, from which they are projected to specific cortical areas by the thalamocortical radiations. Some fibers from the olfactory tubercle, the pyriform cortex and the basolateral amygdaloid nuclei project to the dorsomedial nucleus (DM), but this nucleus does not relay impulses to the primary olfactory cortex (1360, 1467). While portions of the dorsal thalamus serve as primary relay nuclei in various sensory pathways in which impulses are projected to specific regions of the cerebral cortex, the structure and organization of the thalamus indicate that its function is more complex and elaborate than that of a simple relay station. It seems certain that the thalamus is one of the chief sensory integrating mechanism of the neuraxis, but its functions are not limited to this. Abundant evidence indicates that specific parts of the thalamus play a dominant role in the maintenance and regulation of the state of consciousness, alertness and attention, through widespread functional influences upon the activity of the cerebral cortex. The thalamus is concerned not only with general and specific types of awareness, but with certain emotional connotations that accompany, or are associated with, most sensory experiences. Other data suggest that some thalamic nuclei serve as integrative centers for motor functions, since they receive the principal efferent projections from the cerebellum and the corpus striatum.

In terms of physiological functions the thalamus and related neuronal subsystems are concerned with high fidelity transmission of sensory information, with input selection, output tuning, synchronization and desynchronization of cortical activity, parallel processing of information and signal storing and modification (2077).

The Specific Sensory Relay Nuclei. Specific sensory relay nuclei of the thalamus are in the ventral tier of the lateral nuclear group. These include the medial

and lateral geniculate bodies and the two divisions of the ventral posterior nucleus. The medial geniculate body (MGB) receives fibers from the inferior colliculus. The laminated parvicellular part of the nucleus, concerned with audition, projects fibers via the geniculotemporal radiation to the transverse temporal gyrus of Heschl, the *primary auditory area* (Figs. 12-13 and 15-15). The lateral geniculate body (LGB), receiving both crossed and uncrossed fibers of the optic tract, gives rise to the geniculocalcarine fibers, which project in a specific way to the cortex surrounding the calcarine sulcus; this represents the *primary visual area* (Fig. 15-30). As mentioned earlier, the two divisions of the ventral posterior nucleus (VPL and VPM) project to the cortex of the postcentral gyrus. In the postcentral gyrus all parts of the body are represented in a definite sequence (1968); this cortical region is referred to as the *primary somesthetic area* (somatic sensory area I). The sensory representation of the body in the primary somesthetic area (SI) is duplicated in a different sequence at the base of the postcentral gyrus along the border of the lateral sulcus (1963, 2771). This second topographical body representation, known as the *second somatic sensory area* (SS II), receives inputs from cells in the ipsilateral VPLc and from S I bilaterally (331, 812, 1238, 1239, 1241, 1244), but does not receive projections from the posterior thalamic nucleus (331). This cortical area has a representation of different body regions in the form of obliquely oriented cortical strips parallel to the lateral sulcus (812, 2190). Cell columns respond to cutaneous stimulation mainly on contralateral body surfaces (2191). It was previously thought that SS II was concerned in a unique way with pain perception, but this view has been challenged by new evidence (2020, 2190–2192). Ablation experiments indicate that SS II is not essential for somatic discrimination (1891).

The relatively simple impulses from peripheral receptors do not pass through the thalamus without modification. Many of the impulses become synthesized and integrated at a thalamic level before being projected to specific cortical areas. According to Head and Holmes (1062) and Foerster (758), crude sensory modalities such as touch, thermal sense and pain may be injured separately below thalamic levels, but at thalamic levels, and above, they become intimately fused and can no longer be segregated. Thus the sensory cortex probably has little, if any, direct association with peripheral sensory receptors, and is dependent upon the modified and integrated sensory impulses it receives from the thalamus.

The thalamus may represent the neurological substratum of a crude sort of awareness, such as the recognition of touch, temperature and pain, and of the affective quality of sensation (i.e., its pleasantness or unpleasantness). In certain lesions of the thalamus, or of the thalamocortical connections, after a brief initial stage of contralateral anesthesia, pain, crude touch and some thermal sense return. However, tactile localization, two-point discrimination and the sense of position and movement are lost or severely impaired. The sensations recovered are poorly localized and are accompanied by an increase in "feeling tone," most commonly of an unpleasant character. Although the threshold of excitability is raised on the affected side, tactile and thermal stimuli, previously not unpleasant, may evoke disagreeable sensations (dysesthesias), not easily characterized by the patient. Often the patient cannot endure innocuous cutaneous stimulation, yet he cannot tell the nature of the exciting stimulus. Occasionally the reverse occurs: a previously indifferent stimulus evokes a most pleasant feeling. These feeling states may even be induced by other sensations, for instance auditory ones (1061).

There are two aspects to sensation: the discriminative and the affective. In the former, stimuli are compared with respect to intensity, locality and relative position in space and time. These impulses are integrated into perceptions of form, size and texture; movements are judged as to extent, direction and sequence. These aspects of sensation are related primarily to the specific sensory relay nuclei (i.e., VPL and VPM) and the restricted cortical areas to which they project. Within VPL and VPM there is a complete, although distorted, representation of the body in which relationships between the periphery and portions of this complex are very precise. This spec-

ificity is similar to that which exists in the primary sensory cortex. These neurons are modality specific, being concerned mainly with tactile and position sense, and responding to either superficial mechanical stimulation of the skin, mechanical distortion of deep tissues or joint rotation, but not more than one of these.

Many receptors activated by joint movement lie not in the joint capsule but in the muscle stretched by the movement (461). Under certain conditions these receptors may be involved in conscious perception of movement (919). Physiological data indicate that impulses arising from primary endings in muscle spindles (group Ia fibers) are conveyed via relays to the cerebral cortex, but considerable controversy concerns their cortical region of termination and the thalamic relay nuclei involved (1235). Short latency cortical responses can be evoked by stimulation of group Ia muscle afferents in a transitional cortical zone designated as 3a (1904). Area 3a is considered to lie in the depths of the central sulcus between areas 4 and 3, but is difficult to define anatomically (1235). These short latency responses from muscle spindles are considered to reach the thalamus via the posterior column nuclei. Short latency cortical responses from low threshold muscle afferents can be evoked in the primary somesthetic area (SI), the second somatic area (SS II) and area 4, as well as in area 3a (1235). Thalamic inputs to area 4 are independent of those to area 3a and emanate from VPLo and VL. Inputs to the somesthetic cortex arise from VPLc, while those to cortical area 3a could not be separately identified on the basis of thalamic connections (2567). Impulses generated in low threshold stretch receptors probably reach consciousness in area 3a and the primary somesthetic area, but they appear independent of impulses reaching the motor cortex which influence or regulate outflow from the motor cortex. The major suprasegmental structure receiving impulses from stretch receptors is the cerebellum.

"Affective" sensation is concerned with pain, agreeableness and disagreeableness. Pain is a subjective sensation that often is difficult to describe and almost impossible to measure. The localization of different types of pain is often inexact and clinical judgment of its intensity must take into account the personality of the patient. Temperature and many tactile sensations likewise have a marked affective tone. This is especially true for visceral sensations, in which the discriminative element is practically absent. This affective quality, which forms the basis of general bodily well-being or *malaise*, and of the more intense emotional states, is believed to be "appreciated" at the thalamic rather than the cortical level, although it may be profoundly modified and controlled by the latter. The appreciation of pain, crude touch and some thermal sense is retained even after complete destruction of the sensory cortical areas of both sides.

The visual thalamic relay nuclei likewise are organized in a specific manner in which point for point relationships exist between the retina, thalamic nuclei and the visual (striate) cortex. Even though crossed and uncrossed fibers in the optic tract end upon cells in different layers of the LGB, columns of cells in all six layers receive inputs from corresponding points in the retina of each eye related to the contralateral binocular visual field. These columns of cells in different layers correspond to the "lines of projection." Columns of cells in the dorsal nucleus of the LGB all project to a specific loci in the visual cortex. Binocular fusion does not occur in the LGB and cells of this nucleus have receptive fields similar to those of retinal ganglion cells. Geniculocalcarine fibers have a retinotopic projection upon the visual cortex. This relatively undifferentiated visual input is transformed in the cortex in a complex manner that gives individual cortical cells receptive field properties totally different from those of the geniculate neurons, but better suited to detect shapes and patterns (Figs. 19-16 and 19-17).

The auditory thalamic relay nuclei are organized in a similar specific manner. The cellular laminae of the ventral nucleus of the medial geniculate body (MGB), evident only in Golgi preparations, correspond to those of the dorsal nucleus of the LGB. This laminar organization forms the basis for the tonotopic organization in which high frequencies are represented medially and low frequencies laterally. Neurons in the ventral division of the MGB project to the primary auditory cortex, while those in other cytological subdivisions of the MGB project to a belt of cortex surrounding the primary auditory cortex.

The Cortical Relay Nuclei. Cortical relay nuclei of the thalamus receive impulses from specific subcortical structures and project to well defined cortical regions. These nuclei include: (a) the anterior nuclei (b) the ventral lateral nucleus, and (c) the ventral anterior nucleus (in part). The anterior nuclei of the thalamus receive the largest efferent fiber bundle from the hypothalamus, the mammillothalamic tract and direct projections from the hippocampal formation via the fornix (Figs. 15.2, 15-9, and 16-7). These nuclei in turn project to the cingulate gyrus, a cortical area demonstrated to produce a variety of visceral responses upon stimulation (1359, 2671). Impulses from the cingulate gyrus are relayed to the hippocampal formation via the entorhinal area (2094). The hippocampal formation projects to the hypothalamus and to the anterior thalamic nuclei.

Portions of the ventral lateral nucleus of the thalamus receive cerebellar, pallidal and nigra efferent fibers and relay impulses from these sources to the precentral motor cortex. The medial pallidal segment give rise to pallidothalamic fibers that terminate in VLo and in the lateral part of VLm. Nigral efferent fibers from the pars reticulata terminate in medial parts of VLm without overlapping regions receiving pallidal projections. Cerebellar inputs to the ventral lateral nucleus are crossed and widely regarded as terminating in virtually all regions of VL (including "area x"), except VLm. In addition crossed cerebellar efferent fibers terminate in VPLo (441, 1260, 1654, 1708, 2419, 2567). It seems likely that some pallidal and cerebellar efferents may terminate in overlapping fashion in VLo, although evidence suggests that relatively few cerebellar fibers end in this subdivision of VL (1971, 2538, 2567). The extent of the overlap of pallidal and cerebeller efferents in VLo is unknown, as is the precise physiological nature of the interaction of these systems upon their target neurons. Since the ventral lateral nucleus is the principal subcortical structure projecting to the motor cortex, it is apparent that signals conveyed to it have profound effects upon cortical neurons that give rise to impulses that underlie some of the most important aspects of motor function. Neocerebellar disturbances resulting from cerebellar lesions may be the physiological expression of release of the ventral lateral thalamic nucleus from the controlling and regulating influences normally provided by the cerebellum. With respect to the corpus striatum the situation is different in that dyskinesia (disturbances of movement) due to disease processes seems to be dependent upon the integrity of pallidothalamic fibers systems. However, lesions in the ventral lateral nucleus can ameliorate aspects of dyskinesia due to lesions of both the cerebellum and the corpus striatum, presumably by reducing the output of VL to the motor cortex.

Although the distinctive parts of the ventral anterior nucleus receive substantial and nonoverlapping projections from the globus pallidus (VApc) and the pars reticularis of the substantia nigra (VAmc), only part of the cells of this nucleus relay impulses to the cerebral cortex. Cells of VApc which receive some input from VAmc appear to have a widespread projection to the frontal cortex rostral to the precentral motor area (Fig. 15-15). The cortical projection from VAmc to the medial orbitofrontal region is not extensive in distribution (373, 1310). The later projection is considered to be involved in "triggering" of the recruiting response (2610). In addition this rostral ventral tier thalamic nucleus has connections with the intralaminar and dorsomedial thalamic nuclei. Thus the ventral anterior nucleus exhibits some characteristics of both the specific and the nonspecific thalamic nuclei.

As a group the cortical relay nuclei of the thalamus possess common features, although the ventral anterior nucleus presents certain exceptions: (a) all receive substantial projections from specific parts of the neuraxis, (b) all, except for parts of VA, project to well defined cortical areas and (c) all, except VA, undergo extensive cell change following ablation of their cortical projection areas. These nuclei, with the exception of parts of VA, constitute the *specific thalamic relay nuclei*. Low frequency electrical stimulation of individual specific sensory relay nuclei, and certain cortical relay nuclei (i.e., the ventral lateral nucleus), evokes a primary surface potential followed by an augmenting sequence which is limited to the cortical projection area. This response, called the *augmenting responses*, is characterized by: (a) a short latency, (b) diphasic responses which increase in magnitude during the initial four or five stimuli of a repetitive train and (c) localization to the primary cortical projection area of the specific thalamic nucleus stimulated (618).

The Association Nuclei. The association nuclei of the thalamus receive relatively few direct fibers from the ascending systems, but have abundant connections with other diencephalic nuclei. They project largely to association areas of the cerebral cortex in the frontal and parietal lobes and, to a lesser extent, in the occipital and temporal lobes. The principal association nuclei include the dorsomedial nucleus (DM), the lateral dorsal nucleus (LD), the lateral posterior nucleus (LP) and the pulvinar (P) (Fig. 15-13).

The dorsomedial nucleus, the most prominent gray mass of the medial thalamus, is highly developed in primates, especially man (Fig. 15-13). Different portions of this nucleus have connections with the lateral thalamic nuclei, the amygdaloid nuclear complex and temporal lobe neocortex. The pars reticulata of the substantia nigra also has an impressive projection to the paralaminar part of the nucleus (DMpl) and there are profuse reciprocal connections with the granular frontal cortex (Figs. 13-25 and 13-26). It has been suggested that in this nucleus somatic impulses forming the basis for discriminative cortical sensibility are blended with the feeling tone engendered by visceral activities. These somatovisceral impulses are projected to the prefrontal cortex, which constitutes a large, phylogenetically new cortical area highly developed in man. While the signficiance of the prefrontal cortex is not fully understood, it has been regarded as the place where the discriminative cortical activities may be developed.

Large injuries to the frontal lobes of both hemispheres are likely to cause defects in complex associations, as well as changes in behavior, expressed by loss of acquired inhibitions and more direct and excessive emotional responses. Similar alterations in emotional behavior may be produced when the pathways between the dorsomedial nucleus and the frontal cortex are severed (e.g., in frontal lobotomy).

The lateral dorsal and lateral posterior nuclei receive afferent fibers principally from the ventral nuclei and apparently are concerned with complex somesthetic association mechanisms related to various parts of the body. The lateral dorsal nucleus projects upon portions of the limbic and precuneal cortex. The larger lateral posterior nucleus has extensive connections with the association cortex of the superior and inferior parietal lobules, concerned with cognitive and symbolic functions.

The pulvinar, considered as an outgrowth of the lateral posterior nucleus, appears relatively late in phylogenetic development. Development of this huge nuclear mass seems to be correlated with increasing complexity in the integration of somatic and special senses, especially vision and audition. The cortical projections of this thalamic nuclear complex are largely to portions of the posterior parietal and occipitotemporal cortex. The inferior and adjacent lateral pulvinar receive fibers from the superficial layers of the superior colliculus which topographically represent the contralateral visual field (154, 1039, 1941). Both of these divisions of the pulvinar project retinotopically upon the striate (area 17), the parastriate (area 18) and the peristriate (area 19) cortex to layers that do not receive inputs from the lateral geniculate body. This complex linkage implicates these divisions of the pulvinar in an extrageniculate visual pathway (2139). Other divisions of the pulvinar have connections with association cortex of the temporal, parietal and frontal lobes.

The Intralaminar Nuclei. The intralaminar nuclei of the mammalian dorsal thalamus have long constituted an unexplored and poorly understood region. Phylogenetically these nuclei are older than the specific relay nuclei which develop *pari passu* with the cerebral cortex. Although the midline thalamic nuclei show a progressive regression in ascending phylogeny, the intralaminar thalamic nuclei continue to develop in primates and man (1837). Most of these nuclei have been regarded anatomically as having no cortical projections, although they have connections with other thalamic nuclei (1827), the globus pallidus (1313, 1398, 1825) and the striatum (1234, 2055). As previously described, many of the afferent fibers to the intralaminar nuclei ascend from the brain stem in the central tegmental fasciculus, a composite bundle containing predominantly long axons originating from neurons in the reticular formation. Stimulation of the ascending reticular activating system and various kinds of sensory stimuli result in a generalized desynchronization and activation of the electroencephalogram, and behavioral arousal. These phenomena are comparable to those associated with arousal from natural sleep. It is generally accepted that the electroencephalographic (EEG) arousal response, which produces dramatic effects upon cortical activity, is mediated, in part, by the intralaminar nuclei. Physiological studies presumed that impulses producing these changes in cortical activity reached the cortex via a diffuse thalamic projection system (1208, 1210, 1756, 2421), the exact nature of which was ill-defined. Studies utilizing retrograde axonal transport of horseradish peroxidase indicate that the nonspecific cortical projections arise as collaterals of projection fibers from the intralaminar thalamic nuclei; the principal projection from these nuclei is to the neostriatum (1234). Golgi studies also indicate that the principal axons from the centromedian and parafascicular nuclei project to the putamen, and that collaterals of these fibers project to the overlying cortex (2279). Axons from the rostral intralaminar nuclei pass through parts of the ventral anterior nucleus and through the thalamic reticular nucleus to the caudate nucleus. Some of these fibers can be followed into the white matter of the orbitofrontal cortex.

The classical studies of Dempsey and Morison (618, 619) and of Morison and Dempsey (1752) showed that stimulation of the so-called nonspecific thalamic nuclei, and the basal diencephalic region, produced widespread and pronounced effects upon electrocortical activity. The *nonspecific*, or *diffuse*, thalamic nuclei include the intralaminar and midline nuclei and part of the ventral anterior nucleus. Repetitive stimulation of these thalamic nuclei alters spontaneous electrocortical activity over large areas and, under certain conditions, resets the frequency of brain waves by eliciting responses that are time-locked to the thalamic stimulus. The most characteristic effect of stimulating the nonspecific thalamic nuclei is the *recruiting response*. When the frequency of stimulation is in the range of 6 to 12 cycles/sec, predominantly surface negative cortical responses rapidly increase to a maximum (by the fourth to sixth stimulus of the train) and then decrease over a broad area; continued stimulation causes the evoked responses to wax and wane. Stimulation of one of the nonspecific thalamic nuclei causes all others to be activated in a mass excitation (2421). Bilateral cortical responses do not depend upon transmission by fibers of the corpus callosum or anterior commissure, nor does spread from one cortical area to another depend upon intracortical propagation (1208, 1752). Cortical spread involves intrathalamic activities, including conduction across midline gray masses of the thalamus. Although stimulating the nonspecific thalamic nuclei produces changes in electrocortical activity over broad areas, these effects are not indiscriminate or equal in all cortical areas. Responsive cortical zones appear to be relatively specific in the frontal, cingulate, orbital, parietal and occipital association areas. This diffuse thalamic projection system appears capable of exerting a massive influence mainly upon large regions of associate cortex, but the most profound effects are upon the frontal association cortex (2424). The recruiting response has been abolished by lesions, or reversible cryogenic blockade, at three sites: (a) the ventral anterior nucleus, (b) the inferior thalamic peduncle and (c) the orbitofrontal cortex (2350). Stimulation of the nonspecific thalamic nuclei demonstrates that these nuclei also exert a potent influence upon subcortical structures, particularly the thalamic association nuclei, such as the dorsomedial nucleus, the lateral dorsal nucleus, the lateral posterior nucleus and the pulvinar (2424).

The observation of Moruzzi and Magoun (1756) that cortical recruiting responses induced by low frequency stimulation of the nonspecific thalamic nuclei could be reduced, or blocked, by stimulation of the bulbar reticular formation provides evidence that the nonspecific nuclei of the thalamus are within the sphere of influence of the ascending reticular formation. This finding together with anatomical evidence (1824, 2274) supports the thesis that EEG arousal reactions elicited by ascending reticular volleys are mediated, at least in part, via the nonspecific thalamic nuclei.

Some idea of the complex physiological relationship between the brain stem reticular formation and nonspecific thalamic nuclie is provided by the antagonistic effects of reticular activation on the recruiting responses and other varieties of electrocortical synchronization elicited by stimulation of the nonspecific thalamus, as noted above. However, it must be pointed out that electrocortical synchronization also may be obtained by stimulation of caudal as well as rostral regions of the brain stem reticular formation and that, conversely, electrocortical desynchronization may be obtained with high frequency stimulation of nonspecific thalamic nuclei. The overt electroencephalographic effects appear to depend in part on both the frequency and the intensity of stimulation at different sites within the mesencephalic and diencephalic reticular system (1755).

The largest component of the intralaminar nuclei, the centromedian-parafascicular nuclear complex (CM-PF) receives its input mainly from forebrain derivatives. The precentral and premotor cortex project profusely upon these nuclei (31, 1393, 1394). In addition the CM receives a large number of pallidofugal fibers. The fact that the principal projection of CM-PF is to the striatum suggests that this nuclear complex must play an important role in motor function. It would seem that part of the output of the corpus striatum is fed back to the striatum via thalamostriate fibers and that impulses from cortical motor areas could modify this input via fibers projecting to CM-PF. The intralaminar thalamic nuclei have also been considered as components of a nonspecific sensory system and part of a central mechanism concerned with pain (33, 709, 1494, 2233).

It has been suggested that the nuclei of the posterior thalamic complex should be grouped with the intralaminar nuclei (1243). The prefrontal, premotor and precentral cortex project largely to the intralaminar nuclei while the somesthetic and auditory cortex project to nuclei of the posterior thalamic complex. The posterior thalamic nuclei are hypothesized to constitute a posterior extension of the intralaminar thalamic nuclei related to all the cortex on the lateral surface of the hemisphere caudal to area 4, with the exception of areas 17, 18, and 19. Experiments with small lesions indicate almost all cortical areas project fibers to: (a) their respective principal thalamic nucleus, (b) part of the reticular nucleus and (c) either a part of the intralaminar or posterior thalamic nuclei. Further, most afferent fibers to the thalamus, whether part of a sensory system or from some other subcortical structure, project to: (a) one or more principal thalamic nuclei and (b) either a component of the intralaminar or posterior thalamic nuclei, or to both of these. This hypothesis presents evidence of striking similarities between these groups of thalamic nuclei. The visual cortex appears unique in that it does not send or receive fibers from either the intralaminar or posterior thalamic nuclei. It has been suggested that the pretectum, or parts of it might be the equivalent of the intralaminar-posterior thalamic nuclei for the visual cortex.

The thalamus is played upon by two great streams of afferent fibers: the peripheral and the cortical. The former brings sensory impulses from all parts of the body concerning changes in the external and internal environment. The cortical connections link the thalamus with the associative memory mechanism of the pallium and bring it under cortical control. The thalamus has subcortical efferent connections with the hypothalamus and striatum through which the thalamus can influence visceral and somatic effectors. The functional nature of these subcortical efferent thalamic pathways is unknown, but they are considered to serve primarily affective reactions. These pathways, like the thalamus itself, are under the control of the cerebral cortex. Corticothalamic projections usually are considered to exert inhibitory influences upon thalamic activity. It has been suggested that corticothalamic fibers may constitute part of a complex neural mechanism for the selective regulation of the integrative actions of the thalamus, permitting certain subdivisions to function while inhibiting the activity of others.

CHAPTER 16

The Hypothalamus

The current reductionist (cellular) approach in neuroscience has been very successful, but as one approaches the study of complex behaviors it becomes clear that molecular and cellular studies must proceed together with the systems level of analysis. Coghill, in seminal studies on the salamander brain, concluded that the primary function of the nervous system is the maintenance of the integrity of the individual while behavior patterns expand (496). He promulgated the idea that basic brain stem neuronal networks regulated patterns of activity necessary for the nourishment, reproduction and defense of the organism, so that during phylogeny other brain structures could evolve for higher order perception, movement and communication. The region of the mammalian brain that is most important in the coordination of behaviors essential for the maintenance and continuation of the species is the hypothalamus.

The hypothalamus occupies only about 0.5% of the volume of the human brain, yet it plays a major role in the regulation of the release of hormones from the pituitary gland, maintenance of body temperature, and the organization of goal seeking behaviors such as feeding, drinking, mating and aggression. While the coordination of smooth and striated muscles and secretory epithelial cells required to carry out these behaviors is not exclusively controlled by the hypothalamus, this region of the brain is essential for behavioral adjustments to changes in the internal or external environment. For example, aggression or territorial defense may be elicited by specific visual or olfactory stimuli, but the behavior depends upon the hormonal state of the animal (754a). Behaviors such as feeding or aggression can be elicited by electrical stimulation of the hypothalamus, but the particular behavior observed depends upon the test situation (558). The linkage between the lower brain stem, spinal cord and smooth muscles and glands is described in Chapter 8. In this chapter the diencephalic structures acting upon the brain stem and cord will be described. The human hypothalmus appears to follow the same basic developmental sequence seen in lower mammals when due consideration is given to the topographical alterations brought about by the greater development of the temporal lobe in man (1107, 1307).

The hypothalamus is the part of the diencephalon concerned with the central control of visceral, autonomic and endocrine functions, and with affective behavior. The hypothalamus lies in the walls of the third ventricle below the hypothalamic sulci and

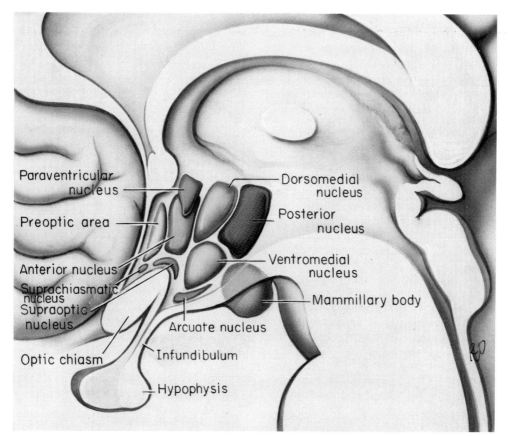

Figure 16-1. Schematic diagram of the medial hypothalamic nuclei. Nuclei in the supraoptic region are in *blue*. The paraventricular and supraoptic nuclei are *dark blue*; the suprachiasmatic and anterior nuclei of the hypothalamus are *light blue*. Nuclei of the middle or tuberal region of the hypothalamus are *yellow*. Nuclei of the caudal or mammillary region are shades of *red*. The preoptic area lies rostral to the anterior hypothalamic region and classically is regarded as a forebrain derivative functionally related to the hypothalamus.

is continuous across the floor of this ventricle (Figs. 2-28 and 16-1).

On the ventral surface of the brain the *infundibulum*, to which the hypophysis is attached, emerges posterior to the optic chiasm (Figs. 2-8, 2-9 and 16-1). A slightly bulging region posterior to the infundibulum is the *tuber cinereum* (Fig. 16-6). The ventral external hypothalamus is bounded anteriorly by the optic chiasm, laterally by the optic tracts and posteriorly by the mammillary bodies (Figs. 2-8, 2-9 and 2-27). This region is roughly diamond shaped and its surface is irregular because of several small protuberances, identified as eminences. The zone forming the floor of the third ventricle is called the *median eminence* of the tuber cinereum. The portion rostral to the infundibular stem is the *anterior median eminence*; the portion posterior to the infundibular stem forms the *posterior median eminence*, which is better developed in man (Figs. 2-8 and 2-9). Paired lateral eminences form well-defined landmarks. The ventral protrusion of the hypothalamus and the third ventricular recess form the infundibulum (Fig. 9-6). The most distal portion of the infundibular process is the neurohypophysis; tissue joining the infundibular process to the median eminence is called the infundibular stem. The median eminence represents the final point of convergence of pathways from the central nervous system upon the peripheral endocrine system (1338). The median eminence is the anatomical site of the interface between brain and the anterior pituitary. Primary capillaries of the hypophysial portal vessels vascularize the median eminence (2048). Ependymal cells lining the floor of the third ventricle have processes that traverse the width of the median eminence and terminate near the portal perivascular space. These cells (tanycytes) in the median eminence appear to be structurally and functionally capable of providing a link between the cerebrospinal fluid (CSF) and the perivascular space of the pituitary portal vessels. The *mammillary bodies* are found posteriorly near the interpeduncular fossa (Figs. 2-8, 2-9, 2-27 and 16-1). The hypothalamus can be described as extending from the region of the optic chiasm to the caudal border of the mammillary bodies. Anteriorly it passes without sharp demarcation into the basal olfactory area (diagonal gyrus of the anterior perforated substance) (Fig. 18-2). The region immediately in front of the optic chiasm, extending rostrally to the lamina terminalis and dorsally to the anterior commissure, is known as the preoptic area (Fig. 16-1). The preoptic area, classically regarded as a forebrain derivative (470), is considered by Kuhlenbeck (1383) to arise from a rostral hypothalamic anlage and to be structurally and functionally a part of the hypothalamus. Caudally the hypothalamus merges imperceptibly into the central gray and tegmentum of the midbrain. The thalamus lies dorsal to the hypothalamus; the subthalamic region is lateral and caudal (Figs. 2-28 and 15-7).

HYPOTHALAMIC CYTOARCHITECTONICS

Pervading the whole hypothalamic area is a diffuse matrix of cells constituting the central gray substance, in which are found a number of more or less distinct nuclear masses. A sagittal plane passing through the anterior column of the fornix roughly separates the medial and lateral hypothalamic areas (Figs. 16-2 and 16-3).

The Lateral Hypothalamic Area. This area is bounded medially by the mammillothalamic tract and the anterior column of the fornix; the medial edge of the internal capsule and the subthalamic region form its lateral boundary (Figs. 16-2 and 16-3). Rostrally this area is continuous with the lateral preoptic nucleus, while caudally it merges with the ventral tegmental area of the midbrain. Rostral and caudal portions of this area are narrow, but the tuberal region is expanded. The lateral hypothalamic area contains several groups of cells, the largest of which is the *tuberomammil-*

lary nucleus which caudally extends lateral and ventral to the mammillary body (1823). The *lateral tuberal nuclei* (nuclei tuberis lateral or tuberales) consists of two or three sharply delimited cell groups which often produce small visible eminences on the basal surface of the hypothalamus (Fig. 15-11). They consist of small, pale, multipolar cells surrounded by a delicate fiber capsule about which are found the large cells of the lateral hypothalamic nucleus (Figs. 16-2 and 16-3).

The Preoptic Region. This region constitutes the periventricular gray of the most rostral part of the third ventricle (Figs. 16-1–16-3). The *preoptic periventricular nucleus* surrounds the walls of the third ventricle in the region of the preoptic recess. The diffusely arranged small cells are poorly differentiated from the ependymal lining. The *medial preoptic nucleus*, composed of predominantly small cells, lies lateral to the preoptic periventricular nucleus and extends ventrally to the optic chiasm (Fig. 16-3).

The preoptic region plays a role in regulating the release of gonadotropic hormones from the anterior lobe of the hypophysis. In the human female, pituitary gonadotropins are released in a cyclic manner, and the duration of the cycle determines the length of the menstrual cycle. In the male, the gonadotropins are released tonically without regularly occurring fluctuations. It is therefore not surprising that there are differences in the functional organization of the preoptic region in the male and female of the species. A morphological expression of this difference has been observed in the preoptic region of the rat, where a nucleus of densely stained cells is larger in the male (927). This nucleus has been termed the "sexually dimorphic nucleus of the preoptic area" (Fig. 16-16). The full ontogenetic development of this nucleus, as well as the male pattern of tonic gonadotropic release, depends upon the presence of testosterone in the circulation during the first week of life. If the testes are removed from the newborn rat, the genetic male will fail to develop the sexually dimorphic nucleus of the preoptic region and will have a female pattern of gonadotropin release at puberty. Conversely, a newborn female given exogenous testosterone will, as an adult, show the male pattern of gonadotropin release.

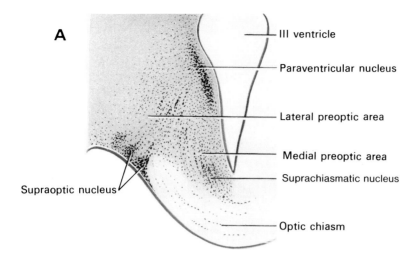

A
- III ventricle
- Paraventricular nucleus
- Lateral preoptic area
- Medial preoptic area
- Suprachiasmatic nucleus
- Supraoptic nucleus
- Optic chiasm

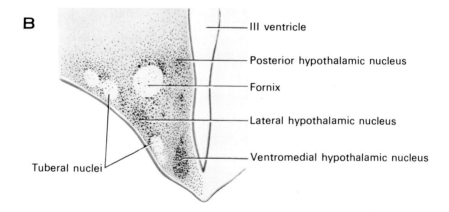

B
- III ventricle
- Posterior hypothalamic nucleus
- Fornix
- Lateral hypothalamic nucleus
- Ventromedial hypothalamic nucleus
- Tuberal nuclei

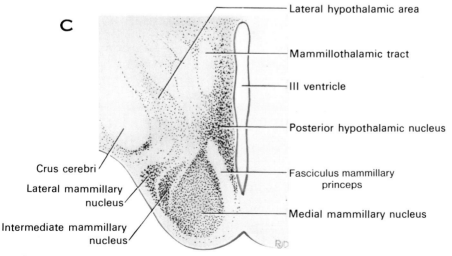

C
- Lateral hypothalamic area
- Mammillothalamic tract
- III ventricle
- Posterior hypothalamic nucleus
- Crus cerebri
- Lateral mammillary nucleus
- Fasciculus mammillary princeps
- Intermediate mammillary nucleus
- Medial mammillary nucleus

Figure 16-2. Drawings of transverse sections through portions of the human hypothalamus: *A*, supraoptic region; *B*, infundibular region; *C*, mammillary region (after Clark et al. (470)).

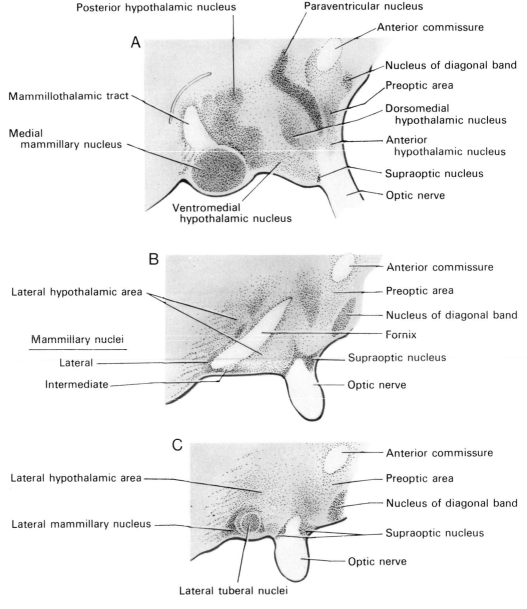

Figure 16-3. Sagittal drawings of the human hypothalamus: *A*, near ventricular surface; *B*, through the anterior column of the fornix; *C*, near lateral border of hypothalamus (after Clark et al. (470)).

The *lateral preoptic nucleus*, rostral to the lateral hypothalamic area, is composed of diffusely dispersed medium-sized cells (Figs. 16-2 and 16-3) and is regarded as the interstitial nucleus of the median forebrain bundle (1383).

Caudal to the preoptic region three hypothalamic regions are recognized. In rostrocaudal sequence these are: (a) an anterior or *supraoptic region*, lying above the optic chiasm and continuous rostrally with the preoptic area, (b) a middle or *tuberal region* and (c) a posterior or *mammillary region*, which is continuous caudally with the central gray of the midbrain (Fig. 16-1).

The Supraoptic Region. This region contains two of the most striking and sharply defined hypothalamic nuclei, the *paraventricular nucleus* and the *supraoptic nucleus*. Cells of the paraventricular nucleus form a vertical plate of densely packed cells immediately beneath the ependyma of the third ventricle, while cells of the supraoptic nucleus straddle the optic tract (Figs. 16-1–16-3 and 16-5). Cells in both these nuclei appear similar. They are larger than cells in the surrounding central gray and stain deeply. The Nissl substance is distributed peripherally, and cytoplasmic inclusions of colloidal material are found which are regarded as the neurosecretory product of these cells. Both of these nuclei send fibers to the posterior lobe of the hypophysis.

When sections of the hypothalamus are stained to reveal cell bodies, some nuclei, or parts of nuclei, contain larger perikarya and are termed the *magnocellular hypothalamic nuclei*. The supraoptic and paraventricular nuclei are the major magnocellular nuclei. The cytological characteristics of supraoptic and paraventricular neurons reflect the synthesis of the peptide oxytocin or the peptide vasopressin (antidiuretic hormone). These peptide hormones are formed in the cell body and conjugated with a larger carrier protein called neurophysin. The carrier protein-hormone conjugate is carried by axoplasmic transport along the axon to the posterior lobe of the pituitary gland where it is released from the axon terminal (309). Individual paraventricular or supraoptic neurons produce either vasopressin or oxytocin (2605) and each cell type also produces a characteristic neurophysin.

The less differentiated central gray in the supraoptic region constitutes an *anterior hypothalamic* nucleus. This nucleus merges imperceptibly with the preoptic area (Figs. 16-1 and 16-3). The *suprachiasmatic nucleus* forms a group of small round cells immediately dorsal to the optic chiasm and close to the ventral part of the third ventricle (Figs. 16-1 and 16-2). This small nucleus receives direct projections from the retina (1732, 1739, 2009) and also indirect visual input from the thalamus (2482). In rodents, destruction of the suprachiasmatic nuclei causes light-entrained circadian rhythms in hormone release or in drinking behavior to become free-running (1666). While the distribution of axons from suprachiasmatic neurons is not well understood, there is some evidence for a projection to the tuberal region of the hypothalamus (2478). In

man, nearly one third of the cells in the suprachiasmatic nucleus show immunoreactivity for vasopressin (2376). However, the axonal projection, and hence the site of release of vasopressin, is not known.

The organum vasculosum lamina terminalis (OVLT) or "supraoptic crest" is a vascular midline circumventricular organ located in the rostral wall of the third ventricle superior to the optic chiasm (see Fig. 1-19). While this structure is found in many vertebrates, it is particularly prominent in rodents and has been proposed as a site at which the peptide, angiotensin II, binds to receptors and initiates drinking (2001).

The Tuberal Region. In this region the hypothalamus reaches its widest extent and the fornix separates the medial and the lateral hypothalamic regions (Figs. 16-2 and 16-6). The medial portion forms the central gray substance of the ventricular wall, in which there may be distinguished a *ventromedial* and a *dorsomedial nucleus*. The ventromedial nucleus, the largest cell group in the tuberal region, has a round or oval shape and is surrounded by a cell-poor zone that helps to delineate its boundaries (Figs. 16-1–16-3). Neurons of the ventromedial nucleus typically have dendrites that extend beyond the borders of the nucleus (1710). The cell-free capsular zone around the nucleus is formed by a dense ring of axons and terminals (Fig. 16-4). The dorsomedial nucleus is a less distinct aggregation of cells that borders the third ventricle (Fig. 16-3). The *arcuate nucleus* (infundibular nucleus) is located in the most ventral part of the third ventricle near the entrance to the infundibular recess, and extends into the median eminence (Fig. 16-1). The small cells of this nucleus are in close contact with the ependyma lining the ventricle. In coronal sections the nucleus has an arcuate shape (1823). In the caudal part of the tuberal region many large oval or rounded cells are scattered in a matrix of smaller ones; collectively they constitute the *posterior hypothalamic nucleus* (Figs. 16-1–16-3). The large cells, especially numerous in man, extend caudally over the mammillary body to become continuous with the central gray of the midbrain.

The Mammillary Region. This region consists of the mammillary bodies and the dorsally located cells of the posterior hypothalamic nucleus (Figs. 15-6, 16-1–16-3

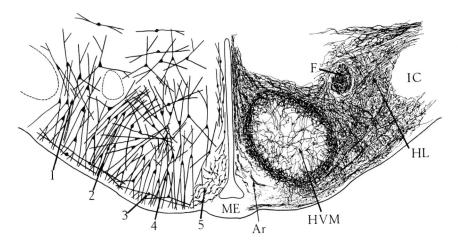

Figure 16-4. A drawing of the tuberal region of the rodent hypothalamus based upon Golgi preparations. On the reader's left the general arrangement of dendrites and axons is shown. *(1)* Dendrites of HL radiate in the mediolateral and dorsoventral directions. *(2)* There is a compression of the dendritic fields of neurons located between F and HVM. *(3)* The dendritic fields of neurons along the hypothalamic surface are generally parallel with the pia. *(4)* The long dendrites of HVM extend in all directions from the nucleus. *(5)* Small bipolar neurons of Ar nestle against the ventricle wall, adjacent to ME. Abbreviations: *Ar* = arcuate nucleus, *F* = Fornix, *HL* = lateral hypothalamic area, *HVM* = hypothalamic ventromedial nucleus, *IC* = internal capsule, *ME* = median eminence. Reproduced with permission from O. E. Millhouse: *Handbook of the Hypothalamus, Vol. I. Anatomy of the Hypothalamus,* edited by P. Morgane and J. Panksepp. Marcel Dekker, New York, 1979.)

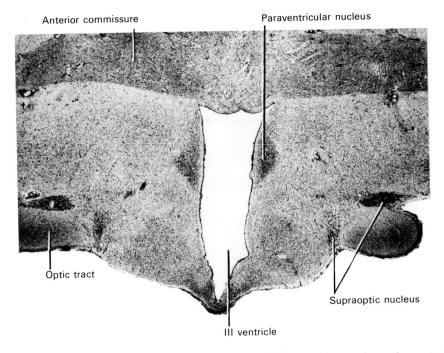

Figure 16-5. Photograph of human hypothalamus at the level of the anterior commissure demonstrating the paraventricular and supraoptic nuclei (Nissl strain).

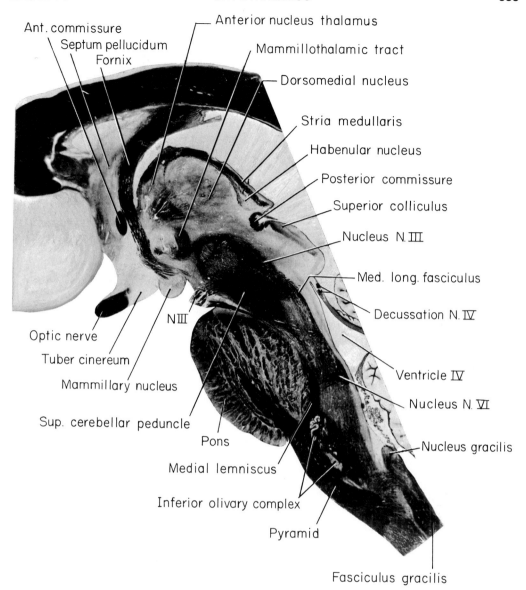

Figure 16-6. Sagittal section of brain stem through the pillar of fornix, the mammillothalamic tract and the stria medullaris (Weigert's myelin stain, photograph).

and 16-6). In man the mammillary body consists almost entirely of the large, spherical *medial mammillary nucleus*, composed of relatively small cells invested by a capsule of myelinated fibers. Lateral to this is the small *intermediate (intercalated) mammillary nucleus* composed of smaller cells (Fig. 16-2). Even further lateral is a well-defined group of large cells, the *lateral mammillary nucleus*, which probably represents a condensation of cells from the posterior hypothalamic nucleus.

The most characteristic features of the human hypothalamus are the sharply circumscribed tuberal nuclei, the large size of the medial mammillary nuclei and the extensive distribution of the large cells in the posterior and lateral hypothalamic areas. Although synthetic descriptions may suggest that all hypothalamic nuclei are well delimited structures, the hypothalamus is broadly continuous with the surrounding gray matter. The transition from hypothalamus to surrounding gray matter is gradual and tissue continuities contain the major afferent and efferent hypothalamic pathways.

Rostrally and laterally the hypothalamus is continuous with the *basal olfactory region*, a large gray mass beneath the rostral part of the lentiform nucleus and the head of the caudate nucleus (Figs. 16-3, 18-2 and A-24). Near the median plane this region extends dorsally, rostral to the anterior commissure, where it becomes the *septal region* (Figs. 18-6 and A-23). Beneath the lentiform nucleus the gray mass extends toward the amygdaloid complex; this region contains cell islands and groups referred to as the *substantia innominata* (Fig. A-22). The rostral part of the substantia innominata lies under the cortex of the anterior perforated substance (Figs. 2-9 and 18-2). The base of the septal region (i.e., the part ventral to the anterior commissure) is continuous with the substantia innominata laterally and with the preoptic region caudally. The dorsal part of the septum forms the septum pellucidum (Figs. 2-5, A-23 and A-24). The septal region contains the *medial septal nucleus*, composed of fairly large neurons, and the *lateral septal nucleus*, which consists of smaller neurons. One of the largest nuclei in this region is the *nucleus accumbens septi* (Fig. A-24), which leans against the base of the septum and is situated medially at the junction of caudate nucleus and putamen.

CONNECTIONS OF THE HYPOTHALAMUS

The hypothalamus, in spite of its small size, has extensive and complex fiber connections. Some fibers are organized into definite and conspicuous bundles, while others are diffuse and difficult to analyze.

The Afferent Connections of the Hypothalamus

The afferent connections of the hypothalamus which have been established are: (a) the *medial forebrain bundle*, a complex group of fibers arising from the basal olfactory regions, the periamygdaloid region and the septal nuclei, that pass to, and through, the lateral preoptic and hypothalamic regions (Figs. 16-7 and 16-8). The bundle is formed, at levels rostral to the anterior commissure, mainly of fibers from the septal region, and in its parasagittal course

receives contributions from the substantia innominata and amygdalopyriform cortex. The bundle is a loose-textured fiber system, in part composed of relatively short fibers, although some longer axons continue caudally into the midbrain tegmentum. The medial forebrain bundle conducts both rostrally and caudally. (b) *Hippocampohypothalamic fibers*, originating from the hippocampal formation, form the fornix and medial corticohypothalamic tract (Figs. 16-6, 16-7, 16-8 and 18-6). In transverse sections at the level of the optic chiasm the medial corticohypothalamic tract appears as a group of myelinated fascicles coursing medial to the fornix. The hippocampal formation projects to the hypothalamus through both the fornix and the medial corticohypothalamic tract. Pyramidal cells from all regions of the hippocampus project to the septum but not to the hypothalamus In degeneration and autoradiographic studies it has been shown that axons reaching the hypothalamus from the temporal lobe originate in the subiculum (see Figs. 16-8, 18-10, 18-12 and 18-13) (1662, 2092, 2095, 2478, 2481). Many of these axons terminate in the cell-free zone surrounding the hypothalamic ventromedial nucleus (HVM) (Fig. 16-4), and others extend caudally to terminate at the level of the medial mammillary nuclei. The general distribution of these fibers corresponds to the location of hypothalamic neurons that selectively concentrate tritiated estradiol (1996, 2460, 2461). Axonal terminals containing epinephrine (1119) or a prolactin-like peptide (830) are also observed in the hypothalamic regions supplied by medial corticohypothalamic tract fibers. The transmitter in medial corticohypothalamic tract terminals has not yet been identified. In the septal region fibers of the fornix form two distinct bundles: (i) a compact fornix column or *postcommissural fornix*, which arches caudal to the anterior commissure, and (ii) a more diffuse *precommissural fornix* (587, 2062). Precommissural fibers are distributed to the septal nuclei, the lateral preoptic region, the nucleus of the diagonal band and the dorsal hypothalamic area (1815). Postcommissural fibers of the fornix project to the medial mammillary nucleus, except for those which leave the bundle and terminate in thalamic nuclei. (c) *Amygdalohypothalamic fibers*, arising from different

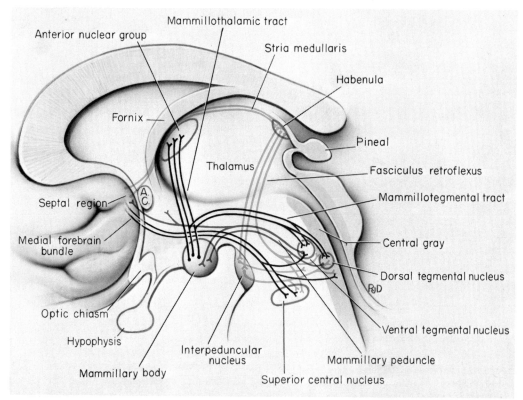

Figure 16-7. Semischematic diagram of limbic pathways interrelating the telencephalon and diencephalon with medial midbrain structures. The medial forebrain bundle and efferent fibers of the mammillary body are shown in *black*. The *medial forebrain bundle* originates from the septal and lateral preoptic regions, traverses the lateral hypothalamic area and projects into the midbrain tegmentum. The *fasciculus mammillary princeps* divides into two bundles, the *mammillothalamic tract* and the *mammillotegmental tract.* Ascending fibers of the *mammillary peduncle*, arising from the dorsal and ventral tegmental nuclei, are shown in *red*; most of these fibers pass to the mammillary body, but some continue rostrally to the lateral hypothalamus, the preoptic region and the medial septal nucleus. Fibers arising from the septal nuclei project caudally in the medial part of the *stria medullaris (blue)* to terminate in the medial habenular nucleus. Impulses conveyed to the habenular nucleus are distributed to midbrain tegmental nuclei via the *fasciculus retroflexus.* (Based on Nauta (1816).)

parts of the amygdaloid nuclear complex (Fig. 2-9) and following distinctive pathways to the hypothalamus, are: (i) the *stria terminalis* (Figs. 15-7 and 15-8), and (ii) the *ventral amygdalofugal pathway* (899). The stria terminalis arises principally from the corticomedial group of the amygdaloid nuclei (Fig. 18-16) and distributes terminals in the medial preoptic area, medial parts of the anterior hypothalamic area and in the ventromedial and arcuate nuclei (650, 1010, 1069, 1815, 1817, 1823). The ventral amygdalofugal pathway arises from the pyriform cortex and the basolateral amygdaloid nuclei and supplies the whole extent of the medial forebrain bundle region, as well as having terminations in the lateral hypothalamic nucleus (Fig. 16-11) (557, 1010,

2090, 2604). (d) *Thalamohypothalamic fibers* that arise chiefly from the midline thalamic nuclei. Fibers from periventricular thalamic nuclei are considered to descend into the dorsal hypothalamic area, but relatively little is known about this system (Fig. 16-10). (e) *Brain stem reticular afferent fibers* ascend to the hypothalamus via: (i) the *mammillary peduncle,* and (ii) the *dorsal longitudinal fasciculus.* The mammillary peduncle arises from the dorsal and ventral tegmental nuclei of the midbrain and projects mainly to the lateral mammillary nucleus (Fig. 16-7). In this course the mammillary peduncle passes rostrally through the rootlets of the third nerve and lies lateral to the interpeduncular nucleus. A few of these fibers ascend in the medial

Limbic brain stem connections

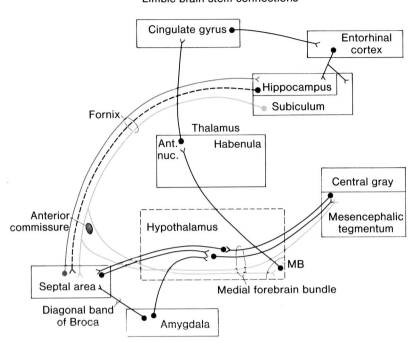

Figure 16-8. Schematic block diagram of major interconnections of structures comprising the "limbic system." Projection fibers arising from the subiculum *(blue)* project via the fornix to the septal area, hypothalamus and mesencephalic tegmentum. Fibers projecting in the fornix from the hippocampus are shown in *black*-dashed lines. Projections from the septal area to the hippocampus are shown in *red. MB* indicates mammillary body.

forebrain bundle beyond the hypothalamus. The ascending component of the dorsal longitudinal fasciculus is formed from cells in the central gray of the midbrain. Fibers in this bundle spread out over caudal and dorsal regions of the hypothalamus where they become part of a periventricular system (1823). Since fibers of this bundle conduct impulses both rostrally and caudally, it may be regarded as a reciprocally organized association system between the hypothalamus and the midbrain central gray (Fig. 16-10). In addition to ascending projections originating in cells of the reticular formation, neurons in the raphe nuclei of the midbrain and the parabrachial nuclei of the pons send axons to the preoptic region and lateral hypothalamus (1556). A discrete group of cells located within the dorsal nucleus of the lateral lemniscus in the rostral pons projects to the ventromedial nucleus. Ascending noradrenergic fibers originating in the nucleus locus ceruleus form a dorsal tegmental bundle which

distributes to the hypothalamus where dense terminal axonal networks can be seen in the dorsomedial and paraventricular nuclei (1497). Afferent fibers to the hypothalamus from the brain stem and amygdala are summarized in diagrammatic form in Figures 16-8 and 16-9. (f) *Retinohypothalamic fibers,* arising from the ganglion cells of the retina, project to the suprachiasmatic nucleus and are thought to convey impulses which lead to photic entrainment of circadian rhythms in the release of gonadotropins and other anterior pituitary hormones (1732, 2262). Although visual input to the hypothalamus had been suspected on the basis of influence of light on neuroendocrine systems (565), light microscopic degeneration studies failed to provide convincing evidence of retinohypothalamic connections. Recently, however, direct retinohypothalamic projections have been demonstrated in autoradiographic and electron microscopic studies. Bilateral retinal projections through the optic nerve to the

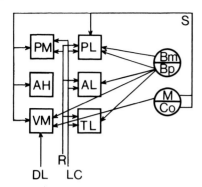

Figure 16-9. A diagrammatic summary of some afferent paths to the hypothalamus which originate from neurons in the pons and amygdala. Abbreviations: *AH*, anterior medial hypothalamic region; *AL*, anterior lateral hypothalamic region; *Bm*, large celled basal nucleus of amygdala; *Bp*, small celled basal nucleus of amygdala; *Co*, cortical nucleus of amygdala; *DL*, dorsal nucleus of lateral lemniscus (pons); *LC*, locus ceruleus (pons); *M*, medial nucleus of amygdala; *PL*, lateral preoptic region; *PM*, medial preoptic region; *R*, raphe nuclei of pons; *S*, stria terminalis; *TL*, lateral hypothalamus, tuberal level; and *VM*, ventromedial nucleus of hypothalamus. (Reproduced with permission from J. Sutin and R. L. McBride: *Handbook of the Hypothalamus, Vol. 1. Anatomy of the Hypothalamus,* edited by P. J. Morgane and J. Panksepp. Marcel Dekker, New York, 1979.)

suprachiasmatic nucleus of the hypothalamus have been shown in several species (1073, 1732, 2545). The retinal neurons terminate on dendrites of suprachiasmatic nucleus cells (1043, 1073, 1739). The suprachiasmatic nucleus also receives indirect visual input. The ventral lateral geniculate nucleus of the rat and cat projects bilaterally to the suprachiasmatic nucleus, by a path through the zona incerta (2142, 2482). Afferent fibers to the ventral lateral geniculate originate in the retina, superior colliculus, and visual cortex (2482).

Opinion is varied concerning *corticohypothalamic fibers,* usually described as arising from portions of the frontal lobe and passing directly to the hypothalamus. The region from which these fibers seem to be described most consistently is the posterior orbital cortex (475, 1818, 2244, 2332, 2672). Descriptions of pallidohypothalamic fibers projecting to the ventromedial nucleus have not been substantiated with silver staining technics (1825).

Sensory information may reach the hypothalamus indirectly by way of corticohypothalamic pathways, but there is no evidence that the hypothalamus receives direct input from the primary sensory regions of the cortex. The cingulate gyrus vocalization area, identified by electrical stimulation, projects to the preoptic region and the dorsomedial hypothalamus along its whole extent, mostly by way of the internal capsule (1780).

Following medial prefrontal cortex lesions in monkeys, preterminal and terminal degeneration is located throughout the rostrocaudal extent of the lateral hypothalamus and in the lateral mammillary nucleus (1465). Frontal granular cortex lesions in monkeys result in degeneration in the lateral, dorsal, and posterior hypothalamic areas (1819). Valverde (2604) reports frontal cortical projections to the lateral hypothalamus in cats.

After lesions of prefrontal cortex in cats, there is heavy degeneration in the dorsomedial nucleus of the thalamus but only sparse degeneration in the lateral hypothalamus (2338). Few hypothalamic units are driven by prefrontal stimulation in cats (685).

Direct thalamohypothalamic pathways are apparently quite sparse; regions of the thalamus receiving sensory information through spinal pathways do not appear to have hypothalamic projections. Although degeneration in the lateral preoptic and hypothalamic regions and substantia innominata is reported following dorsomedial nucleus lesions in monkeys (1818), the rat dorsomedial nucleus does not have a corresponding projection (2339).

Broadly stated, the principal forebrain afferents to the hypothalamus arise from the two phylogenetically oldest cortical areas, the pyriform cortex and the hippocampal formation (Fig. 16-11) (2090). In each instance the cortical projection is reinforced by a corresponding subcortical projection, the amygdala in the case of the pyriform cortex, and the septum in the case of the hippocampal formation. Each of these subcortical nuclei is reciprocally connected with the overlying cortical area. Of the phylogenetically newer cortical areas the cingulate gyrus appears particularly favored to influence the hypothalamus indirectly through the entorhinal cortex and the hippocampal formation. The cingulate

cortex can in turn be influenced by hypothalamic projections to the anterior nuclear
group of the thalamus.

Both the senses of taste and olfaction are
directly involved in the arousal and con-
summatory phases of behavior. While the
gustatory pathway to the hypothalamus
may be multisynaptic, the olfactory system
has relatively direct neuronal connections
with the hypothalamus.

The olfactory bulb and accessory olfactory bulb project to different regions of the
cortical and medial amygdaloid nuclei
(2264, 2349). These amygdaloid nuclei in
turn project directly to the hypothalamus
by way of two fiber tracts, the stria terminalis and the ventral amygdalofugal pathway. In the rat, the dorsal component of
the stria terminalis arises primarily from
the caudal portions of the cortical and medial amygdaloid nuclei and terminates in a
shell around the periphery of the HVM.
The rostral portions of the cortical and
medial amygdaloid nuclei project to the
core of the HVM by way of the ventral
component of the stria (1877). Degeneration studies have shown the stria terminalis
to project also to the preoptic area and
anterior hypothalamus (1070, 1877, 2096,
2604).

The Efferent Connections of the Hypothalamus

The efferent connections of the hypothalamus appear, in part, to be reciprocal
to the afferent systems. There are reciprocal connections in the medial forebrain bundle which provide indirect connections between the lateral hypothalamus and the
hippocampal formation (2091). In addition,
there are hypothalamic projections to the
amygdaloid nuclear complex via both the
stria terminalis (Fig. 18-6) and the ventral
pathway (1556). Reciprocal connections
with the midbrain tegmentum and central
gray are conducted by the dorsal longitudinal fasciculus and via pathways projecting to and from the mammillary bodies. In
addition, there are several efferent hypothalamic pathways which have no counterpart among afferent systems.

The *medial forebrain bundle* conveys
impulses from the lateral hypothalamus
rostrally to the nuclei of the diagonal band
and to the medial septal nuclei (980, 2091),
which in turn send fibers to the hippocampal formation via the fimbria of the fornix
(587). Descending hypothalamic efferents
in the medial forebrain bundle project
through the ventral tegmental region to the
superior central nucleus, the ventral tegmental nucleus and to parts of the central
gray (Fig. 16-7) (980, 1816, 2472). Hypothalamic efferents to the amygdaloid nuclear complex via both the stria terminalis
and the ventral pathway degenerate after
lesions in the medial forebrain bundle (557,
1816, 2501). Fibers from the lateral hypothalamic region appear to follow the ventral
pathway through the substantia innominata to the amygdala, while those that pass
via the stria terminalis arise from more
medial cells (1823).

The *dorsal longitudinal fasciculus* contains descending fibers mostly from medial
and periventricular portions of the hypothalamus, that are distributed to the central
gray of the midbrain and the tectum. Some
descending fibers in this system may extend
to the dorsal tegmental nucleus (Fig. 16-
10). The pathways by which impulses originating in the hypothalamus are relayed to
nuclei in the medulla and spinal cord are
poorly understood. It is presumed that impulses are projected to cells in the reticular
formation which relay the impulses to the
medulla and to spinal levels (Fig. 16-10).
Evidence concerning pupillodilator pathways in the brain stem supports this thesis
(1516).

Mammillary efferent fibers, arising from
the medial mammillary nucleus, and to a
lesser extent from the lateral and intermediate mammillary nuclei, form a well defined bundle, the *fasciculus mammillaris
princeps* (Figs. 16-2 and 16-7). This bundle
passes dorsally for a short distance and
divides into two components: the *mammillothalamic tract* and the *mammillotegmental tract* (Figs. 16-6, 16-7 and A-20). The
mammillothalamic tract contains fibers
from the medial mammillary nucleus which
project to the ipsilateral anteroventral and
anteromedial thalamic nuclei, and fibers
from the lateral mammillary nucleus that
pass bilaterally to the anterodorsal nucleus
(816). Superimposed upon this are direct
projections from the hippocampal formation to the anterior thalamic nuclei via the
fornix (979, 2603). Each of the anterior tha-

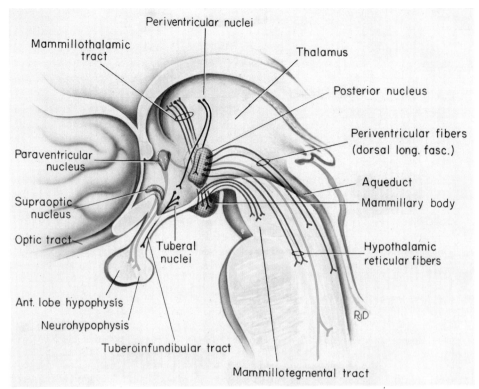

Figure 16-10. Diagram of some of the efferent hypothalamic pathways. Color code is the same as in Figure 16-1. Terminations of the mammillotegmental tract are shown in Figure 16-7.

lamic nuclei in turn projects to subdivisions of the cingulate cortex (Figs. 2-5, 18-6 and 18-17). Thus the main neocortical projection of impulses from the hippocampal formation and subiculum is to the cingulate cortex via postcommissural fibers of the fornix to: (a) the anterior thalamic nuclei and (b) the mammillary body which relays impulses to the anterior thalamic nuclei (Fig. 16-11). Impulses from the cingulate cortex pass back to the hippocampal formation via the entorhinal cortex (2094) (Fig. 16-8). These connections appear to form a closed anatomical circuit. The mamillotegmental tract curves caudally into the midbrain tegmentum. Fibers of this tract terminate in the dorsal and ventral tegmental nuclei (Fig. 16-7).

Hypothalamospinal Fibers. Although it was thought at one time that no efferent axons from the hypothalamus descended beyond the level of the midbrain, new technics have revealed at least two direct paths to the spinal cord and medulla (Figs. 10-23 and 16-11). One path originates in the paraventricular nucleus and projects to laminae I and II of the dorsal horn in the spinal cord and to the nucleus of the solitary tract and dorsal motor nucleus of the vagus in the medulla. Immunocytochemical studies indicate that the spinal portion of this path is made up of mainly oxytocin-containing axons while the medullary projections are predominantly vasopressinergic (1842). Parts of the paraventricular nucleus also project to the intermediolateral cell column of the thoracic cord, but the tracing method employed does not permit identification of the neurotransmitter or neuromodulator involved (1887, 2255). Paraventricular nucleus cells projecting to the spinal cord are largely distinct from those sending axons to the posterior lobe of the pituitary gland (1147, 1887).

A second descending projection to the spinal cord arises in the dorsomedial hypothalamus and zona incerta (187, 190, 2255). These axons may be dopaminergic (187).

Hypothalamocortical Fibers. With retrograde tracing methods it has been shown that hypothalamic projections to the

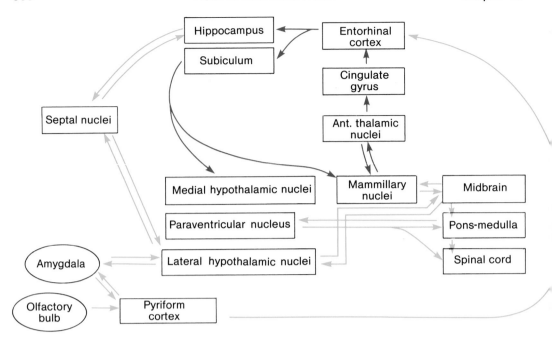

Figure 16-11. A schematic diagram of the principal fiber connections of the hypothalamus. The principal afferents to the hypothalamus from the forebrain arise from two phylogenetically older cortical areas, the *pyriform cortex* and the *hippocampal formation*. Each of these projections is reinforced by a second projection from a related subcortical nuclear mass; this secondary projection arises from the *amygdaloid complex* in the case of the pyriform cortex, and from the *septal nuclei* in the case of the hippocampal formation. Reciprocal connections exist between the hypothalamus and these subcortical nuclei. The cingulate gyrus and the pyriform cortex can exert influences upon the hypothalamus via the entorhinal area and the hippocampal formation. The mammillary nuclei and the hippocampal formation project to the anterior thalamic nuclei which in turn influence activities in the cingulate gyrus. Projection pathways from the mammillary nuclei to the cortex and from the hippocampus and subiculum to the hypothalamus are in *red*. Other connections are shown in *blue* and black. (Modified from Raisman (2090).)

primate motor cortex originate from cells in the ipsilateral lateral hypothalamus and substantia innominata (1309). While the synaptic actions of hypothalamic efferents to the motor cortex are not known, this existence of a path raises the possibility of a direct action of the hypothalamus upon the corticospinal system.

The Supraopticohypophysial Tract. This term is used to designate fibers arising from the supraoptic and paraventricular nuclei that project to the posterior lobe of the hypophysis (967, 2013, 2431) (Figs. 16-5, 16-10 and 16-12). Cells of the supraoptic and paraventricular nuclei are *neurosecretory* and transmit peptides which are liberated at their endings in the neurohypophysis. Following transection of the hypophysial stalk, stainable neurosecretory substance accumulates above the cut, and dis-

appears distally. Electron microscopic studies reveal that the neurosecretory material consists of aggregates of granules, 50 to 200 nm in diameter (206, 207, 1917). The neurosecretory substance, which consists of a carrier protein and the peptide hormone, is liberated near capillaries of the neurohypophysis. While there is evidence which suggests that the supraoptic nucleus is mainly related to vasopressin (antidiuretic hormone) and the paraventricular nucleus to oxytocin (1072, 1873, 2007), both hormones are produced in each nucleus (2605).

The Tuberohypophysial (Tuberoinfundibular) Tract. This tract arises from the tuberal region, mainly from the arcuate nucleus (Fig. 16-1), and can be traced only to the median eminence and the infundibular stem (1058, 2501). According to Szentágothai et al. (2501), these fibers properly

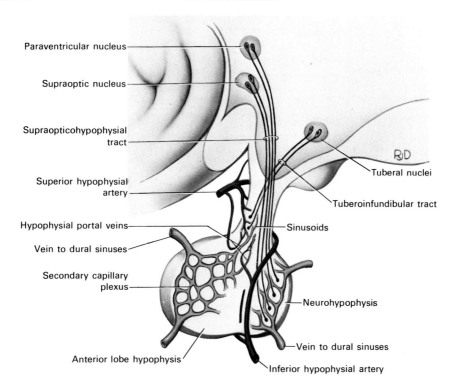

Figure 16-12. Diagram of the hypophysial portal system, the tuberoinfundibular tract and the supraoptico-hypophysial tract. The hypophysis is supplied by the *superior* and *inferior hypophysial arteries*. Branches of these arteries form sinusoidal capillaries about the infundibulum. Blood from the sinusoids passes to the anterior lobe of the hypophysis via the portal vessels which give rise to a second capillary plexus in the anterior lobe. The tuberoinfundibular tract ends in the sinusoids of the infundibular stem and transports neurosecretory substances, called *releasing hormones*, which enter the sinusoids. The *supraopticohypophysial tract* contains fibers from the *supraoptic* and *paraventricular nuclei* which pass to the neurohypophysis. Neurosecretory products of cells in these hypothalamic nuclei are conveyed directly to the neurohypophysis. The supraoptic nuclei are the main source of antidiuretic hormone, while cells of the paraventricular nuclei produce oxytocin.

should be referred to as the tuberoinfundibular tract (figs. 16-10 and 16-12). Although these fibers accompany those of the supraopticohypophysial tract in part of their course, they end upon capillary loops near the sinusoids of the hypophysial portal system (Fig. 16-12). These are fine fibers, but secretory granules can be demonstrated in their axons (provided tissues are not fixed in formalin). Fibers of the tuberoinfundibular tract are assumed to convey "releasing" hormones which are transported to the anterior lobe by the portal vessels where they modulate the synthesis and release of adenohypophysial hormones (1058). Functionally, the tuberoinfundibular tract and the hypophysial portal system establish the neurohumoral link between the hypothalamus and the anterior pitui-

tary. Under stressful conditions neurosecretory granules disappear from nerve fibers, and adrenocorticotropic hormone (ACTH) releasing factor is present in the plasma obtained from portal vessels (2047). The infundibulum also contains high concentrations of acetylcholine (1058), and the cell bodies and fibers of the tuberoinfundibular system contain dopamine (829).

Hypothalamic efferent projections fall into three main categories: (a) those that emerge via the medial forebrain bundle, (b) those concerned with neurosecretion which convey hormones to the neurohypophysis, and releasing hormones to the median eminence and (c) those that arise from the mammillary nuclei which project to the anterior nuclear group of the thalamus and to nuclei in the midbrain tegmentum.

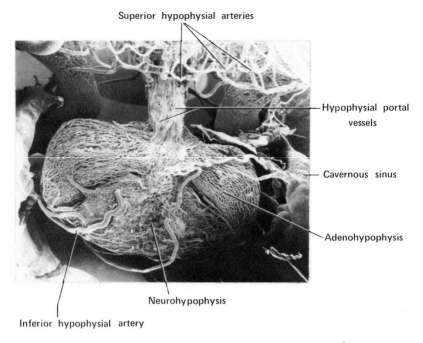

Superior hypophysial arteries

Hypophysial portal vessels

Cavernous sinus

Adenohypophysis

Neurohypophysis

Inferior hypophysial artery

Figure 16-13. Scanning electron micrograph of vascular casts of the pituitary gland, infundibular stalk and median eminence in the monkey. The gland is viewed from its posterior aspect. The hypophysial arteries and the portal system of vessels shown in this figure should be compared with the schematic diagram showing a sagittal view in Figure 16-12. (Reproduced with permission from R. B. Page and R. M. Bergland: *American Journal of Anatomy*, **148**:345–357, 1977.)

HYPOPHYSIAL PORTAL SYSTEM

The hypophysis is supplied by two sets of arteries, both of which arise from the internal carotid artery (Figs. 16-12 and 16-13). The superior hypophysial artery forms an arterial ring around the upper part of the hypophysial stalk; the inferior hypophysial artery forms a ring about the posterior lobe and gives branches to the lower infundibulum. Both of these arteries enter the hypophysial stalk and break up into a number of sinusoids. Blood from these sinusoids collects into vessels which pass into the anterior lobe of the hypophysis. The anterior lobe of the pituitary receives almost all of its blood supply via these vessels. These vessels are referred to as the hypophysial portal vessels (2045). The flow of blood from the hypophysial stalk and median eminence to the anterior lobe of the hypophysis has been demonstrated in living animals (958).

There is considerable evidence that hypothalamic influences upon the anterior lobe of the hypophysis are conveyed by humoral substances, transported along the tuberoinfundibular tract to the sinusoids, that reach the anterior lobe via the portal system (1031, 1033).

The hypothalamus appears intimately concerned with mechanisms that influence the hormonal activity of the anterior lobe and cause the secretion of gonadotropic, ACTH and thyrotropic (TSH) hormones (Fig. 16-14). Electrical stimulation of the hypothalamus can increase the discharges of gonadotropic hormone, TSH and ACTH. Stimulation of the tuberal region in the rabbit has produced ovulation. Direct stimulation of the anterior lobe does not elicit these responses, presumably because the humoral part of this pathway is not electrically excitable. The neurosecretory substances acting upon cells of the anterior lobe are called *releasing hormones*, and are named according to the hormone they release. The releasing hormones are hypophysiotropic neuropeptides which can be studied by immunochemical methods. The pituitary gonadotropins leutinizing hormone (LH) and follicle stimulating hormone (FSH) are regulated by the hypothalamic peptide leutinizing hormone releasing hormone (LHRH). In the human brain LHRH is found in greatest amounts in the infundibular stalk (1868), while in the rat it is most abundant in the tuberal region of the hypothalamus (2700). Section of the pituitary stalk is followed by varying degrees of functional activity of the anterior pituitary and this may be correlated with the degree of preservation, or regenration, of portal vessels at the site of section. If vascular regeneration is prevented by placement of a plate between the cut ends of the stalk, little anterior pituitary function is observed.

SUPRAOPTIC DECUSSATIONS

Dorsal to the optic chiasm several bundles of fine fibers cross the midline. These fiber bundles constitute the supraoptic decussations. Three decussations or commissures are recognized, although little is known concerning their origin, course, termination or function.

The most rostral of these decussations is the anterior hypothalamic commissure (Ganser; Figs. 17-12 and 17-13). Fibers of this commissure are most readily identified as they project ventromedially from Forel's field H and arch over the fibers of the fornix. These fibers pass ventrally in the hypothalamus, cross the midline ventral to the third ventricle and contralaterally fan out into the lateral preopticohypothalamic area (1823). Fibers of the anterior hypothalamic commissure are considered to arise from the reticular formation of the rostral pons and to ascend in association with fibers of the medial longitudinal fasciculus (309a).

Two decussations lie along the dorsal aspect of the optic chiasm, the *dorsal supraoptic decussation* (Meynert) and the *ventral supraoptic decussation* (Gudden; Figs. 15-7, 17-12 and 17-13). The precise origin of both of these bundles is obscure.

CHEMICALLY DEFINED NEURONS AND TRACTS IN THE HYPOTHALAMUS

Many peptides (see Table 4-1) and transmitters can be localized with immunohis-

tochemical and histochemical methods, permitting cell bodies of origin, course of axons and sites of synaptic termination to be studied experimentally. The noradrenergic and dopaminergic systems of neurons have been mentioned in several earlier chapters. When the cell bodies of catecholaminergic neurons (see Chapter 4, p. 104) were first identified, they were designated by the letter A and a numerical subscript (Table 16-1). This designation is used less frequently now, and the catecholaminergic (CA) cell groups are described by conventional descriptive terms such as locus ceruleus or median eminence.

Within the hypothalamus, dopamine-containing cell bodies are found in the arcuate nucleus, dorsomedial nucleus and periventricular zones (Fig. 16-15). Noradrenergic perikarya are not found in the hypothalamus, but terminals arising from CA cells in the pons and medulla are distributed widely, with the most dense plexus in the periventricular zone (1120, 1922). Noradrenergic axons ascending from the pons and medulla form a dorsal and ventral bundle. The dorsal bundle contains fibers arising in the locus ceruleus of the pons destined for the dorsal hypothalamic nuclei. The ventral noradrenergic bundle is composed of fibers arising from medullary neurons with some contributions from pontine CA cells. At the level of the rostral midbrain the ventral and dorsal bundles largely fuse. Most CA axons continue rostrally in the medial forebrain bundle, while others ascend in the periventricular zone. A particularly prominent plexus of CA terminals occurs in the paraventricular nucleus (1575).

The localization and axonal projections of neurons synthesizing the peptides vasopressin and oxytocin have been described earlier in this chapter. The role of these peptides in memory is a subject of active investigation which has already led to the development of new approaches to the cell biology of higher mental function. In a number of behavioral tests vasopressin facilitates and oxytocin diminishes memory consolidation and retrieval. These actions appear to involve different regions of the peptide, for the covalent ring portion of the molecule affects mainly consolidation and the linear part is implicated in memory

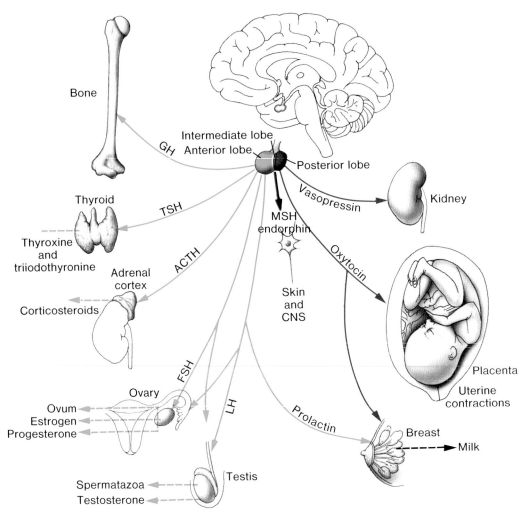

Figure 16-14. Schematic diagram of the target organs upon which pituitary hormones act. Pituitary (hypophysial) hormones are either secreted or controlled by neurons of the hypothalamus. Hormones secreted by cells in the anterior *(blue)* and intermediate lobes *(black)* of the pituitary are regulated by hypothalamic hypophysiotrophic peptides conveyed by the hypophysial portal system. Hormones of the anterior lobe include: (1) growth hormone (GH), (2) thyrotropin (TSH), (3) corticotrophin (ACTH), (4) follicle stimulating hormone (FSH), (5) luteinizing hormone (LH), and (6) prolactin. Melanocyte stimulating hormone (MSH) is derived from cells of the intermediate lobe *(black)* of the pituitary. The posterior (neural) lobe *(red)* of the pituitary contains vasopressin and oxytocin secreted by cells of the supraoptic and paraventricular nuclei of the hypothalamus. These hormones act upon the kidney tubules, the smooth muscle of the uterus and glandular tissue of the breast. (Modified from Schally et al. (2267).)

retrieval (2715). Indirect evidence indicates that vasopressin may interact with noradrenergic synapses to influence memory consolidation.

Elsewhere in this chapter several of the "releasing hormones" have been mentioned. Some of these peptides, as well as several peptides of pituitary origin that originate from a common precursor glyco-

sylated molecule called pro-opiocortin, also have been identified in extrahypothalamic regions of the brain. Their functional significance as possible neurotransmitters or modulators has not yet been established (1367).

The naturally occurring opioid peptide β-endorphin is found in the rat intermediate lobe and adenohypophysis and in the

Table 16-1
Location of Principal Catecholamine Cell Groups[a]

Ventrolateral medulla and lateral reticular nucleus	A_1	NE + E	
Dorsomedial medulla: dorsal vagal nucleus and solitary nucleus	A_2	NE + E	MEDULLA
Ventrolateral medulla and lateral reticular nucleus	A_3	NE	
Lateral pontine	A_4		
Periventricular Region			
Ventrolateral pons medial to N. VII, also dorsolateral to superior olive	A_5	NE	PONS
Locus ceruleus	A_6	NE	
Nucleus subceruleus	A_7	NE	
Midbrain tegmentum dorsolateral to red nucleus	A_8	DA	
Substantia nigra	A_9	DA	MIDBRAIN
Ventral tegmental area	A_{10}	DA	
Periventricular zone of posterior hypothalamus	A_{11}	DA(+NE?)	
Median eminence	A_{12}	DA	
Dorsomedial hypothalamus and zona incerta	A_{13}	DA	HYPOTHALAMUS
Periventricular zone of anterior hypothalamus	A_{14}	DA	
Olfactory bulb	A_{15}	DA	

[a] These major groups of catecholamine-containing cell bodies and the corresponding alphanumeric designation were given by the investigators who first described them in fluorescence histochemical studies. The letter A in the second column refers to "adrenergic" cells numbered according to their position in ascending caudorostral levels of the brain stem and olfactory bulb. In the third column, the subsequent identification of the catecholamine is shown. DA = dopamine, NE = norepinephrine and E = epinephrine. Cells containing the indoleamine serotonin (5-hydroxytryptamine) are not included in this table.

brain. Hypophysectomy does not reduce brain β-endorphin, suggesting an endogenous synthesis within the CNS. β-Endorphin-labeled cell bodies are at the base of the tuberal region of the hypothalamus, and labeled axons are distributed along the ventricular wall extending anteriorly to the level of the anterior commissure. The supraoptic, periventricular, paraventricular and suprachiasmatic nuclei receive abundant β-endorphin-labeled fibers (195). The cells and fibers labeled for β-endorphin are distinct from those labeled by antisera specific for the enkephalins (see Chapter 4).

FUNCTIONAL CONSIDERATIONS

Experimental evidence and clinical observations have demonstrated that the hypothalamus and immediately adjoining regions are related to all kinds of visceral activities. The most diverse disturbances of autonomic functions involving water balance, internal secretion, sugar and fat metabolism and temperature regulation, all can be produced by stimulation or destruction of hypothalamic areas. Even the mechanism for normal sleep may be altered by such lesions. It is established that the hypothalamus is the chief subcortical center for the regulation of both sympathetic and parasympathetic activities. These dual activities are integrated into coordinated responses which maintain adequate internal conditions in the body. It is highly improbable that each of the autonomic activities has its own discrete center in view of the small size of the hypothalamus and the complex nature of these activities. There is a fairly definite topographical organization as regards the two main divisions of the autonomic system. Control of parasympathetic activities is related to the anterior and medial hypothalamic regions. Stimulation of these regions results in increased vagal and sacral autonomic responses, characterized by reduced heart rate, peripheral vasodilatation and increased tonus and motility of the alimentary and vesical walls.

The lateral and posterior hypothalamic regions are concerned with the control of sympathetic responses. Stimulation of this region, especially the posterior portion from which most of the descending efferent fibers arise, activates the thoracolumbar outflow.

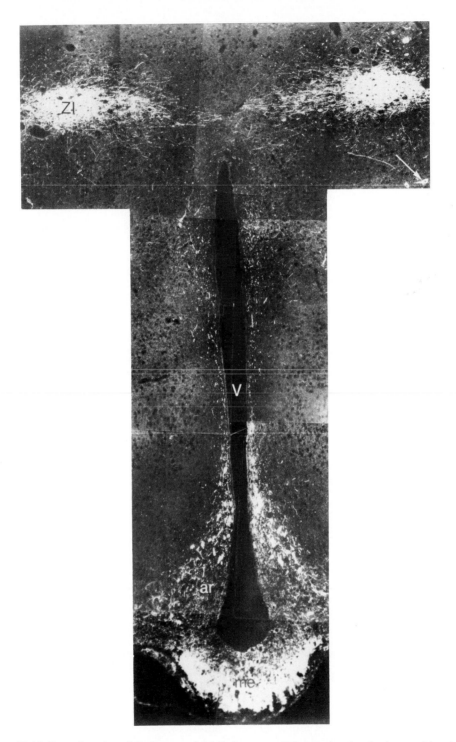

Figure 16-15. Frontal section of the hypo- and subthalamus, medial part, showing the immunohistochemical localization of tyrosine hydroxylase *(TH)*. Oblique section in the frontal plane with the ventral part more cranial than the dorsal part. Fluorescent cell bodies are seen in the arcuate nucleus *(ar)* (A_{12} cell group) and in the zona incerta *(ZI)* (A_{13} cell group). Note the dense plexus of TH-positive fibers in the median eminence *(me)*, especially the external layer. At this level the TH-positive fibers are present in the whole external layer, whereas at a more caudal level the highest concentrations are found in the lateral parts. Note single cell bodies *(arrow)* ventral to the A_{13} cell group. Note also that the ventral TH-positive arcuate cells have a considerably lower intensity than the dorsal TH-positive arcuate- periventricular nerve cells. *V* = third ventricle (magnification ×160). (Reproduced with permission from T. Hökfelt et al.: *Medical Biology*, **54:**427–453, 1976.)

This results in increased metabolic and somatic activities characteristic of emotional stress, combat or flight. These responses are expressed by dilatation of the pupil, piloerection, acceleration of the heart rate, elevation of blood pressure, increases in the rate and amplitude of respiration, somatic struggling movements and inhibition of the gut and bladder. All these physiological correlates of emotional excitement can be elicited when the hypothalamus is released from cortical control. Removal of the cortex, or interruption of the cortical connections with the hypothalamus, induces many of the above visceral symptoms which are collectively designated as "sham rage" (111, 823). On the other hand, destruction of the posterior hypothalamus produces emotional lethargy, abnormal sleepiness and a fall in temperature due to a general reduction of visceral and somatic activities.

The coordination of sympathetic and parasympathetic responses is strikingly shown in the regulation of body temperature. This complex function, involving widespread physical and chemical processes, is mediated by two hypothalamic mechanisms, one concerned with the dissipation of heat and the other with its production and conservation. There is considerable experimental evidence that neurons in the anterior hypothalamus are sensitive to increases in blood temperature, and set in motion the mechanisms for dissipating excess heat. In man this consists mainly of profuse sweating and vasodilatation of the cutaneous blood vessels. These actions permit the rapid elimination of heat by convection and radiation from the surface of the engorged blood vessels, and by the evaporation of sweat. In animals with fur this is supplemented to a considerable degree by rapid, shallow respiratory movements (panting); the heat loss is effected mainly by the rapid warming of successive streams of inspired air. Lesions involving the anterior part of the hypothalamus abolish the neural control of mechanisms concerned with the dissipation of heat and result in hyperthermia. Thus hyperthermia (hyperpyrexia) may result from tumors in, or near, the anterior hypothalamus.

The posterior hypothalamus, on the other hand, is sensitive to conditions of decreasing body temperature, and controls mechanisms for the conservation and increased production of heat. The cutaneous blood vessels are constricted and sweat secretion ceases, so that heat loss is reduced. Simultaneously there is augmentation of visceral activities, and the somatic muscles exhibit shivering. All these activities tremendously increase the processes of oxidation, with a consequent production and conservation of heat. Bilateral lesions in posterior regions of the hypothalamus usually produce a condition in which body temperature varies with the environment (poikilothermia), since such lesions effectively destroy all descending pathways concerned with both the conservation and dissipation of heat.

These two intrinsically antagonistic mechanisms do not function independently but are continually inter-related and balanced against each other to meet the changing needs of the body; the coordinated responses always are directed to the maintenance of a constant and optimum temperature.

The supraoptic nuclei are specifically concerned with the maintenance of body water balance (Figs. 16-2, 16-3, 16-5, 16-10 and 16-12). Destruction of these nuclei, or their hypophysial connections, invariably is followed by the condition known as *diabetes insipidus*, in which there is an increased consumption of fluids (polydipsia) and an increased secretion of urine (polyuria), without an increase in the sugar content. The antidiuretic hormone (vasopressin) is secreted directly by the cells of the supraoptic nuclei. The peptide is conjugated to a carrier protein, neurophysin, and transported to the posterior lobe along the unmyelinated axons of the supraopticohypophysial tract (116). The antidiuretic hormone is stored in the posterior lobe of the pituitary. The production of antidiuretic hormone varies in accordance with changes in the osmotic pressure of the blood. An increase in the osmotic pressure of the blood which supplies the supraoptic nuclei increases the activity of these neurons and the release of antidiuretic hormone. In states of experimental dehydration there is a depletion of the hormone in the posterior lobe and increased secretory activity in the supraoptic nuclei. After reestablishment of water balance, there is a reaccumulation of the hormone in the posterior lobe (1097).

Evidence suggests that the antidiuretic hormone acts specifically on the kidneys rather than on tissues in general (2007). Although the exact mechanism by which the antidiuretic hormone brings about reabsorption of renal water is still under investigation active reabsorption of sodium, chloride and bicarbonate ions is followed by passive reabsorption of water. The antidiuretic hormone also appears to alter the osmotic permeability of water in the distal and collecting tubules of the kidney.

There is evidence that a region of the hypothalamus is responsible for the regulation of water intake. Electrical stimulation of anterior regions of the hypothalamus in goats creates fantastic "thirst" and results in consumption of large volumes of water (63). This is probably part of a more extensive system which regulates the consumption of both food and water. An increase in the osmotic pressure of body fluids may be an effective stimulus for water intake. According to Verney (2617), osmoreceptors probably are situated close to the cells of the supraoptic nucleus which have an abundant blood supply. Localized lesions in the lateral hypothalamus at the level of the ventromedial nucleus in rats cause a reduction in water intake without affecting food intake (2439), but larger lesions in the lateral hypothalamus may cause adipsia as well as aphagia. According to Emmers (708), the lateral hypothalamic area can excite cells of the supraoptic nucleus which in turn inhibit the lateral hypothalamic area in a negative feedback circuit.

The paraventricular nuclei produce the nonapeptide oxytocin, which chemically is related closely to the antidiuretic hormone, but causes contractions of uterine muscle and myoepithelial cells surrounding the alveoli of the mammary gland (1072, 1873).

Tumors of the adenohypophysis may produce symptoms due to (a) their mass effect outside the pituitary or (b) increased or decreased hormonal secretions (2547). As the tumors expand they may compress the optic chiasm or tract and also cause headaches due to traction of the meninges about the sella. The visual field defects typically take the form of a bitemporal hemianopsia, although the visual symptoms vary with the growth pattern of the tumor. Endocrinopathy resulting from hypersecretion can take many forms depending upon the type of cellular hyperplasia. The most commonly observed syndromes involve cells producing excess prolactin (amenorrhea-galactorrhea) growth hormone (acromegaly) and adrenocorticotrophic hormone (Cushing's disease). Improvements in serum hormone radioimmunoassays and neuroradiologic evaluations of the sella and its contents make it possible to diagnose some pituitary microtumors before symptoms appear due to increased tissue mass.

The important role of the hypothalamus in maintaining and regulating the activity of the anterior lobe of the hypophysis has been described in relation to the hypophysial portal system (Fig. 16-12). It should be emphasized that this is a humoral control mechanism in which releasing hormones are transmitted via the portal system (1033). There are no hypothalamic efferent fibers that reach the anterior lobe of the pituitary. The anterior pituitary stands in marked contrast to other endocrine organs, such as the ovary, testis, thyroid and adrenal cortex, which may be transplanted to distant sites and still retain their endocrine functions. The anterior lobe of the pituitary cannot be transplanted to distant locations and retain its function, because it is dependent upon its close relationships with the hypothalamus. The essential hypothalamic structures are the tuberoinfundibular tract and the hypophysial portal system (Fig. 16-12). Thus the hypothalamus is considered the site of elaboration of releasing hormones related to gonadotropic, adrenocorticotropic (ACTH), thyrotropic (TSH) and growth hormones (1033, 2262). Attempts to determine the loci within the hypothalamus concerned with particular releasing hormones suggest that the neural area related to TSH appears to lie on either side of the midline between the paraventricular nucleus and the median eminence (966). Electrical stimulation of the anterior median eminence also results in increased thyroid activity, probably mediated by releasing factors (1034). Similarly, electrical stimulation of the hypothalamus in the rabbit can cause the discharge of gonadotropic hormone (1030, 1605) and of ACTH (972).

While bilateral lesions in almost any region near the base of the hypothalamus will reduce ACTH release, the median eminence-tuberal region was found to have the most important controlling influence (300). It was concluded that control of ACTH secretion lies in a diffuse hypothalamic region rather than in a discrete localized center.

The brain plays an important role in the initiation and coordination of reproductive functions, and these functions are different in the two sexes. The tuberal region of the hypothalamus appears essential for the maintenance of basal levels of gonadotropic hormone, but the integrity of the preoptic area is necessary for the cyclic surge of gonadotropin which precedes ovulation (727, 2096, 2261). Electrical stimulation of the preoptic area, or the corticomedial nuclear group of the amydgaloid complex, produces ovulation in rabbits and cats. The effects of preoptic stimulation are abolished by lesions separating this area from the tuberal hypothalamus, and the effects of amygdaloid stimulation are blocked by section of the stria terminalis. These observations suggest a functional linkage between the amygdala and medial preoptic area via the stria terminalis, and fiber systems from the medial preoptic area to the tuberal region of the hypothalamus. However, the amygdaloid input to the preoptic area is not essential for ovulation, for bilateral destruction of the stria terminalis does not prevent ovulation (305).

Tumors and other pathological processes involving the hypothalamus frequently modify sexual development. Such lesions may be associated with precocious puberty or hypogonadism associated with underdevelopment of secondary sex characteristics. Although hypergonadism has been attributed to tumors of the pineal gland, most tumors of the brain associated with precocious puberty actually involve, or impinge upon, the hypothalamus. The "sexually dimorphic nucleus of the preoptic area" was described on page 554 (see Fig. 16-16). The size of the nucleus depends upon the action of testosterone during a critical period in the maturation of the brain (927). Other morphological features in specific hypothalamic nuclei that are affected by fetal or neonatal exposure to androgens are changes in the size of neuronal nuclei and nucleoli, types of synaptic vesicles and terminals, synaptic organization and dendritic branching patterns (see MacLusky and Naftolin (1553) for review). The mechanisms by which steroid hormones affect the brain to determine sexual behavior and patterns of gonadotropin release are complex. For example, implantation of small quantities of estradiol into the hypothalamic ventromedial nucleus (HVM) of the rat activates feminine sexual behavior. Estradiol has been shown to alter a number of cellular properties in the HVM, including induction of progestin receptors, decrease of the inhibitory neurotransmitter synthetic enzyme glutamic acid decarboxylase, increased muscarinic cholinergic receptor binding and a decrease in the type A monoamine oxidase activity. This example illustrates estrogen regulation of a neurotransmitter, synthetic and degradative enzymes, and neurotransmitter receptors (1562).

It has been known for a long time that certain lesions near the base of the brain are associated with obesity. Localized bilateral lesions in the hypothalamus involving primarily, or exclusively, the ventromedial nucleus in the tuberal region produce *hyperphagia* (1091, 1185, 2438, 2439). Such animals eat voraciously, consuming two or three times the usual amount of food. In addition, most animals with such lesions exhibit savage and vicious behavior. Obesity appears to be the direct result of increased food intake. Lesions destroying portions of the lateral hypothalamic nucleus bilaterally impair, or abolish, the desire to feed in hyperphagic and normal animals (55, 56, 2439). Because lesions in the lateral hypothalamic area concomitantly destroy the medial forebrain bundle, its importance in aphagia was investigated. It was concluded that only lesions in this bundle in the vicinity of the ventromedial nucleus produced aphagia. These data led to the hypothesis that the ventromedial nucleus of the hypothalamus is concerned with *satiety*, while the lateral hypothalamic nucleus is involved in the initiation of feeding. This concept, though useful, has proved too simplistic to incorporate all of the information available about the appetitive and consumatory phases of ingestive behavior. The study of α- and β-adrenergic receptor

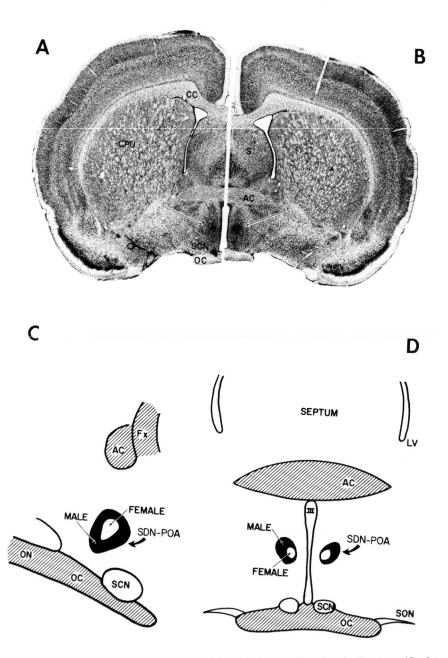

Figure 16-16. Coronal sections through the brain of the adult female *(A)* and male *(B)* rat sacrificed two weeks after gonadectomy; thionine stain. The arrows indicate that portion of the medial preoptic nucleus which exhibits a marked sexual dimorphism. Both at the same magnification. The absence of the suprachiasmatic nucleus *(SCN)* in *B* is an artifact of the plane of tissue sectioning. The localization and magnitude of the sexually dimorphic nucleus of the preoptic area *(SDN-POA)* is shown diagramatically in the parasagittal *(C)* and frontal *(D)* planes. Abbreviations: *AC*, anterior commissure; *CC*, corpus callosum; *CPU*, caudate-putamen; *FX*, fornix; *LV*, lateral ventricle; *OC*, optic chiasm; *S*, septum; *SCN*, suprachiasmatic nucleus; *SON*, supraoptic nucleus; and *III*, third ventricle. (Reproduced with permission from R. A. Gorski et al.: *Brain Research*, **148**:333–346, 1978; and *Advances in Physiological Science*, **15**:121–130, 1981.)

mechanisms in feeding (1464) and electrophysiological studies in alert, behaving animals (1888) have extended the concepts based exclusively upon lesions or knife cuts, and suggest that neural models that can explain feeding behavior may be similar in principle to those used to explain the regulation of blood pressure and respiration.

The hypothalamus is regarded as one of the principal centers concerned with emotional expression. Since it is acknowledged that the physiological expression of emotion is dependent, in part, upon both sympathetic and parasympathetic components of the autonomic nervous system, it is evident that the hypothalamus, intimately relating both of these, probably is involved directly or indirectly in most emotional reactions. As mentioned above, lesions in the ventromedial nucleus of the hypothalamus produce savage behavior and extreme rage reactions (902, 2699). Stimulation of the hypothalamus in unanesthetized cats with implanted electrodes (902, 1090, 1631) provokes responses resembling rage and fear which can be increased by stimuli of graded intensities. These reactions, referred to by some as "pseudo-affective," are "stimulus-bound" in that they are present only during the period of stimulation. Different types of responses are elicited from different parts of the hypothalamus; flight responses are most readily evoked from lateral regions of the anterior hypothalamus, while aggressive responses characterized by hissing, snarling, baring the teeth and biting are seen most commonly with stimulation of the region of the ventromedial nucleus (902, 1795). Because the emotional reactions provoked by electrical stimulation of the hypothalamus are directed, it seems likely that the thalamus, cerebral cortex and many forebrain structures play important roles in these responses. In these reactions the hypothalamus cannot be regarded as a simple efferent mechanism influencing only lower levels of the neuraxis.

Observations that selective stimulation and lesions of the ventromedial hypothalamic nucleus both produce aggressive and savage behavior raises basic questions concerning the mechanisms involved. Studies in the cat suggest that the savage behavior after bilateral lesions of the ventromedial nucleus cannot be assumed to result from a release of inhibitory influences (902). Because animals with bilateral lesions in the ventromedial hypothalamic nuclei never show spontaneous outbursts of aggressive behavior, unless disturbed, and this hyper-irritable state develops gradually, it has been postulated that destruction of these nuclei may lead to a state of supersensitivity similar to that described by Cannon and Rosenblueth (366). Furthermore, it was demonstrated that secondary midbrain lesions involving many structures, including the central gray, the reticular formation and the lemniscal systems, had "taming" effects upon this savage behavior.

Other studies, based upon electrical stimulation of unrestrained animals, indicate that the perifornical region and the central gray of the midbrain play important roles in expression of anger (1176). The fact that hypothalamically induced rage reactions may be blocked by midbrain lesions suggests that certain midbrain structures are essential for the elaboration of aggressive behavior (452). Finally, electrical stimulation of the amygdaloid nuclear complex also produces behavioral changes in which fear and rage are prominent. It appears generally accepted that the morphophysiological substrates of abnormal and aggressive behavior involve, in some differential and selective fashion, predominantly brain structures rostral to the rhombencephalon. This part of the central nervous system contains the neural structures concerned with goal-directed behavior and the motivational and emotional concomitants that make such behavior possible. Impulses generated in sensory systems, the cerebral cortex and still undetermined neural structures may trigger mechanisms that excite visceral and somatic systems whose activities in concert provide the physiological expression of aggressive behavior.

Although hypothalamic lesions produce somnolence resembling normal sleep (347, 2108), the fact that sleep and sleeplike states can be produced by electrical and chemical stimulation in a variety of structures within the brain stem makes it clear that there is no single "sleep center." The intralaminar thalamic nuclei seem to be the pre-eminent structures concerned with inducing sleep. Sleep induced by thalamic stimulation lasts for long periods of time and is comparable to that occurring naturally. The pontine reticular formation and the raphe nuclei constitute a lower center concerned with the triggering of paradoxical sleep (see p. 409).

The intermediolateral cell column of the thoracic cord is the major origin of sympathetic preganglionic neurons. There is a dense innervation of the intermediolateral column by catecholamine containing terminals, but their source in the medulla and pons has not been definitely established (1515). Descending serotonin (5-hydroxytryptamine, 5-HT) containing axons from the raphe nuclei also reach the intermediolateral cell column. Recent anatomical studies have emphasized the close association between visceral receptive cells in the solitary nucleus of the medulla and the hypothalamus (459, 460, 1515, 2485) and between the hypothalamus and the spinal cord (2485). Oxytocin immunoreactivity is seen in terminals of laminae I and II of the dorsal horn and in the intermediolateral cell column (1842). This recent information about connectivity and putative transmitters in visceroceptive and visceromotor regions of the CNS is leading to new experimental approaches in the physiological study of cardiovascular regulatory mechanisms.

CHAPTER 17

The Corpus Striatum

In close relationship to the diencephalon, but separated from it by the internal capsule, are the large nuclear masses that constitute the basal ganglia (Figs. 17-1 and 17-2). The basal ganglia, representing massive subcortical nuclei derived from the telencephalon, consist of two distinctive parts: (a) the corpus striatum, concerned with somatic motor function, and (b) the amygdaloid nuclear complex, regarded as a component of the limbic system.

The *amygdaloid nuclear complex*, phylogenetically the oldest part of the basal ganglia, is known as the *archistriatum*. This structure is located beneath the uncus in the temporal lobe and lies rostral to the inferior horn of the lateral ventricle and the hippocampal formation (Figs. 2-9 and 17-2). This nuclear complex has primarily olfactory inputs and has reciprocal connections with the hypothalamus and prepyriform cortex (1069, 1817, 2060, 2090). Because the amygdaloid nuclear complex is concerned with visceral, endocrine and behavioral functions, it is considered in detail in Chapter 18.

THE CORPUS STRIATUM

The corpus striatum consists of two parts, the neostriatum and the paleostriatum, which lie next to each other, lateral to the internal capsule. The term *neostriatum* refers to two structures partially separated by fibers of the anterior limb of the internal capsule. The two components of the neostriatum, the caudate nucleus and putamen, represent a single anatomical and functional entity which for embryological reasons has a particular configuration. Both portions of the striatum arise from a thickening of the lateral telencephalic vesicle known as the striatal ridge (Fig. 3-15). The neostriatum commonly is referred to as the

579

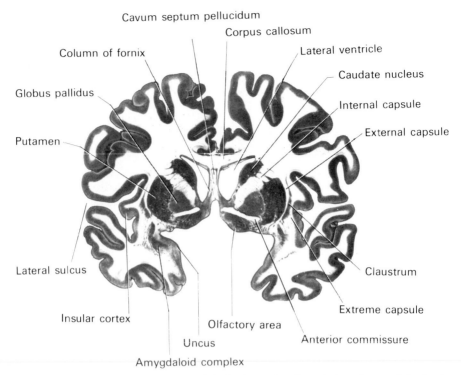

Cavum septum pellucidum
Corpus callosum
Column of fornix
Lateral ventricle
Globus pallidus
Caudate nucleus
Internal capsule
Putamen
External capsule
Lateral sulcus
Claustrum
Insular cortex
Extreme capsule
Olfactory area
Uncus
Anterior commissure
Amygdaloid complex

Figure 17-1. Photograph of a frontal section of the brain passing through the columns of the fornix and the anterior commissure. At this level the putamen and the lateral pallidal segment lie beneath the insular cortex.

striatum. The globus pallidus, forming the smaller, most medial part of the corpus striatum, lies medial to the putamen and lateral to the internal capsule. This portion of the corpus striatum is designated the *paleostriatum*. The globus pallidus plus the putamen are referred to as the *lentiform nucleus*.

The Striatum

The neostriatum consists of two parts, the caudate nucleus and the putamen, which rostrally and ventrally are in continuity.

Caudate Nucleus. The *caudate nucleus*, an elongated "C"-shaped cellular mass, is related throughout its extent to the lateral ventricle. The *head* of the caudate nucleus lies rostral to the thalamus and bulges into the anterior horn of the lateral ventricle (Figs. 2-12, 2-13, 17-4 and 17-5). The body of the caudate nucleus is a slender elongated gray mass that arches along the dorsolateral border of the thalamus, lateral to fibers of the stria terminalis (Figs. 17-2 and 17-4). This portion of the caudate

nucleus is suprathalamic. The *tail* of the caudate nucleus becomes evident caudal to the thalamus where it lies in the roof of the inferior horn of the lateral ventricle (Figs. 2-12, 15-27 and 17-4). The terminal part of the tail of the caudate nucleus comes into relationship with the central nucleus of the amygdaloid nuclear complex (Figs. 17-4 and 18-16).

Putamen. The *putamen*, the largest and most lateral portion of the corpus striatum, lies between the external capsule and the lateral medullary lamina of the globus pallidus (Figs. 2-12, 15-27, 17-1, 17-2, 17-3–17-5). Most of the putamen is situated medial to the insular cortex and is separated from it by the extreme capsule, the claustrum and the external capsule. In transverse sections, the lightly stained putamen is transversed by myelinated fibers coursing ventromedially, which are bundles of striopallidal fibers (Figs. 15-9 and 17-2). Rostrally and ventrally the putamen and head of the caudate nucleus are continuous because fibers of anterior limb of the internal capsule do not extend into this medial region (Fig.

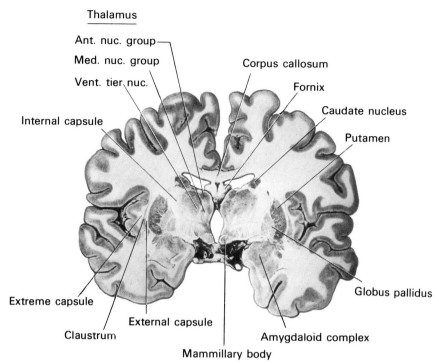

Figure 17-2. Photograph of a frontal section of the brain at the level of the mammillary bodies. In this section the main nuclear groups of the thalamus are identified, and portions of all components of the basal ganglia are present. The amygdaloid nuclear complex lies in the temporal lobe internal to the uncus and ventral to the lentiform nucleus.

17-4). In more dorsal regions, portions of the caudate nucleus and the putamen are connected by a number of slender gray (striatal) bridges passing between fibers of the internal capsule (Figs. 15-9 and 17-3). At levels of the septum pellucidum the nucleus accumbens lies adjacent to medial and ventral portions of the striatum. Autoradiographic studies suggest that the nucleus accumbens is ontogenetically more closely related to the caudate and putamen than to the septal nuclei and the bed nucleus of the stria terminalis (2478). This conclusion is strengthened by data indicating that the nucleus accumbens projects to both the globus pallidus and portions of the substantia nigra.

Cytologically the caudate nucleus and the putamen are considered to be identical. Cells are densely packed, exhibit no laminations or special arrangements and classically are considered to be of two types: (a) small achromatic neurons, and (b) large multipolar neurons with rounded contours and irregularly clumped Nissl substance.

Although small cells were considered to outnumber large cells by ratios of 20:1 or 60:1 (771, 1796), a morphometric and statistical analysis of the human striatum indicated that: (a) the mean numerical density of small striatal neurons is approximately 11,000 cells mm³, while the mean numerical density of the large striatal neurons is about 65 cells/mm³, and (b) the ratio of small to large striatal neurons averages about 170:1, with a range from 130:1 to 258:1 (2288). The putamen on average is about 13% larger than the caudate nucleus in man. Golgi and electron microscopic observations indicate that striatal neurons fall into two categories: (a) those with spiny dendrites, and (b) those with smooth dendrites (14, 634, 787, 789, 1282, 1943).

Spiny neurons, considered the most numerous striatal neuron, are round or oval, have a relatively large nucleus and are surrounded by a narrow rim of cytoplasm containing free ribosomes (634). Seven or eight primary dendrites extending from the soma branch into secondary dendrites which be-

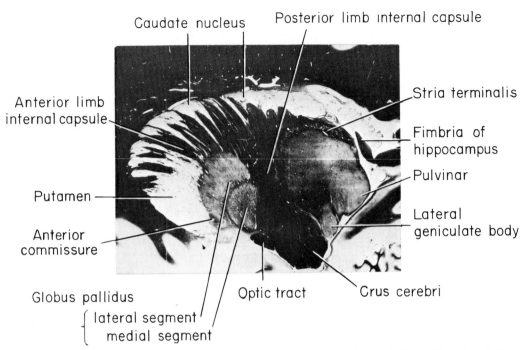

Caudate nucleus

Posterior limb internal capsule

Anterior limb internal capsule

Stria terminalis

Fimbria of hippocampus

Pulvinar

Putamen

Anterior commissure

Lateral geniculate body

Globus pallidus

{ lateral segment

medial segment

Optic tract

Crus cerebri

Figure 17-3. Sagittal section through the corpus striatum, internal capsule and thalamus. Note the relationships of the caudate nucleus to the fibers of the anterior limb of the internal capsule. (Weigert's myelin stain, photograph.)

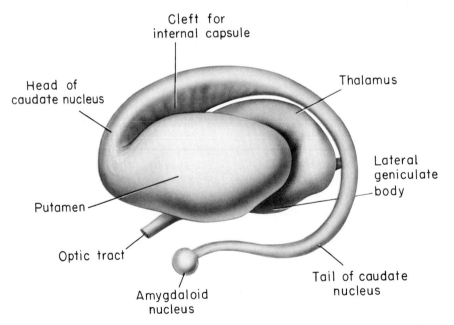

Cleft for internal capsule

Head of caudate nucleus

Thalamus

Lateral geniculate body

Putamen

Optic tract

Tail of caudate nucleus

Amygdaloid nucleus

Figure 17-4. Semischematic drawing of the isolated striatum, thalamus, and amygdaloid nucleus showing: (a) the continuity of the putamen and head of the caudate nucleus rostrally, and (b) the relationships between the tail of the caudate nucleus and the amygdaloid nucleus. The cleft occupied by fibers of the internal capsule is indicated. The anterior limb of the internal capsule is situated between the caudate nucleus and the putamen (Figs. 15-27, 17-3 and 17-5), while the posterior limb of the internal capsule lies between the lentiform nucleus and the thalamus.

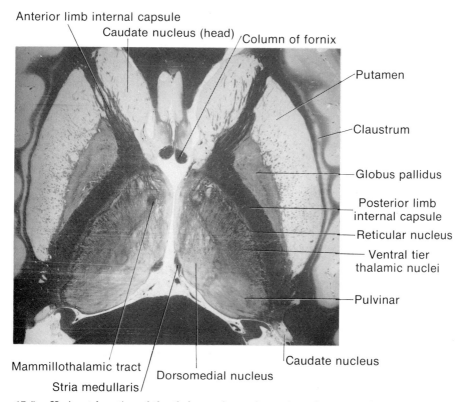

Anterior limb internal capsule

Caudate nucleus (head)

Column of fornix

Putamen

Claustrum

Globus pallidus

Posterior limb internal capsule

Reticular nucleus

Ventral tier thalamic nuclei

Pulvinar

Caudate nucleus

Mammillothalamic tract

Dorsomedial nucleus

Stria medullaris

Figure 17-5. Horizontal section of the thalamus, internal capsule and corpus striatum. (Weigert's myelin stain, photograph.)

come covered with both sessile and pedunculated spines (Figs. 17-6 and 17-7). Cells are close to each other, and there is considerable overlap in the dendritic province of each neuron. It has been estimated that dendrites of spiny neurons radiate into a spheroid space with a diameter of about 300 μm. Two types of spiny striatal neurons described by DiFiglia, Pasik and Pasik (634) have axons emerging from the soma, or a proximal dendrite, that can be followed beyond the dendritic field (Fig. 17-6). Axon collaterals from type I spiny neurons branch at nearly right angles from the parent axon and travel 400 μm before ending. Axons of the larger type II spiny neurons take a straight course in the direction of the pallidum. Data from experimental studies using horseradish peroxidase (HRP) (Fig. 17-8) suggest that axons of spiny neurons constitute the striatal efferent system (969, 1322).

Aspiny striatal neurons of various sizes have a number of smooth dendrites (Fig. 17-7). In most Golgi studies, it has been difficult to identify axons (634, 789). These

neurons are thought to have short axons and to correspond to the large striatal cells seen in Nissl preparations.

On the basis of cytological data now available, it is not possible to provide a complete interpretation of the neuronal organization of the striatum, although there is impressive evidence suggesting that the afferent systems arising from cortex, thalamus and midbrain terminate upon spiny neurons (1281, 1284, 1285, 1286). It is widely accepted that spiny neurons also constitute the striatal output neuron, particularly type II spiny neurons (1943). The role of interneurons (Golgi type II) with short axons, represented by aspiny striatal neurons, is unknown, but it may be inhibitory as in many other sites within the central nervous system.

The striatum contains high concentrations of dopamine (584). Dopamine in the striatum is contained in small granular vesicels in terminal boutons considered to be terminals of nigrostriatal fibers (59, 1127, 1145, 2025, 2598). In addition, the striatum contains glutamate conveyed by cortico-

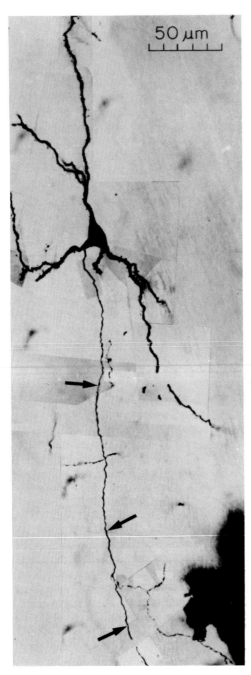

50 μm

Figure 17-6. Photomontage of a *spiny type II* striatal neuron in a Golgi preparation of the monkey. These cells are pyramidal in shape, give rise to four to six primary dendrites with relatively low spine densities and have an axon which emerges from the soma or a proximal dendrite. Axons of these neurons take a straight course and have been followed for 300 μm without narrowing or forming terminal arborizations. The axon (*arrows*) is directed toward the globus pallidus and appears to give rise to collaterals (634). (Full scale, 50 μm.) (Reproduced with permission from M. DiFiglia, P. Pasik and T. Pasik: *Brain Research,* **114:** 245–256, 1976 (634).)

striate fibers (779, 1312, 2393) and serotonin (5-HT) transmitted from the raphe nuclei of the midbrain (1086, 1704, 1878, 2532). Striatal efferent neurons contain γ-aminobutyric acid (GABA) and substance P; GABA is transported to both the globus pallidus and the substantia nigra (1053, 1564, 2082), but substance P is transmitted only to the substantia nigra (841, 1137, 1262).

The Globus Pallidus

This nucleus, forming the smaller and inner part of the lentiform nucleus, lies medial to the putamen throughout most of its extent. The dorsomedial margin of the pallidum borders the posterior limb of the internal capsule. A thin *lateral medullary lamina* lies on the external surface of the pallidum at its junction with the putamen. A *medial medullary lamina* divides the globus pallidus into medial and lateral segments (Figs. 17-2, 17-3, 17-10 and 17-11). A less distinct *accessory medullary lamina* (1398) divides the medial pallidal segment into outer and inner portions which appear to give rise to efferent fibers that have distinctive courses (Fig. 17-10). Some cells of the substantia innominata of Meynert extend dorsally in the medullary laminae of the pallidus (924, 1691). The globus pallidus, phylogenetically older than the striatum, classically is considered to be a telencephalic derivative (1012). Studies of the ontogenetic development of the globus pallidus and subthalamic nucleus suggest that these structures are diencephalic derivatives (2149). During early development the anlage of the corpus subthalamicum and both segments of the pallidum are arranged in a linear fashion with the anlage of the lateral pallidal segment most rostral, that of the subthalamic nucleus most caudal and that of the medial pallidal segment (entopeduncular nucleus) in an intermediate position. In the third month of fetal life the lateral pallidal segment migrates rostrolaterally to contact the medial surface of the putamen. The entopeduncular nucleus follows the lateral pallidal segment rostrolat-

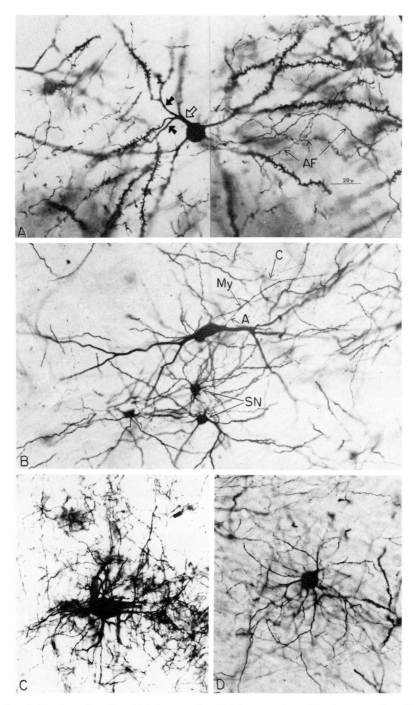

Figure 17-7. *A:* Montage of a spiny striatal neuron in a Golgi preparation of the rhesus monkey. "Boutons en passage" of afferent fibers (*AF*) cross over its dendrites. The *open arrow* and the *closed arrows* indicate the spine-free dendritic trunk and the initial, spine-free dendritic branches, respectively. (Golgi, ×700.) *B:* A large aspiny striatal neuron. *A,* axon; *My,* initial segment of myelin sheath; *C,* axon collateral; *SN,* spiny striatal neurons. (Golgi, ×300.) *C:* A large aspiny neuron in the putamen. (Golgi, ×300.) *D:* A spidery aspiny neuron in the putamen. (Golgi, ×300.) (Courtesy of the late Dr. C. A. Fox of Wayne State University.)

erally and assumes an adjacent medial position, where it is called the medial pallidal segment. The most caudal anlage in this longitudinal hypothalamic zone, the subthalamic nucleus, is pushed medially by invading fibers of the hemispheric stalk and becomes separated from the pallidum by the internal capsule. Anatomical connections between the subthalamic nucleus and the pallidum are maintained during these migrations by fibers which traverse the peduncular part of the internal capsule.

Many bundles of myelinated fibers traverse the globus pallidus, which in fresh preparations give it a paler appearance than the putamen or caudate nucleus. A morphometric analysis of the human globus pallidus indicates that the lateral segment constitutes 70% of the total volume of the pallidum and has cell densities which are greater than those for the medial pallidal segment (2288). However, the mean volume of nerve cells in the medial pallidal segment is 10% higher than in the lateral pallidal segment. Estimates of the total number of pallidal neurons indicate a range of 465,000 to 540,000 for the lateral segment and 143,000 to 171,000 for the medial segment. Golgi studies reveal that pallidal neurons are large ovoid or polygonal cells, 35 to 50 μm in their long axis, with long, thick, relatively smooth dendrites (788). These neurons have dendrites which have been traced for nearly 900 μm and nuclei with irregular contours and deep infoldings. A rich plexus of afferent fibers invests the long dendrites with an array of longitudinal fibers that bear "boutons en passage." The most prevalent synaptic endings contain large ovoid synaptic vesicles 50 nm to 70 nm. The most surprising observation is that in Golgi preparations it is not possible to detect differences in the large neurons in the different pallidal segments. Although axons of large pallidal neurons are difficult to impregnate beyond the initial segment in Golgi preparations, there is no evidence of axon collaterals within the globus pallidus.

THE CLAUSTRUM

This is a thin plate of gray matter lying in the medullary substance of the hemisphere between the lentiform nucleus and the insular cortex, which is separated from these structures by two white laminae, the external capsule medially and the extreme capsule laterally (Figs. 2-12, 15-27, 17-1 and 17-2). Although the claustrum has been considered to be a part of the striatum, it seems likely that it is more closely related to the cerebral cortex. The claustrum consists of two parts, an insular part composed of comparatively large cells underlying the insular cortex, and a temporal part composed of small, loosely arranged cells located between the putamen and temporal lobe (258, 1802). The cerebral cortex projects in a gross topographic fashion upon the claustrum (655, 656, 1802) and it may be the site of convergence of polymodal afferents from the sensory cortex. Observations based upon the retrograde transport of HRP indicate that cells in the claustrum project to widespread regions of the cerebral cortex (1850, 2146). These observations suggest a reciprocal relationship between the claustrum and sensory areas of the cortex. Studies indicate that projections from the striate and peristriate cortex end in restricted dorsolateral regions of the claustrum with evidence of a retinotopic organization (1213, 2321). Comparison of the receptive field properties of claustral neurons with those of visual cortical neurons indicates that most claustral neurons respond best to appropriately oriented bars of light, have little spontaneous activity and respond poorly to stationary light stimuli (2321). Claustral neurons respond equally well to stimulation of either eye, and those dominated by the contralateral eye have receptive fields in the monocular segment of the visual field.

The claustrum is a telencephalic cell group with widespread reciprocal connections with the neocortex. It bears striking and unique resemblances to the thalamus. The corticoclaustral projection arises from pyramidal cells in cortical layer VI, and fibers projected by the claustrum terminate most densely in layer IV of the cortex (1880, 2321). Cells of layer VI of the visual cortex projecting to the claustrum are distinct from those projecting to the lateral geniculate nucleus. The claustrum contains discrete visual and somatosensory subdivisions that have interconnections with corresponding primary sensory areas of the neocortex.

A

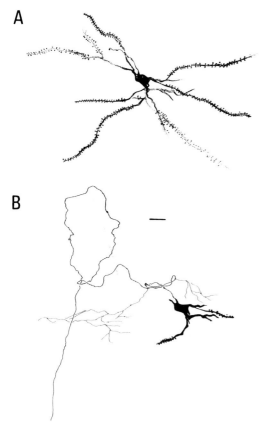

B

—

Figure 17-8.   Drawing of a single spiny striatal neuron injected iontophoretically with horseradish peroxidase to produce a Golgi-like picture of the soma and dendrites. Unlike the usual Golgi preparation, the axon can be followed beyond the proximal segment. *A* shows a reconstruction of the soma and dendritic region and the proximal portion of the axon. *B* is a reconstruction of the soma and part of the axon. The axon follows a coiled and circuitous course and gives rise to two collaterals. This axon was followed for a total distance of 1.5 mm (1340). (Calibration in *B*, 20 μm.) (Reproduced with permission from J. D. Kocsis, M. Sugimori, and S. T. Kitai: *Brain Research*, **124**: 403–413, 1977 (1340).)

STRIATAL CONNECTIONS

Striatal Afferent Fibers

The striatum receives the principal afferent systems projecting to the corpus striatum. Afferent systems arising from the cerebral cortex, the intralaminar thalamic nuclei and the substantia nigra are profuse and topographically organized (Fig. 17-9). In addition, the striatum, or parts of it, receive projections from cells of the dorsal

nucleus of the raphe that convey serotonin (5-HT).

Corticostriate Fibers. Virtually all regions of the neocortex project fibers to the striatum, and all parts of the striatum receive fibers from the cortex (369, 370, 1285). Cortical projections to the striatum are on a simple topographic basis with overlap of terminal fibers in all dimensions. No part of the caudate nucleus or putamen is under the sole influence of one functional area of the neocortex, but the projection from the sensorimotor cortex is more substantial than that from other areas. In the rat, rabbit and cat, the cortex of the frontal region is related to a larger volume of the striatum than is the posterolateral cortex (369, 2682, 2683). In the monkey, as in other mammals, the projection to the striatum from the sensorimotor cortex is substantial, while that for the visual cortex is small. The corticostriate projection from the association cortex of the frontal and parietotemporal lobes in the monkey is greater than in other mammals (1285). Although there are differences in the extent of the striatum to which different areas of the cortex project, most regions of the cortex are connected with both the caudate nucleus and the putamen, evidence which strengthens the concept that the caudate nucleus and the putamen constitute a single structure. In degeneration studies, corticostriate projections from the sensorimotor cortex have been found to be bilateral in the rat, rabbit and cat (371). Contralateral projections from these cortical areas cross the midline in the corpus callosum and enter the caudate nucleus via the subcallosal fasciculus, and the putamen through the external capsule. Autoradiographic studies in the monkey have demonstrated that areas 4 and 6 project bilaterally and symmetrically to the putamen (1231, 1392). Although Cajal (348) considered corticostriate fibers to be collaterals of corticofugal projections destined for lower centers, studies based upon the retrograde transport of horseradish peroxidase (HRP) have clearly demonstrated that these fibers, both ipsilateral and contralateral, arise from cell populations distinct from those that form the corticospinal, corticobulbar, corticopontine, corticorubral and corticothalamic systems (1231, 1245). The corticostriate projection arises from

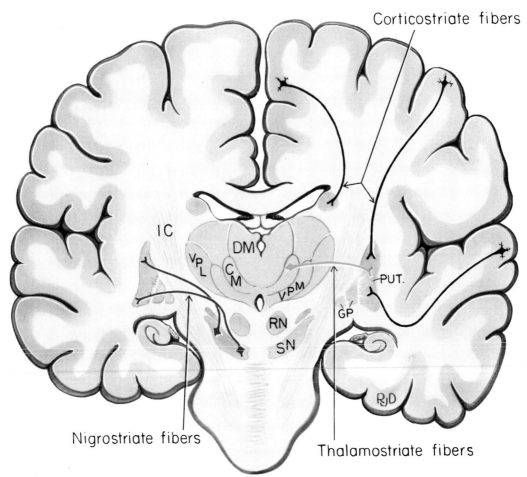

Figure 17-9. Semischematic diagram of the major striatal afferent systems. *Corticostriate projections (black)* arise from broad regions of the cerebral cortex, are topographically organized, and are distributed to both the caudate nucleus and the putamen. Corticostriate fibers arise from pyramidal cells in the upper half of lamina V, and those from area 4 project bilaterally and somatotopically upon the putamen. These projections have glutamate as their neurotransmitter. *Nigrostriatal fibers (red)* arise from cells of the pars compacta of the substantia nigra and convey dopamine to terminals in the caudate nucleus and putamen. *Thalamostriate fibers (blue)* arise largely from the centromedian-parafascicular nuclear complex. Not shown in this diagram are striatal afferents from mesencephalic indolamine cell groups in the median raphe. Cell groups in the median raphe have serotonin as their neurotransmitter. Abbreviations used: CM, centromedian nucleus; DM dorsomedial nucleus; GP, globus pallidus; IC, internal capsule; PUT, putamen; RN, red nucleus; SN, substantia nigra; VPL and VPM, ventral posterolateral and ventral posteromedial thalamic nuclei.

smaller pyramidal cells, 14 to 16 μm in somal diameter, restricted to the upper half of lamina V and constant in size and laminar distribution from area to area. The implication of these studies is that the corticostriate projections are not formed by collaterals of corticospinal, corticobulbar or corticothalamic axons and that interactions of these systems with corticostriate neurons must involve local intracortical circuits.

Tritiated amino acids injected into local-

ized regions of area 4 can be traced autoradiographically to extensive regions of the putamen, while only sparse radioactivity is evident in the caudate nucleus (1392). Silver grains in patch-like arrangements seen bilaterally show a greater density laterally and extend rostrocaudally nearly the length of the putamen. Although these localized grain patterns in the putamen are symmetrical in location, the contralateral patches of radioactivity are less dense, and corticostriate fibers from area 4 are bilateral, symmetrical and topographically organized. The face region of area 4 projects terminals to ventral regions of the putamen, while the leg area projects to dorsal regions; the arm area projects fibers to the region between the face and the leg (1392). The premotor cortex (area 6) projects fibers to both the caudate nucleus and the putamen, while the prefrontal cortex projects predominantly to the caudate nucleus (1394). Labeling in the striatum is heavy, extensive and characterized by a series of strips or clusters of silver grains that separate from each other and rejoin at other sites. Almost all autoradiographic studies of corticostriate projections have emphasized the overlapping nature of terminals arising from different cortical areas (909, 1231, 1392). Corticostriate fibers have glutamate as their neurotransmitter (779, 2393).

Thalamostriate Fibers. Thalamostriate fibers constitute one of the most important groups of afferent fibers passing to the caudate nucleus and putamen (Figs. 17-9 and 17-11). The largest number of these fibers originate from the centromedian-parafascicular nuclear complex (CM-PF), traverse the internal capsule and enter the putamen (1686, 1827, 2055). Other studies demonstrate that the centromedian nucleus projects to both the putamen and the body of the caudate nucleus (231, 1651). None of these fibers project to the globus pallidus or the claustrum. The parafascicular nucleus also has a topographical projection to the putamen and shows a similar organization. Afferent fibers to the caudate nucleus originate from the smaller, more rostral intralaminar thalamic nuclei (medial central, paracentral and lateral central). Available evidence suggests that terminals of thalamostriate fibers have small synaptic vesicles and end exclusively upon the dendritic spines of spiny striatal neurons (787). Studies utilizing the retrograde axonal transport of horseradish peroxidase (HRP) have made it possible to further explore the projections of the intralaminar thalamic nuclei. Injections of HRP into the putamen produced intense labeling of cells in the CM-PF complex and some labeling of cells in posterior parts of the central lateral nucleus (CL), while HRP injections in various cortical areas produced intense labeling of cells in corresponding thalamic relay nuclei and relatively light labeling of cells in portions of the intralaminar nuclei (1234). These results have been interpreted to mean that the intralaminar thalamic nuclei project profusely to the striatum and sparsely and diffusely upon broad regions of the cerebral cortex. Studies of the efferent projections of the intralaminar thalamic nuclei based upon autoradiographic technics stress the dorsoventral and rostrocaudal organization of thalamostriate fibers and indicate that such fibers end in mosaic patterns similar to those established for the corticostriate system (1078). Collaterals of thalamostriate fibers projecting to broad cortical areas end in laminae V and VI.

Nigrostriate Fibers. Evidence concerning nigrostriatal fibers has for a long time been based almost entirely upon retrograde cell changes produced in the substantia nigra following large striatal lesions (744, 745, 1682, 1720). Attempts to trace fiber degeneration from lesions in the substantia nigra to the striatum in Marchi preparations and silver-impregnated material (20, 419, 504, 736) either failed to demonstrate these fibers or indicated that they were sparse. However, the fluorescence technic for the demonstration of monoamines (368, 730) revealed that cells in the pars compacta of the substantia nigra (Fig. 13-22 and 13-23) send axons to the striatum that convey dopamine to their terminals (60, 143, 586, 828, 1127, 2598). Striatal dopamine is stored in varicosities in nerve terminals. Varicosities, both terminal and nonterminal, in the striatum are fine, densely packed and exhibit a diffuse green fluorescence. Dopaminergic fibers form a distinct matrix of fine varicose axons forming thick sworls around both small and large striatal neurons (2340). Nerve terminals containing dopamine have small granular vesicles about 50 nm in diameter (1127). Dopamine is considered to be synthesized in the pigmented cells of the pars compacta. In contrast to nerve terminals in the striatum, the concentrations of dopamine in the large cells of the substantia nigra seem low because the monoamine occurs mainly in the perinuclear cytoplasm. Lesions in the substantia nigra cause conspicuous reductions in striatal dopamine ipsilaterally (60, 828, 1127, 2598). Large striatal lesions produce distinct increases in dopamine in the cells of the pars compacta which decrease as the cells undergo chromatolysis. Most data suggest that dopaminergic fibers exert inhibitory influences upon striatal neurons (196, 1086, 1571, 2340).

Studies in the monkey based upon a modified silver staining method (2721) confirm that nigrostriatal fibers arise exclusively from cells of the pars compacta and are topically arranged (Figs. 13-14, 13-24 and 17-9 and Ref. 413). Nigrostriatal fibers appear organized in a manner reciprocal to that of strionigral fibers (2489–2491). Caudal parts of the substantia nigra project primarily to the putamen, and there is a correspondence between lateral parts of the nigra and dorsal regions of the putamen, and medial parts of the nigra and ventral regions of the putamen (2492). (Fig. 17-21). The medial two-thirds of the pars compacta sends efferents to the head of the caudate nucleus. An inverse relationship exists dorsoventrally between the nigra and the caudate nucleus, in that cells in the ventral part of the pars compacta project to dorsal regions of the caudate nucleus; dorsally situated cells of the pars compacta project to ventromedial regions of the caudate nucleus (2492, 2493). These fibers pass rostrally from the substantia nigra into Forel's field H and then course laterally, dorsal and rostral to the subthalamic nucleus. Nigrostriatal fibers traverse the internal capsule and portions of the globus pallidus *en route* to the putamen (Figs. 13-25 and 17-21).

Striatal Brain Stem Afferents. Serotonin (5-HT) is present in relatively high concentrations in the striatum, where it is believed to act as an inhibitory neurotransmitter (1086, 1704, 1878). Histofluorescent studies have demonstrated several ascending pathways originating from mesencephalic indolamine cell groups in the median raphe (585, 2598). The indolamine cell groups of the median raphe include the dorsal raphe nucleus in the central gray ventral to the cerebral aqueduct at levels of the trochlear nucleus (Figs. 11-15 and 12-30), and the median raphe nucleus, commonly referred to as the superior central nucleus (Fig. 12-25) (201, 649, 1885). Stimulation of the dorsal raphe nucleus strongly inhibits striatal neurons, while the median raphe nucleus inhibits a smaller number of

striatal neurons (1878). An analysis of the distribution of serotoninergic terminals in the striatum of the rat and cat suggests that 5-HT terminals are localized mainly in ventrocaudal regions of the putamen (2532). The density of 5-HT terminals decreases progressively from caudal to rostral levels in the neostriatum. This preferential localization of serotoninergic terminals in ventrocaudal parts of the striatum is in agreement with autoradiographic studies (201, 515). Ascending brain stem afferents from the dorsal and median raphe nuclei appear to modulate neuronal activities in both the striatum and the substantia nigra.

Striatal Efferent Fibers

Striatal efferents project to the globus pallidus and the substantia nigra (Figs. 17-21 and 17-22).

Striopallidal Fibers. Striopallidal fibers are topographically organized in both dorsoventral and rostrocaudal sequences and radiate into various parts of the pallidum like spokes of a wheel (Figs. 15-9 and 17-3). Studies in the monkey (556, 1825, 2490) indicate that putaminopallidal fibers terminate in both pallidal segments. The precommissural part of the putamen appears to project exclusively to the globus pallidus, while other regions of the striatum project to both globus pallidus and substantia nigra (2490). Striopallidal fibers from the caudate nucleus pass ventrally through the internal capsule, while fibers from the putamen project medially into the globus pallidus. Bundles of myelinated striopallidal fibers are most numerous in medial parts of the putamen (Fig. 17-17). These bundles of striopallidal fibers are referred to as Wilson's pencils (2736).

Studies of the termination of striopallidal fibers at the ultrastructural level indicate that pallidal dendrites are studded with axonal terminals ensheathed with glia. Less frequent axosomatic synapses are seen; cell bodies have a wrapping of glial processes except over axon terminals (1283). Although axons of striatal efferent fibers rarely are well impregnated in Golgi preparations, it has been proposed that striatal efferents, traversing the globus pallidus in a radial fashion, emit collaterals to both pallidal segments and enter the "comb" bundle as strionigral fibers (795, 796). This concept assumes a single striatal efferent system supplying both the pallidum and the pars reticulata of the substantia nigra. This thesis, derived from horizontal Golgi sections, is supported by: (a) ultrastructural similarities of pallidal neurons and cells of the pars reticulata, (b) similarities of synaptic terminals in the pallidum and nigra and (c) computer measurements of axis cylinders of "radial" and "comb" bundle fibers (796).

Striopallidal fibers have γ-aminobutyric acid (GABA) as their neurotransmitter (1563, 2082). The globus pallidus is particularly rich in GABA and glutamic acid decarboxylase (GAD), the enzyme that synthesizes GABA (108, 728, 1865). Synaptosomal preparations of the globus pallidus show a high uptake of GABA and a high sodium-independent binding of GABA, which is thought to represent the interaction of GABA with postsynaptic receptors (713).

Strionigral Fibers. Experimental studies have demonstrated that strionigral fibers are topographically organized and end predominantly upon cells of the pars reticulata (1825, 2489–2491). Fibers from the head of the caudate nucleus project to rostral parts of the nigra. Putaminonigral fibers pass to more caudal parts of the nigra and are arranged so that dorsal parts of the putamen project to lateral parts of the nigra, and ventral parts of the putamen are related to medial parts of the nigra.

Studies of afferent projections to the substantia nigra, based upon the retrograde transport of HRP, also indicate that the caudatonigral projection system is arranged topographically (324). All portions of the caudate-putamen except the medial core were found to contain HRP-positive cells. In the positive areas a large percentage of cells were found to participate in this projection, but only medium-sized cells (12 to 20 μm) contained the enzyme (324, 969). In autoradiographic studies, terminals of strionigral fibers were restricted to the pars reticulata (1313).

Strionigral fibers are of two types, those that convey GABA to terminals in the pars reticulata (728, 1865), and fibers that contain substance P (596, 841). Neurons in all parts of the striatum transmit GABA to nigral terminals in the pars reticulata. Only

rostral portions of the striatum give rise to an independent parallel strionigral projection that conveys substance P to particles in nerve terminals in the pars reticulata.

Strionigral and nigrostriatal fibers appear to be reciprocally organized, although one or more local circuit neurons may be interposed within the striatum (1813). Nigrostriatal fibers convey dopamine, and strionigral fibers transport GABA and substance P to their terminals. Both dopamine and GABA serve inhibitory functions, while substance P is excitatory.

PALLIDAL CONNECTIONS

Pallidal Afferent Fibers

Established projections to the globus pallidus arise from two structures, the striatum and the subthalamic nucleus. Unlike the striatum, the globus pallidus does not receive afferents from the cerebral cortex, thalamic nuclei or the substantia nigra. In studies of corticostriate projections, most authors either sidestep or ignore reference to pallidal afferents from the cortex (369, 371, 1285, 2683), but a few authors report no evidence of such fibers (1989, 1994, 2682). While questions must remain concerning the existence of corticopallidal fibers, there is excellent autoradiographic evidence that the motor cortex has no projection to any part of the globus pallidus (1392). *Striopallidal* fibers distributed to both pallidal segments have been discussed under striatal connections.

Subthalamopallidal Fibers. Subthalamopallidal fibers project ventrolateral through the peduncular part of the internal capsule as a number of small fascicles and enter the medial pallidal segment, from which site they are distributed to both pallidal segments (398, 419, 1339, 2712). Autoradiographic studies of the subthalamopallidal projection in the monkey indicates that these fibers are topographically organized and terminate in arrays parallel to the medullary laminae of the pallidum (398, 1812). A retrograde transport study using HRP indicated that subthalamopallidal fibers arise exclusively from the caudal and medial two-thirds of the subthalamic nucleus and project most profusely upon the medial pallidal segment (Fig. 17-18, *A* and *B*) (395). Cells in the lateral third of the

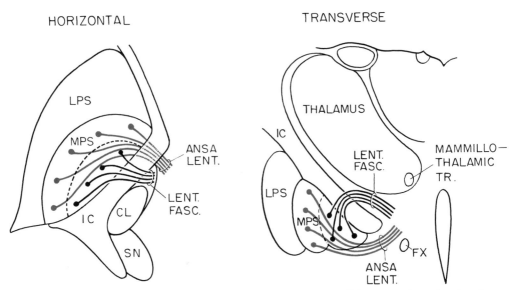

HORIZONTAL   TRANSVERSE

Figure 17-10. Diagramatic representation of the origin and course of pallidothalamic fibers forming the *ansa lenticularis* and *lenticular fasciculus*. Fibers of the ansa lenticularis (*red*) arise from the outer portion of the medial pallidal segment (lateral to the accessory medullary lamina, *dashed line*) and course rostrally, ventrally and medially. Fibers of the lenticular fasciculus (black) arise from the inner portion of the medial pallidal segment (medial to the accessory medullary lamina, *dashed line*) and course dorsally and medially through the fibers of the internal capsule (1398). Abbreviations used: CL, subthalamic nucleus; FX, fornix; IC, internal capsule; LPS, lateral pallidal segment; MPS, medial pallidal segment; SN, substantia nigra.

subthalamic nucleus do not project to either pallidal segment. Considerable evidence indicates that single cells in the subthalamic nucleus project to both the globus pallidus and the pars reticulata of the substantia nigra (1339, 1344, 1812).

Pallidofugal Fiber Systems

Pallidofugal fiber systems represent the principal efferent system of the corpus striatum. Impulses from nuclei projecting upon the globus pallidus are ultimately transmitted from the pallidum by an intricate pallidofugal fiber system. Pallidal efferent fibers can be divided into four main bundles: (a) the *ansa lenticularis*, (b) the *lenticular fasciculus*, (c) the *pallidotegmental fibers* and (d) the *pallidosubthalamic fibers* (Figs. 17-10–17-13 and 17-15). The first three of these arise exclusively from the medial pallidal segment (Figs. 17-10–17-13 and 17-15; and Refs. 389, 419, 1313, 1825 and 2112). Pallidosubthalamic fibers arise exclusively from the lateral pallidal segment (Figs. 17-10 and 17-18C and D and Refs. 395, 398 and 1554). Pallidofugal fibers are arranged in a rostrocaudal sequence

with the ansa lenticularis most rostral, the lenticular fasciculus in an intermediate position and pallidosubthalamic fibers most caudal.

The Ansa Lenticularis. Fibers of the ansa lenticularis arise primarily from lateral portions of the medial segment of the globus pallidus and form a well-defined bundle on the ventral surface of the pallidum (Figs. 17-10–17-12). Fibers sweep ventromedially and rostrally around the posterior limb of the internal capsule and then course posteriorly to enter Forel's field H.

The Lenticular Fasciculus. Fibers of the lenticular fasciculus arise largely from the inner part of the medial pallidal segment, issue from the dorsomedial margin of the pallidum, slightly caudal to the ansa lenticularis, and traverse ventral parts of the internal capsule in a number of small fascicles (Figs. 17-10, 17-11 and 17-13). These fibers cross through the internal capsule immediately rostral to the subthalamic nucleus and form a relatively discrete bundle ventral to the zona incerta (Fig. 17-13). Although most of the lenticular fasciculus lies rostral to the subthalamic nucleus,

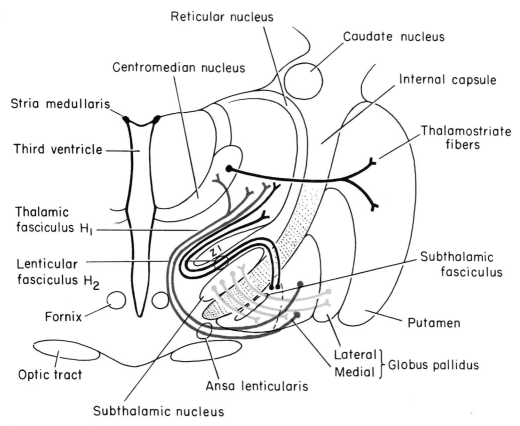

Figure 17-11. Schematic diagram of pallidofugal fiber systems in a transverse plane. Fibers of the ansa lenticularis (*red*) arise from the outer portion of the medial pallidal segment, pass ventrally, medially and rostrally around the internal capsule and enter the prerubral field. Fibers of the lenticular fasciculus (H_2, *black*) issue from the dorsal surface of inner part of the medial pallidal segment, traverse the posterior limb of the internal capsule, and pass medially dorsal to the subthalamic nucleus to enter the prerubral field. The ansa lenticularis and the lenticular fasciculus merge in the prerubral field (field H of Forel, not labeled here) and project dorsolaterally as components of the thalamic fasciculus (H_1). Fibers of the thalamic fasciculus (H_1) pass dorsal to the zona incerta (*ZI*). The subthalamic fasciculus (*blue*) consists of pallidosubthalamic fibers arising from the lateral pallidal segment, and subthalamopallidal fibers that terminate in arrays parallel to the medullary lamina in both pallidal segments. Both components of the subthalamic fasciculus traverse the internal capsule. Thalamostriate fibers from the centromedian nucleus (*black*) project to the putamen, as part of a feedback system. Compare with Figs. 17-9, 17-10 and 17-15.

some fibers of this bundle course along the dorsal capsule of this nucleus. Fibers of the lenticular fasciculus are referred to as Forel's field H_2. While fibers of the lenticular fasciculus pursue a distinctive course through the internal capsule, they pass medially and caudally to join fibers of the ansa lenticularis in Forel's field H (prerubral field). The majority of the fibers of the lenticular fasciculus (H_2) and the ansa lenticularis merge in Forel's field H and ultimately enter the thalamic fasciculus (Forel's field H_1) located dorsal to the zona incerta (Figs. 17-11 and 17-13).

Investigations of the origin of pallidothalamic fibers in the monkey indicate that fibers emerging via the ansa lenticularis and the lenticular fasciculus arise from specific portions of the medial pallidal segment (389, 1398). These data indicate that fibers of the ansa lenticularis arise predominantly from the outer part of the medial pallidal segment (i.e., from that part of the medial pallidal segment lateral to the accessory medullary lamina). These fibers course rostrally, ventrally and medially, and traverse portions of the inner pallidal segment (Fig. 17-10). Fibers of the lenticular fasciculus

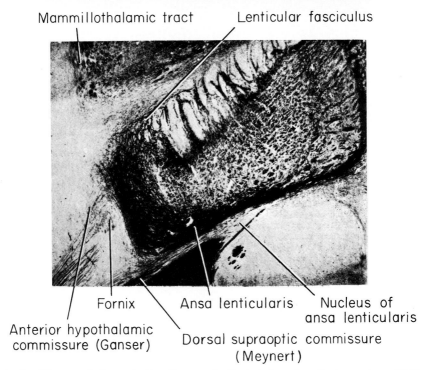

Mammillothalamic tract   Lenticular fasciculus

Fornix   Ansa lenticularis   Nucleus of ansa lenticularis

Anterior hypothalamic commissure (Ganser)   Dorsal supraoptic commissure (Meynert)

Figure 17-12. Photograph demonstrating the ansa lenticularis in a decorticate monkey. All fibers of the internal capsule have degenerated, so that pallidofugal fibers sweeping medially around the internal capsule are especially prominent. (Weigert's myelin stain.) (Reproduced with permission from F. A. Mettler: *Neuroanatomy*, C. V. Mosby Company, St. Louis, 1948 (1688).)

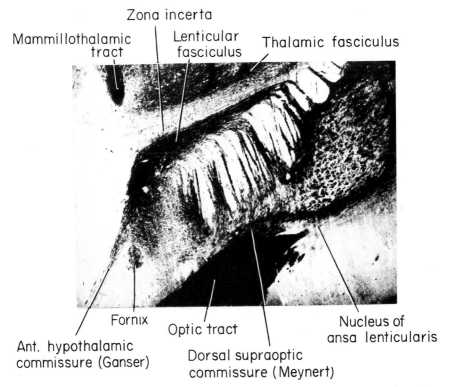

Zona incerta

Mammillothalamic tract   Lenticular fasciculus   Thalamic fasciculus

Fornix   Optic tract   Nucleus of ansa lenticularis

Ant. hypothalamic commissure (Ganser)   Dorsal supraoptic commissure (Meynert)

Figure 17-13. Photograph demonstrating the lenticular fasciculus in a decorticate monkey. Fibers of this bundle can be seen passing through the degenerated internal capsule. At this level, immediately rostral to the subthalamic nucleus, the lenticular fasciculus lies on the inner aspect of the internal capsule ventral to the zona incerta. (Weigert's myelin stain.) (Reproduced with permission from F. A. Mettler: *Neuroanatomy*, C. V. Mosby Company, St. Louis, 1948 (1688)

arise largely from the inner pallidal segment (i.e., from the portion medial to the accessory medullary lamina). These fibers course dorsally, rostrally and medially and traverse the peduncular part of the internal capsule (Fig. 17-10).

The Thalamic Fasciculus. Pallidofugal fibers from Forel's field H pass rostrally and laterally along the dorsal surface of the zona incerta where they form part of the thalamic fasciculus (Figs. 17-11 and 17-13). Most of the pallidothalamic fibers in the lenticular fasciculus merely make a tight "C"-shaped loop around the medial part of the zona incerta and enter the thalamic fasciculus (Figs. 17-11, 17-15 and 17-22). The thalamic fasciculus is a complex bundle containing pallidothalamic fibers, as well as dentatothalamic fibers which ascend through the prerubral region. Fibers of this composite bundle pass dorsolaterally over the zona incerta to enter parts of the rostral ventral tier thalamic nuclei. In the region dorsal to the zona incerta, where fibers of this bundle are distinct and separate from those of the lenticular fasciculus (Figs. 17-11 and 17-13), the thalamic fasciculus is designated as bundle H_1 of Forel. Pallidofugal fibers in the thalamic fasciculus project rostrally and dorsally into the ventral anterior (VApc) and ventral lateral (VLo and VLm) thalamic nuclei (Figs. 15-14, 17-14A and 17-15). Some of the pallidofugal fibers separate from the thalamic fasciculus and course dorsally, caudally and medially to enter the centromedian (CM) nucleus of the thalamus (Figs. 17-11 and 17-14B). In their course, these latter fibers pass through portions of the ventral posteromedial (VPM) nucleus of the thalamus. Fibers projecting to the centromedian nucleus may be collaterals of fibers passing to the rostral ventral tier thalamic nuclei (1825). Dentatothalamic fibers coursing with the thalamic fasciculus pass to the ventral lateral (VLc, VLo) and ventral posterolateral, (VPLo) thalamic nuclei but some of these cerebellar efferent fibers also project to the more rostral intralaminar nuclei.

Studies of pallidothalamic fibers in the monkey indicate that this projection to the rostral ventral tier thalamic nuclei (i.e., VApc, VLo and VLm) is topographically organized in three cardinal dimensions (1313, 1398). Rostral parts of the medial pallidal segment project predominantly to

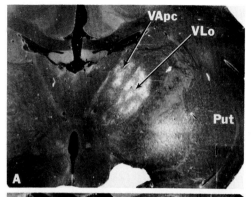

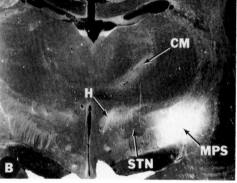

Figure 17-14. Dark field photomicrographs of sections through the diencephalon in a monkey demonstrating transport of [³H] amino acids from the medial pallidal segment (*MPS*) to thalamic nuclei. In *A*, transported radioactive label is distributed in a patchy fashion to the pars oralis of the ventral lateral (*VLo*) and to the principal part of the ventral anterior nuclei (*VApc*) of the thalamus. *B* shows the central region of the injection in the medial pallidal segment (*MPS*) and modest transport of the label to the centromedian nucleus (*CM*) of the thalamus. Radioactive label also is seen in Forel's field H and in lateral parts of the subthalamic nucleus (*STN*). *Put*, indicates putamen. (Cresyl violet, ×3.5.)

parts of VApc, while caudal parts of this pallidal segment project primarily to VLo. There also is a dorsoventral and mediolateral correspondence in the pallidal projection to VApc and VLo which exhibits some overlap. Pallidothalamic projections to the centromedian nucleus (CM) terminate predominantly in rostral and medial regions.

Thus the thalamic fasciculus contains two distinct afferent systems projecting to different the rostral ventral tier thalamic nuclei: (a) fibers from the contralateral dentate nucleus (Fig. 14-16), and (b) fibers from the ipsilateral medial pallidal segment (Figs. 17-11, 17-14, 17-15 and 17-22). These projections have been described as overlap-

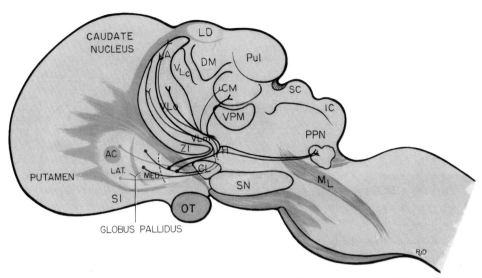

Figure 17-15. Schematic diagram of the efferent projections and terminations of pallidofugal fibers arising from the medial and lateral pallidal segments shown in a sagittal plane. Fibers of the ansa lenticularis (*red*) and lenticular fasciculus (*black*) merge in a field H of Forel. The bulk of these fibers pass in the thalamic fasciculus to the ventral lateral (*VLo* and *VLm*) and ventral anterior (*VA*) thalamic nuclei. Some fibers separate from the thalamic fasciculus and pass to the centromedian (*CM*) nucleus (Fig. 17-11). Descending pallidotegmental fibers from the medial pallidal segment terminate upon cells of the pedunculopontine nucleus (*PPN*) (Fig. 17-19c). Pallidosubthalamic fibers arising from the lateral pallidal segment (*blue*) project only to the subthalamic nucleus (*CL*). Other abbreviations: *AC*, anterior commissure; *DM*, dorsomedial nucleus; *H*, Forel's field H; *IC*, inferior colliculus; *LD*, lateral dorsal nucleus; *ML*, medial lemniscus; *OT*, optic tract; *Pul*, pulvinar; *SC*, superior colliculus; *SI*, substantia innominata; *SN*, substantia nigra; *VLc*, ventral lateral nucleus, pars caudalis; *VPM*, ventral posteromedial nucleus; *ZI*, zona incerta.

ping in the ventral lateral (VLo) nucleus and distinctive with respect to the intralaminar thalamic nuclei. Some investigators indicate relatively few cerebellar efferent fibers terminate in VLo (1971, 2538, 2567). Fibers from the deep cerebellar nuclei projecting to the intralaminar thalamic nuclei end in the central lateral nucleus, while the globus pallidus projects fibers exclusively to the centromedian nucleus. The degree of integration of cerebellar and pallidal impulses in the ventral lateral (VLo) nucleus of the thalamus is unknown. It is highly significant that the ventral lateral nucleus of the thalamus projects upon the motor cortex (area 4).

A small number of pallidal efferent fibers, emerging from the union of the lenticular fasciculus and the ansa lenticularis, pass ventromedially over the columns of the fornix toward the hypothalamus. These fibers are intermingled with those of the anterior hypothalamic decussation (Fig. 17-13; Gan-

ser's commissure) but have not been traced to hypothalamic terminations. These fibers, previously regarded as pallidohypothalamic projections, loop back to join the principal bundle of pallidofugal fibers in their projection to thalamic nuclei (1825). A small number of pallidofugal fibers are distributed to cells in Forel's field H or the prerubral field (Fig. 15-7) (1931, 2765). No pallidofugal fibers project to the red nucleus or the zona incerta.

Pallidohabenular Fibers. The medial pallidal segment gives rise to several smaller projections, among which is a distinctive pallidohabenular bundle (401a, 1825). These fibers separate from the ansa lenticularis and lenticular fasciculus near the apex of the pallidum, course dorsally and rostrally, through and around the medial part of the internal capsule, and enter the stria medullaris. Fibers course caudally in the stria medullaris to the lateral habenular nucleus (Fig. 15-6). Autoradiographic

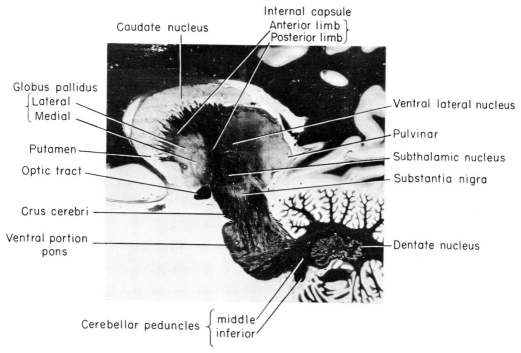

Figure 17-16. Sagittal section through the corpus striatum, thalamus, upper brain stem and cerebellum. Relationships between the corpus striatum, the subthalamic nucleus and the substantia nigra are evident. (Weigert's myelin stain, photograph.)

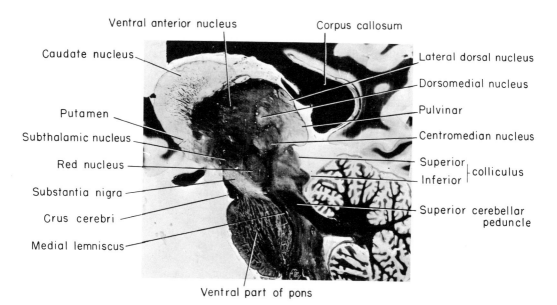

Figure 17-17. Sagittal section through medial regions of the corpus striatum, thalamus and upper brain stem, showing the relationships of caudate nucleus and putamen as well as those of the subthalamic nucleus, the red nucleus and the substantia nigra. (Weigert's myelin stain, photograph.)

studies in the cat stress the substantial nature of this bundle and the diverse routes followed by different components (1438, 1811). Injections of HRP confined to the lateral habenular nucleus in the rat label large numbers of cells in the entopeduncular nucleus (the homologue of the primate medial pallidal segment) and lesser numbers of cells in the lateral hypothalamus, the nuclei of the diagonal band, the substantia innominata and the lateral preoptic area (1079, 1438).

The habenular nuclear complex is an epithalamic structure considered to be an integral part of the limbic system. In the habenular complex the enzyme glutamic acid decarboxylase (GAD) is contained in terminals about cells of the lateral nucleus (928a). Sources of GABA-ergic fibers projecting to the lateral habenular nucleus are multiple and include pallidohabenular fibers and fibers in the stria medullaris. Histofluorescent, histochemical and sensitive microassay technics reveal several neurotransmitters and their synthesizing enzymes in the habenular nuclei; these include catecholamines, serotonin, choline acetyltransferase, acetylcholine and substance P, in addition to GAD. It has been suggested that projections of the medial pallidal segment to the lateral habenular nucleus may be involved in a circuitry that functions in conjunction with the limbic system (1811).

Pallidonigral Fibers. Most of the evidence supporting a pallidonigral pathway has been based upon the retrograde transport of HRP from the substantia nigra to the lateral segment of the globus pallidus (324, 969, 1263, 1554). Retrograde transport studies suggest that most pallidonigral fibers terminate in the pars reticulata of the nigra. Autoradiographic studies in the rat employing 6-hydroxydopamine (6-OHDA) to produce degeneration in cells of the pars compacta suggest that pallidonigral fibers terminate preferentially upon dopaminergic cells in the substantia nigra (1051). Pallidonigral fibers are considered to have GABA as their neurotransmitter (1053, 1563). These fibers are distinguished from strionigral fibers, which also have GABA as their neurotransmitter, by their termination upon cells of the pars compacta.

Pallidotegmental Fibers. This small group of descending pallidofugal fibers (Figs. 17-15 and 17-20), derived from the medial segment of the globus pallidus (1398, 1825), becomes identifiable as a separate bundle dorsomedial to the subthalamic nucleus. This bundle descends along the ventrolateral border of the red nucleus. In the caudal midbrain tegmentum these fibers sweep dorsolaterally to terminate upon large cells of the pedunculopontine nucleus (Figs. 13-3 and 17-19C). No pallidofugal fibers descend to more caudal regions of the brain stem.

Although the pedunculopontine nucleus receives its largest input from the medial pallidal segment, it also receives projections from the cerebral cortex (1042, 1411) and the substantia nigra (140, 398, 1066, 1141, 1729, 1730). Projections of the pedunculopontine nucleus appear to be mainly ascending; the largest number of ascending fibers project to the pars compacta of the substantia nigra, although small numbers of fibers project to the medial pallidal segment and the subthalamic nucleus (Fig. 17-20) (140, 395, 398, 627, 948, 1729, 1844). Connections between the pedunculopontine nucleus and the substantia nigra are not reciprocal in the strict sense, since nigrotegmental fibers arise from cells of the pars reticulata and ascending projections from the pedunculopontine nucleus end upon cells of the pars compacta (140, 1729, 1730). The functional nature of this mesencephalic loop circuit is unknown, but it may provide pathways which modulate the activities of nigral and pallidal neurons. No pallidofugal fibers pass to the red nucleus or the zona incerta.

The Subthalamic Fasciculus. The subthalamic fasciculus consists of pallidofugal fibers that pass through the internal capsule to enter the subthalamic nucleus, and of fibers from the subthalamic nucleus that project back to the globus pallidus. *Pallidosubthalamic fibers,* arising only from the lateral segment of the globus pallidus, project upon cells of the subthalamic nucleus (395, 398, 401a, 419, 1825, 2112). These fibers are topographically organized. Pallidosubthalamic fibers traverse ventromedial and caudal parts of the internal capsule, caudal to both the ansa lenticularis and the lenticular fasciculus (Figs. 17-11 and 17-15). *Subthalamopallidal fibers* traverse the same part of the internal capsule in the opposite direction and are dis-

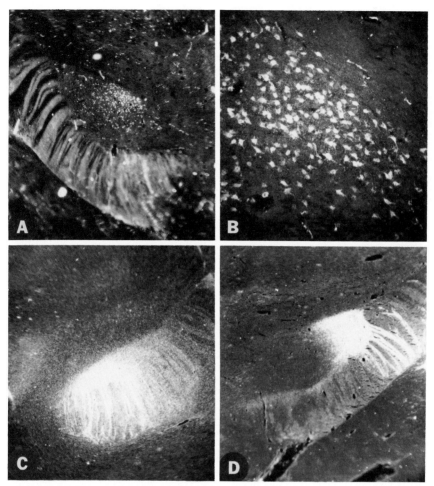

Figure 17-18. Dark field photomicrographs of the subthalamic nucleus in the monkey, demonstrating connections with the globus pallidus. *A* and *B* show retrograde transport of horseradish peroxidase to cells of the subthalamic nucleus following injections of the enzyme into the central part of the lateral pallidal segment. (×18, ×80.) *C* and *D* are autoradiographs of [³H] amino acids transported from the lateral pallidal to the subthalamic nucleus. Fibers from the rostral part of the lateral pallidal segment (LPS) project to medial part of the nucleus (*C*), while the portion LPS flanking the medial pallidal segment projects to the lateral third of the nucleus. (×18, ×6.) (Reproduced with permission from M. B. Carpenter, R. R. Batton, III, S. C. Carleton and J. T. Keller: Journal of Comparative Neurology, **197:** 579–603, 1981 (395).)

tributed to both pallidal segments (395, 398, 419, 1812).

THE SUBTHALAMIC REGION

The subthalamic region lies ventral to the thalamus, medial to the internal capsule and lateral and caudal to the hypothalamus (Figs. 2-28, 15-6, 15-7 and 17-11). Nuclei found within the subthalamic region include the subthalamic nucleus, the zona incerta and the nuclei of the tegmental fields of Forel (nucleus campi Foreli, Forel's field H). Prominent fiber bundles passing through this region include the ansa lenticularis, the lenticular fasciculus (Forel's field H₂), the thalamic fasciculus (Forel's field H₁) and the subthalamic fasciculus.

The Subthalamic Nucleus. The subthalamic nucleus (*corpus Luysi*), located on the inner surface of the peduncular portion of the internal capsule, has the shape of a thick biconvex lens (Figs. 2-28, 15-6, 15-7, 15-11, 15-12, 17-11, 17-15–17-17 and A-20). Caudally the medial part of the nucleus overlies rostral portions of the substantia nigra. (Fig. 15-16).

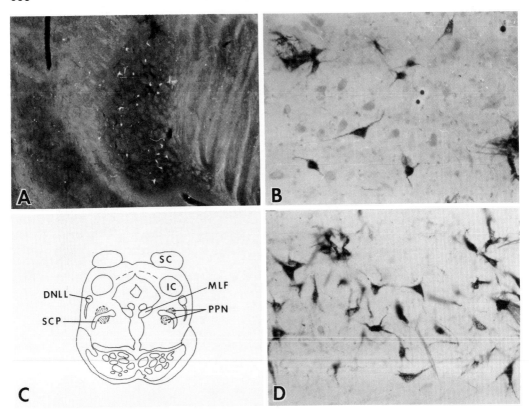

Figure 17-19. Connections of the pedunculopontine nucleus (*PPN*) in the monkey demonstrated by the retrograde transport of horseradish peroxidase (HRP). An injection of HRP into the pedunculopontine nucleus, shown diagrammatically in *C*, has retrogradely labeled cells in caudal parts of the medial pallidal segment (*A*) and the pars reticulata of the substantia nigra (*B*). Cells of the pedunculopontine nucleus in *C* lie on both sides of the superior cerebellar peduncle (*SCP*) at caudal midbrain levels. *D*, photomicrograph of retrograde transport of HRP to cells of the pedunculopontine nucleus following an injection of the substantia nigra. Other abbreviations: *DNLL*, dorsal nucleus of lateral lemniscus; *IC*, inferior colliculus; *MLF*, medial longitudinal fasciculus; *SC*, superior colliculus. (*A*, dark field, ×12.) (*B*, ×128.) (*D*, ×128.) (Reproduced with permission from M. B. Carpenter, S. C. Carleton, J. T. Keller and P. Conte: *Brain Research*, **224**: 1–29, 1981 (398).)

The subthalamic nucleus is considered to be derived from the dorsocaudal part of the lateral hypothalamic cell column (1381, 1385). Richter (2149) describes the subthalamic nucleus as arising from the "subthalamic longitudinal zone," along with both segments of the pallidum. The anlage of the corpus Luysi, caudal to that of both pallidal segments, is said to mature before either the globus pallidus or the substantia nigra. Neurons of the subthalamic nucleus are relatively large and have large nuclei containing chromatin and a massive nucleolus. Cells are multipolar, round and pyramidal in shape. Fusiform cells are seen near the margins of the nucleus, oriented parallel to capsular fibers. All cells contribute to an extremely rich neuropil, and there are mediolateral differences in cell size and concentrations (771, 1341). Cells in medial regions of the nucleus are smaller but more concentrated.

Golgi studies of the primate subthalamic nucleus reveal two varieties of principal neurons, and local interneurons (2089). Principal neurons have been referred to as radiating and elongated fusiform types. Radiating neurons have a few delicate somatic spines and five to eight dendritic trunks which give rise to branched, tapering dendrites. Dendrites of these cells are thinner than those of pallidal and nigral neurons. Fusiform neurons, less numerous than those of the radiating type, are found mainly near the capsule of the nucleus. Dendrites of local circuit neurons are dis-

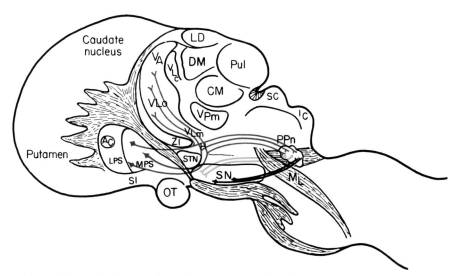

Figure 17-20. Schematic diagram of pallidotegmental (*red*) and nigrotegmental (*black*) projections in a sagittal plane. Pallidotegmental fibers arise from the medial pallidal segment (*MPS*), separate from pallidothalamic fibers in medial parts of Forel's field H and terminate upon cells of the pedunculopontine nucleus (*PPn*) at caudal midbrain levels. Cells of the pars reticulata of the substantia nigra (*SN*) project as nigrotegmental fibers to PPn. Ascending fibers from PPn (*blue*) project mainly to the pars compacta of the substantia nigra, although a small number of fibers project to subthalamic nucleus (*STN*) and the medial pallidal segment (*MPS*) (based on Refs. 140, 395, 627, 1729 and 1730). Other abbreviations are listed in the legend for Figure 17-21.

posed in mediolateral and rostrocaudal directions.

The nucleus has a café-au-lait color in fresh sections, and a rich blood supply derived from branches of the posterior communicating, posterior cerebral and anterior choroidal arteries (770). The subthalamic nucleus has a consistent distribution in mammals; it is rudimentary in carnivores but well developed in primates. While the nucleus is small in the monkey, its relative size is essentially the same as in man (216, 2712).

Connections of the Subthalamic Nucleus. Because of the deep position of the subthalamic nucleus, it has been singularly difficult to determine its connections. Afferent projections to the subthalamic nucleus are derived from the precentral motor cortex and other regions of the frontal lobe, the lateral segment of the globus pallidus and the pedunculopontine nucleus. Autoradiographic studies in the monkey reveal that the precentral motor cortex projects somatotopically upon a restricted lateral part of the subthalamic nucleus (1041). In

this projection, fibers from the face area terminate laterally within the nucleus, while fibers from the leg area end in a more medial region. Less substantial projections from the premotor and prefrontal cortex end in more medial parts of the subthalamic nucleus (1394, 1395). Electron microscopic studies indicate that cortical influences upon subthalamic nucleus neurons are mediated by thin myelinated and unmyelinated axons that terminate in small round boutons on spines and small dendrites (2202). Attempts to determine the lamina of origin of corticosubthalamic projections in the cat and monkey by retrograde transport of HRP have been inconclusive (1554, 2161). HRP injections in the subthalamic nucleus have resulted in the retrograde labeling of only a few cortical neurons.

The lateral pallidal segment is the source of the largest number of subcortical afferents to the subthalamic nucleus (395, 398, 401a, 627, 1554, 1825). Cells in the lateral pallidal segment are arranged in arrays parallel to the lateral medullary lamina and in the monkey have a rostrocaudal organiza-

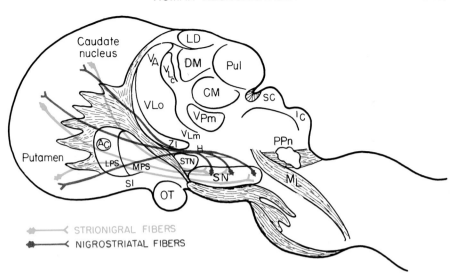

Figure 17-21. Schematic diagram of the strionigral feedback system in a sagittal plane. Strionigral fibers (*blue*) project topographically upon cells of the pars reticulata of the nigra and have GABA and substance P as neurotransmitters. Cells of the pars compacta of the nigra give rise to reciprocally arranged nigrostriatal fibers (*red*) which convey dopamine to specific loci within the striatum. Abbreviations: *AC*, anterior commissure; *CM*, centromedian nucleus; *H*, Forel's field H; *IC*, inferior colliculus; *LD*, lateral dorsal nucleus; *LPS*, lateral pallidal segment; *MD*, dorsomedial nucleus; *ML*, medial lemniscus; *MPS*, medial pallidal segment; *OT*, optic tract; *PPn*, pedunculopontine nucleus; *Pul*, pulvinar; *SC*, superior colliculus; *SI*, substantia innominata; *SN*, substantia nigra; *STN*, subthalamic nucleus; *VA*, ventral anterior nucleus; *VLc*, *VLo* and *VLm*, ventral lateral nucleus, pars caudalis, pars oralis and pars medialis, respectively; *VPm*, ventral posterior medial nucleus; *ZI*, zona incerta.

tion in which fibers from: (a) the rostral division of the lateral pallidal segment (i.e., the part rostral to the medial medullary lamina) project to the medial two-thirds of the subthalamic nucleus, and (b) the central division of the lateral pallidal segment (i.e., the part lateral to the medial medullary lamina) project to the lateral third of the nucleus (395, 398, 401a). These fibers traverse the medial pallidal segment and the peduncular part of the internal capsule in passage to the subthalamic nucleus. Retrograde transport studies using HRP in the cat suggest a mediolateral topographical relationship between the subthalamic nucleus and the lateral pallidal segment (1554).

A small number of afferent fibers to the subthalamic nucleus arise from the pedunculopontine nucleus (398, 1729, 1730, 1844, 2161).

Efferent fibers from the subthalamic nucleus traverse the internal capsule, enter caudal parts of the medial pallidal segment and radiate into all parts of the globus

pallidus. Autoradiographic studies reveal the massive nature of this projection and indicate that subthalamopallidal fibers are arranged in arrays parallel to the medullary laminae of the pallidum (398, 1812). Retrograde transport studies using HRP indicate the topographical organization of this projection (395). Cells in medial and caudal parts of the subthalamic nucleus project mainly to the medial pallidal segment, while cells in the central third of the nucleus project to the lateral pallidal segment. Few cells in the lateral third of the subthalamic nucleus project to any part of the globus pallidus. The observation that subthalamic afferent and efferent fibers terminate and arise in different parts of the nucleus suggest that this relatively small structure is not homogeneous and that reciprocal circuits between the lateral pallidal segment and the subthalamic nucleus probably involve interneurons.

Subthalamic nucleus neurons also project fibers to the pars reticulata of the substantia nigra (620, 1263, 1812, 2712). A flu-

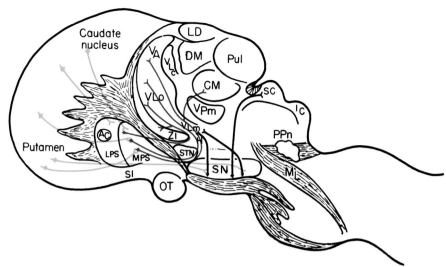

Figure 17-22. Schematic diagram of the major efferent systems of the corpus striatum. *Striopallidal* (*blue*) and *strionigral* (*blue*) fibers project to both segments of the globus pallidus and to the pars reticulata of the substantia nigra (*SN*). Striopallidal fibers have GABA as their neurotransmitter, while strionigral fibers are of two types (Fig. 17-21). *Pallidothalamic fibers* (*red*) arise from the medial pallidal segment and project to the ventral lateral (*VLo* and *VLm*), ventral anterior (VApc) and centromedian (*CM*) thalamic nuclei. The ventral lateral nucleus of the thalamus (*VLo*) projects upon the motor complex. *Nigrothalamic fibers* (*black*) arise from cells of the pars reticulata and project to the medial part of ventral lateral nucleus (VLm). Not shown on this diagram are nigral projections to the magnocellular part of the ventral anterior nucleus (VAmc) and to the dorsomedial nucleus (DMpl) (see Fig. 13-25). Nigrotectal projections (*black*) also arise from the pars reticulata of the substantia nigra. Pallidothalamic and nigrothalamic fibers collectively constitute the major efferent systems of the corpus striatum. Abbreviations are the same as in Fig. 17-21.

orescence retrograde double-labeling study in the rat suggests that single subthalamic nucleus neurons project fibers to both the globus pallidus and the substantia nigra (1344). Because the subthalamic nucleus projects to both the globus pallidus and the pars reticulata of the substantia nigra, it could modulate the activities of neurons which collectively constitute the output system of the entire corpus striatal complex.

In man, relatively discrete lesions in the subthalamic nucleus, usually hemorrhagic, give rise to violent, forceful and persistent choroid movements, referred to as *hemiballism*. These unusually violent involuntary movements occur contralateral to the lesion and involve primarily axial and proximal musculature of the upper and lower extremities, although they may involve the facial and cervical musculature as well (1200, 1618, 1622, 2253, 2710).

Zona Incerta. The zona incerta is a strip of gray matter situated between the thalamic and lenticular fasciculi (Figs. 15-7, 17-11, 17-13 and 17-15). It is a diffuse cell group which laterally is continuous with the thalamic reticular nucleus. This zone receives corticofugal fibers from the precentral cortex. Studies in the rat, based upon the retrograde transport of HRP, suggest that neurons of the zona incerta project to portions of the red nucleus, the superior colliculus and the pretectal area (2144).

The lenticular fasciculus, ansa lenticularis and thalamic fasciculus constitute the largest and best-defined fibers of passage in the subthalamic region. Scattered along and between the fibers of the ansa lenticularis are strands of cells which collectively constitute the so-called *nucleus of the ansa lenticularis* (2155).

Forel's Field H. Forel's field H (*prerubral field*) contains pallidofugal fibers and scattered cells which constitute the nucleus of the prerubral field (nucleus campi Foreli). The nuclei of the prerubral field (Figs. 15-7, 15-11 and 17-15), together with similar cells scattered along pallidofugal pathways, have been referred to collectively as the *subthalamic reticular nucleus.*

FUNCTIONAL CONSIDERATIONS

Over 70 years ago, Wilson (2735) introduced the term "extrapyramidal" motor system in his classic description of hepatolenticular degeneration, a familial disorder of copper metabolism characterized by degeneration of the striatum, cirrhosis of the liver, flapping tremor, muscular rigidity and a golden-brown pigmentation of the cornea (i.e., the Kayser-Fleischer ring). Although Wilson failed to define this term, it has been used widely with many interpretations. Literally the term extrapyramidal includes the entire central nervous system except for the corticospinal system. It is interesting that this phylogenetically older motor system has been defined with respect to the corticospinal system, even though the latter is present only in mammals. The convenience of the term extrapyramidal was that it grouped together, under a single designation, the corpus striatum and an unspecified array of brain stem considered to serve a somatic motor function. Common usage of this term has lead to the implication that the corpus striatum and a poorly defined group of brain stem nuclei constituted a complete and independent motor unit. More detailed anatomical, physiological and pharmacological data from studies based upon sophisticated and reliable research technics make it clear that the so-called extrapyramidal system is not an independent motor unit.

In reptiles and birds the neopallium is rudimentary, and descending fibers from the cortex are few in number. The corpus striatum, on the other hand, is an older part of the forebrain found in all vertebrates. The paleostriatum, comparable to the globus pallidus, is already well developed in fish. It receives mainly olfactory impulses and gives rise to the "basal forebrain bundle" which discharges into the thalamus, hypothalamus and midbrain (i.e., a lateral forebrain bundle). This bundle probably is homologous with the ansa lenticularis and lenticular fasciculus of mammals. In reptiles and birds the neostriatum receives impulses mainly from the thalamus. The stria-

tal complex in birds becomes highly differentiated and forms the most massive forebrain structure. In animals without a cortex, or with a poorly developed one, the corpus striatum is the most important forebrain center. Largely instinctive activities, such as locomotion, defense, feeding and courting, depend upon the integrity of the striatum. Motor activities in submammalian forms are highly stereotyped and resemble well-patterned reflex movements. These activities in avian forms are practically unaffected by ablations of the primitive cortex, but they are severely impaired by lesions of the corpus striatum (2200). Thus in submammalian forms the diencephalon and corpus striatum together constitute the highest sensorimotor integrating mechanism of the forebrain. The thalamus of such animals represents the receptive center; the corpus striatum and hypothalamus are related respectively to motor and visceral control.

With the evolution of the neopallium in mammals the functions of the corpus striatum become subordinated to those of the cerebral cortex. However, the old motor system continues to be utilized for the more or less automatic movements concerned with postural adjustments, defensive reactions and feeding. Many mammals are able to perform their normal activities after destruction of both pyramidal tracts. Even chimpanzees recover sufficiently to feed themselves and to execute movements of walking and climbing. Whether the human striatum has similar functions is disputed. Destruction of the corticospinal tract in man causes a far more complete and lasting paralysis, but the grosser movements are affected less severely and show remarkable recovery. According to Wilson (2738), the corpus striatum maintains a postural background for voluntary activities, reinforcing and steadying movements, but is incapable of initiating such movements.

The two distinctive components of the corpus striatum (i.e., the neostriatum and the paleostriatum) are structurally and functionally related mainly, but not exclusively, to two brain stem nuclei, the substantia nigra and the subthalamic nucleus. The neostriatum (i.e., the caudate nucleus and putamen) has massive projections to the globus pallidus and reciprocal connections with the distinctive cytological divisions of the substantia nigra (409, 413, 1813, 1825, 2489–2493). Fibers in each limb of the apparent feedback circuit between the neostriatum and the substantia nigra have distinctive neurotransmitters (1127, 1145, 1563, 1564, 2082, 2598). The paleostriatum (i.e., globus pallidus) consists of two cytologically identical segments, but each segment has different efferent projections. The lateral pallidal segment has a form of reciprocal connections with the subthalamic nucleus (395, 398, 401, 419, 1313, 1554). Pallidosubthalamic projections have a mediolateral laminar origin and are arranged in rostrocaudal sequence (398, 1554). However, these reciprocal connections do not appear to be on a point-for-point basis. The medial pallidal segment gives rise to major efferent systems projecting to thalamic nuclei and the midbrain tegmentum (i.e., the pedunculopontine nucleus). The striatum, representing the receptive component of the corpus striatum, receives a large number of afferent from the cerebral cortex, the thalamus and the midbrain (390). Striatal afferents arise from: (a) small pyramidal cells in the upper half of lamina V in extensive regions of the cerebral cortex and have glutamate as their neurotransmitter (779, 1231, 1245, 1312, 2393), (b) the intralaminar thalamic nuclei (1078, 1234, 1651, 1814), (c) cells of the pars compacta of the substantia nigra that convey dopamine (828, 2025, 2598) and (d) the dorsal raphe nucleus of the midbrain which has serotonin as its neurotransmitter (201, 1704, 1878, 2532). The medial pallidal segment, and the pallidofugal fiber systems arising from it, constitute the principal, but not the exclusive, output system of the corpus striatum. Pallidothalamic fibers project upon the ventral anterior (VApc), the ventral lateral (VLo and VLm) and the centromedian (CM) thalamic nuclei (1398). Impulses passing to the ventral lateral (VLo) nucleus are relayed to the motor cortex. Output from the striatum, via synaptic linkages in the pars reticulata of the substantia nigra, impinges upon different thalamic nuclei, the ventral anterior, pars magnocellularis (VAmc), the ventral lateral pars medialis (VLm) and the paralaminar part of the dorsomedial nucleus (390, 409, 413, 2492–2493). Thus the major output systems of the corpus striatum are: (a) pallidothalamic fibers and (b) synaptically linked strionigral and nigrothalamic

fibers. These output systems terminate upon distinctive thalamic nuclei which can modify the activity of cortical neurons. Overwhelming evidence suggests that the corpus striatum and anatomically related nuclei exert their influences upon motor function via impulses projected to the cerebral cortex by neurons in the rostral ventral tier thalamic nuclei. Impulses from the cerebral cortex concerned with motor function are conveyed to spinal levels via the corticospinal tract. Because most fibers of the corticospinal tract decussate at medullary levels, disturbances of motor function, due to pathological processes involving the corpus striatum and related nuclei, are manifest contralateral to the lesion.

Although no fibers from the corpus striatum, subthalamic nucleus or substantia nigra project directly to spinal levels, both the medial pallidal segment and the pars reticulata of the substantia nigra give rise to fibers that terminate in midbrain structures. A pallidotegmental bundle descends to caudal midbrain levels where fibers terminate upon cells of the pedunculopontine nucleus (395, 419, 1313, 1398, 1825). The pedunculopontine nucleus also receives projections from the pars reticulata of the substantia nigra (140, 398, 1066, 1729, 1730). It is of interest that the pedunculopontine nucleus receives subcortical inputs from structures that receive striatal efferents, namely the medial pallidal segment and the substantia nigra. The major efferent projections of the pedunculopontine nucleus are to the pars compacta of the substantia nigra (140, 398) and the medial pallidal segment (395). Cells of the pars reticulata of the substantia nigra also project profusely upon the deep and middle gray layers of the caudal two-thirds of the superior colliculus (736, 949, 952, 1212, 2162). Nigrotectal fibers appear topographically organized. It is of interest that the frontal eye field projects to both the superior colliculus and the paralaminar part of the dorsomedial nucleus (DMpl), both of which receive inputs from the pars reticulata (1395, 2299).

Clinically, two basic types of disturbances are associated with diseases of the corpus striatum. These disturbances are: (a) various types of abnormal involuntary movements, collectively referred to as *dyskinesia*, and (b) disturbances of muscle tone. Types of dyskinesia occurring in association with these diseases include *tremor, athetosis, chorea* and *ballism*.

Tremor. Tremor, the most common form of dyskinesia, is a rhythmical, alternating, abnormal involuntary activity having a relatively regular frequency and amplitude. A major clinical criterion used to describe and classify different tremors is whether the tremor occurs "at rest" or during voluntary movement. The type of tremor commonly seen in paralysis agitans (parkinsonism), involving primarily the digits, the head and the lips, occurs during the absence of voluntary movement. During the course of voluntary movements the tremor ceases. Tremor classically associated with cerebellar lesions becomes evident during voluntary and associated movements and ceases when the patient is "at rest." Although this criterion is of importance in clinical neurology, it is acknowledged that tremor "at rest" and tremor during voluntary movement sometimes occur together in various degrees in association with diseases involving primarily either the corpus striatum, or the cerebellum. Tremor also is seen in association with weakness (paresis), emotional excitement and as a side effect of a variety of drugs. In general, tremor is exaggerated when the patient is anxious, self-conscious or exposed to cold. Tremor disappears during sleep and under general anesthesia.

Athetosis. Athetosis (1016) is the term used to designate slow, writhing, vermicular involuntary movements involving particularly the extremities. It may also involve axial muscle groups and the muscles of the face and neck. The movements blend with each other to give the appearance of a continuous mobile spasm. Athetoid movements involving primarily the axial musculature produce severe torsion of the neck, shoulder girdle and pelvic girdle. This form of the disturbance, referred to as *torsion spasm* or *torsion dystonia*, is considered as a variant (36, 1201) of athetosis; differences between torsion dystonia and athetosis are considered to be due largely to inherent mechanical differences between axial and appendicular musculature.

Chorea. Chorea is a brisk, graceful series of successive involuntary movements of considerable complexity which resemble fragments of purposeful voluntary movements. These movements involve primarily the distal portions of the extremities, the muscles of facial expression, the tongue and the deglutitional musculature. Most forms of choreoid activity are associated with hypotonus. Sydenham's chorea occurs in childhood in association with rheumatic heart disease, and most patients recover from the chorea in a relatively short time. Huntington's chorea is a hereditary disorder characterized by choreiform movements and progressive dementia. Although sporadic cases occur, the disorder is inherited as a Mendelian dominant.

Ballism. Ballism, a violent, forceful flinging movement, involves primarily the proximal appendicular musculature and muscles about the shoulder and pelvic girdles. It represents the most violent form of dyskinesia known. Ballism is almost invariably associated with discrete lesions in the subthalamic nucleus or its connections. The dyskinesia occurs contralateral to the lesion and is associated with marked hypotonus.

Although athetosis, chorea and ballism each present distinguishing features, basic resemblances among these forms of dyskinesia are greater than their differences (380, 449, 1690, 2737). Characteristics common to these dyskinesias include: (a) variable amplitude and frequency, (b) occurrence of movements in immediate and delayed sequence, (c) variations in the duration of single movements and (d) a highly integrated, complex activity pattern. While each of these types of involuntary motor activity is specialized to a degree, there are indications that athetosis, chorea and ballism may form a spectrum of choreoid activity in which athetosis and ballism represent extreme forms possessing distinguishing characteristics.

Although it is customary to associate increased muscle tonus with most syndromes of the corpus striatum, this is not always found. The initial symptom of paralysis agitans is frequently a rigidity of the muscles, which gradually increases over a period of years. The augmentation of muscle tone is not selective, as in hemiplegia, but is present to a nearly equal degree in antagonistic muscle groups (i.e., in both flexor and extensor muscles). The rigidity in the early stages can be demonstrated by passively flexing or extending the muscles of the extremities, or by attempting to rotate the hand in a circular fashion at the wrist.

These movements are interrupted by a series of jerks, referred to as *cogwheel phenomenon*. In later stages of the disease, rigidity may be so severe as to completely incapacitate the patient. Athetosis usually is associated with variable degrees of paresis and spasticity. It is suggested that the slow, writhing character of this dyskinesia may be due in part to the spasticity. Although muscle tone is increased greatly during athetoid movements and persists after the completion of the movement, muscle tone may thereafter gradually diminish (1087). Chorea and ballism usually are associated with variable degrees of hypotonus (1618).

Neural Mechanisms Involved in Dyskinesia

The various types of dyskinesia and excesses of muscle tone associated with diseases of the basal ganglia are regarded as positive disturbances, since they involve an excess of neural activity and the expenditure of energy (1619). Such disturbances cannot arise directly from destruction of specific neural structures but must represent the functional capacity of surviving intact structures. According to this thesis, which is supported by experimental and clinical data, positive disturbances (i.e., tremor, athetosis, chorea and ballism) are believed to be the result of *release phenomena*. A lesion in one structure removes the controlling and regulating influences which that structure previously exerted upon an associated neural mechanism, and thus leads to overactivity of the second intact neural structure. This theory forms the basis for neurosurgical attempts to alleviate and abolish dyskinesia and excesses of muscle tone without producing paresis.

However, not all of the disturbances associated with diseases of the basal ganglia can be regarded as positive phenomena, particularly in paralysis agitans. Patients with paralysis agitans also exhibit a mask-like face, infrequent blinking of the eyes, a slow dysarthric speech, a stooped posture, a slow shuffling gait, loss of associated movements (e.g., swing of the arms while walking), slowness of movement (bradykinesia) and general poverty of movement. Some patients may have excessive secretion of saliva, unusual oiliness of the skin, difficulty in holding the head erect and disturbances of equilibrium. The negative symptoms of parkinsonism largely concern disorders of postural fixation, equilibrium, locomotion, phonation and articulation (1618, 1623, 1624). Negative symptoms are considered to be deficits due to loss of function of destroyed neural structures.

Clinicopathological studies of most forms of dyskinesia categorized as extrapyramidal indicate widespread neuropathological changes. In these disorders the corpora striata suffer severe pathological alterations, but specific brain stem nuclei and parts of the cerebral cortex also may be affected. In paralysis agitans, pathological changes most consistently affect the substantia nigra, but significant alterations may be found also in the globus pallidus, the cerebral cortex and the brain stem reticular formation (150, 625, 1064). In the parkinsonian syndrome there is a virtual absence of dopamine in the neostriatum and substantia nigra (1145, 2011). In this syndrome there is a decreased ability of the affected brain tissues to form dopamine. Dopamine, formed in the large cells of the pars compacta of the nigra, is conveyed to the neostriatum via nigrostriatal fibers and stored in terminals. The manner in which dopamine is liberated in the striatum is unknown. Neurophysiological evidence indicates that dopamine has an inhibitory effect upon single neurons (1145), which suggests that in parkinsonism there may be an impairment of neostriatal inhibition, which normally acts upon pallidal neurons. In this sense the dyskinesia and increased muscle tone seen in parkinsonism may be regarded as release phenomenon (i.e., a removal of inhibitory influences). The above rationale forms the basis for giving L-Dopa in the treatment of parkinsonism. This compound passes the blood-brain barrier and is a precursor of dopamine (Fig. 1-17). L-Dopa can be given in smaller dosages when used with a peripheral decarboxylase inhibitor which prevents systemic decarboxylation of L-dopa to dopamine (1608).

Athetosis most frequently is associated with pathological processes involving the striatum and cerebral cortex, although lesions are sometimes found in the globus pallidus and thalamus (376). Hemiathetosis may develop after a hemiparesis, or in association with it, as a consequence of a necrotizing cerebrovascular lesion destroying portions of the internal capsule and striatum. Athetoid activity occurs contralateral to the lesion.

With respect to chorea, there is relatively little information available, except that concerning chronic progressive chorea, or Huntington's chorea. This hereditary disease is characterized by an insidious onset in adult life. Pathological changes are widespread but have a special predilection for the cerebral cortex and striatum. A study of postmortem brain tissue in a large series of patients dying with Huntington's chorea (181) demonstrated that striatal neurons have reduced concentrations of glutamic acid decarboxylase (GAD), γ-aminobutyric acid (GABA) and choline acetyltransferase (ChAc), the enzyme which synthesizes acetylcholine. Glutamic acid decarboxylase (GAD) is the enzyme responsible for the biosynthesis of GABA and is localized mainly in inhibitory neurons which release GABA as their transmitter (1193). In these same patients, concentrations of tyrosine hydroxylase (T-H) and dopamine were normal in the corpus striatum. The most consistent lesion in Huntington's chorea appears to be a loss of GABA-containing neurons in the corpus striatum, along with a loss of some cholinergic neurons. It is well known that L-dopa given in large doses to patients with Parkinson's disease may cause choreiform movements to appear. L-Dopa also tends to exacerbate choreiform activity in patients with Huntington's chorea. The most effective drugs for ameliorating choreiform dyskinesia are those which deplete catecholamines, such as reserpine, and dopamine receptor antagonists. It thus seems that the presence of normal dopaminergic systems in association with reduced availability of GABA (and often acetylcholine) may be the key neuropharmacological feature of Huntington's chorea (181). Clinical attempts to overcome the presumed GABA and acetylcholine deficiencies by administering GABA-mimetic drugs or inhibitors of acetylcholine hydrolysis have so far met with only limited success (2330, 2331). In order for such approaches to be successful, GABA and acetylcholine receptors must be unaltered by the disease. Synaptic receptor binding and enzyme assays based upon frozen tissue from postmortem brains of patients with Huntington's chorea indicated that: (a) GAD activity was reduced 68% in the pu-

tamen, 62% in the globus pallidus and 66% in the substantia nigra, (b) the density of GABA receptor binding sites was normal in the putamen and globus pallidus and almost doubled with the substantia nigra, and (c) the density of muscarinic cholinergic and serotonin receptor binding sites was greatly reduced (712). The increased density of GABA receptor binding sites in the substantia nigra may reflect a reduction (shrinkage) in the total volume of this nucleus or a "denervation suprasensitivity" accompanying degeneration of GABA terminals of strionigral fibers. These findings support the suggestion that dopaminergic cells in the substantia nigra and their dendrites have a high density of GABA receptors. Reported failures of GABA, or the GABA agonist imidazoleacetic acid, to benefit patients with this form of chorea may be explained by inability of these agents to cross the blood-brain barrier in sufficient concentrations.

The biochemical changes which characterize Huntington's (chorea) disease in humans can be mimicked in the rat by striatal injections of kainic acid, an analogue of glutamate (1629, 2292). After injections of 2 µg of kainic acid, the activities of glutamic acid decarboxylase (GAD) and choline acetyltransferase were reduced 80%, whereas the activity of tryosine hydroxylase was increased 80%. In contrast, the striatal content of dopamine and the synaptosomal uptake of dopamine were unchanged. The neurotoxic effects of kainic acid appear related to the excessive stimulation of glutamate receptors that results in degeneration which occurs first in the cell somata and proceeds to the dendrites, small axons and terminal boutons (1052, 2292). Myelinated and unmyelinated axons terminated in, and passing through the region of, the injection site show no signs of degeneration. Studies of the long-term effects of striatal kainic acid lesions indicate marked striatal atrophy, unilateral ventricular dilatation and reductions in the activities of GABA-ergic and cholinergic neurons which are not as severe as those reported in Huntington's disease (2789).

Ballism appears to be the only form of dyskinesia resulting from a discrete lesion. The lesion, usually hemorrhagic, is confined to the subthalamic nucleus or its immediate connections (2710).

Attempts to produce dyskinesia in experimental animals by creating lesions in the corpus striatum have been notoriously unsuccessful (1488, 1681a, 2736). Experimental attempts to provoke dyskinesia in animals by striatal or pallidal lesions have been criticized on the basis of Meltzer's (1664) principle of physiological safety. This principle states that in biological organisms, more tissue is found in individual organs and structures than is required for the maintenance of their essential functions. If this principle is applied to the neuraxis, it would seem to mean that a lesion cannot be expected to produce the symptoms and signs characteristic of a specific tissue deficit unless the amount of destruction includes some of the irreducible minimum necessary for normal function. Failure to produce athetoid or choreoid activity in animals by striatal lesions has been said to be due to the rather limited volumes of tissue destroyed. This explanation does not appear valid in all cases. Wilson (2736) succeeded in destroying selectively virtually the entire putamen in the monkey without producing dyskinesia. The experiments of Mettler (1681a) indicate that large bilateral striatal lesions produce forced progression and cursive hyperkinesia but no dyskinesia. This form of hyperactivity implies that the striatum normally may inhibit other neural mechanisms subserving motor function.

Unilateral lesions of the globus pallidus in monkeys produce minimal disturbances of motor function. Bilateral lesions of the globus pallidus, inflicted simultaneously, produce profound hypokinesis, loss of associated movements and disturbances of posture. Bizarre and enforced postures are maintained for long periods of time, with only feeble or ineffective attempts to establish a normal attitude. These animals bear certain striking resemblances to patients with paralysis agitans, but there is no tremor or rigidity. Evidence suggests that the globus pallidus makes a positive contribution to motor function, and may in some way be involved in all forms of dyskinesia because: (a) it is the source of the principal output of the corpus striatum, and (b) it is the only part of the corpus striatum that projects to thalamic nuclei which in turn project to the motor cortex (1398). The validity of this thesis is demonstrated by the gratifying amelioration of various forms of dyskinesia, in selected patients, following stereotaxic lesions produced in either the globus pallidus or the ventral lateral (VLo) nucleus of the thalamus (519, 522, 1801, 2403, 2404, 2781). Destruction of portions of the globus pallidus (i.e., medial pallidal segment) appears most effective in relieving contralateral rigidity in paralysis agitans, while thalamic lesions (ventral lateral nucleus) are often most successful in alleviating contralateral tremor. Similar clinical evidence indicates that lesions in these locations can ameliorate dystonia (520, 521, 524), chorea (2402) and ballism (67, 520, 1625, 2197, 2510).

The only form of dyskinesia, other than cerebellar tremor, produced in experimental animals which resembles that occurring in man is that resulting from discrete lesions in the subthalamic nucleus. In the monkey, violent choreoid and ballistic activity occurs contralateral to localized lesions in the subthalamic nucleus, which: (a) destroy approximately 20% of the nucleus, and (b) preserve the integrity of surrounding pallidofugal fiber systems (421, 2712). Injections of kainic acid in the subthalamic nucleus made with a micropipette produce similar dyskinesia which appears several days after surgery (1015). This experimental form of abnormal involuntary activity has been referred to as *subthalamic dyskinesia*.

Both clinical and experimental studies suggest somatotopic relationships between the portions of the subthalamic nucleus destroyed and the portions of the body exhibiting dyskinesia (399, 2253, 2254). In the monkey, subthalamic dyskinesia involves the contralateral lower extremity most frequently and most severely, and involvement of the facial, glossal, deglutitional and cervical musculature was never observed. Dyskinesia in the lower extremity was associated with destruction of the rostral part of the subthalamic nucleus, while dyskinesia, predominantly in the upper extremity, was related to lesions in caudal parts of the nucleus. Somatotopic terminations of cortical projections from area 4, based upon autoradiography, indicate that corticofugal fibers end mainly in the lateral half of the subthalamic nucleus, with the face represented laterally and the lower extremity medially (1041).

Studies of subthalamic dyskinesia in the monkey indicate that it can be abolished contralaterally without producing paresis by lesions destroying: (a) portions of the medial segment of the globus pallidus, (b) the lenticular fasciculus or (c) the ventral lateral nucleus of the thalamus (421). This form of dyskinesia can be abolished, but with concomitant paresis, by ablations of the contralateral motor cortex (area 4), or by surgical section of the ipsilateral corticospinal tract at high cervical spinal levels (383, 401, 408). No significant modification of this form of dyskinesia in the monkey results from: (a) ablation of area 6, (b) destruction of the centromedian nucleus or (c) large lesions in the red nucleus or the substantia nigra (396, 408, 2454). Selective partial cordotomies in animals with this form of dyskinesia indicate that surgical interruption of the rubrospinal, vestibulospinal and reticulospinal tracts has little or no effect upon ipsilateral dyskinesia (401). Multiple dorsal root sections (i.e., dorsal rhizotomy), virtually abolishing afferent input from an entire extremity, cause an increase in amplitude of the dyskinesia (2428). This increase in amplitude appears to be due to loss of kinesthetic sense and loss of muscle tone.

These experimental results have been interpreted to mean that the subthalamic nucleus normally exerts inhibitory and regulating influences upon the globus pallidus. A lesion in the subthalamic nucleus releases the globus pallidus from this controlling influence; removal of this controlling influence is expressed physiologically by bursts of irregular, forceful, large amplitude ballistic movements on the opposite side of the body. Impulses from the globus pallidus reach the ipsilateral motor cortex via the ventral lateral (VLo) nucleus of the thalamus. Dyskinesia occurs contralaterally because impulses responsible for this dyskinesia are conveyed to segmental levels of the spinal cord via the corticospinal tract (401), and most fibers of this system decussate at medullary levels. These experimental results, relative to the effects of pallidal and thalamic lesions, have been confirmed upon human ballism (1625, 2197, 2510).

Attempts to abolish various forms of dyskinesia and excesses of muscle tone by surgery are based on the thesis that these disturbances are the physiological expression of release phenomena. This implies that disease or pathological alterations of certain neural structures has removed inhibitory influences normally acting upon other intact neural structures, and that this overactivity, or excessive function of intact structures, is responsible for the dyskinesia.

Physiological studies done under barbiturate anesthesia in cats reveal two cell types in the subthalamic nucleus: (a) regularly spontaneously active cells, designated as type "A," and (b) quiescent cells, designated as type "B" (2586). Type "A" cells are inhibited by pallidal stimulation, but type "B" cells respond to the same stimulus with long-latency, high-frequency bursts of spikes. Under local anesthesia, type "B" cells are spontaneously active, while type "A" cells fire irregularly, preceding inhibition evoked by pallidal stimulation. These data suggest that both excitatory and inhibitory impulses from the globus pallidus project upon the subthalamic nucleus; barbiturates appear to preferentially block the excitatory pathway. Electron microscopic evidence indicates that terminal boutons of most pallidosubthalamic fibers end upon dendrites of subthalamic nucleus neurons (1794).

Stimulation of the subthalamic nucleus in the cat suppresses the firing of cells in the entopeduncular nucleus (i.e., the feline equivalent of the medial pallidal segment) in both barbiturate-anesthetized and cerveau isolé cats (1439). Although this neural mechanism appears similar to that hypothesized for the primate, the projection of the entopeduncular nucleus upon the rostral ventral tier thalamic nuclei is smaller in the cat and appears to lack the topographic features seen in the monkey (1438). Physiological studies are in agreement with anatomical data that most subthalamic nucleus neurons send branched axons to both the globus pallidus and the pars reticulata of the substantia nigra (620). Subthalamonigral projections are monosynaptic and considered to be excitatory (1014). There is thus clear evidence that the cells of the subthalamic nucleus can influence neurons of both the globus pallidus and pars reticulata which collectively give rise to the efferent systems of the corpus striatum. Histochemical data indicate lesions of the lateral pallidal segment produce significant reductions in glutamic acid decarboxylase

(GAD), the enzyme that synthesizes GABA (777). The reduction in GAD within the subthalamic nucleus appears regional and related to the size and position of the pallidal lesion. The reduction in GAD appears greatest in lateral parts of the subthalamic nucleus which receive the major pallidal input (395, 398).

Although subthalamic dyskinesia in the monkey represents a unique form of dyskinesia, it may share underlying common features with other forms of dyskinesia. Thus in these strikingly different forms of dyskinesia the basic mechanism may be the same, namely the removal of inhibitory influences which normally act upon the medial segment of the globus pallidus.

The fact that the medial and lateral segments of the globus pallidus have unique connections suggests that they may have distinctive functions. The medial pallidal segment may be involved in all forms of dyskinesia due to pathological involvement of the corpus striatum, since it gives rise to the major efferent system which connects with thalamic relay nuclei. For this reason, lesions in the medial pallidal segment ameliorate most forms of the basal ganglia dyskinesia. Evidence from pathological studies suggests that extensive bilateral destruction of the lateral pallidal segment may provoke choreoid dyskinesia (418a). It has been postulated that the dyskinesia associated with such lesions is due to the interruption of pallidal efferent fibers, most of which project to the subthalamic nucleus (1934).

There is abundant evidence that the cerebral cortex must play an important role in neural mechanisms of dyskinesia. It is well known that almost all forms of abnormal involuntary movement cease during sleep and are abolished by general anesthesia. Most forms of dyskinesia are exaggerated in situations where the patient becomes self-conscious, overly anxious or excited. The fact that ablations of motor cortex and interruption of the corticospinal tract at various locations abolish dyskinesia suggests that impulses from centers considered to be responsible for dyskinesia must be transmitted to segmental levels via the corticospinal tract (311, 312, 401). These observations imply that the so-called extrapyramidal system is not a complete and independent motor entity.

CHAPTER 18

Olfactory Pathways, Hippocampal Formation and Amygdala

RHINENCEPHALON

The term *rhinencephalon* refers to the olfactory brain. Although some authors use this term broadly to include those regions of the brain concerned with both the reception and integration of olfactory information, not all regions of the brain in which responses can be recorded upon olfactory stimulation are concerned exclusively with olfactory sense. Higher order pathways of the olfactory system are complex and subject to modifying influences from many sources. Some of these regions have lost their original olfactory specificity. For this reason use of the term "rhinencephalon" should be restricted to those structures of the central nervous system that receive fibers from the olfactory bulb (267). In this strict sense the rhinencephalon includes the olfactory bulb, tract, tubercle and striae, the anterior olfactory nucleus, parts of the amygdaloid complex and parts of the prepyriform cortex. The term rhinencephalon, in this restricted sense, is equivalent to the *paleopallium* or primitive olfactory lobe (2604). Although the rhinencephalon is large and conspicuous in the lower vertebrates, including many macrosmatic mammals, in

man it is overshadowed and comparatively reduced by the tremendous development of the *neopallium*. The *archipallium*, the oldest cortical derivative, is represented by the hippocampal formation, the dentate gyrus, the fasciolar gyrus and the indusium griseum (supracallosal gyrus). The hippocampal formation reaches its greatest development in microsmatic man and is well formed in certain anosmatic aquatic mammals (e.g., porpoise, whale).

OLFACTORY PATHWAYS

Olfactory Receptors. The olfactory membrane is a yellowish brown patch of specialized epithelium in the upper posterior part of the nasal cavity. Olfactory receptors are located in this membrane (Fig. 18-1). Slender sensory cells scattered among supporting cells in the olfactory epithelium have two processes, a coarse peripheral one, passing to the surface, and a fine central one, projecting through the basement membrane. From the coarse peripheral processes a variable number of fine olfactory hairs arise. The delicate central processes, which constitute the unmyelinated *olfactoria fila*, converge to form small fascicles and pass from the nasal cavity via foramina in the cribriform plate of the eth-

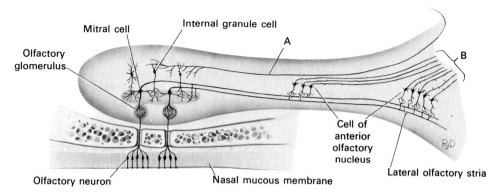

Figure 18-1. Diagram of the olfactory bulb and tract showing relationships of the olfactory receptors and neurons in the nasal mucosa with cells in the olfactory bulb. Cells of the anterior olfactory nucleus form scattered groups caudal to the olfactory bulb. Centrally projecting fibers from the anterior olfactory nucleus are labeled *B*, while a fiber from the contralateral anterior olfactory nucleus is labeled *A* (after Cajal (348)).

moid bone. These exceedingly small fibers, have a very slow conduction rate and enter the ventral surface of the olfactory bulb (Figs. 18-1 and 18-2). The olfactory fila, representing the central processes of bipolar cells in the olfactory epithelium, collectively constitute the olfactory nerve (N. I).

Morphologically the olfactory epithelium represents a primitive type of sensory cell and supports the thesis that olfaction is phylogenetically the oldest and most primitive of all senses (270). The extent of the olfactory area in the nasal cavity varies greatly in different animals. Although there is some degree of histological differentiation of olfactory receptor cells, attempts to distinguish morphologically distinct types have been unsuccessful (468, 1533).

The olfactory receptor is a bipolar neuron with a lifespan of 30–40 days, depending upon the species. New axons are continually growing into the olfactory bulb and forming new synapses. When the olfactory fibers are surgically cut as they enter the olfactory bulb (1728), olfactory receptor axons can regenerate and form new synapses in the glomeruli of the olfactory bulb. The normal cyclic loss and formation of olfactory receptor axons and their synapses upon mitral cells, and the demonstration of post-traumatic regeneration in primates, offers hope that a means can be devised to minimize scar tissue formation and permanent deafferentation of the bulb in humans with anosmia due to fractures of the cribriform plate.

In addition to receptors in the olfactory

epithelium, chemosensory cells are found in most mammalian species in the vomeronasal organ, a bilateral, elongated and flattened tubular structure in the nasal septum. The central processes of vomeronasal sensory cells project to the accessory olfactory bulb, forming a separate path to higher olfactory structures. In man, there is no accessory olfactory bulb, and the evidence for the presence of the vomeronasal organ is equivocal (2782). The vomeronasal system is mentioned because of its sensitivity to olfactory stimuli produced by substances with low volatility which evoke or facilitate reproductive behavior in rodents (2065, 2782).

Olfactory Bulb. This flattened ovoid body resting on the cribriform plate of the ethmoid bone is the terminal "nucleus" of the olfactory nerve (Figs. 18-1 and 18-2). The paired olfactory bulbs are parts of the central nervous system evaginated from the telencephalon. Most of the fibers of the olfactory nerve enter the anterior tip of the olfactory bulb. Structurally the olfactory bulb has a laminar organization, but in man this is difficult to demonstrate. Within the gray matter of the olfactory bulb are several types of nerve cells, the most striking of which are the large, triangular *mitral cells,* so named because of their resemblance to a bishop's mitre (Figs. 18-1, 18-3 and 18-4). Primary olfactory fibers synapse with the brushlike terminals of vertically descending dendrites of the mitral cells to form the *olfactory glomeruli* (2074) (Fig. 18-3). Smaller cells of the olfactory bulb, known

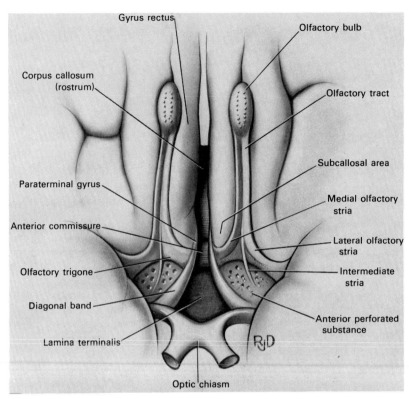

Figure 18-2. Diagram of olfactory structures on the inferior surface of the brain. The optic nerves and chiasm have been retracted caudally to expose the olfactory area.

as *tufted cells,* have a number of dendrites, one of which participates in the formation of the glomerulus. The number of glomeruli and mitral cells is rather modest with respect to the large number of receptor cells, suggesting an extensive convergence of impulses (46). *Granule cells* of various sizes are found throughout the olfactory bulb but are most dense toward the center of the bulb, forming the granular cell layer (Fig. 18-3) (2073). Granule cells have no axons, and their dendrites have dendritic spines, or gemmules, which form dendrodendritic synapses with mitral cells. The morphological features of these junctions suggest dual synapses; one from granule cell to mitral cell, and one from mitral cell to granule cell (Fig. 18-3). This arrangement is called a reciprocal synapse (see p. 118). Granule cells inhibit mitral cells, and the mitral cells appear to excite the granule cells (872). Iontophoresis, autoradiography and immunohistochemistry experiments indicate that γ-aminobutyric acid (GABA) may be the inhibitory transmitter released by gran-

ule cells (1007, 1570, 2143). Although the arrangement of afferent fibers in the olfactory bulb does not appear to be localized in any patterned way (478), a regional organization of olfactory nerve projections to the olfactory bulb has been demonstrated in mammals (18, 467, 469). Localized lesions in different regions of the olfactory epithelium produce degeneration in specific regions of the glomerular layer (1420). Groupings of glomeruli show marked variations in the intensity of degeneration and some normal glomeruli are present in regions containing degeneration. It has been suggested that a selective projection from receptors in small regions of the olfactory epithelium to specific glomeruli, or groups of glomeruli, could provide the anatomical basis for selective responses to odors. Axons of mitral and tufted cells enter the olfactory tract as *secondary olfactory fibers* (Figs. 18-1 and 18-3).

Caudal to the olfactory bulb are scattered groups of neurons, intermediate in size between mitral and granule cells, that form

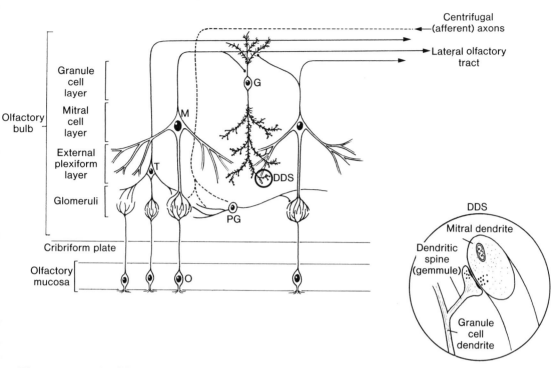

Figure 18-3. A simplified schematic diagram of the major classes of cells in the olfactory bulb. The sensory receptors (*O*) in the olfactory mucosa are illustrated at the bottom of the figure. The central process of the receptor enters the olfactory bulb and synapses upon a dendritic tuft of a mitral cell to form a complex called a glomerulus. Axons of mitral cells (*M*) pass centrally to form the lateral olfactory tract. Mitral axons also have recurrent collaterals which synapse upon granule cells. The granule cells (*G*) have no axons. Their external dendrites have dendritic spines which form reciprocal dendrodendritic synapses (*DDS* and insert) on mitral dendrites. Periglomerular cells (*PG*) represent several morphological types of cells linking mitral cell glomeruli. Tufted cells (*T*) are morphologically similar to mitral cells, but their cell bodies are dispersed throughout the external plexiform layer.

the *anterior olfactory nucleus* (Figs. 18-1 and 18-4). Some cells of this loosely organized nucleus are found along the olfactory tracts near the base of the hemisphere. Dendrites of these cells pass among the fibers of the olfactory tract, from which they receive impulses. Axons of the cells of the anterior olfactory nucleus pass centrally, cross in the anterior part of the anterior commissure and enter the contralateral anterior olfactory nucleus and olfactory bulb (Fig. 18-4) (1521, 2060, 2604).

The olfactory bulb receives a monaminergic innervation, with serotonin (5-hydroxytryptamine, 5-HT) terminals synapsing upon periglomerular cell dendrites in glomeruli and norepinephrine varicosities distributed throughout the granular and external plexiform layers (1006). At least 10% of the periglomerular cells, and some tufted cells, show tyrosine hydroxylase immuno-

reactivity. Several lines of evidence indicate that these cells synthesize dopamine as their transmitter.

The dipeptide carnosine (β-alanyl-L-histidine) normally occurs in relatively high concentration in the olfactory bulb and mucosa. Deafferentation of the bulb results in a marked reduction of carnosine content (1602). While binding kinetics suggest a ligand-receptor type of interaction (1106), there is no unequivocal electrophysiological evidence that carnosine is a neurotransmitter or modulator in the olfactory bulb.

Olfactory Tract. This tract passes toward the anterior perforated substance and divides into well defined *lateral* and *medial olfactory striae*. A thin covering of gray substance over the olfactory striae composes the *lateral* and *medial olfactory gyri* (Figs. 18-2 and 18-4). The lateral olfactory stria and gyrus pass along the lateral mar-

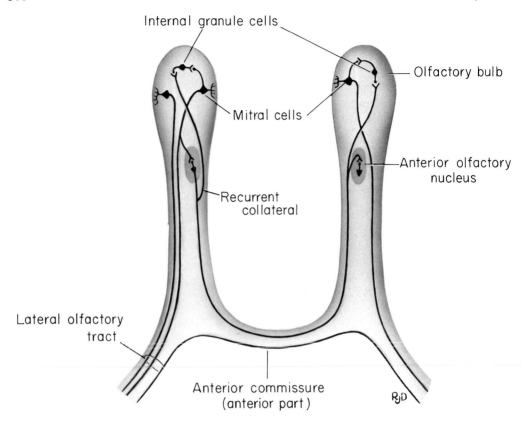

Figure 18-4. Schematic diagram of interconnections of the olfactory bulbs and anterior olfactory nuclei. Collaterals of mitral cell axons synapse upon apical dendrites of pyamidal-shaped cells of the anterior olfactory nuleus. These cells give rise to fibers that cross in the anterior part of the anterior commissure (Fig. 18-9) and synapse upon cells in the contralateral anterior olfactory nucleus and internal granule cells in the olfactory bulb. Recurrent collaterals of axons of the anterior olfactory nuclei project back to the ipsilateral olfactory bulb to terminate upon internal granule cells, which can in turn activate mitral cells. The principal axons of mitral cells enter the lateral olfactory tract. (Based on Valverde (2604).)

gin of the anterior perforated substance to reach the prepyriform region (Figs. 18-5 and 18-6). Fibers of the lateral olfactory stria arising in the olfactory bulb give collaterals to the anterior olfactory nucleus and the anterior perforated substance (which corresponds to the olfactory tubercle in macrosmatic animals). These fibers terminate in the prepyriform cortex and in the corticomedial part of the amygdaloid nuclear complex (44, 474, 2060). Terminations of these fibers are axodendritic in relation to pyramidal cells of the plexiform layer of the prepyriform cortex and axosomatic in the corticomedial part of the amygdaloid nuclear complex (44, 2060). Terminations also are present in the nucleus of

the lateral olfactory tract and in parts of the anterior amygdaloid nucleus. The prepyriform cortex and the periamygdaloid area, which receive fibers from the lateral olfactory stria, constitute the *primary olfactory cortex.* Olfaction appears unique among the sensory systems in that impulses in this system reach the cortex without being relayed by thalamic nuclei.

Olfactory Lobe. This lobe makes its appearance in the 2nd month as a narrow longitudinal bulge on the basal surface of the developing cerebral hemisphere, ventral and medial to the basal ganglia (Fig. 3-11 *A*). It is demarcated from the lateral surface of the pallium by the *rhinal sulcus* (Fig. 2-9), and soon differentiates into an-

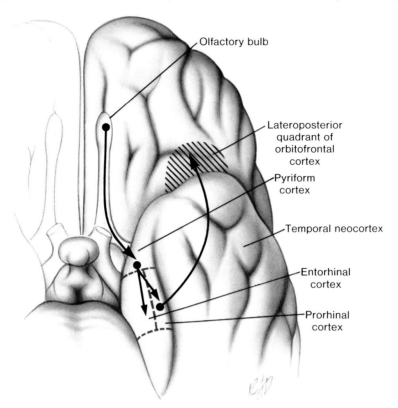

Figure 18-5. Diagram of the inferior surface of the frontal and temporal lobes of a primate brain showing olfacto-frontal connections. The lateroposterior quadrant of the orbitofrontal cortex receives olfactory information which is relayed from the lateral entorhinal area (prorhinal cortex). The lateral entorhinal area receives olfactory information indirectly from the pyriform cortex. (Based upon the studies of Potter and Nauta (2049).)

terior and posterior portions. The anterior portion, at first containing an extension of the lateral ventricle, elongates into a tubular stalk which becomes solid by the end of the 3rd month, and forms the rudiment of the olfactory tract and bulb. The posterior portion differentiates into the olfactory area (anterior perforated substance) and certain other olfactory structures closely related to the anteromedial portion of the temporal lobe, collectively known as the *pyriform lobe*.

At the point of division of the olfactory tract into lateral and medial olfactory striae, there is a rhomboid-shaped region, bounded by the olfactory trigone and the optic tract, known as the *anterior perforated substance* (Figs. 2-9, 18-2 and 18-8). This region is studded with numerous perforations made by entering blood vessels (Fig. 20-10). The posterior border of this region, near the optic tract, has a smooth

appearance and forms an oblique band, the *diagonal band of Broca* (Fig. 18-2). In macrosmatic animals, especially those with well developed snouts or muzzles, the rostral portion of the area is marked by a prominent elevation, the *olfactory tubercle* (Fig. 18-6). Only rudiments of this structure are present in man. The region of the olfactory tubercle receives fibers from the olfactory bulb (996, 2303), the anterior olfactory nucleus, the amygdaloid nuclear complex and temporal neocortex (1112). It projects fibers into the stria medullaris and the medial forebrain bundle.

The medial olfactory stria extends toward the medial hemispheric surface and becomes continuous with a small cortical field known as the *subcallosal area* (parolfactory area), located beneath the rostrum of the corpus callosum (Figs. 18-2 and 18-6). This area is limited in front by the anterior parolfactory sulcus, while behind

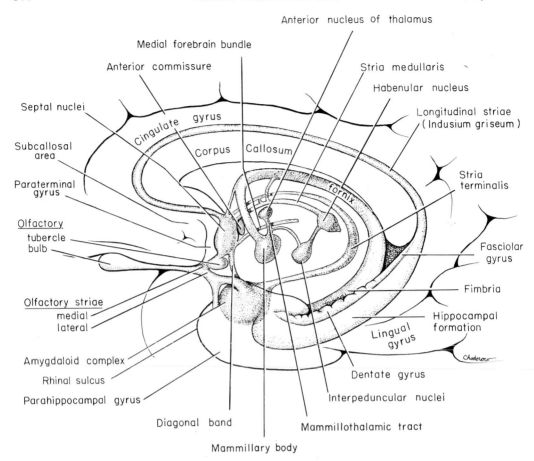

Figure 18-6. Semischematic drawing of rhinencephalic structural relationships as seen in medial view of the right hemisphere. Both deep and superficial structures are indicated. (Modified from a drawing by Krieg (1365).)

it is separated by the posterior parolfactory sulcus from another strip of cortex, the *paraterminal gyrus* (subcallosal gyrus), which is closely applied to the rostral lamina of the corpus callosum (Fig. 18-6).

The subcallosal area and the paraterminal gyrus together constitute the *septal area* (paraterminal body). The term septal area refers to the cortical part of this region. The subcortical part of the septal region consists of the *medial* and *lateral septal nuclei*, which are found rostral to the anterior commissure (Fig. 18-6). The medial septal nucleus becomes continuous with the nucleus and tract of the diagonal band (Fig. 18-2) and thus establishes connections with the amygdaloid nuclear complex (Fig. 18-6). The lateral septal nucleus appears continuous over the anterior commissure with scattered neurons of the septum pellucidum. The septal nuclei receive a large number of afferent fibers from the hippocampal formation via the fornix (1815, 1816, 2090) and some fibers from the amygdaloid complex. The medial septal nucleus also receives fibers from the medial midbrain reticular formation; these fibers ascend in the mammillary peduncle (Fig. 18-7) and continue rostrally in the medial forebrain bundle (979, 980, 1824). It is uncertain whether the septal nuclei receive olfactory impulses. Evidence suggests that fibers from the olfactory tubercle passing to the septal region are largely nonolfactory. Efferent fibers from the septal nuclei enter the medial part of the stria medullaris and pass to the habenular nucleus (Figs. 18-6 and 18-7). In addition, axons from these nuclei enter the medial forebrain bundle to be distributed caudally to the entire lateral extent of the hypothalamic region (Fig. 16-10); some fibers of this group extend into the midbrain

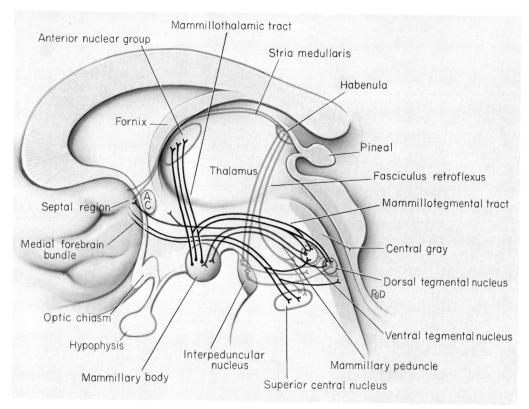

Figure 18-7. Semischematic diagram of limbic pathways inter-relating the telencephalon and diencephalon with medial midbrain structures. The medial forebrain bundle and efferent fibers of the mammillary body are shown in *black*. The *medial forebrain bundle* originates from the septal and lateral preoptic regions, traverses the lateral hypothalamic area and projects into the midbrain tegmentum. The mammillary princeps fasciculus divides into two bundles, the *mammillothalamic tract* and the *mammillotegmental tract*. Ascending fibers of the *mammillary peduncle*, arising from the dorsal and ventral tegmental nuclei, are shown in *red*; most of these fibers pass to the mammillary body, but some continue rostrally to the lateral hypothalamus, the preoptic regions and the medial septal nucleus. Fibers arising from the septal nuclei project caudally in the medial part of the *stria medullaris* (*blue*) to terminate in the medial habenular nucleus. Impulses conveyed by this bundle are distributed to midbrain tegmental nuclei via the fasciculus retroflexus. (Based on Nauta (1816).)

tegmentum (1815, 1816). The medial septal nucleus projects fibers back to the hippocampal formation via the fornix (587, 2090). The studies of Nauta (1815, 1816) indicate that the septal region constitutes a nodal area in the limbic projection system through which primary hippocampal and amygdaloid projections appear to overlap. Two distinct and separate pathways originating from this region conduct impulses to the midbrain tegmentum. These tracts are: (a) the stria medullaris which synapses upon the habenular nuclei (which in turn give rise to the fasciculus retroflexus), and (b) the medial forebrain bundle (Fig. 18-7).

The *pyriform lobe* consists of the lateral olfactory stria, the uncus and the anterior part of the parahippocampal gyrus. The rostral part of the parahippocampal gyrus is rolled inward and upward as a consequence of the tremendous development of the neopallium. The rostromedial protrusion of this gyrus is the *uncus* (Figs. 2-9 and 18-8). The shallow rhinal sulcus, a rostral continuation of the collateral sulcus, separates the anterior part of the parahippocampal gyrus from the more lateral neocortex (Figs. 2-5, 2-9 and 18-10). In man the caudal limits of this area are indistinct, and it is uncertain how much of the parahippocampal area should be included.

The pyriform lobe, so named because of its pear shape in certain species, is divided into several regions. These include the *pre-*

pyriform, the *periamygdaloid* and the *entorhinal* areas. The prepyriform area, often referred to as the lateral olfactory gyrus, extends along the lateral olfactory stria to the rostral amygdaloid region (Fig. 18-6). Since it afferent fibers are derived from the lateral olfactory stria, it is regarded as an olfactory relay center. The periamygdaloid area is a small region dorsal and rostral to the amygdaloid nuclear complex; it is intimately related to the prepyriform area. The entorhinal area, the most posterior part of the pyriform lobe, corresponds to area 28 of Brodmann and constitutes a major portion of the anterior parahippocampal gyrus in man (Fig. 19-5). This area, relatively large in primates and in man, is composed of a six-layered cortex of a transitional type. The entorhinal cortex does not receive direct fibers from the olfactory bulb or tract (348, 474, 785, 1173, 2060).

The prepyriform cortex projects fibers to the entorhinal cortex (area 28), the basal and lateral amygdaloid nuclei, the lateral preoptic area, the nucleus of the diagonal band, the medial forebrain bundle and to parts of the dorsomedial nucleus of the thalamus (2060). The *entorhinal cortex* is regarded as a secondary *olfactory cortical area* (Figs. 18-5, 18-13 and 19-5). Although it has been generally thought that no lateral olfactory tract fibers project to the entorhinal cortex without synapsing in the prepyriform cortex, recent evidence indicates some direct connections exist (1352). Efferent fibers from the entorhinal cortex are projected to the hippocampal formation, and to the anterior insular and frontal cortex via the uncinate fasciculus. No fibers from the prepyriform cortex pass to the hippocampal formation.

Monkeys with lesions of the lateroposterior quadrant of the orbitofrontal cortex (Fig. 18-5) are unable to learn to discriminate between two odors (2512). The pyriform cortex receives an olfactory input, and projects to the medial (magnocellular) subdivision of the dorsomedial thalamic nucleus which has a major efferent projection to the orbitofrontal cortex. Electrical stimulation of the olfactory bulb evokes potentials in the lateroposterior orbitofrontal cortex in monkeys with extensive damage to the thalamus, so some other path must also exist. While the anatomical data are limited, the lateral entorhinal cortex appears to form a major link between olfactory regions of the temporal and frontal lobes (Fig. 18-5) (2049).

Different parts of the amygdaloid nuclear complex receive olfactory inputs. Direct projections from the olfactory bulb pass to the corticomedial amygdaloid nuclei, while indirect, but substantial, olfactory impulses pass to the basal and lateral amygdaloid nuclei, via relays in the prepyriform cortex. It is of interest that direct and indirect olfactory pathways to the amygdaloid complex terminate in different components.

Clinical Considerations. The ability of the human nose, in concert with the brain, to discriminate thousands of different odor qualities is well known, but the physiological and psychological bases for such discriminations are unknown. Olfactory discrimination does not appear to be based upon morphologically distinct types of receptors, but there is some evidence that certain odors may be distinguished by their relative effectiveness in stimulating particular regions of the olfactory epithelium (1420, 1772). Current theories suggest that spatial and temporal factors probably play important roles in the neural coding of olfactory responses (1762). Other evidence indicates that the sense of smell is based upon the geometry of molecules (53). Two optical isomers, molecules identical in every respect except that one is the mirror image of the other, may have different odors. Seven primary odors have been distinguished (i.e., camphoraceous, musky, floral, pepperminty, ethereal (ether-like), pungent and putrid) and are considered to be equivalent to the three primary colors because every known odor can be produced by appropriate mixtures of primary odors. Molecules with the same primary odor appear to have particular configurations, and these configurations are thought to fit appropriately shaped receptors in olfactory nerve endings. Some molecules may fit more than one receptor in different fashions and these are considered to signal a complex odor.

From a clinical viewpoint the importance of the olfactory system is slight in man, since this special sense plays a less essential role than in lower vertebrates. In certain instances valuable clinical information can be obtained by testing olfactory sense by appropriate methods. Olfaction is tested in each nostril separately by having the patient inhale or sniff nonirritating volatile oils or liquids with characteristic odors. Substances which stimulate gustatory end organs, or peripheral endings of the trigeminal nerve in the nasal mucosa, are not appropriate for testing olfaction. Comparisons between the two sides are of great importance. While the olfactory nerves are rarely the seat of disease, they frequently are involved by disease or injury of adjacent structures. Fractures of the cribriform plate of the ethmoid bone or hemorrhage at the base of the frontal lobes may cause tearing of the olfactory filaments. The olfactory nerves may be involved as a consequence of meningitis or abscess of the frontal lobe. Unilateral anosmia may be of important diagnostic significance in localizing intracranial neoplasms, especially meningiomas of the sphenoidal ridge or olfactory groove. Hypophysial tumors affect the olfactory bulb and tract only when they extend above the sella turcica. Olfactory "hallucinations" frequently are a consequence of lesions involving or irritating the parahippocampal gyrus, the uncus or adjoining areas around the amygdaloid nuclear complex. The olfactory sensations which these patients experience usually are described as disagreeable in character and may precede a generalized convulsion. Such seizures are referred to as "uncinate fits."

ANTERIOR COMMISSURE

The anterior commissure crosses the midline as a compact fiber bundle immediately in front of the anterior columns of the fornix (Figs. 2-13, 2-14, 15-2, 18-6–18-8 and A-25). Proceeding laterally it splits into two portions. The small anterior, or olfactory portion, greatly reduced in man, loops rostrally and connects the gray substance of the olfactory tract on one side with the olfactory bulb of the opposite side (Fig. 18-9). Fibers in this part of the anterior commissure arise from the anterior olfactory nucleus, cross to the opposite side and project to the contralateral anterior olfactory nucleus and to granule cells in the olfactory bulb (Fig. 18-4). It has been suggested (2057) that these centrifugal fibers may subserve reflex control of activity in the olfactory bulb, and in principle may be comparable to the efferent system to sensory nuclei at spinal levels.

The larger posterior portion forms the bulk of the anterior commissure. From its central region fibers of the anterior commissure pass laterally and backward through the most inferior parts of the lateral segment of the globus pallidus and putamen, a relationship most obvious in sagittal sections of the brain (Figs. 17-3, A-31 and A-32). Further laterally the fibers of the anterior commissure enter the external capsule and come into apposition with the inferior part of the claustrum. On entering the external capsule the fibers of the commissure twist so that posterior fibers pass ventrally. Fibers of the posterior portion of the anterior commissure mainly interconnect the middle temporal gyri, although some pass into the inferior temporal gyrus (791). Similar findings have been reported in physiological studies in the monkey (1561) and in the chimpanzee (99). The findings of Whitlock and Nauta (2705), who used silver impregnation methods, appear similar to those of Fox and his associates.

THE HIPPOCAMPAL FORMATION

The hippocampal formation is laid down in the embryo on the medial wall of the hemisphere along the hippocampal fissure, immediately above and parallel to the choroidal fissure, which marks the invagination of the choroid plexus into the ventricle (Fig. 3-15). With the formation of the temporal lobe, both these fissures are carried downward and forward, each forming an arch extending from the region of the interventricular foramen to the tip of the inferior horn of the lateral ventricle (Fig. 3-17). The various parts of the hippocampal arch do not develop to the same extent. The upper or anterior portion of the hippocampal fissure is invaded by the crossing fibers of the corpus callosum and ultimately becomes the callosal fissure, which separates this massive commissure from the overlying pallium. The corresponding part of the hippocampal formation, which lies above the corpus callosum, undergoes little differentiation; in the adult it forms a thin vestigial convolution, the *indusium griseum* (Figs. 2-10, 18-6 and 18-8). The lower temporal portion of the arch, which is not affected by the corpus callosum, differentiates into the main structures of the hippocampal for-

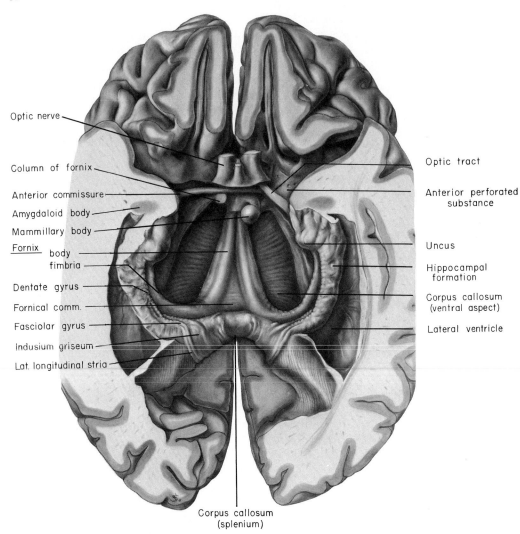

Optic nerve

Column of fornix

Anterior commissure

Amygdaloid body

Mammillary body

Fornix
  body
  fimbria

Dentate gyrus

Fornical comm.

Fasciolar gyrus

Indusium griseum

Lat. longitudinal stria

Optic tract

Anterior perforated
  substance

Uncus

Hippocampal
  formation

Corpus callosum
  (ventral aspect)

Lateral ventricle

Corpus callosum
(splenium)

Figure 18-8. Dissection of the inferior surface of the brain showing the configuration of the fornix, the hippocampal formation, the dentate gyrus and related structures. (Reproduced with permission from F. A. Mettler: *Neuroanatomy,* Ed. 2, The C. V. Mosby Co., St. Louis, 1948.)

mation. The hippocampal fissure deepens, and the invaginated portion, which bulges deeply into the inferior horn, becomes the *hippocampus*, while the lips of the fissure give rise to the *dentate* and the *parahippocampal gyri*. The relationships of these structures are best illustrated in a frontal section through this area, or in special dissections (Figs. 18-8, 18-9 and 18-10). Proceeding from the collateral sulcus, the *parahippocampal gyrus* extends to the hippocampal fissure, where it dips into the ventricle to form the *hippocampal formation*.

The latter curves dorsally and medially and, on reaching the medial surface, curves inward again to form a semilunar convolution, the *dentate gyrus* or *fascia dentata* (Figs. 18-11 and 18-12). The whole ventricular surface of the hippocampal formation is covered by a white layer, the *alveus*, which is composed of axons from cells of the hippocampus (Figs. 18-10–18-12). These fibers converge on the medial surface of the hippocampus to form a flattened band, the *fimbria*, lying medial to the hippocampus and the dentate gyrus. Fibers from the al-

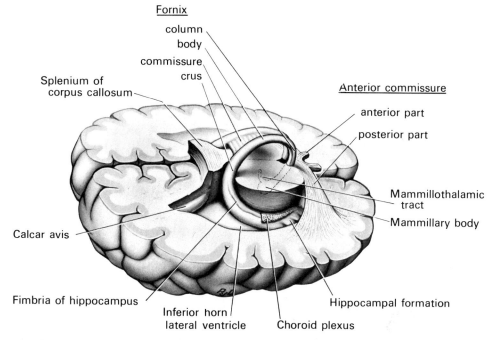

Figure 18-9. Drawing of a brain dissection showing the hippocampal formation, the fornix system and the anterior and posterior parts of the anterior commissure. In this drawing postcommissural fibers of the fornix are shown projecting only to the mammillary body.

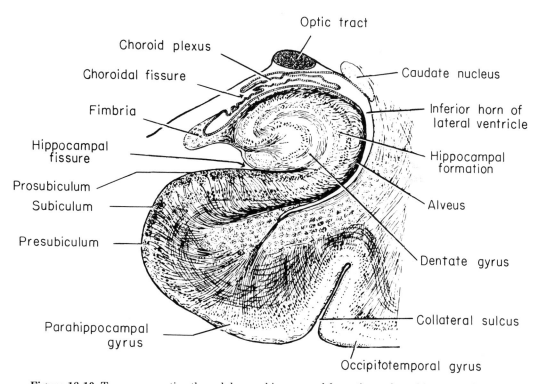

Figure 18-10. Transverse section through human hippocampal formation and parahippocampal gyrus.

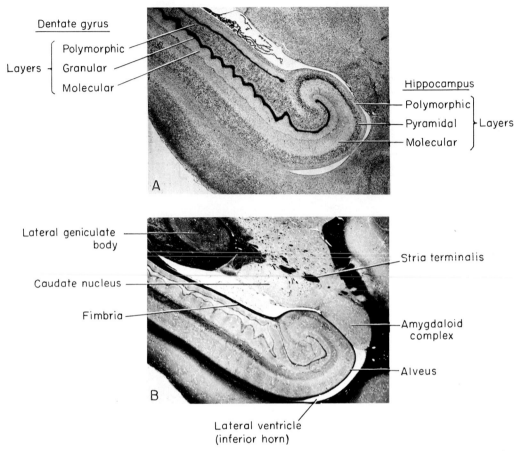

Figure 18-11. Sagittal sections through the hippocampal formation and dentate gyrus in the rhesus monkey showing the relationships of these structures to the inferior horn of the lateral ventricle, the neostriatum and the amygdaloid nuclear complex. In *A*, the cellular layers of the hippocampal formation and dentate gyrus are identified. In *B*, the alveus, fimbria, tail of the caudate nucleus, stria terminalis, amygdaloid complex and part of the lateral geniculate body are identified (*A*, Nissl stain, ×8; *B*, Weil stain, ×9).

Figure 18-12. Hippocampal region in the rhesus monkey in horizontal section showing the respective layers of the hippocampal formation and dentate gyrus. *A*, Nissl stain, photograph ×20. In *B*, the borders of the layers and sectors of the hippocampal formation are designated according to Lorente de Nó (1528, 1530). Abbreviations used are: *28a*, entorhinal area; *CA4-2*, hilus fasciae dentatae; *49*, parasubiculum; *27*, presubiculum; *str. gran.*, stratum granulosum; *str. lac-mol.*, stratum lacunosum-moleculare; *str. mol.*, stratum moleculare; *st. or.*, stratum oriens; *str. pyr.*, stratum pyramidale; *str. rad.*, stratum radiatum; *supra* and *infra*, suprapyramidal and infrapyramidal limbs of the stratum granulosum; *lpi*, lamina principalis interna; *lpe*, lamina principalis externa. (The assistance of Dr. J. B. Angevine of the University of Arizona, College of Medicine, and Dr. R. S. Nowakowski, University of Mississippi Medical Center, is acknowledged for delimiting the cytoarchitectonic boundaries.)

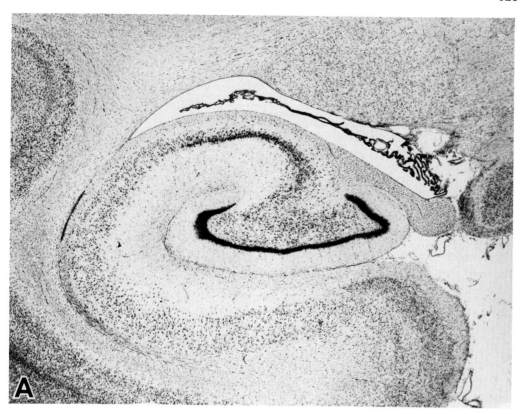

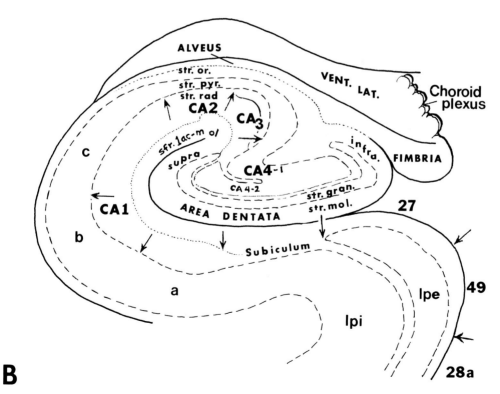

veus entering the fimbria constitute the beginning of the fornix system (Figs. 18-6, 18-8 and 18-9). The free thin border of the fimbria is directly continuous with the epithelium of the choroidal fissure, which lies immediately above it. The choroid plexus, invaginated into the ventricle along this fissure, partly covers the hippocampus (Fig. 18-10). The superior portion of the parahippocampal gyrus adjoining the hippocampal fissure is known as the *subiculum*, and the area of transition between it and the parahippocampal gyrus, as the *presubiculum* (Fig. 18-10).

On the basis of phylogenetic observations, the cerebral cortex can be divided into an older portion, the *allocortex*, and a newer part, the *neocortex*. The allocortex consists, in turn, of the *archicortex* and *paleocortex*. The presubiculum, subiculum, prosubiculum, hippocampal formation and dentate gyrus have an archicortical structure, while the pyriform cortex is paleocortical. The larger inferior portion of the parahippocampal gyrus, which is bounded by the collateral sulcus (Fig. 2-5 and 2-9), has the structure of neocortex.

The dentate gyrus, hippocampus proper (also called cornu ammonis) and subiculum all develop from the embryonic hippocampal formation. The term "hippocampal formation" has been used in varied ways by different authors to describe the adult temporal lobe structures. In this discussion we use the terms hippocampal formation and hippocampus interchangeably to refer only to that region between the subiculum and the dentate gyrus.

When the hippocampal fissure is opened up, the *dentate gyrus* is seen as a narrow, notched band of cortex between the hippocampal fissure below and the fimbria above (Fig. 18-8). In sagittal sections (Fig. 18-11) the relationships between the hippocampal formation, the dentate gyrus, the amygdaloid nucleus and the inferior horn of the lateral ventricle can be readily appreciated. Traced backward, the gyrus accompanies the fimbria almost to the splenium of the corpus callosum. There it separates from the fimbria, loses its notched appearance, and as the delicate *fasciolar gyrus*, passes on to the superior surface of the corpus callosum (Fig. 18-8). It spreads out into a thin gray sheet representing a vestigial convolution, the *indusium griseum* or *supracallosal gyrus* (Figs. 18-6 and 18-8). Imbedded in the indusium griseum are two slender bands of myelinated fibers which appear as narrow longitudinal ridges on the superior surface of the corpus callosum. These are the *medial* and *lateral longitudinal striae* (*Lancisii*), which constitute the white matter of these vestigial convolutions (Figs. 2-10 and 18-8). The indusium griseum and the longitudinal striae extend the whole length of the corpus callosum, pass over the genu and become continuous with the paraterminal gyrus, which is in turn prolonged into the diagonal band of Broca (Fig. 18-2). Traced forward, the dentate gyrus extends into the notch between the uncus and hippocampal gyrus. Here it makes a sharp dorsal bend and passes as a smooth band across the inferior surface of the uncus. This terminal portion is known as the *band of Giacomini*, and the part of the uncus lying posterior to it often is designated as the *intralimbic gyrus*.

The cortical zones from the parahippocampal gyrus through the presubiculum, the subiculum and the prosubiculum to the hippocampal formation and the dentate gyrus show a gradual transition from a six- to three-layered cellular organization (Figs. 18-10 and 18-12). Although the entorhinal region (area 28) is six-layered cortex, it represents a transitional form not typical of neocortex. In more medial cortical areas certain layers of the entorhinal cortex drop out and undergo rearrangement, so that the cortex of the *hippocampal formation* has only three fundamental layers. These are the *polymorphic layer*, the *pyramidal layer* and the *molecular layer* (Fig. 18-11). Several secondary laminae are formed by the arrangement of axons and dendrites of cells within the fundamental layers. Immediately beneath the ependyma of the ventricle is the alveus. Recognized laminae passing inward from the alveus are: (a) the stratum oriens, (b) the stratum pyramidale, (c) the stratum radiatum, (d) the stratum lacunosum and (e) the stratum moleculare (Figs. 18-12 and 18-14). The last three laminae are considered to correspond to the molecular layer of the neocortex (1528, 1530). The most characteristic layer of the hippocampal formation is the pyramidal layer consisting of large and small pyramidal and Golgi type II cells (Fig. 18-13). *Large* and *small pyramidal cells* exhibit

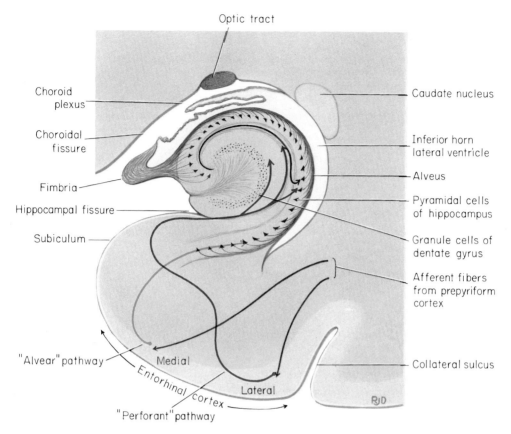

Figure 18-13. Semischematic diagram of the hippocampal formation, dentate gyrus and entorhinal area. In the dentate gyrus only the granular layer is indicated. In the hippocampal formation only pyramidal cells and their axons projecting into the alveus are shown. Afferent fibers from prepyriform cortex projecting to the entorhinal cortex are shown in *black*. Projections of the entorhinal cortex to the hippocampal formation follow two pathways: (a) the lateral region gives rise to fibers which follow the so-called "perforant" pathway (*red*), and (b) the medial region gives rise to fibers which follow the so-called "alvear" pathway (*blue*). Axons of pyramidal cells in the hippocampal formation entering the alveus pass to the fimbria of the hippocampus. The dentate gyrus gives rise to fibers that project only to the hippocampal formation. (Based on Lorente de Nó (1530) and a schematic diagram by Peele(1960).)

many morphological differences, especially in dendritic development. Some of the cells are described as double pyramids because of the rich dendritic plexuses arising from both poles (Fig. 4-5*J*). Basal and apical dendrites of the pyramidal cells enter adjacent layers, while axons of these cells pass through the stratum oriens to enter the alveus (Fig. 18-13). *Hippocampal basket cells*, similar to the pyramidal cells, are found mainly near the border between the stratum pyramidale and the stratum oriens (2094). Their axons do not enter the alveus, but loop back through the stratum radiatum to form a dense basket plexus about pyramidal cell bodies. The stratum oriens,

containing fibers and polymorphic cells, has been divided into outer and inner zones. Cells of the outer zone distribute axons to the molecular layer. Cells of the inner zone send some axons into the alveus, while others ramify within this layer or pass into the pyramidal layer. The stratum radiatum is made up largely of interlacing and branching processes which appear to radiate from the bordering pyramidal layer. The stratum lacunosum and stratum moleculare, sometimes considered as a single lamina, contain a rich plexus of fibers from other layers.

Although the architectonics of the hippocampal formation is uniform throughout its extent, there are variations in cell mor-

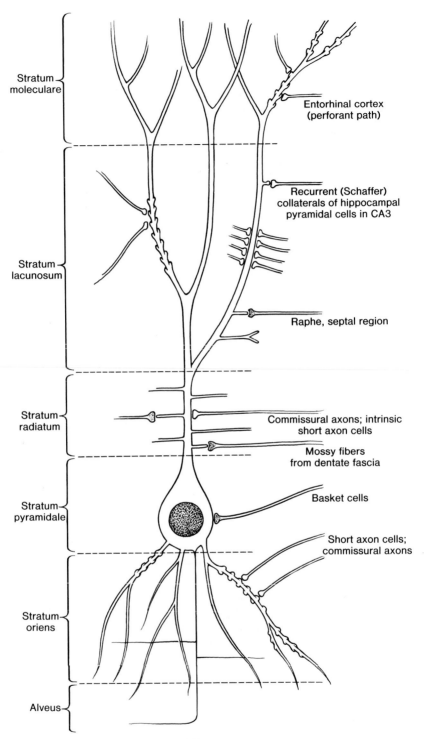

Stratum moleculare

Entorhinal cortex (perforant path)

Recurrent (Schaffer) collaterals of hippocampal pyramidal cells in CA3

Stratum lacunosum

Raphe, septal region

Stratum radiatum

Commissural axons; intrinsic short axon cells

Mossy fibers from dentate fascia

Basket cells

Stratum pyramidale

Short axon cells; commissural axons

Stratum oriens

Alveus

Figure 18-14. A schematic drawing of a CA1 sector hippocampal pyramidal neuron indicating the regions of the cell which receive specific afferent inputs. Specific cell layers of the hippocampal formation can be related to specific parts of the pyramidal cell and are shown on the readers left. Afferent inputs from several sources are indicated on the readers right. Afferent fibers synapse in specific locations upon dendritic shafts, dendritic spines, the cell body and the basal dendrites of the pyramidal cell.

phology, differences in the relative development of various cortical regions and differences in the pathways followed by various fiber systems. On the basis of these differences Lorente de Nó (1530) subdivided the hippocampal formation into sectors designated as CA1, CA2, CA3 and CA4. The letters "CA" are derived from *cornu monis*, an older descriptive term applied to the hippocampus because of its resemblance, when seen in cross-section, to a mythological figure with a ram's horn (1696). The position of these various sectors is shown in Figure 18-12.

The *dentate gyrus*, like the hippocampus, consists of three layers: a *molecular layer*, a *granular layer* and a *polymorphic layer* (Figs. 18-11 and 18-12). Layers of the dentate gyrus are arranged in a "U"-shaped configuration in which the open portion is directed toward the fimbria in transverse sections (Figs. 18-10 and 18-13). Thus layers are present on both sides of sector CA3 of the hippocampus which extends into the hilus of the dentate gyrus. The molecular layer of the dentate gyrus is continuous with that of the hippocampus in the depths of the hippocampal fissure. The granular layer, made up of closely arranged spherical or oval neurons, gives rise to axons which pass through the polymorphic layer to terminate upon dendrites of pyramidal cells in the hippocampus. Dendrites of granule cells enter mainly the molecular layer. Cells of the polymorphic layer are of several types, including modified pyramidal cells and so-called basket cells. The dentate gyrus does not give rise to fibers passing beyond the hippocampal formation (2095).

The *area dentata* (188) is bounded by imaginary lines extending from the tip of the pyramidal cell layer of the hippocampus to the extremities of the granular layer of the dentate gyrus (Fig. 18-12). Within this line is the hilus of the fascia dentata containing polymorphic neurons; this region has been designated as sector CA4 by Lorente de Nó. The term *fascia dentata* applies only to the molecular and granular layers of the areas dentata.

Histochemical studies provide further clues to the operation of the hippocampus. Acetylcholinesterase (AChE) is found in the terminals of the cholinergic septohippocampal projection (588, 1484, 1485, 1663).

Some AChE containing cell bodies are found within the hilus of the area dentata and scattered throughout the pyramidal cell layer, but most of the enzyme is confined to axon terminals.

The noradrenergic innervation of the hippocampus originates in cells of the locus ceruleus in the pons. These fibers reach the hippocampus by ascending through the caudal septal region, the postcommisural fornix and fornix. Other afferent axons from the locus ceruleus course over the corpus callosum to enter the hippocampus superiorly and caudally. Within the hippocampus the noradrenergic varicosities are most numerous in the hilar region of the dentate gyrus (1498a). A less dense plexus of noradrenergic axons occupies the strata lacunosum and moleculare of sectors CA1 and CA3.

The mossy fiber terminals arising from dentate granule cells have a high concentration of zinc. While the significance of this is not known, it provides a convenient marker for mossy fiber synapses.

Leu- and met-enkephalin immunoreactive axons form two distinct projection systems in the rat hippocampus (842). One emerges from the hilar region of the dentate gyrus and terminates as large, mossy fiber-like boutons on proximal apical dendrites of hippocampal pyramidal cells. The second enkephalin containing group of axons follows the course of the perforant path from the lateral entorhinal cortex to the hippocampus.

Studies of the hippocampal region utilizing autoradiographic technics (74) have provided new information concerning the development and migration of neurons in this cortical region. This technic is based upon the injection of tritiated thymidine into pregnant animals, which becomes incorporated into the DNA of premitotic cells. ^{3}H-Thymidine remains in the nuclei of those daughter cells which no longer divide, providing a radioactive label in neuroblasts. This makes it possible to study the proliferation and migration of neuroblasts destined for various parts of the brain. Studies of neurogenesis show that active displacement and migration of neurons is the rule. Neurons in all components of the hippocampal formation but one arise in a general, but not rigid, "inside-out" sequence. The outstanding exception in this cortical region is the granular layer of the dentate gyrus. Granule cells originating prenatally, or perinatally, migrate to the granular layer in an "outside-in" pattern, and postnatally granule cells arise by proliferation of deeply situated neuroblasts in the granular layer itself.

This "inside-out" sequence of neuron origin applies to the majority of cells in most cortical areas. Thus neurons arising late in gestation, and destined for superficial locations in a given cortical area, must traverse an extensive population of neurons which originated at earlier times. This same sequence of cell differentiation has been demonstrated in the hippocampal formation in human embryos (1174).

Even though the hippocampal formation has in the past been considered as an important olfactory center, there is no decisive evidence to support this concept (261). The anatomical connections of this structure indicate that it does not receive fibers from the olfactory bulb or the anterior olfactory nucleus (474, 794, 2217) and suggest that it is largely an effector structure.

Afferent fibers to the hippocampal formation arise mainly from the entorhinal area (348, 1528, 1530), a portion of the pyriform lobe which does not receive many direct olfactory fibers. Fibers from the entorhinal area (area 28) are distributed to the dentate gyrus and hippocampus in their entire posterior portion (1530). Fibers arising from the medial part of the entorhinal area follow the so-called "alvear path" to enter the hippocampus from its ventricular surface (Fig. 18-13). These fibers are distributed to the deep layer of the subiculum and to sector CA1 of the hippocampus (Fig. 18-14). Fibers from the lateral parts of the entorhinal cortex pursue the so-called "perforant path" and traverse the subiculum (Fig. 18-13). These fibers are distributed to the dentate gyrus and all sectors of the hippocampus except CA4. Afferent fibers following these pathways establish synaptic contacts with dendrites of pyramidal cells in the hippocampus (Fig. 18–14), and granule cells in the dentate gyrus.

Other afferent fibers to the hippocampal formation have been described. The medial septal nucleus projects fibers via the fimbria (587) to sectors CA3 and CA4 of the hippocampus and to the dentate gyrus. The cingulum (Figs. 2-10 and 2-19), a massive fiber bundle derived from cells of the cingulate cortex, projects to the presubiculum and the entorhinal area (Fig. 18-15) (2094), but not to the hippocampal formation. Since the entorhinal area projects to the hippocampus proper, these findings imply that impulses from the cingulate cortex are relayed to the hippocampus via the entorhinal area. Although it has been postulated that the indusium griseum contributes fibers to the hippocampus, these fibers are not numerous. In addition, some fibers crossing in the hippocampal commissure may interconnect the two hippocampi. None of these afferent pathways to the hippocampal formation appears to transmit olfactory impulses. The pyriform cortex gives rise to deep and superficial pathways that project to the lateral entorhinal cortex, but no fibers that pass directly to the hippocampal formation (2060). A polysynaptic olfactory path involving the lateral entorhinal cortex and fascia dentata has been suggested by electrophysiological studies (2734).

Fornix. This band of white fibers constitutes the main efferent fiber system of the hippocampal formation, including both projection and commissural fibers (Figs. 18-8 and 18-9). It is composed of axons from the large pyramidal cells of the hippocampus and subiculum (1661, 1662, 2223, 2480, 2481) which spread over the ventricular surface as the *alveus* and then converge to form the *fimbria*. Proceeding backward, the fimbriae of the two sides increase in thickness. On reaching the posterior end of the hippocampus, they arch under the splenium of the corpus callosum as the *crura* of the fornix, at the same time converging toward each other. In this region a number of fibers pass to the opposite side, forming a thin sheet of crossing fibers, the *fornical commissure* (hippocampal commissure, or psalterium), a structure rather poorly developed in man (Figs. 18-8 and 18-9). The two crura then join to form the *body of the fornix*, which runs forward under the corpus callosum to the rostral margin of the thalamus (Fig. 15-2). Here the bundles separate again, and as the *anterior columns of the fornix*, arch ventrally in front of the interventricular foramina and caudal to the

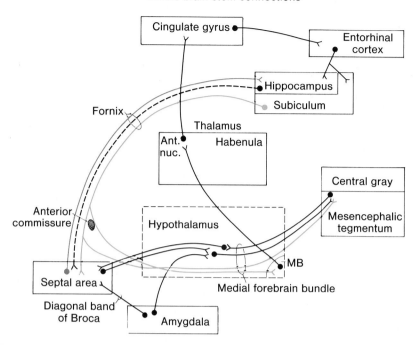

Figure 18-15. Schematic block diagram of major inter-connections of structures comprising the "limbic system." Projection fibers arising from the subiculum (*blue*) project via the fornix to the septal area, hypothalamus and mesencephalic tegmentum. Fibers projecting in the fornix from the hippocampus are shown in *black*-dashed lines. Projections from the septal area to the hippocampus are shown in *red. MB* indicates mammillary body.

anterior commissure. The fimbriae, thin bands of fibers situated laterally, accompany the fornices throughout most of their extent (Figs. 18-8 and 18-9), but rostrally they become incorporated within the main bundles as the latter form the anterior columns of the fornix. Approximately half of the fibers descend caudal to the anterior commissure as the *postcommissural fornix* (587, 2062). Remaining fibers of the fornix pass rostral to the anterior commissure as the *precommissural fornix.*

Postcommissural fornix fibers traverse the hypothalamus *en route* to the mammillary body, but in their course give off fibers to the thalamus (Fig. 15-2). Fornix fibers passing directly to the mammillary body terminate mainly in the medial nucleus. Fibers leaving the postcommissural fornix rostral to the hypothalamus are distributed mainly to the anterior and the rostral intralaminar thalamic nuclei (979, 1815, 2603).

According to Powell et al. (2062), the anterior nuclei of the thalamus receive as many direct fibers from the fornix as from the mammillothalamic tract. Some postcommissural fornix fibers descend caudally beyond the mammillary bodies to enter the midbrain tegmentum (979, 1815, 1816). Anterograde tracing studies in the rat show that axons in the postcommissural fornix destined for the hypothalamus originate from cell bodies in the subicular cortex and not from hippocampal pyramidal cells (Fig. 18-15) (1662, 2481).

Precommissural fornix fibers, constituting a less compact bundle than the postcommissural fibers, are distributed to the septal nuclei, the lateral preoptic area, the anterior part of the hypothalamus and the nucleus of the diagonal band (1815). Part of these direct fibers, continuing beyond these nuclei, are distributed to rostral parts of the midbrain central gray. The latter fibers represent a direct hippocampo-mesencephalic projection (Fig. 18-15) (1816). Caudally continuing fibers of the precommissural fornix are joined by numerous fibers from the septal nuclei to form a large part of one of the most massive roots of the medial forebrain bundle (Zuckerkandl's "olfactory bundle of Ammon's horn").

Detailed studies (2095, 2481) provide data concerning the differential origin and distribution of hippocampal efferent fibers contained in the fornix and fimbria. *Precommissural fornix fibers* arise from the posterior part of CA1 and from sector CA3. These precommissural fibers terminate ipsilaterally in the medial septal nuclei, and bilaterally in the lateral septal nuclei and the diagonal band nuclei. The dentate gyrus does not have an extrahippocampal projection.

The above anatomical connections indicate the complex pathways by which impulses from the hippocampal formation can be projected to different parts of the neuraxis. Thus both direct and indirect pathways connect the hippocampal formation with certain thalamic nuclei (i.e., the anterior and the intralaminar), the hypothalamus and the midbrain reticular formation (Fig. 18-7). The anterior nucleus of the thalamus in turn projects to the cingulate gyrus, from which impulses can reach the hippocampus via the cingulum and the entorhinal cortex. This path is known as the *Papez circuit*, after the neuroanatomist who first perceived its possible role in affective and emotional behaviors (1929) (Fig. 18-7). Another path emphasized in generalizations about the fornix and limbic system is that described by Nauta (1816) (Fig. 18-15). The anatomical arrangement of *Nauta's limbic-midbrain circuit* suggests a role for the hippocampus in correlation of activity in the septal region, hypothalamus and midbrain. The fornix bundle is anatomically organized into two separate components: (a) cells of the subiculum send axons through both the postcommissural fornix to the hypothalamus and the precommissural fornix to the septal region, and (b) cells of the hippocampus proper send axons through the precommissural fornix to the septal nuclei.

Hippocampal pyramidal cells and dentate granule cells give rise to commissural projections to the contralateral hippocampal formation. Many cells have an axon with one branch which may be intrinsic or exit via the fornix and a collateral branch to the hippocampus on the opposite side of the brain (2486).

Functional Considerations. Although the hippocampal formation is a large structure and considerable information is available concerning its anatomical connections and microphysiology, relatively little is known about its function. Abundant anatomical and physiological evidence indicates that the hippocampus has no significant olfactory function (261). Comparative anatomists have long known that development of the hippocampus in mammals does not proceed parallel to the development of olfaction. The hippocampus and dentate gyrus are well developed in anosmatic cetaceans that lack olfactory bulbs and nerves (8, 2150). Animal experiments have shown that olfactory discrimination is not affected by ablations of the hippocampus (2476, 2477), and that olfactory-conditioned reflexes persist after removal of the hippocampus (41, 42).

Localized lesions in the hippocampus and local stimulation of this structure in conscious cats tend to produce similar phenomena (955). Behavioral changes observed in these animals resemble those occurring in psychomotor epilepsy, and it seems likely that the abnormal fears, hyperesthesia and pupillary dilatation seen may represent fragments of a seizure. The behavioral changes noted initially after lesions tend to disappear within several weeks, but recur at a later time. The hippocampus is recognized as having an exceedingly low threshold for seizure activity, (955, 959, 1550, 1551). Seizure discharges spread from the hippocampus to other parts of the limbic lobe and ultimately to the neocortex.

Considerable evidence indicates that the hippocampus and infratemporal cortex may be concerned with recent memory (959). Relatively large bilateral lesions of the hippocampus (137, 647, 895, 2305, 2619) are associated with profound impairment of memory for recent events and with relatively mild behavioral changes, such as persistent inactivity, indifference and loss of initiative. Memory for remote events usually is unaffected. Although general intellectual functions may remain at a fairly high level, these patients demonstrate an inability to learn new facts and skills. These findings are in accord with those found after bilateral resection of the medial parts of the temporal lobe. According to Scoville and Milner (2305), lesions of the most anterior portion of the temporal lobe do not impair memory; impairment of memory occurs only when the lesions extend far enough posteriorly to involve the hippocampal formation, the dentate gyrus and parts of the parahippocampal gyrus. It is generally felt that loss of memory occurs only if lesions of the hippocampal formation and parahippocampal gyrus are bilateral (1967), but some patients may show mild verbal disorders or disturbances of memory following resections of parts of the temporal lobe of the dominant hemisphere. In these cases unsuspected lesions of the opposite hippocampus have been thought to be present. Some evidence suggests that in certain cases of senile dementia, characterized mainly by loss of memory, the most prominent lesions are found in the hippocampus. Experimental studies (1892, 2434) in the monkey indicate that bilateral removals of the amygdaloid complex and portions of the hippocampus impair memory and learning that depend upon visual and auditory discriminations. The type of behavioral test used to measure retention following temporal lobe lesions is very important. When rhesus monkeys are tested for their ability to discriminate between pairs of visual stimuli presented concurrently, anterior inferotemporal cortex lesions impair learning. This is also true when the lesions extend more deeply to include the hippocampus. With the extension of the lesions into the hippocampus, the animals show an additional impairment of learning for tactile stimuli (1760). These complexities in analyzing the involvement of the hippocampus and other temporal lobe structures in mechanisms of memory make it difficult to draw broad generalizations from the experimental and clinical literature related to lesions (1143).

In rats, bilateral destruction of the hippocampus, the fornix and mammillary bodies produces a severe disturbance in maze learning (1251a). Chronic single hippocampal neuron recordings in freely behaving rats indicate that these cells encode the animals' specific position in its environment (1866). It has been hypothesized that the hippocampus contains an internal "cognitive map" of behaviorally significant features of the environment (1867). Single unit recordings in the rabbit hippocampus show a high correlation between pyramidal cell discharge in CA1 and CA3 and the acquisition of a conditioned response (162).

Much more information is needed about the location of neurons that are essential for learning a specific task before it will be possible to understand the mechanisms of learning. It can be reasonably argued from the available literature that memory and learning are distributed processes, involving neuron assemblies in many regions of the brain. If this is the case, progress on the problem of memory will require new strategies to relate biophysical and biochemical events at the cellular level (1264) to the properties of distributed neuronal networks (526).

Even though the fornix contains many of the efferent fibers from the hippocampal formation, evidence that interruption of these fibers produces memory loss is meager. No discernible deficits of memory have been reported after section of both fornices in the monkey (846, 1760) or in man (29, 30, 641). One human case reported by Sweet et al. (2487) showed severe and lasting memory loss, apathy and lack of spontaneity following section of both columns of the fornix to facilitate removal of a tumor in the third ventricle. It seems that the hippocampal connections with the entorhinal cortex (2223) are important for associative learning involving more than one modality (1760).

Korsakoff's syndrome (amnestic confabulatory syndrome), appearing as a sequel to Wernicke's encephalopathy and probably caused by a thiamine deficiency associated with alcoholism, is characterized by severe impairment of memory, without clouding of consciousness, confusion and confabulatory tendencies. Lesions in this syndrome almost always involve the mammillary bodies and adjacent areas (2488). However, it has been suggested that the amnesia of Korsakoff's syndrome is present only if there is additional involvement of the thalamus (2618).

Although it is not possible to further define the functions of the hippocampus, there are suggestions that it also may be concerned with: (a) emotional reactions or control of emotions, (b) certain visceral activities, and (c) regulation of reticular activating influences upon the cerebral cortex (956). Particularly prominent among concepts relating the hippocampal formation to emotion is the theory proposed by Papez (1929), which attempts to provide an anatomical basis for emotion. Realizing that the term "emotion" denotes both subjective feelings and the expression of these feelings by appropriate autonomic and somatic responses, Papez concluded, as have others, that the cortex is essential for subjective emotional experience and that emotional expression must be dependent upon the integrative actions of the hypothalamus. He expressed the belief that the hippocampal formation and its principal projection system, the fornix, provide one of the main pathways by which impulses from the cortex reach the hypothalamus (Figs. 15-2, 16-10 and 16-11). Impulses reaching the hypothalamus could be projected caudally through the brain stem to effector structures, as well as rostrally to thalamic, and ultimately cortical levels. Electrical stimulation of the hippocampus produced infrequent reports of mental phenomena in patients with partial complex seizures (psychomotor epilepsy) during evaluation for therapeutic resection of the temporal lobe. The varied experiential responses were often associated with afterdischarges evoked by the stimulus, and therefore may be due to activity in distant structures. The nature of the experiences reported included alimentary sensations and memory-like hallucinations and seemed to correlate with the patients' personality characteristics rather than electrode location (1009).

It has been supposed by many investigators that short and long term learning and memory must be related to morphological or functional changes in synapses. The association of the hippocampal formation with learning, together with its highly ordered arrangement of cells and input axons (Fig. 18-14), has led to a large number of experiments dealing with neuronal plasticity. Brief repetitive stimulation of fornix or entorhinal afferent axons leads to a prolonged increase in the responsivity of hip-

pocampal pyramidal cells or dentate granule cells (191, 357). Depending upon the conditions of the experiment, the excitability change may last several hours and is associated with phosphorylation of a 40,000 dalton protein in the synaptic plasma membrane (306).

The hippocampus also shows reactive synaptogenesis following interruption of some of its afferent fiber systems. This morphological plasticity has been studied extensively in the dentate gyrus following interruption of perforant path fibers from the entorhinal cortex (538, 539). Unilateral entorhinal cortex ablation leads, over a period of weeks, to the formation of new synapses in the denervated area of the ipsilateral dentate gyrus. Many of the new synapses are formed by growth of collaterals from axons originating in the contralateral entorhinal cortex, and by sprouting of septohippocampal axons. Like the original perforant path projection, the newly formed synapses may sustain long term potentiation following repetitive stimulation (2733).

AMYGDALOID NUCLEAR COMPLEX

The amygdaloid nuclear complex is a gray mass situated in the dorsomedial portion of the temporal lobe, in front of, and partly above the tip of the inferior horn of the lateral ventricle (Figs. 2-9, 2-15, 18-6, 18-8, 18-11 and 18-16). It is covered by a rudimentary cortex and caudally is continuous with the uncus of the parahippocampal gyrus (Figs. 2-5, 2-9, 2-19 and 18-16).

The amygdaloid complex usually is divided into two main nuclear masses, a corticomedial nuclear group and a basolateral nuclear group (570, 571, 900, 2604). A central nucleus is regarded as a separate subdivision, but sometimes is included as part of the corticomedial nuclear group. In man the *corticomedial nuclear group* constitutes a dorsal or dorsomedial part of the complex due to a medial rotation of the temporal lobe. Nuclear subdivisions of the corticomedial group include: (a) the anterior amygdaloid area, (b) the nucleus of the lateral olfactory tract, (c) the medial amygdaloid nucleus, and (d) the cortical amygdaloid nucleus. The nucleus of the lateral olfactory tract is the least well developed of the amygdaloid nuclei in man. The anterior amygdaloid area, representing the most ros-

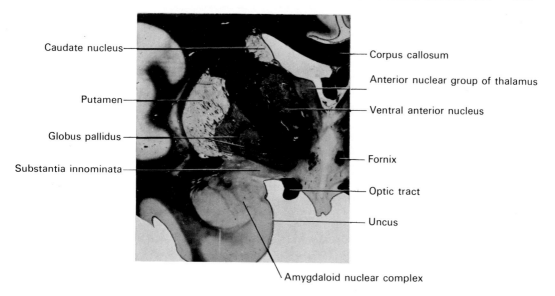

Caudate nucleus

Putamen

Globus pallidus

Substantia innominata

Corpus callosum

Anterior nuclear group of thalamus

Ventral anterior nucleus

Fornix

Optic tract

Uncus

Amygdaloid nuclear complex

Figure 18-16. Photograph of transverse section through the thalamus, corpus striatum and amygdaloid nuclear complex (Weil stain).

tral part of the amygdaloid complex, is rather poorly differentiated (785). The corticomedial amygdaloid nuclear group lies closest to the putamen and tail of the caudate nucleus.

The largest and best differentiated part of the amygdaloid complex in man is the *basolateral nuclear group*. Subdivisions of this nuclear group are: (a) the lateral amygdaloid nucleus, (b) the basal amygdaloid nucleus, and (c) an accessory basal amygdaloid nucleus. The amygdaloid complex is related medially to the area olfactoria and laterally to the claustrum, while dorsally it is hidden partially by the lentiform nucleus. Caudally the amygdaloid complex is in contact with the tail of the caudate nucleus, which sweeps rostrally in the roof of the inferior horn of the lateral ventricle (Figs. 2-12, 17-4 and 18-11). The amygdaloid complex is found in all mammals and has been homologized with the olfactory striatum (archistriatum) of submammalian forms.

Among the afferent connections of the amygdaloid complex, olfactory fibers are the best established. Fibers originating in the olfactory bulb project via the lateral olfactory tract to terminate in the cortico-medial nuclear group (12, 45, 474, 900, 2060). No fibers from the lateral olfactory tract appear to enter the basolateral nu-

clear group. The basolateral amygdaloid nuclei receive an indirect olfactory input via relays in the prepyriform cortex (2060, 2604). Thus nearly all parts of the amygdaloid nuclear complex receive either direct or indirect olfactory pathways. The central nuclear group appears to be the exception.

While amygdala neurons respond to olfactory stimuli in the rat (346), there is some controversy regarding man. Recordings have been made from depth electrodes implanted in the amygdala of patients with temporal lobe epilepsy being evaluated for amygdalotomy. There is agreement that olfactory stimuli produce a short latency "spindle" in the focal electrical activity (1170, 1171), but no discharge of action potentials is observed in single unit recordings (1008). Whether the "spindles," which have a characteristic power spectrum, are specific to olfactory stimuli or signal mechanical activation of the olfactory mucosa by inspired air remains to be determined.

Experimental evidence indicated important diencephalic projections to the amygdala that follow pathways which parallel efferent systems. Fibers arising in the rostral half of the hypothalamus pass via the stria terminalis and pathways ventral to the basal ganglia (ventral amygdalopetal) to all amygdaloid nuclei, except the central nucleus (557, 2131, 2501). This diencephalic input to the amygdaloid nuclear complex passes to all nuclei which receive direct or indirect olfactory afferents.

The amygdala also receives fibers from neocortical areas (1417). Neocortical projections from the temporal lobe and cingulate gyrus to the basolateral and lateral nuclei of the amygdala have been described in the monkey (1088, 1924, 2705). There appears to be reciprocal relationships between the amygdala and these neocortical areas (1362, 1576, 1817). The orbitofrontal cortex also has been described as a source of afferent fibers to the amygdala (2604), and van Alphen (49) found a limited number of afferent fibers from parietal, occipital and temporal areas that pass to the lateral amygdaloid nucleus via the posterior limb of the anterior commissure. Frontal lobe association cortex receives both direct and indirect projections from the basolateral and basomedial amygdaloid nuclei in the rhesus monkey. The direct path ends in the orbital cortex and anterior cingulate gyrus. The amygdala also sends axons to the magnocellular part (DMmc) of the dorsomedial thalamic nucleus (1656, 2046) which in turn projects to the same region of the orbitofrontal cortex receiving the direct amygdalocortical fibers. A similar amygdalothalamic path exists in the rat but not in the cat (1361).

Anatomical evidence concerning nonolfactory sensory afferents to the amygdaloid complex is meager, although electrophysiological studies suggest such connections. Evoked potentials can be elicited in the amygdaloid complex in response to stimulation of nearly all sensory receptors (862, 1577). These responses are recorded mainly in the basolateral nuclear group. Impulses originating from distant parts of the body surface, as well as impulses concerned with different sensory modalities, were found to converge upon the same cells (900). Additional subcortical structures projecting afferent fibers to the amygdaloid complex include the brain stem reticular formation (1577), and the pyriform cortex (785).

The amygdala receives noradrenergic afferents from the locus ceruleus and dopaminergic afferents from the region of the ventral tegmental area and substantia nigra in the midbrain (1498a, 2598). Dopamine containing terminals are densest in the central nucleus, but also innervate the lateral and basolateral nuclei. Noradrenergic varicosities are distributed in a similar manner, being most prominent in the central nucleus. The catecholamine (dopamine and norepinephrine) axons reach the amygdala through both the stria terminalis and ventral paths.

Acetylcholinesterase and choline acetyltransferase are found in highest concentration in the posterior lateral and basolateral nuclei and the nucleus of the lateral olfactory tract. There is some species variation in enzyme distribution, but this appears to reflect the difficulty in identifying boundaries of nuclei rather than a difference in the pattern of cholinergic innervation of the amygdala (149).

The peptides enkephalin, substance P and somatostatin have been localized mainly to the central and medial nuclei (148, 694, 714, 973).

In the rhesus monkey, opiate receptors are distributed widely throughout the amygdala (1419). The locations of enkephalin and opiate receptors generally parallel each other, but there are some regions, such as the amygdala, in which differences occur.

Aside from afferents originating in the hypothalamus and preoptic region (see below), the amygdala receives fibers from the brainstem raphe and parabrachial nuclei (1911, 2608, 2787). Axons from both of these brainstem regions, which also project to the hypothalamus (1556), converge upon the central and parts of the basolateral nuclei of the amygdala.

Stria Terminalis (*stria semicircularis*). This is the most prominent efferent pathway from the amygdaloid nuclear complex (Figs. 2-24, 2-28, 15-5, 15-7, 15-8, 17-3 and 18-6). Most, but not all, of the fibers in this bundle originate from the corticomedial part of the amygdaloid complex (557, 785, 1010, 1417, 1877, 2090, 2604). Fibers of the stria terminalis arch along the entire medial border of the caudate nucleus near its junction with the thalamus (Fig. 15-8). Rostrally these fibers pass into and terminate in the nuclei of the stria terminalis located lateral to the columns of the fornix and dorsal to the anterior commissure (1070, 1877). This is the most massive termination of the stria terminalis. Part of these fibers, which belong to the postcommissural part of the stria terminalis, also end in the anterior hypothalamic nucleus, and some of the fibers may join the medial forebrain bundle. Fibers of the precommissural part of the stria terminalis terminate in the medial preoptic area and continue caudally to end in a cell-poor zone surrounding the ventromedial hypothalamic nucleus (650, 1010, 1069, 1070, 1877). The axons of the stria terminalis which terminate in the ventromedial hypothalamic nucleus originate in basomedial and corticomedial nuclei of the amygdala (1556) (Fig. 18-18). These amygdaloid nuclei also receive an input from the vomeronasal organ (2093).

The Ventral Amygdalofugal Projection. This projection, considered to arise from both the basolateral amygdaloid nuclei and the pyriform cortex, emerges from the dorsomedial part of the amygdala and spreads medially and rostrally beneath the lentiform nucleus (557, 899, 1817). These fibers pass through the substantia innominata (Figs. 18-16 and A-22) and enter the lateral preoptic and hypothalamic areas, the septal region and the nucleus of the diagonal band (Broca). Evidence in the rat suggests that fibers in this projection arise mainly from the periamygdaloid cortex (1468, 2604); some evidence suggests that ventral amygdalofugal fibers are unique to higher mammals.

Amygdalofugal fibers, bypassing the preoptic region and hypothalamus, enter the inferior thalamic peduncle (Fig. 15-10) and project to the magnocellular part of the dorsomedial nucleus of the thalamus (786, 1361, 1817, 2046). It has been suggested that these fibers arise from the basolateral amygdaloid nuclei, but Valverde (2604) reports they arise chiefly from the anterior amygdaloid area. Fibers with this course are joined by projections arising from temporal neocortex (Fig. 15-14). There is conflicting evidence concerning reciprocal connections between the dorsomedial nucleus of the thalamus and the amygdala (1817, 1656).

Functional Considerations. Even though the amygdaloid complex receives an olfactory input, the importance of this complex for olfactory sensation is uncertain. Most evidence suggests that the amygdaloid complex cannot be closely related to olfaction since it is well developed in anosmatic aquatic mammals, and bilateral destruction of it does not impair olfactory discrimination (42, 2476).

Electrical stimulation and ablation of the amygdaloid nuclear complex in animals have produced a wide variety of behavioral, visceral, somatic and endocrine changes (900, 1250, 1552, 2312). The most pronounced behavioral changes are elicited by stimulation in unanesthetized animals. The most common response to amygdaloid stimulation under such conditions is an "arrest" reaction in which all spontaneous activities cease as the animal assumes an attitude of aroused attention. This response is indistinguishable from the arousal reaction obtained from brain stem reticular formation stimulation and is associated with cortical desynchronization (737, 2600). The "arrest" reaction appears as the initial phase of flight and defense reactions obtained by amygdaloid stimulation. Flight (fear) and defensive (rage and aggression) reactions, termed agonistic behavior, have been elicited from different regions of the amygdaloid complex (2600). In the amygdaloid complex the intensity of the electrical current determines the intensity of the response, but unlike similar hypothalamic stimulation, the response builds up gradually and always outlasts the period of stimulation (2792). The reactions of fear and rage can be intense and are associated with pupillary dilatation, piloerection, growling, hissing and unmistakable signs of emotional involvement and participation of the autonomic nervous system. Electrical stimulation of the stria terminalis, or of the ventral amygdalofugal fibers, produces components of the defense reaction, but lesions of the stria terminalis do not alter the responses obtained by stimulating the amygdala (1100). After lesions completely interrupting the ventral amygdalofugal projections, defense reactions can no longer be obtained by stimulating the amygdaloid complex (2792). These findings suggest that the basolateral part of the amygdaloid complex may play an important role in defense reactions. In man stimulation of the amygdaloid region sometimes produces feelings of fear, confusional states, disturbances of awareness and anmesia for events taking place during the stimulation (738, 901,

1779). Although rage is the most common behavioral response to amygdaloid stimulation in animals, it rarely is associated with temporal lobe seizures or deep stimulation of the temporal lobe in man (901). On a few occasions rage has been elicited by amygdaloid stimulation in man (1065, 1604).

Electrical stimulation of the amygdala may enhance or suppress certain forms of attack behavior elicited by concurrent stimulation of the hypothalamus in cats (757). In these experiments low intensity stimulation of the amygdala alone produced no behavioral effects. Hypothalamic stimulation alone produced a form of predatory attack only when an appropriate object was present in the test chamber. When lateral amygdaloid nucleus and hypothalamic stimulation were applied together, the latency of attack was shortened (facilitated). Medial amygdala stimulation lengthened the latency (i.e., inhibits attack).

Visceral and autonomic responses resulting from amygdala stimulation include alterations of respiratory rate, rhythm and amplitude, as well as inhibition of respiration. The most common response of amygdala stimulation in unanesthetized animals is an acceleration of the respiratory rate associated with a reduction in amplitude (1250). Inhibition of respiration in animals and man has been elicited particularly from ventral parts of the amygdala (1251, 2312). Cardiovascular responses involve both increases and decreases in arterial blood pressure and alterations of heart rate. Pressor responses appear to predominate following amygdala stimulation in unanesthetized animals (2129). Gastrointestinal motility and secretion may be inhibited or activated, and both defecation and micturition may be induced. Piloerection, salivation, pupillary changes and alterations of body temperature can occur. These responses are both sympathetic and parasympathetic in nature.

Somatic responses obtained by stimulation of the amygdaloid complex include turning of the head and eyes to the opposite side, and complex rhythmic movements related to chewing, licking and swallowing. It is of interest that the varied somatic and autonomic effects of electrical stimulation of the amygdaloid complex constitute an insignificant part of the syndrome produced by lesions in this complex.

Endocrine responses to stimulation of the amygdaloid nuclear complex include the release of ACTH and gonadotrophic hormone, and lactogenic responses. As might be expected, stimulation of amygdaloid areas that produce arousal and emotional responses also produce increased adrenocortical hormone output (1250, 2800). Bilateral lesions in the medial amygdaloid nuclei produce an elevation of serum levels of ACTH (697) presumably due to release of an inhibitory influence upon the secretion of ACTH (223, 697). More extensive damage to the amygdala or its hypothalamic projection system may attenuate, but not abolish corticosteroid responses (2800). Stimulation of the corticomedial division of the amygdala may induce ovulation; this response is abolished by transection of the stria terminalis (726, 2312, 2611). The corticomedial nuclei of the amygdala have many estrogen concentrating neurons in females, and constitute part of a system of such cells which extends into other limbic and hypothalamic structures (1997). The amygdala also has been implicated in the regulation of luteinizing (LH) and follicle-stimulating (FSH) hormone release, but evidence is somewhat conflicting (1250). However, evidence is quite clear that the amygdala participates with the hypothalamus in the control and regulation of hypophysial secretions.

Bilateral lesions, fairly well confined to the amygdaloid complex, in monkeys and cats consistently produce disturbances of emotional behavior (57, 900, 954, 957, 1250, 2021, 2069, 2544). The animals become placid and display no reactions of fear, rage or aggression. Previously dominant and abusive animals become tame and do not retaliate to the threats or molestations of other animals. Hypersexuality has been noted as a prominent feature in some experimental studies (957, 2287), but not in all. There are some indications that hypersexual behavior may occur only when the lesions concomitantly involve the pyriform cortex, since amygdaloid lesions sparing this region do not alter sexual behavior. In most instances hypersexual behavior following bilateral lesions develops after a latent period of several weeks. Castration will prevent hypersexuality, or cause it to disappear, following bilateral amygdalectomy (2287), but this should not necessarily be interpreted as indicating that an increased production of sex hormone is the basic cause of hypersexuality in these animals (900) or even that the behavior represents a specific increase in copulatory behavior. It appears that the temporal lobe lesions produce a more general change in approach and withdrawal behavior (86).

In a number of studies, all in cats, removal of the amygdala has led to increased aggressiveness (113, 114, 957). Cats displaying postoperative rage frequently developed seizures which were considered to play a role in the savage behavior. Theoretically, the aggressive savage behavior is caused by removal of structures exerting inhibitory influences, but their identification has been elusive.

Observations in man concerning the effects of bilateral lesions in the amygdaloid complex indicate that these lesions cause a decrease of aggressive and assaultive behavior (960, 2044, 2304). Reports concerning stereotaxic lesions in the amygdaloid complex in man (1799, 1800) suggest that such lesions produce a marked reduction in emotional excitability and tend to normalize the social behavior and adaptation of individuals with severe behavior disturbances. Unilateral lesions in some cases proved sufficient to bring about definite improvement. Small bilateral lesions did not produce signs and symptoms suggestive of the Klüver-Bucy syndrome. The *Klüver-Bucy syndrome* is characterized by conversion of wild, intractable animals (monkeys) to docile beasts which show no evidence of fear, rage or aggression (1335). In addition, these animals display apparent "psychic blindness," a compulsion to examine objects visually, tactually and orally, bizarre sexual behavior and certain changes in dietary habits. These animals appear unable to distinguish between food and potentially dangerous objects. Almost all objects are examined, smelled and mouthed; if the object is not edible, it is discarded. Hypersexuality is characterized by the indiscriminate partnerships sought with both male and female animals. Tendencies to explore objects orally and docile behavior persist for years in these animals (1333). The Klüver-Bucy syndrome has been described in man following large bilateral removals of portions of the temporal lobe (2534, 2535) and following temporal lobe meningoencepha-

litis (1607).

The amygdaloid complex also plays an important role in food and water intake. Depending on their location, bilateral ablations of the amygdala may result in striking hyperphagia, or in hypophagia. Lesions of the basolateral nucleus of the amygdala result in hyperphagia (775), while stimulation of this part of the amygdala produces an arrest of feeding behavior (776). It has been postulated that this part of the amygdaloid complex inhibits the lateral hypothalamic area, which is regarded as the feeding center of the hypothalamus (1250, 1889).

The corticomedial part of the amygdaloid complex is a facilitatory area concerned with food intake. Stimulation of this region produces increases in food intake, as does stimulation of the stria terminalis (2188, 2189). The amygdala appears to exert its influence upon feeding by modulating the activity of hypothalamic mechanisms (2473) (Fig. 18-18). As might be expected, the effects of amygdaloid lesions are less severe than those involving the hypothalamus. Hypophagia is produced by bilateral lesions of the corticomedial amygdaloid nucleus and is more severe in the rat than in the cat; it is not found in the monkey (1331).

LIMBIC SYSTEM

On the medial surface of the cerebral hemisphere, a large arcuate convolution formed primarily by the cingulate and parahippocampal gyri surrounds the rostral brain stem and interhemispheric commissures (Fig. 2-5). These gyri, which encircle the upper brain stem, constitute what Broca (257) referred to as the *grand lobe limbique*.

Limbic Lobe. The limbic lobe includes the subcallosal, cingulate and parahippocampal gyri, as well as the underlying hippocampal formation and dentate gyrus (Fig. 18-17). From a phylogenetic and cytoarchitectural point of view, the limbic lobe consists of *archicortex* (hippocampal formation and dentate gyrus), *paleocortex* (pyriform cortex of the anterior parahippocampal gyrus), and *juxtallocortex* or *mesocortex* (cingulate gyrus). The latter represents a type of cortex that is transitional between allocortex and neocortex. Some authors in addition have included the cortex of the posterior orbital surface of the

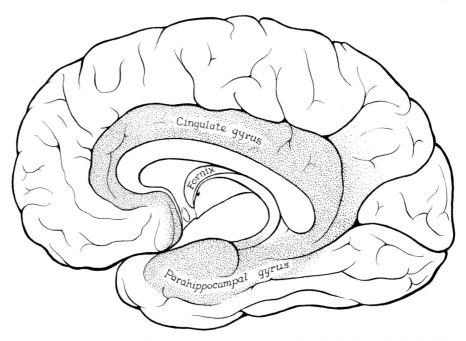

Figure 18-17. Drawing of the medial surface of the hemisphere. *Shading* indicates the limbic lobe which encircles the upper brain stem. Although the cortical areas designated as the limbic lobe have some common structural characteristics, the extent to which they form a functional unit is not clear.

frontal lobe, the anterior insular region and the temporal polar region, because of cytoarchitectural and functional similarities. One of the striking features of the limbic lobe is the constancy of its gross and microscopic structure throughout phylogeny, compared with that of the expanding neopallium which surrounds it. Although the cortical areas designated as the limbic lobe have some common structural characteristics, the extent to which they form a functional unit is not understood.

An even more extensive and inclusive designation is the *limbic system*. This term is used to include all components of the limbic lobe (Fig. 18-17) as well as associated subcortical nuclei (Fig. 18-6), such as the amygdaloid complex, septal nuclei, hypothalamus, epithalamus, anterior thalamic nuclei and parts of the basal ganglia (1549). Nauta (1816) regards the medial tegmental region of the midbrain as part of the limbic system, since anatomical connections, both ascending and descending, relate this region to the hippocampal formation and the amygdaloid complex. Despite the heterogeneity and diffuse nature of the so-called limbic system, there are compelling obser-

vations that structures comprising this system are related by a neural circuitry that gives rise to a subcortical continuum that begins in the septal area and extends in a paramedian zone through the preoptic region and hypothalamus into the rostral mesencephalon. In this view the hypothalamus is regarded as the central part of this system which suggests the term "septo-hypothalamo-mesencephalic continuum" (1820). The principal pathways inter-relating the thalamic nuclei and the brain stem reticular formation with the hippocampus and amygdaloid complex appear to come together in this region (Figs. 18-6 and 18-7).

The role of the cerebral cortex in the subjective aspects of emotion has been emphasized repeatedly, yet the neocortex appears to have relatively few hypothalamic connections and comparatively little autonomic representation. The intimate relationship of the limbic lobe with the hypothalamus, and the inclusion of these neural structures within the limbic system, have caused many authors to refer to the limbic system as the "visceral brain (1549)." Papez's proposed mechanism of emotion,

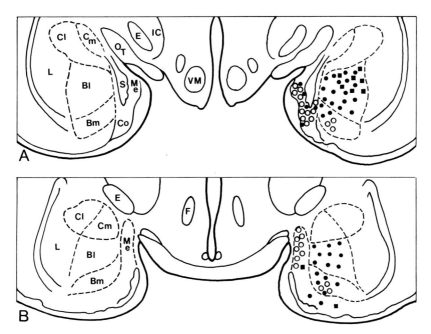

Figure 18-18. Diagrams of the amygdala of the cat at the level of the tuberal region (*A*) and the optic chiasm (*B*). The major nuclear boundaries are shown with *dashed lines*. On the right side of the diagrams are the locations of cell bodies labeled by retrograde transport of horseradish peroxidase injected into three locations in the hypothalamus: ○, ventromedial nucleus; ■, lateral hypothalamus; ●, preoptic area (modified from Sutin and McBride, '79 (2474)). Abbreviations: *Bl*, basolateral nucleus of amygdala (magnocellular); *Bm*, basomedial nucleus of amygdala (parvicellular); *Cl*, central amygdaloid nucleus, lateral part; *Cm*, central amygdaloid nucleus, medial part; *Co*, cortical nucleus of amygdala; *E*, entopeduncular nucleus (part of corpus striatum); *F*, fornix; *IC*, internal capsule; *L*, lateral nucleus of amygdala; *Me*, medial nucleus of amygdala; *VM*, ventromedial nucleus of hypothalamus; *S*, stria terminalis.

which implicated structures of the limbic system, received experimental support from the studies of Klüver and Bucy (1335) on monkeys deprived of parts of both temporal lobes.

Various visceral, somatic and behavioral responses also are obtained by electrical stimulation of the anterior cingulate cortex and the orbital-insular-temporal cortex. Elevation, as well as depression, of arterial blood pressure results from electrical stimulation of these regions in experimental animals (58, 1251). Points from which pressor and depressor effects can be obtained frequently are only a few millimeters apart; most authors report that declines in blood pressure are more frequent and of greater magnitude. Effects upon arterial pressure do not appear to be secondary to associated respiratory changes. Other autonomic responses obtained in experimental animals include inhibition of peristalsis in the pyloric antrum, pupillary dilatation, salivation

and bladder contraction. Perhaps the most striking effect of stimulating these regions is profound inhibition of respiratory movements (2365), which involves mainly the inspiratory phase of the respiratory cycle. Acceleration of respiratory movements, produced most readily in the dog, can be elicited by stimulating portions of the cingulate gyrus posterior to the zone yielding maximum inhibitory effects.

Somatic effects obtained by stimulating the anterior cingulate and orbital-insular-temporal cortex include: (a) inhibition of spontaneous movements, (b) inhibition and facilitation of cortically induced and reflex movements, and (c) chewing, licking and swallowing movements. Inhibition of spontaneous movements is associated with muscular relaxation and inhibition of respiration. Cortically induced movements appear to be more readily facilitated than spinal reflexes.

Neither unilateral nor bilateral ablations

of the cingulate cortex, or of the cortex of the orbital-insular-temporal polar region, appear to disturb basic somatomotor or autonomic functions to any marked degree. These ablations do not alter: (a) voluntary or reflex motor performance, (b) muscle tone, or (c) respiratory, cardiovascular or gastrointestinal functions.

Experiments have shown that electrical stimulation of certain parts of the limbic system via implanted electrodes in unanesthetized rats, cats and monkeys produces self-stimulation behavior (238, 1871). In these studies the experimental arrangement is such that the animals can deliver an electrical stimulus to localized areas of their own brains by pressing a pedal or bar. Self-stimulations of the septal region, the anterior preoptic area and the posterior hypothalamus by bar pressing may be at rates as high as 5000/hr in the rat (1870). The behavior seen in these situations, where the only reward is an electric shock to a localized region of the brain, suggests that the stimulus may provide a primary reinforcement. Repeated self-stimulation may occur in the monkey from electrodes implanted in a variety of subcortical sites, such as the head of the caudate nucleus, the amygdaloid complex, the medial forebrain bundle and the midbrain reticular formation (238). Self-stimulation of certain regions of the thalamus and hypothalamus may produce avoidance reactions, but these regions appear relatively small in number compared to those in which stimulation is rewarding.

There is general agreement that the limbic lobe and system occupy central positions in the neural mechanisms that govern behavior and emotion. The components of the limbic system appear to have their main afferent and efferent relationships with two great functional realms, the neocortex and the autonomic and endocrine systems. Among the most prominent neocortical connections are the fibers of the cingulum which arise from the cingulate cortex (Figs. 2-10 and 2-19) and project to the entorhinal cortex along with fibers from other neocortical areas. The entorhinal cortex is a major site of convergence of cortical inputs to the hippocampal formation. Stated broadly and simply, impulses generated in sensory systems, the cerebral cortex and the limbic system appear to activate mechanisms that in turn excite visceral and somatic effectors whose activities provide the physiological expression of behavior and emotion.

The *nucleus accumbens*, which lies ventral to the caudate nucleus, receives afferent fibers from the basolateral nucleus of the amygdala and appears to link limbic structures with the basal ganglia (968, 1826). Anatomical considerations have led Mesulam and Geschwind (1679) to propose that nucleus accumbens may be part of a limbic-inferior parietal lobule circuit concerned with mechanisms of attention in man and sub-human primates.

The functions of the so-called limbic system are complex and multiple, and the functions of the separate parts may be expressed through distinctive neural structures. Visceral functions appear to predominate in the amygdaloid complex, the anterior cingulate gyrus and the cortex of the orbital-insular-temporal region. Amygdaloid efferent fibers contained in the stria terminalis and the ventral amygdalofugal pathways projecting to the septal region, the preoptic region and portions of the hypothalamus mediate most of the responses produced by stimulation of the amygdaloid complex (Fig. 18-18). However, it must be recalled that amygdalofugal fibers also project to the dorsomedial nucleus of the thalamus via the inferior thalamic peduncle and to specific cortical regions (1817). Although the limbic system has been referred to as the "visceral brain," there are some parts of the system in which no visceral function has been demonstrated. In addition certain somatic functions appear to be intermingled inseparably with visceral functions.

CHAPTER 19

The Cerebral Cortex

STRUCTURE OF THE CORTEX

The cerebral cortex develops from the telencephalon which in early stages of histogenesis resembles other parts of the embryonic neural tube. The suprastriatal portion of the early telencephalic vesicle is composed of three concentric zones in its smooth-surfaced (lissencephalic) stage: (a) a *germinal zone* surrounding the lateral ventricle, (b) the *intermediate zone* which becomes the white matter of the cerebral hemispheres, and (c) a *marginal zone* which becomes the cortical zone or plate. The original columnar epithelial cells extend through all zones (2337). At the end of the 2nd month cells migrate from the intermediate zone into the marginal zone, where they form a superficial gray layer, the *cerebral cortex*. As the cerebral cortex gradually thickens by the addition and differentiation of the migrating cells, it assumes a laminated appearance. As cells become organized into horizontal layers, between the 6th and 8th months, six such layers may be distinguished (301). The deeper pyramidal layer, rich in cells, forms layers II to VI, while the outermost layer, composed mostly of fibers, becomes the molecular layer (I). Cells formed at the same time tend to remain in the same layer, and newly formed cells migrate through these layers to more superficial locations (77). This "inside-out" sequence of neuronal migration applies to the majority of cortical cells. This six-layered cellular arrangement is characteristic of the entire neopallial cortex, which is referred to as *neocortex, isocortex* (2625) or *homogenetic cortex* (301). The *paleopallium* (olfactory cortex) and the *archipallium* (hippocampal formation and dentate gyrus) do not show six layers in either the developing or adult stage. The paleopallium and archipallium together constitute the *allocortex* or *heterogenetic cortex*.

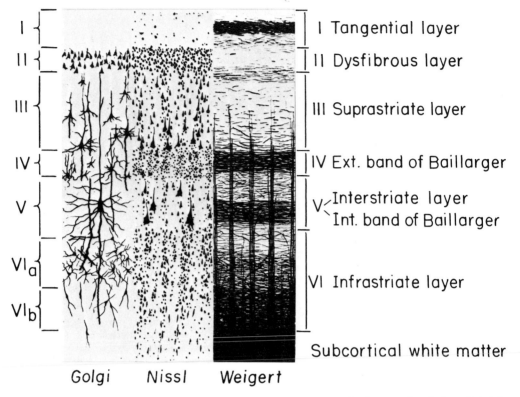

I Tangential layer
II Dysfibrous layer
III Suprastriate layer
IV Ext. band of Baillarger
V Interstriate layer
Int. band of Baillarger
VI Infrastriate layer

Subcortical white matter

Golgi   Nissl   Weigert

Figure 19-1. The cell layers and fiber arrangement of the human cerebral cortex (semischematic) (after Brodmann (301)).

The cerebral cortex has an area of approximately 2200 cm² (2.5 sq ft), only one-third of which is on the free surface; the remaining cerebral cortex is hidden in the depths of the sulci. The thickness of the cortex varies from about 4.5 mm in the precentral gyrus to about 1.5 mm in the depths of the calcarine sulcus. The cortex is always thickest over the crest of a convolution and thinnest in the depth of a sulcus. It has been estimated that besides nerve fibers, neuroglia and blood vessels, the cerebral cortex contains nearly 14 billion neurons (682).

The cerebral cortex contains: (a) *afferent fibers* and *terminals* from other parts of the nervous system (e.g., thalamocortical fibers), (b) *association* and *commissural neurons* whose axons inter-relate cortical regions of the same or opposite hemisphere, and (c) *projection neurons* whose axons conduct impulses to other parts of the neuraxis (e.g., corticospinal, corticoreticular or corticopontine fibers). Most projection fibers arise from the deeper layers of the cortex, while the association and commissural fibers arise mainly from the more superficial ones (1245). A striking feature of pallial structure is the relatively small number of projection fibers compared with the enormous number of cortical neurons.

Cortical Cells and Fibers. Although the cerebral cortex contains an enormous number of cells, the number of cell types is small (507). The principal types of cells found in the cortex are pyramidal, stellate and fusiform neurons (Figs. 4-5, 19-1 and 19-2).

The pyramidal cells, which are most characteristic of the cortex, have the form of an isosceles triangle whose upper pointed end is continued toward the surface of the brain as the *apical dendrite*. Besides the apical dendrite, a number of more or less horizontally running *basal dendrites* spring from the cell body and arborize in its vicinity. The axon emerges from the base of the cell and descends toward the medullary substance, either terminating in the deeper layers of the cortex, or entering the white

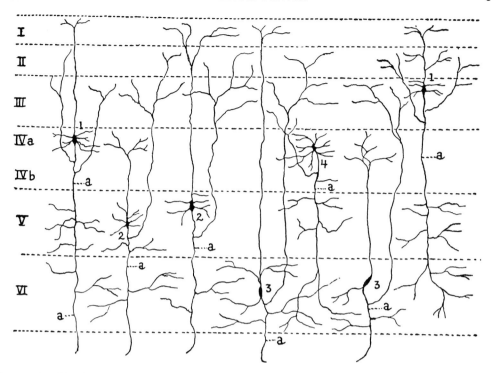

Figure 19-2. The dendritic and axonal branchings of several types of cortical neurons with descending axons. Semischematic. *1*, Pyramidal cells of superficial layers; *2*, pyramidal cells from ganglionic layer; *3*, spindle cells; *4*, stellate cells; *a*, axon. (Based on data by Cajal (348) and Lorente de Nó (1531).)

matter as a projection, or association fiber. Pyramidal cells have large vesicular nuclei, prominent Nissl granules and usually are classified as small, medium and large. The height of the cell body varies from 10 to 12 µm for the smaller neurons to 45 or 50 µm for the larger ones. The giant pyramidal cells of Betz, found in the precentral gyrus, may be more than 100 µm in height.

The *stellate* or *granule cells* are small, polygonal or triangular in shape and have dark-staining nuclei and scanty cytoplasm. These cells, ranging from 4 to 8 µm, have a number of dendrites passing in all directions and a short axon which ramifies close to the cell body (Golgi type II). Other larger stellate cells have longer axons which may enter the medullary substance. Some resemble pyramidal cells in that they have an apical dendrite which extends to the surface. These cells are known as *stellate or star pyramidal cells* (1531). Stellate cells are found throughout all layers of the cortex but are especially numerous in layer IV.

The *fusiform cells* are found mainly in the deepest cortical layer, with their long

axis vertical to the surface. The two poles of the cell are continued into dendrites; the lower dendrites arborize within the layer, while the upper ones ascend toward the surface. The axon arises from the middle or lower part of the cell body, and enters the white matter as a projection fiber. The large fusiform cells have been classified as "modified pyramidal" cells (2329).

Other cell types found in the cortex are the *horizontal cells of Cajal*, and the *cells with ascending axons*, known as the *cells of Martinotti* (*M* in Fig. 19-3). The former are small fusiform cells found in the most superficial cortical layer; their long axons run horizontally for considerable distances and arborize within that layer. Martinotti cells, present in practically all cortical layers, are small triangular cells whose axons are directed toward the surface. Some fibers arborize in the same layer; others send collaterals to a number of layers.

Fibers in the cerebral cortex are disposed both radially and tangentially. The former are arranged in delicate radiating bundles running vertically from the medullary sub-

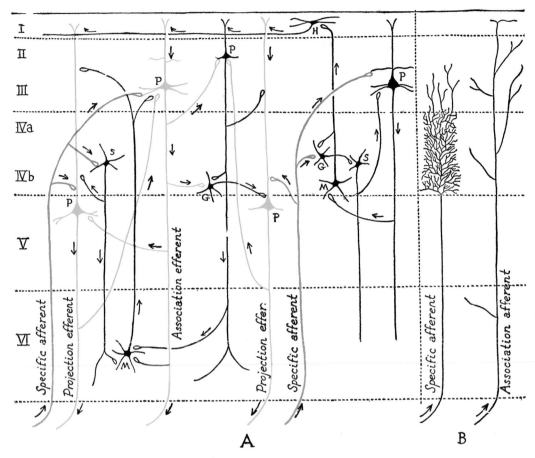

Figure 19-3. (*A*) Diagram showing some of the intracortical circuits. Synaptic junctions are indicated by *loops*. *Red*, Afferent thalamocortical fibers; *blue*, efferent cortical neurons; *black*, intracortical neurons; *G*, granule cell; *H*, horizontal cell; *M*, Martinotti cell; *P*, pyramidal cell; *S*, stellate cell. (*B*) Mode of termination of afferent cortical fibers. (Based on data by Lorente de Nó (1531).)

stance toward the cortical surface (Fig. 19-1). They include the axons of pyramidal, fusiform and stellate cells, which leave the cortex as projection or association fibers, and the entering afferent and association fibers, which terminate within the cortex. Ascending axons of the Martinotti cells likewise have a vertical course.

The tangential fibers run horizontal to the cortical surface. They are composed principally of: (a) the terminal branches of the afferent and association fibers, (b) the axons of the horizontal and granule cells and (c) the terminal branches of collaterals from the pyramidal and fusiform cells. The horizontal fibers represent, in large part, the terminal portions of the radial fibers, which bend horizontally to come into synaptic relation with cortical cells. The tan-

gential fibers are not distributed evenly throughout the cortex. They are concentrated at varying depths into horizontal bands separated by layers with relatively few fibers (Fig. 19-1). The two most prominent bands, known as the *bands of Baillarger*, are visible to the naked eye as delicate white stripes in sections of the fresh cortex.

The Cortical Layers. In sections stained by the Nissl method, cell bodies are not uniformly distributed, but are arranged in superimposed horizontal layers. Each layer is distinguished by the types, density and arrangements of its cells. In preparations stained for myelin, a similar lamination is visible; in this case it is determined primarily by the disposition of the horizontal fibers, which differ in amount and density for each cellular layer (Fig. 19-1). In the neopallial cortex or isocortex, which forms 90% of the hemispheric surface, six fundamental layers are recognized (301); some of these layers are divided into sublayers. In the neocortex the following layers are distinguished in passing from the pial surface to the underlying white matter: I, molecular; II, external granular; III, external pyramidal; IV, internal granular; V, internal pyramidal; and VI, multiform.

I. The *molecular layer* contains cells with horizontal axons and Golgi type II cells. Within it are the terminal dendritic ramifications of the pyramidal and fusiform cells from the deeper layers, and the axonal endings of Martinotti cells. These dendritic and axonal branches form a fairly dense tangential fiber plexus (Fig. 19-1).

II. The *external granular layer* consists of numerous closely packed small granule cells whose apical dendrites terminate in the molecular layer and whose axons descend to the deeper cortical layers. This layer is poor in myelinated fibers.

III. The *external pyramidal layer* is composed mainly of well formed pyramidal neurons. Two sublayers are recognized: a superficial layer of medium-sized pyramids, and a deeper layer of larger ones. Their apical dendrites go to the first layer, while most of their axons enter the white matter, chiefly as association or commissural fibers (1245, 2499). Intermingled with the pyramidal neurons are granule and Martinotti cells. In the most superficial part of the layer a number of horizontal myelinated fibers constitute the band of Kaes-Bechterew.

IV. The *internal granular layer* is composed chiefly of closely packed stellate cells, many of which have short axons ramifying within the layer. Other larger cells have descending axons which terminate in deeper layers, or may enter the white substance. The whole layer is premeated by a dense horizontal plexus of myelinated fibers, forming the external band of Baillarger (Fig. 19-1).

V. The *internal pyramidal layer* consists of medium-sized and large pyramidal neurons intermingled with granule and Martinotti cells. The apical dendrites of the larger pyramids ascend to the molecular layer; dendrites of the smaller pyramids

ascend only to layer IV, or may even arborize within this layer (Figs. 19-2 and 19-3). Axons of these cells enter the white matter chiefly as projection fibers, although a small number of callosal fibers are furnished by the smaller pyramidal cells. The horizontal fiber plexus in the deeper portion of this layer constitutes the internal band of Baillarger.

VI. The *multiform* or *fusiform layer* contains predominantly spindle-shaped cells whose long axes are perpendicular to the cortical surface. Like the pyramidal neurons of layer V, the spindle cells vary in size; the larger ones send dendrites into the molecular layer, while the dendrites of the smaller ones ascend only to layer IV, or arborize within the fusiform layer. The dendrites of many pyramidal and spindle cells from layers V and VI come into direct relation with the endings of sensory thalamocortical fibers, which ramify chiefly in the internal granular layer. Axons of the spindle cells enter the white substance mainly as projection fibers. Some of the short arcuate association fibers connecting adjacent convolutions are furnished by the deep stellate cells of layer VI (1531). The multiform layer may be divided into an upper sublayer of densely packed larger cells, and a lower one of loosely arranged small cells. The whole layer is pervaded by fiber bundles which enter or leave the medullary substance (Fig. 19-3).

Besides the horizontal cellular lamination, the cortex also exhibits a vertical radial arrangement of the cells, which gives the appearance of slender vertical cell columns extending the thickness of the cortex (Figs. 19-9 and 19-10). This vertical lamination, quite distinct in the parietal, occipital and temporal lobes, is practically absent in the frontal lobe. The columnar arrangement of cells in the cerebral cortex appears to be determined largely by the mode of termination of corticocortical afferents rather than specific sensory afferents (2499). Corticocortical afferents are distributed throughout all layers of the cortex in columnar modules 200 to 300 μm in diameter, while terminals of specific sensory afferents usually are restricted to layer IV. It is remarkable that columnar units of corticocortical afferents are all nearly the same size and have dimensions similar to physiologically identified columnar units in the specific sensory cortex (909, 1154, 1763, 1843a, 2499). The arrangement into vertical cell columns is produced by the radial fibers of the cortex, just as the horizontal lamination is largely determined by the distribution of the tangential fibers.

The internal granular layer, which receives the main specific afferent projections and is best developed in the primary sensory areas, has been used to distinguish supragranular and infragranular layers. The *supragranular layers* (II and III) are the last to arise, the most highly differentiated and the most extensive in man (1254). These layers are considered to be concerned mainly with associative cortical functions. The *infragranular layers* (V and VI), well developed in all mammals, give rise to subcortical projection fibers concerned with efferent mechanisms. The supragranular layers are not present in the archipallium or paleopallium.

Interrelation of Cortical Neurons. The structure of the cerebral cortex as seen in Nissl or myelin sheath stained sections is incomplete, for these stains reveal only the type and arrangement of cell bodies, or the course and distribution of myelinated fibers. These methods give no information regarding terminal dendritic and axonal arborizations, which contain the synaptic junctions through which nerve impulses are transmitted. An understanding of the neuronal relationships, and of intracortical circuits, can be obtained from: (a) classic Golgi studies, (b) electron microscopic studies of various types of synaptic relationships and (c) electron microscopic reconstructions of clearly identified Golgi-stained neurons. With the Golgi technic the distribution of dendritic and axonal terminals has been studied by a number of investigators, notably Cajal (348). Lorente de Nó (1531) has given a detailed account for the elementary pattern of cortical organization that is applicable to the parietal, temporal and occipital isocortex. The arrangement of the axonal and dendritic branchings forms one of the most constant features of cortical organization. Most cortical interneurons also are highly specific with respect to their pattern of axonal arborizations and their synaptic contacts with other cortical neurons which form local networks.

The afferent fibers to the cortex include projection fibers from the thalamus, association fibers from other cortical areas of the same hemisphere and commissural fibers from the opposite side. The thalamocortical fibers, especially the specific afferent ones from the ventral tier thalamic nuclei and the geniculate bodies, pass unbranched to layer IV (Figs. 10-1, 10-6, 10-7, 12-27, 14-17, 15-14 and 15-15). Here the axons form a dense terminal plexus (507); some of the fibers extend to layer III where they arborize (Fig. 19-3*B*). Specific afferent fibers in layer IV establish both axodendritic and axosomatic synapses upon stellate neurons which are fantastically profuse on some cells (Fig. 19-4) (507). Estimates of the number of synaptic contacts upon neurons in the motor and visual cortex in the monkey indicate as many as 60,000 synapses per neuron in the motor area and 5600 in the striate cortex (560). In addition these cells receive synaptic contacts from intracortical neurons.

Fibers of the so-called nonspecific thalamocortical system, related to the intralaminar thalamic nuclei and indirectly to the ascending reticular activating system, also reach the cerebral cortex. The intralaminar thalamic nuclei, which project mainly to the striatum, project diffuse collateral fibers to broad regions of the cerebral cortex (1234). The potent effects of the stimulation of the intralaminar thalamic and the brain stem reticular formation upon electrocortical activity probably are mediated by these diffuse collateral projections. These collateral projections to the cerebral cortex appear the same as the nonspecific cortical afferent fibers with diffuse connections described previously by Lorente de Nó (1531). According to Jasper (1209a), the synaptic termination of fibers of this nonspecific system in the cortex is chiefly axodendritic and widely distributed in all layers, but the principal physiological effects appear to be within the superficial layers. The recruiting response, recorded from the surface of the cerebral cortex, is regarded as a reflection of dendritic electrical activity, which implies that it is a graded response not dependent on the all-or-none firing of cortical cells (2079a).

Commissural fibers arise from cells in all cortical regions and interconnect homolo-

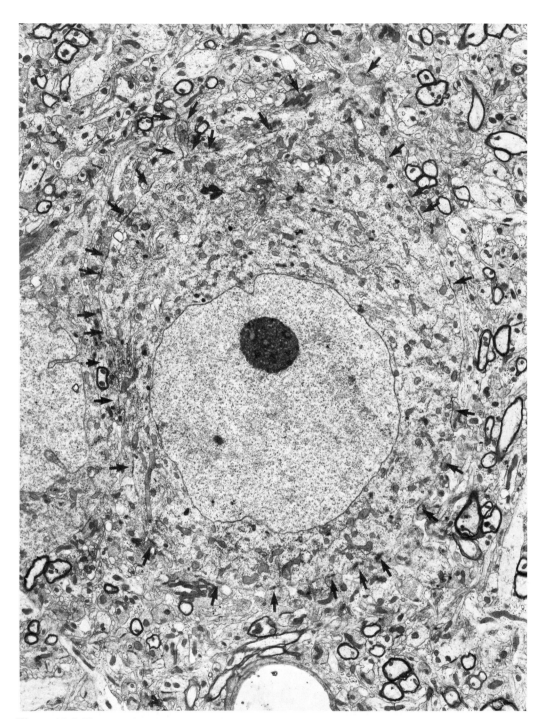

Figure 19-4. Electron micrograph of a stellate cell in the fourth layer of the striate cortex of the cat. *Arrows* indicate the large number of synaptic contacts (×5000). (Courtesy of Dr. Marc Colonier, School of Medicine, Laval University and Elsevier Publishing Company, Amsterdam.)

gous cortical areas. The majority of these fibers pass in the corpus callosum although some are found in the anterior commissure and the hippocampal commissure. Small injections of horseradish peroxidase (HRP) confined to a small cortical field results in retrograde labeling of cells in a small focus in the homologous site in the contralateral hemisphere. Exceptions to this generalization are found in the regions of the primary motor (area 4) and somesthetic cortex (S I) that represent the hand and foot (1233, 1245, 1269), in the visual cortex, area 17 (1160, 2761, 2763, 2794) and in parts of the auditory cortex (629). Commissural cells retrogradely labeled by HRP are large pyramidal cells in deep parts of layer III (1245). Cortical afferents from commissural neurons extend throughout all cortical layers and give off collaterals that fill a column about 200 to 300 μm in diameter (2499). Not all callosal fibers terminate in the entire columnar space and some collaterals terminate preferentially in particular layers. Similar studies of association fibers in the same hemisphere indicate that most of these fibers arise form the supragranular layers (1245). Ipsilateral corticocortical fibers arise from cells in more superficial parts of layer III and from parts of layer II. Terminal branches of association fibers are distributed mainly to layers III and IV but they have been identified in deeper layers as well (1236).

The cortical neurons may be grouped into cells with descending, ascending, horizontal and short axons. The last three types provide only intracortical connections (Fig. 19-3). The cells with descending axons (pyramidal, fusiform and larger stellate cells) furnish all the efferent projection and association fibers, and their axonal collaterals form extensive intracortical connections. Some descending axons which do not reach the medullary substance have only intracortical branches.

The pyramidal cells of layers II, III and IV have a similar pattern of dendritic and axonal branchings (Fig. 19-2). They have a number of basilar dendrites which arborize in the same layer, and an apical dendrite which ends in the molecular layer. Their descending axons in part terminate in the deeper layers of the cortex and, in part, are continued as association or callosal fibers.

They give off a few recurrent collaterals to their own layers, chiefly II and III, and numerous horizontal collaterals to layers V and VI, where they contribute to the horizontal plexuses.

The pyramidal and fusiform cells of layers V and VI have a characteristic pattern of dendritic and axonal branchings. All the pyramidal cells of layer V give off basilar dendrites to their own layer and an apical dendrite which extends to the molecular layer. There are, however, medium-sized pyramidal neurons, whose apical dendrites terminate in layer IV, and short pyramidal cells, whose dendrites all ramify in layer V (Fig. 19-2). The spindle cells of layer VI have similar branches. Axons of pyramidal and spindle neurons, and some of deep stellate cells are continued as projection fibers. All these axons send horizontal collaterals to layers V and VI, where they contribute to the horizontal plexuses, especially those of layer V (internal band of Baillarger). In addition, one or more recurrent collateral ascends unbranched to arborize in layers II and III, and some even extend to the molecular layer (Fig. 19-2).

The horizontal laminar arrangement of the cerebral cortex has served as one of the major criteria used to map the cortex into distinctive cytoarchitectonic areas, but it also serves to segregate different efferent projections from the cortex. Recent studies indicate that each of the major efferent pathways emanating from sensory-motor cortex has a specific laminar or sublaminar origin (1245). The somata of the majority of cells whose axons are distributed intracortically (both ipsilaterally and contralaterally) lie in the supragranular layers (layers II and III). Cortical neurons whose axons are projected to subcortical structures are located in the infragranular layers, particularly layer V. In the supragranular layers, cells whose axons are distributed ipsilaterally as corticocortical fibers lie superficial to cells projecting axons to the cortex of the opposite hemisphere, and cells with shorter axons tend to lie superficial to those with longer axons. In the infragranular layers the somata of corticostriate neurons lie in the most superficial part of layer V while somata giving rise to corticospinal and corticotectal fibers are in the deepest part of the same layer. Somata of neurons giving rise to corticorubral, corticopontine and corticobulbar fibers lie in intermediate regions of layer V, between corticostriate and corticospinal neurons. Layer VI of the cortex contains the somata of cells that give rise to corticothalamic projections. Cells giving rise to a particular set of efferent connections are of nearly the same size and do not vary in their laminar distribution. Only neurons giving rise to corticospinal fibers show great variation in cell size. Cells of particular efferent systems occur in single or multiple strips oriented mediolaterally across the cortex.

Functional Columnar Organization. Although the most striking feature of Nissl-stained sections of the cerebral cortex is its horizontal lamination, physiological studies of the somatic sensory and visual cortex indicate that a vertical column of cells, extending across all cellular layers, constitutes the elementary functional cortical units (1156, 1157, 1763, 2064). This conclusion is supported by the following evidence: (a) neurons of a particular vertical column are all related to the same, or nearly the same, peripheral receptive field, (b) neurons of the same vertical column are activated by the same peripheral stimulus, and (c) all cells of a vertical column discharge at more or less the same latency following a brief peripheral stimulus. The topographical pattern present on the cortical surface extends throughout its depth. Studies of the visual (striate) cortex demonstrate similar discrete functional columns extending from the pial surface to the white matter that are responsive to a specific kind of retinal stimulation in the form of long narrow rectangles of light ("slits"), dark bars against a light background, or straight-line borders, all of which have a particular axis of orientation (1156, 1157). Microelectrode recordings indicate that functional columns of cells are arranged radially, perpendicular to the cortical layers. Columns display variations in size and cross-sectional area but most fall within the 200 to 500 μm range (1157). The receptive field axis of orientation varies in a continuous manner as the surface of the cortex is traversed. Columns of cells in the striate cortex are of two types, ocular dominance columns and orientation columns (2717, 2718). Ocular dominance columns receive their input predominantly

from one eye, while orientation columns are concerned with the receptive field axis (Fig. 19-20).

Anatomically an elementary functional unit of the cortex, represented by a column of cells, must contain the afferent, efferent and internuncial fiber systems necessary for the formation of a complete cortical circuit (1843a). In the basic columnar units the internal circuitry must vary with differences in cytoarchitecture. The convergence of specific afferents upon cells in the columnar unit appears to imprint a specific sensory modality which is relayed by intracortical connections to other cells in the column. The complex axonal branching suggests that intracortical circuits involve cells in all parts of the column. These vertical circuits are interconnected by short neuronal links, represented primarily by the short axons of granule cells. Through these short links, cortical excitation may spread horizontally and involve a progressively larger number of vertical units (Fig. 19-3). Thus a specific afferent fiber may not only fire vertical columns of cells in its immediate vicinity, but may reach other units through Golgi type II cell relays. These vertical units are fundamentally similar in all mammals. However, the columns of cells with short relays increase in complexity in the higher forms, especially man. According to Cajal the unique morphological feature of the human cortex is the enormous number of Golgi type II cells, considered to interrelate vertical cell columns.

The cerebral cortex has been envisaged as a mosaic of columnar units of remarkably similar internal structure (2499). In addition to the functional columnar arrangement described in the sensory cortical areas, there are corticocortical columns delineated primarily by the pattern of termination of association and commissural fibers. The columnar units of corticocortical afferents are of the same general size as those of the functional columns of the sensory cortex. In the corticocortical columns there is a convergence of afferent fibers from multiple modular units that create a vast mosaic of cortical connections. Neurons within the cortical column are conceived of as being arranged in microcolumns, smaller than the larger units, concerned primarily with the vertical connec-

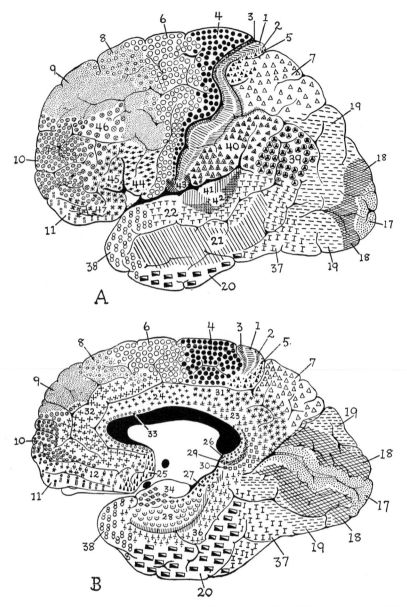

Figure 19-5. Cytoarchitectural map of human cortex. (*A*) Convex surface; (*B*) medial surface (after Brodmann (301)).

tivity within each column. Excitatory inputs from the thalamus and other cortical areas are considered to be processed through a column-oriented circuitry composed of both excitatory and inhibitory neurons. Most interneurons in the cerebral cortex are highly specific with respect to: (a) the neurons from which they receive inputs, (b) the arborization pattern of their axons, and (c) the specific sites at which they establish synapses on other neurons. The vast majority of stellate, or granular

cells belong to the heterogeneous group, referred to as Golgi type II cells, which do not project fibers beyond the cerebral cortex. Many unresolved problems remain concerning synaptic relationships of cells within the cortex, but electron microscopic evidence, based upon the types of synaptic contact, suggests that the majority of cortical interneurons are excitatory (asymmetrical synapses with spherical synaptic vesicles). Interneurons identified as putative inhibitory cells in the cortex constitute only

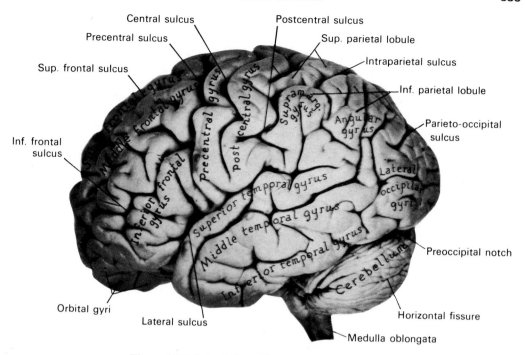

Figure 19-6. Lateral view of human brain (photograph).

a minority of the known interneuron types. Both excitatory and inhibitory influences within the cerebral cortex are exerted upon selected segments of pyramidal cells that represent the principal cortical output neurons.

CORTICAL AREAS

The cerebral cortex does not have a uniform structure. It has been mapped and divided into a number of distinctive areas that differ from each other in total thickness, in the thickness and density of individual layers and in the arrangement of cells and fibers. In certain areas the structural variations are so extreme that the basic six-layered pattern is practically obscured. Such areas are termed *heterotypical cortex*, as opposed to *homotypical*, which describes cortex in which the six layers are easily distinguished (301). Differences in the arrangements and types of cells, as well as the patterns of myelinated fibers, have been used to construct several fundamentally similar maps of the cortex composed of distinctive cytological areas (Fig. 19-5). Campbell (356) described some 20 cortical areas; Brodmann (301) increased the number to 47, and von Economo (682)

to 109; the Vogts (2625) parcelled the human cerebral cortex into more than 200 areas. Even the last number is apparently insufficient, since other investigators have found a number of distinctive cytoarchitectural areas in regions previously considered homogeneous (138, 2219). The brain map of Bailey and von Bonin (98) utilizes various colors to distinguish distinctive cytoarchitectural features. These authors felt that the concept of absolutely sharp areal boundaries has been carried to absurd lengths and that most brain maps failed to properly represent transitional areas. Brodmann's chart, which is the most widely used for reference, is shown in Figure 19-5. This cytoarchitectural map of the human cortex can be compared with the lateral view of the brain shown in Figure 19-6.

According to von Economo (682), all cortical structure is reducible to five fundamental types, based primarily on the relative development of granule and pyramidal cells. Types 2, 3 and 4, known respectively as the frontal, parietal and polar types, are homotypical and constitute by far the largest part of the cortex. Types 1 (agranular) and 5 (granulous) are heterotypical and limited to smaller specialized regions (Figs. 19-7 and 19-8).

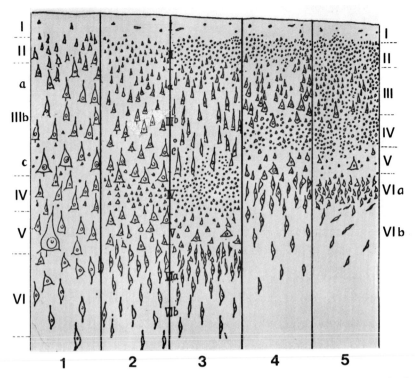

Figure 19-7. The five fundamental types of cortical structure: *1*, agranular; *2*, frontal; *3*, parietal; *4*, polar; *5*, granulous (koniocortex) (after Economo (682)).

Agranular type cortex (type 1) is distinguished by its thickness and the virtual absence of granule cells (Figs. 19-7 and 19-9, *A* and *B*). Pyramidal cells of layers III and V are well developed and large. Even the smaller cells in layers II and IV are predominantly pyramidal-shaped, making it difficult to distinguish individual layers. The agranular type cortex is represented classically by the cortex of the precentral gyrus.

Frontal type cortex (type 2) is relatively thick and shows six distinct layers. Pyramidal cells of layers III and V are large and well developed, as are the spindle cells of layer VI (Fig. 19-7). Although the granular layers are distinct, they are narrow and composed of loosely arranged small triangular cells.

Parietal type cortex (type 3) is characterized by even more distinctive cortical layers due to the greater thickness and cell density of the granular layers (Figs. 19-7 and 19-10, *A* and *B*). In this type of cortex, the pyramidal layers are thinner and their cells are smaller and more irregularly arranged.

Polar type cortex (type 4), found near the frontal and occipital poles, is characterized by its thinness, its well developed granular layers and its comparative wealth of cells.

Granulous type cortex or *koniocortex* (type 5) is extremely thin and is composed mainly of densely packed granule cells (Figs. 19-7 and 19-10C). These are found not only in layers II and IV, but the other layers, especially layer III, show large numbers of such small cells and a consequent reduction of the pyramidal cells. The most striking example of this type is the calcarine cortex (Fig. 19-10C).

The general distribution of these five types of cortex is shown in Figure 19-8. The agranular type cortex covers the caudal part of the frontal lobe in front of the central sulcus, the anterior half of the gyrus cinguli and the anterior portion of the insula. A narrow strip also is found in the retrosplenial region of the gyrus cinguli and

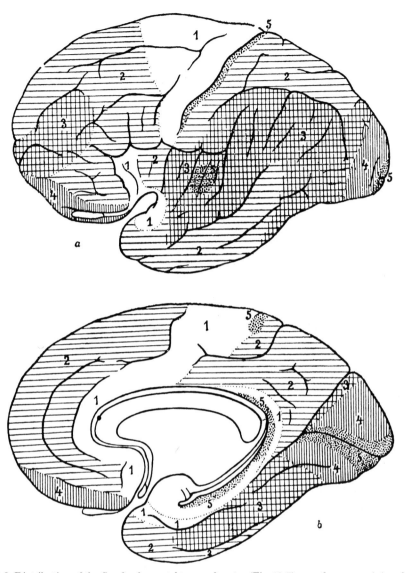

Figure 19-8. Distribution of the five fundamental types of cortex (Fig. 19-7) over the convex (*a*) and the medial (*b*) surfaces of the hemisphere: *1*, agranular; *2*, frontal; *3*, parietal; *4*, polar; *5*, granulous (koniocortex) (after Economo (682)).

is continued along the parahippocampal gyrus and uncus. Since the chief efferent fiber systems arise from these regions, especially from the precentral gyrus, the agranular cortex may be considered as efferent or motor type cortex (Figs. 10-13 and 11-30). The koniocortex may be regarded as primarily sensory in character, since it is found only in the areas receiving the specific sensory thalamocortical projections. These areas include the anterior wall of the postcentral gyrus, the banks of the calcarine

sulcus and the transverse temporal gyri (Heschl; Figs. 2-10 and 12-13).

By far the largest part of the hemispheric surface is covered by homotypical cortex. Frontal type cortex is spread over the larger anterior part of the frontal lobe, the superior parietal lobe, the precuneus and most of the middle and inferior temporal gyri. Parietal type cortex includes chiefly the inferior parietal lobule, the superior temporal gyrus, the occipitotemporal gyrus and the anterior convex parts of the occipital

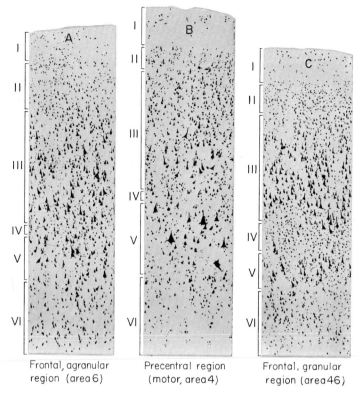

Figure 19-9. Cytoarchitectural pictures of several representative cortical areas (after Campbell (356)).

lobe. Polar type cortex, as the name implies, covers the frontal and occipital poles. The thalamic connections of these areas are mainly with the association nuclei, such as the dorsomedial, lateral dorsal, lateral posterior and the pulvinar.

Practically every part of the cerebral cortex is connected with subcortical centers by afferent and efferent projections. Strictly speaking there are no circumscribed cortical areas which are purely associative or projective in character. However, there are regions from which the more important descending tracts arise, which directly or through intercalated centers reach the lower motor neurons for the initiation and control of both somatic and visceral activities (1965). These primarily efferent or motor areas, from which muscular movements can be elicited by electrical stimulation, are concentrated chiefly in the precentral part of the frontal lobe. Similarly those cortical regions which receive direct thalamocortical sensory fibers from the ventral tier thalamic nuclei and from the geniculate

bodies represent the primary receptive or sensory areas. The remaining cortical areas which constitute the largest part of the cerebral cortex in man are referred to as "association areas." Although the primary sensory and motor areas are predominant in lower mammals in that they constitute unusually large parts of the neocortex, there is considerable intermingling of functions. In higher mammals, the primary sensory and motor areas become more specific, and there is an absolute increase in the association cortex (2771). Afferent fibers to the association areas are derived from association nuclei of the thalamus and from primary sensory areas of the cortex.

SENSORY AREAS OF THE CEREBRAL CORTEX

Primary Sensory Areas. The localized regions to which impulses concerned with specific sensory modalities are projected constitute the primary sensory areas of the cerebral cortex. Although certain aspects of sensation probably enter consciousness at

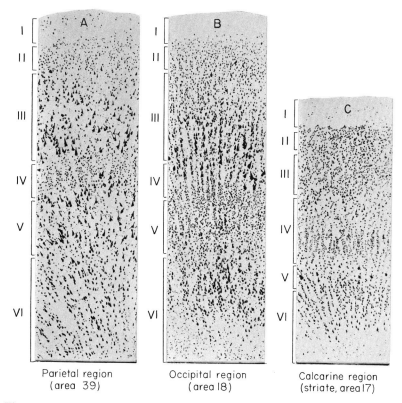

Figure 19-10. Cytoarchitectural picture of several cortical areas (after Campbell (356)).

thalamic levels, the primary sensory areas are concerned especially with the integration of sensory experience and with the discriminative qualities of sensation. With the exception of olfaction, impulses involved in all forms of sensation reach localized areas of the cerebral cortex via thalamocortical projections. The organization of the thalamus is such that all of the specific sensory relay nuclei are located caudally in the ventral tier (Figs. 15-14 and 15-15). The cortical projections of the specific sensory relay nuclei are to localized areas in the parietal, occipital and temporal lobes. Although there is probably a primary cortical receptive area for each sensory modality, each modality is not represented separately, and the primary sensory areas for some forms of sensation are poorly defined. Established primary sensory areas in the cerebral cortex are: (a) the *somesthetic area*, consisting of the postcentral gyrus and its medial extension in the paracentral lobule (areas 3, 1 and 2), (b) the *visual* or *striate area*, located along the lips of the

calcarine sulcus (area 17), and (c) the *auditory area*, located on the two transverse gyri (Heschl; areas 41 and 42; see Figs. 2-5, 2-7, 2-10, 12-13, 15-15 and 19-5). The *gustatory area* appears to be localized to the most ventral part (opercular) of the postcentral gyrus (area 43). The primary *olfactory area*, consisting of the allocortex of the prepyriform and periamygdaloid regions, is not assigned numbers under the Brodmann parcellation. A vestibular projection to the human cerebral cortex has not been established.

Secondary Sensory Areas. The primary sensory areas of the cerebral cortex undoubtedly receive the principal projections of the specific sensory relay nuclei of the thalamus, and are the focal regions in the cerebral cortex where specific sensory modalities are most extensively and critically represented. Evidence suggests that near each primary receptive area there are cortical zones which may receive sensory inputs directly from the thalamus, from the primary sensory area or from both (812,

1159). These cortical zones, adjacent to primary sensory areas, but outside of the principal projection area of the specific sensory relay nuclei of the thalamus, are referred to as the *secondary sensory areas*. Secondary areas have been defined and mapped in experimental animals by recording evoked potentials in response to peripheral stimulation (16, 17, 1159, 2019, 2543, 2697, 2775, 2778). Studies of these secondary sensory areas indicate that sequential representation of parts of the body, or of the tonotopic pattern in the case of the auditory areas, is not the same as in the primary areas (2218, 2771). The secondary sensory areas are smaller than the primary sensory areas, and the order of representation is the reverse, or different from that found in the primary areas. Evidence suggests that ablations of secondary sensory areas produce relatively minor sensory disturbances compared with those resulting from ablations of primary sensory areas. In the monkey ablations of the secondary somatic area do not appear to interfere with the performance tests based upon somesthetic discrimination (1891).

Secondary sensory areas, defined primarily in experimental animals, include: (a) a *second somatic sensory area* (somatic sensory area II; SS II), located ventral to the primary sensory and motor areas along the superior lip of the lateral sulcus (2190, 2708, 2771) (Figs. 19-13 and 19-14); (b) a *secondary auditory area* (auditory area II; A II), located ventral to the primary auditory area (auditory area I) in the cat (10, 1675, 1838, 2218); and (c) a *secondary visual area* (visual area II; V II), described in the rabbit, cat and monkey (48, 1159, 2511, 2543, 2592, 2770) as anterolateral to visual area I, and identical to the area defined anatomically as area 18 (Fig. 19-13). A second somatic sensory area has been demonstrated in man (1968), stimulation of which produces various sensations in the upper and lower extremities. Representation of the extremities is chiefly contralateral, although ipsilateral representation also is present. In man no cortical representation for the face, tongue, mouth or throat has been found in SS II. Because of the intimate functional relationships between the primary and secondary sensory areas, these will be discussed together.

The Primary Somesthetic Area (S I). The cortical area subserving general somatic sensibility, superficial as well as deep, is located in the postcentral gyrus and in the posterior part of the paracentral lobule. Histologically the gyrus is composed of three narrow strips of cortex (areas 3, 1, 2) which differ in their architectural structure (Figs. 19-5 and 19-11). In the postcentral region there is a definite anteroposterior gradient of morphological change, but the gradient is not uniformly gradual. The anterior part, area 3, is clearly distinguishable from the posterior part; areas 1 and 2 show more gradual morphological changes. Area 3 lies along the posterior wall of the central sulcus; its transition with area 4 anteriorly is not sharp and most of it lies in the depths of the central sulcus (Fig. 19-11). The cortex of area 3 is characterized by its thinness and by the fact that layers II, III and IV tend to fuse with each other (2063) and are composed of densely packed granule cells (682). Areas 1 and 2, forming, respectively, the crown and posterior wall of the postcentral gyrus, have a six-layered structure characteristic of homogenetic cortex (Fig. 19-11). The most marked differences between area 3 and area 1 are found in layer III; cells in layer III all become pyramidal in shape and there is a reduction in cell density. The transition from area 1 to area 2 is not sharply defined, but is characterized by an increase in the thickness of the cortex and an increase in the number of large pyramidal cells in layers III and V. The transition from area 2 to areas 5 and 7 is gradual; in the latter areas layers II and IV are sharply demarcated and a pronounced columnar arrangement of cells is seen (Fig. 19-5).

The postcentral gyrus receives the thalamic projections from the ventral posterior nuclei (VPL and VPM), which relay impulses from the medial lemniscus, the spinothalamic tracts, the secondary trigeminal tracts and ascending gustatory pathways from the nucleus of the solitary fasciculus. The majority of the cells of the ventral posterior nuclei project to area 3. Area 1, however, receives the exclusive projections of about 30% of the cells in these nuclei, but it also receives collaterals of fibers passing to area 3. Most of the fibers projecting to area 2 appear to be collaterals

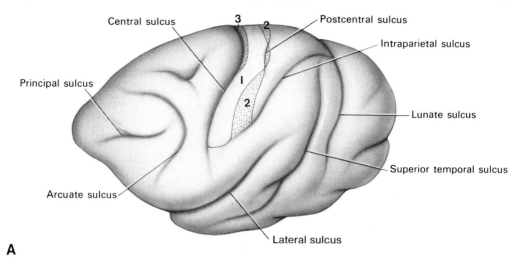

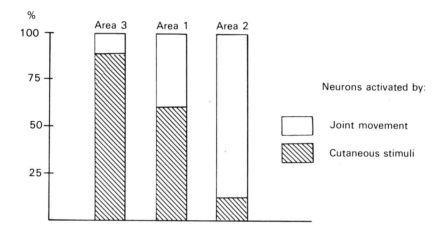

B

Figure 19-11. (*A*) Diagram of the lateral surface of the monkey cerebral hemisphere showing the extent of the three areas which compose the primary somesthetic cortex, Area 3, which forms the posterior wall of the central sulcus, is hidden, except for a small dorsomedial region indicated in the diagram. Areas 1 and 2 form the crown and posterior wall of the postcentral gyrus. (*B*) Bar graph indicating the relative prevalence in each cytoarchitectural area of the postcentral gyrus of neurons activated by cutaneous stimuli and joint movement. (Based upon Powell and Mountcastle (2063) and Mountcastle and Powell (1769).)

of fibers passing primarily to areas 3 and 1. Although most of the information concerning thalamocortical projections is based upon retrograde cellular degeneration (473, 477, 2178, 2651), studies of discrete lesions in the ventral posterior thalamic nuclei reveal that coarse fibers project profusely to area 3 while fibers projecting to areas 1 and 2 are of fine caliber and distribute terminals sparsely throughout these two areas (1241, 1244). Autoradiographic studies of the projections of the ventral posterior thalamic nuclei confirm the substantial projection to area 3, but do not resolve the question concerning collateral projections to areas 1 and 2 (1227). Because neurons in area 3

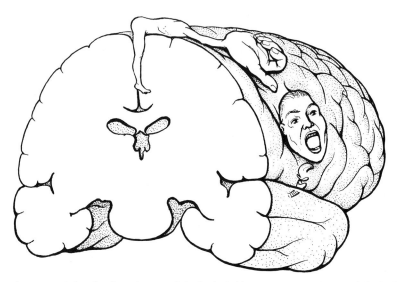

Figure 19-12. Somatotopic localization of parts of the body in the motor cortex. Parts of the body are drawn in proportion to the extent of their cortical representation. The resulting disproportionate figure is called the motor "homunculus." A similar pattern of localization with respect to somesthetic sense is found in the postcentral gyrus (after Penfield and Rasmussen (1968)).

respond preferentially to light tactile stimuli and cells in areas 1 and 2 are excited mainly by deep stimuli and joint movement, it would be expected that different populations of thalamic neurons would project to areas 3, 1 and 2 (2063, 2696). In the somatosensory cortex most of the thalamic afferents terminate in layer IV, but some end in deep parts of layer III (1227).

The various regions of the body are represented in specific portions of the postcentral gyrus, the pattern corresponding to that of the motor area (Fig. 19-12). Thus the face area lies in the most ventral part, while above it are the sensory areas for the hand, arm, trunk, leg and foot in the order named; the lower extremity extends into the paracentral lobule (Fig. 2-5). The cortical areas representing the hand, face and mouth regions are disproportionally large. The digits of the hand, particularly the thumb and index finger, are well represented. The cortical area related to sensations from the face occupies almost the entire lower half of the postcentral gyrus; the upper part of the face is represented above, while the lips and mouth are represented below. The tongue and pharyngeal region are localized in more ventral areas. The distorted representation of the body surface in the primary sensory area has been said to reflect the peripheral innerva-

tion density. Those regions of the body with higher densities of receptor elements have extensive cortical representation, while those regions with relative few receptors have a minimal representation. According to Penfield, sensations from intra-abdominal structures are represented near the opercular surface of the postcentral gyrus. Most of our information concerning the pattern of representation in the somesthetic cortex in man has been obtained from stimulating this region in patients operated upon under local anesthesia (1963, 1965, 1968). In attempts to present a readily apparent visual pattern of the sequence of sensory representation in the cerebral cortex, Penfield has drawn the "sensory homunculus" relating different parts of the body to appropriate areas of the cortex. The "sensory homunculus" corresponds to the "motor homunculus" (Fig. 19-12).

Using the evoked potential technic, Adrian (17) found that touch, pressure and movements were the only stimuli which evoked well marked responses in the contralateral postcentral gyrus in the cat. No responses were observed to pain or thermal stimuli. Pressure applied to a foot produced a sustained discharge which increased in frequency as the pressure was increased and gradually declined with a constant stimulus. Tactile stimuli produced brief discharges that were not sustained. The fact that one cortical locus frequently could be activated by touching hairs within a relatively large skin area indicates a considerable degree of convergence. This convergence of pathways in the sensory cortex was observed also by Marshall et al. (1614). Cortical responses were evoked contralaterally from all stimuli, except in the face area, where some ipsilateral responses were recorded.

Physiological studies (1769, 2064) in the monkey indicate that the majority of neurons in the postcentral gyrus are activated by mechanical stimulation, and are selectively excited by stimulation of receptors within either skin or deep tissues, but not by stimulation of both (Fig. 19-11). Over 90% of the neurons in area 2 are related to receptors in deep tissues of the body, while the majority of neurons in area 3 are activated only by cutaneous stimuli; different neurons in area 1 are related to either cutaneous or deep receptors. This differential representation of sensory modalities appears closely correlated with the gradient of morphological change that characterizes these three cytoarchitectural areas. Further evidence (1770) indicates that afferent impulses from receptors in joint capsules and pericapsular tissues, stimulated by joint movement, are conveyed by the posterior columns, the medial lemniscus and thalamic relay neurons to particular cell columns in the postcentral gyrus (Fig. 10-1). Impulses conveyed by this system subserve position sense and kinesthesis.

Stretch receptors in muscle and tendons probably do not provide information useful in the perception of joint position; furthermore, most of the afferent impulses from stretch receptors are projected to the cerebellum (1900, 1903). However, the rostral margin of the primary somesthetic area, designated as area 3a, has been shown to be a preferential receiving zone for impulses conveyed by group Ia fibers from muscle spindles (1904). It is not clear whether area 3a is a distinct cortical field, a component of the sensory or motor cortex, or a true transitional zone (1235). An anatomical definition of area 3a is difficult in the cat and monkey, and in the monkey its structure varies from place to place. The known medullary relay centers for group I muscle af-

ferents are in the rostral part of the nuclei gracilis and cuneatus; autoradiographic data indicate that these nuclei project only to the ventral posterolateral nucleus pars caudalis (VPLc) (2567). The above findings suggest that VPLc may project to the posterior part of so-called area 3a. This region is probably best considered a part of the somesthetic cortex, but many unresolved questions remain concerning how impulses from stretch receptors may be utilized for conscious perception of limb positions and movement.

Studies of cell columns of the postcentral gyrus responsive to cutaneous stimuli (1770) indicate that receptive fields on the body surface are constant. The size and position of the receptive fields are not changed by variations in the depth of anesthesia. Furthermore, there is no evidence that the position of the stimulus within the receptive field is coded in terms of the temporal characteristics of the response. The majority of cortical neurons driven by cutaneous stimuli adapt quickly to steady stimuli. The above observations pertain only to the somatic afferent system composed of primary dorsal root afferents in the posterior columns, lemniscal fibers arising from the posterior column nuclei and thalamocortical fibers arising from the ventral posterolateral nucleus (VPLc). Within the overall map of the primary somatosensory area a precise mapping of individual dermatomes has been described, so that each dermatome is represented in serial order in topographical relationship with neighboring dermatomal areas (2696). Individual dermatomal areas show considerable overlap. This is a system of great synaptic security, poised for action at high frequency levels, and possessing the neural attributes required for discriminatory functions.

Although fibers of the spinothalamic tract project to the ventral posterolateral nucleus of the thalamus, fibers of this system also project bilaterally upon portions of the intralaminar and posterior thalamic nuclei (210, 213, 232, 331, 1230, 1302, 1658, 2707). Thus impulses conducted in the anterolateral part of the spinal cord terminate upon multiple thalamic nuclei. Cells of the ventral posterior nucleus project to areas 3, 1 and 2 (S I) as well as to the second somatic

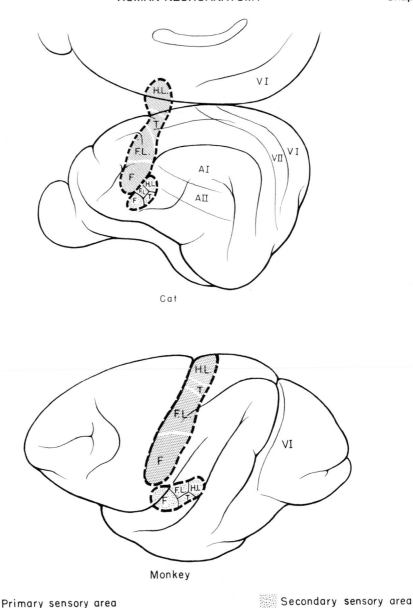

Cat

Monkey

░ Primary sensory area   ░ Secondary sensory area

Figure 19-13. Diagrams of the primary and secondary sensory areas in the cortex of the cat and monkey. Somatotopic representation of different parts of the body are indicated in the primary and secondary somatic sensory areas: *F*, face area; *T*, trunk; *FL*, forelimb; *HL*, hindlimb. Primary and secondary auditory (*AI* and *A II*) and visual (*VI* and *VII*) areas in the cat brain are shown. The medial aspect of the cat brain is represented above (after Woolsey (2771)). See more detailed diagram (Fig. 19-14) of the second somatic area (SS II) in the monkey based upon carefully controlled anatomical and physiological data.

area (SS II) (Figs. 19-13 and 19-14), a sensory area located along the superior bank of the lateral sulcus (1238, 1239, 1241, 1244). Both of these cortical projections are topographically organized. The second somatic area (SS II) also receives topographically ordered projections from both the ipsilateral and contralateral primary sensory area (S I) which coincides with the thalamic projection from the ventral posterior nuclear complex (1238, 1239).

Cells of the posterior thalamic nucleus (Fig. 15-18) differ from those of the ventral posterior complex in that they are described as only crudely place and modality specific. Most of these thalamic neurons

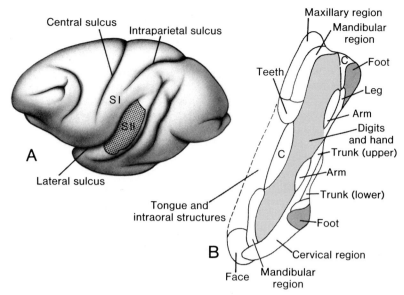

Figure 19-14. Diagrams of the position and somatotopic organization of the second somatic area (*SS II*) in *Macacus cynomologus*. Most of SS II lies buried in the depths of the lateral sulcus and has been identified on the basis of its cytoarchitecture and connections with the ventrobasal complex and projections from the primary somesthetic cortex (*S I*). In *A*, SS II is shown in a flattened view on the cortical surface. In *B*, the body representation in SS II is outlined as determined from recordings in awake monkeys. Different regions of the body are represented by a series of oblique strips parallel to the lateral sulcus, with the face and intraoral structures most rostral. The area in *blue* represents the digits and hand, while the areas in *red* represent the foot. Areas designated *C* are regions with poorly defined receptive fields. (Based on Robinson and Burton (2190).)

have large receptive fields, frequently bilateral, and are considered to respond to high threshold noxious stimuli (2019). Early experimental evidence suggested that cells of the posterior thalamic nucleus projected most of their fibers to the second somatic area (SS II) and that this area might be concerned with perception of pain (1338a, 1652, 2708). Recent autoradiographic studies indicate that the medial part of the posterior thalamic nucleus which receives most of the somatic afferent fibers projects to a retroinsular cortical area caudal to SS II (331). At one time it was thought that this projection might overlap portions of SS II. Recent physiological studies of the response properties of SS II in the monkey that are in good agreement with the anatomical definition of this area indicate that neurons in this area respond to somatic stimuli similar to those recorded in S I (2190). However, cortical cells with properties similar to those of the posterior thalamic nuclei have been observed in a small percentage of cells in the postcentral gyrus of the monkey (1770).

Microelectrode multiunit mapping of the primary somatosensory cortex in the monkey suggests that the representation of the body surface may be far more complex than indicated by earlier studies (1673). This study suggests two large systematic representations of the body surface each of which is activated by low threshold stimuli. One representation of the body surface is coextensive with area 3 and the other with area 1. Each of these somatotopic transformations of the skin surface has some discontinuities where adjoining skin surfaces are not represented. While the two fields of cutaneous representation are basically similar and are approximate mirror images of each other, they differ in size and in the relative proportion of cortex devoted to the representation of various body parts. Because the proportions in each representation differ, both cannot be simple reflections of peripheral innervation density. Area 2 appears to contain a systematic representation of deep body structures. These observations suggest that each of three distinctive cytoarchitectonic areas that compose the postcentral gyrus may represent different aspects of somatic sensation in unique ways.

Stimulation of the postcentral gyrus in man produces sensations described by the patient as numbness, tingling or a feeling of electricity. Occasionally the patient may report a sensation of movement in a particular part of the body, although no actual movement is observed. A sensation of pain is rarely produced by these stimulations. Sensations described are referred to contralateral parts of the body, except in response to stimulation of the cortical area for the face. Evidence suggests that the face and tongue are represented bilaterally. It is of interest that essentially the same sensations can be elicited by stimulating the precentral gyrus. According to Penfield and Rasmussen (1968), 25% of the locations giving sensory responses are in the precentral gyrus, but the ratio of sensory responses obtained from the postcentral gyrus to those from the precentral gyrus varies in different parts of the sensory sequence. Sensation referable to the eyes is obtained, almost exclusively, by stimulating the precentral gyrus, while sensation in the lips is associated almost invariably with stimulation of the postcentral gyrus. Sensory responses are reported only rarely with stimulation at points greater than 1 cm from the central sulcus. That stimulation of the precentral gyrus still produces sensory responses after removal of the postcentral gyrus indicates that these responses are not dependent upon the postcentral gyrus or collateral fibers to it. Even though sensation can be produced by stimulating the precentral gyrus, ablation of it produces no clinically detectable sensory deficits.

There are other observations which suggest that the somesthetic cortical area is not limited to the postcentral gyrus, but may include portions of the superior and inferior parietal lobules. The clinical observations of Foerster (762) indicate that destructive processes in the superior parietal lobule are followed by sensory disturbances similar to those associated with lesions of the postcentral gyrus. Other authors (1968) report no detectable somatic sensory deficits following cortical removals of large parts of the superior and inferior lobules in the nondominant hemisphere, although

their patient tended to ignore the contralateral hand and had difficulty performing complex maneuvers with it.

Available evidence indicates that position sense and kinesthesis are represented only contralaterally. Whether the discriminative aspects of tactile sensibility are represented bilaterally in the human cortex is not known definitely. Clinically the sensory deficits caused by lesions in the postcentral gyrus are detectable only on the opposite side of the body.

The sensory cortex is not concerned primarily with the recognition of crude sensory modalities, such as pain, thermal sense and mere contact. These apparently enter consciousness at the level of the thalamus, and their appreciation is retained even after complete destruction of the sensory area. "The sensory activity of the cortex . . . endows sensation with three discriminative faculties. These are: (a) recognition of spatial relations, (b) a graduated response to stimuli of different intensity, (c) appreciation of similarity and difference in external objects brought into contact with the surface of the body" (1061). Hence in lesions of the primary somesthetic area there is loss of appreciation of passive movement, of two-point discrimination and of ability to differentiate various intensities of stimuli. In severe lesions the patient, although aware of the stimulus and its sensory modality, is unable to locate accurately the point touched, to gauge the direction and extent of passive movement and to distinguish between different weights, textures or degrees of temperature; as a result, he is unable to identify objects by merely feeling them (astereognosis). The more complicated the test, the more evident the sensory defect becomes.

Second Somatic Sensory Area (SS II). As described in experimental animals, somatic sensory area II lies along the superior bank of the lateral sulcus and extends posteriorly into the parietal lobe (2771). In the monkey the greater part of SS II lies buried in the lateral sulcus (1238, 1239, 1241). Representation of the various parts of the body is depicted in reverse sequence to that found in the primary somesthetic area, and the regions of the two face areas are adjacent (Fig. 19-13). Parts of the body are described as being represented bilaterally in the SS II, although contralateral representation predominates. In unanesthetized monkeys two distinct portions of SS II were identified physiologically: (a) an anterior part described as responding to bilateral low threshold somatic stimuli in which body regions were arranged in the sequence of their dermatomes, and (b) a posterior region responding to nociceptive stimuli, related to asymmetrical receptive fields and lacking a definite topographic organization (2708).

There have been considerable discrepancies concerning the boundaries, the somatotopic representation and the modality representation in SS II in different animals suggesting that this area is not easily defined physiologically (2190–2192, 2708, 2771). The cortical area defined as SS II in the strict anatomical sense is the area on the superior bank of the lateral sulcus (or buried in it) that receives afferents from: (a) the ventral posterior nucleus of the thalamus (331, 1241, 1244) and (b) both the ipsilateral and contralateral primary somesthetic cortex (S I) (812, 1238, 1239). In physiological studies in subprimates, using these criteria SS II has been found to be a well-defined, somatotopically organized area that responds to relatively small contralateral receptive field (426, 1000, 2076). Reexamination of the somatotopic organization of SS II in the monkey using both anatomical and physiological methods suggests that the different body regions are represented in successive, obliquely oriented cortical strips parallel with the lateral sulcus (812, 2190). Neurons with trigeminal receptive fields were found rostrally in SS II and responded to bilateral stimuli (Fig. 19-14). Regions representing the hand were posterior to the face area and formed the largest component; regions related to the arm, trunk and hind limbs follow in a rostrocaudal sequence. These cortical strips representing various parts of the body in sequence in SS II do not form a precise topological map of the body surface as depicted in the figurines for S I and SS II.

In addition to the SS II, there are a number of small areas in the parietal and insular cortex that respond in various ways to cutaneous stimulation (2191). Of these the retroinsular area seems especially significant because it receives projections from the medial part of the posterior thalamic nucleus (331). Physiological observations indicate that cells in the retroinsular cortex are activated only from small, well-defined contralateral receptive fields located in the hand and foot (2190). These findings raise important questions concerning the notion that cells in the posterior thalamic nucleus (Fig. 15-18) may be specifically involved in relaying impulses concerned with pain and noxious stimuli to regions of the cerebral cortex (2019). These elegant and carefully anatomically controlled studies cast doubt upon the concept that impulses concerned with painful and noxious stimuli are relayed to SS II or the retroinsular cortex via the posterior thalamic nucleus. It has been suggested that some of the response characteristics attributed to neurons in SS II may be those of cells in neighboring cortical areas, perhaps the area referred to as 7b in the inferior parietal lobule (2190).

The efferent cortical connections of the SS II are with the primary somesthetic cortex (S I) and with the motor and supplementary motor areas within the same hemisphere (1236, 1238). Thus connections between SS II and S I are reciprocal. The most remarkable feature of these connections between somatic sensory areas is the interlocking nature of the topographical subdivisions. Parts of the S I, the SS II and the motor cortex related to the same periphery are interconnected. Commissural connections also exist for the somatic sensory cortex. The S I has connections with its counterpart and with SS II on the opposite side; SS II projects to its counterpart on the opposite side, but only to the region of S I which represents perioral regions (1239). Only the S I projects to parietal cortex and this projection is restricted to area 5.

The SS II has been described in man, but face, mouth and tongue regions have not been identified, presumably because of proximity to the primary face area (1968). Stimulation of somatic sensory area II in the unanesthetized patient produces sensations in the extremities similar to those obtained by stimulating the primary somesthetic cortex.

The Primary Visual Area. Area 17, located in the walls of the calcarine sulcus

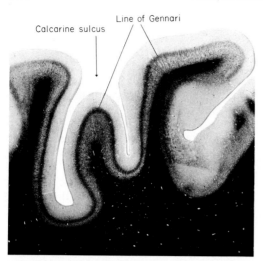

Calcarine sulcus　　Line of Gennari

Figure 19-15. Frontal section through calcarine cortex (area striata) showing extent of line of Gennari (Weigert's myelin stain, photograph).

and adjacent portion of the cuneus and lingual gyrus, represents the primary visual area. It occasionally extends around the occipital pole on to the lateral surface of the hemisphere (Figs. 15-15 and 19-5). The exceedingly thin cortex of this area (1.5 to 2.5 mm) is the most striking example of the heterotypical granulous cortex (type 5). Layers II and III are narrow and contain numerous small pyramidal cells that are hardly larger than typical granule cells (Fig. 19-10*C*). Layer IV, which is very thick, is subdivided by a light band into three sublayers (Fig. 19-20). The upper and lower sublayers are packed with small granule cells. In the middle, lighter layer, fewer small cells are scattered between the large stellate cells (giant stellate cells of Meynert). This light layer is occupied by the greatly thickened outer band of Baillarger, known here as the *band of Gennari* (Fig. 19-15). This band, visible to the naked eye in sections of the fresh cortex, has given this region the name *area striata* (Figs. 19-15 and 19-20). Layer V is relatively narrow and poor in small cells, but scattered among these cells are isolated large pyramidal cells which may reach a height of 60 μm (Fig. 19-10*C*).

The visual cortex receives the geniculocalcarine tract, whose course and exact projection have been discussed in an earlier chapter (Fig. 15-30). Geniculocalcarine fibers pass in the *external sagittal stratum*

(Fig. 15-31) which is separated from the wall of the inferior and posterior horns of the lateral ventricle by the *internal sagittal stratum*, and by fibers of the corpus callosum designated as the *tapetum* (Fig. 2-21). Fibers of the internal sagittal stratum are corticofugal fibers passing from the occipital lobe to the superior colliculus and the lateral geniculate body (848, 1129, 1273, 2732, 2760). The optic radiation projects topographically upon the striate cortex so that cells in: (a) the medial half of the lateral geniculate body, representing upper retinal quadrants (lower quadrants of the visual field) project to the superior bank of the calcarine sulcus, and (b) the lateral half of the lateral geniculate body (upper quadrants of the visual field) project to the inferior bank of the calcarine sulcus (Figs. 15-24 and 15-30).

The macular fibers terminate in the caudal third of the calcarine area, and those from the paracentral and peripheral retinal areas end in respectively more rostral portions. The representation of the macular area in the occipital cortex appears relatively large compared with the macular area of the lateral geniculate body (Figs. 15-24, 15-25 and 15-30).

Because some unilateral lesions of the visual cortex result in a sparing of macular vision, certain authors have suggested that the macula is represented bilaterally. Anatomical evidence supports the thesis that parts of each macular area are represented only in the visual cortex of one hemisphere, since unilateral lesions of the visual cortex result in retrograde cell changes, or cell loss, only in the ipsilateral lateral geniculate body. Clinically, sparing of macular vision associated with vascular lesions involving the occipital cortex usually is attributed to collateral circulation provided by branches of the middle cerebral artery (Fig. 20-7). Following occlusion of the posterior cerebral artery, these collateral vessels frequently may be sufficient to preserve some macular vision. Similar collateral circulation apparently is not present in the cortical area representing paracentral and peripheral parts of the retina. Complete unilateral destruction of the visual cortex in man produces a contralateral homonymous hemianopia in which there is blindness in the ipsilateral nasal field and the contralateral temporal field. Thus a lesion in the right visual cortex produces a left homonymous hemianopsia (Figs. 15-30 and 15-32). Lesions involving portions of the visual cortex, such as the inferior calcarine cortex, produce an *homonymous quadrantanopsia*, in which blindness results in the superior half of the visual field contralaterally. Homonymous hemianopsia can result from lesions involving all fibers of either the optic tract or the optic radiations (Fig. 15-32C), but lesions in these locations tend to be incomplete and the visual field defects in the two eyes are rarely identical. Frequently patients are unaware of homonymous hemianopsia and complain of bumping into people and objects on the side of the visual field defect. Bilateral destruction of the striate areas causes total blindness in man, but other mammals, such as dogs and monkeys, retain the ability to distinguish light intensities after ablations of the visual cortex (892, 1332, 2372).

An image falling upon the retina initiates a tremendously complex process that results in vision. The transformation of a retinal image into a perceptual image occurs partly in the retina but mostly in the brain. An impressive series of elegant studies by Hubel and Wiesel in the cat and monkey have provided the first real insight into the functional organization of the visual cortex.

The receptive field of a cell in the visual system is defined as the region of the retina (or visual field) over which one can influence the firing of that cell. In the retina the receptive field comprises those receptor sets (i.e., rods and cones) and other retinal neurons which influence the firing of one retinal ganglion cell. Receptive fields of retinal ganglion cells are circular, vary somewhat in size and are of two types: (a) those with an "on" (excitatory) center and an "off" (inhibitory) surround, and (b) those with an "off" (inhibitory) center and an "on" (excitatory) surround (1375). It is well known that retinal ganglion cells fire at a fairly steady rate even in the absence of stimulation. An "on" response is characterized by an increased firing rate of the cell to a light stimulus; in an "off" response the cell's firing rate diminishes when the light stimulus decreases. The physiological basis for the "on" and "off" retinal responses are

the concentric receptive fields with either an "on" or "off" center and the reverse type of surround (Fig. 19-16). Illuminating the entire retina diffusely does not affect retinal ganglion cells as strongly as a small circular spot of light that covers only the excitatory center of the receptive field.

Cells of the lateral geniculate body are of two types and have physiological characteristics similar to retinal ganglion cells, in that: (a) each cell is driven from a circumscribed retinal region (receptive field), and (b) each receptive field has either an "on" or "off" center with an opposing surround (1155). Lateral geniculate neurons are more specialized than retinal ganglion cells in that they are more sensitive to the differences in retinal illumination than to the illumination itself. Cells in different laminae of the lateral geniculate body are driven from receptive fields in one eye, either ipsilaterally or contralaterally, depending upon the uncrossed or crossed connections. In the lateral geniculate body, few, if any, cells are influenced binocularly (1155). Visual processing by the brain begins in the lateral geniculate body.

The striate cortex, anatomically far more complex than the retina or lateral geniculate body, does not have cells with concentric receptive fields. Cells of the striate cortex show marked specificity in their responses to restricted retinal stimulation (1154, 1156, 1157, 1161). The most effective stimulus shapes are long narrow rectangles of light ("slits"), dark bars against a light background ("dark bars") and straight line borders separating areas of different brightness ("edges"). A given cell responds vigorously when an appropriate stimulus is shone on its receptive field, or moves across it, provided the stimulus is presented in a specific orientation. This orientation is referred to as the "*receptive field axis of orientation*," and it is critical and constant for any particular cell, but it differs for other cells in the locations. Cells with the same receptive field axis of orientation are arranged in columns extending from the cortical surface to the white matter.

The cortical columns of the striate cortex may be looked upon as the structural expression of the necessity to code more than two variables. The two surface coordinates (eccentricity from fovea and dis-

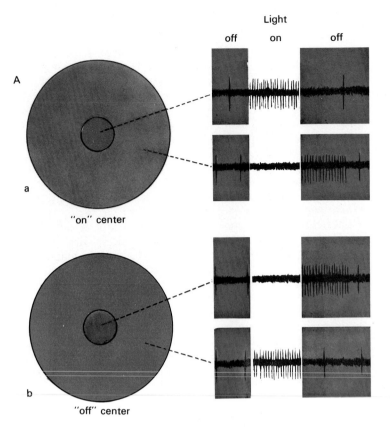

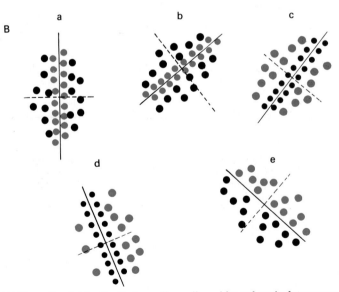

Figure 19-16. (*A*) Receptive fields of retinal ganglion cells and lateral geniculate neurons are concentric with either an "on" (excitatory) center and an "off" (inhibitory) surround, or the reverse. In *a*, a spot of light (red) filling the "on" center causes the cell to fire vigorously. If the spot of light strikes the surrounding "off" zone, firing of the neuron is suppressed until the light is turned off. In *b*, the responses of a cell with an "off" center and an "on" surround are the reverse. (*B*) Simple cells of striate cortex receive their input from sets of lateral geniculate neurons whose "on" or "off" centers are arranged in straight lines. The receptive field axis of orientation varies for simple cells, as in *a*, *b* and *c*, with excitatory areas represented by *red* dots and inhibitory areas by *black* dots. Although simple cells always have excitatory and inhibitory areas parallel and in a straight line, these areas may be asymmetrical as in *d* and *e*. (Based on Hubel and Wiesel (1156).)

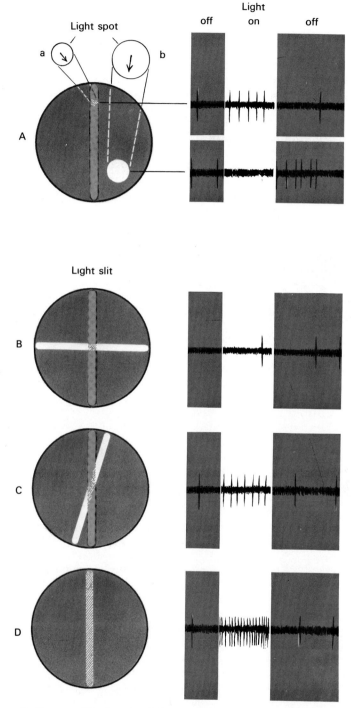

Figure 19-17. Schematic diagram of the functional characteristics of "simple" cells in the striate cortex. In *A*, a small circular spot of light (*a*) shone on the excitatory part of the receptive field (*red*) of a simple cortical cell produces a weak response. A larger spot of light (*b*) shone on the inhibitory surround produces no response. Small spots of light (*a*) produce vigorous responses in retinal ganglion cells and lateral geniculate neurons. The receptive field of the simple cell shown above is similar to *a* in Figure 19-16B. A narrow slit of light shone perpendicular to the receptive field axis of orientation (*red*) in *B*. produces virtually no response. Tilting the slit of light as in *C*. produces a weak response, while a vertical slit of light, as in *D*, which corresponds to receptive field axis of the simple striate cell, produces a vigorous response (after Hubel (1152)).

tance above or below the horizontal meridian) are used for topographical representation of the visual fields. Engrafted upon this representation are two more variables in columnar form concerned with receptive-field orientation and ocular dominance. The topographical representation of the retinae upon the striate cortex is primary and for each position in the visual field there is neuronal machinery for each orientation and for each eye (1164). In the monkey striate cortex there exist two independent and overlapping systems of columns referred to as orientation columns and ocular dominance columns (1161). Ocular dominance columns are parallel sheets or slabs arranged perpendicular to the cortical surface which are subdivided into a mosaic of alternating left eye and right eye stripes 250 to 500 μm in width (1163). Orientation columns are an order of magnitude smaller than the ocular dominance columns (Fig. 19-20). The horizontal distance corresponding to a complete cycle of orientation columns, representing a rotation through 180°, appears to be roughly equal to a set of left plus right ocular dominance columns with a thickness of 0.5 to 1 mm (1165).

Orientation Columns. The visual cortex is subdivided into discrete columns extending from the surface to the white matter; all cells within each column have the same receptive field axis of orientation. The many varieties of cells in the striate cortex have been grouped into two main functional types, but it is apparent that other subtypes or varieties also exist. The main functional cell types are referred to as *"simple"* and *"complex."*

"Simple" type cells respond to slits of light having the proper receptive field axis of orientation. A slit of light oriented vertically in the visual field may activate a given "simple" cell, whereas the same cell will not respond, although other cells will, if the orientation of the slit of light is moved out of the vertical position. The retinal region over which a "simple" type cell can be influenced is, like the receptive fields of retinal and geniculate cells, divided into "on" and "off" areas (Fig. 19-16). In "simple" cells these "on" areas are not circular but are narrow rectangles, adjoined on each side by larger "off" regions. The magnitude of the "on" response depends

upon how much of the rectangular region is covered by the stimulating light. A narrow slit of light that just fills the elongated "on" region produces a powerful "on" response; stimulation with a slit of light having a different orientation produces a weaker response, because it includes part of the antagonistic "off" regions. A slit of light at right angles to the optimum orientation for a particular cell usually produces no response (Fig. 19-17). Thus a large spot of light covering the whole retina evokes no response in "simple" cortical cells, because "on" and "off" effects balance. A particular cortical cell's optimum receptive field axis of orientation appears to be a functional property built into the cells by its anatomical connections. The receptive field axis of orientation differs from one cell column to the next, and may be vertical, horizontal or oblique. There is no evidence that any one orientation is more common than any other.

Evidence (1156) suggests that "simple" cells receive their impulses directly from the lateral geniculate body. Presumably a typical "simple" cell receives an input from a large number of lateral geniculate neurons whose "on" centers are arranged in a straight line which corresponds to the receptive field orientation of the "simple" cell (Fig. 19-16*B*). Thus for each area of the retina stimulated, each line, and each orientation of the stimulus, there is a particular set of "simple" striate cortical cells that respond. Changing any of the stimulus arrangements will cause an entirely new and different population of "simple" striate cells to respond.

"Complex" type cells, like "simple" cells, respond best to "slits," "bars" or "edges," provided the orientation is suitable. Unlike "simple" cells, these cells respond with sustained firing as the slits of light are moved across the retina, preserving the same receptive field axis of orientation (1156). These cells have peculiar characteristics in that a slit of light with the appropriate receptive field axis of orientation can cause cells to fire vigorously as it moves across the retina in one direction, but reversing the direction of movement of the light stimulus may diminish the response. Although "complex" cells in the striate cortex have some characteristics similar to those of simple cells, their receptive fields cannot be mapped into antagonistic "on" and "off" regions. It is believed that a "complex" cell receives its input from a large number of "simple" cells, all of which have the same receptive field axis of orientation. Combined physiological and anatomical studies have shown that most "simple" cells in the striate cortex are stellate cells located in layer IV (Fig. 19-20); the majority of "complex" and "hypercomplex" cells are pyramidal neurons lying in layers superficial or deep to layer IV (1161, 1280). "Hypercomplex" cells have the properties of two or more "complex" cells from which they are believed to receive their input. Most cells in layer IV are driven by only one eye while cells in other layers are driven binocularly (1161). There are a few cells in layer III of the striate cortex that have a center-surround field organization, but their behavior is much more complex than cells in the lateral geniculate body.

These findings imply that a vast network of intracortical connections relate "simple" and "complex" cells in the striate cortex in a very specific fashion, and that similar arrangements must exist for all receptive field axes of orientations. Since columns of cells constitute the fundamental functional units of the cortex, each small region of the visual field must be represented in the striate cortex many times, in column after column of cells with different receptive field orientations.

Attempts have been made to determine the geometry and sequence of the orientation columns in the monkey striate cortex (1164). Orientation columns appear to have the form of narrow slabs, as do ocular dominance columns. The arrangement of the columns is highly ordered and recordings made along a tangential microelectrode penetration show that the preferred orientations of cells change in a systematic fashion, in either a clockwise or counterclockwise direction with advancement of the electrode (A in Fig. 19-20). There is a continuous variation in the preferred orientation with horizontal distance along the cortex but the highly ordered sequences of small variations occasionally are broken by abrupt shifts. When the electrode crosses from a right-eye region to a left-eye region, there is no noticeable disturbance in the sequence of orientation columns which suggests a degree of independence for the two systems (Fig. 19-20). The horizontal distance along the cortex corresponding to a complete cycle of orientation columns, representing rotations through 180°, is said to be of the same size as a set of left and right ocular dominance columns (0.5 to 1 mm). The principal finding is that orientation columns are arranged with great regularity so that a probe moving along the cortex horizontally generally can be expected to encounter all values of orientation in a regular sequence before any one value is repeated (1165). In young monkeys deprived of vision by suturing the eyelids closed, the same highly ordered sequence of orientation columns is found in the striate cortex (1164). This finding indicates that the orientation column system is innately determined and not the result of early visual experience.

Ocular Dominance Columns. Recording from single cells at various levels of the visual system offers a direct means of determining the site of convergence of impulses from the two eyes. In the lateral geniculate body, the first point at which convergence is at all likely, binocularly influenced cells have not been observed (1155); further anatomical findings have provided no evidence that crossed and uncrossed optic tract fibers overlap in layers of the lateral geniculate body (850, 1056, 1094). It has long been recognized that the primary visual cortex receives projections via the lateral geniculate body from both eyes. In early studies in the cat it was noted that about 80% of cells in the striate cortex were influenced independently by the two eyes (1156). The receptive fields of all binocularly influenced cortical cells occupy corresponding sites in the two retinas (Fig. 15-23). In a binocularly influenced cell the two receptive fields have the same organization and axis of orientation, and a summation occurs when corresponding parts of the two retinas are stimulated simultaneously in the same fashion. In the monkey binocular convergence in area 17 is delayed beyond what are probably the first and second synaptic stages (1161, 1166). The bulk of the projections of the lateral geniculate body terminate in deep parts of layer IV where they are segregated into a series

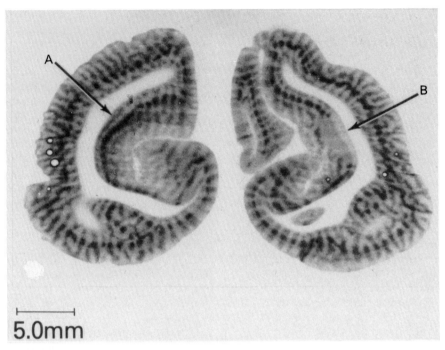

Figure 19-18. Autoradiographic mapping of the visual system in the monkey using 2-[¹⁴C]deoxyglucose. Coronal sections of the striate cortex in an animal with the right eye occluded. The alternate dark and light striations, each 0.3 to 0.4 mm in width, represent ocular dominance columns. These columns are darkest in a band which corresponds to layer IV, but they extend the entire thickness of the cortex. *Arrows A* and *B* point to regions without ocular dominance columns; these regions receive only monocular input. The region indicated by *arrow A* is contralateral to the occluded eye. The region indicated by *arrow B* is ipsilateral to the occluded eye and shows no evidence of radioactivity. Both arrows indicate loci believed to be the cortical representation of the blind spots. (Courtesy of Dr. Louis Sokoloff, Laboratory of Cerebral Metabolism, National Institute of Mental Health, Bethesda, Maryland; reproduced with permission from C. Kennedy et al.: *Proceedings of the National Academy of Sciences, U.S.A.*, **73:** 4230–4234, 1976.)

of parallel alternating stripes, one set connected with the left eye and the other to the right eye. Although input to deep parts of layer IV is essentially monocular, ocular dominance columns extend vertically from the pial surface to the white matter, and also show alternate preference for left and right eyes (Figs. 19-18–19-20). This columnar arrangement is demonstrated by vertical electrode penetrations of the striate cortex in which there is no change in eye preference (*B* in Fig,. 19-20). In tangential penetrations of the striate cortex, the electrode moves from a region in which one eye gives the best response to an adjacent region where the other eye dominates (1166). In layer IV the responses are strictly monocular, while cells in other layers respond binocularly, but with definite dominance by one eye. In the binocular representation of area 17 there is no evidence that the widths of the ocular dominance columns inner-

vated by the ipsilateral or contralateral eye are different. The width of a set of right and left ocular dominance columns range from 0.5 to 1 mm (1165). As mentioned earlier ocular dominance columns are larger than orientation columns and a set of right-left ocular dominance columns appears to correspond to a complete cycle of orientation columns representing a rotation of receptive field axes through 180° (Fig. 19-20). The striate cortex is organized into both vertically and horizontal systems. The vertical or columnar system is concerned with retinal position, line orientation, ocular dominance and perhaps detection of direction of movement; these functional features are mapped in sets of superimposed, but independent mosaics (Figs. 19-18 and 19-19). The horizontal system segregates cells of different orders of complexity. Cells of the lowest order (simple cells), located in layer IV, are driven monocularly, while those of higher orders (complex and hyper-complex), located in the other layers, are driven by impulses from both eyes (Fig. 19-20).

Ocular dominance columns in the striate cortex have been demonstrated by a variety of neuroanatomical technics. After a discrete lesion in a single layer of the lateral geniculate body, degenerated fibers can be traced to a region of the striate cortex where bands of degenerated fibers in layer IV (250 to 500 μm) are separated from interbands of the same extent free of degeneration (1163). Combined physiological studies and a reduced silver staining method show that the boundaries of ocular dominance columns correspond with a mosaic pattern of dark bands seen in tangential sections of the striate cortex (1470). Autoradiographic methods, using the principal of transneuronal transport or 2-[^{14}C]deoxyglucose as a metabolic marker to measure glucose utilization, also reveal the characteristic pattern of ocular dominance columns (Figs. 19-18 and 19-19) (1291, 2718). Based upon physiological evidence two regions of the striate cortex should not contain ocular dominance columns: (a) the region representing the blind spot of the retina and (b) the cortical region representing the monocular temporal crescent of the visual field. These regions of striate cortex, receiving only monocular visual inputs, have been identified with the 2-[^{14}C]deoxyglucose metabolic mapping technic and other autoradiographic methods (Figs. 19-18, 19-19, 19-21 and 19-22). The area of the optic disc in the nasal half of each retina transmits no visual impulses to the contralateral striate cortex; this region of striate cortex receives its sole input from the temporal half of the ipsilateral retina. When an animal is deprived of vision in the right eye and the 2-[^{14}C]deoxyglucose method is employed as a metabolic marker: (a) the left striate cortex shows the striped pattern of ocular dominance columns, except in the representation of the blind spot where metabolic activity is evidenced by a continuous band of isotope uptake, and (b) the right striate cortex shows a similar pattern of striped columns but no evidence of metabolic activity or isotope in the cortical area representing the blind spot (Figs. 19-18, 19-21 and 19-22). The cortical area representing the monocular crescent of the right

visual field, which lies in the left striate cortex, would not contain isotope because all of its afferent input is crossed.

Visual Deprivation. Physiological studies in very young, visually inexperienced kittens and monkeys deprived of all vision from birth by visual occluders, have shown that responses in the striate cortex are similar to those of the adult animal with respect to receptive field organization and functional architecture (1158, 2717). The visual system in the cat is immature at birth and this immaturity appears to contribute to sluggish cortical responses and less precisely defined orientation columns. In the visually naive young monkey orientation columns are as highly ordered as in the adult. These observations suggest that the connections responsible for the highly organized behavior of cells in the visual cortex must be present at birth and develop even in the absence of patterned visual experience. Thus the development of orientation specificity in the striate cortex in these two species appears to be genetically determined. The surprising finding in young monkeys deprived of binocular vision for a few weeks after birth was the marked reduction in number of cells in the striate cortex that could be influenced by both eyes. This finding suggested that deprivation of binocular vision for a few weeks after birth may result in deterioration of innate cortical connections subserving binocular vision.

Unilateral visual deprivation, accomplished by suturing the eyelids closed or placing a contact occluder over the cornea, in very young kittens results in marked histological changes in the layers of lateral geniculate body receiving fibers from the deprived eye, but no obvious histological changes in the retina, optic nerves, superior colliculi or striate cortex (2716). Similar visual deprivation in older kittens or in adult animals produced less severe, or no detectable, histological changes in the lateral geniculate body. In young kittens most of the geniculate neurons with inputs from the deprived eye had abnormal receptive fields, and the overall activity of cells in these layers was diminished. Single unit recordings from the striate cortex in these animals indicated that the majority of cortical cells were driven only from the normal eye (2716). Kittens deprived from birth for

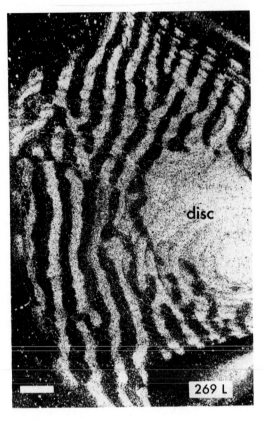

Figure 19-19. Autoradiographic montage of tangential sections of area 17 on the left in a monkey (269) whose right eye was removed as an adult. The left eye was injected 4 months later with [³H]proline. The montage shows the normal mosaic pattern of ocular dominance columns with uniformly labeled bands alternating with unlabeled bands. The uniformly labeled area (*disc*) represents the monocular area which covers the blind spot (optic disc) of the enucleated right eye (bar equals 1 mm). (Courtesy of Dr. David Hubel and Allan R. Liss, Inc., New York; reproduced with permission from S. LeVay et al.: *Journal of Comparative Neurology*, **191:** 1–51, 1980.)

2 to 3 months showed profound visual defects in the deprived eye, although pupillary light reflexes were normal. Thus, monocular visual deprivation in kittens from birth can result in severe visual defects and unresponsiveness of cortical neurons to stimulation of the deprived eye. Physiological defects following unilateral visual deprivation appear to result from disruption of cortical connections present from birth.

Studies of the development of ocular dominance columns in normal and visually deprived monkeys indicate that these columns are only partially formed at birth (1166, 1471). Ocular dominance columns develop rapidly during the first 6 weeks of life and after this time show the adult type columnar segregation. The process of left and right eye segregation of afferent fibers in layer IV of the striate cortex occurs in the presence or absence of visual experience. Monocular visual deprivation during the first six postnatal weeks causes the afferent fibers associated with the open eye to form greatly expanded ocular dominance columns in the deep parts of layer IV, while dominance columns for the closed eye appear shrunken. Thus monocular visual deprivation in very young monkeys causes a redirection of cortical afferents into sets of columns of unequal width. The eye preference of neurons in layers of the striate cortex superficial and deep to layer IV also changes as a consequence of monocular deprivation. In young animals deprived of vision bilaterally, cells in upper and lower layers of the striate cortex responding binocularly are greatly reduced (2717). Monocular eyelid suture in the adult animal does not result in detectable anatomical or physiological defects in the striate cortex (1471). These studies indicate normal visual binocular experience, particularly in the first six weeks of life, is necessary for the maintenance of cortical connections beyond the deep parts of layer IV of the striate cortex that subserve binocular vision.

Secondary Visual Areas. A second visual area (visual area II) has been mapped in the rabbit, cat and monkey by recording the potentials evoked by photic stimulation of the retina (2511, 2543, 2770). Visual area

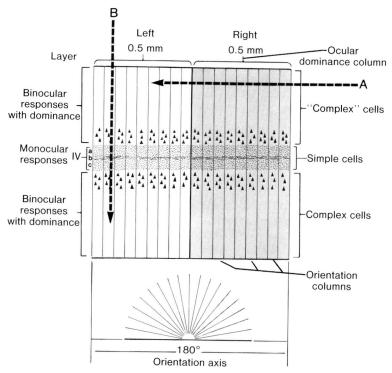

Figure 19-20. Schematic representation of the organization of ocular dominance and orientation columns in the striate cortex. Ocular dominance columns (0.25 to 0.5 mm) are an order of magnitude larger than orientation columns and a pair of left-right ocular dominance columns (0.5 to 1 mm) are roughly equal to a set of orientation columns representing a complete cycle of orientations through 180°. Input from the lateral geniculate to layer IV is strictly monocular and consists of a series of parallel and alternating stripes—one for the left eye and one for the right eye. Most of the cells in layer IV are "simple" cells. Binocularly influenced cells are predominantly "complex" cells in layers above and below layer IV. A recording electrode inserted tangential to the pial surface, as in *arrow A*, will detect responses to successive stimuli with different orientations, first with right eye dominance and then with left eye dominance. A recording electrode inserted vertically, as in *B*, will indicate responses only to stimuli presented in one axis of orientation. About 50% of the cells above and below layer IV will respond to binocular stimuli, but with consistent left dominance. When the electrode is in layer IV, monocular responses will be recorded. (Based on Hubel and Wiesel (1164) and Hubel et al. (1166).)

II is a smaller mirror image representation of the primary visual area, located anterolaterally, which appears to be anatomically identical to area 18 in the cat (Fig. 19-13). Lateral to visual areas I and II is a third systematic projection of the contralateral visual field (visual area III), which in the cat appears to be identical with area 19 (1159).

Area 18 is six-layered granular cortex which lacks the band of Gennari and rostrally merges with area 19 without distinct demarcation (Figs. 19-5 and 19-10*B*). Large pyramidal cells in the third layer of area 18 are useful in establishing its medial and lateral borders and coarse, irregular, often oblique fibers are seen in the deep cortical layers in myelin-stained sections (1159). Otsuka and Hassler (1910) have provided a comprehensive study of the visual areas in the cat. Area 18 interrelates areas 17 and 19 of the same and opposite hemispheres by association and commissural fibers.

The retinotopic organization of area 18 indicates that the border between areas 17 and 18 corresponds to the representation of the vertical meridian of the visual hemifield (contralateral half of the visual field). Thus as successive recordings are made moving from area 17 to area 18 there is a reversal of the receptive fields (i.e., from peripheral to central followed by a central to periph-

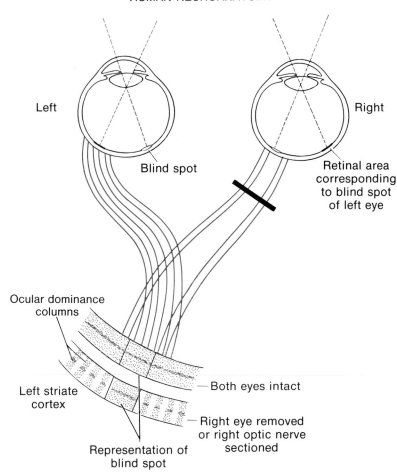

Figures 19-21 and 19-22. Schematic diagrams demonstrating the ocular dominance columns and the blind spot in the striate cortex with the 2-[^{14}C]deoxyglucose metabolic mapping technic in the monkey. In the animal with an intact visual system silver grains are distributed throughout the striate cortex with greatest concentrations in layer IV; neither the blind spot or ocular dominance columns can be demonstrated. Following removal of the right eye, or section of the right optic nerve (*heavy black line*), silver grains are distributed evenly in the representation of the blind spot on the left (*A* in Fig. 19-18 and Fig. 19-21) but no isotope is evident in the blind spot on the right (*B* in Fig. 19-18 and Fig. 19-22). Other regions of the striate cortex demonstrated ocular dominance columns on both sides. Fibers from the ipsilateral temporal retina normally cover the blind spot of the opposite eye. (Courtesy of Dr. Louis Sokoloff, National Institute of Mental Health, N.I.H.)

eral sequence) about the vertical meridian. The isoelevation lines running through both areas 17 and 18 are roughly perpendicular to the representation of the vertical meridian (1159, 2592). Visual area II (area 18) represents roughly the central 50° of the visual hemifield which corresponds to the binocular overlap zone in the cat. In area 19 (visual area III) the visual hemifield is represented basically as a mirror image of area 18 and the vertical meridian for area 19 lies on its lateral border. If a recording electrode were moved lateral from the bor-

der of areas 17 and 18 successive lateral positions in area 18 would represent more peripheral regions of the visual field; when the medial border of area 19 is reached the visual receptive fields would begin to move centrally toward the vertical meridian. The manner in which the contralateral visual hemifield is represented in areas 18 and 19 has been referred to as a second order transformation which means that some adjacent points in the visual field are not represented by adjacent points on the cortex (47, 48).

Cells of the dorsal division of the lateral

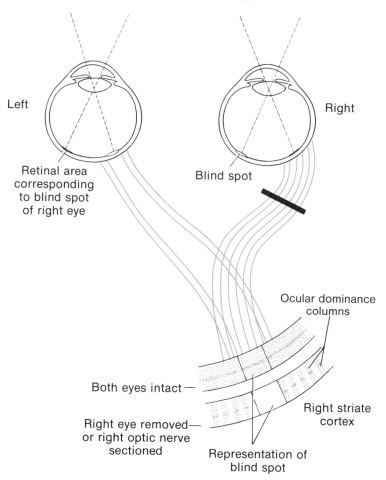

Left

Retinal area
corresponding
to blind spot
of right eye

Right

Blind spot

Ocular dominance
columns

Both eyes intact —

Right eye removed—
or right optic nerve
sectioned

Representation of
blind spot

Right striate
cortex

Figure 19-22

geniculate nucleus (LGB) project mainly upon area 17 but some fibers also reach areas 18 and 19 (691, 851, 875, 898, 1130, 1840, 2731, 2762). Larger cells in the dorsal nucleus of the LGB project to area 18, while cells of all sizes project to area 17 (875, 1130); some of the larger cells may project collaterals to both areas 17 and 18. The inferior pulvinar and the adjacent part of the lateral pulvinar each contains a representation of the contralateral visual hemifield and project retinotopically upon areas 18 and 19, where fibers end upon cortical layers IV, III, and I, and upon the striate cortex (area 17) where fibers end upon the supragranular layers (155, 2139, 2224). Fibers projecting to area 18 and 19 from these parts of the pulvinar appear to constitute important links in the extrageniculate vis-

ual projection. In addition area 17 has been demonstrated to project association fibers to area 18 and 19 (1159, 1628). Although there are few commissural connections between area 17 in the two hemispheres, both anatomical and physiological findings indicate that commissural fibers interconnect the junctional region at the border between areas 17 and 18 (1160, 1628, 2761, 2763, 2794). These fibers arise mainly from the cells in layer III. In both the cat and the macaque monkey cells situated at the boundary between areas 17 and 18 functionally represent the vertical meridian of the visual hemifield. There is reason to believe that the vertical meridian of the visual field is bilaterally represented in the visual cortex because of commissural connections. This bilateral representation insures a uniform visual field free of interruptions along the vertical midline (1160, 2761).

Cells in visual areas II and III, like those in visual area I, respond best to slits, dark bars and edges which have a specific orientation (1159). The majority (over 90%) of cells in visual area II are "complex" and over half of the cells in visual area III are "complex"; other cells in these areas, referred to as "hypercomplex", demonstrate more elaborate response properties. Both visual areas II and III are organized in columns, extending from the surface to the white matter, containing both "complex" and "hypercomplex" cells, all of which have the same receptive field orientation. These cells, however, differ in the precise position and arrangement of receptive fields. Hypercomplex cells have been divided into two types: (a) lower order hypercomplex cells which behave as though their input was derived from two sets of complex cells, one excitatory and one inhibitory, and (b) higher order hypercomplex cells which behave as though they receive their input from a large number of lower order hypercomplex cells. In visual area II, 5 to 10% of the cells were lower order hypercomplex cells, while in visual area III they comprised about half of the cells.

In visual area III there are columns in which some cells have one receptive field orientation, others with an orientation at 90 degrees to the first, and still others, which respond to both of these orientations. The majority of cells in visual areas II and III are driven from both eyes. Thus there appears to be as much binocular representation in visual areas II and III as in visual area I.

A separate representation of the contralateral visual hemifield (visual area II) adjacent to the primary visual (striate) cortex and with a common vertical meridian (junction of areas 17 and 18) has been found in every mammalian species studied (2592). The fact that all mammals appear to have an area 18 suggests that this area may be homologous in different species, although all connections may not be identical. In contrast representation of the contralateral visual hemifield in visual area III (area 19) has not been found in all species and its organization differs from species to species. Although the function(s) of area 19 are

elusive, area 18 appears ideally suited for processing visual information concerned with stereoscopic depth perception and may play a special role in the analysis of retinal disparities (1162, 2592). Area 18 contains a representation of the entire binocular visual field and usually not much more.

The Primary Auditory Area. In man this area (areas 41 and 42) is located on the two transverse gyri (Heschl) which lie on the dorsal surface of the superior temporal convolution. The primary auditory area is buried in the floor of the lateral sulcus (Figs. 2-7, 2-10, 2-13 and 19-5). The middle part of the anterior transverse gyrus constitute the principal auditory receptive areas (area 41). Remaining parts of the posterior transverse gyrus and adjacent portions of the superior temporal gyrus compose area 42, which is largely an auditory association area. In order to visualize these gyri in an intact brain, it is necessary to separate widely the banks of the lateral sulcus (Fig. 2-7). These two cortical areas are cytoarchitecturally distinct. Although area 41 is typical koniocortex, resembling that of areas 3 and 17, it is relatively thick (3 mm) and distinguished by the thickness of the granular layers. Granular cells are arranged in perpendicular columns. Area 42 is six-layered cortex of the parietal type (type 3, Fig. 19-7), distinguished by a number of large pyramidal cells in layer III.

The auditory area receives geniculotemporal fibers (auditory radiation) from the medial geniculate body (Fig. 2-10). The auditory radiation reaches its cortical projection site by passing through the sublenticular portion of the internal capsule (Fig. 15-28). The greater part of the auditory radiation projects to area 41, although fibers also project to area 42.

One of the characteristic features of the auditory system in the brain stem is the large number of relay nuclei involved in the central transmission of auditory signals (Fig. 12-13). Each of these relay nuclei is subject to descending influences from higher levels that can influence or modify synaptic activities at various levels. In spite of the large number of auditory relay nuclei and multiple sites at which fibers of this ascending system partially cross to the opposite side, the tonotopic localization present in the cochlea is preserved in all major relay nuclei (27, 1676, 1828, 2209, 2211, 2232, 2703). Portions of the auditory spectrum are represented in a tonotopic fashion in each of the three distinctive cochlear nuclei (2209) and in two of the major divisions of the inferior colliculus (Fig. 13-4) (27, 1676, 2232). The ventral laminated part of the medial geniculate body (MGB) also has a tonotopic organization in which high frequencies are represented medially and low frequencies laterally (26, 840, 974). The principal projection of the central nucleus of the inferior colliculus is to the ventral laminated nucleus of the MGB (429, 1374, 1735, 1743, 1874, 2194). The ventral laminated nucleus of the MGB (Fig. 15-19) gives rise to fibers of the auditory radiation which terminate in the primary auditory cortex where there is a spatial representation of tonal frequencies (429, 1838, 1875, 2087, 2750). These fibers passing to the primary auditory cortex constitute the *core projection* (Figs. 19-23 and 19-24).

The medial geniculate body also has two other divisions which are not laminated and receive inputs from the lateral tegmental area, the inferior colliculus and several diverse structures (429, 1243, 1374, 1735, 1874). These divisions of the MGB, referred to as dorsal and medial (magnocellular) (1743), project ipsilaterally via the auditory radiation to at least five cytoarchitectonic areas forming a cortical belt around the primary auditory area (1838, 1875, 2087, 2750). Fibers arising from the nonlaminated parts of the medial geniculate body passing to the secondary auditory areas constitute the *belt projection* (270, 2087, 2750). There appears to be very little overlap of the auditory projections to the belt area surrounding the primary auditory cortex except for the projection arising from the caudal part of the medial division of the MGB (1875). The medial magnocellular division appears to project to the entire cortical area receiving fibers from the medial geniculate body, although the laminar distribution of fibers in the cortex is different. The caudal part of the medial nucleus projects primarily upon layer VI, while other subdivisions of the MGB project primarily upon cells in layer IV and to parts of layer III.

In the cat two auditory areas were defined originally on the lateral aspect of the

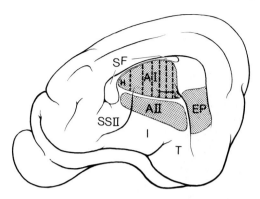

Figure 19-23. Schematic diagram of the auditory areas in the cat. The primary auditory area AI has a tonotopic organization with high frequencies (*H*) represented rostrally and low frequencies (*L*) caudally. The dashed vertical lines represent isofrequency bands. The primary auditory area is surrounded by a belt of secondary auditory cortex designated as *SF*, suprasylvian fringe, partially in the depth of the suprasylvian sulcus, *EP*, the posterior ectosylvian area, *A II*, the secondary auditory area, *SS II*, the second somatic area, *I*, the insular area and *T*, the temporal area. (Based upon Woolsey (2772) and Merzenich et al. (1675).)

hemisphere below the suprasylvian sulcus by recording evoked potentials from auditory stimuli (2778). These auditory areas, designated auditory area I (A I) and auditory area II (A II) were both considered to be tonotopically organized (Fig. 19-23). In the more dorsal auditory area (A I) responses from the basal turn of the cochlea (high frequencies) were represented rostrally while responses from stimulating apical regions of the cochlea (low frequencies) were recorded from caudal regions. In the second auditory area (A II), situated ventral to A I, the order of cochlear representation was considered to be the reverse (Fig. 19-23). An additional auditory area in the posterior ectosylvian (EP) region was described subsequently which included parts of A II (9, 10). The pattern of tonotopic localization in these and surrounding areas has been studied in detail and has been found to be much more complex than the initial concept of dual cortical auditory areas (2772).

Microelectrode studies of the frequency representation in A I indicate a series of isofrequency strips oriented vertically in

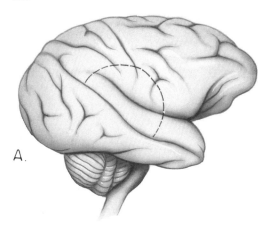

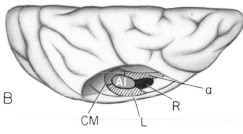

Figure 19-24. (*A*) Drawing of the lateral aspect of the rhesus monkey brain with dashed line indicating region excised to expose the superior temporal plane. (*B*) Dorsal view of the right hemisphere exposing the auditory region in the superior temporal plane. In the primary auditory area, A I (*blue*) low frequencies are represented rostrally and laterally and high frequencies are represented caudally and medially. The area designated R (black) has a cytoarchitecture similar to A I, an orderly representation of the auditory spectrum and responds vigorously to auditory stimuli. Auditory areas *A I* and *R* are surrounded by a belt of secondary auditory cortex (*shaded*) designated as *a, L,* and *CM*. (Based on Merzenich and Brugge (1672), Imig et al. (1182).)

which high frequencies are represented rostrally and low frequencies caudally (1674, 1675). In A I there is an orderly representation of frequencies and of cochlear place, in which the basal coils of the cochlea are represented rostrally and the apical region caudally. On an axis perpendicular to the vertical strips (i.e., longitudinal axis of the hemisphere) best-frequencies change as a simple function of cortical location. Isofrequency strips across the cortex are of nearly constant width, but a disproportionally

large cortical surface is devoted to higher octaves (Fig. 19-23). This larger representation of high octaves has been considered to be related to greater innervation densities in the basal coils of the cochlea (2407). On the basis of response characteristics and cytoarchitecture there appear to be at least five secondary auditory fields bordering A I (Fig. 19-23). These areas in the cat have been designated as: (a) the suprasylvian fringe (SF), (b) the posterior ectosylvian area (EP), (c) A II, (d) the insulotemporal area and (e) parts of the SS II (1675, 1838). In A II no clear evidence of a tonotopic representation could be established because of the broad tuning curves of its neurons. The tonotopic representation in SF and in EP appears the reverse of that seen in A I (2772, 2773). Neurons in the field rostral to A I appear sharply tuned and there is a reversal of frequency progression in passing from A I into this region (1675). Anatomical studies indicate that A I receives its input from the ventral laminated part of the MGB, while A II receives most of its fibers from the medial magnocellular nucleus (1838). The other secondary areas receive their inputs from nonlaminated parts of the MGB and constitute the belt projection (1838, 2087, 2750).

Some single unit studies of the auditory cortex in the unanesthetized cat have raised doubts concerning its tonotopic organization (483, 717, 724, 725, 911, 912, 2703). These investigators found many units did not respond to tones, even though they responded to complex sounds. A number of cortical units responded over such a wide frequency range that it was impossible to assign any particular frequency to them, although other units could be assigned a characteristic frequency. While high frequencies were located anteriorly in A I, low frequencies seemed to be distributed throughout the auditory cortex. Discrepancies between these and previously cited studies suggest important differences in the locations of recording sites, the depth at which the recordings were made and possibly the effects of anesthesia. Cortical surface landmarks are regarded as unreliable and the response characteristics in the superficial cortical layers may differ from those in deep layers (1675). Some authors suggest that units concerned with specific frequencies decrease at higher levels of the auditory system (483).

Since studies of the somesthetic and visual cortex indicate that a vertical column of cells constitutes the elementary functional unit, it might be expected that a similar arrangement would exist in the auditory cortex. A study based upon the functional architecture of the auditory cortex in unanesthetized cats has indicated that: (a) units responsive to noise bursts are randomly distributed, (b) different regions respond to a high or low proportion of click stimuli which do not follow the direction of vertical columns, and (c) narrowly tuned units are aligned with vertical cell columns which tend to occur in clusters (1). The functional architecture of the auditory cortex appears similar to that of the visual and somesthetic cortex in that cells in the same cell column share the same functional properties. The functional columns in the auditory cortex appear less discrete, do not have such sharp boundaries and are considered to be much smaller units than in other sensory areas. Other studies indicate that the isofrequency strips oriented across the primary auditory cortex probably represent, or are composed of, isofrequency cell columns (1675). In these columns units throughout the depth of the cortex respond to the same frequency. Both binaural and monaural cell columns have been described (1181). With the exception of some neurons responding only to binaural stimulation, monaural responses were classified as contralateral dominant, ipsilateral dominant or equidominant. Most neurons in the same perpendicular column display the same aural dominance and binaural interaction.

Studies of the auditory cortex in the monkey have revealed a rather precise tonotopic organization (1182, 1672). In these studies the best frequencies at different cortical depths were averaged because of the small variations within individual penetrations. The primary auditory area in the monkey lies caudally on the superior surface of the superior temporal gyrus and can be exposed by resection of the overlying parietal cortex (Fig. 19-24). Best frequencies in the full auditory range for the monkey were represented in an orderly fashion in the primary auditory area in a cytoarchitectonic field coextensive with the kon-

iocortex. Lowest frequencies were represented rostrally and laterally, whereas highest frequencies were found caudally and medially (Fig. 19-24). A cortical region immediately rostral to the A I has a cytoarchitecture similar to that of A I and appears to respond as vigorously to acoustic stimulation (1182). This rostral field is smaller than A I but contains a complete and orderly representation of the audible frequency spectrum with lower frequencies represented rostral and higher frequencies represented in progressively more caudal and medial regions (Fig. 19-24). The A I and the field rostral to it, designated R, appear to constitute the central core of the auditory cortex in the monkey. The primary auditory cortex in the monkey is surrounded by a belt of auditory cortex which is not cytoarchitectonically uniform and can be parcelled into several divisions. This cortical belt, which represents the secondary auditory areas, has been divided topographically into three, or more, auditory fields (Fig. 19-24). In the fields which form this cortical belt, units are less responsive to acoustic stimulation and the frequency organization is more complex than in A I or R. The organization and tonotopic localization in the A I appears to be very similar in monkeys, apes and man. Within this field low frequencies are represented rostrolaterally and higher frequencies extend caudomedially.

Electrical stimulation of the cortical areas in the temporal lobe near the primary auditory area (i.e., areas 42 and 22) in man produces sounds described as the noise of a cricket, a bell or a whistle. These sounds are elementary tones which may be high or low pitched, continuous or interrupted, but always are devoid of complicated or changing qualities (1968). Most of these auditory responses are referred to the contralateral ear.

One of the distinctive features of the auditory system, in contrast to other sensory systems, is the large number of actual and potential sites at which impulses from one side can be transmitted to contralateral relay nuclei. The largest and most important fiber crossing is in the trapezoid body, but others also are present (Fig. 12-13), including fibers from auditory cortical areas that cross in the corpus callosum (1681).

The commissural connections of the auditory cortex in the cat project to homologous areas in the opposite hemisphere (629). A I projects contralaterally to A I and A II, while A II sends fibers only to A II. Within each subdivision of the auditory cortex there are some areas which receive only small numbers of terminal fibers; the region of A I representing the low frequency range is a clear example. Auditory commissural connections differ greatly from those of the visual cortex (area 17) which are absent except near the border of area 18. Association fibers in the auditory cortex of the cat reciprocally interconnect primary and secondary areas with each other (630).

Physiological studies (11, 2225, 2778) indicate that each cochlea is represented bilaterally in the auditory cortex, although some slight differences exist between the two sides. Rosenzweig (2225) demonstrated that although the cortical effects of stimulating each ear separately are nearly the same, significant differences occur when the position of the stimulus is varied with respect to the ears during bilateral stimulation. When the sound is presented on one side, the cortical response is greatest in the contralateral hemisphere. If the sound is presented in a median plane, the cortical activity in the two hemispheres is equal. These studies suggest a correlation between auditory localization and differential responses in the auditory cortex. There are considerable variations in the size and convolutional patterns of Heschl's gyrus in the two hemispheres; the gyrus on the left is frequently unpaired, larger and longer than on the right side (683, 2756).

Because audition is represented bilaterally at a cortical level, unilateral lesions of the auditory cortex cause only a partial deafness. The deficits, however, are bilateral, and the greatest loss is contralateral. According to Penfield and Evans (1964), removal of one temporal lobe impairs sound localization on the opposite side, especially judgment of the distance of sounds. Clinically, unilateral lesions of the auditory cortex are difficult to recognize. Experimental studies indicate that bilateral ablations of auditory areas I, II and EP in the cat do not abolish auditory localization of sound in space, although discriminations of this kind are impaired (1829, 1830). Sound lo-

calization in space is most critically impaired by bilateral ablations of AI (2451). Bilateral ablations of the auditory cortical areas reportedly have little or no effect on the ability of cats to discriminate changes in frequency (336, 1698, 1829). Following bilateral ablations of auditory areas I, II and EP, and somatic area II, cats could not relearn to discriminate changes in frequency, but could discriminate changes in sound intensity (1698). Although ability to localize sound in space depends to a degree upon the auditory cortex, it is not affected by section of the corpus callosum and is affected very little by section of the commissure of the inferior colliculus, but it is severely affected by section of the trapezoid body (1219, 1829).

Brodmann's area 22, bordering the primary auditory area (Fig. 19-5) and representing typical six-layered isocortex, receives fibers from areas 41 and 42 and has connections with areas of the parietal, occipital and insular cortex (98a, 2462, 2463). Lesions of area 22 in the dominant hemisphere, or bilateral lesions produce word deafness or sensory aphasia (see p. 703). Although patients with these lesions can hear, they cannot interpret the meaning of sounds, especially speech. This form of sensory aphasia usually is associated with lesions in the posterior part of area 22.

The Gustatory Area. Clinical and experimental evidence indicates that taste sensibility probably is represented in the parietal operculum (area 43) and in the adjacent parainsular cortex (Fig. 19-5) (96, 220, 221, 1950, 1968). Ablations of the precentral and postcentral opercula in the monkey and chimpanzee reportedly cause a loss of taste. Similar lesions involving the anterior insular cortex, the postcentral operculum and the anterior supratemporal cortex in the monkey impair taste sensibility (96). Stimulations of the parietal operculum (1963) and adjacent insular cortex (1968) in conscious patients produce gustatory sensations.

Physiological studies in the rat, cat and squirrel monkey indicate that taste impulses conveyed by the chorda tympani and glossopharyngeal nerves are projected to the most medial and caudal part of the ventral posteromedial (VPMpc) nucleus of the thalamus (193, 705, 710). In the rat this projection is bilateral and symmetrical; in the cat and squirrel monkey this projection is ipsilateral. Anatomical findings in the rat indicate that rostral portions of the nucleus of the solitary fasciculus, which receive primary gustatory afferents, project ipsilaterally to a "pontine taste area" in the rostral pons in the region of the parabrachial nuclei (1847, 1848). Cells in the parabrachial nuclei in turn project bilaterally upon VPMpc, as well as to regions of the hypothalamus and ventral forebrain structures (1846, 1848, 2145). In the monkey cells in rostral regions of the nucleus of the solitary fasciculus project fibers ipsilaterally to VPMpc while cells in slightly more caudal regions of this nucleus project fibers ipsilaterally to both the parabrachial nuclei and VPMpc (Figs. 11-22 and 15-17) (141). Lesions destroying VPMpc produce gustatory deficits in the monkey (198, 1951) and goat (64). Thalamic cell groups subserving taste are located medially and are separated spatially from neurons related to other sensory modalities of the tongue (193, 707, 710, 1849).

In the rat unilateral ablations of the cortical area in which potentials can be evoked by stimulating the chorda tympani and glossopharyngeal nerves (i.e., the parietal operculum) did not impair taste discrimination (157). Bilateral ablations of this area produced a partial loss of taste. Ablations of this cortical taste area produced retrograde degeneration of thalamic neurons confined to the most medial, parvocellular subdivision of the ventral posteromedial (VPMpc) nucleus. In an extensive study of thalamic projections to the insular and opercular cortex in the monkey, it was established that VPMpc (Fig. 15-16) projects to the parietal operculum and the insular cortex (2178). The gustatory representation in the cerebral cortex is adjacent to the somesthetic area for the tongue, but is separated from the nongustatory lingual area (156, 845, 1849). The cortical gustatory area lies ventral and rostral to the somesthetic representation of the tongue in sensory cortex and appears to have little overlap. Thus, gustatory impulses projecting to a distinctive part of the ventral posteromedial nucleus of the thalamus (VPMpc) also have a separate representation in the parietal operculum.

Vestibular Representation. In the cerebral cortex vestibular sense is poorly defined in comparison with other sensory modalities. In man, electrical stimulation of portions of the superior temporal gyrus, particularly regions rostral to the auditory area, provoke sensations of turning movements, referred to as *vertigo* (1968). These sensations are mild compared with the vertigo produced by direct stimulation of the labyrinth. Less distinct illusions of body movement have been reported following stimulation of parietal cortex (1962).

Physiological studies in the monkey indicate that vestibular nerve stimulation or angular acceleration of the head about a vertical axis evokes short latency responses in thalamic nuclei. These responses are not affected by cerebellectomy, but are abolished by vestibular nerve section. Direct stimulation of the vestibular nerve evokes responses contralaterally in the ventral posterior inferior (VPI; Fig. 15-16) and the ventral posterolateral (pars oralis, VPLo) thalamic nuclei (605–607, 1489). Angular acceleration of the head activates variable numbers of neurons in these thalamic nuclei ipsilaterally and contralaterally, depending on the direction of rotation (339, 340, 1584). Thalamic units responding to angular acceleration were not numerous and were intermingled with cells activated only by touch, pressure or joint movement (339). Activity recorded in thalamic neurons in alert monkeys was very similar to that seen in the vestibular nuclei and suggested that these thalamic neurons constituted a relay in a vestibular pathway to the cortex (340). The further observation that the discharge pattern of thalamic neurons in VPLo and VPI was related only to angular acceleration and not to oculomotor behavior (i.e., saccades, smooth pursuit or fixation) strengthened the thesis that they are vestibular relay neurons (1584). Autoradiographic studies reveal that vestibulothalamic projections in the monkey are bilateral and terminate in VPLo and to a lesser extent in adjacent regions of VPI and VLc (1423). The vestibular projection to the thalamus is small compared with that to the oculomotor nuclei and terminals in VPLo occur in small patches throughout the nucleus. Most, but not all, fibers ascending to the thalamus course outside of the medial longitudinal fasciculus (MLF).

Vestibulothalamic fibers appear to arise largely from the lateral, medial and superior vestibular nuclei (513, 1355, 1423, 2123). Because thalamic neurons responding to vestibular inputs are few in number, scattered over several subdivisions of the thalamus and are intermingled with cells activated by somatosensory input (i.e., kinesthetic sense and pressure) evidence for a specific vestibular relay nucleus in the thalamus is not strong (339, 607, 1489).

In the monkey the primary cortical projection area of the vestibular nerve was found to be in the postcentral gyrus near the lower end of the intraparietal sulcus (800, 1349). This projection area, near the face region of S I, has a different cytoarchitecture than area 2 and has been designated as area 2v (801). Antidromic stimulation has indicated that cells in VPI project to area 2v (605, 606, 800, 801). Many neurons in cortical area 2v show bimodal inputs in that they receive both vestibular and deep somatic afferents (2296). This observation has suggested a convergence of vestibular and somatosensory afferents that subserve conscious orientation in space. The degree of integration of vestibular and somatosensory inputs in thalamic nuclei is unclear (1489). Stimulation of the vestibular nerve also has evoked responses in area 3a which lies in the depths of the central sulcus between areas 4 and 3 (801, 1863). It is uncertain as to whether input to area 3a is derived from VPLo but it has been suggested that vestibular and muscle afferents (group Ia) may converge in area 3a. Although the location of the vestibular sensory area in the human brain is unknown, data from experimental studies indicate it may be buried in the cortex near the anterior part of the intraparietal sulcus, a region which corresponds to area 2v in the monkey (801). Vestibular representation in the cerebral cortex appears to be bilateral and lacks the modality specificity which characterizes other primary sensory areas.

CORTICAL AREAS CONCERNED WITH MOTOR FUNCTION

Corticofugal fibers arise from all regions of the cerebral cortex. These projections convey impulses concerned with motor function, modifications of muscle tone and reflex activity, modulation of sensory input and alterations of awareness and the state of consciousness. Corticofugal fibers, originating largely from the deeper layers of the cerebral cortex, can be grouped under the following designations: (a) corticospinal, (b) corticoreticular, (c) corticopontine, (d) corticothalamic, (e) corticostriate and (f) corticonuclear, a composite grouping of fibers that project to brain stem nuclei at different levels (e.g., corticosubthalamic, corticorubral, corticotectal and projections to various sensory and cerebellar relay nuclei). The somata of the cells of origin of particular corticofugal fiber systems have a specific laminar or sublaminar distribution (1245). Corticospinal neurons lie in the deepest part of layer V, occur in definite clusters and show great variation in cell size, particularly in area 4. Corticostriate cells form the smallest group of pyramidal cells in layer V and are concentrated in the superficial part of this layer. Corticopontine, corticobulbar and corticorubral neurons lie in middle regions of layer V. The majority of corticothalamic cells are found in layer VI, but some of these neurons are located in deep parts of layer V. The somata of cortical association and commissural neurons lie in the supragranular layers of the cortex; association neurons giving rise to ipsilateral corticocortical projections are superficial (layers II and III) to neurons giving rise to commissural connections (layer III). These observations based upon retrograde transport of HRP indicate that cells contributing to distinctive fiber systems occur in single or multiple strips 0.5 to 1 mm wide oriented mediolaterally across the cortex.

The Primary Motor Area. Area 4 of Brodmann, commonly designated as the motor area, is located on the anterior wall of the central sulcus and adjacent portions of the precentral gyrus (Figs. 19-5 and 19-6). Broad at the superior border of the hemisphere, where it spreads over a considerable part of the precentral gyrus, it narrows inferiorly and, at the level of the inferior frontal gyrus, is practically limited to the anterior wall of the central sulcus. On the medial surface of the hemisphere it comprises the anterior portion of the paracentral lobule (Fig. 2-5). The unusually thick cortex of the motor area (3.5 to 4.5 mm) is agranular in structure, and its ganglionic layer contains the giant pyramidal cells of Betz, whose cell bodies may reach a height of 60 to 120 μm (Figs. 4-6 and 19-9B). These cells are largest in the paracentral lobule, and smallest inferiorly in the opercular region. The density of Betz cells varies in different parts of area 4 (1442). Approximate percentages of Betz cells in different topographical subdivisions of area 4 are: 75% in the leg area, 18% in the arm area and 7% in the face area. Approximately 34,000 giant pyramidal cells with cross-sectional areas between 900 and 4100 μm^2 have been counted in area 4 in the human brain (1442, 1443). Cytoarchitecturally area 4 represents a modification of the typical six-layered isocortex in which the pyramidal cells in layers III and V are increased in number and the internal granular layer is obscured. For this reason the cortex is called agranular.

The rostral border of area 4 has been distinguished physiologically as a distinct subdivision, referred to as area 4S (1101, 1102). Ablation of this narrow strip of cortex along the rostral border of area 4 in the monkey was said to produce a transient spastic paralysis, and stimulation of this area was reported to inhibit extensor muscle tone. Subsequent studies indicated that area 4S was one of a number of cortical areas from which suppressor effects of a questionable character were said to be obtained in response to stimulation (663). This subdivision cannot be distinguished from other parts of area 4 anatomically and it is not regarded as a separate entity.

The corticospinal tract, which is considered ultimately to transmit impulses for highly skilled volitional movements to lower motor neurons, arises in large part from area 4. The larger corticospinal fibers are probably the axons of giant pyramidal cells, for these cells undergo chromatolysis following section of the pyramid (1133, 1480). Since the number of fibers in the human corticospinal tract at the level of the pyramid is approximately 1,000,000, axons of the giant cells of Betz could account for only a little over 3% of these fibers, assuming that each cell gives rise to a single corticospinal fiber (1442). The fiber spectrum of the human corticospinal tract indicates about 30,000 fibers with diameters between 9 and 22 μm (1447, 1449, 1450), supporting the view that these fibers are the parent axons of the giant pyramidal cells. Approximately 90% of the fibers of

the corticospinal tract range from 1 to 4 μm in diameter. Of the total number of fibers in the tract, about 40% are poorly myelinated. The more numerous small fibers of the corticospinal tract arise from smaller cells in this and other cortical regions. Interruption of the corticospinal tract reportedly also gives rise to chromatolytic cell changes in small pyramidal cells in the III and V layers, not only in area 4, but also in areas 3, 1, 2 and 5 (1480). Data concerning the cortical areas which contribute fibers to the corticospinal tract and the extent of their individual contributions are variable and incomplete. Ablations of area 4 in the monkey cause degeneration of 27 to 40% of the corticospinal tract, including virtually all of the large myelinated fibers (1443, 1447). Other authors have reported smaller percentages of degenerated fibers after similar ablations (999), but none report complete degeneration of the corticospinal tract (1684, 2695). Ablations of parietal cortex (areas 3, 1, 2, 5 and 7) also produce degeneration of myelinated fibers in the corticospinal tract (1714, 1959). Combined ablations of the precentral and postcentral gyri cause degeneration of 50 to 60% of the fibers in the corticospinal tract (1443, 1444, 2241). A quantitative study of the origin of corticospinal fibers in the monkey based on silver staining methods (2241) indicates that virtually all fibers of the corticospinal tract arise from area 4, area 6 and parts of the parietal lobe. Approximate percentages of corticospinal fibers arising from these areas are as follows: (a) area 4, 31%; (b) area 6, 29%; and (c) parietal lobe, 40%. Complete decortication, or hemispherectomy, causes all fibers of the corticospinal tract to degenerate in man (1448) and in the monkey (1684, 2241).

Retrograde transport studies in the monkey using HRP indicate that corticospinal fibers arise from cells widely distributed in the sensorimotor cortex, all of which are located in layer V (540, 1245). Labeled corticospinal neurons in the deep parts of layer V are found in areas 6, 4, 3a, 3, 1, 2, 5 and in SS II. Although these neurons show great variation in size, all are pyramidal cells; apical and basal dendrites are well outlined by HRP granules. The largest cells are seen in area 4, while smaller cells, more nearly the same size, are evident in other areas. Cells giving rise to corticospinal projections

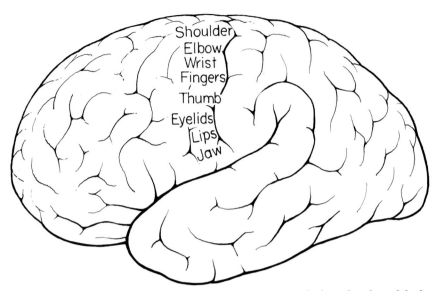

Figure 19-25. Representation of parts of the body in the motor area on the lateral surface of the hemisphere. According to Scarff (2265), the leg usually is represented only in the anterior part of the paracentral lobule.

occur in clusters aligned to form strips oriented mediolaterally across the cortex. These studies do not support the earlier hypothesis that "slow" conducting corticospinal axons arise from pyramidal cells in layer III. Autoradiographic data suggest that major differences exist in the pattern of terminal labeling in the spinal gray following injections of different cytoarchitectonic areas (541). Isotope injected into cortical areas 3, 1, 2 and 5 label terminals in parts of the posterior horn which correspond to Rexed's laminae III and IV, while injections into areas 4 and 3a label terminals largely in Rexed's lamina VII, but with extensions into regions of spinal motor neurons. No corticospinal neurons project into Rexed's laminae I and II. It is generally accepted that some corticospinal neurons end directly upon anterior horn cells in the brachial and lumbosacral enlargements in the monkey (1408, 1500). These corticospinal fibers arise from cells in area 4. Physiological studies of the branching of corticospinal fibers into the spinal cord indicate some axons innervate more than one spinal segment, but that axons supplying motor pools innervating distal limb muscles have fewer collaterals (2328). This arrangement is considered to be related to discrete contraction of individual distal limb muscles.

Electrical stimulation of the motor area evokes discrete isolated movements on the opposite side of the body. Usually the contractions involve the functional muscle groups concerned with a specific movement, but individual muscles, even a single interosseus, may be contracted separately. While the pattern of excitable foci is nearly the same for all mammals, the number of such foci, and hence the number of discrete movements, is increased greatly in man. Thus flexion or extension at a single finger joint, twitchings at the corners of the mouth, elevation of the palate, protrusion of the tongue and even vocalization, expressed in involuntary cries or exclamations, all may be evoked by careful stimulation of the proper areas. Charts of motor representation, which are in substantial agreement, have been furnished by a number of investigators (763, 764, 1963, 1965, 1968, 2265). These data concerning the human brain were collected during neurosurgical procedures in which patients were operated upon under local anesthesia (Fig. 19-25). The location of centers for specific movements may vary from individual to individual, but the orderly sequence of motor representation appears constant (e.g., the point which on stimulation produces a movement of the pharynx always lies nearer to the lateral sulcus than points producing movement of the lips). Ipsilateral movements have not been observed in man, but bilateral responses occur in the muscles of the eyes, face, tongue, jaw, larynx and pharynx. According to Penfield and Boldrey (1963), the center for the pharynx (swallowing) lies in the most inferior opercular portion of the precentral gyrus; it is followed, from below upward, by centers for the tongue, jaw, lips, larynx, eyelid and brow, in the order named (Fig. 19-12). Next come the extensive areas for finger movements, the thumb being lowest and the little finger highest; these are followed by areas for the hand, wrist, elbow and shoulder. Finally, in the most superior part, are the centers for the hip, knee, ankle and toes. The last named are situated at the medial border of the hemisphere and extend into the paracentral lobule, which also contains the centers for the anal and vesicle sphincters (Fig. 19-12).

There has been considerable controversy regarding the location of representation of the lower extremity, due mainly to difficulties in stimulating the medial surface. According to Foerster (763), the paracentral lobule (Fig. 2-5) contains foci related to the foot, the toes, the bladder and the rectum. Penfield and Boldrey (1963) reported leg movements in 23 cases produced by stimulation of superior portions of the precentral gyrus, but Scarff (2265) was unable to elicit any leg movements by stimulating the lateral surface of the hemisphere. According to Scarff (2265) the leg, as a rule, is represented only on the medial surface of the hemisphere (i.e., in the paracentral lobule). This upward shift of the motor area, which appears unique to man, is considered to be due to the great expansion of cortical areas on the lateral surface of the hemisphere representing the tongue, mouth, lips, face and upper extremity (Fig. 19-25).

The movements elicited by electrical stimulation of the motor cortex probably are not equivalent to voluntary movements, although they are interpreted as "volitional" by the patient. These movements are never skilled movements, comparable to complex acquired movements, but consist largely of either simple flexions or extensions at one or more joints. The threshold in different topographical parts of area 4 varies. The region representing the thumb appears to have the lowest threshold, while the face area has the highest threshold. Excessive stimulation of area 4 produces either a focal seizure, or one resembling a Jacksonian convulsion.

The classical view of the somatotopic organization in the motor cortex is a single continuous, distorted representation of the body parts within the primary motor area. This organization most frequently is represented by the motor homunculus or its equivalent (Fig. 19-12). This concept of motor cortical representation has been extrapolated from studies in which movements have been produced by surface stimulation in a variety of animals and in man (Fig. 19-25). The summation of cortical representation depicted in a single line drawing is regarded as an oversimplification because it rarely takes into account the extent of overlap of various body regions which is a characteristic feature of the motor cortex (2777). Studies indicating a double representation of the body surface within cytoarchitectonic areas 3 and 1 in the monkey (1673) have raised questions concerning multiple representations of body parts in the regions of overlap in the primary motor cortex (2449). The possibility of multiple representation of the body in motor cortex has been explored in the squirrel monkey in which none of the primary motor area is buried in the central sulcus (2449). Microstimulation at depths coincident with layer V revealed a discrete double representation of the hand and wrist with the second hand zone located rostrally. Although all regions of the motor cortex have not been explored in detail, the possibility of dual representation of motor function appears to have some foundation, although it seems unlikely that these systems could be entirely independent. Earlier physiological studies have indicated that repetitive microstimulation at various depths in the motor cortex can either facilitate or inhibit monosynaptic reflexes (88). Although stimulation can change the excitability of a given pool of lower motor neurons, there is as yet no evidence that cells in the motor cortex are organized into functional cell columns as reported in the somesthetic and visual cortex (1229).

Ablations of the motor cortex in mammals produce increasingly greater neurological deficits at progressively higher levels of the phylogenetic scale (2658). In the cat removals of the motor cortex, or even hemidecortication, do not impair the animal's ability to walk upon recovery from anesthesia. Ablations of area 4 in the monkey produce a contralateral flaccid paralysis, marked hypotonia and areflexia. Within a relatively short time myotatic reflexes reappear, along with withdrawal responses to nociceptive stimuli (824). Recovery of movement begins in the proximal musculature and progresses distally, but the digits tend to remain permanently paralyzed. Studies in the monkey confirm these findings, except that recovery of motor function in the distal parts of the extremity was as rapid as that in proximal parts (2568). Although considerable improvement of motor function occurred, skilled movements were performed slowly and with some deliberation. Atrophy present in the paretic limbs during the period of greatest disuse disappeared after maximal functional recovery. No significant spasticity developed in these animals. Other results (624, 626) differ from the above in that some degree of spasticity accompanied the paretic manifestations after all lesions of the precentral gyrus in the monkey. Relatively mild spasticity, developed first in proximal muscle groups, was described as most enduring following total ablations.

Because the precentral gyrus gives rise to a large number of nonpyramidal fibers, and is the source of only a part of the corticospinal tract, it is instructive to compare the motor deficits described above with those which follow surgical section of the pyramids. Selective pyramidotomy in the monkey and chimpanzee, accomplished by an anterior approach, produces a contralateral paresis which is somewhat more severe in the chimpanzee than in the monkey (2564, 2565). In neither animal is the paresis so severe that the effected limbs are useless. The relatively stereotyped movements of progression are impaired, and there is a severe poverty of movement. The usage which survives is stripped of all the finer qualities which contribute to the skill, precision and versatility of motor performance. Although remaining stereotyped movements are useful, execution of purposeful movements appears to require deliberation and critical attention. Pyramidotomy is associated with hypotonia and loss of superficial abdominal and cremasteric reflexes.

The myotatic reflexes are increased in threshold and somewhat pendular. Tonic neck reflexes are absent, and clonus does not occur. A forced grasp reflex is prominent and may be so severe as to interfere with climbing. In the chimpanzee, a persistent and enduring Babinski sign can be elicited. Observations on monkeys with bilateral pyramidal lesions by Lawrence and Kuypers (1458) also indicate that considerable recovery of independent limb movements occurs, but recovery of individual finger movements never returns. All movements are slower and the muscles fatigue is more rapidly than in normal animals. These findings indicate that corticospinal pathways conduct impulses concerned with speed and agility of movement, and fractionation of movements, as exemplified by individual finger movements. Motor function remaining after bilateral pyramidotomy must be mediated by brain stem pathways projecting to spinal levels. These findings have been confirmed in young monkeys (1457). Relatively independent finger movements are not present in young monkeys until approximately 8 months of age; such finger movements develop gradually in parallel with the spinal connections of the corticospinal system. Following bilateral pyramidal tract lesions a few weeks after birth, relatively independent finger movements failed to develop in a 3-year period of observation.

Lesions of the motor cortex in man produce neurological deficits similar to those described in the primate, although anatomical details are not so precise. Since conclusions based upon pathological lesions of various types are difficult to interpret, reliable data are limited to instances in which all, or parts, of the precentral gyrus have been removed surgically (310, 313, 763, 1968). Ablations limited to the "arm" or "leg" area of the precentral gyrus result in a paralysis of a single limb (i.e., monoplegia). The ultimate loss of movement is always greatest in the distal muscle groups, but motor recovery in the affected limb usually is more complete than that associated with nearly total lesions of the motor area (310). Immediately after complete or partial lesions of the precentral gyrus, there is a flaccid paralysis of the contralateral limbs or limb, marked hypotonia and loss

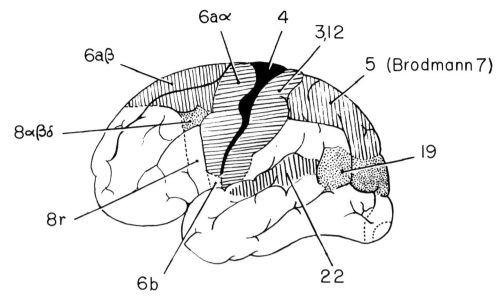

Figure 19-26. The areas of electrically excitable cortex on the lateral surface of the human brain. The motor area is shown in *black*, and the so-called "extrapyramidal areas" of the frontal lobe are *hatched* except for the eye fields, which are *stippled* (after Foerster (764)).

of superficial and myotatic reflexes. Within a relatively short time the Babinski sign can be elicited. The myotatic reflexes generally return early in an exaggerated form. There are differences of opinion concerning whether removals of area 4 in man result in a permanent spastic paralysis (310, 313, 763, 1968). According to Bucy (310), the spasticity is not severe and is less intense than that commonly associated with hemiplegias resulting from large capsular lesions. Although there is considerable restitution of function in proximal muscle groups, relatively little recovery of skilled motor function occurs in the smaller distal muscles of the extremities. The neural mechanisms underlying this partial recovery of function are not known.

The Premotor Area. This area (area 6) lies immediately in front of the motor area, runs dorsoventrally along the lateral aspect of the frontal lobe and is continued on the medial surface to the sulcus cinguli (Fig. 19-5). Near the superior border it is quite broad and includes the caudal portion of the superior frontal gyrus. Inferiorly the premotor area narrows, and near the operculum it is limited to the precentral gyrus. Its histological structure resembles that of

the motor area; it is composed principally of large well formed pyramidal cells, but there are no giant cells of Betz (Fig. 19-9A). Pyramidal cells in layers III and V and the narrowness of layer IV make it difficult to distinguish an internal granular layer. For this reason area 6, like area 4, is referred to as agranular frontal cortex. Area 6 has been subdivided into various portions, as shown in Figure 19-26 (764). According to this parcellation, area 6aα lies immediately rostral to area 4 along the convexity of the hemisphere, while area 6aβ occupies the region of the superior frontal gyrus on both the lateral and medial surfaces of the hemisphere. A small area designated 6b lies in front of the face area.

Electrical stimulation of area 6aα in man produces responses similar to those obtained from area 4, although stronger currents are required (760, 763). It is probably that area 6aα discharges via the corticospinal tract. Stimulation of area 6aβ elicits more general movement patterns characterized by rotation of the head, eyes and trunk to the opposite side, and synergic patterns of flexion or extension in the contralateral extremities. These general movement patterns appear independent of area

4, since they can be obtained after its removal. Portions of area 6aβ on the medial aspect of the hemisphere are considered to constitute part of the *supplementary motor area*. Stimulation of area 6b is reported to produce rhythmic coordinated movements of a complex type involving facial, masticatory, laryngeal and pharyngeal musculature.

Unilateral ablations of area 6, including portions on the medial aspect of the hemisphere, produce transient grasp reflexes in the monkey (2147). Bilateral removals of area 6 produce more enduring grasp reflexes (1288, 2695). Unilateral destruction of area 6aβ in man produces little or no motor deficit (763). Evidence in man and monkey emphasizes that only lesions involving the supplementary motor areas produce grasping phenomena (715, 2569). Ablations of area 6, not involving the precentral or supplementary motor areas, do not produce paresis, grasp reflexes or hypertonia.

Studies in the monkey have suggested that combined ablations of areas 4 and 6 produce a contralateral spastic paralysis (825, 1287, 1288). Similar findings were reported in man following ablations of area 6, which undoubtedly included parts of area 4, as well as so-called area 4S (1289). Attempts to clarify these results by Hines (1102) indicated the removal of area 4S in the monkey produced only a temporary paresis, but a permanent increase in tone in the contralateral antigravity muscles. Ablations of the posterior part of area 4 result in a contralateral flaccid paresis. These studies suggested that ablation of area 4S probably was responsible for the release phenomena expressed as spasticity. Subsequent investigations (2569) have explained the spasticity resulting from combined lesions of areas 4 and 6 on the basis of simultaneous destruction of precentral and supplementary motor areas. This same investigator has shown that bilateral removals of area 4S in the monkey do not produce spasticity until the lesions encroach upon the supplementary motor area.

Inputs to the Motor Cortex. Although impulses generated in neurons of the motor cortex are responsible for movement, changes in muscle tone and certain cortical reflex responses, these motor activities are initiated by inputs that arise from the thalamus, other cortical regions and peripheral receptors. Particular potent drives upon the primary motor cortex are conveyed by fibers arising from thalamic nuclei (i.e., the ventral lateral, VLc and VLo, and the ventral posterolateral, pars oralis, VPLo) (612, 2170, 2445, 2446, 2567). Crossed cerebellar projections, via largely the dentate nucleus project preferentially to VLc and VPLo, while uncrossed pallidothalamic fibers project to VLo (1313, 1398, 1825, 1971, 2538, 2567). Neurons of the ventral lateral nucleus show increased activity prior to any movement suggesting that these neurons play a role in initiating activity in muscles concerned with control of posture and discrete limb movements (2446). The premotor area appears to receive projections from the ventral anterior, the ventral lateral (VLc) and from area X (i.e., the most medial part of VL) (373, 1310, 2178, 2445). Retrograde transport studies indicate that thalamic neurons which project to the motor and premotor cortex are distinct and separate from those that project to somatic sensory areas (1241, 1310, 2445). Electron microscopic evidence in the cat indicates that fibers from VL projecting to the motor cortex make synaptic terminations largely in three cortical layers: (a) upper third of layer I (18%), (b) layer III (66%) and (c) layer VI (13%) (2450). Fibers terminating directly in layer V were relatively rare (3%). The majority of fibers from VL neurons synapse upon dendritic spines; in layer III this input synapses upon the apical dendrites of motor neurons (Betz cells of layer V) and upon stellate cells (interneurons). Autoradiographic data in the monkey also demonstrates that the largest number of efferents from VL terminate in layer III of area 4 (1227).

The primary motor area also receives inputs from the primary somesthetic area (S I), the second somatic area (SS II), and the supplementary motor area (1236, 1238, 1244). These cortical inputs to the motor area are of an interlocking nature in that somatotopical subdivisions are connected with each other. More recent detailed studies indicate that only area 2 of S I projects directly to area 4 (1232, 2623). Area 2 which receives an input from deep somatic receptors also has connections with area 5 via intracortical fibers in layers III and IV as well as through the white matter. Area 5, difficult to distinguish from area 2, has been shown to project to area 4 and parts of area 6 by anterograde and retrograde transport technics and by antidromic activation (1232, 2448, 2791). These data suggest that area 5 has important influences upon the motor cortex and raise questions concerning the nature of this input. About two-thirds of the neurons in area 5 are activated by passive joint rotation. It has been postulated that area 5 contains the "command apparatus" for limb and hand movements in immediate extrapersonal space (1768). Neurons in area 5 have been observed to discharge only when an animal moves its arm toward a desired object or manipulates an object with its hand. The "command" hypothesis suggests that the cortical pathway from area 5 to area 4 is involved in initiating limb and hand movements.

Physiological studies indicate that the motor cortex receives inputs from both cutaneous and deep receptors (2221, 2719). Impulses from group I muscle afferent have been recorded in cortical area 3a, but it is not known how these impulses influence the motor cortex, because there is no known projection from area 3a to area 4 (1232, 2000). Impulses from joint receptors projecting to area 2 appear to have access to the motor cortex directly and via area 5. It is unclear as to how impulses from cutaneous receptors reach the motor cortex but relays in the postcentral gyrus appear to be involved. Impulses from cutaneous receptors may be involved in mechanisms of instinctive grasping as well as in the startle reaction (2719).

Supplementary Motor Area. Observations by early investigators indicated that motor responses in different parts of the body could be elicited by electrical stimulation of the medial surface of the frontal lobe above the cingulate gyrus and rostral to the primary motor area (1970). This motor area, identified in the human brain, has been designated as the supplementary motor area (1968). The supplementary motor area in man and monkey occupies the medial surface of the superior frontal gyrus rostral to area 4 (Fig. 19-27). Detailed descriptions of somatotopic representation within the supplementary motor area of the

monkey have been provided by Woolsey et al. (2777). The sequential representation of body parts in this area is shown in Figure 19-27. The threshold for stimulation of the supplementary motor area in man and monkeys is slightly higher than for the precentral region. Motor responses obtained from the supplementary motor area are not due to spread of excitation to the primary motor area because they are not significantly altered by: (a) ablation of area 4, or (b) section of the corticospinal tract (1965, 2774).

Stimulation of the supplementary motor area in man produces raising of the opposite arm, turning of the head and eyes and bilateral synergic contractions of the muscles of the trunk and legs. Movements provoked by stimulation of the supplementary motor area have been divided into three types: (a) assumption of postures, (b) maneuvers consisting of a series of complex patterned movements, and (c) infrequent rapid incoordinate movements. The whole pattern of movement seems to be bilateral and synergistic, but most movements are described as tonic contractions of the postural type. Other responses obtained included pupillary dilatation, cardiac acceleration, vocalization and occasional sensory phenomena. Although the visceral responses resemble those commonly obtained from the cingulate gyrus, these are not due to spread of the stimulus. Unilateral ablations of the supplementary motor area in man produce no permanent deficit in the maintenance of posture or movement (1968, 1970).

Systematic studies in the monkey of removals of the supplementary motor area alone, and in combination with the precentral motor area, have produced conflicting results. According to Travis (2568, 2569), unilateral ablations of the supplementary motor area in the monkey produce weak transient grasp reflexes in the contralateral limbs, and moderate bilateral hypertonia of the shoulder muscles, but no paresis. Bilateral simultaneous ablations of this area result in disturbances of posture and tonus, but produce no paresis. Gradually increasing hypertonia, resulting in muscle contracture, develops in a period of 2 to 4 weeks. The hypertonia is mainly in flexor muscles. Myotatic reflexes are hyperactive, and

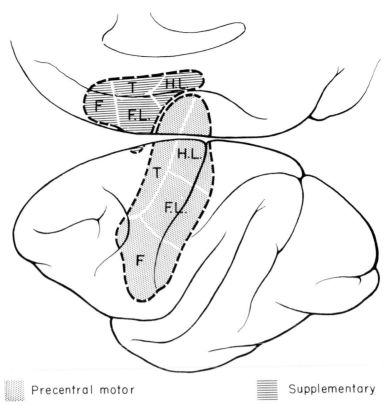

▒ Precentral motor   ≡ Supplementary

Figure 19-27. Diagram of the precentral and supplementary motor areas in the monkey. The somatotopic representation of different parts of the body are shown: *F*, face area; *T*, trunk; *FL*, forelimb; *HL*, hindlimb. The precentral motor area on the lateral convexity extends over onto the medial aspect of the hemisphere; the *outlined area* shown posterior to the central sulcus represents cortex hidden in the depths of the central sulcus. The supplementary motor area, largely on the medial aspect of the hemisphere, is shown *above* (after Travis (2569)).

clonus can be demonstrated. The developed spasticity demonstrates a topographical localization according to the portions of the supplementary motor area removed. These observations could not be confirmed in a similar study by Coxe and Landau (559). Although the ablation method has not yielded specific information concerning the role of the supplementary motor area in motor control, there appears to be agreement that combined lesions of the supplementary and precentral motor areas on the same side result in a spastic rather than a flaccid paresis (253, 626, 2568, 2569, 2570). As mentioned previously, physiological findings concerning the supplementary motor area have been cited to explain the controversy regarding ablations of areas 4 and 6, and the relationships of so-called area 4S to muscle tonus.

Although relatively little is known concerning the functional attributes of the supplementary motor area, the mammalian cerebral cortex seems to possess at least two separate motor areas (2754). Physiological evidence of their respective roles in control of movement are quite different. It has been suggested that the supplementary motor area may serve mainly as a control system for posture (2720). Studies done in conscious, behaving monkeys indicate that neurons in the supplementary motor area are related to movements on both sides of the body, involving equally both distal and proximal musculature (254). These observations imply that the supplementary motor area probably is concerned with more than control of posture. Most of the neurons in the supplementary motor area increase their activity before the onset of movement and large numbers of neurons in this area discharge during particular movements of either arm. Only a small number of cells in this area receive a peripheral sensory input (254, 2754).

The supplementary motor area, as described in man and monkeys has no clear-cut cytoarchitectonic borders and its neural connections are poorly understood. Corticocortical (association) connections are fairly well known and include afferents from the ipsilateral primary sensory area (areas 3, 1, and 2) and from the second somatic area (SS II) (1232, 1238). Reciprocal connections also exist with the ipsilateral primary motor area (area 4), area 3a in the depths of the central sulcus, area 5 and with the superior part of area 6 on the lateral convexity of the hemisphere (1925, 2623). Less well established subcortical projections to the supplementary motor area are derived from the ventral anterior (VA), ventral lateral (VLo, VLc) and the paracentral (PCN) thalamic nuclei (254, 1258, 1310). On the basis of its cortical connections the supplementary motor area has been regarded an area in which sensory impulses converge (1226, 1242). The efferent connections of the supplementary motor area suggests that it plays a direct role in motor control. Cortical efferents project to the primary motor area (area 4) and to lateral portions of area 6 (628, 1242). In addition the supplementary motor area has bilateral projections to the striatum (1231, 1285) and ipsilateral projections to thalamic nuclei (VA, VLo, VLc, VPLo) (628, 2720), the red nucleus and the pontine nuclei. A direct corticospinal projection from the supplementary motor area has been disputed but recent anatomical and physiological studies support the existence of this pathway (173, 254, 1784, 1785). It has been estimated that only 5% of cells in the supplementary motor area project axons into the corticospinal tract. In summary, present data support the concept that the supplementary motor area as a separate cortical motor region that has striking bilateral influences upon motor function of both proximal and distal musculature, but it remains difficult to characterize.

According to Bates (131), stimulation of this motor area in man, following hemispherectomy, induces ipsilateral movements similar to those which can be produced voluntarily.

Cortical Eye Fields. In front of the premotor area is a cortical region particularly concerned with voluntary eye movements. The *frontal eye field* in man occupies principally the caudal part of the middle frontal gyrus (corresponding to parts of area 8, shown in Figs. 19-5 and 19-26) and extends into contiguous portions of the inferior frontal gyrus. The entire frontal eye field does not lie within a single cytoarchitectonic area. Cytoarchitecturally, area 8 is typical six-layered isocortex of the frontal type in which the granular layers are distinct (Fig. 19-7). Electrical stimulation of the frontal eye field in man causes conjugate deviation of the eyes, usually to the opposite side (760, 1968). This cortical field is believed to be a center for voluntary eye movements not dependent upon visual stimuli. The conjugate eye movements commonly are called "movements of command," since they can be elicited by instructing the patient to look to the right or left (488). Some studies in man and primates suggest a double representation of specific eye movements in each frontal eye field (569a, 571, 1466).

The concept of an *occipital eye center* for conjugate eye movements is based upon the fact that stimulation of occipital cortex produces conjugate eye movements to the opposite side, and lesions in this area are associated with transient deviation of the eyes to the side of the lesion. Unlike the frontal eye field, the occipital eye center is not localized to a small area. Eye responses can be obtained from a wide region of the occipital lobe in the monkey, but the lowest threshold is found in area 17 (2659). The occipital eye centers are presumed to subserve movements of the eyes induced by visual stimuli, such as following moving objects. These pursuit movements of the eyes are largely involuntary, although they are not present in young infants. The occipital eye centers, unlike the frontal eye fields, are interconnected by fibers passing in the splenium of the corpus callosum. The threshold for excitation is higher in the occipital lobe than in the frontal eye fields; the latency of responses is longer, and eye movements tend to be smoother and less brisk. Following a lesion of the occipital eye field the patient may have difficulty following a slow moving object, but on command can direct the eyes to a particular location. Eye movements on command are impaired by lesions in the frontal eye field, particularly in the dominant hemisphere.

The pathways by which responses from the frontal and occipital eye fields are mediated, are thought to involve projections to the superior colliculus. Autoradiographic tracing technics indicate that fibers from area 8 project profusely to the stratum zonale, the stratum opticum and the intermediate gray stratum (1395, 1396). These corticofugal fibers terminate in the same layers of the superior colliculus that receive fibers from the retina and striate cortex (1153). Although fibers from the frontal eye field end in the pretectum, none of these fibers project to the pretectal olivary nucleus. None of the corticofugal fibers from the frontal eye field project to the oculomotor nucleus, the accessory oculomotor nuclei or the paramedian pontine reticular formation. The most massive projection of area 8 is to the paralaminar part of the dorsomedial nucleus with which it has reciprocal connections. The most substantial and highly organized projection to the superior colliculus arises from the visual cortex (582, 848, 2732). These fibers mainly enter the stratum opticum via the brachium of the superior colliculus and terminate in superficial layers in a retinotopic pattern (Fig. 13-9). Both retinotectal and corticotectal fibers convey impulses related to central and peripheral parts of the retina. Although the superior colliculus does not project direct fibers to the nuclei of the extraocular muscles, it has projections to both the reticular formation and the accessory oculomotor nuclei (386).

NONPYRAMIDAL CORTICOFUGAL FIBERS

These cortical projections consist largely of corticoreticular, corticopontine, corticothalamic and corticonuclear fibers.

Corticoreticular Fibers. These originate from all parts of the cerebral cortex, but the largest number arise from the motor and premotor areas (2227). Inferior cortical areas (basal) and parts of the cortex on the medial surface of the hemisphere also contribute to the corticoreticular projection,

but few fibers arise from the auditory and visual areas. Corticoreticular fibers descend in association with fibers of the corticospinal tract, but they leave this bundle to enter specific areas of the brain stem reticular formation. The number of corticoreticular fibers is not large and the major part of these fibers terminate in two fairly well circumscribed areas in the medulla and in the pons. The terminal area in the medulla corresponds to the nucleus reticularis gigantocellularis, while the pontine area coincides with the nucleus reticularis pontis oralis (Fig. 10-22). Unilateral cerebral lesions produce an approximately equal distribution of degenerated corticoreticular fibers on both sides of the reticular formation. Some corticoreticular fibers also reach reticular cerebellar relay nuclei, such as the reticulotegmental nucleus, the lateral reticular nucleus and the paramedian reticular nuclei of the medulla.

Corticopontine Fibers. These fibers arise from regions of the frontal, temporal, parietal and occipital regions of the cortex (139, 291–293, 1858). Studies of corticopontine fibers in the monkey indicate that the largest number of fibers arise from areas 4, 3, 1, 2, 5 and parts of the visual cortex (296, 297, 1245). These fibers arise from pyramidal cells in layer V lying superficial to the giant pyramidal cells and are larger than those of other efferent systems except for corticospinal neurons. Corticopontine fibers arising from the visual cortex are from regions representing the peripheral visual field. Contributions to this system from temporal and prefrontal cortex are relatively modest; most of the fibers from the prefrontal areas arise from areas 9 and 8 (90, 291). On reaching the midbrain, the frontopontine tract forms the most medial part of the crus cerebri, and is distributed to the medial pontine nuclei (Fig. 13-1 and 14-21). Corticopontine fibers from the "motor" and "sensory" areas in the cat project in a somatotopical manner onto two longitudinally oriented cell columns in the pontine nuclei (291). One cell column is located medial and one is lateral. Within the medial column, the hindlimb is represented ventrally and the face dorsally, while in the lateral column, the hindlimb is represented caudally and the forelimb rostrally. Thus fibers from particular regions of the cerebral cortex end within columnar zones of pontine nuclei which are separated from each other. Although the synaptic relationships of corticopontine fibers are incompletely known, most of these fibers appear to end only upon dendrites (527). There appears to be considerable overlap in the terminations of corticopontine fibers from some cortical areas. Most corticopontine fibers exert a monosynaptic excitatory action upon pontine neurons (37).

Through the synaptic linkage of corticopontine and pontocerebellar fibers impulses from the cerebral cortex are brought into association with the synaptic and regulating influences of the cerebellum. The patterns of this synaptic linkage are most complex, but there is no doubt that this is the most massive input system to the cerebellum.

Corticothalamic Fibers. A large and impressive group of corticofugal fibers arise from specific regions of the cortex and project upon particular thalamic nuclei. In general, cortical areas receiving projections from particular thalamic nuclei give rise to reciprocal fibers which pass back to the same nuclei. The granular frontal cortex projects primarily to the dorsomedial nucleus of the thalamus, although some fibers pass to the submedial nucleus (466). Particularly prominent among these fibers are those arising from frontal areas 9 and 10. According to Mettler (1685), corticofugal fibers to the dorsomedial nucleus come from areas 11, 10, 9, 8 and 6 in the monkey. Reciprocal connections exist between the prefrontal cortex and the parvicellular part of the dorsomedial nucleus (DMpc) and between the premotor cortex and the paralaminar part of the dorsomedial nucleus (DMpl) (31, 1310). Particularly profuse interconnections relate area 8 and DMpl (1395, 1396, 2299). Most of these fibers reach the thalamus via the anterior limb of the internal capsule.

Fibers from the cingulate gyrus have been described as passing to the anterior nucleus of the thalamus, but cortical projections from this region are not clearly reciprocal to those projected by the anterior thalamic nuclei. Most of these fibers come from the supracallosal part of the cingulate gyrus at the transition of areas 24 and 23 and pass through the anterior thalamic radiation. A larger number of fibers from the cingulate gyrus enter the cingulum (Fig. 2-19) and pass to the entorhinal cortex (2094).

Corticothalamic fibers from the precentral area have long been recognized to project to the ventral lateral nucleus of the thalamus (463, 1103, 1478, 1479, 1687, 2157, 2170, 2615). These projections are more widespread than previously thought in that they pass to VLo, VLm, VLc and VPLo as well as to portions of the intralaminar thalamic nuclei (CM, PCN and CL) (31, 1393, 1883). Cortical projections from area 4 to VLo and VPLo are reciprocal and topographically arranged. The projections from area 4 to VLc are not as impressive as those from area 6 (1394). These data indicate that corticofugal fibers from the precentral gyrus project to thalamic nuclei which receive selective inputs from the deep cerebellar nuclei, the globus pallidus and the substantia nigra. Area 6 projects fibers to VA, VLc, "area X," VPLo and the parafascicular nucleus of the thalamus (1394). In addition the premotor area has a projection to DMpl. In general, the premotor area shows a thalamic projection pattern in different regions related to either the precentral or prefrontal cortex. According to physiological studies inhibitory effects upon VL neurons resulting from stimulation of the motor cortex can be graded by varying the intensity of the stimulation (2170).

Both the precentral and premotor cortex project upon portions of the intralaminar thalamic nuclei; the largest number of these fibers terminate in the centromedian-parafascicular nuclear complex (CM-PF) (31, 92, 1393, 1394, 1837, 1988, 1990, 1992, 2157). The precentral motor cortex sends fibers ipsilaterally primarily to CM, but some fibers reach the same nucleus on the opposite side following isotope injections of the motor face region (1393). Fibers from the premotor cortex project largely to PF, although some may reach the transitional zone with CM. The intralaminar thalamic nuclei, particularly CM-PF, receive substantial projections from the precentral and premotor cortex, but these nuclei project diffusely upon broad regions of the cortex in a fashion that cannot be regarded as reciprocal (1234, 1310).

Efferent fibers from the parietal cortex in the monkey pass by way of the sensory radiations to the thalamic nuclei, from which they receive fibers. Corticothalamic fibers from the primary somesthetic cortex project to the ventral posterolateral (VPL) and posteromedial (VPM) nuclei, and have been described as ending in a somatotopic fashion within these nuclei (1236, 1366, 1959). Both the primary somesthetic area and somatic sensory area II in the cat project in a topographically organized manner upon VPL and VPM. Corticothalamic projections from areas 3, 1 and 2 are confined to the ventrobasal complex, except from small projections to the reticular and central lateral thalamic nuclei (1246). No labeled terminals from these areas project to VPLo, the ventral posterior inferior (VPI), the lateral posterior (LP) or the posterior thalamic nuclei. The ventral posterior thalamic nucleus gives rise to a thalamocortical projection to the somatic sensory cortex and appears to receive a reciprocal corticothalamic projection. It is considered likely that reciprocating corticothalamic fibers may influence the transmission of impulses to the cortex in a way similar to that exerted by corticofugal fibers upon the posterior column nuclei and neurons of the trigeminal nuclear complex. Area 5 of the parietal cortex does not receive fibers from VPM, nor does it project to that thalamic nucleus (1236); this cortical area sends fibers to the lateral posterior and the suprageniculate nuclei (1246).

Fibers from parts of the auditory cortex project back to the medial geniculate body through sublenticular parts of the internal capsule (1364, 1928, 2155, 2668). The cortical projections from the primary and secondary auditory areas are back to the subdivisions of the medial geniculate body (MGB) from which they receive inputs (429, 1875). The primary auditory cortex has reciprocal connections with the ventral laminated part of the MGB; both geniculocortical and corticogeniculate fibers are ipsilateral (631, 782). Although cortical projections to the medial geniculate body do not participate the descending auditory pathways that influence auditory relay nuclei at lower levels of the brain stem, projections from auditory cortex to the inferior colliculus (pericentral nucleus) are involved in this activity (429, 631, 1875, 2195).

The striate cortex, area 17, sends axons to the lateral geniculate body (LGB), the superior colliculus, the pretectum and the inferior pulvinar (875, 1129, 1537). Corticofugal fibers from area 17 project to all layers of the lateral geniculate body. This cortical projection has a retinotopic organization and arises from small and medium-sized pyramidal cells in layer VI (1129, 1537). Cells in the V layer of the striate cortex project to the superior colliculus and the inferior pulvinar. Although corticogeniculate and geniculocortical fibers are topographically organized they are not reciprocal in the true sense since they arise and terminate in different layers of the striate cortex and cells in the magnocellular layers of the LGB have no cortical projection.

While reciprocal relationships exist between the principal thalamic nuclei and their cortical projection sites, a different relationship pertains to the reticular and intralaminar thalamic nuclei. The thalamic reticular nucleus, which forms a nuclear envelope about the lateral and rostral surfaces of the thalamus, receives afferents from almost all areas of the cerebral cortex (370). These corticothalamic fibers are organized so that rostral cortical regions project to rostral parts of the reticular nucleus and posterior cortical regions project to posterior portions of the nucleus. There is no evidence that the reticular nucleus of the thalamus projects to the cerebral cortex (370, 1227, 2276). However, collaterals of fibers from thalamic nuclei, including the intralaminar nuclei, destined for specific cortical areas terminate in particular parts of the reticular nucleus (370, 1227). Corticothalamic fibers passing to a particular thalamic nucleus likewise given collaterals to the same portions of the reticular nucleus as the thalamic nucleus which receives the main cortical projection. Thus the reticular nucleus of the thalamus is strategically situated to sample activity passing between the cerebral cortex and the main thalamic relay nuclei. Cells in particular portions of the reticular nucleus of the thalamus project fibers to the thalamic relay nucleus which provides collateral input. This complex arrangement suggests that the reticular nucleus of the thalamus, composed of heterogeneous cell types, may serve to integrate and modulate intrathalamic activities.

The intralaminar thalamic nuclei, like the thalamic reticular nucleus, receive corticofugal fibers. According to Powell and Cowan (2058), most of the prefrontal cortex projects fibers to the rostral intralaminar thalamic nuclei. The premotor and motor cortex project fibers to centromedian and parafascicular nuclei; parietal and occipital cortex do not project fibers to the intralaminar thalamic nuclei. It has been suggested that the posterior thalamic nuclei may constitute the caudal extension of the intralaminar thalamic nuclei since they are related primarily to cortex on the lateral surface of the hemisphere caudal to area 4 (1243). Most areas of the neocortex project fibers to a particular nucleus of the dorsal thalamus and to either part of the intralaminar or posterior thalamic nuclei. The striate cortex is unique in that it does not project, or receive fibers from, either the intralaminar or posterior thalamic nuclei. The principal projections of the intralaminar nuclei are to the striatum, but thalamostriate fibers give rise to an extensive collateral system that projects diffusely upon broad regions of the cerebral cortex (1234). Comparisons of the differences in the nature of corticothalamic fibers projecting to the intralaminar nuclei and the collateral system from these nuclei passing to the cortex indicate fibers are in no sense reciprocal (31, 1310).

SPREADING DEPRESSION OF CORTICAL ACTIVITY

Certain areas of the cerebral cortex, whose electrical stimulation was said to suppress cortical motor responses, transmission of sensory inputs to the cortex and reduce the amplitude of the EEG were described as suppressor areas (662, 1101, 1102, 1560). The studies, based in part upon strychnine neuronography (662), are now mainly of historical interest. The phenomenon of cortical suppression has been discredited because the suppression observed in stimulating these areas probably is identical with that of the spreading depression of Leão (654, 2352). The latter phenomenon is not restricted to specific cortical areas, but is related to unfavorable experimental conditions. Leão (1462) described a depression of cortical rhythms in the rabbit which spreads slowly outward from the site of a weak mechanical, electrical or chemical stimulus to the cortex. Neither evoked potentials nor motor responses to cortical stimulation could be observed when the depression reached the sensorimotor cortex. Species differences in susceptibility of the cortex to spreading depression have been noted in that depression is more easily produced in the rabbit than the cat, and is seen only occasionally in the monkey. Substantial evidence indicates that cortical depression results from exposure of the brain to less than optimal physiological conditions, such as dehydration, cooling, ischemia or prolonged experimentation (1610–1613). The release of depolarizing substances from cortical neurons is probably involved in spreading depression (2725a). Some process like spreading depression occurs in man following a severe generalized seizure or direct trauma to the cortex.

CONSIDERATION OF CORTICAL FUNCTIONS
Cerebral Dominance

Although the two cerebral hemispheres appear as mirror images, or duplicates of each other, many functions are not represented equally at a cortical level. This appears true even though impulses from receptors on each side of the body seem to project nearly equally, although largely contralaterally, to symmetrical cortical areas, and certain information received in the cortex of one hemisphere can be transferred to the other via interhemispheric commissures (1699). In certain higher functions, believed to be cortical in nature, one hemisphere appears to be the "leading" one and, in this sense, is referred to as the *dominant hemisphere*. The most remarkable feature of cerebral dominance in man is the fact that in the adult the capacity for speech is overwhelmingly controlled by the left hemisphere. There is no known example in any other mammal of a class of learning so predominantly controlled by one half of the brain (870). With respect to most of the higher functions, cerebral dominance appears to be one of degree (2790). According to Henschen (1077), cerebral dominance is most complete in relation to the complex and highly evolved aspects of language. Handedness also is related to cerebral dominance, although its relationship is less clear cut than has been assumed. It seems likely that handedness is a graded characteristic. Left-handedness, in particular, is less definite than right-handedness, and less regularly associated with dominance in either hemisphere. There also appears to be a group of disturbances related to language that are said to be commonly associated with imperfectly developed cerebral dominance. These include the improper development of reading, writing and drawing abilities, poor spatial judgment and imperfect directional control (2790). In true right-handed individuals, the left hemisphere is nearly always dominant and governs language and related processes; the converse of this is not necessarily true. The degree of cerebral dominance appears to vary widely, not only among individuals, but with respect to different functions. Although a degree of "cerebral ambilaterality" would appear to be a distinct advantage with respect to recovery of speech following a unilateral cerebral injury, it appears to carry the risk of possible difficulty in learning to read, spell and draw. The relationship between handedness and speech is perhaps a more natural one than is commonly realized, since some gesturing often accompanies speech and in certain situations may substitute for it. Although most clinicians relate handedness and speech to the dominant hemisphere, Penfield and Roberts (1969) reported that there is no difference in the incidence of aphasia after operation on the left hemisphere between left- and right-handed patients, provided patients with cerebral injury occurring early in life are excluded. With this same exclusion there is said to be no significant difference in the frequency of aphasia after operations on the right hemisphere between right- and left-handed patients. Nevertheless, these authors regard the left hemisphere as dominant for speech regardless of handedness. Cerebral dominance is considered to have a genetic basis, but its hereditary determination probably is not absolute. Pathological and psychological factors also influence handedness, and many determining factors remain unknown.

The dominant hemisphere, usually the left, is primarily concerned with processing language, arithmetic and analytic functions, while the nondominant hemisphere is concerned with spatial concepts, recognition of faces and some elements of music (2398). There is some evidence that ideographic (pictographic) languages may be largely a function of the nondominant hemisphere because of its spatial and pictorial features, while grammatical languages using script depend upon the dominant hemisphere. The visual messages of sign language used by deaf persons appears to be processed primarily in the left hemisphere.

It has been suggested that the normal neonate in a sense has a split-brain because the corpus callosum is incompletely developed and not fully functional (856). Thus interhemispheric communication at birth probably is slight, but it increases with development of the corpus callosum which becomes reasonably complete about the 2nd or 3rd year of life. Until this level of development is reached, each hemisphere may process and record some linguistic information. Hand use probably reinforces hemisphere use, and the development of a special competence in one hemisphere results in a mutual reinforcement that establishes a life pattern. The major differences between the right and left hemispheres concern the analysis of language and the ability to speak. The fact that large left hemisphere lesions in young children do not cause total disruption of speech indicates that the right hemisphere has some linguistic competence. Surgical section of the interhemispheric commissure sheds light on certain problems of cerebral dominance, and indicates that in the adult the left hemisphere speaks for both hemispheres.

Many cortical functions are concerned only with contralateral regions of the body, and unilateral lesions affecting these areas produce disturbances only contralaterally, regardless of cerebral dominance. This appears particularly true of the primary motor and sensory areas. It also is the case with lesions of the parietal cortex which result in *astereognosis*, or inability to recognize the form, size, texture and identity of an object by touch alone. In certain parietal lobe lesions there is evidence that particular deficits occur more commonly in the nondominant hemisphere. One such syndrome is characterized by a disorder of the body image in which the patient: (a) fails to recognize part of his own body, (b) fails to appreciate the existence of hemiparesis, and (c) neglects to wash, shave or cover the part of his body which he denies (564).

Interhemispheric Transfer

Although the corpus callosum is the largest of the interhemispheric commissures, relatively little was known of its functions until recently. The first convincing evidence regarding its function was the demonstration of its importance in interhemispheric transfer of visual discrimination learning in cats with longitudinal section of the optic chiasm (1699). Following section of the optic chiasm and corpus callosum, cats trained with one eye masked were unable to remember simple visual discriminations learned with the first eye. The untrained eye could be trained to make a reverse type of discrimination without interfering with the patterned discrimination learned on the opposite side. This functional independence of the surgically separated cerebral hemispheres with respect to learning, memory and other gnostic activity has been the stimulus for considerable investigation (1764). The results originally suggested that section of the corpus callosum prevented the spread of learning and memory from one hemisphere to the other. It was as if each hemisphere existed independently and had a complete amnesia for the experience of the other (2396). Extension of these transfer studies in the monkey from visual to somesthetic and motor learning (856, 2395, 2396) have indicated that the independence of the surgically separated hemispheres may be less clear-cut than originally supposed. In man and monkey, a subcallosal route may be active in transmitting high-order tactile information. Furthermore, both hemispheres may learn to discriminate simultaneously, one via a contralateral sensory system and the other by an ipsilateral sensory system (856).

Observations of the functional effects of surgical separation of the hemispheres in man (857, 858) by complete transection of the corpus callosum, anterior and hippocampal commissures, and separation of the thalamic adhesion (massa intermedia) have been reported. These patients show a striking functional independence of the gnostic activities of the two hemispheres. Perceptual, cognitive, mnemonic, learned and volitional activities persist in each hemisphere, but each can proceed outside the realm of awareness of the other hemisphere. Subjective experiences of each hemisphere are known to the other only indirectly through lower level and peripheral effects. Disconnection of the hemispheres produces little disturbance of ordinary, daily behavior, temperament or intellect. Functional deficits tend to be compensated for by development of bilateral motor control from each hemisphere, as well as by the bilaterality of some sensory pathways. Information perceived exclusively, or generated exclusively, in the minor (right) hemisphere could not be communicated in speech or in writing; it was expressed entirely by nonverbal responses. There was no detectable impairment of speech or writing with reference to information processed in the major (left) hemisphere. These authors found linguistic expression to be organized almost exclusively in the dominant hemisphere.

In contrast to the above, comprehension of language, both spoken and written, was found to be represented in both hemispheres, with the minor hemisphere less proficient. In an analysis of the visual fields, with fixation assured, subjects verbally described only those small spots of light presented in the right half of the visual field (856). A similar light stimulus present in the left half of the visual field produced no verbal responses. With double field stimulation, only spots of light falling in the right visual field were reported. In these subjects, the visual fields stopped exactly in the midline and no macular sparing was evident. Thus it would appear that no visual information can be transferred from one hemisphere to the other after section of the corpus callosum.

Certain lesions involving portions of the corpus callosum, or association areas of the cortex which give rise to commissural fibers, produce disturbances of higher brain functions collectively recognized as *disconnection syndromes* (868–870). Word blindness without agraphia presumably results from lesions which interrupt fibers from the visual association areas which cross in the splenium of the corpus callosum and project to the left angular gyrus. Pure word deafness may result from subcortical lesions in the left temporal lobe which interrupt the left auditory radiation, as well as callosal fibers from the contralateral auditory region. Similar syndromes manifested by various forms of agnosia or apraxia may result from lesions involving portions of the corpus callosum and association fiber systems.

Sleep

Sleep has been considered a unique passive state, interpreted physiologically as the expression of functional deafferentation of the ascending reticular activating system. The awake state was explained in terms of increased activity of this ascending activating system, while sleep was correlated with passive dampening of this system. Recent advances indicate that sleep is an active, complex neural phenomenon initiated by sleep-inducing structures and mediated, in part, by biochemical transmitters. Sleep is not a single phenomenon, but a series of successive functionally related states, which depend upon different active mechanisms, some of which can be selectively modified or suppressed (1248, 1249, 1330, 1496). In mammals two recurring, distinctive and related sleep states can be readily recognized. These are referred to as slow wave sleep and paradoxical sleep.

Slow wave sleep is characterized in the EEG by synchronized cortical activity consisting of spindles (11 to 16 cycles/sec) and high voltage slow waves. There are no specific behavioral criteria for slow wave sleep because the relationship between synchronized, or slow cortical activity, and sleep behavior is not absolute. During slow wave sleep, tone remains in the neck muscles, spinal reflex activity is present and changes in autonomic activity are minimal. After a time, this state is succeeded by a totally different sleep state, known as paradoxical sleep.

Paradoxical sleep is characterized by an EEG pattern with low voltage fast activity which resembles that of the alert, waking state. This sleep state occurs intermittently after variable periods of slow wave sleep and has precise behavioral criteria: (a) abolition of antigravity muscle tone (especially in cervical muscles), (b) depression of

spinal reflex activity, (c) characteristic autonomic changes (i.e., reduction in blood pressure, bradycardia and irregular respiration), and (d) bursts of rapid eye movements (REM). The fact that paradoxical sleep is "deeper" than slow wave sleep, but associated with an EEG pattern similar to that of the waking state, gave rise to the term paradoxical sleep. REM of 50 to 60/min occur in a stereotyped pattern different from that seen in the waking state. These rapid eye movements are associated with subcortical and cortical activity, which have been termed *pontogeniculo-occipital* (PGO) *activity*. These high voltage phasic activities can be recorded from the pontine reticular formation, the lateral geniculate body and the occipital cortex. This activity occurs transiently during slow wave sleep, and always precedes paradoxical sleep. During paradoxical sleep, PGO waves are fairly constant (about 60 waves/min), and it has been suggested that electrical events are triggering both these activities and the rapid eye movements (1249). Bursts of ascending impulses from the medial and inferior vestibular nuclei have been implicated in the REM occurring during paradoxical sleep (2038, 2042). Median rates of spontaneous discharge of units in these nuclei were two to four times higher during desynchronized sleep than during quiet waking. Lesions in the medial and inferior vestibular nuclei abolish the bursts of REM, but desynchronized sleep is still characterized by low voltage, fast activity in the EEG. The conclusion drawn is that the medial and inferior vestibular nuclei represent the causal link leading to activation of the extraocular motor nuclei which are responsible for the bursts of REM. So-called REM sleep (paradoxical sleep) occurs periodically during a night of sleep, with longer periods during the latter part of the night. If the subject is awakened during or immediately after a period of rapid eye movements, 80% of the subjects will report that they have been dreaming, and can relate the content of the dream (1496).

Advances in neuroanatomy, neurophysiology and neuropharmacology concerning the biogenic amines have provided a more complete understanding of their role in sleep states (1248, 1249). In the cat reserpine, which depletes both serotonin and norepinephrine, produces a tranquil state and suppresses both slow wave and paradoxical sleep for different periods of time. Most monoamine oxidase (MAO) inhibitors have a suppressive effect upon paradoxical sleep and increase slow wave sleep. Histofluorescence technics have demonstrated that most serotonin-containing neurons are located in the raphe system (740, 2598), and norepinephrine-containing neurons are located principally in the locus ceruleus (585, 2598). Inhibition of serotonin synthesis at the level of tryptophane hydroxylase leads to total insomnia which is reversible; injections of the immediate precursor of serotonin (5-hydroxytryptophane) causes a return to normal sleep. Nearly total destruction of serotonin-containing neurons in the raphe system also produces insomnia. Pharmacological studies suggest that serotonin may be most intimately associated with slow wave sleep, but many intricate facets of the sleep process are still poorly defined.

The relationship between slow wave sleep and paradoxical sleep is not simple, but it has been suggested that serotonergic neurons involved in slow wave sleep may act as part of the priming mechanism for triggering paradoxical sleep (1249). Serotonergic neurons triggering paradoxical sleep are located in caudal regions of the pontine raphe (Fig. 11-15), since lesions at this level severely depress paradoxical sleep relative to slow sleep. The structures responsible for paradoxical sleep, however, lie outside of the raphe system, and have been thought to include the locus ceruleus (Fig. 12-31 and 12-32). Cells of the locus ceruleus contain norepinephrine and monoamine oxidase. Monamine oxidase inhibitors and bilateral lesions of the locus ceruleus have been described as selectively suppressing paradoxical sleep (1249). Recent studies of lesions in the locus ceruleus in cats, found to greatly diminish norepinephrine in the cerebral cortex, did not suppress paradoxical sleep (1224). These observations have cast doubts upon the role of the locus ceruleus in triggering paradoxical sleep. Certain cholinergic mechanisms also have been implicated in the mechanism of paradoxical sleep, in that atropine suppresses this form of sleep, while direct injections of acetylcholine in the locus ceruleus produce paradoxical sleep. Thus the complex neuropharmacological events which underlie paradoxical sleep involve a variety of neurotransmitters and neural structures, not all of which are known.

Integrated Cortical Functions

The most striking feature of the human cerebral cortex is its elaborate neural mechanisms for complex correlations, sensory discriminations and the utilization of former reactions. The principal function of these mechanisms may be termed *associative memory* and the reactions they use, *mnemonic* (memory) *reactions*. In man, the acquired changes which occur in the cortex after birth permit the neurons to alter subsequent stimuli reaching the cortex. This ability to retain, modify and reuse neuronal networks probably provides the basis of memory, of personal experience and of individually acquired neural mechanisms. Other animals also utilize individual experience to "learn." However, it is doubtful if any animal other than man summates experience by transmitting it to other individuals and new generations. The symbolization necessary for this summation probably requires the pallial mechanism for associative memory. It has been estimated that the cerebral cortex contains nearly 14 billion nerve cells, and the largest number of these may be utilized for the above activities.

In a general way, the central sulcus divides the brain into a posterior receptive portion and an anterior portion related closely to efferent or motor functions. The posterior part contains all the primary receptive areas, except that for olfaction, which receive specific sensory impulses from the lower centers of the brain stem and spinal cord. Hence, this large region receives inputs indirectly from the peripheral sensory receptors. Impulses entering these primary areas produce sensations of a sharply defined character, such as distinct vision and hearing, sharply localized touch and accurate sensations of position and movement. However, these sensations probably have not attained the perceptual level necessary for the recognition of an object. This requires the integration of primary stimuli with other neural information. The regions in immediate contact with the receptive centers, known as *parasensory areas*, serve for the combination and elaboration of the primary impulses into more complex sensory perceptions which can be recalled under appropriate conditions. . In the more distant association areas the various sensory fields overlap (e.g., the inferior parietal lobule and adjacent portions of the occipital and temporal lobes). In these areas the combinations are still more complex and are expressed as multisensory perceptions of a higher order. Thus tactile and kinesthetic impulses are built up into perceptions of form, size and texture (stereognosis). Visual impulses similarly are compounded into perceptions of visual object recognition. Hence any object comes to be represented ultimately by a constellation of memories compounded from several sensory channels which are dependent upon previous experience. When sensory impulses initiated by feeling, or seeing, an object excite these memory networks, the object is "recognized" (i.e., remembered as having been seen or felt before). This arousal of the associative mnemonic complexes by cortical afferents may be termed "gnosis," and it forms the basis of understanding and knowledge. Disorders of this mechanism caused by lesions in the association areas are known as gnostic disturbances or *agnosias*. The tactile, visual or auditory events evoked in the cortex no longer arouse the appropriate memories; hence the object and its uses appear unfamiliar and strange. When such gnostic disturbances involve the far more complicated associative mechanisms underlying the comprehension of language, they form part of a complex known as the *aphasias*. Closely related to both agnosia and aphasia is another group of disorders characterized by difficulty in performing learned complex or skilled movements even though no paralysis, sensory loss or ataxia is present. These disorders, which affect the motor side of higher sensory-motor integration, are referred to as the *apraxias*. There are only two ways in which a patient can show that he recognizes an object: (a) by naming the object or describing its use, and (b) by demonstrating its use. Thus, agnosia in part underlies both aphasia and apraxia. If the patient can demonstrate the use of an object, but is unable to name or describe it, he has an aphasia. If he can name or describe an object, but does not know how to use it, he has an apraxia.

Agnosia. The term agnosia means a failure to recognize. Various types of agnosias have been defined according to the particular sensory modality effected. Of the many types of agnosia classified on this basis with respect to both objects and space, three may properly be considered here, namely, *tactile agnosia, visual agnosia* and *auditory agnosia*.

Tactile agnosia is a failure to recognize objects by means of tactile and kinesthetic-sensibilities when both of these sensory modalities are normal in the part of the body being tested. Astereognosis is the inability to recognize objects owing to sensory impairment at a cortical level. According to Brain (239), tactile agnosis is associated especially with lesions of the supramarginal gyrus in the left cerebral hemisphere, which probably is the dominant hemisphere for tactile recognition.

Visual agnosia is a failure to recognize objects that cannot be attributed to a defect of visual acuity or to intellectual impairment. Although a patient with visual agnosia is unable to recognize an object by sight, he may recognize it by other sensibilities, and he can still recognize people. The disability usually is limited to small objects and varies somewhat from day to day. In some instances the visual agnosia may extend to surroundings; it then is associated with spatial disorientation. Lesions associated with visual agnosia involve the lateral visual association areas in the dominant hemisphere. The term *alexia* denotes a special form of visual agnosia in which the patient is unable to read because he fails to recognize written or printed words. Lesions in this syndrome interrupt pathways conveying impulses from the visual cortex of both sides to the angular gyrus of the left hemisphere.

Auditory agnosia is the term used to describe the condition in which a patient with unimpaired hearing fails to recognize or distinguish what he hears. This type of agnosia may involve speech, musical sounds or familiar noises, such as the telephone bell or running water. One form of auditory agnosia, known as word deafness, constitutes a type of receptive aphasia. Lesions associated with auditory agnosia involve parts of the superior temporal convolution posteriorly (area 22) in the dominant hemisphere; these disturbances are more severe when the injury is bilateral.

Aphasia. This disorder is characterized by receptive and expressive disturbances in the use of symbols and signs to communicate. It results from organic neural lesions involving cerebral memory mechanisms for language without impairment of cortical or subcortical structures essential for the relay of impulses, or the innervation of speech organs (i.e., the muscles of the larynx, tongue, and lips). The aphasias usually are divided into two basic types: receptive (sensory) and expressive (motor). In receptive aphasia the disturbance involves an impairment in the appreciation of the meanings of both spoken and written words. Expressive aphasia is characterized by impairment or lack of ability to express thoughts in a meaningful way in speech or writing. Less severe forms of expressive aphasia may involve primarily the incorrect choice of words or grammatical confusion. The division of the aphasias into two types suggests a more clear cut distinction than our understanding permits, since common disturbances of memory and language must be involved in both types. While relatively pure receptive or expressive forms of aphasia do occur, mixed varieties are the most common. Certain patients with severe expressive forms of aphasia may be capable of making meaningful gestures which suggest some degree of thought comprehension.

It is extremely difficult to locate precisely the site, or sites, of lesions which result in different forms of aphasia. Most evidence suggests that the disorder is associated with lesions involving the posterior temporoparietal region, and the so-called Broca's area (portions of the pars opercularis and triangularis of the inferior frontal gyrus) in the dominant hemisphere (239, 1969). Penfield and Roberts (1969) report that any large lesion in the posterior temporoparietal region involving the cortex and underlying projection areas of the thalamus causes a severe aphasia. Although Broca's speech area has long been considered the cortical site of lesions in expressive aphasia, several observers have questioned its significance (1216, 1603 1689). According to these authors, this area can be sacrificed in the adult without eventual loss of normal speech. Penfield and Roberts (1969) also suggest that it is less important than the posterior temporoparietal region.

Apraxia. The inability to perform certain learned complex movements, in the absence of paralysis, sensory loss or disturbance of coordination, is known as apraxia. Since complex voluntary movements require the utilization of cerebral processes in formulating the nature of the act to be performed, movements of this nature are considered separate from those which are more or less automatic. Formulation of these movement complexes is largely unconscious and appears to depend upon memory constellations of similar acts previously performed. Complex learned movement patterns are organized in space and time, and follow sequences requiring close attention. Multiple sensory systems contribute to the skill of these movement patterns. Apraxia has been regarded as a disorganization of the underlying complex movement patterns. Many varieties of apraxia have been proposed as distinct entities, although some tend to have common features.

Kinetic apraxia is characterized by an inability to execute fine acquired motor movements; there is no paresis, and automatic and associated movements can be carried out. This disturbance may be confined to one limb. It has been interpreted as an expressive defect, most frequently associated with lesions of the precentral cortex. The defect usually occurs contralateral to the lesion (609).

Ideomotor apraxia is caused by an interruption of pathways between the centers for formulation of a motor act and the motor areas necessary for its execution. Although the patient may know what he wants to do, he is unable to do it. He can perform many complex acts automatically, but he may fail to perform the same acts on command. Spontaneous gestures may be normal. Ideomotor apraxia is often bilateral and affects the extremities equally. It is said to be associated with lesions of the parietal lobe, particularly the supramarginal gyrus, in the dominant hemisphere.

Ideational apraxia is the term used to describe loss of ability to formulate the ideational plan for the execution of the components of a complex act. While simple isolated movements may be performed normally, the component movements of a complex act are not synthesized into a purposeful plan and individual movements may be performed in a faulty sequence. Since kinesthetic memory and appreciation of the act to be performed are defective, ideational apraxia may be a variety of agnosia. This form of apraxia has been considered to result from lesions in the dominant parietal lobe, or in the corpus callosum (871), but frequently it is associated with rather diffuse pathological processes.

Constructional apraxia is a disorder characterized by loss of visual guidance, impairment of the visual image and disturbances of revisualization. A patient suffering from this form of apraxia is unable to reproduce simple geometric figures by drawing or by the arrangement of blocks. Although this form of apraxia is included with expressive disorders of motor function, it is rarely a pure motor disorder. As a rule the patient is unaware of his inability to perceive spatial relationships. This variety of apraxia appears to be related to interruption of pathways between the occipital and parietal cortex (564).

Curious combinations of agnosia and apraxia occur as a consequence of lesions involving primarily the inferior parietal lobe, usually in the dominant hemisphere (564, 867). This syndrome is characterized by: (a) finger agnosia, (b) right-left disorientation, (c) agraphia or dysgraphia, and (d) acalculia or dyscalculia. Patients suffering from this syndrome have difficulty in differentiating their fingers, in naming the individual fingers and in pointing to particular fingers. Right-left disorientation, unlike finger agnosia, may affect all parts of the body, as well as inanimate objects and other individuals. The disturbance in writing does not extend to copying, which can be accomplished without difficulty. Inability to solve arithmetical problems is most evident with written figures, but it involves mental calculations as well.

Prefrontal Cortex

The frontal lobe rostral to area 6 represents a relatively late phylogenetic acquisition which is well developed only in primates, especially in man. These areas of cortex, including that on the orbital surface, are referred to as the prefrontal cortex. Areas of cortex on the lateral convexity of the brain (particularly areas 9 and 10) receive a large number of fibers from the dorsomedial nucleus of the thalamus, which may bring impulses from certain autonomic centers. These areas are connected by the cingulum and the uncinate fasciculus with anterior portions of the temporal lobe and, directly or indirectly, with parietal and adjacent occipitotemporal association areas. In the prefrontal region, cortical activities are influenced by the activities of medial nuclear groups of the thalamus, which appear associated with more primitive affective components of consciousness, and probably play an important role in emotional responses. Russell (2242) believes that the prefrontal areas are not primarily concerned with memory or general intelligence, but rather with the establishment and conditioning of emotional reactions. They are of great importance during childhood and the growing years, when behavioral patterns are being formed. Emotional reactions become less prominent after maturity, when behavior patterns have become established.

A procedure known as prefrontal *lobotomy* or *leucotomy* was used widely some years ago in attempts to modify the behavior of severely psychotic patients. The basic operation involved bilateral sectioning of the fiber connections to and from the prefrontal area. Lobotomy, introduced by Moniz (1724), was performed in the United States and elsewhere in the 1940's (805). This neurosurgical procedure permitted many institutionalized patients to return home and even to resume their former activities. Moreover, a considerable number of lobotomies were performed for the relief of chronic intractable pain of organic origin when other measures, such as massive doses of narcotics and even cordotomy, had proved of no avail (733, 805, 2266). After the operation, the patient no longer complained spontaneously of pain and no longer appeared to be in distress, although when asked patients acknowledged that pain was still present. Relief apparently was due to removal of the anxiety and fear usually associated with pain. Since prefrontal lobotomy, and numerous technical variations of it (961, 1689), was performed on a large number of patients, it afforded an opportunity to study the associated intellectual and behavioral effects of these lesions.

The results of numerous lobotomies have been critically discussed in a number of publications (623, 805, 1942). These studies are difficult to evaluate because of lack of agreement concerning the extent of the changes in behavior and intellect. Most striking are the alterations in emotional behavior, which were characterized by Freeman and Watts as a lessening of "consciousness of the self," and a narrowing of the patient's mental horizon to the immediate present and to his own person. The patient was easily amused, careless in personal habits, unconcerned in social relations and little affected by criticism. His emotional reactions were abrupt, transient and superficial, and they often were accompanied by outspoken tactlessness. Pain and hardship were not associated with anxiety, nor was there much concern about financial or domestic difficulties. There was inability to gauge or appreciate the gravity of a situation and to maintain a responsible attitude toward it. These were the most enduring changes which could be attributed to the operation, and they probably were responsible for the successful abolition of morbid anxiety and obsessional states (805).

Intellectual damage is especially difficult to evaluate. General memory returns rapidly, and standard psychometric tests are accurately performed. Nearly all agree that the capacity for abstract thought is reduced and that the patient develops a more concrete attitude. Easy distractibility is common, judgment is poor and initiative is reduced. Mental concentration and the capacity for sustained intellectual effort are impaired, especially with respect to solving complex problems. The most reliable data concerning the effects of lobotomy upon intelligence are those obtained from nonpsychotic patients in whom this procedure was done for relief of pain. On the basis of thorough studies of patients before and after operation, Rylander (2243) concluded that intellectual and emotional deterioration may be severe. The results of the operation necessarily depend upon the intelligence of the patient and the extent of the operative procedure. This conclusion appears to be supported by others (1353).

Other forms of prefrontal lobe surgery, such as topectomy and orbitofrontal lobotomy, were not reported to produce such severe impairment of intellectual function (961, 1422). The fact that the extent of intellectual deterioration following prefrontal lobotomy cannot be measured in specific terms reflects the exceedingly complex nature of what is called intellect and suggests that the criteria used to evaluate it may not be adequate. The unpredictable effects of the procedure upon intellect and severe personality changes associated with the irreversible nature of surgery have caused this procedure to be rarely used.

In spite of the difficulties in evaluating the behavior changes and the intellectual alterations of prefrontal lobotomy, some patients were considered to have benefited from the operation. Perhaps the greatest problem, and one of the reasons why this form of psychosurgery is now rarely done, was the difficulty in determining preoperatively which patients might be expected to be improved by it. Another important factor in the decline of psychosurgery was the introduction of the tranquilizing drugs which have facilitated the treatment of severe behavioral disorders.

The human nervous system has evolved slowly, and although many of the details of its anatomical structure appear firmly established, concepts concerning the functional significance and interrelation of its various subdivisions change as a result of continuing research. Many so-called "electronic brains" have been constructed which can perform certain functions faster and more efficiently than the human brain. The more complex the performed function, the more elaborate the programming of the computer must be. "Electronic brains" are impressive in appearance and function; yet they do not approach in versatility or scope the fantastic potentialities of the human brain. The human brain is unique in that it provides its own programming; in fact, it is programmed throughout life by daily experiences. It seems likely that "electronic brains" will in the future perform many more of the functions now performed by human brains, but this change must be regarded as a redistribution of labor. The "electronic brain" is after all only one of the expressions of the ingenuity of the human brain.

CHAPTER 20

Blood Supply of the Central Nervous System

The central nervous system is metabolically one of the most active systems of the body. Its metabolism depends almost entirely upon the aerobic combustion of glucose. Since there is little storage of glucose or oxygen in the brain, even brief interference with cerebral circulation can cause permanent neurological or mental disturbances. Neural tissue deprived of an adequate blood supply undergoes necrosis. Impairment of local or regional blood supply constitutes the most common cause of central nervous system lesions. The duration of consciousness after complete cessation of brain circulation is less than 10 sec.

Estimates of cerebral blood flow based on the nitrous oxide method of Kety and Schmidt (1305) indicate a normal blood flow of about 50 ml/100 g of brain tissue per min. Thus a brain of average weight has a normal blood flow of about 750 ml/min. The mean oxygen consumption in the normal conscious individual is about 3.3 ml/100 g of brain tissue, or about 46 ml/min for the entire brain. Thus the brain, constituting about 2% of the body weight, requires about 17% of the normal cardiac output and consumes about 20% of the oxygen utilized by the entire body. Since the brain is not a homogeneous organ, the metabolic activity and nutritive requirements of various regions differ greatly. This differential functional activity of neuronal systems under various conditions can be demonstrated autoradiographically and mapped quantitatively by injections of 2-[^{14}C]deoxyglucose which passes the blood-brain barrier and is partially metabolized by active neurons before it is trapped within these cells (1290, 1291, 2017). This technic has revealed surprisingly detailed features of neuronal activity under controlled conditions. (Figs. 19-18, 19-21 and 19-22). Examples of this mapping technic are described in Chapter 19, page 673.

If adequate circulation is not maintained to local regions of the brain or spinal cord, the neural tissue deprived of its blood sup-

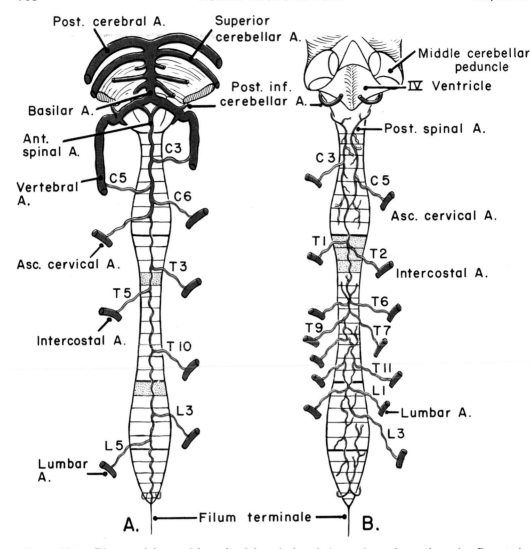

Figure 20-1. Diagram of the arterial supply of the spinal cord. *A*, anterior surface and arteries; *B*, posterior surface and arteries. Vulnerable segments of the spinal cord are *stippled*. *Letters* and *numbers* indicate most important radicular arteries. (Based on the work of Bolton (215), Suh and Alexander (2466), and Zulch (2802).

ply undergoes softening, necrosis and degeneration. Vascular lesions most commonly result from disease of the cerebral vessels (arteriosclerosis) which leads to thrombosis of particular vessels. Occlusions of cerebral vessels due to embolism may result from fragments of blood clots, fat, tumor or, in some instances, air bubbles. Hemorrhage into the brain or meninges may result from pathological changes in cerebral vessels. One of the most common causes of spontaneous hemorrhage into the brain and the subarachnoid space is rupture of abnormal sacculations (aneurysms), most of which are of congenital origin. Lo-

calized neural lesions resulting from interruptions of blood supply often can be correlated with specific sensory and motor changes which are characteristic for different cerebral vessels.

BLOOD SUPPLY OF THE SPINAL CORD

The spinal cord is supplied by: (a) branches of the *vertebral arteries* that descend, and (b) multiple *radicular arteries* derived from segmental vessels (Fig. 20-1). As the vertebral arteries ascend along the anterolateral surfaces of the medulla, each gives rise to two paired descending vessels:

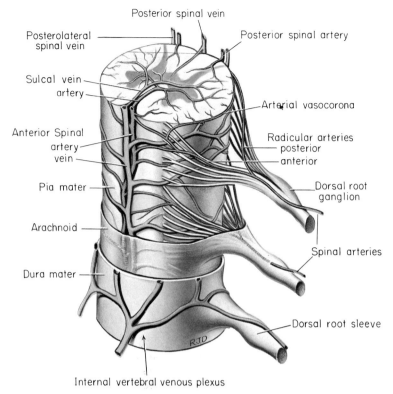

Posterior spinal vein

Posterolateral spinal vein

Posterior spinal artery

Sulcal vein
artery

Arterial vasocorona

Anterior Spinal
artery
vein

Radicular arteries
posterior
anterior

Pia mater

Dorsal root ganglion

Arachnoid

Spinal arteries

Dura mater

Dorsal root sleeve

RJD

Internal vertebral venous plexus

Figure 20-2.   Blood supply and venous drainage of the spinal cord, shown with respect to the meninges and internal structure.

(a) posterior spinal artery, and (b) the anterior spinal artery.

Posterior Spinal Arteries. Paired posterior spinal arteries descend on the posterior surface of the spinal cord medial to the dorsal roots (Fig. 20-1*B*). These arteries receive variable contributions from the posterior radicular arteries and form two longitudinal plexiform channels near the dorsal root entry zone. At certain sites these spinal arteries become so small that they appear discontinuous. These vessels and their small branches supply the posterior third of the spinal cord (2590).

Anterior Spinal Arteries. The paired anterior spinal arteries unite to form a single descending midline vessel that supplies midline rami to the lower medulla and sulcal branches that enter the anterior median fissure of the spinal cord (Figs. 20-1*A* and 20-2). The continuity of the anterior spinal artery is dependent upon anastomotic branches which it receives from the anterior radicular arteries (2466). The anterior radicular arteries join the anterior spinal artery by branching gently upward or sharply downward. Where two anterior radicular arteries reach the same level of the spinal cord, they form a diamond-shaped configuration. The anterior and posterior spinal arteries are anastomotic channels extending the length of the spinal cord which receive branches from the radicular arteries. Branches of the vertebral arteries provide the principal blood supply of virtually the entire cervical spinal cord. In the thoracic region the anterior spinal artery may narrow to such an extent that it may not form a functional anastomosis if the radicular arteries are occluded above or below. The caudal end of the anterior spinal artery communicates with an arterial ring that encircles the conus medullaris.

Radicular Arteries. Radicular arteries are derived from segmental vessels (i.e., ascending cervical, deep cervical, intercostal, lumbar and sacral arteries), pass through the intervertebral foramina and divide into *anterior* and *posterior radicular arteries* which provide the principal blood supply of thoracic, lumbar, sacral and coccygeal spinal segments (Figs. 20-1 and 20-2). In the thoracic and lumbar regions of the spinal cord, radicular arteries are situated most frequently on the left side, while in the cervical region the spinal cord is supplied equally from both sides. Radicular arteries course along the ventral surface of the spinal root that they accompany (Fig. 20-2). Where the epineurium blends with the dura mater, the radicular arteries enter the subarachnoid space. A single radicular artery may become either an anterior or posterior radicular artery, or divide to form both (2590). Small twigs leave the arteries to supply the dura mater and the spinal roots that they accompany.

The *anterior radicular arteries* contributing to the anterior spinal artery vary from 2 to 17, but most commonly number between 6 and 10. The cervical spinal cord receives from 0 to 6 anterior radicular arteries, while the thoracic cord receives 2 to 4 and the lumbar cord has 1 or 2. In the lumbar region one anterior radicular artery is appreciably larger than all others; this vessel is known as the *artery of Adamkiewicz*, or the artery of the lumbar enlargement (1460). This large radicular artery accompanies a lower thoracic or upper lumbar spinal root most frequently on the left side. The greatest distance between radicular arteries is seen in the thoracic spinal segments, which means the occlusion of one radicular artery may seriously compromise the circulation in this region of the spinal cord (1083).

The *posterior radicular arteries*, numbering between 10 and 23, divide on the posterolateral surface of the spinal cord and join the paired posterior spinal arteries. These vessels are most consistent on the left side, but the predominance is not as evident as with the anterior radicular arteries.

The anterior spinal artery gives rise to a number of sulcal branches which enter the anterior median fissure and alternately pass to the right or left, except for an occasional sulcal artery that divides into right and left branches (878) (Fig. 20-2). Central branches arising from the anterior spinal artery are most numerous in the cervical and lumbar regions and are of larger caliber (1045). Sulcal branches of the anterior spinal artery supply the anterior horn, the lateral horn,

the central gray and the basal part of the posterior horn. These branches also supply the anterior and lateral funiculi. Branches of the posterior spinal arteries supply the posterior gray horns and the posterior funiculi (Fig. 20-2). Peripheral portions of the lateral funiculi receive small branches from the *arterial vasocorona* formed by the anastomosis of surface vessels.

The blood supply of the spinal cord may be jeopardized in certain transitional regions where its arterial supply is derived from more than one source. For example, the cervical segments are supplied primarily by branches of the vertebral artery and to a lesser extent by small branches of the ascending cervical artery. The upper segments of the thoracic spinal cord, on the other hand, are dependent upon the radicular branches of the intercostal arteries. If one or more of the parent intercostal vessels are compromised by injury or ligature, segments of the spinal cord T1 to 4 could not be adequately maintained by the small sulcal branches of the anterior spinal artery (Fig. 20-1A). For this reason, thoracic segments T1 to 4, particularly T4, are considered vulnerable areas in the distribution of the anterior spinal artery (2802). The occlusion of one intercostal artery in a vulnerable region can result in spinal cord infarction. This clinical picture may be seen in association with dissecting aneurysms of the aorta or as a complication of surgery on the aorta where more than one intercostal artery has been occluded (2591). Spinal cord segment L1 is another vulnerable region. The posterior surface of the cord most susceptible to vascular insult is also in segments T1 to 4 (Fig. 20-1B). Such vascular injuries may result in necrosis of an entire segment and produce neurological symptoms comparable to complete cord transection.

Spinal Veins. Veins draining the spinal cord have a general distribution similar to that of spinal arteries. Anterior longitudinal venous trunks consist of anteromedian and anterolateral veins (Fig. 20-2). Sulcal veins entering the anteromedian vein drain anteromedial portions of the spinal cord; each sulcal vein drains regions on both sides of the spinal cord. Anterolateral regions of the spinal cord drain into anterolateral veins and into the *venous vasocorona*. The *anteromedian* and *anterolateral spinal veins*

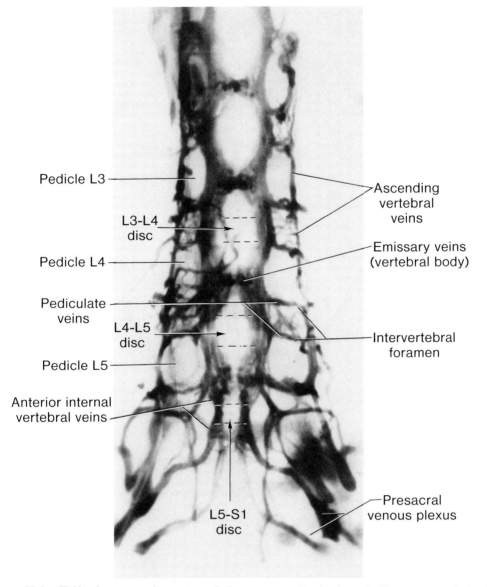

Pedicle L3

L3-L4 disc

Pedicle L4

Pediculate veins

L4-L5 disc

Pedicle L5

Anterior internal vertebral veins

L5-S1 disc

Ascending vertebral veins

Emissary veins (vertebral body)

Intervertebral foramen

Presacral venous plexus

Figure 20-3. Epidural venogram done retrograde from one ascending lumbar vein. Venogram reveals details of the internal vertebral venous plexus, including ascending vertebral veins, emissary veins from vertebral body, pediculate veins at the superior and inferior margins of the intervertebral foramina, the anterior internal vertebral veins and the presacral venous plexus. The pedicles of L3, L4 and L5 vertebrae are well outlined, and the approximate position of the intervertebral discs at three levels are indicated by *dashed lines*. (Courtesy of Drs. Daniel Hottenstein and Keith Himes, Holy Spirit Hospital, Camp Hill, Pa.)

are drained by 6 to 11 anterior radicular veins which empty into the epidural venous plexus. One large radicular vein in the lumbar region is referred to as the *vena radicularis magna* (2466); other smaller radicular veins are distributed along the spinal cord.

Posterior longitudinal venous trunks, consisting of a *posteromedian vein* and

paired *posterolateral veins*, drain the posterior funiculus, the posterior horns (including their basal regions) and the white matter in the lateral funiculi adjacent to the posterior horn (Fig. 20-2). The posterior longitudinal veins are drained by 5 to 10 posterior radicular veins that enter the epidural venous plexus. The longitudinal veins are connected with each other by coronal

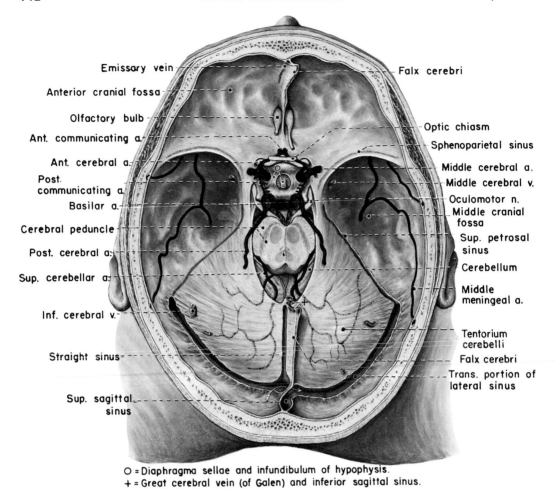

O = Diaphragma sellae and infundibulum of hypophysis.
+ = Great cerebral vein (of Galen) and inferior sagittal sinus.

Figure 20-4. Cranial cavity after brain was removed to demonstrate relationship of the cerebral arterial circle, adjacent neural structures, and reflections of the dura mater. (Reproduced with permission from R. C. Truex and C. E. Kellner: *Detailed Atlas of the Head and Neck*, Oxford University Press, New York, 1948 (2582).)

veins (venous vasocorona) which encircle the spinal cord.

The *internal vertebral venous plexus* (epidural venous plexus), located between the dura mater and the vertebral periosteum (Fig. 20-3), consists of two or more anterior and posterior longitudinal venous channels which extend from the region of the clivus (Fig. 20-20) within the skull to the sacral region (568). At each intervertebral space there are connections with thoracic, abdominal and intercostal veins, as well as with the external vertebral venous plexus. Since there are no valves in this spinal venous network, blood flowing in these channels may pass directly into the systemic venous system. When intra-abdominal pressure is increased, venous blood

from the pelvic plexus passes upward in the internal vertebral venous system. When the jugular veins are obstructed, blood leaves the skull via this plexus. The importance of the continuity of this venous plexus with the prostatic plexus has been noted and cited as a route by which neoplasms may metastasize (133). Epidural venograms reveal many details of the internal vertebral venous plexus and usually fill the pediculate veins which outline the superior and inferior margins of the intervertebral foramina (Fig. 20-3).

BLOOD SUPPLY OF THE BRAIN

The entire brain is supplied by two pairs of arterial trunks, the internal carotid arteries and the vertebral arteries. On the left

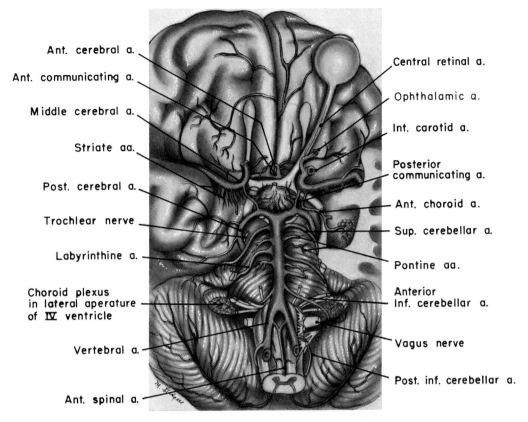

Figure 20-5. Formation and branches of the arterial circle on the inferior surface of the brain. The relationships of the arterial circle to structures on the base of the skull are shown in Figure 20-4.

the common carotid artery arises directly from the aortic arch; the right common carotid is one of the two branches which arises from the bifurcation of the brachiocephalic artery. The common carotid artery bifurcates at the upper level of the thyroid cartilage forming the internal and external carotid arteries.

Internal Carotid Artery

The internal carotid artery can be divided into four segments: cervical, intrapetrosal, intracavernous and cerebral portion (supraclinoid). The *cervical segment*, which has no branches, extends from the bifurcation of the common carotid to the point where the vessel enters the carotid canal in the petrous bone. The *intrapetrosal segment* of this vessel is surrounded by dense bone. The *intracavernous segment* of the internal carotid artery lies close to the medial wall of the cavernous sinus, courses nearly horizontally, and bears important relationships to cranial nerves III, IV, V and VI which are within this sinus

(Fig. 20-21). The *cerebral portion* of the internal carotid begins as the artery emerges from the cavernous sinus and passes medial to the anterior clinoid process (Fig. 20-4). This portion of the artery usually extends upward and backward toward its bifurcation, but variations are common. The intracavernous and cerebral portions of the internal carotid artery are referred to as the "carotid siphon" by neuroradiologists (demonstrated but unlabeled in Fig. 20-8; Ref. 2520). Although all major branches of the internal carotid artery arise from the cerebral portion of this vessel, numerous small branches are given off from the intrapetrosal and intracavernous portions. These include branches to the tympanic cavity (caroticotympanic), the cavernous and inferior petrosal sinuses, the trigeminal ganglion and the meninges of the middle fossa.

Major branches of the internal carotid artery, originating from the cerebral portion, are the ophthalmic, posterior communicating and anterior choroidal arteries

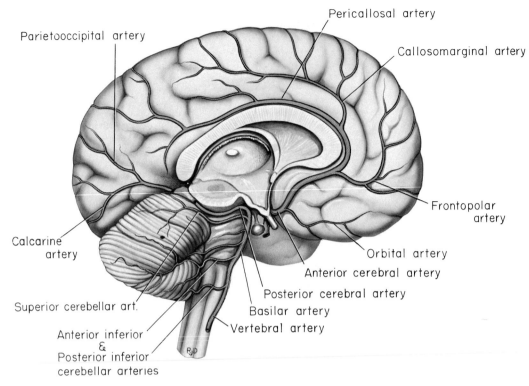

Parietooccipital artery

Pericallosal artery

Callosomarginal artery

Frontopolar artery

Calcarine artery

Orbital artery

Anterior cerebral artery

Posterior cerebral artery

Superior cerebellar art.

Basilar artery

Vertebral artery

Anterior inferior
&
Posterior inferior
cerebellar arteries

RJD

Figure 20-6. Principal arteries on the medial surface of the cerebrum, shown together with the arteries of the brain stem and cerebellum.

(Figs. 20-4 and 20-5). The *ophthalmic artery* enters the orbit through the optic foramen, ventral and lateral to the optic nerve. The *posterior communicating artery* arises from the dorsal aspect of the carotid siphon and passes posteriorly and medially to join the posterior cerebral artery (Fig. 20-5). The *anterior choroidal artery* usually arises from the internal carotid artery distal to the posterior communicating artery and passes backward across the optic tract and then laterally to enter the choroidal fissure in the temporal lobe (Figs. 20-5 and 20-10) (410). Lateral to the optic chiasm the internal carotid artery divides into its two terminal branches: the smaller *anterior cerebral artery* and the larger *middle cerebral artery*, which is regarded as the direct continuation of the internal carotid artery.

Most of the arterial blood within the internal carotid artery is distributed by the more mobile branches of the anterior and middle cerebral arteries. The rostral parts of the brain normally supplied by these two arteries are the anterior half of the thalamus, the corpus striatum, the corpus callosum, most of the internal capsule, the medial and lateral surfaces of the frontal and parietal lobes and the lateral surface of the temporal lobe (Figs. 20-5–20-7).

Vertebral Artery

The vertebral arteries originate as the first branch of the subclavian artery on each side, enter the foramina transversaria of the sixth cervical vertebra and ascend in the foramina in all higher cervical vertebrae. This artery curves posteriorly around the superior articular process of the atlas, passes forward and medially to pierce the atlanto-occipital membrane and dura and enters the posterior fossa through the foramen magnum (Fig. 20-14). The cervical part of the vertebral artery gives rise to spinal and muscular branches. Thin radicular branches of the vertebral artery pass through the intervertebral foramina to supply the meninges and portions of the cervical spinal cord (Fig 20-1). The relationships of the two vertebral arteries to the anterior and posterior surfaces of the caudal brain stem are shown in Figures 1-4, 1-

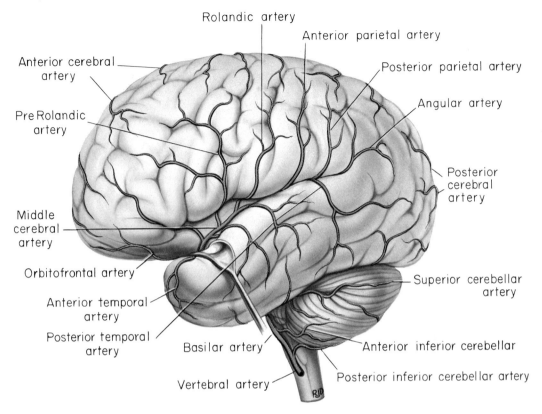

Figure 20-7.   Principal arteries on the lateral surface of the cerebrum and cerebellum.

10, 20-1 and 20-5. The two vertebral arteries unite at the caudal border of the pons to form the basilar artery (Figure 20-15). Branches of these three arteries normally provide the sole arterial blood supply of the cervical spinal cord, medulla, pons, midbrain and cerebellum, and in addition they supply posterior portions of the thalamus, the occipital lobe and the medioinferior surfaces of the temporal lobe (Fig. 20-5). The slender labyrinthine branch of the basilar artery follows the course of the vestibulocochlear nerve and nourishes internal ear structures through its vestibular and cochlear rami (Fig. 20-5).

Cerebral Arterial Circle

The cerebral arterial circle (Willis) is an arterial wreath encircling the optic chiasm, the tuber cinereum and the interpeduncular region formed by anastomotic branches of the internal carotid artery and the most rostral branches of the basilar artery (Figs. 20-4, 20-5 and 20-10). This arterial circle is formed by anterior and posterior commu-

nicating arteries and proximal portions of the anterior, middle and posterior cerebral arteries. The *anterior cerebral arteries* run medially and rostrally toward the interhemispheric fissure; in the region rostral to the optic chiasm these two arteries are joined by a short connecting vessel, the *anterior communicating artery*. At the rostral border of the pons the basilar artery bifurcates forming the two *posterior cerebral arteries*. The *posterior communicating arteries* arise from the internal carotid arteries and anastomose with proximal portions of the posterior cerebral arteries. The posterior cerebral arteries give rise to numerous small branches that enter the interpeduncular fossa and hypothalamus, while the main vessels pass laterally, rostral to the root fibers of the oculomotor nerve, and encircle part of the mesencephalon before passing above the tentorium cerebelli (Figs. 20-4 and 20-5). The cerebral arterial circle formed by the anastomoses of these vessels is said to equalize blood flow to various parts of the brain, but normally there is little exchange of blood between the right and left halves of the arterial circle because of the equality of blood pressure. Alterations of blood flow in the arterial circle undoubtedly occur following occlusion of one or more of the arteries contributing to the circle. However, the communicating arteries of the arterial circle often form functionally inadequate anastomoses which account for the high incidence of serious disturbances in blood flow following unilateral occlusion or compression of the internal carotid artery, especially in elderly individuals.

Relationships of the arterial circle and its branches to the inferior surface of the brain and the origins of the respective cranial nerves are shown in Figure 20-5. The *in situ* surgical relationships of the arterial circle to the base of the skull following removal of the brain can be appreciated by comparing Figure 20-4 with the relationships illustrated in Figure 20-5.

From the arterial circle and the main cerebral arteries (anterior, middle and posterior) two types of branches arise: the *central* or *ganglionic*, and the *cortical* or *circumferential*. The central and cortical arteries form two distinct systems. The *central* arteries arise from the circle of Willis and the proximal portions of the three cerebral arteries, dip perpendicularly into the brain substance and supply the diencephalon, corpus striatum and internal capsule (Fig. 20-10). For a long time these penetrating vessels have been referred to as terminal or end arteries. Studies by Scharrer (2270) indicate that the vast majority of arteries in the brains in lower animals are end arteries, but in the human brain there are no end arteries. Precapillary anastomoses have been observed in man and animals, but these anastomoses usually are not sufficient to maintain adequate circulation if a major vessel is occluded suddenly. Thus occlusion of one of these arteries produces a softening in the area deprived of an adequate blood supply. The anterior and posterior choroidal arteries, respectively, branches of the internal carotid and posterior cerebral arteries, may be included in this group.

The larger *cortical* branches of each cerebral artery enter the pia mater, where they form a superficial plexus of more or less freely anastomosing vessels, which in some places may be continuous with the plexuses derived from the other main arteries. From these plexuses arise the smaller terminal arteries which enter the brain substance at right angles and run for variable distances. The shorter ones arborize in the cortex, while the longer ones supply the more deeply placed medullary substance of the hemisphere. Owing to the anastomoses of the larger cortical branches, the occlusion of one of these vessels is compensated to a variable extent by the blood supply from neighboring branches, although such collateral circulation is rarely sufficient to prevent brain damage. The great majority of vascular occlusions occur in the cerebral vessels before they enter the substance of the brain. Areas of the cerebral cortex, internal capsule, or basal ganglia which lie between the territorial distributions of two primary arteries are the sites most severely involved after vascular injury (1692). The degree of brain damage is variable and depends upon several factors (e.g., site of injury, amount of vascular overlap and confluence and the rapidity with which an occlusion develops).

Cortical Branches

The cortical branches of the cerebral hemisphere are derived from the anterior, middle and posterior cerebral arteries.

Anterior Cerebral Artery. The anterior cerebral artery originates at the bifurcation of the internal carotid artery, passes rostromedially, dorsal to the optic nerve, and approaches the corresponding artery of the opposite side with which it connects via the anterior communicating artery (Figs. 20-5, 20-6 and 20-10). The artery enters the interhemispheric fissure, passes upward on the medial surface of the hemisphere, curves around the genu of the corpus callosum and continues posteriorly on the superior surface of the corpus callosum. The first part of the anterior cerebral artery lies close to the optic chiasm and gives rise to the smaller anterior communicating artery dorsal to the optic chiasm. The first part of both the anterior cerebral and the anterior communicating arteries gives rise to perforating arteries that enter the anterior perforated substance (Figs. 2-9, 18-2 and 20-10), the optic chiasm, the region of the optic tract, the anterior region of the hypothalamus and the septum pellucidum (1974). Other branches of the anterior cerebral artery include: (a) the medial striate artery, (b) orbital branches, (c) the frontopolar artery, (d) the callosomarginal artery, and (e) the pericallosal artery. The pericallosal artery may be considered as the terminal part of the anterior cerebral artery.

The *medial striate artery* (recurrent artery of Heubner) may arise either proximal or distal to the anterior communicating artery (1459, 1909, 1974), but courses caudally and laterally to enter the anterior perforated substance. This vessel supplies the anteromedial part of the head of the caudate nucleus, adjacent parts of the internal capsule and putamen and parts of the septal nuclei (Figs. 20-10, 20-12 and 20-13). The medial striate artery is said to anastomose with the lenticulostriate arteries and surface branches of the anterior and middle cerebral arteries (1266) and frequently gives rise to several branches supplying the inferior surface of the frontal lobe (1974, 1975).

Orbital branches of the anterior cerebral artery arise from the ascending portion of this vessel just below the corpus callosum. These branches extend forward to supply the orbital and medial surfaces of the frontal lobe (Figs. 20-5 and 20-6). A *frontopolar branch* of the anterior cerebral artery is given off as the anterior cerebral artery curves around the genu of the corpus callosum (Fig. 20-6). Two or three branches of the frontopolar artery supply medial parts of the frontal lobe and extend laterally on reaching the convexity of the hemisphere. A major branch of the anterior cerebral artery, the *callosomarginal artery*, arises distal to the frontopolar artery and passes backward and upward in the callosomarginal sulcus, dorsal to the cingulate gyrus (Fig. 20-6). Branches of this artery supply the paracentral lobule and parts of the cingulate gyrus (1459). The *pericallosal artery*, as the terminal branch of the anterior cerebral artery, continues caudally along the dorsal surface of the corpus callosum; its terminal branches supply the precuneus (2251). Anomalies of the anterior cerebral artery occur in about 25% of brains; these include unpaired arteries and instances where branches are given off to the contralateral hemisphere (109, 1974, 1975). Occlu-

sion of the trunk of one anterior cerebral artery produces a contralateral hemiplegia which is greatest in the lower limb. Obstruction of both anterior cerebral arteries is associated with bilateral paralysis, especially in the lower limbs, and impaired sensation that mimics spinal cord disease.

Middle Cerebral Artery. The middle cerebral artery, the continuation of the internal carotid artery, passes laterally over the anterior perforated substance to the lateral cerebral fossa between the temporal lobe and the insula (Fig. 20-7). This artery, the largest and most complex of the cerebral arteries, divides into a number of large branches in the insular region which course upward and backward; as these arteries reach the uppermost portions of the insula, they reverse their course abruptly (180° turns) and pass downward to the lower margin of the lateral sulcus (874). The course of the branches of the middle cerebral artery in the insular region is of great importance in the interpretation of cerebral angiograms (2520). In the insular region, 5 to 8 branches of the middle cerebral artery lie within what is called the Sylvian triangle. The Sylvian point (or apex) is established angiographically by the most posterior branch of the middle cerebral artery to emerge from the lateral sulcus. The inferior margin of the Sylvian triangle is formed by the lower branches of the middle cerebral artery, while the superior margin is formed by looping branches of this artery that are reversing their course (Fig. 20-8). Displacement of branches of the middle cerebral artery in the Sylvian triangle by mass lesions can be detected readily in cerebral angiograms, and the direction of displacement provides important information concerning localization of these lesions.

Branches of the middle cerebral artery emerge from the lateral sulcus and are distributed in a "fanlike" fashion over the lateral convexity of the hemisphere. These cortical branches supply lateral portions of the orbital gyri, the inferior and middle frontal gyri, large parts of the precentral and postcentral gyri, the superior and middle temporal gyri, including the temporal pole. The largest cortical branches appear to supply the temporo-occipital and angular areas (874). The cortical arteries arise from stem arteries and supply individual cortical

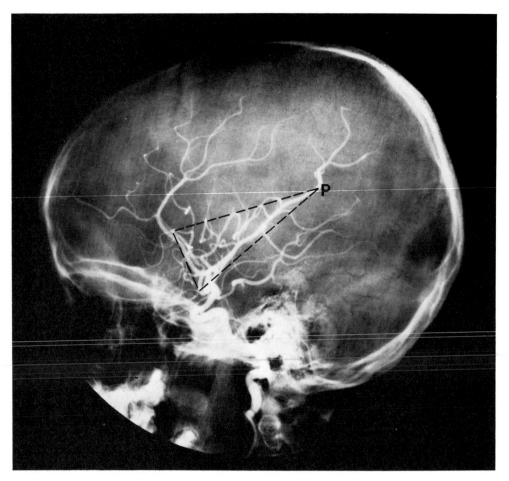

Figure 20-8. Cerebral angiogram demonstrating the Sylvian triangle. There are 5 to 8 branches of the *middle cerebral artery* on the surface of the insula. As they course upward, they reach the deepest portion of the sulcus formed by the junction of the insula and the frontoparietal operculum. Upon reaching this point, the middle cerebral branches change direction and proceed downward a short distance to emerge from the lateral sulcus (Sylvian fissure). The points of reversal can be identified in the angiogram, and a line drawn from the most anterior to the most posterior point (*P*) forms the upper margin of the Sylvian triangle. The inferior margin of the triangle is a line from the most posterior point (the angiographic Sylvian point, *P*) to the anterior extremity of the middle cerebral artery. The anterior border is a line drawn from the rostral extremity of the middle cerebral artery to the first turn of the opercular branch. The triangle contains branches of the middle cerebral artery as they are disposed on the insula. (Reproduced with permission from J. M. Taveras and the late E. H. Wood: *Diagnostic Neuroradiology*, Williams & Wilkins, 1976 (2520).)

regions. In general, one or two cortical arteries pass to each cortical region supplied. The cortical branches to the frontal, anterior temporal and anterior parietal regions are smaller than those to the posterior parietal, posterior temporal and temporo-occipital regions, but they are more numerous.

Branches of the middle cerebral artery include: (a) the lenticulostriate arteries, (b) the anterior temporal artery, (c) the orbitofrontal artery, (d) pre-Rolandic and Ro-

landic branches, (e) anterior and posterior parietal branches, and (f) a posterior temporal branch which extends caudally to supply lateral portions of the occipital lobe.

The first branches to arise from the middle cerebral artery are the *lenticulostriate arteries* which enter the anterior perforated substance (Figs. 18-2 and 20-10). These vessels will be considered with the central or ganglionic branches. The next branches to arise from the middle cerebral artery are the anterior temporal artery and the orbitofrontal artery (Fig. 20-7). The *anterior temporal artery* frequently anastomoses with temporal branches of the posterior cerebral artery, while the *orbitofrontal artery* may anastomose with the frontopolar branch of the anterior cerebral artery. Ascending branches of the middle cerebral artery, given off more distally, include *pre-Rolandic branches*, a *Rolandic branch*, an *anterior parietal* (or post-Rolandic) *branch* and a *posterior parietal branch*. A *posterior temporal branch* extends backwards to supply lateral portions of the occipital lobe. The angular branches supplying the angular gyrus constitute the terminal part of the middle cerebral artery.

The extensive territory nourished by the middle cerebral artery includes the motor and premotor areas, the somesthetic and auditory projection areas and the integrative association areas of the parietal lobe. Occlusion of the middle cerebral artery near the origin of its cortical branches, when not fatal, produces a contralateral hemiplegia most marked in the upper extremity and face, and a contralateral sensory loss of the cortical type, in which there may be astereognosis and inability to distinguish between stimuli of different intensities. When the left or dominant hemisphere is involved, severe aphasic disturbances, may be present (page 703).

Posterior Cerebral Arteries. The posterior cerebral arteries, formed by the bifurcation of the basilar artery, pass laterally around the crus cerebri (Figs. 20-4–20-6). After receiving anastomoses from the posterior communicating arteries, these arteries continue along the lateral aspect of the midbrain and then pass dorsal to the tentorium to course on the medial and inferior surfaces of temporal and occipital lobes (Figs. 20-14 and 20-15). Branches of the posterior cerebral artery extend onto the lateral surfaces of the hemisphere to supply part of the inferior temporal gyrus, variable portions of the occipital lobe and portions of the superior parietal lobule (Figs. 20-6, 20-7, 20-14 and 20-15). Branches of the posterior cerebral artery also are distributed to the brain stem, the choroid plexus of the third and lateral ventricles and to regions of the cerebral cortex (2793).

The posterior cerebral artery divides into two main branches, the posterior temporal (temporo-occipital) and the internal occip-

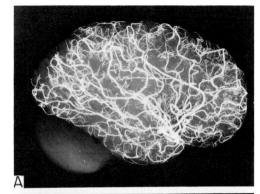
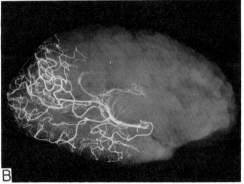

Figure 20-9. Roentgenograms of fresh cadaver brains in which cerebral vessels have been injected with radiopaque material. *A*, injections of the anterior, middle and posterior cerebral arteries. *B*, injection of the posterior cerebral artery. Note the filling of the thalamoperforating branches. (Courtesy of Dr. Harry A Kaplan.)

ital arteries. The *posterior temporal artery* (Fig. 20-15) gives off an anterior temporal branch which supplies anterior portions of the inferior surface of the temporal lobe and frequently anastomoses with branches of the anterior temporal artery derived from the middle cerebral artery (Figs. 20-6 and 20-9*B*). The largest branches of the posterior temporal artery reach the lateral surface of the hemisphere immediately anterior to the preoccipital notch (2793). More posterior branches of this vessel supply the occipitotemporal and lingual gyri. The *internal occipital artery* divides into the *parieto-occipital artery* and the *calcarine artery*, both of which supply different regions on the medial aspect of the occipital lobe and portions of the splenium of the corpus callosum (Figs. 20-6 and 20-14). Thus the cortical branches of the posterior cerebral artery supply the medial and inferior sur-

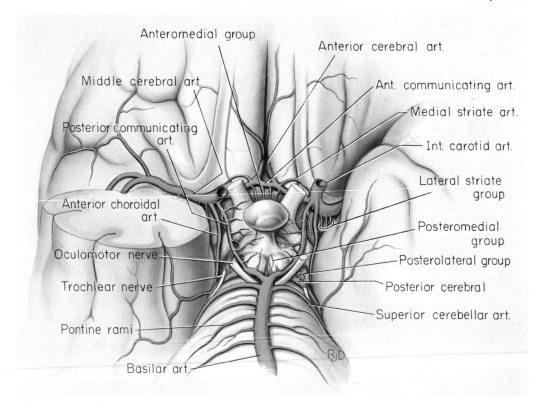

Figure 20-10. The cerebral arterial circle at the base of the brain, showing the distribution of the ganglionic branches. These vessels form *anteromedial, posteromedial, posterolateral* and *lateral striate* arterial groups. The *medial striate* and *anterior choroidal arteries* also are shown.

faces of the occipital lobe and the inferior surface of the temporal lobe, except for the temporal pole (Figs. 20-6 and 20-9*B*). Branches of these arteries extend onto the lateral surface of the brain and supply the inferior temporal gyrus and variable portions of the lateral occipital region; some of the branches from the medial surface supply a considerable part of the superior parietal lobule. In these regions, branches of the posterior cerebral artery anastomose with marginal branches of the anterior and middle cerebral arteries (Fig. 20-7). The calcarine branch of the posterior cerebral artery is of major importance because it supplies the primary visual cortex (Figs. 20-6 and 20-14). The extensive anastomoses mentioned above appear to explain why occlusion of the posterior cerebral artery rarely produces softening (encephalomalacia) in the total distribution of this vessel. Occlusion of the posterior cerebral artery produces a contralateral homonymous hemianopsia (Fig. 15-32), frequently with

sparing of macular vision. Anastomoses between branches of the middle and posterior cerebral arteries in the region of the occipital pole probably account for the preservation of macular vision.

The introduction of cerebral angiography as a diagnostic technic in clinical neurology (1722, 1723) emphasized the great importance of the anatomical distribution, course and variations of individual cerebral vessels. This technic, based upon the injection of radiopaque solutions into the internal carotid or vertebral arteries, permits the taking of serial roentgenograms during various phases of the passage of the radiopaque solution through cerebral vessels. Cerebral angiography is particularly useful in localizing aneurysms and vascular malformations, and often it provides specific information concerning occlusive vascular disease and space-occupying intracranial masses. Cerebral aneurysms are mostly of congenital origin and appear to arise frequently from vessels on the inferior surface

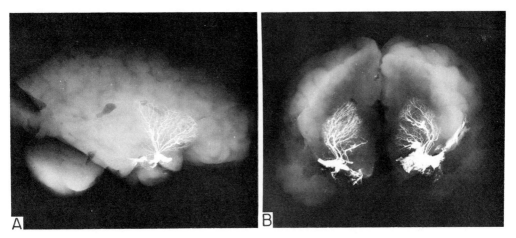

Figure 20-11.   Roentgenograms of fresh cadaver brains in which individual arteries have been injected with radiopaque material. *A* and *B* are lateral and frontal views, respectively, of the deep ganglionic branches of the *middle cerebral artery* that penetrate the brain in the anterior perforated substance. (Courtesy of Dr. Harry A. Kaplan.)

of the brain. Although it has been stated that aneurysms arise only at the point of bifurcation of an artery, Dandy (592) found that many were not associated with arterial branching. Vascular malformations are of many types: Arteriovenous malformations are characterized by an abnormal nest of blood vessels in which there are direct anastomoses of arteries and veins. Cerebral angiography is of importance in diagnosing occlusive vascular disease in the internal carotid (both cervical and intracranial portions) and in the vertebral and basilar arteries, as well as in the trunk of the middle cerebral artery (Figs. 20-8, 20-14 and 20-15). It is more difficult to ascertain the presence of vascular occlusions in the distal branches of the anterior, middle and posterior cerebral arteries (2519) because of direct end-to-end anastomoses between branches of these vessels on the surface of the brain. While intracerebral hemorrhage cannot be distinguished angiographically from cerebral edema or other avascular space-occupying lesions, intracranial hemorrhage sometimes can be localized on the basis of occlusion of certain vessels and displacement of cerebral vessels. Certain highly vascular brain tumors may produce what is called a "tumor stain" in the cerebral angiogram.

While cerebral angiography provides invaluable diagnostic information, it is unusual for the contrast medium to permeate the very small terminal arteries (Fig. 20-8).

Injection of the internal carotid artery usually permits visualization of the main branches of the anterior and middle cerebral arteries on the side of the injection. A radiographic technic for studying individual cerebral vessels and their branches in fresh cadaver brains has been developed by Kaplan (1265–1267) and has been used extensively to study cerebral vessels (2251). The exquisite detail which can be brought out by this method is demonstrated in Figures 20-9 and 20-11.

The Central Branches

Central or Ganglionic Arteries. The central or ganglionic arteries which supply the diencephalon, corpus striatum and internal capsule are arranged in four general groups: anteromedial, anterolateral, posteromedial and posterolateral (Fig. 20-10).

The *anteromedial arteries* arise from the domain of the anterior cerebral and anterior communicating arteries, but some twigs come directly from the terminal portion of the internal carotid (Fig. 20-10). They enter the most medial portion of the anterior perforated space and are distributed to the anterior hypothalamus, including the preoptic and suprachiasmatic regions.

The *posteromedial arteries*, which enter the tuber cinereum, mammillary bodies and interpeduncular fossa, are derived from the most proximal portion of the posterior cerebral, and from the whole extent of the

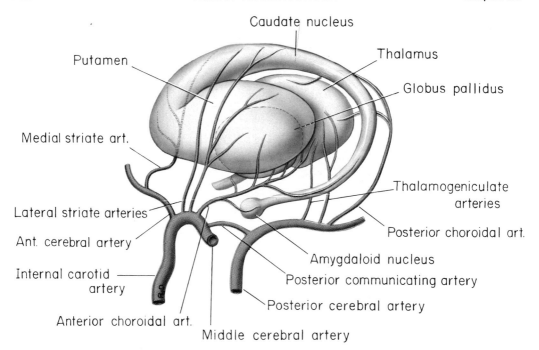

Figure 20-12. Diagrammatic representation of the arterial supply of the corpus striatum and thalamus. (Modified from Aitken (24).)

posterior communicating arteries (Fig. 20-10). Some twigs come directly from the internal carotid artery just before its bifurcation. A rostral and caudal group may be distinguished. The rostral group supplies the hypophysis, infundibulum and tuberal regions of the hypothalamus. A number of vessels, the *thalamoperforating arteries*, penetrate more deeply and are distributed to the anterior and medial portions of the thalamus (Figs. 20-9*B* and 20-14). The caudal group supplies the mammillary region of the hypothalamus, the subthalamic region, and sends small branches to the medial nuclei of the thalamus. Other vessels from the caudal group are distributed in the midbrain to the rapheal region of the tegmentum, the red nucleus and medial portions of the crus cerebri.

The *posterolateral (thalamogeniculate) arteries* arise more laterally from the posterior cerebral arteries (Figs. 20-10 and 20-12). They penetrate the lateral geniculate body and supply the larger caudal half of the thalamus, including the geniculate bodies, the pulvinar and most of the lateral nuclear mass.

The *anterolateral (striate) arteries*, which pierce the anterior perforated substance, arise mainly from the initial portion of the middle cerebral artery and, to a lesser extent, from the anterior cerebral artery (Figs. 20-5 and 20-10). As a rule, those from the anterior cerebral artery supply the rostroventral portion of the head of the caudate nucleus and adjacent portions of the putamen and internal capsule. The rest of the putamen, caudate nucleus and anterior limb of the internal capsule are supplied by branches from the middle cerebral artery, except the most caudal tip of the putamen and the tail of the caudate nucleus (Figs. 20-11 and 20-12). These branches also nourish lateral parts of the globus pallidus and dorsal portions of the posterior limb of the internal capsule. In some instances all the striate arteries may be derived from the middle cerebral artery. One of the striate arteries, described as the cerebral vessel most prone to rupture, has been called the "artery of cerebral hemorrhage" (Charcot). Such an artery usually cannot be distinguished anatomically. While it appears doubtful that the striate arteries supply parts of the thalamus, vessels, referred to as lenticulo-optic arteries, have been described. The central perforating branches arising from the middle cerebral artery are

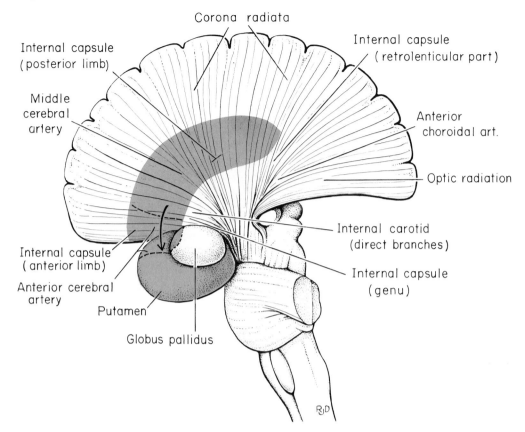

Figure 20-13.   Diagram of the blood supply of the internal capsule and corpus striatum. The putamen and globus pallidus are shown rotated ventrally away from the internal capsule. Regions supplied by branches of the *middle* and *anterior cerebral arteries* are shown in *red*; portions of the internal capsule and corpus striatum supplied by the *anterior choroidal artery* and in *yellow*. Direct branches of the *internal carotid artery* supply the genu of the internal capsule (Based on Alexander (36).)

shown radiographically in injected specimens in Figure 20-11.

Choroidal Arteries. The anterior and posterior choroidal arteries may be regarded as distinctive central branches.

The *anterior choroidal artery* usually arises from the internal carotid artery distal to the origin of the posterior communicating artery, but it may arise from the middle cerebral artery (410). This artery passes backward across the optic tract, to which it usually gives a few small branches, and then courses laterally toward the medial surface of the rostral part of the temporal lobe (Figs. 20-10 and 20-12). The vessel passes into the inferior horn of the lateral ventricle through the choroidal fissure where it supplies the choroid plexus. The anterior choroidal artery also supplies the hippocampal formation, portions of both segments of the globus pallidus (i.e., lateral parts of the medial pallidal segment and medial parts of the lateral pallidal segment), a large ventral part of the posterior limb of the internal capsule and the entire retrolenticular portion of the internal capsule (Fig. 20-13). Smaller branches of this vessel supply parts of the amygdaloid nuclear complex, ventral portions of the tail of the caudate nucleus and extreme posterior parts of the putamen. A few branches of this artery enter lateral portions of the thalamus (1268). Alexander (36) considered the anterior choroidal artery as a vessel highly susceptible to thrombosis because of its long subarachnoid course and its relatively small caliber. It appears significant that the globus pallidus and hippocampal formation, two of the most vulnerable structures of the brain, are both supplied by this artery.

The *posterior choroidal arteries* arising from the posterior cerebral artery (Fig. 20-12) consist of one medial posterior choroidal artery and at least two lateral posterior choroidal arteries (843). The medial posterior choroidal artery arises from the proximal part of the posterior cerebral artery, curves around the midbrain and reaches the region lateral to the pineal body. This vessel gives off branches to the tectum, the choroid plexus of the third ventricle and the superior and medial surfaces of the thalamus (Fig. 20-9*B*). The lateral posterior choroidal arteries arise from the posterior cerebral artery as this vessel encircles the brain stem. These vessels penetrate the choroidal fissure where they anastomose with branches of the anterior choroidal artery (410, 664).

BLOOD SUPPLY OF CORPUS STRIATUM INTERNAL CAPSULE AND DIENCEPHALON

The *striatum* is nourished mainly by the lateral striate arteries derived from the middle cerebral artery (Figs. 20-12 and 20-13). Rostromedial parts of the head of the caudate nucleus are supplied by the medial striate artery (Heubner), while the tail of the caudate nucleus and caudal parts of the putamen receive branches of the anterior choroidal artery. The lateral segment of the globus pallidus is supplied by branches of both the lateral striate and anterior choroidal arteries (1693). The lateral part of the medial pallidal segment receives branches from the anterior choroidal artery, while branches of the posterior communicating artery nourish the most medial portions of this pallidal segment.

The *internal capsule*, both anterior and posterior limbs, is supplied primarily by the lateral striate branches of the middle cerebral artery (Fig. 20-13). The medial striate artery supplies a rostromedial part of the anterior limb of the internal capsule. As a rule, the genu of the internal capsule receives some direct branches from the internal carotid artery (36), while ventral parts of the posterior limb and its entire retrolenticular part are supplied by branches of the anterior choroidal artery (2251).

The *thalamus* is nourished mainly by branches of the posterior cerebral artery (Figs. 20-9*B*, 20-10 and 20-12). *Thalamoperforating branches*, referred to as the posteromedial arteries, course dorsally and medially to supply chiefly medial and anterior regions of the thalamus (769, 2251). These arteries, arising from the most medial part of the posterior cerebral artery and from the terminal part of the basilar artery, course dorsally into the diencephalon and nourish paraventricular regions of the hypothalamus and medial regions of the thalamus (861, 1025). These perforating arteries can be visualized in vertebral angiograms (Fig. 20-14) and may be displaced, deformed or stretched by space-occupying lesions or enlargement of the third ventricle. *Thalamogeniculate branches*, referred to as the posterolateral arteries, supply the pulvinar and the lateral nuclei of the thalamus. These arteries arise from the posterior cerebral artery as it winds around the crus cerebri and from the choroidal arteries (410, 1461). The *medial posterior choroidal artery* supplies the choroid plexus of the third ventricle and superior and medial portions of the thalamus. The *inferior thalamic arteries* arise from the posterior communicating artery and from the bifurcation of the basilar artery. These arteries course rostrally and dorsally and enter inferior portions of the thalamus (1461). The inferior thalamic arteries supply regions of the thalamus rostral to the territory of the thalamoperforating arteries.

The anterior *hypothalamus* and preoptic region receive their blood supply from the anteromedian ganglionic arteries. Remaining portions of the hypothalamus and the subthalamic region are supplied by branches of the posteromedian group derived from the posterior cerebral and posterior communicating arteries.

VERTEBRAL BASILAR SYSTEM

With the exception of the most rostral portions of the crus cerebri, the entire blood supply of the medulla, pons, mesencephalon and cerebellum is derived from the vertebral basilar system.

Vertebral Artery. Each vertebral artery, as it passes over the anterior surface of the medulla, gives rise to: (a) a *posterior spinal artery*, (b) an *anterior spinal artery*, (c) a large *posterior inferior cerebellar artery*, and (d) a *posterior meningeal artery*. The two vertebral arteries unite to form the basilar artery at the caudal border of the pons. This large vessel passes rostrally in the basilar sulcus and bifurcates at the upper border of the pons, forming the posterior cerebral arteries (Figs. 20-1, 20-5, 20-6, 20-14 and 20-15).

Basilar Artery. The basilar artery gives rise to: (a) the *anterior inferior cerebellar arteries*, (b) the *labyrinthine arteries*, (c) *numerous paramedian* and *circumferential pontine rami*, and (d) the *superior cerebellar arteries* (Figs. 20-1, 20-5, 20-6 and 20-10). The *posterior cerebral arteries*, representing the terminal branches of the basilar artery, furnish the main blood supply to the midbrain via branches which arise from proximal portions of these vessels. The labyrinthine arteries do not supply the brain stem, but pass laterally through the internal auditory meati (Fig. 20-5).

Vertebral angiography is more difficult to perform than carotid angiography because this artery is smaller and contained within a bony canal. Many of the branches of the vertebral and basilar arteries are small and difficult to identify angiographically, but the posterior inferior cerebellar, the anterior inferior cerebellar, the superior cerebellar and the posterior cerebral arteries usually can be seen. Both posterior cerebral arteries are filled by contrast media following injection of one vertebral artery (Figs. 20-14 and 20-15).

Medulla and Pons. The medulla and pons are supplied by the anterior and posterior spinal arteries, and by branches of the vertebral, basilar and the posterior inferior cerebellar arteries. Minor contributions also may be made by the *superior* and the *anterior inferior cerebellar arteries* (Fig. 20-5). There is great variation in the extent of the areas supplied by each vessel, as well as considerable overlapping of adjacent fields. These variations are due in part to the different levels of origin of the anterior spinal arteries, and to the varying level of fusion of the two vertebrals into the basilar artery. Not uncommonly one or another artery may be missing altogether, and its place is taken by the vessel supplying the adjacent territory. Since the vascular supply of this region has considerable clinical importance, the main structures normally supplied by the various arteries are summarized briefly (Figs. 20-16 and 20-17).

The *posterior spinal artery* supplies the gracile and cuneate fasciculi and their nuclei, and the caudal and dorsal portions of the inferior cerebellar peduncle (Figs. 20-1 and 20-17). There are numerous anastomoses between branches of the posterior spinal and the posterior inferior cerebellar arteries (664). When the posterior spinal artery on one side is missing, its territory is taken over by the posterior inferior cerebellar artery. Branches of the posterior spinal artery also supply parts of the nucleus of the solitary tract, the vagal nuclei and portions of the spinal trigeminal nucleus. Small branches of this artery with a superficial course may penetrate the taenia to supply the area postrema.

The *anterior spinal artery* supplies the medial structures of the medulla, including the pyramids, pyramidal decussation, medial lemniscus, medial longitudinal fasciculus, predorsal bundle and hypoglossal nucleus, except its most cephalic portion. In addition, the artery supplies the medial accessory olive, the most caudal portions of the solitary nucleus and fasciculus and the dorsal motor nucleus of the vagus. Medullary branches arising from the anterior spinal artery increase in size and number from caudal to rostral levels. The larger and longer branches pass in the medial raphe between the medial lemnisci (Fig. 20-17*C*), and their terminal rami reach the floor of the fourth ventricle. Smaller, shorter branches of the anterior spinal artery run obliquely through the medial lemnisci to enter the medial reticular formation and medial parts of the inferior olivary nuclear complex (664). In the upper medulla the distribution of the anterior spinal artery is reduced gradually, and it is replaced by branches of the vertebral and basilar arteries (Fig. 20-17).

The *bulbar branches of the vertebral artery* arise as a series of rami that enter the brain stem in relation to rootlets of the glossopharyngeal, vagus and accessory nerves. The most densely vascularized lateral medullary region lies dorsal to the inferior olivary complex; this region contains numerous small arteries and veins on the surface which penetrate deeply into the medulla (Fig. 20-17*B*). The inferior rami arise directly from the vertebral artery, enter the medulla between the rootlets of the accessory nerve, and supply the region between the inferior olivary nuclear complex

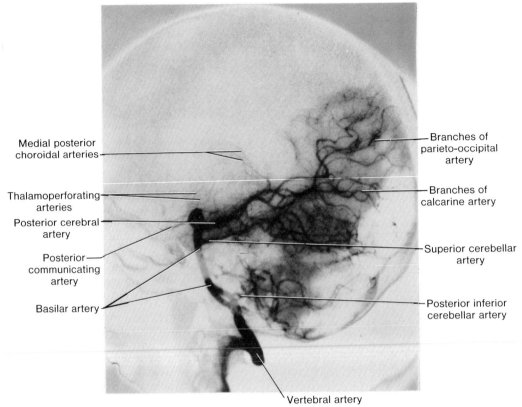

Medial posterior choroidal arteries

Thalamoperforating arteries

Posterior cerebral artery

Posterior communicating artery

Basilar artery

Branches of parieto-occipital artery

Branches of calcarine artery

Superior cerebellar artery

Posterior inferior cerebellar artery

Vertebral artery

Figure 20-14. Lateral projection of a vertebral angiogram demonstrating major branches of the vertebral basilar system. (Courtesy of Drs. Daniel Hottenstein and Keith Himes, Holy Spirit Hospital, Camp Hill, Pa.)

and the inferior cerebellar peduncle (Figs. 20-16C and 20-17C). A larger and more important group of rami enter the lateral surface of the medulla in relation to the glossopharyngeal and vagus nerves. These direct branches of the vertebral artery normally supply the pyramids at the lower border of the pons, the most cephalic part of the hypoglossal nucleus, and large parts of the inferior olivary nucleus, including the dorsal accessory olive. These arteries also supply olivocerebellar fibers traversing the reticular formation, portions of the dorsal motor nucleus of the vagus, and the solitary nucleus and fasciculus. At the level of the pyramidal decussation the most caudal branches are distributed to practically the whole lateral region of the medulla lying between the pyramids and the fasciculus cuneatus. Two types of arteries enter the medulla. Short arteries supply small branches to the spinal trigeminal, spinotha-

lamic and spinocerebellar tracts, while long arteries supply deeper regions. Some of the long arteries reach the floor of the fourth ventricle (Fig. 20-16C). The medullary region supplied by these branches includes structures involved in the lateral medullary syndrome (104, 2433).

The *posterior inferior cerebellar artery* supplies the lateral medullary region rostral to that supplied by direct bulbar branches of the vertebral artery (Fig. 20-16). This retro-olivary region contains the spinothalamic and rubrospinal tracts, the spinal trigeminal nucleus and tract, the nucleus ambiguus, the dorsal motor nucleus of the vagus, and the emerging fibers of these nuclei. This artery also supplies ventral parts of the inferior cerebellar peduncle. Descending central autonomic tracts are found in this area of the medulla.

The ventral portion of the pons receives arterial blood from three series of branches,

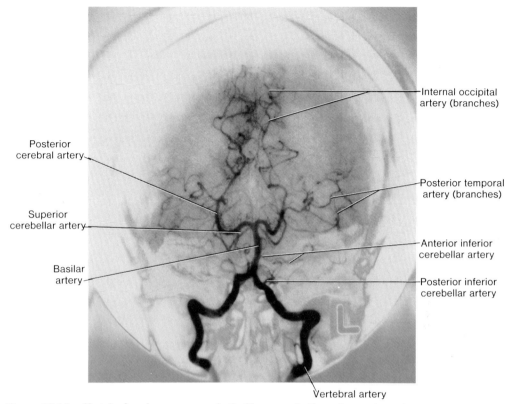

Posterior
cerebral artery

Superior
cerebellar artery

Basilar
artery

Internal occipital
artery (branches)

Posterior temporal
artery (branches)

Anterior inferior
cerebellar artery

Posterior inferior
cerebellar artery

Vertebral artery

Figure 20-15.   Vertebral angiogram as seen in the Towne projection using a subtraction technic. (Courtesy of Drs. Daniel Hottenstein and Keith Himes, Holy Spirit Hospital, Camp Hill, Pa.)

all derived from the *basilar artery* (Figs. 20-16–20-18). These arterial branches are grouped into: (a) paramedian, (b) short circumferential, and (c) long circumferential.

Paramedian arteries leave the dorsal surface of the parent vessel to supply the most medial pontine area, including the pontine nuclei and the corticopontine, corticospinal and corticobulbar tracts. Smaller arterial twigs also penetrate dorsally to supply the most ventral part of the pontine tegmentum, including a portion of the medial lemniscus. Obstruction of the paramedian arteries usually is followed by hemiplegia (or a quadriplegia); pseudobulbar palsy, including dysarthria and dysphagia; transitory hemianesthesia; paresis of conjugate eye movements with deviation of the eyes to the side opposite the lesion (798); or bilateral ophthalmoplegia (1633).

Short circumferential arteries supply a wedge of tissue along the anterolateral pontine surface (Fig. 20-17). Neural structures

in this intermediate area of the pons include a variable number of fibers of the corticospinal tract and medial lemniscus, the pontine nuclei and pontocerebellar fibers and part of the nuclei and fibers of the trigeminal and facial nerves. Some of the circumferential branches may ascend to supply part of the superior cerebral peduncle. Obstruction of the short circumferential arteries on one side may result in ipsilateral cerebellar symptoms, contralateral hemianesthesia and disturbances of the sympathetic system, including an ipsilateral Horner's syndrome.

Long circumferential arteries pass laterally on the anterior surface of the pons to anastomose with smaller branches of the anterior inferior cerebellar and superior cerebellar arteries (Figs. 20-16 and 20-17). The long circumferential and *anterior inferior cerebellar arteries* supply most of the tegmentum in the caudal portion of the pons, whereas the long circumferential and

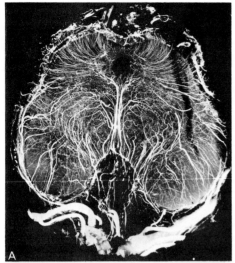

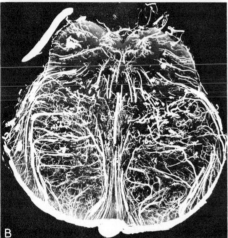

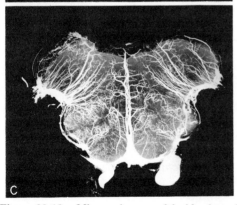

Figure 20-16. Microangiograms of the blood supply of the midbrain, pons and medulla made from 4-mm-thick injected specimens. In the midbrain (*A*) the tegmentum is supplied mainly by branches of the *posterior cerebral* and *superior cerebellar arteries*, but it also receives contributions from the paramedian and both long and short circumferential arteries. The upper pons (*B*) receives paramedian and circumfer-

superior cerebellar arteries supply a similar area in the more rostral levels of the pons. Important neural structures within this area of vascular distribution are the nuclei of cranial nerves III to VIII, the spinal trigeminal nucleus and tract, the medial longitudinal fasciculus, the medial lemniscus, the spinothalamic and spinocerebellar tracts, the superior cerebellar peduncle and the reticular formation. Obstruction of these vessels may produce injury to one or more of the cranial nerves mentioned, paresis of conjugate eye movements, contralateral hemianesthesia, ipsilateral cerebellar symptoms, nystagmus and sympathetic disturbances. Alterations in the individual's sensorium may increase until coma supervenes owing to anoxia or hemorrhage into the pontine tegmentum.

Complete or partial thrombosis of the basilar artery may occur suddenly and is accompanied by severe headache, vomiting and loss of consciousness. Complete thrombosis is generally fatal, although recoveries have been observed after partial occlusion (1054). Insufficiency of the basilar arterial system is characterized by varying signs and symptoms occurring in transient episodes over a period of months or years. Vertigo is fairly common as are dysarthria, dysphagia, diplopia, nystagmus and varying degrees of paresis on one or both sides (879). Thrombosis of the basilar artery was once considered of purely academic interest. Today it is of practical importance as well, for it can be diagnosed and distinguished from basilar insufficiency (Figs. 20-14 and 20-15). The symptoms of basilar artery occlusion (usually bilateral) are due to massive pontine damage and include a deep comatose state, generalized loss of muscular tone (flaccidity of limbs), dilated or pinpoint pupils that do not react to light and loss of superficial abdominal reflexes. Increased muscle tone and Babinski responses may be present within a variable period of time after such vascular accidents. There is often an intermingling of symptoms, depending upon the level, branches

ential branches from the *basilar artery*, as well as branches of the *superior cerebellar artery* distributed to dorsal regions. The vascular pattern in the upper medulla (*C*) should be compared with the diagram of Figure 20-17. (Courtesy of Dr. O. Hassler (1046).)

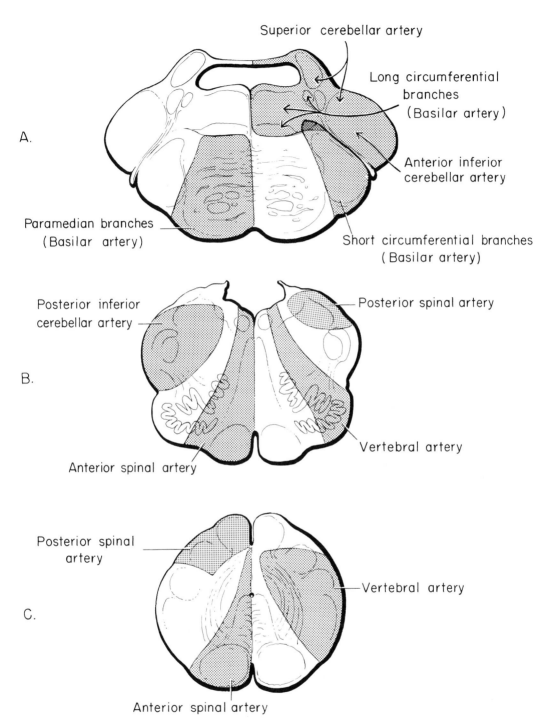

Figure 20-17.   Diagrams of the arterial supply of the medulla and pons. Medullary levels shown are through the posterior column nuclei (*C*) and the inferior olivary nuclear complex (*B*). (Based on Stopford (2442, 2443).) The pons (*A*) is supplied by paramedian and circumferential branches of the basilar artery, Frantzen and Olivarius (798).

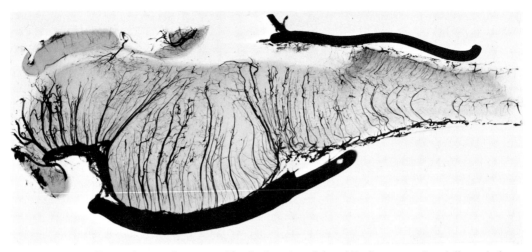

Figure 20-18. Microangiogram of a 4-mm midsagittal section of the midbrain, pons and medulla made from an injected specimen. Paramedian arteries form different angles with the basilar artery at various levels. In the caudal midbrain and upper pons, they are inclined caudally; in the upper medulla and caudal pons, these vessels are inclined rostrally. (Courtesy of Dr. O. Hassler (1046).)

involved and degree of arterial occlusion. For example, thrombosis of the rostral part of the basilar artery, near its bifurcation into the two posterior cerebral arteries, may result only in bilateral visual field defects.

The venous drainage of the hindbrain has been demonstrated by stereomicroangiography (1046). The paramedian veins which run near the midline to the ventral surface of the brain stem are inclined caudally in the upper pons but are nearly perpendicular to the axis of the brain stem in more caudal regions. At the junction of pons and medulla a conspicuously large vein consistently drains the floor of the fourth ventricle. Veins draining ventral portions of the pons usually empty into paired longitudinal venous plexuses several millimeters lateral to the basilar artery. However, in some instances these veins enter a single unpaired vein situated between the basilar artery and the brain stem parenchyma. In the lower medulla, posterior veins are larger than the anterior veins and penetrate deeper regions. Although the veins of the hindbrain seldom accompany the arterial branches in the same vascular sheath, the intraparenchymatous venous angioarchitecture resembles the arterial pattern. Anastomoses between intraparen-

chymatous veins occur mainly at the capillary level. Large veins draining the choroid plexus of the fourth ventricle, most of the pons, and the upper medulla, empty into the sigmoid sinus, or the superior or inferior petrosal sinuses. Veins draining caudal parts of the medulla empty into the anterior and posterior spinal veins (1046).

Mesencephalon. The blood supply of the mesencephalon is derived from branches of the basilar artery, although branches of the internal carotid may also contribute (Figs. 20-14, 20-16 and 20-18). The main vessels supplying this portion of the brain stem include: (a) the *posterior cerebral artery*, (b) the *superior cerebellar artery*, (c) branches of the *posterior communicating artery*, and (d) branches of the *anterior choroidal artery* (Figs. 20-1, 20-4–20-6 and 20-10). Branches from these arteries may be grouped, as in the case of the pons, into: (a) *paramedian arteries*, which nourish structures on both sides of the midline, and (b) *circumferential arteries*, both long and short, which wind laterally around the crus cerebri and supply lateral and dorsal regions of the midbrain (Fig. 20-16A).

Paramedian branches are derived from the posterior communicating artery, from the basilar bifurcation and from proximal portions of the posterior cerebral arteries. These vessels form an extensive plexus in the interpeduncular fossa (Fig. 20-10) and enter the brain stem in the posterior perforated substance. They supply the rapheal region, the oculomotor complex, the medial longitudinal fasciculus, the red nucleus, medial parts of the substantia nigra and the crus cerebri. Vascular lesions involving paramedian arterial branches at midbrain levels frequently produce a *superior alternating hemiplegia*, characterized by ipsilateral oculomotor disturbances and a contralateral hemiplegia (Weber's syndrome). This syndrome results from lesions involving portions of the crus cerebri and fibers of the oculomotor nerve. A less frequent lesion in the paramedian tegmental zone destroys portions of the red nucleus, the superior cerebellar peduncle and intra-axial rootlets of the oculomotor nerve (Benedikt's syndrome).

Short circumferential branches arise in part from both the interpeduncular plexus and from proximal portions of the posterior cerebral and superior cerebellar arteries. These arteries supply central and lateral parts of the crus cerebri, the substantia nigra and lateral portions of the midbrain tegmentum (Fig. 20-16). In the rostral mesencephalon some branches of the anterior choroidal artery are distributed to the interpeduncular fossa. Long circumferential arteries arise primarily from the posterior cerebral artery. The most important of these is the *quadrigeminal* or *collicular artery* which encircles the lateral surface of the midbrain and provides the main blood supply to the superior and inferior colliculi. Other vessels contributing to the blood supply of the tectum are branches of the medial posterior choroidal artery and the superior cerebellar artery.

Angiographic studies (1047) of the arterial pattern of the human brain stem clearly demonstrate the distribution of paramedian and circumferential arteries in the upper pons and midbrain (Figs. 20-16 and 20-17). Sagittal sections show that paramedian arteries entering the brain stem at various levels do so at different angles. At the junction of pons and medulla, these vessels are directed forward at an oblique angle, while at rostral pontine levels these vessels course obliquely in a caudal direction (Fig. 20-18).

Numerous veins of the mesencephalon arise from capillaries and, in general, run near the arteries but not directly with them. These veins form an extensive peripheral plexus in the pia and are collected by the basal veins which drain into either the great cerebral vein (Galen) or the internal cerebral veins (Figs. 20-23 and 20-24).

Cerebellum. Each half of the cerebellum is supplied by one superior and two inferior cerebellar arteries passing, respectively, to the superior and inferior surfaces of the cerebellum (Figs. 20-6 and 20-14).

The *posterior inferior cerebellar artery* arises from the vertebral artery, courses rostrolaterally along the surface of the medulla and then curves upward onto the inferior surface of the cerebellum. This vessel supplies the inferior vermis, especially the uvula and nodulus, as well as the cerebellar tonsil and the inferolateral surface of the cerebellar hemisphere. Medial branches of this artery supply portions of the choroid plexus of the fourth ventricle.

The *anterior inferior cerebellar artery* is usually the most caudal large vessel arising from the basilar artery (Fig. 20-5), but it is highly variable both in its origin and area of distribution (1268). This artery most frequently arises as a single vessel, courses caudally and laterally around the pons toward the cerebellopontine angle and comes into close relationship with both the facial and vestibulocochlear nerves (1627). After crossing the nerves in the cerebellopontine angle, the artery courses laterally above the flocculus to reach the inferior surface of the cerebellum where it supplies the pyramis, tuber, flocculus and portions of the inferior surface of the cerebellar hemisphere. It also sends branches to the deep portion of the corpus medullare and the dentate nucleus. In some cases, the flocculus and portions of the tonsil and biventer lobule may be supplied by an inconstant middle inferior cerebellar artery. Nerve-related branches of the anterior inferior cerebellar artery frequently supply tumors and arteriovenous malformations arising in the cerebellopontine angle. An internal auditory artery arising from this vessel appears quite constant, and occlusion of the anterior inferior cerebellar artery frequently produces nausea, vomiting, deafness, a facial paralysis and cerebellar disturbances (1627).

The *superior cerebellar artery* arises from the rostral part of the basilar artery and encircles the brain stem near the pontomesencephalic junction (Fig. 20-10). This vessel passes caudal to the oculomotor and trochlear nerves and rostral to the trigeminal nerve. In its proximal portion the artery courses medial to the free edge of the tentorium cerebelli (Fig. 20-4), but distally it passes beneath the tentorium, making it the most rostral of the infratentorial arteries (Fig. 20-6). The superior cerebellar artery gives off perforating, precerebellar and cortical branches (1026). Perforating branches of the artery penetrate the interpeduncular fossa, the crus cerebri and portions of the superior and middle cerebellar peduncles. Precerebellar branches supply the colliculi and the superior medullary velum. The cortical branches are divided into vermian, hemispheric and marginal arteries. These branches supply the superior (tentorial) and petrosal surfaces of the cerebellum and in some instances the region of the horizontal fissure (marginal branches). The hemispheric arteries give rise to numerous branches which extend deeply into the cerebellum; these vessels supply the middle and superior cerebellar peduncles, the intrinsic cerebellar nuclei and the superior medullary velum. Smaller branches supply portions of the choroid plexus of the fourth ventricle.

The veins have a course generally similar to that of the arteries. A superior and an inferior median vein drain the respective portions of the vermis, adjacent paravermal regions and the deep cerebellar nuclei. The superior vein terminates in the *great cerebral vein (Galen)*, while the inferior vein drains into the straight and transverse sinuses (Fig. 20-24). Superior and inferior lateral veins drain blood from the hemispheres and flocculi to the transverse, and, in part, to the superior and petrosal sinuses.

ARTERIES OF THE DURA

The cranial dura mater is supplied by a number of meningeal arteries derived from several sources. The largest and most important is the *middle meningeal artery*, which supplies most of the dura and practically its entire calvarial portion. It is a branch of the maxillary artery which enters the cranial cavity through the foramen spinosum and then divides into an anterior and a posterior branch (Figs. 1-3 and 20-4). Each of the branches runs outward and upward and extends toward the superior sagittal sinus, giving off numerous branches which run forward and backward. A small *accessory meningeal artery* which may arise from the maxillary artery, or the middle meningeal artery, enters the middle fossa through the oval foramen. This vessel supplies the dura of the middle fossa and the trigeminal ganglion. Meningeal branches from the intracavernous portion of the internal carotid artery also supply the dura of the middle fossa.

The dura of the anterior and the posterior fossae also receives a number of arteries, known respectively as the *anterior* and *posterior meningeal rami* or *arteries*. The anterior meningeal rami, usually two in number, are branches of the anterior and posterior ethmoidal arteries. The dura of the posterior fossa is supplied by a variable number of posterior meningeal arteries. These include: (a) one or more meningeal branches from the occipital artery entering through the jugular and hypoglossal foramina, (b) meningeal branches of the vertebral artery reaching the posterior fossa through the foramen magnum, and (c) several branches of the ascending pharyngeal artery entering through the foramen lacerum and hypoglossal canal.

CEREBRAL VEINS AND VENOUS SINUSES

Venous Sinuses of the Dura Mater

The cerebral veins of the brain do not run together with the arteries. Emerging as fine branches from the substance of the brain, they form a pial plexus from which the larger venous channels or cerebral veins arise. These veins run in the pia for a variable distance, pass through the subarachnoid space and empty into a system of intercommunicating endothelium-lined channels, the *sinuses of the dura mater*. The dural venous sinuses are located between the meningeal and periosteal layers of the dura (Figs. 1-1-1-4 and 20-4). The walls of these sinuses, unlike those of other veins, are composed of the tough fibrous tissue of the dura; hence, they exhibit a greater tautness and do not collapse when sectioned. The various venous sinuses converge at the internal occipital protuberance into two transversely running sinuses (Figs. 1-1 and 1-3), one for each side, which enter the jugular foramen to form the internal jugular vein. Besides draining the blood from the brain, the venous sinuses communicate with the superficial veins of the head by a number of small vessels which perforate the skull as *emissary veins* (Fig. 20-19).

The *superior sagittal sinus* extends from the foramen cecum to the internal occipital protuberance, lying along the superior border of the falx cerebri. It progressively increases in caliber as it proceeds caudally (Figs. 1-1 and 20-19). In its middle portion it gives off a number of lateral diverticula, the *venous lacunae*, into which the arachnoid villi protrude (Fig. 1-12).

The *inferior sagittal sinus* extends caudally along the free border of the falx. On reaching the anterior border of the tentorium, it is joined by the *great cerebral vein (Galen)*, which drains the deep structures of the brain, and the two veins form the *sinus rectus* (Figs. 1-3 and 20-19). The sinus rectus runs backward and downward along the line of attachment of the falx and tentorium and joins the superior sagittal sinus near the internal occipital protuberance (Figs. 20-4 and 20-20).

The two *transverse sinuses* arise from the confluens sinuum and pass laterally and forward in a groove in the occipital bone (Figs. 1-3 and 20-4). At the occipitopetrosal junction each sinus curves downward and backward as the sigmoid sinus. The *sigmoid sinus* is drained by the internal jugular vein (Fig. 20-19).

The *confluens sinuum* is formed by the union of the superior sagittal, straight and transverse sinuses. A small unpaired *occipital sinus* from the region of the foramen magnum ascends in the falx cerebelli (Figs. 1-1 and 20-20) and joins the confluens. The confluens is asymmetrical and shows many individual variations (Fig. 1-3 and *arrow* in Fig. 20-4). In relatively few cases is there an actual union of the four sinuses. Most often the superior sagittal sinus turns to the right to become continuous with the right transverse sinus, while the straight sinus bends to the left as the left transverse sinus (Fig. 1-1). In general, the venous blood of the superior cerebral veins and the superior

sagittal, right transverse and right sigmoid sinuses is drained by the right internal jugular vein. Most of the venous blood of the Galenic vein, the straight sinus, left transverse and left sigmoid sinuses usually is drained by the left internal jugular vein.

The *cavernous sinus* is a large irregular space located on each side of the sphenoid sinus, sella turcica and pituitary gland that extends from the superior orbital fissure to the petrous portion of the temporal bone (1029). It is a network of intercommunicating venous channels enclosing the internal carotid artery, the oculomotor, trochlear and abducens nerves, and the ophthalmic division of the trigeminal nerve (Fig. 20-21). The oculomotor, trochlear and the first division of the trigeminal nerve lie between dural leaves of the lateral wall of the cavernous sinus. The abducens nerve lies within the sinus, adjacent to the intracavernous portion of the carotid artery. The cavernous sinus of each side is connected with the other by venous channels which pass anterior and posterior to the hypophysis, and by the *basilar venous plexus* (Figs. 20-20 and 20-21). The latter venous plexus extends along the basilar portion of the occipital bone as far caudally as the foramen magnum where it communicates with the venous plexuses of the vertebral canal (Figs. 20-20 and 20-21). The venous ring, surrounding the hypophysis and composed of the two cavernous sinuses and their connecting channels, often is designated as the *circular sinus*. Each cavernous sinus likewise may be regarded as a confluens sinuum. Rostrally it receives the two ophthalmic veins through the orbital fissure and the small *sphenoparietal sinus*, which runs along the under surface of the lesser wing of the sphenoid (Figs. 20-4 and 20-21). Posteriorly it empties into the superior and inferior petrosal sinuses, through which it is connected, respectively, with the transverse sinus and the bulb of the internal jugular vein (Figs. 20-20 and 20-21).

In the adult the sphenoid sinus separates the cavernous sinuses on the two sides and, in addition, separates the pituitary gland from the nasal cavity. The increasing use of the transsphenoidal approach to tumors of the sellar region has created a need for detailed anatomy of this region (818). Three structures producing prominent bulges in

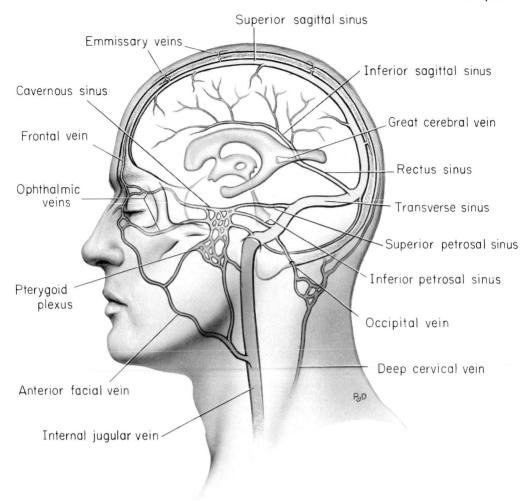

Figure 20-19.   The dural sinuses and their principal connections with extracranial veins. Intracranial venous sinuses and veins are *light blue*; extracranial veins are *dark blue*.

the lateral wall sphenoid sinus are: (a) the optic nerves, (b) the carotid arteries and (c) the maxillary branches of the trigeminal nerve. The bone in the lateral wall of the sphenoid sinus, separating it from the carotid artery and the cavernous sinus, is thin, and extreme care must be taken to avoid injury to this region which offers the potential for neural and arterial damage.

The dural sinuses communicate with the extracranial veins by a number of emissaries (Fig. 20-19). Thus the superior sagittal sinus is connected with the frontal and nasal veins and the emissaries of the foramen cecum (Fig. 20-4). It also sends a *parietal emissary* to the superficial temporal vein. The confluens sinuum usually gives off an

occipital emissary to the occipital vein, which is connected also with the transverse sinus by the larger *mastoid emissary* (Fig. 20-19). Smaller emissaries from the sigmoid sinus pass through the condyloid and hypoglossal foramina and communicate with vertebral and deep cervical veins. The cavernous sinus, besides receiving the ophthalmic veins, is connected with the internal jugular vein and with the pterygoid and pharyngeal plexuses by fine venous nets which pass through the oval, spinous, lacerated, carotid and jugular foramina.

Cerebral Veins

The cerebral veins which, like the dural sinuses, are devoid of valves, usually are

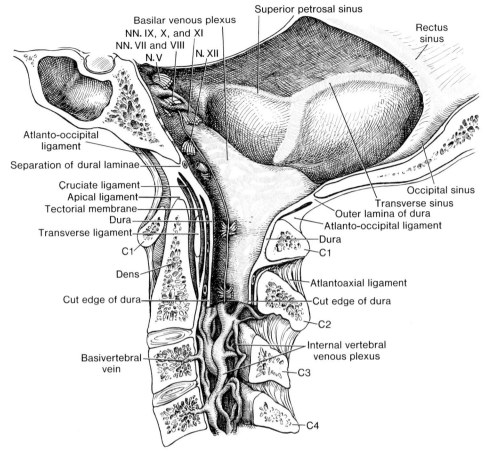

Figure 20-20.   Drawing of a sagittal view of the base of the skull and upper cervical vertebrae, showing ligaments, the dural venous sinuses and the internal vertebral venous plexus at the foramen magnum. Communications of the internal vertebral venous plexus with the basilar plexus are indicated. (Reproduced with permission from F. A. Mettler: *Neuroanatomy*, C. V. Mosby Company, St. Louis, 1948 (1688).)

divided into superficial and deep groups. The superficial cerebral veins drain the blood from the cortex and subcortical medullary substance and empty into the superior sagittal sinus or into the several basal sinuses (Fig. 20-22). The deep veins, draining the deep medullary substance, the basal ganglia and dorsal portions of the diencephalon, ultimately terminate in the internal and great cerebral veins (Figs. 20-23 and 20-24). While the two groups of veins are anatomically distinct, they are interconnected by numerous anastomotic channels, both intracerebral and extracerebral. Thus large surface areas can be drained through the great cerebral vein (Galen). Conversely, territories supplied by deep cerebral veins may be drained, when necessity arises, by

surface vessels. This anastomotic venous arrangement facilitates the drainage of capillary beds by shifting the blood from one area to another and readily equalizes regional increases in pressure due to occlusion or other factors. As a result, the occlusion of even a large vein, if not too rapid, will produce only slight transitory effects. When occlusion or increase in pressure occurs suddenly, there will be marked hyperemia and often extensive hemorrhages, as in birth injuries and occasionally in cases of adult thrombosis (2282, 2294).

Superficial Cerebral Veins. Superficial cerebral veins arise from the cortex and subcortical medullary substance, anastomose freely in the pia and form a number of large vessels which empty into the var-

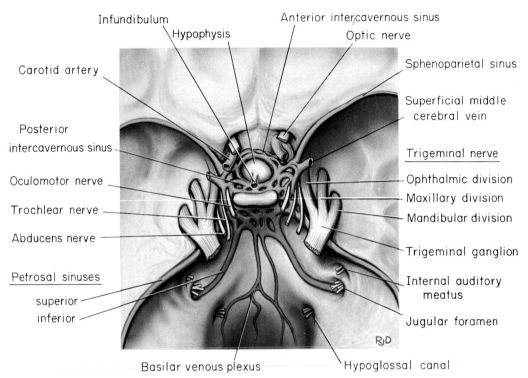

Figure 20-21.   The cavernous sinus, its venous connections and related structures.

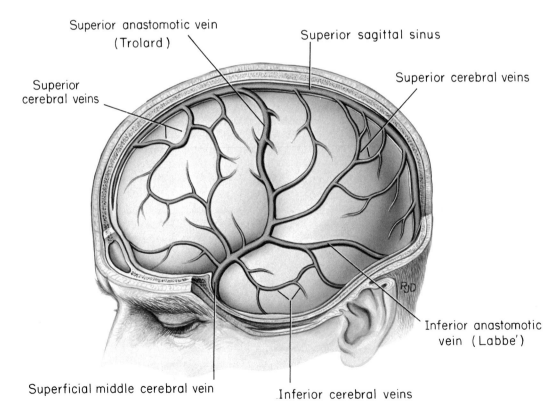

Figure 20-22.   The external cerebral veins on the convexity of the hemisphere.

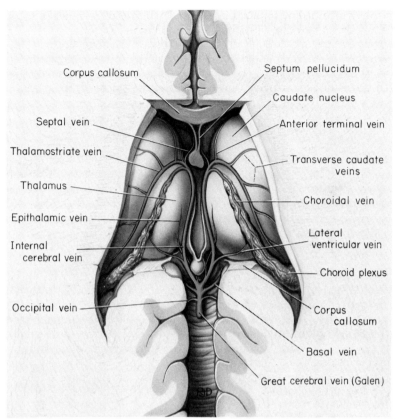

Figure 20-23.   The internal cerebral veins and their tributaries. (Modified from Schwartz and Fink (2294).)

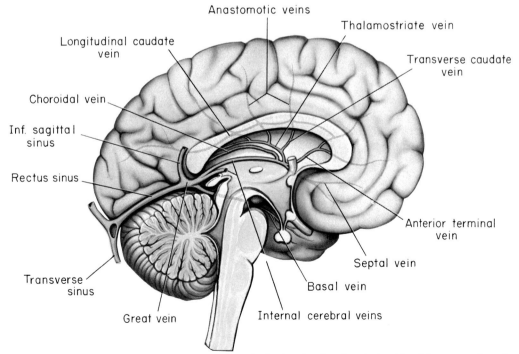

Figure 20-24.   Midsagittal view of the internal cerebral veins showing the relationship of the great vein to the rectus sinus. (Modified from Schlesinger (2282).)

ious sinuses. They include the superior and inferior cerebral veins and the superficial middle cerebral vein.

The *superior cerebral veins*, about 10 to 15 in number, collect blood from the convex and medial surfaces of the brain and open into the superior sagittal sinus, or its venous lacunae (Fig. 20-22). Many of them, especially the larger posterior ones, run obliquely forward through the subarachnoid space and enter the sinus. The direction of blood flow in these veins, as they enter the superior sagittal sinus, is opposite to that in the sinus. Some veins on the medial surface of the brain drain into the inferior sagittal sinus.

The *inferior cerebral veins* drain the basal surface of the hemisphere and the inferior portion of its lateral surface. Those on the lateral surface of the hemisphere empty into the *superficial middle cerebral vein* which runs along the lateral sulcus and terminates in the cavernous or sphenoparietal sinus (Figs. 20-4, 20-21 and 20-22). The middle vein receives anastomotic branches from the superior cerebral veins, and in many cases two of these channels become quite prominent. These are the *superior anastomotic vein (Trolard)* and the *inferior anastomotic vein (Labbé)*, which connect the superficial middle cerebral vein, respectively, with tributaries of the superior sagittal and the transverse sinuses.

On the inferior surface, the small inferior cerebral veins, arising from extensive pial plexuses, drain in part into the basal sinuses. Those from the tentorial surface of the hemisphere empty into the transverse and superior petrosal sinuses (Figs. 20-4 and 20-21). Veins from the anterior temporal lobe and from the interpeduncular regions drain partly into the cavernous and sphenoparietal sinuses, while some veins from the orbital region join the superior or the inferior sagittal sinus.

In addition, large cortical areas, especially on the inferior and medial surfaces of the brain, are drained by a number of vessels which empty into the great cerebral vein (Figs. 20-23 and 20-24). These are anastomotic veins which connect the superficial and deep venous systems. The more important ones include the occipital vein, the basal vein (Rosenthal) and the posterior callosal vein. Veins of this group are best considered in relation to the deep cerebral veins.

Deep Cerebral Veins. The deep cerebral veins of major importance are: (a) the internal cerebral veins, (b) the basal vein (Rosenthal), and (c) the great cerebral vein (Galen).

The *internal cerebral veins* consist of two paired veins, situated just lateral to the midline in the tela chloroidea of the roof of the third ventricle (velum interpositum; Figs. 20-23 and 20-24). The veins begin in the region of the interventricular foramina and extend caudally over the superior and medial surface of the thalamus. Caudally the veins enter the upper part of the quadrigeminal cistern where they join to form the great vein (Galen). Veins draining into the internal cerebral vein on each side include: (a) the thalamostriate vein (terminal vein), (b) the choroidal vein, (c) the septal vein, (d) the epithalamic vein, and (e) the lateral ventricular vein (Fig. 20-23).

The *thalamostriate vein* runs forward in the terminal sulcus at the junction of the thalamus and caudate nucleus. This vein receives the *anterior terminal vein* which drains the ventricular surface of the head of the caudate nucleus. Numerous *transverse caudate veins* join the thalamostriate throughout its course (Figs. 20-23 and 20-24). Distally the transverse caudate veins extend over the caudate nucleus to the lateral angle of the ventricle where they enter the adjacent white matter. In this area the smaller tributaries form the *longitudinal caudate veins* (Fig. 20-24). The latter veins divide at acute angles into a number of branches which fan out into the white matter, as a rule following the fibers of the corpus callosum (Figs. 20-24–20-26). Some of the shorter branches drain the deep capillary plexuses of the white matter. Longer branches of these veins, extending almost to the cortex, may be regarded as intracerebral anastomotic channels connecting ventricular and surface veins. In addition, the transverse and longitudinal caudate veins give rise to another group of branches known as the *superior striate veins* (Figs. 20-26 and 20-27). These veins pass ventrally through and around the caudate nucleus, perforate the internal capsule and break up into a number of smaller vessels which drain the dense capillary plexus of the len-

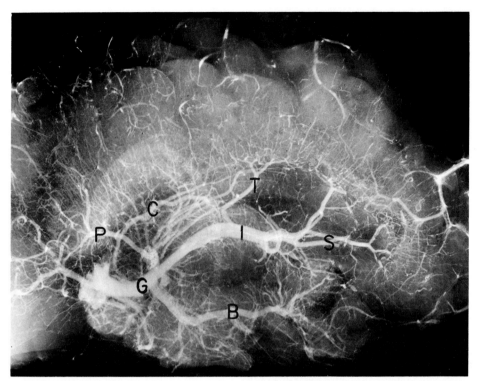

Figure 20-25.   Angiographic appearance of the deep venous system in one intact cerebral hemisphere. *Letters* indicate the following: *S*, septal vein: *T*, thalamostriate vein; *I*, internal cerebral vein; *B*, basal vein; *C*, choroidal vein; *G*, great cerebral vein (Galen); and *P*, occipital vein (vein of the posterior horn). (Courtesy of Dr. O. Hassler (1044).)

tiform nucleus (Fig. 20-26). This capillary plexus is drained from below by the *inferior striate veins* which converge upon the anterior perforated substance and enter the deep middle vein.

The *choroidal vein* runs along the lateral border of the choroid plexus and distally extends into the inferior horn of the lateral ventricle (Fig. 20-23). This tortuous vessel drains portions of the choroid plexus and adjacent hippocampal regions. The choroid plexus also is drained by the choroidal branch of the basal vein and, to a lesser extent, through the lateral ventricular vein.

The *septal vein* drains the septum pellucidum and rostral portions of the corpus callosum. Distally, branches of this vein extend beneath the head of the caudate nucleus into the medullary substance at the base of the frontal lobe (Figs 20-23 and 20-24). The septal vein joins the internal cerebral vein in the region of the interventricular foramen.

The *epithalamic vein* is a small vessel which drains the dorsal part of the diencephalon. This vein enters the internal cerebral vein, or the great cerebral vein, near their junction. Blood from ventral portions of the thalamus and from the hypothalamus is drained by vessels which pass ventrally into the pial venous plexus of the interpeduncular fossa. From this plexus venous blood is conveyed into the cavernous or sphenoparietal sinuses or into tributaries of the basal vein.

The *lateral ventricular vein* courses over the superior caudal surface of the thalamus (Fig. 20-23) and enters the internal cerebral vein as this vessel joins the great cerebral vein. Occasionally this vein terminates directly in the great cerebral vein. Distally the lateral ventricular vein extends over the surface of the thalamus and the tail of the caudate nucleus and enters the medullary substance near the angle of the lateral ventricle. Small branches of this vein arise from the choroid plexus and from the white matter of the parahippocampal gyrus.

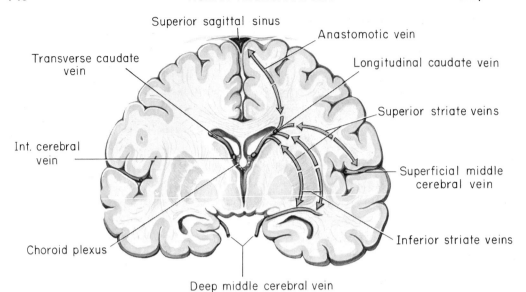

Figure 20-26. Transverse section through the brain of the rhesus monkey, showing diagrammatically the connections between deep and superficial veins. (Modified from Schlesinger (2282).)

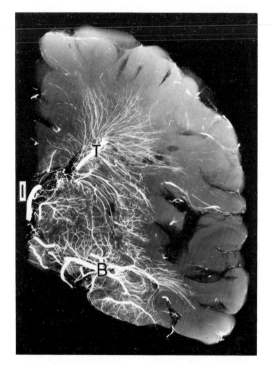

Figure 20-27. Angioarchitecture of the deep cerebral venous system as shown in a 1-cm-thick coronal section. Anastomoses between deep and superficial veins are evident. *Letters* indicate the following: *T*, terminal vein; *B*, basal vein; *I*, internal cerebral vein. Compare with Figure 20-26. (Courtesy of Dr. O. Hassler (1044).)

The *great cerebral vein* (Galen) receives the two internal cerebral veins, the two basal veins, the two occipital veins and the posterior callosal vein (Figs. 20-23–20-25). This very short vein extends posteriorly beneath the splenium of the corpus callosum and empties into the anterior part of the rectus sinus. The walls of this vein are delicate and easily torn, even in the adult.

The *basal vein* (Rosenthal) arises near the medial aspect of the anterior part of the temporal lobe where it receives tributaries from the medial surface and temporal horn (Figs. 20-24 and 20-25). This vein receives the anterior cerebral vein, the deep middle cerebral vein and the inferior striate veins. The *anterior cerebral vein* accompanies the anterior cerebral artery and drains the orbital surface of the frontal lobe, anterior portions of the corpus callosum and rostral parts of the cingulate gyrus. The *deep middle cerebral vein*, situated inferiorly in the depths of the lateral sulcus, drains insular and adjacent opercular cortex. The *inferior striate veins* drain ventral portions of the corpus striatum, emerge through the anterior perforated substance and empty into the deep middle cerebral vein (Figs. 20-25–20-27). In the region of the anterior perforated substance these veins unite with the basal vein which courses caudally around the crus cerebri to join the great cerebral vein. The basal vein receives additional tributaries from the interpeduncular region, the midbrain and the inferior horn of the lateral ventricle. The hypothalamus and ventral portions of the thalamus also are drained by the basal veins.

The *occipital vein*, which drains the inferior and medial surface of the occipital lobe and adjacent parietal regions, empties directly into the great cerebral vein (Fig. 20-23). The posterior callosal vein, which extends around the splenium of the corpus callosum, enters the anterior part of the great cerebral vein. This vein drains the posterior part of the corpus callosum and adjacent medial surfaces of the brain.

Angiographic studies (2520) of cerebral veins made by serial roentgenograms reveal that the superficial frontal veins fill slightly before the parietal veins. The deep veins usually are the last to fill, and they retain sufficient concentrations of radiopaque material to be visualized for a longer time. From the standpoint of diagnostic radiology, the deep cerebral veins are more important than the superficial veins which exhibit extremely variable configurations. Visualization of the thalamostriate vein and some of its major tributaries can provide information concerning the position and size of the lateral ventricle.

The deep veins are concerned primarily with the drainage of the ventricular surface, the choroid plexuses, the deep medullary substance, the caudate nucleus and the dorsal portions of the lentiform nucleus and thalamus. All these structures also can be drained by surface vessels through numerous intracerebral and extracerebral anastomotic veins.

Bibliography

1. ABELES, M., AND GOLDSTEIN, M. H., JR. 1970. Functional architecture in cat primary auditory cortex: Columnar organization and organization according to depth. J.Neurophysiol., **33**: 172–187.
2. ABERCROMBIE, M., AND JOHNSON, M. L. 1947. The effect of reinnervation on collagen formation in degenerating sciatic nerves of rabbits. J. Neurol. Neurosurg. Psychiatry, **10**: 89–92.
3. ACHESON, A. L., ZIGMOND, M. J., AND STRICKER, M. 1980. Compensatory increase in tyrosine hydroxylase activity in rat brain after intraventricular injections of 6-hydroxydopamine. Science **207**: 537–540.
4. ADAL, M. N., AND BARKER, D. 1965. Intramuscular branching of fusimotor fibres. J. Physiol. (Lond.), **177**: 288–299.
5. ADAMS, C. W. M. 1965. Disorders of neurons and neuroglia. In C. W. M. ADAMS (Editor), *Neurohistochemistry.* Elsevier Publishing Company, Amsterdam, Ch. 10, pp. 403–436. (See also, Ch. 1–8, pp. 1–332.)
6. ADAMS, C. W. M., IBRAHIM, M. Z. M., AND LEIBOWITZ, S. 1965. Demyelination, In C. W. M. ADAMS (Editor), *Neurohistochemistry.* Elsevier Publishing Company, Amsterdam, Ch. 11, pp. 437–487.
7. ADAMS, J. C. 1979. Ascending projections to the inferior colliculus. J. Comp. Neurol., **183**: 519–538.
8. ADDISON, W. H. F. 1915. On the rhinencephalon of *Delphinus delphis.* J. Comp. Neurol., **25**: 497–522.
9. ADES, H. W. 1943. A secondary acoustic area in the cerebral cortex of the cat. J. Neurophysiol., **6**: 59–64.
10. ADES, H. W. 1959. Central auditory mechanisms. In J. FIELD (Editor), *Handbook of Physiology*, Section I, Vol. I. American Physiol Society, Washington, D. C., Ch. 24, pp. 585–613.
11. ADES, H. W., AND BROOKHART, J. M. 1950. The central auditory pathway. J. Neurophysiol., **13**: 189–205.
12. ADEY, W. R., AND MEYER, M. 1952. Hippocampal and hypothalamic connexions of the temporal lobe in the monkey. Brain, **75**: 358–384.
13. ADEY, W. R., SEGUNDO, J. P., AND LIVINGSTON, R. B. 1957. Corticofugal influences on intrinsic brain stem conduction in cat and monkey. J. Neurophysiol., **20**: 1–16.
14. ADINOLFI, A. M., AND PAPPAS, G. D. 1968. The fine stucture of the caudate nucleus of the cat. J. Comp. Neurol., **133**: 167–184.
15. ADRIAN, E. D. 1931. The messages in sensory nerve fibres and their interpretation. Proc. R. Soc. B, **109**: 1–18.
16. ADRIAN, E. D. 1940. Double representation of the feet in the sensory cortex of the cat. J. Physiol. (Lond.), **98**: 16P–18P (abstract).
17. ADRIAN, E. D. 1941. Afferent discharges to the cerebral cortex from peripheral sense organs. J. Physiol. (Lond.), **100**: 159–191.
18. ADRIAN, E. D. 1942. Olfactory reactions in the brain of the hedgehog. J. Physiol. (Lond.), **100**: 459–473.
19. ADRIAN, E. D. 1943. Afferent areas in the cerebellum connected with the limbs. Brain, **66**: 289–315.
20. AFIFI, A., AND KAELBER, W. W. 1965. Efferent connections of the substantia nigra in the cat. Exp. Neurol., **11**: 474–482.
21. AGHAJANIAN, G. K., FOOTE, W. E., AND SHEARD, M. H. 1968. Lysergic acid diethylamide: Sensitive neuronal units in the midbrain raphe. Science, **161**: 706–708.
22. AGHAJANIAN, G. K., HAIGLER, H. J., AND BENNETT, J. L. 1975. Amine receptors in the CNS. III. 5-Hydroxytryptamine in brain. In L. L. IVERSON, S. D. IVERSON, AND S. H. SNYDER (Editors), *Handbook of Psychopharmacology*, Ed. 6. Plenum Press, New York, pp. 63–96
23. AHLQUIST, R. P. 1948. A study of the adrenotropic receptors. Am. J. Physiol.,**153**: 586–600.
24. AITKEN, H. F. 1909. A report on the circulation of the lobar ganglia made to Dr. James B. Ayer (with a postscript by J. B. Ayer, M.D.). Boston Med. Surg. J., **160**: Suppl. 18.
25. AITKIN, L. M. AND WEBSTER, W. R. 1971. Tonotopic organization in the medial geniculate body of the cat. Brain Res., **26**: 402–405.
26. AITKIN, L. M., AND WEBSTER, W. R. 1972. Medial geniculate body of the cat: Organization and responses to tonal stimuli of neurons in the ventral division. J. Neurophysiol., **35**: 365–380.
27. AITKIN, L. M., WEBSTER, W. R., VEALE, J. L., AND CROSBY, D. C. 1975. Inferior colliculus. I. Comparison of response properties of neurons in central, pericentral and external nuclei of adult cat. J. Neurophysiol., **38**: 1196–1207.
28. AKAIKE, T., FANARDJIAN, V. V., ITO, M., AND OHNO, T. 1973. Electrophysiological analysis of vestibulospinal reflex pathways of rabbit. II. Synaptic actions upon spinal neurones. Exp. Brain Res., **17**: 497–515.
29. AKELAITIS, A. J. 1943. Study of language function (tactile and visual lexia and graphia) unilaterally following section of the corpus callosum. J. Neuropathol. Exp. Neurol., **2**: 226–262.
30. AKELAITIS, A. J., RISTEEN, W. A., HERREN, R. Y., AND VAN WAGENEN, W. P. 1942. Studies on corpus callosum: Contribution to study of dyspraxia and apraxia following partial and complete section of corpus callosum. Arch. Neurol. Psychiatry, **47**: 971–1008.
31. AKERT, K., AND HARTMANN-VON MONAKOW, K. 1980. Relationships of precentral, premotor and prefrontal cortex to the mediodorsal and intralaminar nuclei of the monkey, thalamus. Acta Neurobiol. Exp. (Warsz.), **40**: 7–25.
32. AKERT, K., POTTER, H. D., AND ANDERSON, J. W. 1961. The subfornical organ in mammals. I. Comparative and topographical anatomy. J. Comp. Neurol., **116**: 1–14.
33. ALBE-FESSARD, D., AND KRUGER, L. 1962. Duality of unit discharge from cat centrum medianum in response to natural and electrical stimulation. J. Neurophysiol., **25**: 3–20.
34. ALBE-FESSARD, D., LEVANTE, A., AND LAMOUR, Y. 1974. Origin of spinothalamic tract in monkeys. Brain Res., **65**: 503–509.
35. ALBE-FESSARD, D., AND ROUGEUL, A. 1958. Activités d'origine somesthésique évoquées sur le cortex nonspécifique du chat anesthésié au chloralose: Rôle du centre médian du thalamus. Electroencephalogr. Clin.

Neurophysiol., **10:** 131–152.

36. ALEXANDER, L. 1942. The vascular supply of the striopallidum. Proc. Assoc. Res. Nerv. Ment. Dis., **21:** 77–132.

37. ALLEN, G. I., KORN, H., OSHIMA, T., AND TOYAMA, K. 1975. The mode of synaptic linkage in the cerebroponto-cerebellar pathway of the cat. II. Responses of single cells in the pontine nuclei. Exp. Brain Res., **24:** 15–36.

38. ALLEN, W. F. 1919. Application of the Marchi method to the study of the radix mesencephalica trigemini in the guinea pig. J. Comp. Neurol., **30:** 169–216.

39. ALLEN, W. F. 1925. Identification of the cells and fibers concerned in the innervation of the teeth. J. Comp. Neurol., **39:** 325–343.

40. ALLEN, W. F. 1927. Experimental-anatomical studies on the visceral bulbospinal pathway in the cat and guinea pig. J. Comp. Neurol., **42:** 393–456.

41. ALLEN, W. F. 1940. Effects of ablating the frontal lobes, hippocampi, and occipito-parieto-temporal (excepting pyriform areas) lobes on positive and negative olfactory conditioned reflexes. Am. J. Physiol., **128:** 754–771.

42. ALLEN, W. F. 1941. Effect of ablating the pyriform-amygdaloid areas and hippocampi on positive and negative olfactory conditioned reflexes and on conditioned olfactory differentiation. Am. J. Physiol., **132:** 81–92.

43. ALLEY, K. R., BAKER, R., AND SIMPSON, J. I. 1975. Afferents to the vestibulocerebellum and the origin of the visual climbing fibers in the rabbit. Brain Res., **98:** 582–589.

44. ALLISON, A. C. 1953. The morphology of the olfactory system in the vertebrates. Biol. Rev., **28:** 195–244.

45. ALLISON, A. C. 1954. The secondary olfactory areas in the human brain. J. Anat., **88:** 481–488.

46. ALLISON, A. C., AND WARWICK, R. 1949. Quantitative observations on the olfactory system of the rabbit. Brain, **72:** 186–197.

47. ALLMAN, J. M. 1977. Evolution of the visual system in the early primates. In J. M. SPRAGUE AND A. EPSTEIN (Editors), *Progress in Physiological Psychology*, Vol. 7. Academic Press, New York, pp. 1–53.

48. ALLMAN, J. M., AND KAAS, J. H. 1974. The organization of the second visual area (VII) in the owl monkey: A second order transformation of the visual hemifield. Brain Res., **76:** 247–265.

49. ALPHEN, H. A. W. VAN. 1969. The anterior commissure of the rabbit. Acta anat. (Basel), **74:** Suppl. 57, 9–111.

50. ALTMAN, J. 1966. Proliferation and migration of undifferentiated precursor cells in the rat during postnatal gliogenesis. Exp. Neurol., **16:** 263–278.

51. ALTMAN, J., AND CARPENTER, M. B. 1961. Fiber projections of the superior colliculus in the cat. J. Comp. Neurol., **116:** 157–178.

52. AMBROGI, L. P. 1960. *Manual of Histologic and Special Staining Technics*, Ed. 2. McGraw-Hill Book Company, Inc., New York, pp. 157–174.

53. AMOORE, J. E., JOHNSTON, J. W., JR., AND RUBIN, M. 1964. The stereochemical theory of odor. Sci. Am., **210:** 42–49.

54. AMOROSO, E. C., BELL, F. R., AND ROSENBERG, H. 1954. The relationship of the vasomotor and respiratory regions in the medulla oblongata of the sheep. J. Physiol. (Lond.), **126:** 86–95.

55. ANAND, B. K., AND BROBECK, J. R. 1951. Hypothalamic control of food intake in rats and cats. Yale J. Biol. Med., **24:** 123–140.

56. ANAND, B. K., AND BROBECK, J. R. 1951a. Localization of a "feeding center" in the hypothalamus of the rat. Proc. Soc. Exp. Biol. Med., **77:** 323–324.

57. ANAND, B. K., AND BROBECK, J. R. 1952. Food intake and spontaneous activity of rats with lesions in the amygdaloid nuclei. J. Neurophysiol., **15:** 421–430.

58. ANAND, B. K., AND DUA, S. 1956. Circulatory and respiratory changes induced by electrical stimulation of limbic system (visceral brain). J. Neurophysiol., **19:**

393–400.

59. ANDÉN, N.-E., CARLSSON, A., DAHLSTRÖM, A., FUXE, K., HILLARP, N.-Å., AND LARSSON, K. 1964. Demonstration and mapping out of nigro-neostriatal dopamine neurons. Life Sci., **3:** 523–530.

60. ANDÉN, N.-E., DAHLSTRÖM, A., FUXE, K., LARSSON, K., OLSON, L., AND UNGERSTEDT, U. 1966. Ascending monoamine neurons to the telencephalon and diencephalon. Acta Physiol. Scand., **67:** 313–326.

61. ANDERSON, M. E., AND YOSHIDA, M. 1977. Electrophysiological evidence for branching nigral projections to the thalamus and the superior colliculus. Brain Res., **137:** 361–364.

62. ANDERSON, M. E., AND YOSHIDA, M. 1980. Axonal branching patterns and location of nigrothalamic and nigrocollicular neurons in the cat. J. Neurophysiol., **43:** 883–895.

63. ANDERSSON, B. 1957. Polydipsia, antidiuresis and milk ejection caused by hypothalamic stimulation. In H. HELLER (Editor), *Neurohypophysis*. Butterworths Scientific Publications, London, pp. 131–140.

64. ANDERSSON, B., AND JEWELL, P. A. 1957. Studies on the thalamic relay for taste in the goat. J. Physiol. (Lond.), **139:** 191–197.

65. ANDERSSON, S. 1962. Projection of different spinal pathways to the second somatic sensory area in cat. Acta Physiol. Scand., **56:** Suppl. 194, 1–74.

66. ANDREW, J., AND NATHAN, P. W. 1964. Lesions of the anterior frontal lobes and disturbances of micturition and defecation. Brain, **87:** 233–262.

67. ANDY, O. J., AND BROWN, J. S. 1960. Diencephalic coagulation in the treatment of hemiballismus. Surg. Forum Clin. Cong. Am. Coll. Surgeons, **10:** 795–799.

68. ANGAUT, P. 1969. The fastigio-tectal projections: An anatomical experimental study. Brain Res., **13:** 186–189.

69. ANGAUT, P. 1970. The ascending projections of the nucleus interpositus posterior of the cat cerebellum: An experimental anatomical study using silver impregnation methods. Brain Res., **24:** 377–394.

70. ANGAUT, P., AND BOWSHER, D. 1965. Cerebello-rubral connexions in the cat. Nature, **208:** 1002–1003.

71. ANGAUT, P., AND BOWSHER, D. 1970. Ascending projections of the medial (fastigial) nucleus: An experimental study in the cat. Brain Res., **24:** 49–68.

72. ANGAUT, P., AND BRODAL, A. 1967. The projection of the "vestibulocerebellum" onto the vestibular nuclei in the cat. Arch. Ital. Biol., **105:** 441–479.

73. ANGELETTI, P. U., ANGELETTI, R. H., FRAZIER, W. A., AND BRADSHAW, R. A. 1973. Nerve growth factor. In D. J. SCHNEIDER, R. H. ANGELETTI, R. A. BRADSHAW, A. GRASSO and B. W. MOORE (Editors), *Proteins of the Nervous System*. Raven Press, New York, pp. 133–154.

74. ANGEVINE, J. B. JR. 1965. Time of neuron origin in the hippocampal region: An autoradiographic study in the mouse. Exp. Neurol., **2:** (suppl), 1–70.

75. ANGEVINE, J. B., JR., LOCKE, S., AND YAKOVLEV, P. I. 1962. Limbic nuclei of thalamus and connections of limbic cortex. IV. Thalamocortical projection of the ventral anterior nucleus in man. Arch. Neurol., **7:** 518–528.

76. ANGEVINE, J. B., JR., MANCALL, E. L., AND YAKOVLEV, P. I. 1961. *The Human Cerebellum. An Atlas of Gross Topography in Serial Sections*. Little, Brown & Company, Boston., 137 pp.

77. ANGEVINE, J. B., JR., AND SIDMAN, R. L. 1961. Autoradiographic study of cell migration during histogenesis of the cerebral cortex in the mouse. Nature, **192:** 766–768.

78. ANTONETTY, C. M., AND WEBSTER, K. E. 1975. The organisation of the spinotectal projection: An experimental study in the cat. J. Comp. Neurol., **163:** 449–465.

79. APPELBERG, B. 1960. Localization of focal potentials evoked in the red nucleus and ventrolateral nucleus of the thalamus by electrical stimulation of the cerebellar nuclei. Acta Physiol. Scand., **51:** 356–370.

80. APTER, J. T. 1946. Eye movements following strychninization of the superior colliculus of cats. J. Neuro-

physiol., **9:** 73–86.

81. ARDUINI, A., AND ARDUINI, M. G. 1954. Effect of drugs and metabolic alterations on brain stem arousal mechanisms. J. Pharmacol. Exp. Ther., **110:** 76–85.

82. AREY, L. B. 1938. The history of the first somite in human embryos. Carnegie Inst. Washington, Contrib. Embryol., **27:** 233–269.

83. ARIËNS KAPPERS, J. 1971. The pineal organ: An introduction. In G. E. W. WOLSTENHOLME and J. KNIGHT (Editors), *The Pineal Gland.* Churchill Livingston, Edinburgh, pp. 1–23.

84. ARIMATSU, Y., SETO, A. AND AMANO, T. 1981. An atlas of α-bungarotoxin binding sites and structures containing acetylcholinesterase in the mouse central nervous system. J. Comp. Neurol., **198:** 603–631.

85. ARMSTRONG, D. M., AND SCHILD, R. F. 1979. Spinoolivary neurons in the lumbo-sacral cord of the cat demonstrated by retrograde transport of horseradish peroxidase. Brain Res., **168:** 176–179.

86. ARONSON, L. R., AND COOPER, M. L. 1979. Amygdaloid hypersexuality in male cats reexamined. Physiol. Behav., **22:** 257–265.

87. ARONSON, L. R., AND PAPEZ, J. W. 1934. Thalamic nuclei of *Pithecus (Macacus) rhesus.* II. Dorsal thalamus. Arch. Neurol. Psychiatry, **32:** 27–44.

88. ASANUMA, H., AND SAKATA, H. 1967. Functional organization of a cortical efferent system examined with focal depth stimulation in cats. J. Neurophysiol., **30:** 35–54.

89. ÅSTRÖM, K. E. 1967. On the early development of the cortex in fetal sheep. In C. G. BERNHARD and J. P. SCHADÉ (Editors), *Developmental Neurology, Progress in Brain Research,* Vol. 26. Elsevier Publishing Company, New York, pp. 1–59.

90. ASTRUC, J. 1971. Corticofugal connections of area 8 (frontal eye field) in *Macaca mulatta.* Brain Res., **33:** 241–256.

91. ATWEH, S. F., AND KUHAR, M. J. 1977. Autoradiographic localization of opiate receptors in rat brain. I. Spinal cord and lower medulla. Brain Res., **124:** 53–67.

92. AUER, J. 1956. Terminal degeneration in the diencephalon after ablation of frontal cortex in the cat. J. Anat., **90:** 30–41.

93. AXELROD, J., WURTMAN, R. J., AND SNYDER, S. H. 1965. Control of hydroxyindole-o-methyl transferase activity in the rat pineal gland by environmental lighting. J. Biol. Chem., **240:** 949–955.

94. BABKIN, B. P. 1950. Significance of the double innervation of the salivary glands. In B. P. BABKIN (Editor), *Secretory Mechanism of the Digestive Glands,* Ed. 2. P. B. Hoeber Company, New York, Ch. 27, pp. 733–766.

95. BACSIK, R. D., AND STROMINGER, N. L. 1973. The cytoarchitecture of the human anteroventral cochlear nucleus. J. Comp. Neurol., **147:** 281–290.

96. BAGSHAW, M. H., AND PRIBRAM, K. H. 1953. Cortical organization in gustation (*Macaca mulatta*). J. Neurophysiol., **275 16:** 499–508.

97. BAILEY, P. 1948. *Intracranial Tumors,* Ed. 2. Charles C Thomas, Publisher, Springfield, Ill., p. 212.

98. BAILEY, P., AND VON BONIN, G. 1951. *The Isocortex of Man.* University of Illinois Press, Urbana, 301 pp.

98a. BAILEY, P., VON BONIN, G., GAROL, H. W., AND McCULLOCH, W. S. 1943. Functional organization of temporal lobe of monkey (*Macaca mulatta* and chimpanzee (*Pan satyrus*). J. Neurophysiol., **6:** 121–128.

99. BAILEY, P., GAROL, H. W., AND McCULLOCH, W. S. 1941. Cortical origin and distribution of corpus callosum and anterior commissure in the chimpanzee (*Pan satyrus*). J. Neurophysiol., **4:** 564–571.

100. BAK, I. J. 1967. The ultrastructure of the substantia nigra and caudate nucleus of the mouse and the cellular localization of catecholamines. Exp. Brain Res., **3:** 40–57.

101. BAK, I. J., CHOI, W. B., HASSLER, R., USUNOFF, K. G., AND WAGNER, A. 1975. Fine structural synaptic organization of the corpus striatum and substantia nigra in rat and cat. In C. CAINE, T. N. CHASE, AND A. BARBEAU (Editors), *Dopamine Mechanisms, Advances in Neurology,* Vol. 9. Raven Press, New York, pp. 15–41.

102. BAKAY, L. 1952. Studies of blood-brain barrier with radioactive phosphorus. Arch. Neurol. Psychiatry, **68:** 629–640.

103. BAKAY, L. 1953. Studies on blood-brain barrier with radioactive phosphorus. III. Embryonic development of the barrier. Arch. Neurol. Psychiatry, **70:** 30–39.

104. BAKER, A. B. 1961. Cerebrovascular disease. IX. The medullary blood supply and the lateral medullary syndrome. Neurology (Minneap.), **11:** 852–861.

105. BAKER, J. R. 1960. *Cytological Technique. Methuen's Monographs on Biological Subjects.* John Wiley and Sons, New York.

106. BAKER, R. 1977. Anatomical and physiological organization of brain stem pathways underlying the control of gaze. In R. BAKER AND A. BERTHOZ (Editors) *Control of Gaze by Brain Stem Neurons: Developments in Neuroscience,* Vol. 1. Biomedical Press, Amsterdam, pp. 207–222.

107. BAKER, R., AND HIGHSTEIN, S. M. 1975. Physiological identification of interneurons and motoneurons in the abducens nucleus. Brain Res., **91:** 292–298.

108. BALCOM, G. J., LENNOX, R. H., AND MEYERHOFF, J. L. 1975. Regional δ-aminobutyric acid levels in rat brain determined by microwave fixation. J. Neurochem., **24:** 609–613.

109. BAPTISTA, A. P. 1963. Studies on the arteries of the brain. II. The anterior cerebral artery: Some anatomic features and their clinical implication. Neurology (Minneap.), **13:** 825–835.

110. BÁRÁNY, E. H. 1972. Inhibition of hippurate and probenecid of *in vitro* uptake of iodipamide and o-iodohyppurate: A composite uptake system for iodipamide in choroid plexus, kidney cortex and anterior uvea of several species. Acta Physiol. Scand., **86:** 12–27.

111. BARD, P. 1939. Central nervous mechanisms for emotional behavior patterns in animals. Proc. Assoc. Res. Nerv. Ment. Dis., **19:** 190–218.

112. BARD, P. 1963. Regulation of the systemic circulation. In V. B. MOUNTCASTLE (Editor), *Medical Physiology,* Ed. 12, Vol. I. C. V. Mosby Company, St. Louis, Ch. 11, pp. 178–208.

113. BARD, P., AND MOUNTCASTLE, V. B. 1948. Some forebrain mechanisms involved in expression of rage with special reference to suppression of angry behavior. Proc. Assoc. Res. Nerv. Ment. Dis., **27:** 362–404.

114. BARD, P., AND RIOCH, D. M. 1937. A study of 4 cats deprived of neocortex and additional portions of the forebrain. Bull. Johns Hopkins Hosp., **60:** 73–147.

115. BARGMANN, W. 1966. Neurosecretion. Int. Rev. Cytol., **19:** 183–201.

116. BARGMANN, W., HILD, W., ORTHMANN, R., AND SCHIEBLER, T. H. 1950. Morphologische und experimentelle Untersuchungen über das hypothalamischhypophysäre System. Acta neuroveg., I: 233–275.

117. BARKER, D. 1948. The innervation of the musclespindle. Q. J. Microscop. Sci., **89:** 143–186.

118. BARKER, D. 1967. The innervation of mammalian skeletal muscle. In A. V. S. DE REUCK AND J. KNIGHT (Editors), *Myotatic, Kinesthetic and Vestibular Mechanisms.* Little, Brown and Company, Boston, pp. 3–15.

119. BARKER, D., AND COPE, M. 1962. The innervation of individual intrafusal muscle fibres. In D. BARKER (Editor), *Symposium on Muscle Receptors.* Hong Kong University Press, Hong Kong, pp. 263–269.

120. BARKER, S. H., AND GELLHORN, E. 1947. Influence of suppressor areas on afferent impulses. J. Neurophysiol., **10:** 133–138.

121. BARNES, S. 1901. Degenerations in hemiplegia: With special reference to a ventrolateral pyramidal tract, the accessory fillet and Pick's bundle. Brain, **24:** 463–501.

122. BARNES, W. T., MAGOUN, H. W., AND RANSON, S. W. 1943. The ascending auditory pathway in the

brain stem of the monkey. J. Comp. Neurol., **79:** 129–152.

123. BARR, M. L. 1939. Some observations on the morphology of the synapse in the cat's spinal cord. J. Anat., **74:** 1–11.

124. BARR, M. L., BERTRAM, L. F., AND LINDSAY, H. A. 1950. The morphology of the nerve cell nucleus according to sex. Anat. Rec., **107:** 283–297.

125. BARRINGTON, F. J. F. 1921. The relation of the hind brain to micturition. Brain, **44:** 23–53.

126. BARTON, A. A., AND CAUSEY, G. 1958. Electron microscopic study of the superior cervical ganglion. J. Anat., **92:** 399–407.

127. BASBAUM, A. I. 1976. Opiate and stimulus-produced analgesia: Functional anatomy of a medullospinal pathway. Proc. Natl. Acad. Sci. U. S. A., **73:** 4685–4688.

128. BASBAUM, A. I., CLANTON, C. H., AND FIELDS, H. L. 1976. Opiate and stimulus-produced analgesia: Functional anatomy of medullospinal pathways. Proc. Natl. Acad. Sci. U. S. A., **73:** 4685–4688.

129. BASBAUM, A. I. CLANTON, C. H., AND FIELDS, H. L. 1978. Three bulbospinal pathways from the rostral medulla of the cat: An autoradiographic study of pain modulating systems. J. Comp. Neurol., **178:** 209–224.

130. BASBAUM, A. I., AND FIELDS, H. L. 1979. The origin of descending pathways in the dorsolateral funiculus of the spinal cord of the cat and rat: Further studies on the anatomy of pain modulation. J. Comp. Neurol., **187:** 513–532.

131. BATES, J. A. V. 1953. Stimulation of the medial surface of the human cerebral hemisphere after hemispherectomy. Brain, **76:** 405–447.

132. BATINI, C., CORVISIER, J., DESTOMBES, J., GIOANNI, H., AND EVERETT, J. 1976. The climbing fibers of the cerebellar cortex, their origin and pathway in cat. Exp. Brain Res., **26:** 407–422.

133. BATSON, O. V. 1940. The function of the vertebral veins and their role in the spread of metastases. Ann. Surg., **112:** 138–149.

134. BATTON, R. R., III, AND CARPENTER, M. B. 1978. Central projections of the vestibulocochlear nerve in the monkey: An autoradiographic study. Anat. Rec., **190:** 334.

135. BATTON, R. R., III, JAYARAMAN, A., RUGGIERO, D., AND CARPENTER, M. B. 1977. Fastigial efferent projections in the monkey: an autoradiographic study. J. Comp. Neurol., **174:** 281–306.

136. BEALL, J. E., MARTIN, R. F., APPLEBAUM, A. E., AND WILLIS, W. D. 1976. Inhibition of primate spinothalamic tract neurons by stimulation of the nucleus raphe magnus. Brain Res., **114:** 328–333.

137. VON BECHTEREW, W. V. 1900. Demonstration eines Gehirns mit Zerstörung der vorderen und inneren Theile der Hirnrinde beider Schläfenlappen. Neurol. Zentralbl., **19:** 990–991.

138. BECK, E. 1929. Die myeloarchitektonische Felderung des in der Sylvischen Furche gelegenen Teiles des menschlichen Schläfenlappens. J. Phychol. Neurol., **36:** 1–21.

139. BECK, E. 1950. The origin, course and termination of the prefronto-pontine tract in the human brain. Brain, **73:** 368–391.

140. BECKSTEAD, R. M., DOMESICK, V. B., AND NAUTA, W. J. H. 1979. Efferent connections of the substantia nigra and ventral tegmental area in the rat. Brain Res., **175:** 191–217.

141. BECKSTEAD, R. M., MORSE, J. R., AND NORGREN, R. 1980. The nucleus of the solitary tract in the monkey: Projections to the thalamus and brain stem nuclei. J. Comp. Neurol., **190:** 259–282.

142. BECKSTEAD, R. M., AND NORGREN, R. 1979. An autoradiographic examination of the central distribution of the trigeminal, facial, glossopharyngeal and vagal nerves in the monkey. J. Comp. Neurol., **184:** 455–472.

143. BÉDARD, P., LAROCHELLE, L., PARENT, A., AND POIRIER, L. J. 1969. The nigrostriatal pathway: A correlative study based on neuroanatomical and neurochemical criteria in the cat and monkey. Exp. Neurol., **25:** 365–377.

144. BEHNSEN, G. 1926. Farbstoffversuche mit Trypanblau an der Schranke zwischen Blut und Zentralnervensystem der washsenden Maus. Munch. Med. Wochenschr., **73:** 1143–1147.

145. Behnsen, G. 1927. Ueber die Farbstoffspeicherung im Zentralnervensystem der weissen Maus in verschiedenen Alterszuständen. Z. Zellforsch. Mikrosk. Anat., **4:** 515–572.

146. BÉKÉSY, G. VON. 1960. *Experiments in Hearing.* McGraw-Hill Book Company, New York.

147. BELL, C. C., AND DOW, R. S. 1967. Cerebellar circuitry. Neurosci. Res. Program Bull., **5:** (no. 2) 121–222.

148. BEN-ARI, Y., LE GAL LA SALLE, G., AND KANAZAWA, I. 1977. Regional distribution of substance P within the amygdaloid complex and bed nucleus of the stria terminalis. *Neurosci. Lett.,* **4:** 299–302.

149. BEN-ARI, Y., ZIGMOND, R. E., SHUTE, C. C. D., AND LEWIS, P. R. 1977. Regional distribution of choline acetyltransferase and acetylcholinesterase within the amygdaloid complex and stria terminalis system. Brain Res., **120:** 435–445.

150. BENDA, C. E., AND COBB, S. 1942. On the pathogenesis of paralysis agitans (Parkinson's disease). Medicine, **21:** 95–142.

151. BENDER, M. B., AND SHANZER, S. 1964. Oculomotor pathways defined by electrical stimulation and lesions in the brain stem of the monkey. In M. B. BENDER (Editor), *The Oculomotor System.* Harper and Row, New York, pp. 81–140.

152. BENDER, M. B., AND WEINSTEIN, E. A. 1944. Effects of stimulation and lesion of the median longitudinal fasciculus in the monkey. Arch. Neurol. & Psychiatry, **52:** 106–113.

153. BENDER, M. B., AND WEINSTEIN, E. A. 1950. The syndrome of the median longitudinal fasciculus. Proc. Assoc. Res. Nerv. Ment. Dis., **28:** 414–420.

154. BENEVENTO, L. A., AND FALLON, J. H. 1975. The ascending projections of the superior colliculus in the rhesus monkey. (*Macaca mulatta*). J. Comp. Neurol., **160:** 339–362.

155. BENEVENTO, L. A., AND REZAK, M. 1976. The cortical projections of the inferior pulvinar and adjacent lateral pulvinar in the rhesus monkey (*Macaca mulatta*): An autoradiographic study. Brain Res., **108:** 1–24.

156. BENJAMIN, R. M. 1963. Some thalamic and cortical mechanisms of taste. In Y. ZOTTERMAN (Editor), *Olfaction and Taste.* Macmillian Company, New York, pp. 309–329.

157. BENJAMIN, R. M., AND AKERT, K. 1959. Cortical and thalamic areas involved in taste discrimination in the albino rat. J. Comp. Neurol., **111:** 231–260.

158. BENTIVOGLIO, M., VAN DER KOOY, D., AND KUYPERS, H. G. J. M. 1979. The organization of the efferent projections of the substantia nigra in the rat: A retrograde fluorescent double labeling study. Brain Res., **174:** 1–17.

159. BENTIVOGLIO, M., KUYPERS, H. G. J. M., CATSMAN-BERREVOETS, C. E., LOEWE, H., AND DANN, O. 1980. Two new fluorescent retrograde neuronal tracers which are transported over long distances. Neurosci. Lett., **18:** 25–30.

160. BERGER, H. 1929. Ueber das Elektrenkephalogramm des Menschen. Arch. Psychiatr. Nervenkr., **87:** 527–570.

161. BERGER, H. 1930. Ueber das Elektrenkephalogramm des Menschen. J. Psychol. Neurol., **40:** 160–179.

162. BERGER, T. W., AND THOMPSON, R. F. 1978. Identification of pyramidal cells as critical elements in hippocampal neuronal plasticity during learning. Proc. Natl. Acad. Sci. U. S. A., **75:** 1572–1576.

163. BERKE, J. J. 1960. The claustrum, the external capsule, and the extreme capsule of the *Macaca mulatta*. J. Comp. Neurol., 115: 297–331.

164. BERKLEY, K. J., AND HAND, P. J. 1978. Projections to the inferior olive of the cat. II. Comparisons of input from the gracile, cuneate and the spinal trigeminal nuclei. J. Comp. Neurol., 180: 253–264.

165. BERKLEY, K. J., AND WORDEN, I. G. 1978. Projections to the inferior olive of the cat. I. Comparisons of input from the dorsal column nuclei, the lateral cervical nucleus, the spino-olivary pathways, the cerebral cortex and the cerebellum. J. Comp. Neurol., 180: 237–252.

166. BERN, H. A., AND KNOWLES, F. G. W. 1966. Neurosecretion. In L. M. MARTINI AND W. F. GANONG (Editors), *Neuroendocrinology*. Academic Press, New York, Ch. 5, pp. 139–186.

167. BERNHARD, C. G. 1954. The corticospinal system. In D. NACHMANSOHN AND H. H. MERRITT (Editors), *Nerve Impulse*, Transactions of the Fifth Conference, J. Macy, Jr. Foundation, New York, pp. 95–134.

168. BERNHARD, C. G., AND BOHM, E. 1954. Cortical representation and functional significance of the cortico-motoneuronal system. Arch. Neurol. Psychiatry, 72: 473–502.

169. BERNHARD, C. G., KOLMODIN, G. M., AND MEYERSON, B. A. 1967. On the prenatal development of function and structure in the somesthetic cortex of the sheep. In C. G. BERNHARD AND J. P. SCHADÉ (Editors), *Developmental Neurology, Progress in Brain Research*, Vol. 26. Elsevier Publishing Company, New York, pp. 78–91.

170. BERNHAUT, M., GELLHORN, E., AND RASMUSSEN, A. T. 1953. Experimental contributions to problem of consciousness. J. Neurophysiol., 16: 21–35.

171. BERRY, C. M., ANDERSON, F. D. AND BROOKS, D. C. 1956. Ascending pathways of the trigeminal nerve in cat. J. Neurophysiol., 19: 144–153.

172. BERRY, C. M., KARL, R. S., AND HINSEY, J. C. 1950. Course of spinothalamic and medial lemniscal pathways in the cat and rhesus monkey. J. Neurophysiol., 13: 149–156.

173. BERTRAND, G. 1956. Spinal efferent pathways from the supplementary motor area. Brain, 79: 461–473.

174. BERTRAND, G. L., BLUNDELL, J., AND MUSELLA, R. 1965. Electrical exploration of the internal capsule and neighboring structures during stereotaxic procedures. J. Neurosurg., 22: 333–343.

175. BESSOU, P., EMONET-DÉNAND, F., AND LAPORTE, Y. 1963. Occurrence of intrafusal muscle fibre innervation by branches of slow A motor fibres in the cat. Nature, 198: 594–595.

176. VAN BEUSEKOM, G. T. 1955. *Fibre Analysis of the Anterior and Lateral Funiculi of the Cord in the Cat*. Eduard Ijdo N. V., Leiden, pp. 1–136.

177. BEVAN, S., AND STEINBACH, J. H. 1977. The distribution of α-bungarotoxin binding sites on mammalian skeletal muscle developing in vivo. J. Physiol. (Lond.), 267: 195–213.

178. BIGNAMI, A., AND DAHL, D. 1974. Astrocyte-specific protein and neuroglial differentiation: An immunofluorescence study with antibodies to the glial fibrillary acidic protein. J. Comp. Neurol., 153: 27–38.

179. BINDSLEV, N., TORMEY, J. McD., PIETRAS, R. J., AND WRIGHT, E. M. 1974. Electrically and osmotically induced changes in permeability and structure of toad urinary bladder. Biochim. Biophys. Acta, 332: 286–297.

180. BINKLEY, S. 1979. A timekeeping enzyme in the pineal gland. Science, 240: 66–71.

181. BIRD, E. D., AND IVERSEN, L. L. 1974. Huntington's chorea: Post-mortem measurements of glutamic acid decarboxylase, choline acetyltransferase and dopamine in the basal ganglia. Brain, 97: 457–472.

182. BISHOP, G. A., McCREA, R. A., LIGHTHALL, J. W., AND KITAI, S. T. 1979. An HRP and autoradiographic study of the projection from the cerebellar cortex to the nucleus interpositus anterior and nucleus interpositus posterior of the cat. J. Comp Neurol., 185: 735–756.

183. BISHOP, P. O., KOZAK, W., LEVICK, W. R., AND VAKKUR, G. J. 1962. The determination of the projection of the visual field on to the lateral geniculate nucleus in the cat. J. Physiol. (Lond.), 163: 503–539.

184. BISHOP, T. W., HEINBECKER, P., AND O'LEARY, J. L. 1933. The function of non-myelinated fibers of the dorsal roots. Am. J. Physiol., 106: 647–669.

185. BISSETTE, G., MARBERG, P., NEMEROTT, C. B., AND PRANGE, A. J. JR. 1978. Neurotensin, a biologically active peptide. Life Sci., 23: 2173–2182.

186. BJÖRKLUND, A., OWMAN, C., AND WEST, K. A. 1972. Peripheral sympathetic innervation and serotonin cells in the habenular region of the rat brain. Z. Zellforsch. Mikrosk. Anat., 127: 570–579.

187. BJÖRKLUND, A., AND SKAGERBERG, G. 1979. Evidence for a major spinal cord projection from the diencephalic A 11 dopamine cell group in the rat using transmitter-specific fluorescent retrograde tracing. Brain Res., 177: 170–175.

188. BLACKSTAD, T. W. 1956. Commissural connections of the hippocampal region in the rat, with special reference to their mode of termination. J. Comp. Neurol., 105: 417–538.

189. BLEIER, R. 1971. The relations of ependyma to neurons and capillaries in the hypothalamus: A Golgi-Cox study. J. Comp. Neurol., 142: 439–464.

190. BLESSING, W. W., AND CHALMERS, J. P. 1979. Direct projection of catecholamine (presumably dopamine) containing neurons from hypothalamus to spinal cord. Neurosci. Lett., 11: 35–40.

191. BLISS, T., AND LØMO, T. 1973. Long lasting potentiation of synaptic transmission in the dentate area of the anesthetized rabbit following stimulation of the perforant path. J. Physiol. (Lond.), 232: 331–356.

192. BLIX, M. 1884. Experimentelle Beiträge zur Lösung der Frage über die specifische Energie der Hautnerven. Z. Biol. (München), 20: 141–156.

193. BLOMQUIST, A. J., BENJAMIN, R. M., AND EMMERS, R. 1962. Thalamic localization of afferents from the tongue in squirrel monkey (*Saimiri sciureus*). J. Comp. Neurol., 118: 77–87.

194. BLOOM, F. E., AND BARRNETT, R. J. 1966. Fine structural localization of noradrenaline in vesicles of autonomic nerve endings. Nature, 210: 599–601.

195. BLOOM, F. E., BATTENBERG, E., ROSSIER, J., LING, N., AND GUILLEMIN, R. 1978. Neurons containing β endorphin in rat brain exist separately from those containing enkephalin: Immunocytochemical studies. Proc. Natl. Acad. Sci. U. S. A., 75: 1591–1595.

196. BLOOM, F. E., COSTA, E., AND SALMOIRAGHI, G. C. 1965. Anesthesia and responsiveness of individual neurons of the caudate nucleus of the cat to acetylcholine, norepinephrine and dopamine administered by microelectrophoresis. J. Pharmacol. Exp. Ther., 150: 244–252.

197. BLOOM, F. E., HOFFER, B. J., AND SIGGINS, G. R. 1971. Studies on norepinephrine-containing afferents to Purkinje cells of rat cerebellum. I. Localization of the fibers and their synapses. Brain Res., 25: 501–521.

198. BLUM, M., WALKER, A. E., AND RUCH, T. C. 1943. Localization of taste in the thalamus of *Macaca mulatta*. Yale J. Biol. Med., 16: 175–192.

199. BLUM, P. S., DAY, M. J., CARPENTER, M. B., AND GILMAN, S. 1979. Thalamic components of the ascending vestibular system. Exp. Neurol., 64: 587–603.

200. BLUNT, J. J., WENDELL-SMITH, C. P., PAISLEY, P. B. AND BALDWIN, F. 1967. Oxidative enzyme activity in macroglia and axons of cat optic nerve. J. Anat., 101: 13–26.

201. BOBILLIER, P., PETITJEAN, F., SALVERT, D., LIGIER, M., AND SEGUIN, S. 1975. Differential projections of the nucleus raphe dorsalis and nucleus raphe centralis as

revealed by autoradiography. Brain Res., **85:** 205–210.

202. BOBILLIER, P., SEGUIN, S., PETITJEAN, F., SALVERT, D., TOURET, M., AND JOUVET, M. 1976. The raphe nuclei of the cat brain stem: A topographical atlas of their efferent projections as revealed by autoradiography. Brain Res., **113:** 449–486.

203. BODIAN, D. 1936. A new method for staining nerve fibers and nerve endings in mounted paraffin sections. Anat. Rec., **65:** 89–97.

204. BODIAN, D. 1937. The structure of the vertebrate synapse: A study of the axon endings on Mauthner's cell and neighboring centers in the goldfish. J. Comp. Neurol., **68:** 117–160.

205. BODIAN, D. 1962. The generalized vertebrate neuron. Science, **137:** 323–326.

206. BODIAN, D. 1963. Cytological aspects of neurosecretion in opossum neurohypophysis. Bull. Johns Hopkins Hosp., **113:** 57–93.

207. BODIAN, D. 1966. Herring bodies and neuro-apocrine secretion in the monkey: An electron microscopic study of the fate of the neurosecretory product. Bull. Johns Hopkins Hosp., **118:** 282–326.

208. BODIAN, D. 1967. Neurons, circuits and neuroglia. In G. C. QUARTON, T. MELNECHUK, AND F. O. SCHMITT (Editors), *The Neurosciences. A Study Program.* Rockefeller University Press, New York, pp. 6–24.

209. BOESTEN, A. J. P., AND VOOGD, J. 1975. Projections of the dorsal column nuclei and the spinal cord on the inferior olive in the cat. J. Comp. Neurol., **161:** 215–238.

210. BOIVIE, J. 1970. Terminations of the cervicothalamic tract in the cat: An experimental study with silver impregnation methods. Brain Res., **19:** 333–360.

211. BOIVIE, J. 1971. The terminations of the spinothalamic tract in the cat: An experimental study with silver impregnation methods. Exp. Brain Res., **12:** 331–353.

212. BOIVIE, J. 1978. Anatomical observations on the dorsal column nuclei, their thalamic projection and the cytoarchitecture of some somatosensory thalamic nuclei in the monkey. J. Comp. Neurol., **178:** 17–48.

213. BOIVIE, J. 1979. An anatomical reinvestigation of the termination of the spinothalamic tract in the monkey. J. Comp. Neurol., **186:** 343–370.

214. BOK, S. T. 1928. Das Rückenmark. In W. VON MÖLLENDORFF (Editor), *Handbuch der mikroskopischen Anatomie des Menschen.* Julius Springer, Berlin, pp. 478–578.

215. BOLTON, B. 1939. The blood supply of the human spinal cord. J. Neurol. Psychiatry, **2:** 137–148.

216. VON BONIN, G., AND SHARIFF, G. A. 1951. Extrapyramidal nuclei among mammals. J. Comp. Neurol., **94:** 427–438.

217. BORG, E. 1973. On the neuronal organization of the acoustic middle ear reflex: A physiological and anatomical study. Brain Res., **49:** 101–123.

218. BORISON, H. L., AND WANG, S. C. 1949. Functional localization of central coordinating mechanisms for emesis in cat. J. Neurophysiol., **12:** 305–313.

219. BORISON, H. L., AND WANG, S. C. 1953. Physiology and pharmacology of vomiting. Pharmacol. Rev., **5:** 193–230.

220. BÖRNSTEIN, W. S. 1940. Cortical representation of taste in man and monkey. I. Functional and anatomical relations of taste, olfaction and somatic sensibility. Yale J. Biol. Med., **12:** 719–736.

221. BÖRNSTEIN, W. S. 1940a. Cortical representation of taste in man and monkey. II. Localization of cortical taste area in man and method of measuring impairment of taste in man. Yale J. Biol. Med., **13:** 133–156.

222. BOS, J., AND BENEVENTO, L. A. 1975. Projections of the medial pulvinar to orbital cortex and frontal eye fields in the rhesus monkey (*Macaca mulatta*). Exp. Neurol., **49:** 487–496.

223. BOVARD, E. W., AND GLOOR, P. 1961. Effect of amygdaloid lesions on plasma corticosterone response of the albino rat to emotional stress. Experientia, **17:** 521.

225. BOWDEN, D. M., GERMAN, D. C., AND POYNTER, W. D. 1978. An autoradiographic, semistereotaxic mapping of major projections from locus coeruleus and adjacent nuclei in *Macaca mulatta*. Brain Res., **145:** 257–276.

226. BOWDEN, R. E. M., AND GUTMANN, E. 1944. Denervation and re-innervation of the human voluntary muscle. Brain, **67:** 273–313.

227. BOWDEN, R. E. M., AND MAHRAN, Z. Y. 1956. The functional significance of the pattern of innervation of the muscle quadratus labii superioris of the rabbit, cat and rat. J. Anat., **90:** 217–227.

228. BOWMAN, J. P., AND SLADEK, J. R. 1973. Morphology of the inferior olivary complex of the rhesus monkey (*Macaca mulatta*). J. Comp. Neurol., **152:** 299–316.

229. BOWSHER, D. 1957. Termination of the central pain pathway: The conscious appreciation of pain. Brain, **80:** 606–622.

230. BOWSHER, D. 1958. Projections of the gracile and cuneate nuclei in *Macaca mulatta*: An experimental degeneration study. J. Comp. Neurol., **110:** 135–155.

231. BOWSHER, D. 1966. Some afferent and efferent connections of the parafascicular-center median complex. In D. P. PURPURA AND M. D. YAHR (Editors), *The Thalamus.* Columbia University Press, New York, pp. 99–108.

232. BOWSHER, D. 1961. The termination of secondary somatosensory neurons within the thalamus of *Macaca mulatta*: An experimental degeneration study. J. Comp. Neurol., **177:** 213–227.

233. BOYCOTT, B. B., AND WÄSSLE, H. 1974. The morphological types of ganglion cells of the domestic cat's retina. J. Physiol. (Lond.), **240:** 397–419.

234. BOYD, I. A. 1962. The nuclear-bag fibre and nuclear-chain fibre systems in the muscle spindles of the cat. In D. BARKER (Editor), *Symposium on Muscle Receptors.* Hong Kong University Press, Hong Kong, pp. 185–190.

235. BOYD, I. A. 1962a. The structure and innervation of the nuclear-bag fibre system and the nuclear-chain fibre system in mammalian muscle spindles. Philos. Trans. R. Soc. Lond. (Biol.), **245:** 81–136.

236. BOYD, J. D. 1960. The embryology and comparative anatomy of the melanocyte. In A. ROOK (Editor), *Progress in the Biological Sciences in Relation to Dermatology.* Cambridge University Press, London, pp. 3–14.

237. BRADLEY, W. E., AND CONWAY, C. J. 1966. Bladder representation in the pontine-mesencephalic reticular formation. Exp. Neurol., **16:** 237–249.

238. BRADY, J. V. 1960. Temporal and emotional effects related to intracranial electrical self-stimulation. In S. R. RAMEY AND D. S. O'DOHERTY (Editors), *Electrical Studies on the Unanesthetized Brain.* Paul B. Hoeber, Inc., New York, Ch. 3, pp. 52–77.

239. BRAIN, R. 1961. *Speech Disorders. Aphasia, Apraxia and Agnosia.* Butterworths, London, 184 pp.

240. BRAITENBERG, V., AND ATWOOD, R. P. 1958. Morphological observations on the cerebellar cortex. J. Comp. Neurol., **109:** 1–27.

241. BRAUS, H. 1932. In C. ELZE (Editor), *Anatomie des Menschen* (Vol. 3). Verlag von J. Springer, Berlin.

242. BRAWER, J. R., MOREST, D. K., AND KANE, E. C. 1974. The neuronal architecture of the cochlear nucleus of the cat. J. Comp. Neurol., **155:** 251–300.

243. BRAZIER, M. A. B. 1954. The action of anaesthetics on the nervous system, with special reference to the brain stem reticular system. In J. F. DELAFRESNAYE (Editor), *Brain Mechanisms and Consciousness* (Symposium). Blackwell Scientific Publications, Oxford, pp. 163–193.

244. BREMER, F. 1922. Contributions à l'étude de la physiologie du cervelet. La fonction inhibitrice du palaeocérébellum. Arch. Int. Physiol. Biochim., **19:** 189–226.

245. BREMER, F. 1936. Nouvelles recherches sur le mécanisme du sommeil. C. R. Soc. Biol. (Paris), **122:** 460–

464.

246. BREMER, F. 1937. L'activité cérébrale au cours du sommeil et de la narcose: Contribution à l'étude du mecanisme du sommeil. Bull. Acad. R. Med., Belg., **2:** 68–86.

247. BREMER, F. AND TERZUOLO, C. 1954. Contribution à l'étude des mécanismes physiologiques du maintien de l'activité vigile du cerveau: Interaction de la formation réticulée et de l'écorce cérébrale dans le processus du réveil. Arch. Int. Physiol. Biochim., **62:** 157–178.

248. BRENDLER, S. J. 1968. The human cervical myotomes: Functional anatomy studied at operation. J. Neurosurg., **28:** 105–111.

249. BRIGHTMAN, M. W. 1965. The distribution within the brain of ferritin injected into cerebrospinal fluid compartments. I. Ependymal distribution. J. Cell Biol., **26:** 99–123.

250. BRIGHTMAN, M. W., AND PALAY, S. L. 1963. The fine structure of ependyma in the brain of the rat. J. Cell Biol., **19:** 415–439.

251. BRIGHTMAN, M. W., AND REESE, T. S. 1969. Junctions between intimately apposed cell membranes in the vertebrate brain. J. Cell Biol., **40:** 648–677.

252. BRIGHTMAN, M. W., REESE, T. S., AND FEDER, N. 1970. Assessment with the electronmicroscope of the permeability to peroxidase of cerebral endothelium and epithelium in mice and sharks. In C. CRONE AND N. A. LASSEN (Editors), *Capillary Permeability.* Academic Press, New York, pp. 468–476.

253. BRINKMAN, J., AND KUYPER, H. G. J. M. 1973. Cerebral control of contralateral and ipsilateral hand and finger movements in the split-brain rhesus monkey. Brain, **96:** 653–674.

254. BRINKMAN, C., AND PORTER, R. 1979. Supplementary motor area in the monkey: Activity of neurons during performance of a learned motor task. J. Neurophysiol., **42:** 681–709.

255. BRIZZEE, K. R., AND NEAL, L. M. 1954. A re-evaluation of the cellular morphology of the area postrema in view of recent evidence for a chemoreceptor function. J. Comp. Neurol., **100:** 41–62.

256. BROADWELL, R. D., OLIVER, C., AND BRIGHTMAN, M. W. 1980. Neuronal transport of acid hydrolases and peroxidase within the lysosomal system of organelles: Involvement of agranular reticulum-like cisterns. J. Comp. Neurol., **190:** 519–532.

257. BROCA, P. 1878. Anatomie comparée circonvolutions cérébrales: Le grand lobe limbique et la scissure limbique dans la série des mammifères. Rev. Anthropol. ser. 2, **1:** 384–498.

258. BROCKHAUS, H. 1940. Die Cyto-und Myeloarchitektonik des Cortex claustralis und des Claustrum beim menschen. J. Psychol. Neurol., **49:** 249–348.

259. BRODAL, A. 1940. Experimentelle Untersuchungen über die olivocerebellare Lokalisation. Z. Gesamte Neurol. Psychiatry, **169:** 1–153.

260. BRODAL, A. 1941. Die Verbindungen des Nucleus cuneatus externus mit dem Kleinhirn beim Kaninchen und bei der Katze: Experimentelle Untersuchungen. Z. Gesamte Neurol. Psychiatry, **171:** 167–199.

261. BRODAL, A. 1947. The hippocampus and the sense of smell. Brain, **70:** 179–222.

262. BRODAL, A. 1948. The origin of the fibers of the anterior commissure in the rat: Experimental studies. J. Comp. Neurol., **88:** 157–205.

263. BRODAL, A. 1949. Spinal afferents to the lateral reticular nucleus of the medulla oblongata in the cat: An experimental study. J. Comp. Neurol., **91:** 259–295.

264. BRODAL, A. 1953. Reticulo-cerebellar connections in the cat: An experimental study. J. Comp. Neurol., **98:** 113–153.

265. BRODAL, A. 1954. Afferent cerebellar connections. In J. JANSEN AND A. BRODAL (Editors). *Aspects of Cerebellar Anatomy.* J. G. Tanum, Oslo, Ch. 2, pp. 82–188.

266. BRODAL, A. 1957. *The Reticular Formation of the Brain Stem. Anatomical Aspects and Functional Correlations.* Charles C Thomas, Publisher, Springfield, Ill., 87 pp.

267. BRODAL, A. 1963. General discussion of the terminology of the rhinencephalon. In W. BARGMANN AND J. P. SCHADÉ (Editors), *The Rhinencephalon and Related Structures, Progress in Brain Research,* Vol. 3. Elsevier Publishing Company, Amsterdam, pp. 237–244.

268. BRODAL, A. 1974. Anatomy of the vestibular nuclei and their connections. In H. H. KORNHUBER (Editor), *Handbook of Sensory Physiology: Vestibular System.* Springer-Verlag, Berlin, Vol. 6, pp. 239–352.

269. BRODAL, A. 1976. The olivocerebellar projection in the cat as studied with the method of retrograde axonal transport of horseradish peroxidase. II. The projection of the uvula. J. Comp. Neurol., **166:** 417–426.

270. BRODAL, A. 1981. *Neurological Anatomy in Relation to Clinical Medicine,* Ed. 3. Oxford University Press, New York.

271. BRODAL, A., AND BRODAL, P. 1971. The organization of the nucleus reticularis tegmenti pontis in the cat in the light of experimental anatomical studies of its cerebral cortical afferents. Exp. Brain Res., **13:** 90–110.

272. BRODAL, A., AND COURVILLE, J. 1973. Cerebellar corticonuclear projection in the cat. Crus II. An experimental study with silver methods. Brain Res., **50:** 1–23.

273. BRODAL, A., AND GOGSTAD, A. C. 1954. Rubrocerebellar connections: An experimental study in the cat. Anat. Rec., **118:** 455–486.

274. BRODAL, A., AND GOGSTAD, A. C. 1957. Afferent connexions of the paramedian reticular nucleus of the medulla oblongata in the cat: An experimental study. Acta Anat. (Basel), **30:** 133–151.

275. BRODAL, A., AND HODDEVIK, G. H. 1978. The pontocerebellar projection to the uvula in the cat. Exp. Brain Res., **32:** 105–116.

276. BRODAL, A., AND HØIVIK, B. 1964. Site and mode of termination of primary vestibulo-cerebellar fibres in the cat. Arch. Ital. Biol., **102:** 1–21.

276a. BRODAL, A., AND JANSEN, J. 1946. The ponto-cerebellar projection in the rabbit and cat. J. Comp. Neurol., **84:** 31–118.

277. BRODAL, A., LACERDA, A. M., DESTOMBES, J., AND ANGAUT, P. 1972. The pattern of the projection of the intracerebellar nuclei onto the nucleus reticularis tegmenti pontis in the cat: An experimental anatomical study. Exp. Brain Res., **16:** 140–160.

278. BRODAL, A., AND POMPEIANO, O. 1957. The vestibular nuclei in the cat. J. Anat., **91:** 438–454.

279. BRODAL, A., AND POMPEIANO, O. 1957a. The origin of ascending fibers of the medial longitudinal fasciculus from the vestibular nuclei: An experimental study in the cat. Acta Morphol. Neerl. scand., **1:** 306–328.

280. BRODAL, A., POMPEIANO, O., AND WALBERG, F. 1962. *The Vestibular Nuclei and Their Connections, Anatomy and Functional Correlations.* Charles C Thomas, Publisher, Springfield, Ill.

281. BRODAL, A., AND ROSSI, G. F. 1955. Ascending fibers in brain stem reticular formation of cat. Arch. Neurol. Psychiatry, **74:** 68–87.

282. BRODAL, A., SZABO, T., AND TORVIK, A. 1956. Corticofugal fibers to sensory trigeminal nuclei and nucleus of solitary tract. J. Comp. Neurol., **106:** 527–555.

283. BRODAL, A., AND SZIKLA, G. 1972. The termination of the brachium conjunctivum descendens in the nucleus reticularis tegmenti pontis: An experimental study in the cat. Brain Res., **39:** 337–351.

284. BRODAL, A., TABER, E., AND WALBERG, F. 1960. The raphe nuclei of the brain stem in the cat. II. Efferent connections. J. Comp. Neurol., **114:** 239–259.

285. BRODAL, A., AND TORVIK, A. 1954. Cerebellar projection of paramedian reticular nucleus of medulla oblongata in the cat. J. Neurophysiol., **17:** 484–495.

286. BRODAL, A., AND TORVIK, A. 1957. Über den Ursprung der sekundären vestibulo-cerebellaren Fasern

bei der Katze. Eine experimentell-anatomische Studie. Arch. Psychiatr., **195:** 550–567.

287. BRODAL, A., AND WALBERG, F. 1952. Ascending fibers in the pyramidal tract of cat. Arch. Neurol. Psychiatry, **68:** 755–775.

288. BRODAL, A., AND WALBERG, F. 1977. The olivocerebellar projection in the cat studied with the method of retrograde axonal transport of horseradish peroxidase. IV. The projection to the anterior lobe. J. Comp. Neurol., **172:** 85–108.

288a. BRODAL, A., AND WALBERG, F. 1982. A re-evaluation of the question of ascending fibers in the pyramidal tract. Brain Res., **232:** 271–281.

289. BRODAL, A., WALBERG, F., AND BLACKSTAD, T. 1950. Termination of spinal afferents to inferior olive in cat. J. Neurophysiol., **13:** 431–454.

290. BRODAL, A., WALBERG, F., AND HODDEVIK, E. G. 1975. The olivocerebellar projection in the cat studied with the method of retrograde axonal transport of horseradish perioxidase. J. Comp. Neurol., **164:** 449–470.

291. BRODAL, P. 1968. The corticopontine projection in the cat. I. Demonstration of a somatotopically organized projection from the primary sensorimotor cortex. Exp. Brain Res., **5:** 212–237.

292. BRODAL, P. 1972. The corticopontine projection from the visual cortex in the cat. I. The total projection and the projection from area 17. Brain Res., **39:** 297–317.

293. BRODAL, P. 1972a. The corticopontine projection from the visual cortex in the cat. II. The projection from areas 18 and 19. Brain Res., **39:** 319–335.

294. BRODAL, P. 1972b. The corticopontine projection in the cat: The projection from the auditory areas. Arch. Ital. Biol., **110:** 119–144.

295. BRODAL, P. 1975. Demonstration of a somatotopically organized projection onto the paramedian lobule and the anterior lobe from the lateral reticular nucleus: An experimental study with the horseradish peroxidase method. Brain Res., **95:** 221–239.

296. BRODAL, P. 1978. Principles of organization of the monkey corticopontine projection. Brain Res., **148:** 214–218.

297. BRODAL, P. 1978a. The corticopontine projection in the rhesus monkey: Origin and principles of organization. Brain, **101:** 251–283.

298. BRODAL, P., MARSALA, J., AND BRODAL, A. 1967. The cerebral cortical projection to the lateral reticular nucleus in the cat, with special reference to the sensorimotor cortical area. Brain Res., **6:** 252–274.

299. BRODAL, P., AND WALBERG, F. 1977. The pontine projection to the cerebellar anterior lobe: An experimental study in the cat with retrograde transport of horseradish peroxidase. Exp. Brain Res., **29:** 233–248.

300. BRODISH, A. 1964. Role of the hypothalamus in the regulation of ACTH release. In E. BAJUSZ AND G. JASMIN (Editors), *Major Problems in Endocrinology.* S. Karger, Basel.

301. BRODMANN, K. 1909. *Vergleichende Lokalisation lehre der Grosshirnrinde in ihren Prinzipien dargestellt auf Grund des Zellenbaues.* J. A. Barth, Leipzig, 324 pp.

302. BROOKS, V. B., KOZLOVSKAYA, I. B., ATKIN, A., HORVATH, F. E., AND UNO, M. 1973. Effects of cooling dentate nucleus on tracking-task performance in monkeys. J. Neurophysiol., **36:** 974–995.

303. BROUWER, B., AND ZEEMAN, W. P. C. 1926. The projection of the retina in the primary optic neuron in monkeys. Brain, **49:** 1–35.

304. BROWN, J. O., AND MCCOUCH, G. P. 1947. Abortive regeneration of the transected spinal cord. J. Comp. Neurol., **87:** 131–138.

305. BROWN-GRANT, K., AND RAISMAN, G. 1972. Reproductive function in the rat following selective destruction of afferent fibres to the hypothalamus from the limbic system. Brain Res., **46:** 23–42.

306. BROWNING, M., DUNWIDDIE, T., BENNETT, W., GISPEN, W., AND LYNCH, G. 1979. Synaptic phosphoproteins: Specific changes after repetitive stimulation of the hippocampal slice. Science, **203:** 60–62.

307. BROWNSON, R. H. 1956. Perineuronal satellite cells in the motor cortex of aging brains. J. Neuropathol. Exp. Neurol., **15:** 190–195.

308. BROWNSTEIN, M. J., PALKOVITZ, M., SAAVEDRA, J. M., AND KIZER, J. S. 1975. Tryptophan hydroxylase in the rat brain. Brain Res., **97:** 163–166.

309. BROWNSTEIN, M. J., RUSSELL, J. T., AND GAINER, H. 1980. Synthesis, transport and release of posterior pituitary hormones. Science, **207:** 373–378.

309a. BUCHER, V. M., AND BÜRGI, S. M. 1953. Some observations on the fiber connections of the di- and mesencephalon in the cat; III. The supraoptic decussations. J. Comp. Neurol., **98:** 355–379.

310. BUCY, P. C. 1949. Effects of extirpation in man. In P. C. BUCY (Editor), *The Precentral Motor Cortex,* Ed. 2. University of Illinois Press, Urbana, Ch. 14, pp. 353–394.

311. BUCY, P. C. 1957. Principes physiologiques et résultats des interventions neurochirurgicales dans les affections dites extrapyramidales. I. Relationship of the "pyramidal tract" and abnormal involuntary movements. In *Premier Congrès International des Sciences Neurologiques. Première Journée Commune, Bruxelles, Juillet, 1957.* Pergamon Press, London, pp. 101–107.

312. BUCY, P. C. 1958. The cortico-spinal tract and tremor. In W. S. FIELDS (Editor), *Pathogenesis and Treatment of Parkinsonism.* Charles C Thomas, Publisher, Springfield, Ill., Ch. XI, pp. 271–293.

313. BUCY, P. C. 1959. The surgical treatment of abnormal involuntary movements. Neurologia medico-chirurgica, **1:** 1–15.

314. BUCY, P. C. 1959a. The basal ganglia and skeletal muscular activity. In G. SCHALTENBRAND AND P. BAILEY (Editors), *Introduction to Stereotaxis, with an Atlas of the Human Brain,* Vol. I. Georg Thieme, Stuttgart, pp. 331–353.

315. BUEKER, E. D. 1948. Implantation of tumors in the hind limb field of the embryonic chick, and the developmental response of the lumbosacral nervous system. Anat. Rec., **102:** 369–389.

316. BULL, J. W. D. 1961. Use and limitations of angiography in the diagnosis of vascular lesions of the brain. Neurology (Minneap.) **11:** 80–85.

317. BULL, J. W. D., AND SUTTON, D. 1949. The diagnosis of paraphysial cysts. Brain, **72:** 487–516.

318. BULLOCK, T. H., AND HORRIDGE, G. A. 1965. *Structure and Function in the Nervous Systems of Invertebrates,* Vols. 1 and 2. W. H. Freeman and Company, San Francisco.

319. BUNGE, M. B., BUNGE, R. P., AND PAPPAS, G. D. 1962. Electron microscopic demonstration of connections between glia and myelin sheaths in the developing mammalian central nervous system. J. Cell Biol., **12:** 448–453.

320. BUNGE, M. B., BUNGE, R. P., PETERSON, E. R., AND MURRAY, M. R. 1967. A light and electron microscope study of long term organized cultures of rat dorsal root ganglia. J. Cell Biol., **32:** 439–466.

321. BUNGE, M. B., BUNGE, R. P., AND RIS, H. 1961. Ultrastructural study of remyelination in an experimental lesion in adult cat spinal cord. J. Biophys. Biochem. Cytol., **10:** 67–94.

322. BUNGE, M. B. 1968. Glial cells and the central myelin sheath. Physiol. Rev., **48:** 197–251.

323. BUNGE, R. P., AND GLASS, P. M. 1965. Some observations on myelin-glial relationships and on the etiology of the cerebrospinal fluid exchange lesion. Ann. New York Acad. Sci., **122:** 15–28.

324. BUNNEY, B. S., AND AGHAJANIAN, G. K. 1976. The precise localization of nigral afferents in the rat as determined by a retrograde tracing technique. Brain Res., **117:** 423–435.

325. BUNT, A. H., HENDRICKSON, A. E., LUND, J. S., LUND, R. D., AND FUCHS, A. F. 1975. Monkey retinal ganglion cells: Morphometric analysis and tracing of axonal projections with a consideration of the peroxidase technique. J. Comp. Neurol., **164:** 265–286.

326. BURDE, R. M., AND LOEWY, A. D. 1980. Central origin of oculomotor parasympathetic neurons in the monkey. Brain Res., **198:** 434–439.

327. VAN BUREN, J. M., AND BORKE, R. C. 1972. *Variations and Connections of the Human Thalamus.* Springer-Verlag, New York, 2 vols.

328. BURGEN, A. S. V., AND EMMELIN, N. G. 1961. Innervation of the glandular elements. In A. S. V. BURGEN AND N. G. EMMELIN (Editors), *Physiology of the Salivary Glands.* Williams & Wilkins, Baltimore, Ch. III, pp. 38–71.

329. BURGI, S., AND BUCHER, V. M. 1960. *Markhaltige Faserverbindungen im Hirnstamm der Katze.* Julius Springer Verlag, Berlin.

330. BURTON, H., AND CRAIG, A. D. JR. 1979. Distribution of trigeminothalamic projection cells in the cat and monkey. Brain Res., **161:** 515–521.

331. BURTON, H., AND JONES, E. G. 1976. The posterior thalamic region and its cortical projection in new world and old world monkeys. J. Comp. Neurol., **168:** 249–302.

332. BURTON, H., AND LOEWY, A. D. 1976. Descending projections from the marginal cell layer and other regions of the monkey spinal cord. Brain Res., **116:** 485–491.

333. BURTON, H., AND LOEWY, A. D. 1977. Projections to the spinal cord from medullary somatosensory relay nuclei. J. Comp. Neurol., **173:** 773–792.

334. BURTON, H., AND McFARLANE, J. J. 1973. The organization of the seventh lumbar spinal ganglion in the cat. J. Comp. Neurol., **149:** 215–232.

335. BUSCH, H. F. M. 1961. *An Anatomical Analysis of the White Matter in the Brain Stem of the Cat.* Thesis, University of Leiden. Te Assen Bij Van Gorcum and Company, N.V., Leiden, 116 pp.

336. BUTLER, R. A., DIAMOND, I. T., AND NEFF, W. D. 1957. Role of auditory cortex in discrimination of changes in frequency. J. Neurophysiol., **20:** 108–120.

337. BÜTTNER, U., BÜTTNER-ENNEVER, J. A., AND HENN, V. 1977. Vertical eye movement related unit activity in the rostral mesencephalic reticular formation of the alert monkey. Brain Res., **130:** 239–252.

338. BÜTTNER, U., AND FUCHS, A. F. 1973. Influence of saccadic eye movements and unit activity in simian lateral geniculate and pregeniculate nuclei. J. Neurophysiol., **36:** 127–141.

339. BÜTTNER, U., AND HENN, V. 1976. Thalamic unit activity in the alert monkey during natural vestibular stimulation. Brain Res., **103:** 127–132.

340. BÜTTNER, U., HENN, V., AND OSWALD, H. P. 1977. Vestibular-related neuronal activity in the thalamus of the alert monkey during sinusoidal rotation in the dark. Exp. Brain Res., **30:** 435–444.

341. BÜTTNER-ENNEVER, J. 1977. Pathways from the pontine reticular formation to structures controlling horizontal and vertical eye movements in the monkey. In R. BAKER AND A. BERTHOZ (Editors), *Control of Gaze by Brain Stem Neurons: Developments in Neuroscience,* Vol. 1. Elsevier-North Holland Biomedical Press, Amsterdam, pp. 89–98.

342. BÜTTNER-ENNEVER, J. A., AND BÜTTNER, U. 1978. A cell group associated with vertical eye movements in the rostral mesencephalic reticular formation of the monkey. Brain Res., **151:** 31–47.

343. BÜTTNER-ENNEVER, J. A., AND HENN, V. 1976. An autoradiographic study of the pathways from the pontine reticular formation involved in horizontal eye movements. Brain Res., **108:** 155–164.

344. BYSTRZYCKA, E. K. 1980. Afferent projections to the dorsal and ventral respiratory nuclei in the medulla oblongata of the cat studied by the horseradish peroxidase technique. Brain Res., **185:** 59–66.

345. CABOT, J. B., WILD, J. M., AND COHEN, D. H. 1979. Raphe inhibition of sympathetic preganglionic neurons. Science, **203:** 184–186.

346. CAIN, D. P., AND BINDRA, D. 1972. Responses of amygdala single units to odors in the rat. Exp. Neurol., **35:** 98–110.

347. CAIRNS, H. 1952. Disturbances of consciousness with lesions of the brain-stem and diencephalon. Brain, **75:** 109–146.

348. CAJAL, S. RAMÓN Y. 1909, 1911. *Histologie du système nerveux de l'homme et des vertébres.* Norbert Maloine, Paris. 2 vols.

349. CAJAL, S. RAMÓN Y. 1913. Sobre un nuevo proceder de impregnación de la neuroglia y sus resultados en los centros nerviosos del hombre y animales. Trab. Lab. Invest. Biol. Univ. Madrid, **11:** 219–237.

350. CAJAL, S. RAMÓN Y. 1916. El proceder del oro-sublimado para la coloración de la neuroglia. Trab. Lab. Invest. Biol. Univ. Madrid, **14:** 155–162.

351. CAJAL, S. RAMÓN Y. 1928. *Degeneration and Regeneration of the Nervous System,* Vol. I. Translation by R. M. May. Oxford University Press, London, pp. 27–40.

352. CALNE, D. B., AND PALLIS, C. A. 1966. Vibratory sense: A critical review. Brain, **89:** 723–746.

353. CAMMERMEYER, J. 1947. Is the human area postrema a neuro-vegetative nucleus? Acta Anat. (Basel), **2:** 294–320.

354. CAMMERMEYER, J. 1965. Histiocytes, juxtavascular mitotic cells and microglia cells during retrograde changes in the facial nucleus of rabbits of varying age. Ergeb. Anat. Entwickl.-Gesch., **38:** 195–229.

355. CAMMERMEYER, J. 1966. Morphological distinctions between oligodendrocytes and microglial cells in the rabbit cerebral cortex. Am. J. Anat., **118:** 227–448.

356. CAMPBELL, A. W. 1905. *Histological Studies on the Localisation of Cerebral Function.* Cambridge University Press, New York, 360 pp.

357. CAMPBELL, B., AND SUTIN, J. 1959. Organization of cerebral cortex. IV. Postetanic potentiation of hippocampal pyramids. Am. J. Physiol., **196:** 330–334.

358. CAMPBELL, J. B., BASSETT, C. A. L., HUSBY, J., AND NOBACK, C. R. 1957. Regeneration of adult mammalian spinal cord. Science, **126:** 929.

359. CAMPBELL, J. B., BASSETT, C. A. L., HUSBY, J., AND NOBACK, C. R. 1958. Axonal regeneration in the transected adult feline spinal cord. Surg. Forum, Clin. Cong. Am. Coll. Surgeons, **8:** 528–532.

360. CAMPBELL, M. F. 1957. Neuromuscular uropathy. In M. F. CAMPBELL (Editor) *Principles of Urology.* W. B. Saunders Company, Philadelphia, Ch. 9, pp. 337–378.

361. CAMPOS-ORTEGA, J. A., GLEES, P., AND NEUHOFF, V. 1968. Ultrastructural analysis of individual layers in the lateral geniculate body of the monkey. Z. Zellforsch. Mikrosk. Anat., **87:** 82–100.

362. CANNON, W. B. 1929. *Bodily Changes in Pain, Hunger, Fear and Rage. An Account of Recent Researches into the Function of Emotional Excitement.* D. Appleton and Company, New York.

363. CANNON, W. B. 1939. A law of denervation. Am. J. Med. Sci., **98:** 737–750.

364. CANNON, W. B., AND ROSENBLUETH, A. 1933. Studies on activity in endocrine organs: Sympathin E and sympathin I. Am. J. Physiol., **104:** 557–574.

365. CANNON, W. B., AND ROSENBLUETH, A. 1937. *Autonomic Neuro-Effector Systems.* Macmillan Company, New York.

366. CANNON, W. B., AND ROSENBLUETH, A. 1949. *The Supersensitivity of Denervated Structures.* Macmillan Company, New York.

367. CARLSSON, A. 1965. Drugs which block the storage of 5-hydroxytryptamine and related amines. In O. EICHLER AND A. FARAH (Editors), *Handbuch der experimentellen Pharmakologie,* Vol. 19. Springer, Heidelberg, pp. 529–592.

368. CARLSSON, A., FALCK, B., AND HILLARP, N. Å. 1962. Cellular localization of brain monoamines. Acta physiol. scand., **56** (suppl. 196): 1–28.

369. CARMAN, J. B., COWAN, W. M., AND POWELL, T. P. S. 1963. The organization of corticostriate connexions in the rabbit. Brain, **86:** 525–562.

370. CARMAN, J. B., COWAN, W. M., AND POWELL, T. P. S. 1964. Cortical connexions of the thalamic reticular nucleus. J. Anat., **98:** 587–598.

371. CARMAN, J. B., COWAN, W. M., POWELL, T. P. S., AND

WEBSTER, K. E. 1965. A bilateral corticostriate projection. J. Neurol. Neurosurg. Psychiatry, **28**: 71–77.

372. CARMEL, P. W. 1968. Sympathetic deficits following thalamotomy. Arch. Neurol., **18**: 378–387.

373. CARMEL, P. W. 1970. Efferent projections of the ventral anterior nucleus of the thalamus in the monkey. Am. J. Anat., **128**: 159–184.

374. CARMEL, P. W., AND STEIN, B. M. 1969. Cell changes in sensory ganglia following proximal and distal nerve section in the monkey. J. Comp. Neurol., **135**: 145–166.

375. CARPENTER, F. W. 1918. Nerve endings of sensory type in the muscular coat of the stomach and small intestine. J. Comp. Neurol., **29**: 553–560.

376. CARPENTER, M. B. 1950. Athetosis and the basal ganglia. Arch. Neurol. Psychiatry, **63**: 875–901.

377. CARPENTER, M. B. 1956. A study of the red nucleus in the rhesus monkey. Anatomic degenerations and physiologic effects resulting from localized lesions of the red nucleus. J. Comp. Neurol., **105**: 195–250.

378. CARPENTER, M. B. 1957. Functional relationships between the red nucleus and the brachium conjunctivum. Physiologic study of lesions of the red nucleus in monkeys with degenerated superior cerebellar brachia. Neurology (Minneap.), **7**: 427–437.

379. CARPENTER, M. B. 1957a. The dorsal trigeminal tract in the rhesus monkey. J. Anat., **91**: 82–90.

380. CARPENTER, M. B. 1958. The neuroanatomical basis of dyskinesia. In W. S. FIELDS (Editor), *Pathogenesis and Treatment of Parkinsonism*. Charles C Thomas, Publisher, Springfield, Ill., Ch. 2, pp. 50–85.

381. CARPENTER, M. B. 1959. Lesions of the fastigial nuclei in the rhesus monkey. Am. J. Anat., **104**: 1–34.

382. CARPENTER, M. B. 1960. Fiber projections from the descending and lateral vestibular nuclei in the cat. Am. J. Anat., **107**: 1–22.

383. CARPENTER, M. B. 1961. Brain stem and infratentorial neuraxis in experimental dyskinesia. A. M. A. Arch. Neurol., **5**: 504–524.

384. CARPENTER, M. B. 1966. The ascending vestibular system and its relationship to conjugate horizontal eye movements. In R. J. WOLFSON (Editor), *The Vestibular System and Its Diseases*. University of Pennsylvania Press, Philadelphia, pp. 68–98.

385. CARPENTER, M. B. 1967. Ventral tier thalamic nuclei. In D. WILLIAMS (Editor), *Modern Trends in Neurology*, Vol. 4. Butterworths, London, pp. 1–20.

386. CARPENTER, M. B. 1971. Upper and lower motor neurons. In J. A. DOWNEY AND R. C. DARLING (Editors), *Physiological Basis of Rehabilitation Medicine*. W. B. Saunders Company, Philadelphia, Ch. 1, pp. 3–27.

387. CARPENTER, M. B. 1971a. Central oculomotor pathways. In P. BACH-Y-RITA *et al.* (Editors), *The Control of Eye Movements*. Academic Press, New York, Ch. 4, pp. 67–103.

388. CARPENTER, M. B. 1978. *Core Text of Neuroanatomy*. Williams & Wilkins, Baltimore, 269 pp.

389. CARPENTER, M. B. 1976. Anatomical organization of the corpus striatum and related nuclei. In M. D. YAHR (Editor), *The Basal Ganglia*. Raven Press, New York, pp. 1–36.

390. CARPENTER, M. B. 1981. Anatomy of the corpus striatum and brain stem integrating systems. In V. BROOKS (Editor), *Handbook of Physiology*, Section 1, Vol. II, *Motor Control*. American Physiological Society, Washington, D. C., Ch. 19, pp. 947–995.

391. CARPENTER, M. B., ALLING, F. A., AND BARD, D. S. 1960. Lesions of the descending vestibular nucleus in the cat. J. Comp. Neurol., **114**: 39–50.

392. CARPENTER, M. B., BARD, D. S., AND ALLING, F. A. 1959. Anatomical connections between the fastigial nuclei, the labyrinth and the vestibular nuclei in the cat. J. Comp. Neurol., **111**: 1–26.

393. CARPENTER, M. B., AND BATTON, R. R., III. 1980. Abducens internuclear neurons and their role in conjugate horizontal gaze. J. Comp. Neurol., **189**: 191–209.

394. CARPENTER, M. B., AND BATTON, R. R., III. 1982. Connections of the fastigial nucleus in the cat and monkey. In S. L. PALAY AND V. CHAN-PALAY (Editors), *The Cerebellum-New Vistas*. Exp. Brain Res. (suppl. 6), Springer-Verlag, Berlin., pp. 250–295.

395. CARPENTER, M. B., BATTON, R. R. III, CARLETON, S. C. AND KELLER, J. T. 1981. Interconnections and organization of pallidal and subthalamic nucleus neurons in the monkey. J. Comp. Neurol., **197**: 579–603.

396. CARPENTER, M. B., AND BRITTIN, G. M. 1958. Subthalamic hyperkinesia in the rhesus monkey. Effects of secondary lesions in the red nucleus and brachium conjunctivum. J. Neurophysiol., **21**: 400–413.

397. CARPENTER, M. B., BRITTIN, G. M., AND PINES, J. 1958. Isolated lesions of the fastigial nuclei in the cat. J. Comp. Neurol., **109**: 65–90.

398. CARPENTER, M. B., CARLETON, S. C., KELLER, J. T., AND CONTE, P. 1981. Connections of the subthalamic nucleus in the monkey. Brain Res., **224**: 1–29.

399. CARPENTER, M. B., AND CARPENTER, C. S. 1951. Analysis of somatotopic relations of the corpus Luysi in man and monkey. J. Comp. Neurol., **95**: 349–370.

400. CARPENTER, M. B., AND CORRELL, J. W. 1961. Spinal pathways mediating cerebellar dyskinesia in the rhesus monkey. J. Neurophysiol., **24**: 534–551.

401. CARPENTER, M. B., CORRELL, J. W., AND HINMAN, A. 1960. Spinal tracts mediating subthalamic hyperkinesia. Physiological effects of partial selective cordotomies upon dyskinesia in the rhesus monkey. J. Neurophysiol., **23**: 288–304.

401a. CARPENTER, M. B., FRASER, R. A. R., AND SHRIVER. J. E. 1968. The organization of pallidosubthalamic fibers in the monkey. Brain Res., **11**: 522–559.

402. CARPENTER, M. B., AND HANNA, G. R. 1961. Fiber projections from the spinal trigeminal nucleus in the cat. J. Comp. Neurol., **117**: 117–132.

403. CARPENTER, M. B., AND HANNA, G. R. 1962. Effects of thalamic lesions upon cerebellar dyskinesia in the rhesus monkey. J. Comp. Neurol., **119**: 127–148.

404. CARPENTER, M. B., HARBISON, J. W., AND PETER, P. 1970. Accessory oculomotor nuclei in the monkey. Projections and effects of discrete lesions. J. Comp. Neurol., **140**: 131–154.

405. CARPENTER, M. B., AND McMASTERS, R. E. 1963. Disturbances of conjugate horizontal eye movements in the monkey. II. Physiological effects and anatomical degeneration resulting from lesions in the medial longitudinal fasciculus. Arch. Neurol., **8**: 347–368.

406. CARPENTER, M. B., AND McMASTERS, R. E. 1964. Lesions of the substantia nigra in the rhesus monkey: Efferent fiber degeneration and behavioral observations. Am. J. Anat., **114**: 293–320.

407. CARPENTER, M. B., McMASTERS, R. E., AND HANNA, G. R. 1963. Disturbances of conjugate horizontal eye movements in the monkey. I. Physiological effects and anatomical degeneration resulting from lesions of the abducens nucleus and nerve. Arch. Neurol., **8**: 231–247.

408. CARPENTER, M. B., AND METTLER, F. A. 1951. Analysis of subthalamic hyperkinesia in the monkey with special reference to ablations of agranular cortex. J. Comp. Neurol., **95**: 125–158.

409. CARPENTER, M. B., NAKANO, K., AND KIM, R. 1976. Nigrothalamic projections in the monkey demonstrated by autoradiographic techniques. J. Comp. Neurol., **165**: 401–416.

410. CARPENTER, M. B., NOBACK, C. R., AND MOSS, M. L. 1954. The anterior choroidal artery. Its origins, course, distribution and variations. Arch. Neurol. Psychiatry, **71**: 714–722.

411. CARPENTER, M. B., AND NOVA, H. R. 1960. Descending division of the brachium conjunctivum in the cat: A cerebello-reticular system. J. Comp. Neurol., **114**: 295–305.

412. CARPENTER, M. B., AND PETER, P. 1970/71. Accessory oculomotor nuclei in the monkey. J. Hirnforsch., **12**: 405–418.

413. CARPENTER, M. B., AND PETER, P. 1972. Nigrostriatal and nigrothalamic fibers in the rhesus monkey. J. Comp. Neurol., **144:** 93–116.

414. CARPENTER, M. B., AND PIERSON, R. J. 1973. Pretectal region and the pupillary light reflex: An anatomical analysis in the monkey. J. Comp. Neurol., **149:** 271–300.

415. CARPENTER, M. B., STEIN, B. M., AND PETER, P. 1972. Primary vestibulocerebellar fibers in the monkey: Distribution of fibers arising from distinctive cell groups of the vestibular ganglia. Am. J. Anat., **135:** 221–250.

416. CARPENTER, M. B., STEIN, B. M., AND SHRIVER, J. E. 1968. Central projections of spinal dorsal roots in the monkey. II. Lower thoracic, lumbosacral and coccygeal dorsal roots. Am. J. Anat., **123:** 75–118.

417. CARPENTER, M. B., AND STROMINGER, N. L. 1964. Cerebello-oculomotor fibers in the rhesus monkey. J. Comp. Neurol., **123:** 211–230.

418. CARPENTER, M. B., AND STROMINGER, N. L. 1965. The medial longitudinal fasciculus and disturbances of conjugate horizontal eye movements in the monkey. J. Comp. Neurol., **125:** 41–66.

418a. CARPENTER, M. B., AND STROMINGER, N. L. 1966. Corticostriate encephalitis and paraballism in the monkey. Arch. Neurol., **14:** 241–253.

419. CARPENTER, M. B., AND STROMINGER, N. L. 1967. Efferent fibers of the subthalamic nucleus in the monkey: A comparison of the efferent projections of the subthalamic nucleus, substantia nigra and globus pallidus. Am. J. Anat., **121:** 41–72.

420. CARPENTER, M. B., STROMINGER, N. L., AND WEISS, A. H. 1965. Effects of lesions in the intralaminar thalamic nuclei upon subthalamic dyskinesia: A study in the rhesus monkey. Arch. Neurol., **13:** 113–125.

421. CARPENTER, M. B., WHITTIER, J. R., AND METTLER, F. A. 1950. Analysis of choreoid hyperkinesia in the rhesus monkey: Surgical and pharmacological analysis of hyperkinesia resulting from lesions in the subthalamic nucleus of Luys. J. Comp. Neurol., **92:** 293–332.

422. CARREA, R. M. E., AND GRUNDFEST, H. 1954. Electrophysiological studies of cerebellar inflow. I. Origin, conduction and termination of ventral spino-cerebellar tract in monkey and cat. J. Neurophysiol., **17:** 208–238.

423. CARREA, R. M. E., AND METTLER, F. A. 1947. Physiologic consequences following extensive removals of the cerebellar cortex and deep cerebellar nuclei and effect of secondary cerebral ablations in the primate. J. Comp. Neurol., **87:** 169–288.

424. CARREA, R. M. E., REISSIG, M., AND METTLER, F. A. 1947. The climbing fibers of the simian and feline cerebellum. J. Comp. Neurol., **87:** 321–365.

425. CARREA, R. M. E., VOLKIND, R., FOLINS, J. C., COSARINSKY, D., SUAREZ, A. M., AND ALFONSO, J. 1970. Some physiological and statistical observations on single unit activity of the feline inferior olive. In W. S. FIELDS AND W. D. WILLIS (Editors), *The Cerebellum in Health and Disease.* Warren H. Green, Inc., St. Louis, Ch. 7, pp. 201–216.

426. CARRERAS, M., AND ANDERSSON, S. A. 1963. Functional properties of neurons of the anterior ectosylvian gyrus of the cat. J. Neurophysiol., **26:** 100–126.

427. CASAGRANDE, V. A., HARTING, J. K., HALL, W. C., AND DIAMOND, I. T. 1972. Superior colliculus of the tree shrew: A structural and functional subdivision into superficial and deep layers. Science, **177:** 444–447.

428. CASPERSON, T. 1950. *Cell Growth and Cell Function, a Cytological Study.* W. W. Norton and Company, New York, 185 pp.

429. CASSEDAY, J. H., DIAMOND, I. T., AND HARTING, J. K. 1976. Auditory pathways to the cortex in *Tapaia glis.* J. Comp. Neurol., **166:** 303–340.

430. CASTIGLIONI, A. J., GALLAWAY, M. C., AND COULTER, J. D. 1978. Spinal projections from the midbrain in the monkey J. Comp. Neurol., **178:** 329–346.

431. DE CASTRO, F. 1923. Contribution á la connaissance de l'innervation du pancréas. Y a-t-il des conducteurs specifigues pour les ilots de Langerhans, pour les acini glandulaires et pour les vaisseaux. Trav. Lab. Rech. Biol., Univ. Madrid., **21:** 423–457.

432. CAUNA, N. 1965. The effects of aging on the receptor organs of the human dermis. In W. MONTAGNA (Editor), *Advances in Biology of Skin,* Vol. 6. *Aging.* Pergamon Press, New York, pp. 63–69.

433. CAUNA, N. 1966. Fine structure of the receptor organ and its probable functional significance. In A. V. S. DEREUCK AND J. KNIGHT (Editors), *Touch, Heat and Pain.* Ciba Foundation Symposium. Little, Brown and Company, Boston, pp. 117–127.

434. CAUNA, N., AND MANNAN, G. 1958. The structure of human digital Pacinian corpuscles (Corpuscula lamellosa) and its functional significance. J. Anat., **92:** 1–20.

435. CAUNA, N., AND MANNAN, G. 1959. Development and postnatal changes of digital Pacinian corpuscles (Corpuscula lamellosa) in the human hand. J. Anat., **93:** 271–286.

436. CAUNA, N., AND MANNAN, G. 1961. Organization and development of the preterminal nerve pattern in the palmar digital tissues of man. J. Comp. Neurol., **117:** 309–328.

437. CAUSEY, G. 1960. *The Cell of Schwann.* E. and S. Livingston Ltd., Edinburgh.

438. CHAMBERS, W. W., AND SPRAGUE, J. M. 1955. Functional localization in the cerebellum. I. Organization in longitudinal corticonuclear zones and their contribution to the control of posture, both extrapyramidal and pyramidal, J. Comp. Neurol., **103:** 105–130.

439. CHAMBERS, W. W., AND SPRAGUE, J. M. 1955a. Functional localization in the cerebellum. II. Somatotopic organization in cortex and nuclei. Arch. Neurol. Psychiatry, **74:** 653–680.

440. CHANG, M. M., AND LEEMAN, S. E. 1970. The isolation of a sialogic peptide from bovine hypothalamic tissue and its characterization as substance P. J. Biol. Chem., **245:** 4784–4790.

440a. CHANG, M. M. LEEMAN, S. W., AND NIALL, H. D., 1971. Amino acid sequence of substance P. Nature Lond. New Biol., **232:** 86–87.

441. CHAN-PALAY, V. 1977. *Cerebellar Dentate Nucleus: Organization, Cytology and Transmitters.* Springer-Verlag, Berlin.

442. CHAN-PALAY, V. 1978. Paratrigeminal nucleus. I. Neurons and synaptic organization. J. Neurocytol., **4:** 405–418.

443. CHAN-PALAY, V. 1978a. Paratrigeminal nucleus. II. Identification and interrelations of catecholamine axons, indoleamine axons and substance P immunoreactive cells in neuropil. J. Neurocytol., **4:** 419–442.

444. CHAN-PALAY, V. 1978b. Morphological correlates for transmitter synthesis, transport, release, uptake and catabolism: A study of serotonin neurons in the nucleus paragigantocellularis lateralis. In F. FONNUM (Editor), *Amino Acids as Chemical Transmitters.* Plenum Publishing Corporation, New York, pp. 1–30.

445. CHAN-PALAY, V., AND PALAY, S. L. 1970. Interrelations of basket cell axons and climbing fibers in the cerebellar cortex of the rat. Z. Anat. Entwickl.-Gesch., **132:** 191–227.

446. CHAN-PALAY, V., AND PALAY, S. L. 1971. The synapse *en marron* between Golgi II neurons and mossy fibers in the rat's cerebellar cortex. Z. Anat. Entwickl.-Gesch., **133:** 274–287.

447. CHAN-PALAY, V., AND PALAY, S. L. 1971a. Tendril and glomerular collaterals of climbing fibers in the granular layer of the rat's cerebellar cortex. Z. Anat. Entwickl.-Gesch., **133:** 247–273.

448. CHANG, M. M., LEEMAN, S. E., AND NIALL, H. D. 1971. Amino acid sequence of substance P. Nature, **232:** 86–87.

449. CHARCOT, J. M. 1879. *Lectures on the Diseases of the Nervous System.* Translated by G. Sigerson. Henry

C. Lea, Philadelphia, 390 pp.

450. CHEATHAM, M. L., AND MATZKE, H. A. 1966. Descending hypothalamic medullary pathways in the cat. J. Comp. Neurol., **127:** 369–380.

451. CHEUNG, W. Y. 1980. Calmodulin plays a pivotal role in cellular regulation. Science, **207:** 19–27.

452. CHI, C. C., AND FLYNN, J. P. 1971. Neuroanatomical projections related to biting attack elicited from hypothalamus in cats. Brain Res., **35:** 49–66.

453. CHRISTENSEN, B. N., AND PERL, E. R. 1970. Spinal neurons specifically excited by noxious or thermal stimuli: Marginal zone of the dorsal horn. J. Neurophysiol., **33:** 293–307.

454. CHRISTOFF, N. ANDERSON, P. J., NATHANSON, M., AND BENDER, M. B. 1960. Problems in anatomic analysis of lesions of the median longitudinal fasciculus. A. M. A. Arch. Neurol., **2:** 293–304.

455. CHU, L. W. 1954. Cytological study of anterior horn cells isolated from human spinal cord. J. Comp. Neurol., **100:** 381–413.

456. CHU, N.-S., AND BLOOM, F. E. 1973. Norepinephrine-containing neurons: Changes in spontaneous discharge patterns during sleeping and waking. Science, **179:** 908–910.

457. CHU, N. S., AND BLOOM, F. E. 1974. The catecholamine-containing neurons in the cat dorsolateral pontine tegmentum: Distribution of the cell bodies and some axonal projections. Brain Res., **66:** 1–21.

458. CHUNG, K., AND COGGESHALL, R. E. 1979. Primary afferent axons in the tract of Lissauer in the cat. J. Comp. Neurol., **186:** 451–464.

459. CIRIELLO, J., AND CALARESU, F. R. 1980. Autoradiographic study of ascending projections from cardiovascular sites in the nucleus tractus solitarii in the cat. Brain Res., **180:** 448–453.

460. CIRIELLO, J., AND CALARESU, F. R. 1980a. Monosynaptic pathway from cardiovascular neurons in the nucleus tractus solitarii to the paraventricular nucleus in the cat. Brain Res., **193:** 529–533.

461. CLARK, F. J., AND BURGESS, P. R. 1975. Slowly adapting receptors in cat knee joint: Can they signal angle? J. Neurophysiol., **38:** 1448–1463.

462. CLARK, W. E. L. 1926. The mammalian oculomotor nucleus. J. Anat., **60:** 426–448.

463. CLARK, W. E. L. 1932. The structure and connections of the thalamus. Brain, **55:** 406–470.

464. CLARK, W. E. L. 1936. The termination of ascending tracts in the thalamus of the macaque monkey. J. Anat., **71:** 1–40.

465. CLARK, W. E. L. 1941. The laminar organization and cell content of the lateral geniculate body in the monkey. J. Anat., **75:** 419–433.

466. CLARK, W. E. L. 1948. The connections of the frontal lobes of the brain. Lancet, **1:** 353–356.

467. CLARK, W. E. L. 1951. The projection of the olfactory epithelium on the olfactory bulb in the rabbit. J. Neurol. Neurosurg. Psychiatry, **14:** 1–10.

468. CLARK, W. E. L. 1956. Observations on the structure and organization of olfactory receptors in the rabbit. Yale J. Biol. Med., **29:** 83–95.

469. CLARK, W. E. L. 1957. Inquiries into the anatomical basis of olfactory discrimination. Proc. R. Soc. Lond. (Biol.), **146:** 299–319.

470. CLARK, W. E. L., BEATTIE, J., RIDDOCH, G., AND DOTT, N. M. 1938. *The Hypothalamus.* Oliver and Boyd, Edinburgh.

471. CLARK, W. E. L., AND BOGGON, R. H. 1933. On the connections of the anterior nucleus of the thalamus. J. Anat., **67:** 215–226.

472. CLARK, W. E. L., AND BOGGON, R. H. 1933a. On the connections of the medial cell group of the thalamus. Brain, **56:** 83–98.

473. CLARK, W. E. L., AND BOGGON, R. H. 1935. The thalamic connections of the parietal and frontal lobes of the brain in the monkey. Philos. Trans. R. Soc. Lond. (Biol.), **224:** 313–359.

474. CLARK, W. E. L., AND MEYER, M. 1947. The terminal connexions of the olfactory tract in the rabbit's brain. Brain, **70:** 304–328.

475. CLARK, W. E. L., AND MEYER, M. 1950. Anatomical relationships between the cerebral cortex and the hypothalamus. Br. Med. Bull., **6:** 341–345.

476. CLARK, W. E. L., AND PENMAN, G. G. 1934. The projection of the retina in the lateral geniculate body. Proc. R. Soc. B, **114:** 291–313.

477. CLARK, W. E. L., AND POWELL, T. P. S. 1953. On the thalamocortical connexions of the general sensory cortex of Macaca. Proc. R. Soc. Lond. (Biol.), **141:** 467–487.

478. CLARK, W. E. L., AND WARWICK, R. T. 1946. The pattern of olfactory innervation. J. Neurol. Neurosurg. Psychiatry, **9:** 101–111.

479. CLARKE, R. H., AND HORSLEY, V. 1905. On the intrinsic fibers of the cerebellum, its nuclei and its efferent tracts. Brain, **28:** 13–29.

480. CLEMENTE, C. D., AND VAN BREEMEN, V. L. 1955. Nerve fibers in the area postrema of cat, rabbit, guinea pig and rat. Anat. Rec., **123:** 65–79.

481. CLEMENTE, C. D., SUTIN, J., AND SILVERSTONE, J. T. 1957. Changes in electrical activity of the medulla on the intravenous injection of hypertonic solutions. Am. J. Physiol., **188:** 193–198.

482. CLIFTON, G. L., COGGESHALL, R. E., VANCE, W. H., AND WILLIS, W. D. 1976. Receptive fields of unmyelinated ventral root afferent fibres in the cat. J. Physiol. (Lond.), **256:** 573–600.

483. CLOPTON, B. M., WINFIELD, J. A., AND FLAMMINO, F. J. 1974. Tonotopic organization: Review and analysis. Brain Res., **76:** 1–20.

484. COBB, J. L. S., AND BENNETT, T. 1969. A study of nexuses in visceral smooth muscle. J. Cell Biol., **41:** 287–297.

485. COBB, S. 1948. *Foundations of Neuro-Psychiatry.* Williams & Wilkins, Baltimore.

486. COERS, C. 1955. Les variations structurelles normales et pathologiques de la jonction neuromusculaire. Acta neurol. (belg.), **55:** 741–866.

487. COERS, C., AND WOOLF, A. L. 1959. *The Innervation of Muscle*: A Biopsy Study. Blackwell Scientific Publications, Oxford.

488. COGAN, D. G. 1956. *Neurology of the Ocular Muscles,* Ed. 2. Charles C Thomas, Publisher, Springfield, Ill.

489. COGAN, D. G., KUBIK, C. S., AND SMITH, W. L. 1950. Unilateral internuclear ophthalmoplegia: Report of eight clinical cases with one postmortem study. Arch. Ophthalmol., **44:** 783–796.

490. COGGESHALL, R. E., APPLEBAUM, M. L., FRAZEN, M., STUBBS, T. B. III, AND SYKES, M. T. 1975. Unmyelinated axons in human ventral roots, a possible explanation for the failure of dorsal rhizotomy to relieve pain. Brain, **98:** 157–166.

491. COGGESHALL, R. E., COULTER, J. D., AND WILLIS, W. D. 1974. Unmyelinated axons in the ventral roots of the cat lumbosacral enlargement. J. Comp. Neurol., **153:** 39–58.

492. COGGESHALL, R. E., AND FAWCETT, D. W. 1964. The fine structure of the central nervous system of the leech, *Hirudo medicinalis.* J. Neurophysiol., **27:** 229–289.

493. COGGESHALL, R. E., AND GALBRAITH, S. L. 1978. Categories of axons in mammalian rami communicantes, part II. J. Comp. Neurol., **181:** 349–360.

494. COGGESHALL, R. E., HANCOCK, M. B., AND APPLEBAUM, M. L. 1976. Categories of axons in mammalian rami communicantes. J. Comp. Neurol., **167:** 105–124.

495. COGGESHALL, R. E., AND ITO, H. 1977. Sensory fibers in ventral roots L7 and S1 in the cat. J. Physiol. (Lond.), **267:** 215–235.

496. COGHILL, G. E. 1929. *Anatomy and the Problem of Behavior.* Cambridge University Press, London.

497. COHEN, B. 1971. Vestibulo-ocular relations. In P. BACH-Y-RITA et al. (Editors), *The Control of Eye Movements.* Academic Press, New York, pp. 105–135.

498. COHEN, B., AND HENN, V. 1972. Unit activity in the pontine reticular formation associated with eye movements. Brain Res., **46:** 403–410.

499. COHEN, B., AND KOMATSUZAKI, A. 1972. Eye move-

ments induced by stimulation of the pontine reticular formation: Evidence for integration in oculomotor pathways. Exp. Neurol., **36** 101–117.

500. COHEN, B., SUZUKI, J. I., AND BENDER, M. B. 1964. Eye movements from semicircular nerve stimulation in the cat. Ann. Otol. Rhinol. Laryngol., **73:** 153–169.

500a. COHEN, B., HOUSEPIAN, E. M., AND PURPURA, D. P. 1962. Intrathalamic regulation of activity in a cerebellocortical projection pathway. Exp. Neurol., **6:** 492–506.

501. COHEN, D., CHAMBERS, W. W., AND SPAGUE, J. M. 1958. Experimental study of the efferent projections from the cerebellar nuclei to the brain stem of the cat. J. Comp. Neurol., **109:** 233–259.

502. COHEN, S. 1960. Purification of a nerve-growth factor promoting protein from the mouse salivary gland and its neuro-cytotoxic antiserum. Proc. Natl. Acad. Sci. U. S. A., **46:** 302–311.

503. COIL, J. D., AND NORGREN, R. 1979. Cells of origin of motor axons in the subdiaphragmatic vagus of the rat. J. Auto. Nerv. Syst., **1:** 203–211.

504. COLE, M., NAUTA, W. J. H., AND MEHLER, W. R. 1964. The ascending efferent projections of the substantia nigra. Trans. Am. Neurol. Assoc., **89:** 74–78.

505. COLLINS, W. F., NULSEN, F. E., AND RANDT, C. T. 1960. Relation of peripheral nerve fiber size and sensation in man. Arch. Neurol., **3:** 381–385.

506. COLLINS, P., and WOOLAM, D. H. M. 1979. The ventricular surface of the subcommisural organ: A scanning and transmission electron microscopic study. J. Anat., **129:** 623–631.

507. COLONNIER, M. 1967. The fine structural arrangement of the cortex. Arch. Neurol., **16:** 651–657.

508. COLONNIER, M. 1968. Synaptic patterns on different cell types in the different laminae of the cat visual cortex: An electron microscopic study. Brain Res., **9:** 268–287.

509. COLONNIER, M. L., AND GUILLERY, R. W. 1964. Synaptic organization in the lateral geniculate nucleus of the monkey. Z. Zellforsch. Mikrosk. Anat., **62:** 333–355.

510. COMBS, C. M. 1949. Fiber and cell degeneration in the albino rat brain after hemidecortication. J. Comp. Neurol., **90:** 373–402.

511. COMBS, C. M. 1956. Bulbar regions related to localized cerebellar afferent impulses. J. Neurophysiol., **19:** 285–300.

512. CONDÉ, F., AND CONDÉ, H. 1973. Etude de la morphologie des cellules due noyau rouge du chat par la methode de Golgi-Cox. Brain Res., **53:** 249–271.

513. CONDÉ, F., AND CONDÉ, H. 1978. Thalamic projections of the vestibular nuclei in the cat as revealed by retrograde transport of horseradish peroxidase. Neurosci. Lett., **9:** 141–146.

514. CONRAD, B., AND BROOKS, V. B. 1974. Effects on dentate cooling on rapid alternating arm movements. J. Neurophysiol., **37:** 792–804.

515. CONRAD, L. C. A., LEONARD, C. A., AND PFAFF, D. W. 1974. Connections of the median and dorsal raphe nuclei in the rat: An autoradiographic and degeneration study. J. Comp. Neurol., **156:** 179–206.

516. CONTRERAS, R. J., GOMEZ, M. M., AND NORGREN, R. 1980. Central origins of cranial nerve parasympathetic neurons in the rat. J. Comp. Neurol., **190:** 373–394.

517. COOPER, E. R. A. 1946. The development of the substantia nigra. Brain, **69:** 22–33.

518. COOPER, E. R. A. 1946a. The development of the human red nucleus and corpus striatum. Brain, **69:** 34–43.

519. COOPER, I. S. 1956. *Neurosurgical Alleviation of Parkinsonism.* Charles C Thomas, Publisher, Springfield, Ill.

520. COOPER, I. S. 1957. Relief of juvenile involuntary movement disorders by chemopallidectomy. J. A. M. A., **164:** 1297–1301.

521. COOPER, I. S. 1959. Dystonia musculorum deformans

alleviated by chemopallidectomy and chemopallidothalamectomy. A. M. A. Arch. Neurol. Psychiatry, **81:** 5–19.

522. COOPER, I. S. 1960. Neurosurgical relief of intention tremor due to cerebral disease and multiple sclerosis. Arch. Phys. Med. Rehabil., **41:** 1–4.

523. COOPER, I. S. 1960a. Neurosurgical alleviation of intention tremor of multiple sclerosis and cerebellar disease. N. Engl. J. Med., **263:** 441–444.

524. COOPER, I. S., AND BRAVO, G. J. 1958. Anterior choroidal artery occlusion, chemopallidectomy and chemothalamectomy in parkinsonism: A consecutive series of 700 operations. In W. S. FIELDS (Editor), *Pathogenesis and Treatment of Parkinsonism.* Charles C Thomas, Publisher, Springfield, Ill., Ch. XV, pp. 325–352.

525. COOPER, I. S., AND POLOUKHINE, N. 1959. Neurosurgical relief of intention (cerebellar) tremor. J. Am. Geriatr. Soc., **7:** 443–445.

526. COOPER, L. N. 1981. Distributed memory in the central nervous system: Possible test of assumptions in visual cortex. In F. O. SCHMITT, F. G. WORDEN, G. ADELMAN, AND S. G. DENNIS (Editors), *The Organization of the Cerebral Cortex.* MIT Press, Cambridge, Mass., pp. 479–503.

527. COOPER, M. H., AND BEAL, J. A. 1978. The neurons and the synaptic endings in the primate basilar pontine gray. J. Comp. Neurol., **180:** 17–42.

528. COOPER, S., AND DANIEL, P. M. 1949. Muscle spindles in human extrinsic eye muscles. Brain, **72:** 1–24.

529. COOPER, S., DANIEL, P. M., AND WHITTERIDGE, D. 1953. Nerve impulses in the brainstem of the goat: Short latency responses obtained by stretching the extrinsic eye muscles and the jaw muscles. J. Physiol. (Lond.), **120:** 471–490.

530. COOPER, S., DANIEL, P. M., AND WHITTERIDGE, D. 1953a. Nerve impulses in the brainstem of the goat: Responses with long latencies obtained by stretching the extrinsic eye muscles. J. Physiol. (Lond.), **120:** 491–513.

531. COOPER, S., DANIEL, P. M., AND WHITTERIDGE, D. 1955. Muscle spindles and other sensory endings in the extrinsic eye muscles: The physiology and anatomy of these receptors and their connections with the brain stem. Brain, **78:** 564–583.

532. COOPER, S., AND SHERRINGTON, C. S. 1940. Gower's tract and spinal border cells. Brain, **63:** 123–134.

533. COPENHAVER, W. M. 1964. *Bailey's Textbook of Histology,* Ed. 15. Williams & Wilkins, Baltimore, 633 pp.

534. COPENHAVER, W. M., BUNGE, R. P. AND BUNGE, M. B. 1971. *Bailey's Textbook of Histology,* Ed. 16. Williams & Wilkins, Baltimore.

535. CORBIN, K. B. 1940. Observations on the peripheral distribution of fibers arising in the mesencephalic nucleus of the fifth cranial nerve. J. Comp. Neurol., **73:** 153–177.

536. CORBIN, K. B., AND HARRISON, F. 1940. Function of the mesencephalic root of the fifth cranial nerve. J. Neurophysiol., **3:** 423–435.

537. CORNING, H. K. 1922. Lehrbuch der topographischen Anatomie für Studierende und Ärzte. J. F. Bergmann, Munich, pp. 609–614.

538. COTMAN, C., GENTRY, C., AND STEWARD, O. 1977. Synaptic replacement in dentate gyrus after unilateral entorhinal lesion: electron microscopic analysis of extent of replacement of synapses by remaining entorhinal cortex. J. Neurocytol., **6:** 455–464.

539. COTMAN, C. W., AND NADLER, J. V. 1978. Reactive synaptogenesis in the hippocampus. In C. W. COTMAN (Editor), *Neuronal Plasticity.* Raven Press, New York, pp, 227–265.

540. COULTER, J. D., EWING, L., AND CARTER, C. 1976. Origin of primary sensorimotor cortical projections to lumbar spinal cord of cat and monkey. Brain Res., **103:** 366–372.

541. COULTER, J. D., AND JONES, E. G. 1977. Differential distribution of corticospinal projections from individual cytoarchitectonic fields in the monkey. Brain Res., **129:**

335–340.

542. COURVILLE, J. 1966. Rubrobulbar fibres to the facial nucleus and the lateral reticular nucleus (nucleus of the lateral funiculus): An experimental study in the cat with silver impregnation methods. Brain Res., 1: 317–337.

543. COURVILLE, J. 1966a. Somatotopical organization of the projection from the nucleus interpositus anterior of the cerebellum to the red nucleus: An experimental study in the cat with silver impregnation methods. Exp. Brain Res., 2: 191–215.

544. COURVILLE, J. 1966b. The nucleus of the facial nerve: The relation between cellular groups and peripheral branches of the nerve. Brain Res., 1: 338–354.

545. COURVILLE, J. 1975. Distribution of olivocerebellar fibers demonstrated by a radioautographic tracing method. Brain Res., 95: 253–263.

546. COURVILLE, J., AUGUSTINE, J. R., AND MARTEL, P. 1977. Projections from the inferior olive to the cerebellar nuclei in the cat demonstrated by retrograde transport of horseradish peroxidase. Brain Res., 130: 405–419.

547. COURVILLE, J., AND BRODAL, A. 1966. Rubrocerebellar connections in the cat: An experimental study with silver impregnation methods. J. Comp. Neurol., 126: 471–485.

548. COURVILLE, J., AND COOPER, C. W. 1970. The cerebellar nuclei of Macaca mulatta: A morphological study. J. Comp. Neurol., 140: 241–254.

549. COURVILLE, J. AND DIAKIW, N. 1976. Cerebellar corticonuclear projection in the cat: The vermis of the anterior and posterior lobes. Brain Res., 110: 1–20.

550. COURVILLE, J., DIAKIW, N., AND BRODAL, A. 1973. Cerebellar corticonuclear projection in the cat: The paramedian lobule: An experimental study with silver methods. Brain Res., 50: 25–45.

551. COURVILLE, J., AND FARACO-CANTIN, F. 1978. On the origin of the climbing fibers of the cerebellum: An experimental study in the cat with an autoradiographic tracing method. Neuroscience, 3: 797–809.

552. COURVILLE, J., AND OTABE, S. 1974. The rubro-olivary projection in the Macaque: An experimental study with silver impregnation methods. J. Comp. Neurol., 158: 497–494.

553. COUTEAUX, R. 1958. Morphological and cytochemical observations on the postsynaptic membrane at motor end plates and ganglionic synapses. Exp. Cell Res., 5: (suppl): 294–322.

554. COWAN, W. M., AND CUÉNOD, M. 1975. The use of axonal transport for study of neuronal connections: A retrospective survey. In The Use of Axonal Transport for Studies of Neuronal Connectivity. Elsevier Scientific Publishing Company, Amsterdam, pp. 2–23.

555. COWAN, W. M., GOTTLIEB, D. I., HENDRICKSON, A. E., PRICE, J. L., AND WOOLSEY, T. A. 1972. The autoradiographic demonstration of axonal connections in the central nervous system. Brain Res., 37: 21–51.

556. COWAN, W. M., AND POWELL, T. P. S. 1966. Striopallidal projection in the monkey. J. Neurol. Neurosurg. Psychiatry, 29: 426–439.

557. COWAN, W. M., RAISMAN, G., AND POWELL, T. P. S. 1965. The connexions of the amygdala. J. Neurol. Neurosurg. Psychiatry, 28: 137–151.

558. COX, V. C., AND VALENSTEIN, E. S. 1969. Distribution of hypothalamic sites yielding stimulus-bound behavior. Brain Behav. Evol., 2: 359–376.

559. COXE, W. S., AND LANDAU, W. M. 1965. Observations upon the effect of supplementary motor cortex ablation in the monkey. Brain, 88: 763–772.

560. CRAGG, B. G. 1967. The density of synapses and neurones in the motor and visual areas of the cerebral cortex. J. Anat., 101: 639–654.

561. CRAIG, A. D. JR. 1978. Spinal and medullary input to the lateral cervical nucleus. J. Comp. Neurol., 181: 729–743.

562. CRAIG, A. D., JR., AND BURTON, H. 1979. The lateral cervical nucleus in the cat: Anatomical organization of cervicothalamic neurons. J. Comp. Neurol., 185: 329–346.

563. CRAIG, A. D., JR., AND TAPPER, D. N. 1978. Lateral cervical nucleus in the cat: Functional organization and characteristics. J. Neurophysiol., 41: 1511–1534.

564. CRITCHLEY, M. 1953. The Parietal Lobes. Edward Arnold, London, 479 pp.

565. CRITCHLOW, V. 1963. The role of light in the neuroendocrine system. In A. V. NALBANDOV (Editor), In Advances in Neuroendocrinology. University of Illinois Press, Urbana, pp. 377–402.

566. VAN CREVEL, H., AND VERHAART, W. J. C. 1963. The rate of secondary degeneration in the central nervous system. I. The pyramidal tract of the cat. J. Anat., 97: 429–449.

567. VAN CREVEL, H., AND VERHAART, W. J. C. 1963a. The rate of secondary degeneration in the central nervous system. II. The optic nerve of the cat. J. Anat., 97: 451–464.

568. CROCK, H. V., AND YOSHIZAWA, H. 1977. The Blood Supply of the Vertebral Column and Spinal Cord in Man. Springer-Verlag, Berlin, 130 pp.

569. CRONE, C. 1963. The permeability of capillaries in various organs as determined by use of the "indicator diffusion" method. Acta Physiol. Scand., 58: 292–305.

569a. CROSBY, E. C. 1953. Relation of brain centers to normal and abnormal eye movements in a horizontal plane. J. Comp. Neurol., 99: 437–480.

570. CROSBY, E. C., AND HUMPHREY, T. 1941. Studies of the vertebrate telencephalon. II. The nuclear pattern of the anterior olfactory nucleus, tuberculum olfactorum and the amygdaloid complex in adult man. J. Comp. Neurol., 74: 309–352.

571. CROSBY, E. C., HUMPHREY, T., AND LAUER, E. W. 1962. Correlative Anatomy of the Nervous System. Macmillan Company, New York, 731 pp.

572. CROUSE, G. S., AND CUCINOTTA, A. J. 1965. Progressive neuronal differentiation in the submandibular ganglia of a series of human fetuses. J. Comp. Neurol., 125: 259–272.

573. CROWE, S. J. 1935. Symposium on tone localization in the cochlea. Ann. Otol. Rhinol. Laryngol., 44: 737–837.

574. CSERR, H. F. 1971. Physiology of the choroid plexus. Physiol. Rev., 51: 273–311.

575. CUELLO, A. C., AND KANAZAWA, I. 1978. The distribution of substance P immunoreactive fibers in the rat central nervous system. J. Comp. Neurol., 178: 129–156.

576. CULLHEIM, S., AND KELLERTH, J.-O. 1978. Morphological study of the axons and recurrent axon collaterals of cat sciatic α motoneurons after intracellular staining with horseradish peroxidase. J. Comp. Neurol., 178: 537–558.

577. CULLHEIM, S., KELLERTH, J.-O., AND CONRADI, S. 1977. Evidence for direct synaptic interconnections between cat spinal α-motoneurons via the recurrent axon collaterals: A morphological study using intracellular injection of horseradish peroxidase. Brain Res., 132: 1–10.

578. CULLING, C. F. A. 1963. Handbook of Histopathological Techniques, Ed. 2. Butterworths, London, pp. 348–375.

579. CUMMINGS, J. F., AND PETRAS, J. M. 1977. The origin of spinocerebellar pathways. I. The nucleus cervicalis centralis of the cranial cervical spinal cord. J. Comp. Neurol., 173: 655–692.

580. CURRIER, R. D., GILES, C. L., AND DEJONG, R. N. 1961. Some comments on Wallenberg's lateral medullary syndrome. Neurology (Minneap.), 11: 778–791.

581. CUTLER, R. W. P., LORENZO, A. V., AND BARLOW, C. F. 1967. Changes in blood-brain permeability during pharmacologically induced convulsions. Prog. Brain Res., 29: 367–384.

582. CYNADER, M., AND BERMAN, N. 1972. Receptive-field organization of monkey superior colliculus. J. Neurophysiol., **35:** 187–201.

583. DAHLSTRÖM, A. 1965. Observation on the accumulation of noradrenaline in the proximal and distal parts of peripheral adrenergic nerves after compression. J. Anat., **99:** 677–689.

584. DAHLSTRÖM, A. 1971. Regional distribution of brain catecholamines and serotonin. Neurosci. Res. Program Bull., **9:** 197–205.

585. DAHLSTRÖM, A., AND FUXE, K. 1964. Evidence for the existence of monoamine-containing neurons in the central nervous system. I. Demonstration of monoamines in the cell bodies of brain stem neurons. Acta Physiol. Scand., **62** (suppl. 232): 1–55.

586. DAHLSTRÖM, A., AND FUXE, K. 1965. Evidence for the existence of monoamines in the central nervous system. II. Experimentally induced changes in the intraneuronal amine levels of bulbospinal neuron systems. Acta Physiol. Scand., **64** (suppl. 247): 1–36.

587. DAITZ, H. M., AND POWELL, T. P. S. 1954. Studies of the connections of the fornix system. J. Neurol. Neurosurg. Psychiatry, **17:** 75–82.

588. DAJAS, F., SILVEIRA, R., AND ECHAGUE, A. 1979. Microdensitometry of acetylcholinesterase in subfields of the hippocampal pyramidal layer and fascia dentata. Acta Anat. (Basel), **103:** 344–350.

589. DALE, H. H. 1914. The action of certain esters and ethers of choline, and their relation to muscarine. J. Pharmacol. Exp. Ther., **6:** 147–190.

590. DALE, H. 1935. Pharmacology and nerve endings. Proc. R. Soc. Med., **28:** 319–332.

591. DANDY, W. E. 1933. *Benign Tumors in the Third Ventricle of the Brain.* Charles C Thomas, Publisher, Springfield, Ill.

592. DANDY, W. E. 1947. *Intercranial Arterial Aneurysms.* Comstock Publishing Company, Ithaca, N. Y., 147 pp.

593. DARIAN-SMITH, I., AND MAYDAY, G. 1960. Somatotopic organization within the brain stem trigeminal complex of the cat. Exp. Neurol., **2:** 290–309.

594. DARIAN-SMITH, I., AND YOKOTA, T. 1966. Corticofugal effects on different neuron types within the cat's brain stem activated by tactile stimulation of the face. J. Neurophysiol., **29:** 185–206.

595. DAVIDOFF, L. M., AND DYKE, C. G. 1951. *The Normal Encephalogram,* Ed. 3. Lea and Febiger, Philadelphia, pp. 167–170.

596. DAVIES, J., AND DRAY, A. 1976. Substance P in the substantia nigra. Brain Res., **107:** 623–627.

597. DAVIS, C. L. 1923. Description of a human embryo having 20 paired somites. Contrib. Embryol., **15:** 1–51.

598. DAVIS, D. 1957. *Radicular Syndromes With Emphasis on Chest Pain Simulating Coronary Disease.* Year Book Medical Publishers, Inc., Chicago, pp. 17–160.

599. DAVIS, H. 1961. Some principles of sensory receptor action. Physiol. Rev., **41:** 391–416.

600. DAVSON, H. 1960. Intracranial and intraocular fluids. In J. FIELD (Editor), *Handbook of Physiology,* Section 1, Vol. III, *Neurophysiology.* American Physiological Society, Washington, D. C., Ch. 71, pp. 1761–1788.

601. DAVSON, H. 1967. *Physiology of the Cerebrospinal Fluid.* Little, Brown and Company, Boston.

602. DAVSON, H. 1976. The blood-brain barrier: Review lecture. J. Physiol. (Lond.), **255:** 1–28.

603. DAVSON, H., AND BRADBURY, M. 1965. The extracellular space of the brain. In E. D. P. DEROBERTIS AND R. CARREA (Editors), *Biology of Neuroglia, Progress in Brain Research,* Vol. 15. Elsevier Publishing Company, Amsterdam, pp. 124–134.

604. DAWSON, N. J., HELLON, R. F., AND HUBBARD, J. I. 1980. Cell responses evoked by tooth pulp stimulation above the marginal layer of the cat's trigeminal nucleus caudalis. J. Comp. Neurol., **193:** 983–994.

605. DEECKE, L., SCHWARZ, D. W. F., AND FREDRICKSON, J. M. 1973. The vestibular thalamus in the Rhesus monkey. Adv. Otorhinolaryngol., **19:** 210–219.

606. DEECKE, L., SCHWARZ, D. W. F., AND FREDRICKSON, J. M. 1974. Nucleus ventroposterior inferior (VPI) as the vestibular thalamic relay in the Rhesus monkey. I. Field potential investigation. Exp. Brain Res., **20:** 88–100.

607. DEECKE, L., SCHWARZ, D. W. F., AND FREDRICKSON, J. M. 1977. Vestibular responses in the rhesus monkey ventroposterior thalamus. II. Vestibuloproprioceptive convergence at thalamic neurons. Exp. Brain Res., **30:** 219–232.

608. DÉJÉRINE, J. 1901. *Anatomie des centres nerveaux,* Vol. 2. J. Rueff, Paris, 720 pp.

609. DEJONG, R. N. 1979. *The Neurological Examination,* Ed. 4. Harper & Row Publishers, New York.

610. DEKABAN, A. 1953. Human thalamus. An anatomical, developmental and pathological study. I. Division of the human adult thalamus into nuclei by use of the cyto-myelo-architectonic method. J. Comp. Neurol., **99:** 639–683.

611. DEKABAN, A. 1954. Human thalamus. An anatomical developmental and pathological study. II. Development of the human thalamic nuclei. J. Comp. Neurol., **100:** 63–97.

612. DEKKER, J. J., KIEVIT, J., JACOBSON, S., AND KUYPERS, H. G. J. M. 1975. Retrograde axonal transport of horseradish peroxidase in the forebrain of the rat, cat and rhesus monkey. In M. SANTINI (Editor), *Prospectives in Neurobiology.* Golgi Centennial Symposium. Raven Press, New York, pp. 201–208.

613. DELL, P. 1952. Corrélations entre le système vegetatif et le système de la vie de relation: Mésencéphale, diencephale et cortex cerebral. J. Physiol. (Paris), **44:** 471–557.

614. DE LONG, M. R. 1971. Activity of pallidal neurons during movement. J. Neurophysiol., **34:** 414–427.

615. DE LONG, M. R., AND STRICK, P. L. 1974. Relation of basal ganglia, cerebellum and motor cortex units to ramp and ballistic movements. Brain Res., **71:** 327–335.

616. DEMPSEY, E. W. 1956. Variations in the structure of mitochondria. J. Biophys. Biochem. Cytol., **2:** (suppl. 4): 305–312.

617. DEMPSEY, E. W., AND LUSE, S. 1958. Fine structure of the neuropil in relation to neuroglia cells. In W. F. WINDLE (Editor), *Biology of Neuroglia.* Charles C Thomas, Publisher, Springfield, Ill., pp. 99–108.

618. DEMPSEY, E. W., AND MORISON, R. S. 1942. The production of rhythmically recurrent cortical potentials after localized thalamic stimulation. Am. J. Physiol., **135:** 293–300.

619. DEMPSEY, E. W., AND MORISON, R. S. 1943. The electrical activity of a thalamocortical relay system. Am. J. Physiol., **138:** 283–298.

620. DENIAU, J. M., HAMMOND, C., CHEVALIER, G., AND FÉGER, J. 1978. Evidence for branched subthalamic nucleus projections to substantia nigra, entopeduncular nucleus and globus pallidus. Neurosci. Lett., **9:** 117–121.

621. DENNIS, J. 1981. Development of the neuromuscular junction: Inductive interactions between cells. Annu. Rev. Neurosci., **4:** 43–68.

622. DENNY-BROWN, D. 1946. Importance of neural fibroblasts in the regeneration of nerve. Arch. Neurol. Psychiatry, **55:** 171–215.

623. DENNY-BROWN, D. 1951. The frontal lobes and their functions. In A. FEILING (Editor), *Modern Trends in Neurology.* Paul B. Hoeber, Inc., New York, pp. 13–89.

624. DENNY-BROWN, D. 1960. Motor mechanisms—Introduction: The general principles of motor integration. In J. FIELD (Editor), *Handbook of Physiology,* Section I, Vol. II. American Physiological Society, Washington, D. C. Ch. 32, pp. 781–796.

625. DENNY-BROWN, D. 1962. *The Basal Ganglia and Their Relation to Disorders of Movement.* Oxford Uni-

versity Press, London.

626. DENNY-BROWN, D., AND BOTTERELL, E. H. 1948. The motor functions of the agranular frontal cortex. Proc. Assoc. Res. Nerv. Ment. Dis., **27**: 235–345.

627. DEVITO, J. L., ANDERSON, M. E., AND WALSH, K. E. 1980. A horseradish peroxidase study of afferent connections of the globus pallidus in *Macaca mulatta*. Exp. Brain Res., **38**: 65–73.

628. DEVITO, J. L., AND SMITH, O. A., JR. 1959. Projections from the mesial frontal cortex (supplementary motor area) to the cerebral hemispheres and brain stem of the *Macaca mulatta*. J. Comp. Neurol., **111**: 261–277.

629. DIAMOND, I. T., JONES, E. G., AND POWELL, T. P. S. 1968. Interhemispheric fiber connections of the auditory cortex in the cat. Brain Res., **11**: 177–193.

630. DIAMOND, I. T., JONES, E. G., AND POWELL, T. P. S. 1968a. The association connections of the auditory cortex of the cat. Brain Res., **11**: 560–579.

631. DIAMOND, I. T., JONES, E. G., AND POWELL, T. P. S. 1969. The projection of the auditory cortex upon the diencephalon and brain stem in the cat. Brain Res., **15**: 305–340.

632. DIETRICHS, E., AND WALBERG, F. 1979. The cerebellar corticonuclear and nucleocortical projections in the cat as studied with antergrade and retrograde transport of horseradish peroxidase. I. The paramedian lobule. Anat. Embryol. (Berl.), **158**: 13–39.

633. DIETRICHS, E., AND WALBERG, F. 1979a. The cerebellar projection from the lateral reticular nucleus as studied with retrograde transport of horseradish peroxidase. Anat. Embryol. (Berl.), **155**: 273–290.

634. DIFIGLIA, M., PASIK, P., AND PASIK, T. 1976. A Golgi study of neuronal types in the neostriatum of monkeys. Brain Res., **114**: 245–256.

635. DIVAC, I., LAVAIL, J. H., RAKIC, P., AND WINSTON, K. R. 1977. Heterogenous afferents to the inferior parietal lobule of the rhesus monkey revealed by the retrograde transport method. Brain Res., **123**: 197–207.

636. DOGIEL, A. S. 1891. Die Nervenendkörperchen (Endkolben, W. Krause) in der Cornea und Conjunctiva Bulbi des Menschen. Arch. Mikrosk. Anat. Entwickl-Gesch., **37**: 602–619.

637. DOGIEL, A. S. 1908. *Der Bau der Spinalganglien des Menschen und der Säugetiere.* Gustav Fischer, Jena.

638. DOHRMANN, G. J. 1970. The choroid plexus: A historical review. Brain Res., **18**: 197–218.

639. DOMESICK, V. B. 1969. Projections from the cingulate cortex in the rat. Brain Res., **12**: 296–320.

640. DOSTROVSKY, J. O., AND HELLON, R. F. 1978. The representation of facial temperature in the caudal trigeminal nucleus of the cat. J. Physiol. (Lond.), **277**: 29–48.

641. DOTT, N. M. 1938. Surgical aspects of the hypothalamus. In W. E. L. CLARK *et al.* (Editors), *The Hypothalamus.* Oliver and Boyd, Edinburgh, pp. 131–185.

642. DOTY, R. W. 1968. Neural organization of deglutition. In C. P. GODE (Editor), *Handbook of Physiology*, Vol. IV, Sect. 6. American Physiological Society, Washington, D. C., pp. 1861–1902.

643. DOW, R. S. 1936. The fiber connections of the posterior parts of the cerebellum in the rat and cat. J. Comp. Neurol., **63**: 527–548.

644. DOW, R. S. 1938. Efferent connections of the flocculonodular lobe in *Macaca mulatta*. J. Comp. Neurol., **68**: 297–305.

645. DOW, R. S., AND MORUZZI, G. 1958. *The Physiology and Pathology of the Cerebellum.* University of Minnesota Press, Minneapolis.

646. DOWLING, J. E., AND BOYCOTT, B. B. 1966. Organization of the primate retina: Electron microscopy. Proc. R. Soc. Lond. (Biol.), **166**: 80–111.

647. DRACHMAN, D. A., AND ARBIT, J. 1966. Memory and the hippocampal complex. II. Is memory a multiple process? Arch. Neurol., **15**: 52–61.

648. DRAY, A., DAVIES, J., OAKLEY, N. R., TONGROACH, P., AND VELLUCCI, S. 1978. The dorsal and medial raphe projections to the substantia nigra in the rat: Electrophysiological, biochemical and behavioural observations. Brain Res., **151**: 431–442.

649. DRAY, A., GONYE, T. J., OAKLEY, N. R., AND TANNER, T. 1976. Evidence for the existence of a raphe projection to the substantia nigra in rat. Brain Res., **113**: 45–57.

650. DREIFUSS, J. J., MURPHY, J. T., AND GLOOR, P. 1968. Contrasting effects of two identified amygdaloid efferent pathways on single hypothalamic neurons. J. Neurophysiol., **31**: 237–248.

651. DROOGLEEVER-FORTUYN, J., AND STEFENS, R. 1951. On the anatomical relations of the intralaminar and midline cells of the thalamus. Electroencephalogr. Clin. Neurophysiol., **3**: 393–400.

652. DROZ, B., AND LEBLOND, C. P. 1963. Axonal migration of proteins in the central nervous system and peripheral nerves as shown by radioautography. J. Comp. Neurol., **121**: 325–346.

653. DROZ, B., RAMBOURG, A., AND KOENIG, H. L. 1975. The smooth endoplasmic reticulum: Structure and role in the renewal of axonal membrane and synaptic vesicles by fast axonal transport. Brain Res., **93**: 1–13.

654. DRUCKMAN, R. 1952. A critique of "suppression" with additional observations in the cat. Brain, **75**: 226–243.

655. DRUGA, R. 1966. Cortico-claustral connections. I. Fronto-claustral connections. Folia Morphol. (Praha), **14**: 391–399.

656. DRUGA, R. 1968. Cortico-claustral connections. II. Connections from the parietal, temporal and occipital cortex to the claustrum. Folia Morphol. (Praha), **16**: 142–149.

657. DUFFY, M. J., MULHALL, D., AND POWELL, D. 1975. Subcellular distribution of substance P in bovine hypothalamus and substantia nigra. J. Neurochem., **25**: 305–307.

658. DUFFY, P. E., GRAF, L., HUANG, Y.-Y., AND RAPPORT, M. M. 1979. Glial fibrillary acidic protein in ependymomas and other brain tumors. J. Neurol. Sci., **40**: 133–146.

659. DUN, N. J. 1980. Ganglionic transmission: Electrophysiology and pharmacology. Fed. Proc., **39**: 2182–2189.

660. DURON, B. 1973. Postural and ventilatory functions of intercostal muscles. Acta Neurobiol. Exp. (Warsz.), **33**: 355–380.

661. DUSSER DE BARENNE, J. G. 1924. Experimental researches on sensory localization in the cerebral cortex of the monkey. Proc. R. Soc. Lond. (Biol.), **96**: 272–291.

662. DUSSER DE BARENNE, J. G., GAROL, H. W., AND MCCULLOCH, W. S. 1942. Physiological neuronography of the corticostriatal connections. Proc. Assoc. Res. Nerv. Ment. Dis., **21**: 246–266.

663. DUSSER DE BARENNE, J. G., AND MCCULLOCH, W. S. 1939. Suppression of motor response upon stimulation of area 4S of the cerebral cortex. Am. J. Physiol., **126**: 482.

664. DUVERNOY, H. M. 1978. *Human Brainstem Vessels.* Springer-Verlag, Berlin.

665. EAGER, R. P. 1963. Efferent cortico-nuclear pathways in the cerebellum of the cat. J. Comp. Neurol., **120**: 81–103.

666. EAGER, R. P. 1963a. Cortical association pathways in the cerebellum of the cat. J. Comp. Neurol., **121**: 381–393.

667. EAGER, R. P. 1965. The mode of termination and temporal course of degeneration of cortical association pathways in the cerebellum of the cat. J. Comp. Neurol., **124**: 243–257.

668. EAGER, R. P., AND BARRNETT, R. J. 1966. Morphological and chemical studies of Nauta-stained degenerating cerebellar and hypothalamic fibers. J. Comp. Neurol., **126**: 487–510.

669. EARLE, K. M. 1952. The tract of Lissauer and its possible relation to the pain pathway. J. Comp. Neurol., **96**: 93–111.

670. Ebbeson, S. O. E. 1968. A connection between the dorsal column nuclei and the dorsal accessary olive. Brain Res., **8**: 393–397.

671. Eccles, J. C. 1959. Neuron physiology—Introduction. In J. Field (Editor), *Handbook of Physiology*, Section I, Vol. I. American Physiological Society, Washington, D. C., Ch. 2, pp. 59–74.

672. Eccles, J. C. 1966. Functional organization of the cerebellum in relation to its role in motor control. In R. Granit (Editor), *Muscular Afferents and Motor Control*. Almquist & Wiksell, Stockholm, pp. 19–36.

673. Eccles, J. C., Eccles, R. M., Iggo, A., and Lundberg, A. 1961. Electrophysiological investigations on Renshaw cells. J. Physiol. (Lond.), **159**: 461–478.

674. Eccles, J. C., Fatt, P., and Koketsu, K. 1954. Distribution of recurrent inhibition among motoneurons. J. Physiol. (Lond.), **126**: 524–562.

675. Eccles, J. C., Ito, M., and Szentágothai, J. 1967. *The Cerebellum as a Neuronal Machine*. Springer Verlag, New York.

676. Eccles, J. C., Llinás, R., and Sasaki, K. 1964. Excitation of cerebellar Purkinje cells by the climbing fibers. Nature, **203**: 245–246.

677. Eccles, J. C., Llinás, R., and Sasaki, K. 1966. The excitatory synaptic action of climbing fibres on the Purkinje cells of the cerebellum. J. Physiol. (Lond.), **182**: 268–296.

678. Eccles, J. C., Llinás, R., and Sasaki, K. 1966a. Parallel fibre stimulation and responses induced thereby in the Purkinje cells of the cerebellum. Exp. Brain Res., **1**: 17–39.

679. Eccles, J. C., Llinás, R., and Sasaki, K. 1966b. The inhibitory interneurones within the cerebellar cortex. Exp. Brain Res., **1**: 1–16.

680. Eccles, J. C., Llinás, R., and Sasaki, K. 1966c. The mossy fibre-granule cell relay of the cerebellum and its inhibitory control by Golgi cells. Exp. Brain Res., **1**: 82–101.

681. von Economo, C. F. 1911. Über dissoziierte Emphindungslähmung bei Ponstumoren und über die zentralen Bahnen des sensiblen Trigeminus. Jahrb. Psychiat. Neurol., **32**: 107–138.

682. von Economo, C. F. 1929. *The Cytoarchitectonics of the Human Cerebral Cortex*. Oxford Medical Publications, London, 186 pp.

683. von Economo, C., and Horn, L. 1930. Über Windungsrelief, Masse und Rindenarchitektonik der Supratemporalfläche, ihre individuellen und ihre Seitenunterschiede. Z. Gesamte Neurol. Psychiatry, **130**: 678–757.

684. von Economo, C. F., and Karplus, J. P. 1909. Zur Physiologie und Anatomie des Mittelhirns. Arch. Psychiatr. Nervenkr., **46**: 275–356.

685. Edinger, H. M., Siegel, A., and Troiano, R. 1975. Effect of stimulation of prefrontal cortex and amygdala on diencephalic neurons. Brain Res., **97**: 17–31.

686. Edwards, S. B. 1972. The ascending and descending projections of the red nucleus in the cat: An experimental study using an autoradiographic tracing method. Brain Res., **48**: 45–63.

687. Edwards, S. B. 1975. Autoradiographic studies of the projections of the midbrain reticular formation: Descending projections of the nucleus cuneiformis. J. Comp. Neurol., **161**: 341–358.

688. Edwards, S. B. 1977. The commissural projection of the superior colliculus in the cat. J. Comp. Neurol., **173**: 23–40.

689. Edwards, S. B., Ginsburgh, C. L., Henkel, C. K., and Stein, B. E. 1979. Sources of subcortical projections to the superior colliculus in the cat. J. Comp. Neurol., **184**: 309–330.

690. Edwards, S. B., and de Olmos, J. S. 1976. Autoradiographic studies of projections of the midbrain reticular formation: Ascending projections of nucleus cuneiformis. J. Comp. Neurol., **165**: 417–432.

691. Edwards, S. B., Rosenquist, A. C., and Palmer, L. A. 1974. An autoradiographic study of ventral lateral geniculate projections in the cat. Brain Res., **72**: 282–

287.

692. Ehringer, H., and Hornykiewicz, D. 1960. Verteilung von Noradrenalin und Dopamin (3-hydroxytyramin) in Gehirn des Menschen und ihr Verhalten bei Erkrankungen dis Extrapiramidalen Systems. Klin Wochenschr., **38**: 1236–1239.

693. Ehrlich, P. 1885. *Das Sauerstoff-Bedürfnis des Organismus. Eine Farbenanalytische Studie*. Herschwald, Berlin, pp. 69–72.

694. Elde, R., Hökfelt, T., Johansson, O., and Terenius, L. 1976. Immunohistochemical studies using antibodies to leucine-enkephalin: Initial observations on the nervous systems of the rat. Neuroscience, **1**: 349–351.

695. Eldred, E., and Fujimori, B. 1958. Relations of the reticular formation to muscle spindle activation. In H. H. Jaspers *et al.* (Editors), *Reticular Formation of the Brain*. Little, Brown and Company, Boston, pp. 275–283.

696. Eldred, E., Granit, R., and Merton, P. A. 1953. Supraspinal control of the muscle spindles and its significance. J. Physiol. (Lond.), **122**: 498–523.

697. Eleftheriou, B. E., Zolovick, A. J., and Pearse, R. 1966. Effects of amygdaloid lesions on pituitary-adrenal axis in the deer-mouse. Proc. Soc. Exp. Biol. Med., **122**: 1259.

698. Elfvin, L. G. 1958. The ultrastructure of unmyelinated fibers in the splenic nerve of the cat. J. Ultrastruct. Res., **1**: 428–454.

699. Eller, T., and Chan-Palay, V. 1976. Afferents to the cerebellar lateral nucleus: Evidence from retrograde transport of horseradish peroxidase after pressure injections through micropipettes. J. Comp. Neurol., **166**: 285–301.

700. Elliott, K. A. C., and Jasper, H. 1949. Measurement of experimentally induced brain swelling and shrinkage. Am. J. Physiol., **157**: 122–129.

701. Elman, R. 1923. Spinal arachnoid granulations with especial reference to the cerebrospinal fluid. Bull. Johns Hopkins Hosp., **34**: 99–104.

702. Elze, C. 1932. Centrales Nervensystem. In H. Braus, *Anatomie des Menschen. Ein Lehrbuch für Studierende und Ärzte*, Vol. III. Julius Springer, Berlin.

703. Emmelin, N. 1967. Nervous control of salivary glands. In C. F. Code (Editor), *Handbook of Physiology*, Section 6, Vol. II, *Secretion*. American Physiological Society, Washington, D. C., Ch. 37, pp. 595–632.

704. Emmelin, N., and Stromblad, B. C. R. 1954. A method of stimulating and inhibiting salivary secretion in man. Acta Physiol. Scand., **31** (suppl. 114): 12–13.

705. Emmers, R. 1964. Localization of thalamic projection of afferents from the tongue in the cat. Anat. Rec., **148**: 67–74.

706. Emmers, R. 1965. Organization of the first and second somesthetic regions (SI and SII) in the rat thalamus. J. Comp. Neurol., **124**: 215–227.

707. Emmers, R. 1966. Separate relays of tactile, thermal and gustatory modalities in the cat thalamus. Proc. Soc. Exp. Biol. Med., **121**: 527–531.

708. Emmers, R. 1973. Interaction of neural systems which control body water. Brain Res., **49**: 323–347.

709. Emmers, R. 1976. Thalamic mechanisms that process a temporal pulse code for pain. Brain Res., **103**: 425–441.

710. Emmers, R., Benjamin, R. M., and Blomquist, A. J. 1962. Thalamic localization of afferents from the tongue in albino rat. J. Comp. Neurol., **118**: 43–48.

711. Englander, R. N., Netsky, M. G., and Adelman, L. S. 1975. Location of human pyramidal tract in the internal capsule—Anatomical evidence. Neurology (Minneap.), **25**: 823–826.

712. Enna, S. J., Bennett, J. P., Byland, D. B., Snyder, S. H., Bird, E. D., and Iverson, L. L. 1976. Alterations of brain neurotransmitter receptor binding in Huntington's chorea. Brain Res., **116**: 531–537.

713. Enna, S. J., Kuhar, M. J., and Snyder, S. H. 1975. Regional distribution of postsynaptic receptor binding for gamma-aminobutyric acid (GABA) in

monkey brain. Brain Res., **93:** 168–174.

714. EPELBAUM, J., ARANCIBIA, L. T., KORDON, C., OTTERSEN, O. P., AND BEN-ARI, Y. 1979. Regional distribution of somatostatin within the amygdaloid complex of the rat brain. Brain Res., **174:** 172–174.

715. ERICKSON, T. C., AND WOOLSEY, C. N. 1951. Observations on the supplementary motor area of man. Trans. Am. Neurol. Assoc., **76:** 50–56.

716. ERLANGER, J., AND GASSER, H. S. 1937. *Electrical Signs of Nervous Activity.* University of Pennsylvania Press, Philadelphia, 221 pp.

717. ERULKAR, S. D., ROSE, J. C., AND DAVIES, P. W. 1956. Single unit activity in the auditory cortex of the cat. Bull. Johns Hopkins Hosp., **99:** 55–86.

718. ESSNER, E., AND NOVIKOFF, A. B. 1960. Human hepatocellular pigments and lysosomes. J. Ultrastruct. Res., **3:** 374–391.

719. VON EULER, C. 1979. On the neural organization of the motor control of the diaphragm. Am. Rev. Respir. Dis., **119:** 45–50.

720. VON EULER, U. S. 1956. *Noradrenaline.* Charles C Thomas, Publisher, Springfield, Ill.

721. VON EULER, U. S. 1961. Neurotransmission in the adrenergic nervous system. *The Harvey Lectures,* Ser. 55. Academic Press, New York, pp. 43–65.

722. VON EULER, U. S. 1966. Catecholamines in nerve and organ granules. In U. S. VON EULER et al. (Editors), *Mechanism of Release of Biogenic Amines.* Pergamon Press, New York, pp. 211–222.

723. VON EULER, U. S., AND GADDUM, J. H. 1931. An unidentified depressor substance in certain tissue extracts. J. Physiol. (Lond.), **72:** 74–87.

724. EVANS, E. F., ROSS, H. F., AND WHITFIELD, I. C. 1965. The spatial distribution of unit characteristic frequency in the primary auditory cortex of the cat. J. Physiol. (Lond.), **179:** 238–247.

725. EVANS, E. F., AND WHITFIELD, I. C. 1964. Classification of unit responses in the auditory cortex of the unanesthetized. J. Physiol. (Lond.), **171:** 476–493.

726. EVERETT, J. W. 1959. Neuroendocrine mechanisms in control of the mammalian ovary. In A. GORBMAN (Editor), *Comparative Endocrinology.* John Wiley & Sons, New York, pp. 168–174.

727. EVERETT, J. W. 1964. Central neural control of reproductive functions of the adenohypophysis. Physiol. Rev., **44:** 373–431.

728. FAHN, S., AND CÔTÉ, L. J. 1968. Regional distribution of δ-aminobutyric acid (GABA) in brain of the rhesus monkey. J. Neurochem., **15:** 209–213.

729. FAHRENKRUG, J., AND SCHAFFALITZKY DE MUCKADELL, D. B. 1978. Distribution of vasoactive intestinal polypeptide (VIP) in the porcine central nervous system. J. Neurochem., **31:** 1445–1451.

730. FALCK, B. 1962. Observations on the possibilities of the cellular localization of monoamines by a fluorescence method. Acta Physiol. Scand., **56**(suppl. 197): 1–25.

731. FALCK, B., HILLARP, N. Å., THIEME, G., AND TORP, A. 1962. Fluorescence of catecholamines and related compounds condensed with formaldehyde. J. Histochem. Cytochem., **10:** 348–354.

732. FALCK, B., AND TORP, A. 1962. A new evidence for localization of noradrenalin in adrenergic nerve terminals. Med. Exp. (Basel), **6:** 169–172.

733. FALCONER, M. A. 1948. Relief of intractable pain of organic origin by frontal lobotomy. Proc. Assoc. Res. Nerv. Ment. Dis., **27:** 706–722.

734. FALCONER, M. A. 1949. Intramedullary trigeminal tractotomy and its place in treatment of facial pain. J. Neurol. Neurosurg. Psychiatry, **12:** 297–311.

735. FARQUHAR, M. G., AND HARTMANN, J. F. 1957. Neuroglial structure and relationships as revealed by electron microscopy. J. Neuropathol. Exp. Neurol., **16:** 18–39.

736. FAULL, R. L. M., AND CARMAN, J. B. 1968. Ascending projections of the substantia nigra in the rat. J. Comp.

Neurol., **132:** 73–92.

737. FEINDEL, W., AND GLOOR, P. 1954. Comparisons of electrographic effects of stimulation of the amygdala and brain stem reticular formation in cats. Electroencephalogr. Clin. Neurophysiol., **6:** 389–402.

738. FEINDEL, W., AND PENFIELD, W. 1954. Localization of discharge in temporal lobe automatism. Arch. Neurol. Psychiatry, **72:** 605–630.

739. FELDBERG, W., AND SHERWOOD, S. L. 1954. Injections of drugs into the lateral ventricle of the cat. J. Physiol. (Lond.), **123:** 148–167.

740. FELTEN, D. L., LATIES, A. N., AND CARPENTER, M. B. 1974. Monamine-containing cell bodies in the squirrel monkey brain. Am. J. Anat., **139:** 153–166.

741. FENSTERMACHER, J. D., AND RALL, D. P. 1973. Physiology and pharmacology of cerebrospinal fluid. In *Pharmacology of the Cerebral Circulation,* Vol. 1. Pergamon Press, Oxford, pp. 35–79.

742. FERGUSON, R. K., AND WOODBURY, D. M. 1969. Penetration of ^{14}C-inulin and ^{14}C-sucrose into brain, cerebrospinal fluid and skeletal muscle of developing rats. Exp. Brain Res., **7:** 181–194.

743. FERNANDEZ, C., GOLDBERG, J. M., AND ABEND, W. K. 1972. Response to static tilts of peripheral neurons innervating otolith organs of the squirrel monkey. J. Neurophysiol., **35:** 978–997.

744. FERRARO, A. 1925. Contributa sperimentale allo studio della substantia nigra normale e dei suoi rapporti con la corteccia cerebrale e con il corpo striato. Arch. Gen. Neurol. Psychiatry, **6:** 26–117.

745. FERRARO, A. 1928. The connections of the pars suboculomotoria of the substantia nigra. Arch. Neurol. Psychiatry, **19:** 177–180.

746. FERRARO, A., AND BARRERA, S. E. 1935. Posterior column fibers and their terminations in the *Macacus rhesus.* J. Comp. Neurol., **62:** 507–530.

747. FERTUCK, H. C., AND SALPETER, M. M. 1976. Quantitation of junctional and extrajunctional acetylcholine receptors by electron microscope autoradiography after ^{125}I α-bungarotoxin binding at mouse neuromuscular junctions. J. Cell Biol., **69:** 144–158.

748. FIELDS, H. L., BASBAUM, A. I., CLANTON, C. H., AND ANDERSON, S. D. 1977. Nucleus raphe magnus inhibition of spinal cord dorsal horn neurons. Brain Res., **126:** 441–454.

749. FINK, D. J., AND GARNOR, H. 1980. Axonal transport of proteins: A new view using *in vivo* covalent labeling. J. Cell Biol., **85:** 175–186.

750. FINK, R. P., AND HEIMER, L. 1967. Two methods for selective silver impregnation of degenerating axons and their synaptic endings in the central nervous system. Brain Res., **4:** 369–374.

751. FINLAY, B. L., SCHNEPS, S. E., WILSON, F. G., AND SCHNEIDER, G. E. 1978. Topography of visual and somatosensory projections to the superior colliculus of the golden hamster. Brain Res., **142:** 223–235.

752. FINLEY, J. C. W., MADERDRUT, J. L., AND PETRUZ, P. 1981. The immunocytochemical localization of enkephalin in the central nervous system of the rat. J. Comp. Neurol., **198:** 541–565.

753. FLECHSIG, P. 1905. Einige Bemerkungen über die Untersuchungsmethoden der Grosshirnrinde, insbesondere des Menschen. Arch. Anat. Entwickl.-Gesch., 337–444.

754. FLOOD, S., AND JANSEN, J. 1961. On the cerebellar nuclei in the cat. Acta Anat. (Basel), **46:** 52–72.

754a. FLOODY, O. R., AND PFAFF, D. W. 1974. Steroid hormones and aggressive behavior: Approaches to the study of hormone sensitive brain mechanisms for behavior. Proc. Assoc. Nerv. Ment. Dis., **52:** 149–185.

755. FLUMERFELT, B. A., OTABE, S., AND COURVILLE, J. 1973. Distinct projections to the red nucleus from the dentate and interposed nuclei in the monkey. Brain Res., **50:** 408–414.

756. FLUUR, E. 1959. Influences of semicircular ducts on extraocular muscles. Acta Otolaryngol. [Suppl.]

(Stockh.), **149:** 1–46.

757. FLYNN, J. P. 1967. The neural basis of aggression in cats. In D. C. GLASS (Editor), *Neurophysiology and Emotion.* Rockefeller University Press and Russell Sage Foundation, New York, pp. 40–60.

758. FOERSTER, O. 1927. *Die Leitungsbahnen des Schmerzgefühles und die chirurgische Behandlung der Schmerzzustände.* Urban and Schwarzenberg, Berlin.

759. FOERSTER, O. 1929. Der Plexus lumbo-sacralis. In O. Bumke and O. Foerster (Editors), *Handbuch der Neurologie,* Suppl., Vol. 2. Julius Springer Verlag, Berlin, pp. 960–970.

760. FOERSTER, O. 1931. The cerebral cortex in man. Lancet, **2:** 309–312.

761. FOERSTER, O. 1933. The dermatomes in man. Brain, **56:** 1–39.

762. FOERSTER, O. 1936. Sensible cortical Felder. In O. BUMKE AND O. FOERSTER (Editors), *Handbuch der Neurologie,* Vol. 6. Julius Springer, Berlin, pp. 358–448.

763. FOERSTER, O. 1936*a.* Motor cortex in man in the light of Hughlings Jackson's doctrines. Brain, **59:** 135–159.

764. FOERSTER, O. 1936*b.* Symptomatologie der Erkrankungen des Grosshirns. Motorische Felder und Bahnen. In O. BUMKE AND O. FOERSTER (Editors), *Handbuch der Neurologie,* Vol. 6. Julius Springer, Berlin, pp. 1–357.

765. FOERSTER, O. 1936*c.* Symptomatologie der Erkrankungen des Rückenmarks und seiner Wurzeln. In O. BUMKE AND O. FOERSTER, (Editors), *Handbuch der Neurologie,* Vol. 5. Julius Springer, Berlin, pp. 1–400.

766. FOERSTER, O., AND GAGEL, O. 1932. Die Vorderseitenstrangdurchschneidung beim Menschen. Eine klinischpathophysiologisch-anatomische Studie. Z. Gesamte Neurol. Psychiatry, **138:** 1–92.

767. FOERSTER, O., GAGEL, O., AND SHEEHAN, D. 1933. Veränderungen an den Endösen im Rückenmark des Affen nach Hinterwurzeldurchschneidung. Z. Anat. Entwickl.-Gesch., **101:** 553–565.

768. FOIX, C. 1921. Les Lésions anatomiques de la maladie de Parkinson. Rev. Neurol. (Paris), **37:** 593–600.

769. FOIX, C., AND HILLEMAND, J. 1925. Les artères de l'axe encéphalique jusqu'au diencéphale inclusivement. Rev. Neurol. (Paris), **44:** 705–739.

770. FOIX, C., AND HILLEMAND, J. 1925. Irrigation de la couche optique. C. R. Soc. Biol. (Paris), **92:** 52–54.

771. FOIX, C., AND NICOLESCO, J. 1925. *Les Noyaux gris centraux et la région mesencephalo-sous-optique.* Masson et Cie, Paris.

772. FOLEY, J. M., KINNEY, T. D., AND ALEXANDER, L. 1942. The vascular supply of the hypothalamus in man. J. Neuropathol. Exp. Neurol., **1:** 265–296.

773. FOLEY, J. O., AND SCHNITZLEIN, H. N. 1957. The contributions of individual thoracic spinal nerves to the upper cervical sympathetic trunk. J. Comp. Neurol., **108:** 109–120.

774. FOLKMAN, J. 1971. Tumor angiogenesis: Theropeutic implications. N. Engl. J. Med., **285:** 1182–1186.

775. FONBERG, E. 1968. The role of the amygdaloid nucleus in animal behaviour. Prog. Brain Res., **22:** 273–281.

776. FONBERG, E., AND DELGADO, J. M. R. 1961. Avoidance and alimentary reactions during amygdala stimulation. J. Neurophysiol., **24:** 651–664.

777. FONNUM, F., GROFOVÁ, I., AND RINVIK, E. 1978. Origin and distribution of glutamate decarboxylase in the nucleus subthalamicus of the cat. Brain Res., **153:** 370–374.

778. FONNUM, F., GROFOVÁ, I., RINVIK, E., STORM-MATHISEN, J., AND WALBERG, F. 1974. Origin and distribution of glutamate decarboxylase in substantia nigra of the cat. Brain Res., **71:** 77–92.

779. FONNUM, F., AND STORM-MATHISEN, J. 1977. High affinity uptake of glutamate in terminals of corticostriate axons. Nature, **266:** 377–378.

780. FONNUM, F., STORM-MATHISEN, J., AND WALBERG,

F. 1970. Glutamate decarboxylase in inhibitory neurons: A study of the enzyme in Purkinje cell axons and boutons in the cat. Brain Res., **20:** 259–275.

781. FONNUM, F., AND WALBERG, F. 1973. An estimate of the concentration of δ-aminobutyric acid and glutamate decarboxylase in the inhibitory Purkinje axon terminals in the cat. Brain Res., **54:** 115–127.

782. FORBES, B. F., AND MOSKOWITZ, N. 1974. Projections of auditory responsive cortex in the squirrel monkey. Brain Res., **67:** 239–254.

783. FORD, D. H. 1976. Blood-brain barrier: A regulatory mechanism. Annu. Rev. Neurosci., **2:** 1–42.

784. FORN, J., AND GREENGARD, P. 1978. Depolarizing agents and cyclic nucleotides regulate the phosphorylation of specific neuronal proteins in rat cerebral cortex slices. Proc. Natl. Acad. Sci. U. S. A., **75:** 5195–5199.

785. FOX, C. A. 1940. Certain basal telencephalic centers in the cat. J. Comp. Neurol., **72:** 1–62.

786. FOX, C. A. 1943. The stria terminalis, longitudinal association bundle and precommissural fornix fibres in the cat. J. Comp. Neurol., **79:** 277–295.

787. FOX, C. A., ANDRADE, A. N., HILLMAN, D. E., AND SCHWYN, R. C. 1971. The spiny neurons in the primate striatum: A Golgi and electron microscopic study. J. Hirnforsch., **13:** 181–201.

788. FOX, C. A., ANDRADE, A. N., LU QUI, I., AND RAFOLS, J. A. 1974. The primate globus pallidus: A Golgi and electron microscopic study. J. Hirnforsch., **15:** 75–93.

789. FOX, C. A., ANDRADE, A. N., SCHWYN, R. C., AND RAFOLS, J. A. 1971/72. The aspiny neurons and the glia in the primate striatum: A Golgi and electron microscopic study. J. Hirnforsch., **13:** 341–362.

790. FOX, C. A., AND BARNARD, J. W. 1957. A quantitative study of the Purkinje cell, dendritic branchlets and their relationship to afferent fibres. J. Anat., **91:** 299–313.

791. FOX, C. A., FISHER, R. R., AND DESALVA, S. J. 1948. The distribution of the anterior commissure in the monkey (*Macaca mulatta*). Experimental studies. J. Comp. Neurol., **89:** 245–277.

792. FOX, C. A., HILLMAN, D. E., SIEGESMUND, K. A., AND DUTTA, C. R. 1967. The primate cerebellar cortex: A Golgi and electron microscope study. In C. A. FOX AND R. S. SNIDER (Editors), *The Cerebellum, Progress in Brain Research,* Vol. 25. Elsevier Publishing Company, Amsterdam, pp. 174–225.

793. FOX, C. A., HILLMAN, D. E., SIEGESMUND, K. A., AND SETHER, L. A. 1966. The primate globus pallidus and its feline and avian homologues: A Golgi and electron microscopic study. In R. HASSLER AND H. STEPHAN (Editors), *Evolution of the Forebrain.* Georg Thieme Verlag, Stuttgart, pp. 237–248.

794. FOX, C. A., McKINLEY, W. A., AND MAGOUN, H. W. 1944. An oscillographic study of olfactory system of cats. J. Neurophysiol., **7:** 1–16.

795. FOX, C. A., AND RAFOLS, J. A. 1975. The radial fibers in the globus pallidus. J. Comp. Neurol., **159:** 177–200.

796. FOX, C. A., RAFOLS, J. A., AND COWAN, W. M. 1975. Computer measurements of axis cylinder diameters of radial fibers and "comb" bundle fibers. J. Comp. Neurol., **159:** 201–224.

797. FOX, C. A., SIEGESMUND, K. A., AND DUTTA, C. R. 1964. The Purkinje cell dendritic branchlets and their relation with the parallel fibers: Light and electron microscopic observations. in M. M. COHEN, AND R. S. SNIDER, (Editors), *Morphological and Biochemical Correlates of Neural Activity.* Harper & Row, New York, Ch. 7, pp. 112–141.

798. FRANTZEN, E., AND OLIVARIUS, B. I. F. 1957. On thrombosis of the basilar artery. Acta Psychiatr. Neurol. Scand., **32:** 431–439.

799. FRASCHINI, F., COLLU, R., AND MARTINI, L. 1971. Mechanisms of inhibitory action of pineal principles on gonadotropin secretion. In G. E. W. WOLSTENHOLME AND J. KNIGHT (Editors), *The Pineal Gland.* Churchill Livingstone, Edinburgh, pp. 259–272.

800. FREDRICKSON, J. M., FIGGE, U., SCHEID, P., AND KORN-

HUBER, H. H. 1966. Vestibular nerve projection to the cerebral cortex of the rhesus monkey. Exp. Brain Res., **2**: 318–327.

801. FREDRICKSON, J. M., KORNHUBER, H. H., AND SCHWARZ, D. W. F. 1974. Cortical projections of the vesitubular nerve. In H. KORNHUBER (Editor), *Handbook of Sensory Physiology*, Vol. 6. Springer-Verlag, Berlin, pp. 565–582.

802. FREEMAN, L. W. 1952. Return of function after complete transection of the spinal cord of the rat, cat and dog. Am. Surg., **136**: 193–205.

803. FREEMAN, W., AND WATTS, J. W. 1947. Retrograde degeneration of the thalamus following prefrontal lobotomy. J. Comp. Neurol., **86**: 65–93.

804. FREEMAN, W., AND WATTS, J. W. 1948. The thalamic projection to the frontal lobe. A. Proc. Assoc. Res. Nerv. Ment. Dis., **27**: 200–209.

805. FREEMAN, W., AND WATTS, J. W. 1949. *Psychosurgery, Intelligence, Emotion and Social Behavior Following Prefrontal Lobotomy for Mental Disorders*, Ed. 2. Charles C Thomas, Publisher, Springfield, Ill., 337 pp.

806. FRENCH, J. D., HERNÁNDEZ-PEON, R., AND LIVINGSTON, R. B. 1955. Projections from cortex to cephalic brain stem (reticular formation) in monkey. J. Neurophysiol., **18**: 74–95.

807. FRENCH, J. D., AND MAGOUN, H. W. 1952. Effects of chronic lesions in central cephalic brain stem of monkeys. A. M. A. Arch. Neurol. Psychiatry, **68**: 591–604.

808. FRENCH, J. D., VERZEANO, M., AND MAGOUN, H. W. 1953. An extralemniscal sensory system in the brain. A. M. A. Arch. Neurol. Psychiatry, **69**: 505–518.

809. FRENCH, J. D., VON AMERONGEN, F. K., AND MAGOUN, H. W. 1952. An activating system in the brain stem of monkey. A. M. A. Arch. Neurol. Psychiatry, **68**: 577–590.

810. FREUND, H.-J. 1973. Neuronal mechanisms of the lateral geniculate body. In R. JUNG (Editor), *Handbook of Sensory Physiology: Central Processing of Visual Information. Part B, Morphology and Function of Visual Centers in the Brain*, Vol. 7, Part 3. Springer-Verlag, Berlin, pp. 177–246.

811. FRIEDE, R. 1961. A histochemical study of DPN-diaphorase in human white matter; with some notes on myelination. J. Neurochem., **8**: 17–30.

812. FRIEDMAN, D. P., JONES, E. G., AND BURTON, H. 1980. Representation pattern in the second somatic sensory area of the monkey cerebral cortex. J. Comp. Neurol., **192**: 21–41.

813. FRIEDMANN, U., AND ELKELES, A. 1932. Weitere Untersuchungen über die Permeabilität der Bluthirnschranke. Z. Gesamte Exp. Med., **80**: 212–234.

814. FRIEND, D. S., AND FARQUHAR, M. G. 1967. Functions of coated vesicles during protein absorption in the rat vas deferens. J. Cell Biol., **35**: 357–376.

815. FRIGYESI, T. L., AND SCHWARTZ, R. 1972. Cortical control of thalamic sensorimotor relay activities in the cat and squirrel monkey. In T. L. FRIGYESI AND M. D. YAHR (Editors), *Corticothalamic Projections and Sensorimotor Activities*. Raven Press, New York, pp. 161–195.

816. FRY, W. J., KRUMINS, R., FRY, F. J., THOMAS, G., BORBELY, S., AND ADES, H. 1963. Origins and distribution of some efferent pathways from the mammillary nuclei of the cat. J. Comp. Neurol., **120**: 195–258.

817. FUCHS, A. 1977. Role of the vestibular and reticular nuclei in the control of gaze: Reticular, prepositus and other internuclear neuronal activity. In. R. BAKER AND A. BERTHOZ (Editors), *Control of Gaze by Brain Stem Neurons: Developments in Neuroscience*. Elsevier North-Holland Biomedical Press, Amsterdam, pp. 341–348.

818. FUJII, K., CHAMBERS, S. M., AND RHOTON, A. L. JR. 1979. Neurovascular relationships of the sphenoid sinus-A microsurgical study. J. Neurosurg., **50**: 31–39.

819. FUJITA, S. 1964. Analysis of neuron differentiation in the central nervous system by tritiated thymidine autoradiography. J. Comp. Neurol., **122**: 311–327.

820. FUKUDA, Y., AND STONE, J. 1974. Retinal distribution and central projections of Y, X and W cells of the cat's retina. J. Neurophysiol., **37**: 749–772.

821. FUKUSHIMA, K., PETERSON, B. W., UCHINO, Y., COULTER, J. D., AND WILSON, V. J. 1977. Direct fastigiospinal fibers in the cat. Brain Res., **126**: 538–542.

822. FULTON, J. F. 1949. *Functional Localization in the Frontal Lobes and Cerebellum*. Clarendon Press, Oxford.

823. FULTON, J. F., AND INGRAHAM, F. D. 1929. Emotional disturbances following experimental lesions of the base of the brain (pre-chiasmal). J. Physiol. (Lond.), **67**: 27–28.

824. FULTON, J. F., AND KELLER, A. D. 1932. *The Sign of Babinski. A Study of the Evolution of Cortical Dominance in Primates*. Charles C Thomas, Springfield, Ill., 165 pp.

825. FULTON, J. F., AND KENNARD, M. A. 1934. A study of flaccid and spastic paralysis produced by lesions of the cerebral cortex in primates. Proc. Assoc. Res. Nerv. Ment. Dis., **13**: 158–210.

826. FULTON, J. F., AND PI-SUÑER, J. 1927-28. A note concerning the probable function of various afferent end-organs in skeletal muscle. Am. J. Physiol., **83**: 554–562.

827. FUXE, K. 1965. Evidence for the existence of monoamine neurons in the central nervous system. IV. Distribution of monoamine nerve terminals in the central nervous system. Acta Physiol. Scand., **64**(suppl. 247): 37–120.

828. FUXE, K., AND ANDÉN, N. E. 1966. Studies on the central monoamine neurons with special reference to the nigro-neostriatal dopamine neuron system. In E. Costa *et al.* (Editors), *Biochemistry and Pharmacology of the Basal Ganglia*. Raven Press, New York, pp. 123–129.

829. FUXE, K., AND HÖKFELT, T. 1970. Central monaminergic systems and hypothalamic function. In L. MARTIN *et al.* (Editors), *The Hypothalamus*. Academic Press, New York, pp. 123–138.

830. FUXE, K., HÖKFELT, T., ENEROTH, P., GUSTAFSSON, J.-Å., AND SKETT, P. 1977. Prolactin-like immunoreactivity: Localization in nerve terminals of rat hypothalamus. Science, **196**: 899–900.

831. FUXE, K., HÖKFELT, T., AND NILSSON, O. 1964. 1964. Observations on the cellular localization of dopamine in the caudate nucleus of the rat. Z. Zellforsch. Mikrosk. Anat., **63**: 701–706.

832. GABE, M., 1966. *Neurosecretion*. Translated by R. Crawford. Pergamon Press, Ltd., Oxford, pp. 427–736.

833. GACEK, R. R. 1961. The efferent cochlear bundle in man. Arch. Otolaryngol., **74**: 690–694.

834. GACEK, R. R. 1977. Location of brain stem neurons projecting to the oculomotor nucleus in the cat. Exp. Neurol., **57**: 725–749.

835. GACEK, R. R. 1978. Location of commissural neurons in the vestibular nuclei of the cat. Exp. Neurol., **59**: 479–491.

836. GACEK, R. R. 1979. Location of abducens afferent neurons in the cat. Exp. Neurol., **64**: 342–353.

837. GACEK, R. R., AND LYON, M. 1974. The localization of vestibular efferent neurons in the kitten with horseradish peroxidase. Acta Otolaryngol. (Stockh.), **77**: 92–101.

838. GADDUM, J. H., AND HAMEED, K. A. 1954. Drugs which antagonize 5-hydroxytryptamine. Br. J. Pharmacol., **9**: 240–248.

839. GALAMBOS, R. 1956. Suppression of auditory nerve activity by stimulation of efferent fibers to cochlea. J. Neurophysiol., **19**: 424–437.

840. GALAMBOS, R., AND ROSE, J. E. 1952. Microelectrode studies on medial geniculate body of the cat. III. Response to pure tone. J. Neurophysiol., **15**: 381–400.

841. GALE, K., HONG, J.-S., AND GUIDOTTI, A. 1977. Presence of substance P and GABA in separate striatonigral neurons. Brain Res., **36**: 371–375.

842. GALL, C., BRECHA, N., KARTEN H. J., AND CHANG, K.-J. 1981. Localization of enkephalin-like immunoreactivity to identified axonal and neuronal populations of the rat hippocampus. J. Comp. Neurol., **198**: 335–350.

843. GALLOWAY, J. R., AND GREITZ, T. 1960. The medial and lateral choroid arteries: An anatomic and roentgenographic study. Acta Radiol. (Stockh.), **53**: 353–356.

844. GAMBLE, H. J. 1964. Comparative electron-microscopic observations on the connective tissues of a peripheral nerve and a spinal nerve root in the rat. J. Anat., **98**: 17–25.

845. GANCHROW, D., AND ERICKSON, R. P. 1972. Thalamocortical relations in gustation. Brain Res., **36**: 289–305.

846. GARCIA-BENGOCHEA, F., CORRIGAN, R., MORGANE, P., RUSSELL, D., AND HEATH, R. 1951. Studies on the function of the temporal lobes: I. The section of the fornix. Trans. Am. Neurol. Assoc., **76**: 238–239.

847. GARDNER E. 1944. The distribution and termination of nerve fibers in the knee joint of the cat. J. Comp. Neurol., **80**: 11–32.

848. GAREY, L. J., JONES, E. G., AND POWELL, T. P. S. 1968. Interrelationships of striate and extrastriate cortex with the primary relay sites of the visual pathway. J. Neurol. Neurosurg. Psychiatry, **31**: 135–157.

849. GAREY, L. J., AND POWELL, T. P. S. 1967. The projection of the lateral geniculate nucleus upon the cortex in the cat. Proc. R. Soc. B, **169**: 107–126.

850. GAREY, L. J., AND POWELL, T. P. S. 1968. The projection of the retina in the cat. J. Anat., **102**: 189–222.

851. GAREY, L. J., AND POWELL, T. P. S. 1971. An experimental study of the termination of the lateral geniculocortical pathway in the cat and monkey. Proc. R. Soc. Lond. (Biol.), **179**: 41–63.

852. GARVEN, H. S. D. 1925. The nerve endings in the Panniculus carnosus of the hedgehog, with special reference to the sympathetic innervation of striated muscle. Brain, **48**: 380–441.

853. GASKELL, W. H. 1916. *The Involuntary Nervous System.* Longmans, Green and Company, London.

854. GASSER, G. 1961 *Basic Neuro-Pathological Technique.* Blackwell Scientific Publications, Oxford, pp. 39–74.

855. GASSER, H. S., AND GRUNDFEST, H. 1939. Axon diameters in relation to the spike dimensions and the conduction velocity in mammalian A fibers. Am. J. Physiol., **127**: 393–414.

856. GAZZANIGA, M. S. 1970. *The Bisected Brain.* Appleton-Century-Crofts, New York.

857. GAZZANIGA, M. S., BOGEN, J. E., AND SPERRY, R. W. 1965. Observations on visual perception after disconnexion of the cerebral hemispheres in man. Brain, **88**: 221–236.

858. GAZZANIGA, M. S., AND SPERRY, R. W. 1967. Language after section of the cerebral commissures. Brain, **90**: 131–148.

859. GEIS, G. S., AND WURSTER, R. D. 1980. Horseradish peroxidase localization of cardiac vagal preganglionic somata. Brain Res., **182**: 19–31.

860. GENIEC, P., AND MOREST, D. K. 1971. The Neuronal architecture of the human posterior colliculus. Acta otolaryngol. [Suppl.] (Stockh.), **295**: 1–33.

861. GEORGE, A. E., SALAMON, G., AND KRICHEFF, I. N. 1975. Pathologic anatomy of the thalmoperforating arteries in lesions of the third ventricle: Part II. Am. J. Roentgenol. Radium Ther. Nucl. Med., **124**: 231–240.

862. GERARD, R. W., MARSHALL W. H., AND SAUL, L. J. 1936. Electrical activity of the cat's brain. Arch. Neurol. Psychiatry, **36**: 675–738.

863. GEREBTZOFF, M. A. 1940. Recherches sur la projection corticale du labyrinthe. I. Des effets de la stimulation labyrinthique sur l'activité électrique de l'écorce cérébrale. Arch. Int. Physiol. Biochim., **50**: 365–378.

864. GEREN, B. B. 1954. The formation from the Schwann cell surface of the myelin in peripheral nerves of chick embryos. Exp. Cell Res., **7**: 558–562.

865. GERSHON, M. D. 1981. The enteric nervous system. Annu. Rev. Neurosci., **4**, 227–272.

866. GERSHON, M. D., AND DREYFUS, C. F. 1977. Serotonergic neurons in the mammalian gut. In F. P. BROOKS AND P. W. EVERS (Editors), *Nerves and the Gut.* Charles B. Slack, Inc., Thorofare, N. J., pp. 197–206.

867. GERSTMANN, J. 1940. Syndrome of finger agnosia: Disorientation for right and left, agraphia and acalculia. Arch. Neurol. Psychiatry, **44**: 398–408.

868. GESCHWIND, N. 1965. Disconnexion syndromes in animals and man. I. Brain, **88**: 237–294.

869. GESCHWIND, N. 1956a. Disconnexion syndromes in animals and man. II. Brain, **88**: 585–644.

870. GESCHWIND, N. 1970. The organization of language and the brain. Science, **170**: 940–944.

871. GESCHWIND, N., AND KAPLAN, E. 1962. A human cerebral deconnection syndrome. Neurology (Minneap.), **12**: 675–685.

872. GETCHELL, T. V., AND SHEPHERD, G. M. 1975. Short-axon cells in the olfactory bulb: Dendrodendritic synaptic interactions. J. Physiol. (Lond.), **251**: 523–548.

873. GEYER, M. A., PUERTO, A., DAWSEY, W. J., KNAPP, S., BULLARD, W. P., AND MANDELL, A. J. 1976. Histologic and enzymatic studies of the mesolimbic and mesotriatal serotoninergic pathways. Brain Res., **106**: 241–256.

874. GIBS, H., CARVER, C. C., RHOTON, A. L., LENKEY, C. AND MITCHELL, R. J. 1981. Microsurgical anatomy of the middle cerebral artery. J. Neurosurg., **54**: 151–169.

875. GILBERT, C. D., AND KELLY, J. P. 1975. The projection of cells in different layers of the cat's visual cortex. J. Comp. Neurol., **163**: 81–106.

876. GILBERT, G. J. 1960. The subcommissural organ. Neurology, **10**: 138–142.

877. GILBERT, G. J., AND GLASER, G. H. 1961. On the nervous system integration of water and salt metabolism. Arch. Neurol., **5**: 179–196.

878. GILLILAN, L. A. 1958. The arterial blood supply of the human spinal cord. J. Comp. Neurol., **110**: 75–103.

879. GILLILAN, L. A. 1964. The correlation of the blood supply to the human brain stem with clinical brain stem lesions. J. Neuropathol. Exp. Neurol., **23**: 78–108.

880. GILLINGHAM, F. J. 1962. Small localized surgical lesions of the internal capsule in the treatment of dyskinesia. Confin. Neurol., **22**: 385–392.

881. GILMAN, S. 1969. The mechanism of cerebellar hypotonia: An experimental study in the monkey. Brain, **92**: 621–638.

882. GILMAN, S., LIEBERMAN, J. S., AND COPACK, P. 1971. A thalamic mechanism of postural control. Int. J. Neurol., **8**: 260–275.

883. GILMAN, S., LIEBERMAN, J. S., AND MARCO, L. A. 1974. Spinal mechanisms underlying the effects of unilateral ablations of area 4 and 6 in monkeys. Brain, **97**: 49–64.

884. GILMAN, S., AND MARCO, L. A. 1971. Effects of medullary pyramidotomy in the monkey. I. Clinical and electromyographic abnormalities. Brain, **94**: 495–514.

885. GIOLLI, R. A., AND GUTHRIE, M. D. 1969. The primary optic projections in the rabbit: An experimental degeneration study. J. Comp. Neurol., **136**: 99–126.

886. GIOLLI, R. A., AND GUTHRIE, M. D. 1971. Organization of subcortical projections of visual areas I and II in the rabbit: An experimental degeneration study. J. Comp. Neurol., **142**: 351–376.

887. GIOLLI, R. A., AND TIGGES, J. 1970. The primary optic pathways and nuclei of primates. In C. R. NOBACK AND W. MONTAGNA (Editors), *The Primate Brain, Advances in Primatology*, Vol. 1. Appleton-Century-Crofts, New York, Ch. 2, pp. 29–54.

888. GIORGI, P. P., AND VAN DER LOOS, H. 1978. Axons

from eyes grafted in Xenopus can grow into the spinal cord and reach the optic tectum. Nature, **275:** 746–748.

889. GLEES, P. 1945. The interrelation of the striopallidum and the thalamus in the macaque monkey. Brain, **68:** 331–346.

890. GLEES, P. 1946. Terminal degeneration within the central nervous system as studied by a new silver method. J. Neuropathol. Exp. Neurol., **5:** 54–59.

891. GLEES, P. 1955. *Neuroglia. Morphology and Function.* Charles C Thomas Publisher, Springfield, Ill.

892. GLEES, P. 1961. *Experimental Neurology.* Oxford University Press, London.

893. GLEES, P. 1961a. Terminal degeneration and transsynaptic atrophy in the lateral geniculate body of the monkey. In R. JUNG AND H. KORNHUBER (Editors), *The Visual System: Neurophysiology and Psychophysics.* Springer-Verlag, Berlin, pp. 104–110.

894. GLEES, P., AND CLARKE, W. E. L. 1941. The termination of optic fibers in the lateral geniculate body of the monkey. J. Anat., **75:** 295–310.

895. GLEES, P., AND GRIFFITH, H. B. 1952. Bilateral destruction of the hippocampus (cornu ammonis) in a case of dementia. Monatsschr. Psychiatr. Neurol., **123:** 193–204.

896. GLEES, P., AND NAUTA, W. J. H. 1955. A critical review of studies on axonal and terminal degeneration. Monatsschr. Psychiatr. Neurol., **129:** 74–91.

897. GLENDENNING, K. K., HALL, J. A., DIAMOND, I. T., AND HALL, W. C. 1975. The pulvinar nucleus of Galago sensgalensis. J. Comp. Neurol., **161:** 419–458.

898. GLICKSTEIN, M., KING, R. A., MILLER, J., AND BERKLEY, M. 1967. Cortical projection from the dorsal lateral geniculate nucleus of cats. J. Comp. Neurol., **130:** 55–76.

899. GLOOR, P. 1955. Electrophysiological studies on the connections of the amygdaloid nucleus in the cat. Electroencephalogr. Clin. Neurophysiol., **7:** 243–264.

900. GLOOR, P. 1960. Amygdala. In J. FIELD (Editor), *Handbook of Physiology,* Section 1, Vol. II. American Physiological Society, Washington, D. C., Ch. 57, pp. 1395–1420.

901. GLOOR, P. 1972. Temporal lobe epilepsy: Its possible contribution to the understanding of the functional significance of the amygdala and of its interaction with neocortical-temporal mechanisms. In B. E. ELEFTHERIOU (Editor), *The Neurobiology of the Amygdala.* Plenum Press, New York, pp. 423–457.

902. GLUSMAN, M. 1974. The hypothalamic "savage" syndrome. Proc. Assoc. Res. Nerv. Ment. Dis., **52:** 52–92.

903. GOBEL, S. 1975. Golgi studies of the substantia gelatinosa neurons in the spinal trigeminal nucleus. J. Comp. Neurol., **162:** 397–416.

904. GOBEL, S. 1978. Golgi studies of the neurons in layer I of the dorsal horn of the medulla (trigeminal nucleus caudalis). J. Comp. Neurol., **180:** 375–394.

905. GOBEL, S. 1978a. Golgi studies of the neurons in layer II of the dorsal horn of the medulla (trigeminal nucleus caudalis). J. Comp. Neurol., **180:** 395–414.

906. GOBEL, S., AND BINCK, J. M. 1977. Degenerative changes in primary trigeminal axons and in neurons in nucleus caudalis following tooth pulp extirpations in the cat. Brain Res., **132:** 347–354.

907. GOBEL, S., AND PURVIS, M. B. 1972. Anatomical studies of the organization of the spinal V nucleus: The deep bundles and the spinal V tract. Brain Res., **48:** 27–44.

908. GOLDBERG, J. M., AND FERNÁNDEZ, C. 1980. Efferent vestibular system in the squirrel monkey: Anatomical location and influence on afferent activity. J. Neurophysiol., **43:** 986–1025.

909. GOLDMAN, P. S., AND NAUTA, W. J. H. 1977. Columnar distribution of cortico-cortical fibres in the frontal association, limbic and motor cortex of the developing Rhesus monkey. Brain Res., **122:** 393–413.

910. GOLDSTEIN, M. 1968. The auditory periphery. In V. B. Mountcastle (Editor), *Medical Physiology,* Ed. 12. C.

V. Mosby Company, St. Louis, Ch. 64, pp. 1465–1498.

911. GOLDSTEIN, M. H., JR., AND ABELES, M. 1975. Note on tonotopic organization of primary auditory cortex in the cat. Brain Res., **100:** 188–191.

912. GOLDSTEIN, M. H., JR., ABELES, M., DALY, R. L., AND MCINTOSH, J. 1970. Functional architecture in cat primary auditory cortex: Tonotopic organization. J. Neurophysiol., **33:** 188–197.

913. GOLGI, C. 1882–1885. Sulla fine anatomia degli organi centrali del sistema nervoso. Riv. Sper. Freniat. Med. Leg., **8:** 165–195, 361–391; **9:** 1–17, 161–192, 385–402; **11:** 72–123, 193–220.

914. GOLGI, C. 1883. Recherches sur l'histologie des centres nerveux. Arch. Ital. Biol., **3:** 285–317; **4:** 92–123.

915. GOLGI, C. 1894. *Untersuchungen über den feineren Bau des centralen und peripherischen Nervensystems.* Gustav Fischer, Jena.

916. GOLGI, C. 1898. Sur la structure des cellules nerveuses. Arch. Ital. Biol., **30:** 60–71.

917. GOMEZ, D. G., CHAMBERS, A. A., DIBENEDETTO, A. T., AND POTTS, D. G. 1974. The spinal cerebrospinal fluid absorptive pathways. Neuroradiology, **8:** 61–66.

918. GOMEZ, D. G., POTTS, D. G., AND DEONARINE, J. 1974. Arachnoid granulations of sheep: Structural and ultrastructural changes with varying pressure differences. Arch. Neurol., **30:** 169–175.

919. GOODWIN, G. M., MCCLOSKEY, D. I., AND MATTHEWS, P. B. C. 1972. Proprioceptive illusions induced by muscle vibration: Contribution by muscle spindles to perception? Science, **175:** 1382–1384.

920. GORDON, B. 1972. The superior colliculus of the brain. Sc. Am., **227:** 72–82.

921. GORDON, G., AND JUKES, M. G. M. 1964. Dual organization of exteroceptive components of the cat's gracile nucleus. J. Physiol. (Lond.), **173:** 263–290.

922. GORDON, G., AND JUKES, M. G. M. 1964a. Descending influences on the exteroceptive organization of the cat's gracile nucleus. J. Physiol. (Lond.), **173:** 291–319.

923. GORDON, G., AND PAINE, P. H. 1960. Functional organization in nucleus gracilis of the cat. J. Physiol. (Lond.), **153:** 331–349.

924. GORRY, J. D. 1963. Studies on the comparative anatomy of the ganglion basale of Meynart. Acta Anat. (Basel), **55:** 51–104.

925. GORSKI, R. A., CSERNUS, V. J., AND JACOBSON, C. D. 1981. Sexual dimorphism in the preoptic area. In B. FLERKÓ, G. SÉTÁLÓ, L. TIMA (Editors), *Advances in Physiological Science,* Vol 15: *Reproduction and Development,* 121–130.

926. GORSKI, R. A., GORDON, J. H. SHRYNE, J. E., AND SOUTHAM, A. M. 1978. Evidence for a morphological sex difference within the medial preoptic area of the rat brain. Brain Res., **148:** 333–346.

927. GORSKI, R. A., HARLAN, R. E., JACOBSON, C. D., SHRYNE, J. E., AND SOUTHAM, A. M. 1980. Evidence for the existence of a sexually dimorphic nucleus in the preoptic area of the rat. J. Comp. Neurol., **193:** 529–539.

928. GOTTLIEB, D. I., AND GLASER, L. 1980. Cellular recognition during neural development. Annu. Rev. Neurosci., **3:** 303–318.

928a. GOTTESFELD, A., MASSARI, V. J., MUTH, E. A., AND JACOBOWITZ, D. M. 1977. Stria medullaris; a possible pathway containing GABAergic afferents to the lateral habenula. Brain Res., **130:** 184–189.

929. GOULD, B. B. 1979. The organization of afferents to the cerebellar cortex in the cat: Projections from the deep cerebellar nuclei. J. Comp. Neurol., **184:** 27–42.

930. GOULD, B. B. 1980. Organization of afferents from the brain stem nuclei to the cerebellar cortex in the cat. Adv. Anat. Embryol. Cell Biol., **62:** 1–90.

931. GOULD, B. B., AND GRAYBIEL, A. M. 1976. Afferents to the cerebellar cortex in the cat: Evidence for an intrinsic pathway leading from the deep nuclei to the cortex. Brain Res., **110:** 601–611.

932. GRAFSTEIN, B. 1977. Axonal transport: the ultracel-

lular traffic of the neuron. In E. R. KANDEL (Editor), *Handbook of Physiology*, Section I: *The Nervous System*, Vol. I, *Cell Biology of Neurons*, Part I. American Physiological Society, Washington, D.C., pp. 691–717.

933. GRAFSTEIN, B., AND LAURENO, R. 1973. Transport of radioactivity from eye to visual cortex in the mouse. Exp. Neurol., **39**: 44–57.

934. GRAFSTEIN, B., MILLER, J. A., LEDEEN, R. W., HALEY, J., AND SPECHT, S. C. 1975. Axonal transport of phospholipid in goldfish optic system. Exp. Neurol., **46**: 261–281.

935. GRAHAM, J. 1977. An autoradiographic study of the efferent connections of the superior colliculus in the cat. J. Comp. Neurol., **173**: 629–654.

936. GRAHAM, R. C., JR., AND KARNOVSKY, M. J. 1966. The early stages of absorption of injected horseradish peroxidase in the proximal tubules of the mouse kidney: Ultrastructural cytochemistry by a new technique. J. Histochem. Cytochem., **14**: 291–302.

937. GRANIT, R. 1955. *Receptors and Sensory Perception*. Yale University Press, New Haven, Conn.

938. GRANIT, R., AND KAADA, B. R. 1952. Influence of stimulation of central nervous structures on muscle spindles in cat. Acta Physiol. Scand., **27**: 130–160.

939. GRANT, G. 1962. Projection of the external cuneate nucleus onto the cerebellum in the cat: An experimental study using silver methods. Exp. Neurol., **5**: 179–195.

940. GRANT, G. 1962a. Spinal course and somatotopically localized termination of the spinocerebellar tracts: An experimental study in the cat. Acta Physiol. Scand. **56**: (suppl. 193): 1–45.

941. GRANT, G., AND REXED, B. 1958. Dorsal spinal root afferents to Clarke's column. Brain, **81**: 567–576.

942. GRAY, E. G. 1961. The granule cells, mossy synapses and Purkinje spine synapses of the cerebellum: Light and electron microscopic observations. J. Anat., **95**: 345–356.

943. GRAY, E. G., AND GUILLERY, R. W. 1961. The basis for silver staining of synapses of the mammalian spinal cord: A light and electron microscope study. J. Physiol. (Lond.), **157**: 581–588.

944. GRAY, E. G., AND GUILLERY, R. W. 1966. Synaptic morphology in the normal and degenerating nervous system. Int. Rev. Cytol. **19**: 111–182.

945. GRAY, J. A. B. 1959. Initiation of impulses at receptors. In J. FIELD (Editor), *Handbook of Physiology*, Section I, Vol. 1. American Physiological Society, Washington, D. C., Ch. 4, pp. 123–145.

946. GRAYBIEL, A. M. 1972. Some extrageniculate visual pathways in the cat. Invest. Ophthalmol., **11**: 322–332.

947. GRAYBIEL, A. M. 1975. Anatomical organization of retinotectal afferents in the cat: An autoradiographic study. Brain Res., **96**: 1–24.

948. GRAYBIEL, A. M. 1977. Direct and indirect preoculomotor pathways of the brainstem: An autoradiographic study of the pontine reticular formation in the cat. J. Comp. Neurol., **175**: 37–78.

949. GRAYBIEL, A. M. 1978. Organization of the nigrotectal connection: An experimental tracer study in the cat. Brain Res., **143**: 339–348.

950. GRAYBIEL, A. M. 1978a. A satellite system of the superior colliculus: The parabigeminal nucleus and its projection to the superficial collicular layers. Brain Res., **145**: 365–374.

951. GRAYBIEL, A. M., AND HARTWIEG, E. A. 1974. Some afferent connections of the oculomotor complex in the cat: An experimental study with tracer techniques. Brain Res., **81**: 543–551.

952. GRAYBIEL, A. M., AND SCIASCIA, T. R. 1975. Origin and distribution of nigrotectal fibers in the cat. Neurosci. Abstr., **1**: 271.

953. GRAZER, F. M., AND CLEMENTE, C. D. 1957. Developing blood-brain barrier to trypan blue. Proc. Soc. Exp. Biol. Med., **94**: 758–760.

954. GREEN, J. D. 1958. The rhinencephalon: Aspects of its relation to behavior and the reticular activating system. In H. H. JASPERS ET AL. (Editors), *Reticular Formation of the Brain*. Henry Ford Hospital International Symposium. Little, Brown and Company, Boston, pp. 607–619.

955. GREEN, J. D. 1960. The hippocampus. In J. FIELD (Editor), *Handbook of Physiology*, Section I, Vol. II. American Physiological Society, Washington, D.C., Ch. 56, pp 1373–1389.

956. GREEN, J. D. 1964. The hippocampus. Physiol. Rev., **44**: 561–608.

957. GREEN, J. D., CLEMENTE, C. A., AND DE GROOT, J. 1957. Rhinencephalic lesions and behavior in cats. J. Comp. Neurol., **108**: 505–545.

958. GREEN, J. D., AND HARRIS, G. W. 1949. Observation of the hypophysioportal vessels of the living rat. J. Physiol. (Lond.), **108**: 359–361.

959. GREEN, J. D., AND SHIMAMOTO, T. 1953. Hippocampal seizures and their propagation. Arch. Neurol. Psychiatry, **70**: 687–702.

960. GREEN, J. R., DUISBERG, R. E. H., AND MCGRATH, W. B. 1951. Focal epilepsy of psychomotor type. A preliminary report of observations on effects of surgical therapy. J. Neurosurg., **8**: 157–172.

961. GREEN, J. R., DUISBERG, R. E. H., AND MCGRATH W. B. 1952. Orbitofrontal lobotomy with reference to effects on 55 psychotic patients. J. Neurosurg., **9**: 579–587.

962. GREENE, J., AND JAMPEL, R. 1966. Muscle spindles in the extraocular muscles of the Macaque. J. Comp. Neurol., **126**: 547–550.

963. GREENGARD, P. 1976. Possible role for cyclic nucleotides and phosphorylated membrane proteins in postsynaptic actions of neurotransmitters. Nature, **260**: 101–108.

964. GREENGARD, P. 1978. *Cyclic Nucleotides, Phosphorylated Proteins and Neuronal Structure*. Raven Press, New York, 124 pp.

965. GREENGARD, P. 1979. Cyclic nucleotides, phosphorylated proteins and the nervous system. Fed. Proc., **38**: 2208–2217.

966. GREER, M. A., AND ERWIN, H. L. 1956. Evidence of separate hypothalamic centers controlling corticotropin and thyrotropin secretion by the pituitary. Endocrinology, **58**: 665–670.

967. GREVING, R. 1935. Makroskopische Anatomie und Histologie des vegetativen Nervensystems. In O. BUMKE AND O. FOERSTER (Editors), *Handbuch der Neurologie*, Vol. 1, Julius Springer, Berlin, pp. 811–886.

968. GROENEWEGEN, H. J., BECKER, N. E. H. M., AND LOHMAN, A. H. M. 1980. Subcortical afferents of the nucleus accumbens septi in the cat, studied with retrograde axonal transport of horseradish peroxidase and bisbenzimid. Neuroscience, **5**: 1903–1916.

969. GROFOVÁ, I. 1975. The identification of striatal and pallidal neurons projecting to substantia nigra: An experimental study by means of retrograde axonal transport of horseradish peroxidase. Brain Res., *91:* 286–291.

970. GROFOVÁ, I., AND RINVIK, E. 1970. An experimental study on the striatonigral projection in the cat. Exp. Brain Res., **11**: 249–262.

971. GROFOVÁ, I., AND RINVIK, E. 1974. Cortical and pallidal projections to the nucleus ventralis lateralis thalami: Electron microscopically studies in the cat. Anat Embryol. (Berl.), **146**: 113–132.

972. DE GROOT, J., AND HARRIS, G. W. 1950. Hypothalmic control of the anterior pituitary gland and blood lymphocytes. J. Physiol. (Lond.), **111**: 335–346.

973. GROS, C., PRADELLES, P., DRAY, F., LE GAL Y DE SALLE, G., AND BEN-ARAI, Y. 1978. Regional distribution of met-enkephalin within the amygdaloid complex and bed nucleus of the stria terminalis. Neurosci. Lett., **10**: 193–196.

974. GROSS, N. B., LIFSCHITZ, W. S., AND ANDERSON, D. J. 1974. The tonotopic organization of the auditory thalamus of the squirrel monkey (*Saimiri sciureus*). Brain Res., **65**: 323–332.

975. GRUNDFEST, H. 1939. The properties of mammalian B fibers. Am. J. Physiol., **127**: 252–262.

976. GRUNDFEST, H. 1940. Bioelectric potentials. Annu. Rev. Physiol., **2**: 213–242.

977. GRUNSTEIN, A. M. 1911. Zur Frage von den Leitungsbahnen des Corpus striatum. Neurol. Zentralbl., **30**: 659–665.

978. GUILLEMIN, R., LING, N., BURGUS, R., BLOOM, F. E., AND SEGAL, D. 1977. Characterization of the endorphins, novel hypothalamic and neurohypophysial peptides with opiate-like activity: Evidence that they induce profound behavioral changes. Psychoneuroendocrinology, **2**: 59–62.

979. GUILLERY, R. W. 1956. Degeneration in the posterior commissural fornix and the mammillary peduncle of the rat. J. Anat., **90**: 350–370.

980. GUILLERY, R. W. 1957. Degeneration in the hypothalamic connexions of the albino rat. J. Anat., **91**: 91–115.

981. GUILLERY, R. W. 1966. A study of Golgi preparations from the dorsal lateral geniculate nucleus of the adult cat. J. Comp. Neurol., **128**: 21–50.

982. GUILLERY, R. W. 1967. A light and electron microscopic study of neurofibrils and neurofilaments at neuroneuronal junctions in the lateral geniculate nucleus of the cat. Am. J. Anat., **120**: 583–604.

983. GUILLERY, R. W. 1970. The laminar distribution of retinal fibres in the dorsal lateral geniculate nucleus of the cat: A new interpretation. J. Comp. Neurol., **138**: 339–369.

984. GUILLERY, R. W., ADRIAN, H. O., WOOLSEY, C. N., AND ROSE, J. E. 1966. Activation of somatosensory areas I and II of the cat's cerebral cortex by focal stimulation of the basoventral complex. In D. P. PURPURA AND M. D. YAHR (Editors), The Thalamus, Columbia University Press, New York, pp. 197–204.

985. GUILLERY, R. W., AND STELZNER, D. J. 1970. The differential effects of unilateral lid closure upon the monocular and binocular segments of the dorsal lateral geniculate nucleus in the cat. J. Comp. Neurol., **139**: 413–422.

986. GULLEY, R. L., AND WOOD, R. L. 1971. The fine structure of the neurons in the rat substantia nigra. Tissue Cell, **3**: 675–690.

987. GUTMANN, E., GUTTMANN, L., MEDAWAR, P. B., AND YOUNG, J. Z. 1942. Rate of regeneration of nerve. J. Exp. Biol., **19**: 14–44.

988. GUTMANN, E., AND YOUNG, J. Z. 1944. The re-innervation of muscle after various periods of atrophy. J. Anat., **78**: 15–43.

989. GUTTMANN, L. 1946. Rehabilitation after injuries to spinal cord and cauda equina. Br. J. Phys. Med. Indus. Hyg., **9**: 162–171.

990. GUTTMANN, L. 1952. Studies on reflex activity of the isolated cord in the spinal man. J. Nerv. Ment. Dis., **116**: 957–972.

991. GWYN, D. G., LESLIE, R. A., AND HOPKINS, D. A. 1979. Gastric afferent to the nucleus of the solitary tract in the cat. Neurosci. Lett., **14**: 13–17.

992. HA, H. 1971. Cervicothalamic tract in the rhesus monkey. Exp. Neurol., **33**: 205–212.

993. HA, H., AND LIU, C. N. 1968. Cell origin of the ventral spinocerebellar tract. J. Comp. Neurol., **133**: 185–205.

994. HA, H., AND MORIN, F. 1964. Comparative anatomical observations of the cervical nucleus, n. cervicalis lateralis, of some primates. Anat. Rec., **148**: 374 (abstract).

995. HABER, L. H., MARTIN, R. F., CHATT, A. B., AND WILLIS, W. D. 1978. Effects of stimulation in nucleus reticularis gigantocellularis on the activity of spinothalamic tract neurons in the monkey. Brain Res., **153**: 163–168.

996. HABERLY, L. B., AND PRICE, J. L. 1977. The axonal projection patterns of the mitral and tufted cells of the olfactory bulb in the rat. Brain Res., **129**: 152–157.

997. HAEFELY, W., HÜRLIMANN, A., AND THOENEN, H. 1965. Relations between the rate of stimulation and the quantity of noradrenaline liberated from the sympathetic nerve endings in the isolated perfused spleen of the cat. J. Physiol. (Lond.), **181**: 48–58.

998. HAGBARTH, K. E., AND KERR, D. I. B. 1954. Central influences on spinal afferent conduction. J. Neurophysiol., **17**: 295–307.

999. HÄGGQVIST, G. 1937. Faseranalytische Studien über die Pyramidenbahn. Acta Psychiatr. Neurol., **12**: 457–466.

1000. HAIGHT, J. R. 1972. The general organization of somatotopic projections to S II cerebral neocortex in the cat. Brain Res., **44**: 483–502.

1001. HAIGLER, H. J., AND AGHAJANIAN, G. K. 1974. Lysergic acid diethylamide and serotonin: A comparison of effects on serotonergic neurons and neurons receiving serotonergic input. J. Pharmacol. Exp. Ther., **188**: 688–699.

1002. HAINES, D. E. 1976. Cerebellar corticonuclear and corticovestibular fibers of the anterior lobe vermis in a prosimian primate (Galago senegalensis). J. Comp Neurol., **170**: 67–96.

1003. HAINES, D. E. 1977. A proposed functional significance of parvicellular regions of the lateral and medial cerebellar nuclei. Brain Behav. Evol., **14**: 328–340.

1004. HAINES, D. E., AND WHITWORTH, R. H. 1978. Cerebellar cortical efferent fibers of the paraflocculus of tree shrew (Tupaia). J. Comp. Neurol., **182**: 137–150.

1005. HAJDU, F., HASSLER, R., AND BAK, I. J. 1973. Electron microscopic study of the substantia nigra and strio-nigral projection in the rat. Z. Zellforsch. Mikrosk. Anat., **146**: 207–220.

1006. HALÁSZ, N., LJUNGDAHL, Å., AND HÖKFELT, T. 1978. Transmitter histochemistry of the rat olfactory bulb. I. Fluorescence histochemical, autoradiographic and electron microscopic localization of monoamines. Brain Res., **154**: 253–272.

1007. HALÁSZ, N., PARRY, D. M., BLACKETT, N. M., LJUNGDAHL, Å., AND HÖKFELT, T. 1981. [^{3}H]γ-aminobutyrate autoradiography of the rat olfactory bulb: Hypothetical grain analysis of the distribution of silver grains. Neuroscience, **6**: 473–479.

1008. HALGREN, E., BABB, T. L., RAUSCH, R., AND CRANDALL, P. H. 1977. Neurons in the human basolateral amygdala and hippocampal formation do not respond to odors. Neurosci. Lett., **4**: 331–335.

1009. HALGREN, E., WALTER, R. D., CHERLOW, D. G., AND CRANDALL, P. H. 1978. Mental phenomena evoked by electrical stimulation of the human hippocampal formation and amygdala. Brain, **101**: 83–118.

1010. HALL, E. A. 1963. Efferent connections of the basal and lateral nuclei of the amygdala in the cat. Am. J. Anat., **113**: 139–151.

1011. HAMILTON, W. J., BOYD, J. D., AND MOSSMAN, H. W. 1962. Human Embryology. Prenatal Development of Form and Function. Williams & Wilkins, Baltimore, Ch. XII, pp. 315–388.

1012. HAMILTON, W. J., AND MOSSMAN, H. W. 1972. Human Embryology. Williams & Wilkins, Baltimore.

1013. HAMLYN, L. H. 1954. The effect of preganglionic section on the neurons of the superior cervical ganglion in rabbits. J. Anat., **88**: 184–191.

1014. HAMMOND, C., DENIAU, J. M., RIZK, A., AND FÉGER, J. 1978. Electrophysiological demonstration of an excitatory subthalamonigral pathway in the rat. Brain Res., **151**: 235–244.

1015. HAMMOND, C., FEGÉR, J., BIOULAC, B., AND SOUTEYRAND, J. P. 1979. Experimental hemiballism in the monkey produced by unilateral kainic acid lesion in corpus Luysii. Brain Res., **171**: 577–580.

1016. HAMMOND, W. A. 1871. A Treatise on Diseases of the Nervous System. D. Appleton and Company, New York, pp. 655–662.

1017. HÁMORI, J., PASIK, T., PASIK, P., AND SZENTÁGOTHAI, J. 1974. Triadic synaptic arrangements and their possible significance in the lateral geniculate nucleus of the monkey. Brain Res., **80**: 379–393.

1018. HÁMORI, J., AND SZENTÁGOTHAI, J. 1966. Identification under the electron microscope of climbing fibers and their synaptic contacts. Exp. Brain Res., **1:** 65–81.

1019. HAMPEL, C. W. 1935. The effect of denervation on the sensitivity to adrenaline of the smooth muscle in the nictitating membrane of the cat. Am. J. Physiol., **61:** 611–621.

1020. HAMPSON, J. L., HARRISON, C. R., AND WOOLSEY, C. N. 1952. Cerebro-cerebellar projections and the somatotopic localization of motor function in the cerebellum. Proc. Assoc. Res. Nerv. Ment. Dis., **30:** 299–316.

1021. HANAWAY, J. 1967. Formation and differentiation of the external granular layer of the chick cerebellum. J. Neurol. Sci., **131:** 1–14.

1022. HANAWAY, J., SCOTT, W. R., AND STROTHER, C. M. 1980. *Atlas of the Human Brain and the Orbit for Computer Tomography*, ed. 2. Warren H. Green, II, Inc. St. Louis.

1023. HANAWAY, J., AND YOUNG, R. R. 1977. Localization of the pyramidal tract in the internal capsule of man. J. Neurol. Sci., **34:** 63–70.

1024. HAND, P. J. 1966. Lumbosacral dorsal root terminations in the nucleus gracilis of the cat: Some observations on terminal degeneration in other medullary sensory nuclei. J. Comp. Neurol., **126:** 137–156.

1025. HARA, K., AND FUJINO, Y. 1966. The thalamoperforate artery. Acta Radiol., **5:** 192–200.

1026. HARDY, D. G., PEACE, D. A., AND RHOTON, A. L. 1980. Microsurgical anatomy of the superior cerebellar artery. Neurosurgery, **6:** 10–27.

1027. HARDY, H., AND HEIMER, L. 1977. A safer and more sensitive substitute for diaminobenzidine in the light microscopic demonstration of retrograde and anterograde axonal transport of HRP. Neurosci. Lett., **5:** 235–240.

1028. HARE, W. K., AND HINSEY, J. C. 1940. Reaction of dorsal root ganglion cells to section of peripheral and central processes. J. Comp. Neurol., **73:** 489–502.

1029. HARRIS, F. S., AND RHOTON, A. L., JR. 1976. Anatomy of the cavernous sinus: A microsurgical study. J. Neurosurg., **45:** 169–180.

1030. HARRIS, G. W. 1948. Electrical stimulation of the hypothalamus and the mechanism of neural control of the adenohypophysis. J. Physiol. (Lond.), **107:** 418–429.

1031. HARRIS, G. W. 1955. *Neural Control of the Pituitary Gland.* Edward Arnold and Company, London.

1032. HARRIS, G. W. 1956. Hypothalamic control of the anterior lobe of the hypophysis. In W. S. FIELDS *et al.* (Editors), *Hypothalamic-Hypophysial Interrelationships* (Symposium). Charles C Thomas, Publisher, Springfield, Ill., pp. 31–42.

1033. HARRIS, G. W., AND GEORGE, R. 1969. Neurohumoral control of the adenohypophysis and regulation of the secretion of TSH, ACTH and growth hormone. In W. HAYMAKER *et al* (Editors), *The Hypothalamus.* Charles C Thomas Publisher, Springfield, Ill., Ch. 10, pp. 326–388.

1034. HARRIS, G. W., AND WOODS, J. W. 1958. The effect of electrical stimulation of the hypothalamus or pituitary gland on thyroid activity. J. Physiol. (Lond.), **143:** 246–274.

1035. HARRISON, J. M., AND HOWE, M. E. 1974. Anatomy of the afferent auditory nervous system in mammals. In W. D. KEIDEL AND W. D. NEFF (Editors), *Handbook of Sensory Physiology*, Vol. III. Springer-Verlag, Berlin, pp. 283–336.

1036. HARTING, J. K. 1977. Descending pathways from the superior colliculus: An autoradiographic analysis in the rhesus monkey (*Macaca mulatta*). J. Comp. Neurol., **173:** 583–612.

1037. HARTING, J. K., CASAGRANDE, V. A., AND WEBER, J. T. 1978. The projection of the primate superior colliculus upon the dorsal lateral geniculate nucleus: Autoradiographic demonstration of intralaminar distribution of tectogeniculate axons. Brain Res., **150:** 593–599.

1038. HARTING, J. K., AND GUILLERY, R. W.

1976. Organization of the retinocollicular pathway in the cat. J. Comp. Neurol., **166:** 133–144.

1039. HARTING, J. K., HALL, W. C., DIAMOND, I. T., AND MARTIN, G. F. 1973. Anterograde degeneration study of the superior colliculus in *Tupaia glis*: Evidence for a subdivision between superficial and deep layers. J. Comp. Neurol., **148:** 361–386.

1040. HARTMANN, J. F. 1956. Electron microscopy of mitochondria in the central nervous system. J. Biophys. Biochem. Cytol., **2** (suppl.): 373–378.

1041. HARTMANN-VON MONAKOW, K., AKERT, K., AND KÜNZLE, H. 1978. Projections of the precentral motor cortex and other cortical areas of the frontal lobe to the subthalamic nucleus in the monkey. Exp. Brain Res., **33:** 395–403.

1042. HARTMANN-VON MONAKOW, K., AKERT, K., AND KÜNZLE, H. 1979. Projections of the precentral and premotor cortex to the red nucleus and other midbrain areas in *Macaca fascicularis*. Exp. Brain Res., **34:** 91–105.

1043. HARTWIG, H. G. 1974. Electron microscopic evidence for a retinohypothalamic projection to the suprachiasmatic nucleus of *Passer domesticus*. Cell Tissue Res., **153:** 88–99.

1044. HASSLER, O. 1966. Deep cerebral venous system in man: A microangiographic study on its areas of drainage and its anastomoses with the superficial cerebral veins. Neurology (Minneap.), **16:** 505–511.

1045. HASSLER, O. 1966a. Blood supply to the human spinal cord. Arch. Neurol., **15:** 302–307.

1046. HASSLER, O. 1967. Venous anatomy of human hindbrain. Arch. Neurol., **16:** 404–409.

1047. HASSLER, O. 1967a. Arterial pattern of human brain stem. Normal appearance and deformation in expanding supratentorial conditions. Neurology (Minneap.), **17:** 368–375.

1048. HASSLER, R. 1939. Zur pathologischen Anatomie des senilen und des parkinsonistischen Tremor. J. Psychol. Neurol., **49:** 193–230.

1049. HASSLER, R. 1950. Über Kleinhirnprojektionen zum Mittelhirn und Thalamus beim Menschen. Dtsch. Z. Nervenh., **163:** 629–671.

1050. HATSCHEK, R. 1907. Zur vergleichenden Anatomie des Nucleus ruber tegmenti. Arb. Neurol. Inst. Wiener Univ., **15:** 89–135.

1051. HATTORI, T., FIBIGER, H. C., AND MCGEER, P. L. 1975. Demonstration of a pallidonigral projection innervating dopaminergic neurons. J. Comp. Neurol., **162:** 487–504.

1052. HATTORI, T., AND MCGEER, E. G. 1977. Fine structural changes in the rat striatum after local injections of kainic acid. Brain Res., **129:** 174–180.

1053. HATTORI, T., MCGEER, P. L., FIBIGER, H. C., AND MCGEER, E. G. 1973. On the source of GABA-containing terminals in the substantia nigra: Electron microscopic autoradiographic and biochemical studies. Brain Res., **54:** 103–114.

1054. HAUGSTED, H. 1956. Occlusion of the basilar artery. Diagnosis by vertebral angiography during life. Neurology (Minneap.), **6:** 823–828.

1055. HAY, E. D., AND REVEL, J. P. 1963. The fine structure of the DNP component of the nucleus: An electron microscope study utilizing autoradiography to localize DNA synthesis. J. Cell Biol., **16:** 29–51.

1056. HAYHOW, W. R. 1958. The cytoarchitecture of the lateral geniculate body in the cat in relation to the distribution of crossed and uncrossed optic fibers. J. Comp. Neurol., **110:** 1–64.

1057. HAYMAKER, W. 1956. *Bing's Local Diagnosis in Neurological Diseases.* C. V. Mosby Company, St. Louis, pp. 57–62 and 105–112.

1058. HAYMAKER, W. 1969. Hypothalamo-pituitary neural pathways and the circulatory system of the pituitary. In W. HAYMAKER *et al.* (Editors), *The Hypothalamus.* Charles C Thomas, Publisher, Springfield, Ill., Ch. 6, pp. 219–250.

1059. HAYMAKER, W., AND WOODHALL, B. 1945.

Peripheral Nerve Injuries: Principles of Diagnosis. W. B. Saunders Company, Philadelphia, 227 pp.

1060. HEAD, H. 1905. The afferent nervous system from a new aspect. Brain, **28:** 99–116.

1061. HEAD, H. 1920. *Studies in Neurology.* Oxford University Press, London. 2 vols.

1062. HEAD, H., AND HOLMES G. 1911. Sensory disturbances from cerebral lesions. Brain, **34:** 102–254.

1063. HEATH, C. J., AND JONES, E. G. 1971. An experimental study of ascending connections from the posterior group of thalamic nuclei in the cat. J. Comp. Neurol., **141:** 397–426.

1064. HEATH, J. W. 1947. Clinicopathologic aspects of Parkinsonian states. Arch. Neurol. Psychiatry, **58:** 484–497.

1065. HEATH, R. G., MONROE, R. R., AND MICKEL, W. 1955. Stimulation of the amygdaloid nucleus in a schizophrenic patient. Am. J. Psychiatry, **111:** 862–863.

1066. HEDREEN, J. C. 1971. Separate demonstration of dopaminergic and nondopaminergic projections of the substantia nigra in the cat. Anat. Rec., **169:** 338.

1067. HEIDARY, H., AND TOMASCH, J. 1969. Neuron numbers and perikaryon areas in the human cerebellar nuclei. Acta Anat. (Basel), **74:** 290–296.

1068. HEIMER, L. 1970. Selective silver-impregnation of degenerating axoplasm. In W. J. H. NAUTA AND S. O. E. EBBESSON (Editors), *Contemporary Research Methods in Neuroanatomy.* Springer-Verlag, New York, pp. 106–131.

1069. HEIMER, L., AND NAUTA, W. J. H. 1967. The hypothalamic distribution of the stria terminalis in the rat. Anat. Rec., **157:** 259.

1070. HEIMER, L., AND NAUTA, W. J. H. 1969. The hypothalamic distribution of the stria terminalis in the rat. Brain Res., **13:** 284–297.

1071. HEINBECKER, P., BISHOP, G. H., AND O'LEARY, J. L. 1936. Functional and histologic studies of somatic and autonomic nerves of man. Arch. Neurol. Psychiatry, **35:** 1233–1255.

1072. HELLER, H. 1966. The hormone content of the vertebrate hypothalamo-neurohypophysial system. Br. M. Bull., **22:** 227–231.

1073. HENDRICKSON, A. E., WAGONER, N., AND COWAN, W. M. 1972. An autoradiographic and electron microscopic study of retino-hypothalamic connections. Z. Zellforsch. Mikrosk. Anat., **135:** 1–26.

1074. HENDRICKSON, A. M., WILSON, M. E., AND TOYNE, M. J. 1970. The distribution of optic nerve fibers in *Macaca mulatta.* Brain Res., **23:** 425–427.

1075. HENDRY, S. H., JONES, E. G., AND GRAHAM, J. 1979. Thalamic relay nuclei for cerebellar and certain related fiber systems in the cat. J. Comp. Neurol., **185:** 679–713.

1076. HENNEMAN, E. 1968. Peripheral mechanisms involved in the control of muscle. In V. B. MOUNTCASTLE (Editor), *Medical Physiology.* C. V. Mosby Company, St. Louis, Ch. 73, pp. 1697–1716.

1077. HENSCHEN, S. E. 1926. On the function of the right hemisphere of the brain in relation to the left in speech, music and calculation. Brain, **49:** 110–123.

1078. HERKENHAM, M. 1978. Intralaminar and parafascicular efferents to the striatum and cortex in the rat: An autoradiographic study. Anat. Rec., **190:** 420.

1079. HERKENHAM, M., AND NAUTA, W. J. H. 1977. Afferent connections of the habenular nuclei in the rat: A horseradish peroxidase study, with a note on the fiber-of-passage problem. J. Comp. Neurol., **173:** 123–145.

1080. HERNÁNDEZ-PEON, R., AND HAGBARTH, K. E. 1955. Interaction between afferent and cortically induced reticular responses. J. Neurophysiol., **18:** 44–55.

1081. HERNDON, R. M. 1964. The fine structure of the cerebellum. II. The stellate neurons, granule cells and glia. J. Cell Biol., **23:** 277–293.

1082. HERNDON, R. M., PRICE, D. L., AND WEINER, L. P. 1977. Regeneration of oligodendroglia during recovery from demyelinating disease. Science, **195:** 693–694.

1083. HERREN, R. Y., AND ALEXANDER, L. 1939. Sulcal and intrinsic blood vessels of human spinal cord. Arch. Neurol. Psychiatry, **41:** 678–687.

1084. HERRICK, C. J. 1948. *The Brain of the Tiger Salamander.* University of Chicago Press, Chicago, pp. 141–142 and 175.

1085. HERRICK, C. J., AND COGHILL, G. E. 1915. The development of reflex mechanisms in Amblystoma. J. Comp. Neurol., **25:** 65–85.

1086. HERZ, A., AND ZIEGLGÄNSBERGER, W. 1968. The influence of microelectrophoretically applied biogenic amines, cholinomimetics and procaine on synaptic excitation in the corpus striatum. Int. J. Neuropharmacol., **7:** 221–230.

1087. HERZ, E. 1931. Die amyostatischen Unruheerscheinungen. J. Psychol. Neurol., **43:** 3–182.

1088. HERZOG, A. G., AND VAN HOESEN, G. W. 1976. Temporal neocortical afferent connections to the amygdala in the rhesus monkey. Brain Res. **115:** 57–70.

1089. HESS, W. R. 1948. *Die Funktionelle Organisation des Vegetativen Nervensystems.* Benno Schwabe and Company, Basel.

1090. HESS, W. R. 1954. *Diencephalon, Autonomic and Extrapyramidal Functions.* Grune & Stratton, Inc., New York, 79 pp.

1091. HETHERINGTON, A. W., AND RANSON, S. W. 1940. Hypothalamic lesions and adiposity in the rat. Anat. Rec., **78:** 149–172.

1092. HEUSER, J. E., AND REESE, T. S. 1977. Structure of the synapse. In E. R. KANDEL (Editor), *Handbook of Physiology, Cellular Biology of Neurons,* Vol. 1, Pt. 1. American Physiological Society, Washington, D. C., pp. 261–294.

1093. HEWITT, W. 1961. The development of the human internal capsule and lentiform nucleus. J. Anat., **95:** 191–199.

1094. HICKEY, T. L., AND GUILLERY, R. W. 1974. An autoradiographic study of retinogeniculate pathways in the cat and the fox. J. Comp. Neurol., **156:** 239–254.

1095. HICKEY, T. L., AND GUILLERY, R. W. 1979. Variability of laminar patterns in the human lateral geniculate nucleus. J. Comp. Neurol., **183:** 221–246.

1096. HIGHSTEIN, S. M. 1977. Abducens and Oculomotor internuclear neurons: Relation to gaze. In R. BAKER AND A. BERTHOZ (Editors) *Control of Gaze by Brain Stem Neurons: Developments in Neuroscience,* Vol 1. Elsevier/North-Holland Biomedical Press, Amsterdam, pp. 153–162.

1097. HILD, W. 1956. Neurosecretion in the central nervous system. In W. S. FIELDS *et al.* (Editors), *Hypothalamic-Hypophysial Interrelationships.* Charles C Thomas, Publisher, Springfield, Ill., pp. 17–25.

1098. HILLARP, N.-Å. 1959. The construction and functional organization of the autonomic innervation apparatus. Acta Physiol. Scand., **46:** (suppl. 157): 1–38.

1099. HILLARP, N-Å. 1960. Peripheral autonomic mechanisms. In J. FIELD. *et al.* (Editors), *Handbook of Physiology,* Sect. I, Vol. II. American Physiological Society, Washington, D. C., Ch. 38, pp. 979–1006.

1100. HILTON, S. M., AND ZBROŻYNA, A. 1963. Defence reaction from the amydala and its afferent connections. J. Physiol. (Lond.), **165:** 160–173.

1101. HINES, M. 1936. The anterior border of the monkey's (*Macaca mulatta*) motor cortex and the production of spasticity. Am. J. Physiol., **116:** 76.

1102. HINES, M. 1937. The "motor" cortex. Bull. Johns Hopkins Hosp., **60:** 313–336.

1103. HINES, M. 1949. Significance of the precentral motor cortex. In P. C. BUCY (Editor), *The Precentral Motor Cortex.* University of Illinois Press, Urbana, Ch. 18, pp. 461–494.

1104. HINMAN, A., AND CARPENTER, M. B. 1959. Efferent fiber projections of the red nucleus in the cat. J. Comp.

Neurol. **113:** 61–82.

1105. HIROSAWA, K. 1968. Electron microscopic studies of pigment granules in the substantia nigra and locus coeruleus of the Japanese monkey (*Macaca fuscata yakui*). Z. Zellforsch. Mikrosk. Anat., **88:** 187–203.

1106. HIRSCH, J. D., GRILLO, M., AND MARGOLIS, F. L. 1978. Ligand binding studies in the mouse olfactory bulb: Identification and characterization of a L-[³H]carnosine binding site. Brain Res., **158:** 407–422.

1107. HIS, W. 1893. Vorschläge zur einteilung des gehirns. Arch. Anat. Entwickl.-Gesch., **17:** 172–179.

1108. HOCHSTETTER, F. 1919. *Beiträge zur Entwicklungsgeschichte des menschlichen Gehirns*, Vol. I. F. Deutcke, Vienna and Leipzig.

1109. HODDEVIK, G. H. 1975. The pontocerebellar projection onto the paramedian lobule in the cat: An experimental study with the use of horseradish peroxidase as a tracer. Brain Res., **95:** 291–307.

1110. HODDEVIK, G. H. 1978. The projection from nucleus reticularis tegmenti pontis onto the cerebellum in the cat: A study using the methods of anterograde degeneration and retrograde axonal transport of horseradish peroxidase. Anat. Embryol., (Berl.), **153:** 227–242.

1111. HODGE, C. J., APKARIAN, A. V., STEVENS, R., VOGELSANG, G., AND WISNICKI, H. J. 1981. Locus coeruleus modulation of dorsal horn unit responses to cutaneous stimulation. Brain Res., **204:** 415–420.

1112. VAN HOESEN, G., MESULAM, M.-M., AND HAAXMA, R. 1976. Temporal cortical projections to the olfactory tubercle in the rhesus monkey. Brain Res., **109:** 375–381.

1113. HOFF, E. C. 1932. Central nerve terminals in the mammalian spinal cord and their examination by experimental degeneration. Proc. R. Soc, Ser. B., **111:** 175–188.

1114. HÖKFELT, T. 1967. The possible ultrastructural identification of tubero-infundibular dopamine-containing nerve endings in the median eminence of the rat. Brain Res., **5:** 121–123.

1115. HÖKFELT, T. 1967a. On the ultrastructural localization of noradrenaline in the central nervous system. Z. Zellforsch. Mikrosk. Anat., **79:** 110–117.

1116. HÖKFELT, T. 1967b. Ultrastructural studies on adrenergic nerve terminals in the albino rat iris after pharmacological and experimental treatment. Acta Physiol. Scand., **69:** 125–126.

1117. HÖKFELT, T., ELDE, R., JOHANSSON, O., TERENIUS, L., AND STEIN, L. 1977. The distribution of enkephalin immunoreactive cell bodies in the rat central nervous system. Neurosci. Lett., **5:** 25–31.

1118. HÖKFELT, T., AND FUXE, K. 1969. Cerebellar monoamine nerve terminals: A new type of afferent fiber to the cerebellar cortex. Exp. Brain Res., **9:** 63–72.

1119. HÖKFELT, T., FUXE, K., GOLDSTEIN, M., AND JOHANSSON, O. 1974. Immunohistochemical evidence for the existence of adrenaline neurons in the rat brain. Brain Res., **66:** 235–251.

1120. HÖKFELT, T., JOHANSSON, O., FUXE, K., GOLDSTEIN, M., AND PARK, D. 1976. Immunohistochemical studies on the localization and distribution of monoamine neuron systems in the rat brain. I. Tyrosine hydroxylase in the mesencephalon and diencephalon. Med. Biol., **54:** 427–453.

1121. HÖKFELT, T., JOHANSSON, O., KELLERTH, J.-O., LJUNGDAHL, Å., NILSSON, G., NYGÅRDS, A., AND PERNOW, B. 1977. Immunohistochemical distribution of substance P. In U. S. VON EULER AND B. PERNOW (Editors), *Substance P.* Raven Press, New York, pp. 117–145.

1122. HÖKFELT, T., KELLERTH, J.-O., NILSSON, G., AND PERNOW, B. 1975. Experimental immunohistochemical studies on the localization and distribution of substance P in cat primary sensory neurons. Brain Res., **100:** 235–252.

1123. HÖKFELT, T., KELLERTH, J.-O., NILLSON, G., AND PERNOW, B. 1975a. Morphological support for a trans-

mitter or modulator role of substance P: Immunohistochemical localization in the central nervous system and in primary sensory neurons. Science, **190:** 889–890.

1124. HÖKFELT, T., AND LJUNGDAHL, A. 1972. Application of cytochemical techniques to the study of suspected transmitter substances in the nervous system. In E. COSTA *etal.* (Editors), *Studies of Neurotransmitters at the Synaptic Level.* Raven Press, New York, pp. 1–36.

1125. HÖKFELT, T. A., LJUNGDAHL, A. TERENIUS, L., ELDE, R., AND NILSSON, G. 1977. Immunohistochemical analysis of peptide pathways possibly related to pain and analgesia: Enkephalin and substance P. Proc. Natl. Acad. Sci. U.S.A., **74:** 3081–3085.

1126. HÖKFELT, T., TERENIUS, T., KUYPERS, H. G. J. M. AND DANN O. 1979. Evidence for enkephalin immunoreactivity neurons in the medulla oblongata projecting to the spinal cord. Neurosci. Lett., **14:** 55–60.

1127. HÖKFELT, T., AND UNGERSTEDT, U. 1969. Electron and fluorescence microscopical studies on the nucleus caudatus putamen of the rat after unilateral lesions of ascending nigro-neostriatal dopamine neurons. Acta Physiol. Scand. **76:** 415–426.

1128. HÖKFELT, T., AND VAN ORDEN, L. S. 1972. Ultrastructure of amine-containing neurons in B. FALCK AND R. Y. MOORE (Editors), *Fluorescence Histochemistry of Biogenic Amines.* Academic Press, New York.

1129. HOLLÄNDER, H. 1974. Projections from the striate cortex to the diencephalon in the squirrel monkey (*Saimiri sciureus*): A light microscopic radioautographic study following intracortical injection of ³H leucine. J. Comp. Neurol., **155:** 424–440.

1130. HOLLÄNDER, H., AND VANEGAS, H. 1977. The projection from the lateral geniculate nucleus onto the visual cortex in the cat: A quantitative study with horseradish peroxidase. J. Comp. Neurol., **173:** 519–536.

1131. HOLMES, G. 1922. The Croonian Lectures on the clinical symptoms of cerebellar disease and their interpretation. Lancet, **1:** 1177–1182.

1132. HOLMES, G. 1939. The cerebellum of man. Brain, **62:** 1–30.

1133. HOLMES, G., AND MAY, W. P., 1909. On the exact origin of the pyramidal tract in man and other mammals. Brain, **32:** 1–43.

1134. HOLMES, G., AND STEWART, T. G. 1908. On the connections of the inferior olive with the cerebellum in man. Brain, **31:** 125–137.

1135. HOLMES, W. 1943. Silver staining of nerve axons in paraffin sections. Anat. Rec., **86:** 157–187.

1136. HOLTZMAN, E., NOVIKOFF, A. B., AND VILLAVERDE, H. 1967. Lysosomes and GERL in normal and chromatolytic neurons of rat ganglion nodosum. J. Cell Biol., **33:** 419–435.

1137. HONG, J. S., YANG H.-Y.T., RACAGNI, G., AND COSTA, E. 1977. Projections of substance P-containing neurons from neostriatum to substantia nigra. Brain Res., **122:** 541–544.

1138. HONGO, T., JANKOWSKA, E., AND LUNDBERG, A. 1969. The rubrospinal tract. I. Effects on alpha-motorneurons innervating hindlimb muscles in cats. Exp. Brain Res., **7:** 344–364.

1139. HONGO, T., JANKOWSKA, E., AND LUNDBERG, A. 1969a. The rubrospinal tract. II. Facilitation of interneuronal transmission in reflex paths to motor neurons. Exp. Brain Res., **7:** 365–391.

1140. HOOKER, D. 1944. *The Origin of Overt Behavior.* University of Michigan Press, Ann Arbor.

1141. HOPKINS, D. A., AND NIESSEN, L. W. 1976. Substantia nigra projections to the reticular formation, superior colliculus and central gray in rat, cat, and monkey. Neurosci. Lett., **2:** 253–259.

1142. HORCH, K. W., TUCKETT, R. P., AND BURGESS, P. R. 1977. A key to the classification of cutaneous mechanoreceptors. J. Invest. Dermatol., **69:** 75–82.

1143. HOREL, J. 1978. The neuroanatomy of amnesia: A critique of the hippocampal memory hypothesis. Brain

101: 403–445.

1144. Hornykiewicz. O. 1962. Dopamin (3-Hydroxytyramin) in Zentralnervensystem und seine Beziehung zum Parkinson-Syndrom des Menschen. Dtsch. Med. Wochenschr., **87**: 1807–1810.

1145. Hornykiewicz, O. 1966. Metabolism of brain dopamine in human parkinsonism: Neurochemical and clinical aspects. In E. Costa et al. (Editors), *Biochemistry and Pharmacology of the Basal Ganglia.* Raven Press, New York, pp. 171–185.

1146. Horstadius, S. 1950. *The Neural Crest.* Oxford University Press, London.

1147. Hosoya, Y., and Matsushita, M. 1979. Identification and distribution of the spinal and hypophyseal projection neurons in the paraventricular nucleus of the rat: A light and electron microscopic study with the horseradish peroxidase method. Exp. Brain Res., **35**: 315–331.

1148. Houk, J., and Henneman, E. 1967. Responses of tendon organs to active contractions of the soleus muscle of the cat. J. Neurophysiol., **30**: 466–481.

1149. Hoyt, W. F., and Luis, O. 1962. Visual fiber anatomy in the infrageniculate pathway of the primate. Arch. Ophthalmol., **68**: 94–106.

1150. Hoyt, W. F., and Luis, O. 1963. The primate chiasm: Details of visual fiber organization studied by silver impregnation techniques. Arch. Ophthalmol., **70**: 69–85.

1151. Hubbard, J. I., and Oscarsson, O. 1962. Localization of the cell bodies of the ventral spinocerebellar tract in lumbar segments of the cat. J. Comp. Neurol., **118**: 199–204.

1152. Hubel, D. H. 1963. The visual cortex of the brain. Sci. Am. **209**: 54–62.

1153. Hubel, D. H., Le Vay, S. and Wiesel, T. N. 1975. Mode of termination of retino-tectal fibers in macaque monkey: An autoradiographic study. Brain Res., **96**: 25–40.

1154. Hubel, D. H., and Wiesel, T. N. 1959. Receptive fields of single neurons in the cat's striate cortex. J. Physiol. (Lond.), **148**: 574–591.

1155. Hubel, D. H., and Wiesel, T. N. 1961. Integrative action in the cat's lateral geniculate body. J. Physiol. (Lond.), **155**: 385–398.

1156. Hubel, D. H., and Wiesel, T. N. 1962. Receptive fields, binocular interaction and functional architecture in the cat's visual cortex. J. Physiol. (Lond.), **160**: 106–154.

1157. Hubel, D. H., and Wiesel, T. N. 1963. Shape and arrangement of columns in cat's striate cortex. J. Physiol. (Lond.), **165**: 559–568.

1158. Hubel, D. H., and Wiesel, T. N. 1963a. Receptive fields of cells in striate cortex of very young, visually inexperienced kittens. J. Neurophysiol., **26**: 994–1002.

1159. Hubel, D. H., and Wiesel, T. N. 1965. Receptive fields and functional architecture in two non-striate visual areas (18 and 19) of the cat. J. Neurophysiol. **28**: 229–289.

1160. Hubel, D. H., and Wiesel, T. N. 1967. Cortical and callosal connections concerned with the vertical meridian of visual fields in the cat J. Neurophysiol., **30**: 1561–1573.

1161. Hubel, D. H., and Wiesel, T. N. 1968. Receptive fields and functional architecture of monkey striate cortex. J. Physiol. (Lond.), **195**: 215–243.

1162. Hubel, D. H., and Wiesel, T. N 1970. Stereoscopic vision in macaque monkey. Nature, **225**: 41–42.

1163. Hubel, D. H., and Wiesel, T. N. 1972. Laminar and columnar distribution of geniculo-cortical fibers in the Macaque monkey. J. Comp. Neurol., **146**: 421–450.

1164. Hubel, D. H., and Wiesel, T. N. 1974. Sequence regularity and geometry of orientation columns in the monkey striate cortex. J. Comp. Neurol., **158**: 267–294.

1165. Hubel, D. H., and Wiesel, T. N. 1974a. Uniformity of monkey striate cortex: A parallel relationship between field size, scatter and magnification factor. J. Comp. Neurol., **158**: 295–306.

1166. Hubel, D. H., Wiesel, T. N., and LeVay, S. 1977. Plasticity of ocular dominance columns in monkey striate cortex. Philos. Trans. R. Soc. Lond. (Biol.), **278**: 377–409.

1167. Hughes, J. 1975. Isolation of an endogenous compound from the brain with pharmacological properties similar to morphine. Brain. Res., *88:* 295–308.

1168. Hughes, J. 1978. Intrinsic factors and the opiate receptor system. Neurosci. Res. Program Bull., **16**: 141–147.

1169. Hughes, J., Smith, T., Kosterlitz, H., Fothergill, L., Morgan, B., and Morris, H. 1975. Identification of two related pentapeptides from the brain with potent opiate agonist activity. Nature, **258**: 577–579.

1170. Hughes, J. R., and Andy, O. J. 1979 The human amygdala. I. Electrophysiological responses to odorants. Electroencephalogr. Clin. Neurophysiol. **46**: 428–443.

1171. Hughes, J. R., and Andy, O. J. 1979a. The human amygdala. II. Neurophysiological correlates of olfactory perception before and after amygdalotomy. Electroencephalogr. Clin. Neurophysiol., **46**: 444–451.

1172. Humason, G. L. 1961. *Animal Tissue Techniques.* W. H. Freeman and Company, San Francisco, pp. 189–217.

1173. Humphrey, T. 1936. The telencephalon of the bat: The non-cortical nuclear masses and certain pertinent fiber connections. J. Comp. Neurol., **65**: 603–711.

1174. Humphrey, T. 1966. Correlations between the development of the hippocampal formation and the differentiation of the olfactory bulbs. Ala. J. Med. Sci., **3**: 235–269.

1175. Humphrey, T. 1968. The development of the human amygdala during early embryonic life. J. Comp. Neurol., **132**: 135–166.

1176. Hunsperger, R. W. 1956. Affektreaktionen auf elektrische Reizung im Hirnstamm der Katze. Helv. Physiol. Pharmacol. Acta, **14**: 70–92.

1177. Hunt, C. C., and Riker, W. K. 1966. Properties of frog sympathetic neurons in normal ganglia and after axon section. J. Neurophysiol., **29**: 1096–1114.

1178. Hunt, J. R. 1915. The sensory field of the facial nerve: A further contribution to the sympatomatology of the geniculate ganglion. Brain **38**: 418–446.

1179. Ibuka, N., Inouye, S. T., and Kawamura, H. 1977. Analysis of sleep-wakefulness rhythms in male rats after suprachiasmatic nucleus lesions and ocular enucleations. Brain Res., **122**: 33–47.

1180. Ikeda, M. 1979. Projections from the spinal and the principal sensory nuclei of the trigeminal nerve to the cerebellar cortex in the cat, as studied by retrograde transport of horseradish peroxidase. J. Comp. Neurol., **184**: 567–585.

1181. Imig, T. J., and Adrian, H. O. 1977. Binaural columns in the primary field (AI) of cat auditory cortex. Brain Res., **138**: 241–257.

1182. Imig, T. J., Ruggero, M. A., Kitzes, L. M., Javel, E., and Brugge, J. F. 1977. Organization of auditory cortex in the owl monkey (*Aotus trivirgatus*). J. Comp. Neurol., **171**: 111–128.

1183. Ingalls, N. W. 1920. A human embryo at the beginning of segmentation with special reference to the vascular system. Contrib. Embryol., **11**: 61–90.

1184. Ingram, W. R. 1940. Nuclear organization and chief connections of the primate hypothalamus. Proc. Assoc. Res. Nerv. Ment. Dis., **20**: 195–244.

1185. Ingram, W. R. 1952. Brain stem mechanisms in behavior, Electroencephalogr. Clin. Neurophysiol., **4**: 397–406.

1186. Ingram, W. R., and Ranson, S. W. 1932. Effects of lesions in the red nuclei in cats. Arch. Neurol. Psychiatry, **28**: 483–512.

1187. Ishii, T., and Friede, R. L. 1968. Tissue binding of tritiated-norepinephrine in pigmented nuclei of human brain. Am. J. Anat., **122**: 139–144.

1188. Ito, M., Obata, K., and Ochi, R. 1966. The origin of cerebellar-induced inhibition of Deiters neurones. II. Temporal correlation between the trans-synaptic activation of Purkinje cells and the inhibition of Deiters neurones. Exp. Brain Res. **2:** 350–364.

1189. ITO, M., AND YOSHIDA, M. 1964. The cerebellar-evoked monosynaptic inhibition of Deiters neurones. Experientia, **20:** 515.

1190. ITO, M., AND YOSHIDA, M. 1966. The origin of cerebellar-induced inhibition of Deiters neurones. I. Monosynaptic initiation of the inhibitory postsynaptic potentials. Exp. Brain Res., **2:** 330–349.

1191. ITO, M., YOSHIDA, M., AND OBATA, K. 1964. Monosynaptic inhibition of the intracerebellar nuclei induced from the cerebellar cortex. Experientia, **20:** 575–576.

1192. ITO, M., YOSHIDA, M., OBATA, K., KAWAI, N., AND UDO, M. 1970. Inhibitory control of intracerebellar nuclei by the Purkinje cell axons. Exp. Brain Res., **10:** 64–80.

1193. IVERSEN, L. L. 1972. The uptake, storage, release and metabolism of GABA in inhibitory nerves. In S. H. SNYDER (Editor) *Perspectives in Neuropharmacology.* Oxford University Press, London, pp. 75–111.

1194. JABBUR, S. J., AND TOWE, A. L. 1961. Cortical excitation of neurones in dorsal column nuclei of cat, including an analysis of pathways. J. Neurophysiol., **24:** 499–509.

1195. JACKSON, I. M. D. 1981. Neural peptides in the cerebrospinal fluid. Adv. Biochem. Psychopharmacol. **28:** 337–356.

1196. JACOBS, B. L., AND TRULSON, M. E. 1979. Mechanisms of action of LSD. Am. Sci., **67:** 396–404.

1197. JACOBS, G. H. 1969. Receptive fields in visual systems. Brain Res., **14:** 553–573.

1198. JACOBSOHN, L. 1908. Über die Kerne des menschlichen Rückenmarks. Abhandlungen der königl. preuss. Akademie der Wissenschaften, p. 72.

1199. JACOBSOHN, L. 1909. Über die Kerne des menschlichen Hirnstamms. Abhandlungen der königl. preuss. Akademie der Wissenschaften, **1:** 1–70.

1200. JAKOB, A. 1923. *Die Extrapyramidalen Erkrankungen.* Julius Springer, Berlin.

1201. JAKOB, A. 1925. The anatomy, clinical syndromes and physiology of the extrapyramidal system. Arch. Neurol. Psychiatry, **13:** 596–620.

1202. JAKOB, A. 1928. Das Kleinhirn. In W. VON MÖLLENDORFF (Editor), *Handbuch der mikroskopischen Anatomie des Menschen,* Vol. IV. Julius Springer, Berlin, pp. 674–916.

1203. JANE, J. A., MASTERTON, R. B., AND DIAMOND, I. T. 1965. The function of the tectum for attention to auditory stimuli in the cat. J. Comp. Neurol., **125:** 165–192.

1204. JANSEN, J. 1933. Experimental studies on the intrinsic fibers of the cerebellum. I. The arcuate fibers. J. Comp. Neurol., **57:** 369–400.

1205. JANSEN, J., AND BRODAL, A. 1940. Experimental studies on the intrinsic fibers of the cerebellum. II. The corticonuclear projection. J. Comp. Neurol., **73:** 267–321.

1206. JANSEN, J., AND BRODAL, A. 1942. Experimental studies on the intrinsic fibers of the cerebellum. The cortico-nuclear projection in the rabbit and in the monkey (*Macacus rhesus*). Norske Vid.-Akad. Avh. Mat.-Naturv., No. 3, 1–50.

1207. JANSEN, J., AND BRODAL, A. 1958. Das Kleinhirn. In W. VON, MÖLLENDORFF (Editor), *Handbuch der mikroskopischen Anatomie des Menschen,* Vol. III. Julius Springer, Berlin, pp. 1–323.

1208. JASPER, H. H. 1949. Diffuse projection systems: The integrative action of the thalamic reticular system. Electroencephalogr. Clin. Neurophysiol., **1:** 405–420.

1209. JASPER, H. H. 1954. Functional properties of the thalamic reticular system. In J. F. DELAFRESNAYE (Editor), *Brain Mechanisms and Consciousness* (Symposium). Blackwell Scientific Publications, Oxford, pp. 374–395.

1209a. JASPER, H. H. 1960. Unspecific thalamocortical relations. In J. FIELD (Editor), *Handbook of Physiology,* Section I, Vol. II. American Physiological Society, Washington, D.C., Ch. 53, pp. 1307–1326.

1210. JASPER, H. H., AJMONE-MARSAN, C., AND STOLL, J. 1952. Corticofugal projections to the brain stem. A. M. A. Arch. Neurol. Psychiatry, **67:** 155–171.

1211. JASPER, H. H., AND BERTRAND, G. 1966. Thalamic units involved in somatic sensation and voluntary and involuntary movements in man. In D. P. PURPURA and M. D. YAHR (Editors), *The Thalamus.* Columbia University Press, New York, pp. 365–384.

1212. JAYARAMAN, A., BATTON, R. R., III, AND CARPENTER, M. B. 1977. Nigrotectal projections in the monkey: An autoradiographic study. Brain Res., **135:** 147–152.

1213. JAYARAMAN, A., AND UPDYKE, B. V. 1979. Organization of visual cortical projections to the claustrum in the cat. Brain Res., **178:** 107–115.

1214. JAYATILAKA, A. D. P. 1965. Arachnoid granulations in sheep. J. Anat., **99:** 315–327.

1215. JAYATILAKA, A. D. P. 1965a. An electron microscopic study of sheep arachnoid granulations. J. Anat., **99:** 635–649.

1216. JEFFERSON, G. 1950. Localization of function in the cerebral cortex. Br. Med. Bull., **6:** 333–340.

1217. JEFFERSON, G. 1958. Discussion: Ch. 2, SCHEIBEL, M. E. and SCHEIBEL, A. B., Substrates for integrative patterns in the reticular core. In H. H. JASPER *et al.* (Editors), *Reticular Formation of the Brain.* Henry Ford Hospital International Symposium. Little, Brown and Company, Boston, pp. 65–68.

1218. JENKINS, T. W., AND TRUEX, R. C. 1963. Dissection of the human brain as a method for its fractionation by weight. Anat. Rec., **147:** 359–366.

1219. JERGER, J. F. 1960. Observations on auditory behavior in lesions of the central auditory pathways. A. M. A. Arch. Otolaryngol., **71:** 797–806.

1220. JESSELL, T. M., AND IVERSEN, L. L. 1977. Opiate analgesics inhibit substance P release from rat trigeminal nucleus. Nature, **268:** 549–551.

1221. JONES, A. E. 1964. The lateral geniculate nucleus of *Ateles ater.* J. Comp. Neurol., **123:** 205–210.

1222. JONES, B. E., BOBILLIER, P., PIN, C., AND JOUVET, M. 1973. The effects of lesions of catecholamine-containing neurons upon monamine content of the brain and EEG and behavioral waking in the cat. Brain Res., **58:** 157–177.

1223. JONES, B. E., HALARIS, A. E., Mc ILHANY, M., AND MOORE, R. Y. 1977. Ascending projections of the locus coeruleus in the rat. I. Axonal transport in central noradrenaline neurons. Brain Res., **127:** 1–22.

1224. JONES, B. E., HARPER, S. T., AND HALARIS, A. E. 1977. Effects of locus coeruleus lesions upon cerebral monamine content, sleep-wakefulness states and the response to amphetamine in the cat. Brain Res., **124:** 473–496.

1225. JONES, B. E., AND MOORE, R. Y. 1977. Ascending projections of the locus coeruleus in the rat. II. Autoradiographic study. Brain Res., **127:** 23–53.

1226. JONES, E. G. 1969. Interrelationships of parieto-temporal and frontal cortex in the rhesus monkey. Brain Res., **13:** 412–415.

1227. JONES, E. G. 1975. Some aspects of the organization of the thalamic reticular complex. J. Comp. Neurol., **162.:** 285–308.

1228. JONES, E. G. 1975a. Lamination and differential distribution of thalamic afferents in the sensory-motor cortex of the squirrel monkey. J. Comp. Neurol., **160:** 167–204.

1229. JONES, E. G. 1981. Anatomy of cerebral cortex: Columnar input-output organization. In F. O. SCHMITT, F. G. WORDEN, G. ADELMAN, AND S. G. DENNIS (Editors), *The Organization of the Cerebral Cortex.* MIT Press, Cambridge, Mass. pp. 199–235.

1230. JONES, E. G., AND BURTON, H. 1974. Cytoarchitecture and somatic sensory connectivity of thalamic nuclei other than the ventrobasal complex in the cat. J. Comp. Neurol., **154:** 395–432.

1231. JONES, E. G., COULTER, J. D., BURTON, H., AND PORTER, R. 1977. Cells of origin and terminal distribution of corticostriatal fibers arising in the sensory-motor cortex of monkeys. J. Comp. Neurol., **173:** 53–80.

1232. JONES, E. G., COULTER, J. D., AND HENDRY, S. H. C. 1978. Intracortical connectivity of architectonic fields in the somatic sensory, motor and parietal cortex of monkeys. J. Comp. Neurol., **181:** 291–348.

1233. JONES, E. G., AND HENDRY, S. H. C. 1980. Distribution of callosal fibers around the hand representation in monkey somatic sensory cortex. Neurosci. Lett., **19:** 167–172.

1234. JONES, E. G., AND LEAVITT, R. Y. 1974. Retrograde axonal transport and the demonstration of non-specific projections to the cerebral cortex and striatum from thalamic intralaminar nuclei in the cat, rat and monkey. J. Comp. Neurol., **154:** 349–378.

1235. JONES, E. G., AND PORTER, R. 1980. What is area 3a? Brain Res. Rev., **2:** 1–43.

1236 JONES, E. G., AND POWELL, T. P. S. 1968. The ipsilateral cortical connexions of the somatic sensory areas in the cat. Brain Res., **9:** 71–94.

1237. JONES, E. G., AND POWELL, T. P. S. 1968a. Projections of the somatic sensory cortex upon the thalamus in the cat. Brain Res., **10:** 369–391.

1238. JONES, E. G., AND POWELL, T. P. S. 1969. Connexions of the somatic sensory cortex of the rhesus monkey. I. Ipsilateral cortical connexions. Brain, **92:** 477–502.

1239. JONES, E. G., AND POWELL, T. P. S. 1969a. Connexions of the somatic cortex of the rhesus monkey. II. Contralateral cortical connexions. Brain, **92:** 717–730.

1240. JONES, E. G., AND POWELL, T. P. S. 1969b. The cortical projections of the ventroposterior nucleus of the thalamus in the cat. Brain Res., **13:** 298–318.

1241. JONES, E. G., AND POWELL, T. P. S. 1970. Connexions of the somatic sensory cortex of the rhesus monkey. III. Thalamic connexions. Brain, **93:** 37–56.

1242. JONES, E. G., AND POWELL, T. P. S. 1970a. An anatomical study of converging sensory pathways within the cerebral cortex of the monkey. Brain, **93:** 793–820.

1243. JONES, E. G., AND POWELL, T. P. S. 1971. An analysis of the posterior group of thalamic nuclei on the basis its afferent connections. J. Comp. Neurol., **143:** 185–216.

1244. JONES, E. G., AND POWELL, T. P. S. 1973. Anatomical organization of the somatosensory cortex. In A. IGGO (Editor), *Handbook of Sensory Physiology*, Vol. 2. Springer-Verlag, Berlin, pp. 579–620.

1245. JONES, E. G., AND WISE, S. P. 1977. Size, laminar and columnar distribution of efferent cells in the sensory-motor cortex of monkeys. J. Comp. Neurol., **175:** 391–438.

1246. JONES, E. G., WISE, S. P., AND COULTER, J. D. 1979. Differential thalamic relationships of sensory-motor and parietal cortical fields in monkeys. J. Comp. Neurol., **183:** 833–881.

1247. JONES, R. M. 1961. *McClung's Handbook of Microscopical Technique*, Ed. 3. Hafner Publishing Company, New York, pp. 346–431.

1248. JOUVET, M. 1967. Neurophysiology of the states of sleep. Physiol. Rev., **47:** 117–177.

1249. JOUVET, M. 1969. Biogenic amines and the states of sleep. Science, **163:** 32–41.

1250. KAADA, B. R. 1972. Stimulation and regional ablation of the amygdaloid complex with reference to functional representations. In B. E. ELEFTHERIOU (Editor), *The Neurobiology of the Amygdala*. Plenum Press, New York, pp. 205–281.

1251. KAADA, B. R., PRIBRAM K. H., AND EPSTEIN, J. A. 1949. Respiratory and vascular responses in monkeys from temporal pole, insula, orbital surface and cingulate gyrus. J. Neurophysiol., **12:** 347–356.

1251a. KAADA B. R., RASMUSSEN, E. W., AND KVEINI, O. 1961. Effects of hippocampal lesions on maze learning and retention in rats. Exp. Neurol., **3:** 333–355.

1252. KAAS, J. H., GUILLERY, R. W., AND ALLMAN, J. M. 1972. Some principles of organization in the dorsal lateral geniculate nucleus. Brain Behav. Evol., **6:** 253–299.

1253. KAAS, J. H., HUERTA, M. F., WEBER, J. T., AND HARTING, J. K. 1977. Patterns of retinal terminations and laminar organization of the lateral geniculate nucleus of primates. J. Comp. Neurol., **182:** 517–554.

1254. KAES, T. 1907. *Die Grosshirnrinde des Menschen in ihren Massen und in ihrem Fasergehalt*, Vol. I. Gustav Fischer, Jena, 64 pp., 92 plates.

1255. KALIA, M. 1977. Neuroanatomical organization of the respiratory centers. Fed. Proc., **36:** 2405–2411.

1256. KALIA, M., AND MESULAM, M.-M. 1980. Brain stem projections of sensory and motor components of the vagus complex in the cat. I. The cervical vagus and nodose ganglion. J. Comp. Neurol., **193:** 435–465.

1257. KALIA, M., AND MESULAM, M.-M. 1980a. Brain stem projections of sensory and motor components of the vagus complex in the cat. II. Laryngeal, tracheobronchial, pulmonary, cardiac, and gastrointestinal branches. J. Comp. Neurol., **193:** 467–508.

1258. KALIL, K. 1975. Thalamo-cortical projections of VA and VL in the rhesus monkey. Neurosci. Abstr., Soc. Neurosci., **1:** 171.

1259. KALIL, K. 1979. Projections of the cerebellar and dorsal column nuclei upon the inferior olive in the rhesus monkey: An autoradiographic study. J. Comp. Neurol., **188:** 43–62.

1260. KALIL, K. 1981. Projections of the cerebellar and dorsal column nuclei upon the thalamus of the rhesus monkey. J. Comp. Neurol., **195:** 25–50.

1261. KANASEKI, T., AND SPRAGUE, J. M. 1974. Anatomical organization of pretectal nuclei and tectal laminae in the cat. J. Comp. Neurol., **158:** 319–338.

1262. KANAZAWA, I., EMSON, P. C., AND CUELLO, A. C. 1977. Evidence for the existence of substance P-containing fibers in striato-nigral and pallido-nigral pathways in rat brain. Brain Res., **119:** 447–453.

1263. KANAZAWA, I., MARSHALL, G. R., AND KELLY, J. S. 1976. Afferents to the rat substantia nigra studied with horseradish peroxidase, with special reference to fibers from the subthalamic nucleus. Brain Res., **115:** 485–491.

1264. KANDEL, E. 1979. Cellular insights into behavior and learning. In *The Harvey Lectures*, Series 73. Academic Press, Inc., New York, pp. 19–92.

1265. KAPLAN, H. A. 1956. Arteries of the brain. Acta Radiol. (Stockh.), **46:** 364–370.

1266. KAPLAN, H. A. 1958. Vascular supply of the base of the brain. In W. S. FIELDS (Editor), *Pathogenesis and Treatment of Parkinsonism*. Charles C Thomas, Publishers, Springfield, Ill., Ch. 6, pp. 138–155.

1267. KAPLAN, H. A. 1961. Collateral circulation of the brain. Neurology (Minneap.), **11:** 9–15.

1268. KAPLAN, H. A., AND FORD, D. H. 1966. *The Brain Vascular System*. Elsevier Publishing Company, Amsterdam, 230 pp.

1269. KAROL, E. A., AND PANDYA, D. N. 1971. The distribution of the corpus callosum in the rhesus monkey. Brain, **94:** 471–486.

1270. KATZ, B. 1966. *Nerve, Muscle and Synapse*. McGraw-Hill Book Company, New York.

1271. KAWAMURA, K. 1975. The pontine projection from the inferior colliculus in the cat: An experimental anatomical study. Brain Res., **95:** 309–322.

1272. KAWAMURA, K., AND BRODAL, A. 1973. The tectopontine projection in the cat: An experimental anatomical study with comments on pathways for teleceptive impulses to the cerebellum. J. Comp. Neurol., **149:** 371–390.

1273. KAWAMURA, S., SPRAGUE, J. M., AND NIIMI, K. 1974. Corticofugal projections from the visual cortices to the thalamus in the cat. J. Comp. Neurol., **158:** 339–362.

1274. KEIBEL, F., AND MALL, F. P. 1912. *Manual of Human Embryology*, Vol. II. J. P. Lippincott Company, Philadelphia, Ch. XIV, pp. 1–144.

1275. KELLER, A. D., AND HARE, W. K. 1934. The rubrospinal tracts in the monkey: Effects of experimental section. Arch. Neurol. Psychiatry, **32:** 1253–1272.

1276. KELLER, A. D., ROY, R. S., AND CHASE, W. P. 1937. Extirpation of the neocerebellar cortex without eliciting so-called cerebellar signs. Am. J. Physiol., 118: 720–733.

1277. KELLER, E. L. 1974. Participation of medial pontine reticular formation in eye movement generation in monkey. J. Neurophysiol., 37: 316–332.

1278. KELLER, J. H., AND MOFFETT, B. C., JR. 1968. Nerve endings in the temporomandibular joint of the Rhesus macaque. Anat. Rec., 160: 587–594.

1279. KELLY, J. P., AND GILBERT, C. D. 1975. The projection of different morphological types of ganglion cells in the cat's retina. J. Comp. Neurol., 163: 65–80.

1280. KELLY, J. P., AND VAN ESSEN, D. C. 1974. Cell structure and function in the visual cortex of the cat. J. Physiol. (Lond.), 238: 515–547.

1281. KEMP, J. 1968. An electron microscopic study of the termination of afferent fibres in the caudate nucleus. Brain Res., 11: 464–467.

1282. KEMP, J. 1968a. Observations on the caudate nucleus of the cat impregnated with the Golgi method. Brain Res., 11: 467–470.

1283. KEMP, J. M. 1970. The termination of striopallidal and strionigral fibers. Brain Res., 17: 125–128.

1284. KEMP, J. M. 1970a. The site of termination of afferent fibers on the neurones of the caudate nucleus. J. Physiol. (Lond.), 210: 17–18.

1285. KEMP, J. M., AND POWELL, T. P. S. 1970. The cortico-striate projection in the monkey. Brain, 93: 525–546.

1286. KEMP, J. M., AND POWELL, T. P. S. 1971. The site of termination of afferent fibres in the caudate nucleus. Philos. Trans. R. Soc. Lond. (Biol.), 262: 429–439.

1287. KENNARD, M. A. 1949. Somatic functions. In P. C. BUCY (Editor), The Precentral Motor Cortex, Ed. 2. University of Illinois Press, Urbana, Ch. 9, pp. 243–276.

1288. KENNARD, M. A., AND FULTON, J. F. 1933. The localizing significance of spasticity, reflex grasping and the signs of Babinski and Rossolimo. Brain, 56: 213–225.

1289. KENNARD, M. A., VIETS, H. R., AND FULTON, J. F. 1934. The syndrome of the premotor cortex in man: Impairment of skilled movement, forced grasping, spasticity and vasomotor disturbances. Brain, 57: 69–84.

1290. KENNEDY, C., DES ROSIERS, M. H., JEHLE, J. W., REIVICH, M., SHARP, F., AND SOKOLOFF, L. 1975. Mapping of functional neural pathways by autoradiographic survey of local metabolic rate with [^{14}C] deoxyglucose. Science, 187: 850–853.

1291. KENNEDY, C., DES ROSIERS, M. H., SAKURADA, O., SHINOHARA, M., REIVICH, M., JEHLE, J. W., AND SOKOLOFF, L. 1976. Metabolic mapping of the primary visual system of the monkey by means of the autoradiographic [^{14}C] deoxyglucose technique. Proc. Natl. Acad. Sci. U. S. A., 73: 4230–4234.

1292. KERR, F. W. L. 1961. Structural relation of the trigeminal spinal tract to upper cervical roots and the solitary nucleus in the cat. Exp. Neurol., 4: 134–148.

1293. KERR, F. W. L. 1962. Facial, vagal and glossopharyngeal nerves in the cat: Afferent connections. Arch. Neurol., 2: 264–281.

1294. KERR, F. W. L. 1963. The divisional organization of afferent fibers of the trigeminal nerve. Brain, 86: 721–732.

1295. KERR, F. W. L. 1969. Preserved vagal visceromotor function following destruction of the dorsal motor nucleus. J. Physiol. (Lond.), 202: 755–769.

1296. KERR, F. W. L. 1970. The organization of primary afferents in the subnucleus caudalis of the trigeminal: A light and electron microscopic study of degeneration. Brain Res., 23: 147–165.

1297. KERR, F. W. L. 1975. Neuroanatomical substrates of nociception in the spinal cord. Pain, 1: 325–356.

1298. KERR, F. W. L. 1975a. Pain: A central inhibitory balance theory, Mayo Clin. Proc., 50: 685–690.

1299. KERR, F. W. L. 1975b. The ventral spinothalamic tract and other ascending systems of the ventral funic-

ulus of the spinal cord. J. Comp. Neurol., 159: 335–356.

1300. KERR, F. W. L. 1978. Segmental circuitry of the spinal cord and nociception. Neurosci. Res. Program Bull., 16: 51–65.

1301. KERR, F. W. L., KRUGER, L. L., SCHWASSMANN, H. O., AND STERN, R. 1968. Somatotopic organization of mechanoreceptor units in the trigeminal nuclear complex of the monkey. J. Comp. Neurol., 134: 127–144.

1302. KERR, F. W. L., AND LIPPMAN, H. H. 1974. The primate spinothalamic tract as demonstrated by anterolateral cordotomy and commissural myelotomy. Adv. Neurol., 4: 147–156.

1303. KERR, F. W. L., AND LYSAK, W. R. 1964. Somatotopic organization of trigeminal-ganglion neurons. Arch. Neurol., 11: 593–602.

1304. KERR, F. W. L., AND PRESHAW, R. M. 1969. Secretomotor function of the dorsal motor nucleus of the vagus. J. Physiol. (Lond.), 205: 405–415.

1305. KETY, S. S., AND SCHMIDT, C. F. 1948. The nitrous oxide method for the quantitative determination of cerebral blood flow in man: Theory, procedure and normal values. J. Clin. Invest., 27: 484–492.

1306. KEY, A., AND RETZIUS, G. 1875. Studien in der Anatomie des Nervensystems und des Bindegewebes. Samson and Wallin, Stockholm.

1307. KEYSER, A. 1979. Development of the hypothalamus in mammals: An investigation into its morphological position during ontogenesis. In P. J. MORGANE AND J. PANKSEPP (Editors), Handbook of the Hypothalamus, Vol. I: Anatomy of the Hypothalamus. Marcel Dekker, Inc., New York, pp. 65–136.

1308. KIEVIT, J., AND KUYPERS, H. G. J. M. 1972. Fastigial cerebellar projections to the ventrolateral nucleus of the thalamus and the organization of the descending pathways. In T. L. FRIGYESI et al. (Editors), Corticothalamic Projections and Sensorimotor Activities. Raven Press, New York, pp. 91–111.

1309. KIEVIT, J., AND KUYPERS, H. G. J. M. 1975. Basal forebrain and hypothalamus connections to frontal and parietal cortex in the rhesus monkey. Science, 187: 660–663.

1310. KIEVIT, J., AND KUYPERS, H. G. J. M. 1977. Organization of the thalamo-cortical connexions to the frontal lobe in the rhesus monkey. Exp. Brain Res., 29: 299–322.

1311. KILLAM, K. F., AND KILLAM, E. K. 1958. Drug action on pathways involving the reticular formation. In H. H. JASPER et. al. (Editors), Reticular Formation of the Brain. Henry Ford Hospital International Symposium. Little, Brown and Company, Boston, Ch. 4, pp. 111–122.

1312. KIM, J.-S, HASSLER, R., HAUG, P., AND KWANG-SE-PAIK 1977. Effect of frontal cortical ablation on striatal glutamic acid level in rat. Brain Res., 132: 370–374.

1313. KIM, R., NAKANO, K., JAYARAMAN, A., AND CARPENTER, M. B. 1976. Projections of the globus pallidus and adjacent structures: An autoradiographic study in the monkey. J. Comp. Neurol., 169: 263–289.

1314. KIMMEL, D. L. 1959. The cervical sympathetic rami and the vertebral plexus in the human fetus. J. Comp. Neurol., 112: 141–162.

1315. KIMMEL, D. L. 1961. Innervation of the spinal dura mater and dura mater of the posterior cranial fossa. Neurology (Minneap.), 9: 800–809.

1316. KIMMEL, D. L., KIMMEL, C. B., AND ZARKIN, A. 1961. The central distribution of afferent nerve fibers of the facial and vagus nerves in the guinea pig. Anat. Rec., 139: 245.

1317. KIMURA, R., AND WERSÄLL, J. 1962. Termination of the olivo-cochlear bundle in relation to the outer hair cells of the organ of Corti in guinea pig. Acta Otolaryngol. (Stockh.), 55: 11–32.

1318. KING. G. W. 1980. Topology of ascending brainstem projections to nucleus parabrachialis in the cat. J. Comp. Neurol., 191: 615–638.

1319. KING, J. S., BOWMAN, M. H., AND MARTIN, G. F. 1971. The red nucleus of the opossum (Didelphis marsupialis virginiana): A light and electron microscopic study. J. Comp. Neurol., **143:** 157–184.

1320. KING, J. S., SCHWYN, R. C., AND FOX, C. A. 1971. The red nucleus in the monkey (*Macaca mulatta*): A Golgi and an electron microscopic study. J. Comp. Neurol., **142:** 75–108.

1321. KIRKPATRICK, J. B. 1968. Chromatolysis in the hypoglossal nucleus of the rat: An electron microscopic analysis. J. Comp. Neurol., **132:** 189–212.

1322. KITAI, S. T., KOCSIS, J. D., PRESTON, R. J., AND SUGIMORI, M. 1976. Monosynaptic inputs to caudate neurons identified by intracellular injection of horseradish peroxidase. Brain Res., **109:** 601–606.

1323. KITAI, S. T., McCREA, R. A., PRESTON, R. J., AND BISHOP, G. A. 1977. Electrophysiological and horseradish peroxidase studies of precerebellar afferents to the nucleus interpositus anterior. I. Climbing fiber system. Brain Res., **122:** 197–214.

1324. KLATZO, I., MIGUEL, J., TOBIAS, C., AND HAYMAKER, W. 1961. Effects of alpha-particle irradiation on the rat brain, including vascular permeability and glycogen studies. J. Neuropathol. Exp. Neurol., **20:** 459–483.

1325. KLEIN, D. C., AUERBACH, D. A., NAMBOODIRI, A. A., AND WHELER, G. H. T. 1981. Indole metabolism in the mammalian pineal gland. In R. J. REITER (Editor), *The Pineal Gland.* CRC Press, Boca Raton, Fla., Ch. 8, pp. 199–227.

1326. KLEIN, D. C., AND MOORE, R. Y. 1979. Pineal N-acetyltransferase and hydroxyindole-o-methyltransferase: Control by the retinohypothalamic tract and the suprachiasmatic nucleus. Brain Res., **174:** 245–262.

1327. KLEIN, D. C., AND WELLER, J. L. 1970. Indole metabolism in the pineal gland: A circadian rhythm in N-acetyltransferase. Science, **169:** 1093–1095.

1328. KLEIN, D. C., AND WELLER, J. L. 1972. A rapid light-induced decrease in pineal serotonin N-acetyltransferase activity. Science, **177:** 532–533.

1329. KLEIN, D. C., WELLER, J. L., AND MOORE, R. Y. 1971. Melatonin metabolism: Neurol regulation of pineal serotonin N-acetyltransferase. Proc. Natl. Acad. Sci. U. S. A., **68:** 3107–3110.

1330. KLEITMAN, N. 1963. *Sleep and Wakefulness.* University of Chicago Press, Chicago.

1331. KLING, A., AND SCHWARTZ, N. B. 1961. Effects of amygdalectomy on feeding in infant and adult animals. Fed. Proc., **20:** 335.

1332. KLÜVER, H. 1942. Functional significance of the geniculo-striate system. *Biological Symposia*, Vol. 7. J. Cattell Press. Lancaster, Pa., pp. 253–299.

1333. KLÜVER, H. 1952. Brain mechanisms and behavior with special reference to the rhinencephalon. Lancet, **72:** 567–574.

1334. KLÜVER, H., AND BARRERA, E. 1953. A method for the combined staining of cells and fibers in the nervous system. J. Neuropathol. Exp. Neurol., **12:** 400–403.

1335. KLÜVER, H., AND BUCY, P. 1939. Preliminary analysis of functions of the temporal lobes in monkeys. Arch. Neurol. Psychiatry, **42:** 979–1000.

1336. KNEISLEY, L. W., BIBER, M. P., AND LaVAIL, J. H. 1978. A study of the origin of brain stem projections to monkey spinal cord using the retrograde transport method. Exp. Neurol, **60:** 116–139.

1337. KNIGGE, K., JOSEPH, S. A., SLADEK, J. R., JR., HOFFMAN, G., AND SCOTT, D. E. 1980. Structure and function of the endocrine hypothalamus. In P. J. MORGANE AND J. PANKSEPP (Editors), *Physiology of the Hypothalamus.* Marcel Dekker, New York.

1338. KNIGGE, K. M., AND SILVERMAN, A. J. 1973. The anatomy of the endocrine hypothalamus. In R. O. GREEP AND E. B. ASTWOOD (Editors), *Handbook of Physiology*, Sect. 7, Vol. 4: *Endocrinology*, American Physiological Society, Washington D. C. pp. 1–32.

1338a. KNIGHTON, R. S. 1950. Thalamic relay nucleus for the second somatic sensory receiving area in the cerebral cortex of the cat. J. Comp. Neurol., **92:** 183–192.

1339. KNOOK, H. L. 1965. *The Fibre-Connections of the Forebrain.* Van Gorcum and Company, N. V. Assen, The Netherlands, 477 pp.

1340. KOCSIS, J. D., SUGIMORI, M., AND KITAI, S. T. 1977. Convergence of excitatory synaptic inputs to caudate spiny neurons. Brain Res., **124:** 403–413.

1341. KODAMA, S. 1928. Über die sogenannten Basalganglien. II. Pathologischanatomische Untersuchungen mit Bezug auf die sogenannten Basalganglien und ihre Adnexe. Schweiz. Arch. Neurol. Psychiatr., **23:** 38–100; 179–265.

1342. KOELLA, W. P., AND SUTIN, J. 1967. Extra-blood-brain-barrier brain structures. Int. Rev. Neurobiol., **10:** 31–55.

1343. KOELLE, G. B. 1970. Anticholinesterase agents. In L. S. GOODMAN AND A. GILMAN (Editors), *The Pharmacological Basis of Therapeutics.* Macmillan Company, New York, Ch. 22, pp. 442–465.

1344. KOOY, D. VAN DER, AND HATTORI, T. 1980. Single subthalamic nucleus neurons project to both the globus pallidus and substantia nigra in rat. J. Comp. Neurol., **192:** 751–768.

1345. KOOY, D. VAN DER KUYPERS, H. G. J. M., AND CATSMAN-BERREVOETS, C. E. 1978. Single mamillary body cells with divergent axon collaterals: Demonstration by a simple fluorescent retrograde double labeling technique in the rat. Brain Res., *158:* 189–196.

1346. KOPELL, H. P., AND THOMPSON, W. A. L. 1963. *Peripheral Entrapment Neuropathies.* Williams & Wilkins, Baltimore.

1347. KORNELIUSSEN, H. K. 1968. On the ontogenetic development of the cerebellum nuclei, fissures and cortex of the rat with special reference to regional variations in corticogenesis. J. Hirnforsch. **10:** 379–412.

1348. KORNELIUSSEN, H. K. 1972. Histogenesis of the cerebellar cortex and cortical zones. In O. LARSELL AND J. JANSEN (Editors), *The Comparative Anatomy and Histology of the Cerebellum: The Human Cerebellum, Cerebellar Connections and Cerebellar Cortex.* University of Minnesota Press. Mineapolis, pp. 164–174.

1349. KORNHUBER, H. H., FREDRICKSON, J. M., AND FIGGE, U. 1965. Die korticale Projektion der vestibulären Afferenz Beim Rhesusaffen. Pfluegers Arch., **283:** 20.

1350. KORTE, G. E. 1979. The brain stem projection of the vestibular nerve in the cat. J. Comp. Neurol., **184:** 279–292.

1351. KORTE, G. E., AND MUGNAINI, E. 1979. The cerebellar projection of the vestibular nerve in the cat. J. Comp. Neurol., **184:** 265–278.

1352. KOSEL, K. C., VAN HOESEN, G. W., AND WEST. J. R. 1981. Olfactory bulb projections to the parahippocampal area of the rat. J. Comp. Neurol., **198:** 467–482.

1353. KOSKOFF, Y. D., DENNIS, W., LAZOVIK, D., AND WHEELER, E. T. 1948. The psychological effects of frontal lobotomy performed for alleviation of pain. Proc. Assoc. Res. Nerv. Ment. Dis., **27:** 723–753.

1354. KOTCHABHAKDI, N., HODDEVIK, G. H., AND WALBERG, F. 1978. Cerebellar afferent projections from the perihypoglossal nuclei: An experimental study with the method of retrograde transport of horseradish peroxidase. Exp. Brain Res., **31:** 13–29.

1355. KOTCHABHAKDI, N., RINVIK, E., WALBERG, F., AND YINGCHAREON K. 1980. The vestibulothalamic projections in the cat studied by retrograde axonal transport of horseradish peroxidase. Exp. Brain Res., **40:** 405–418.

1356. KOTCHABHAKDI, N., AND WALBERG F. 1977. Cerebellar afferents from neurons in motor nuclei of cranial nerves demonstrated by retrograde axonal transport of horseradish peroxidase. Brain Res., **137:** 158–163.

1357. KOTCHABHAKDI, N., AND WALBERG, F. 1978. Primary vestibular afferent projections to the cerebellum as demonstrated by retrograde axonal transport of horseradish peroxidase. Brain Res., **142:** 142–146.

1358. KOTCHABHAKDI, N., AND WALBERG, F. 1978a. Cerebellar afferent projections from the vestibular nuclei in the cat: An experimental study with the method of retrograde transport of horseradish peroxidase. Exp.

Brain Res., **31:** 591–604.

1359. KREMER, W. F. 1947. Autonomic and somatic reactions induced by stimulation of the cingulate gyrus in dogs. J. Neurophysiol., **10:** 371–379.

1360. KRETTEK, J. E., AND PRICE, J. L. 1974. A direct input from the amygdala to the thalamus and the cerebral cortex. Brain Res., **67:** 169–174.

1361. KRETTEK, J. E., AND PRICE, J. L. 1977. Projections from the amygdaloid complex to the cerebral cortex and thalamus in the rat and cat. J. Comp. Neurol., **172:** 687–722.

1362. KRETTEK, J. E., AND PRICE, J. L. 1977a. Projections from the amygdaloid complex and adjacent olfactory structures to the entorhinal cortex and to the subiculum in the rat and cat. J. Comp. Neurol., **172:** 723–752.

1363. KRIEG, W. J. S. 1932. The hypothalamus of the albino rat. J. Comp. Neurol., **55:** 19–89.

1364. KRIEG, W. J. S. 1947. Connections of the cerebral cortex. I. The albino rat. C. Extrinsic connections. J. Comp. Neurol., **86:** 267–394.

1365. KRIEG, W. J. S. 1953. *Functional Neuroanatomy.* Blakiston Company, New York, 658 pp.

1366. KRIEG, W. J. S. 1954. Connections of the cerebral cortex. II. The macaque. E. The postcentral gyrus. J. Comp. Neurol., **101:** 101–165.

1367. KRIEGER, D. T., AND LIOTTA, A. S. 1979. Pituitary hormones in brain: Where, how and why? Science, **205:** 366–372.

1368. KRUGER, L. 1979. Functional subdivision of the brainstem sensory trigeminal nuclear complex. In J. J. BONICA, J. C. LIEBESKIND, AND D. G. ALBE-FESSARD (Editors), *Proceedings of the Second World Congress on Pain: Advances in Pain Research and Therapy,* Vol. 3. Raven Press, New York, pp. 197–211.

1369. KRUGER, L., AND MAXWELL, D. S. 1966. Electron microscopy of oligodendrocytes in normal rat cerebrum. Am. J. Anat., **118:** 411–436.

1370. KRUGER, L., AND MICHEL, F. 1962. A morphological and somatotopic analysis of single unit activity in the trigeminal sensory complex of the cat. Exp. Neurol., **5:** 139–156.

1371. KRUGER, L., AND MICHEL, F. 1962a. Reinterpretation of the representation of pain based on physiological excitation of single neurons in the trigeminal sensory complex. Exp. Neurol., **5:** 157–178.

1372. KRUGER, L., AND PORTER, P. 1958. A behavioral study of the functions of the Rolandic cortex in the monkey. J. Comp. Neurol., **109:** 439–469.

1373. KRUGER, L., SIMINOFF, R., AND WITKOVSKY, P. 1961. Single neuron analysis of dorsal column nuclei and spinal nucleus of trigeminal in cat. J. Neurophysiol., **24:** 333–349.

1374. KUDO, M., AND NIIMI K. 1978. Ascending projections of the inferior colliculus on the medial geniculate body in the cat studied by anterograde and retrograde tracing techniques. Brain Res., **155:** 113–117.

1375. KUFFLER, S. W. 1953. Discharge patterns and functional organization of mammalian retina. J. Neurophysiol., **16:** 37–68.

1376. KUFFLER, S. W., AND NICHOLLS, J. G. 1977. *From Neuron to Brain: A Cellular Approach to the Function of the Nervous System.* Sinauer Associates, Inc., Sunderland, Mass., pp. 215–216.

1377. KUFFLER, S. W., NICHOLLS, J. G., AND ORKAND, R. K. 1966. Physiological properties of glial cells in the central nervous system of amphibia. J. Neurophysiol., **29:** 768–787.

1378. KUFFLER, S. W., AND POTTER, D. D. 1964. Glia in the leech central nervous system: Physiological properties and neuron-glia relationships. J. Neurophysiol., **27:** 290–320.

1379. KUHAR, M. J., PERT, C. B., AND SNYDER, S. H. 1973. Regional distribution of opiate receptor binding in monkey and human brain. Nature, **245:** 447–450.

1380. KUHAR, M. J., ROTH, R. H., AND AGHAJANIAN, G. K. 1972. Synthesis of catecholamines in the locus

coeruleus from H³-tyrosine *in vivo.* Biochem. Pharmacol., **21:** 2280–2282.

1381. KUHLENBECK, H. 1948. The derivatives of the thalamus ventralis in the human brain and their relation to the so-called subthalamus. Milit. Surg., **102:** 433–447.

1382. KUHLENBECK, H. 1951. The derivatives of thalamus dorsalis and epithalamus in the human brain: Their relation to cortical and other centers. Milit. Surg., **108:** 205–256.

1383. KUHLENBECK, H. 1969. Derivation and boundaries of the hypothalamus, with atlas of hypothalamic grisea. In W. HAYMAKER *et al.* (Editors), *The Hypothalamus.* Charles C Thomas Publisher, Springfield, Ill., Ch. 2, pp. 13–60.

1384. KUHLENBECK, H. 1975. *The Central Nervous System of Vertebrates,* Vol. 4: *Spinal Cord and Deuterencephalon.* S. Karger, Basel, pp. 332–348.

1385. KUHLENBECK, H., AND HAYMAKER, W. 1949. The derivatives of the hypothalamus in the human brain: Their relation to the extrapyramidal and autonomic systems. Milit. Surg., **105:** 26–52.

1386. KUHLENBECK, H., AND MILLER, R. N. 1949. The pretectal region of the human brain. J. Comp. Neurol., **91:** 369–408.

1387. KUHN, R. A. 1949. Topographical pattern of cutaneous sensibility in the dorsal column nuclei of the cat. Trans. Am. Neurol. Assoc., **74:** 227–230.

1388. KUHN, R. A. 1950. Functional capacity of the isolated human spinal cord. Brain, **75:** 1–51.

1389. KUMAZAWA, T. E., PERL, E. R., BURGESS, P. R., AND WHITEHORN, D. 1975. Ascending projections from marginal zone (lamina I) neurons of the spinal dorsal horn. J. Comp. Neurol., **162:** 1–12.

1390. KÜNZLE, H. 1973. The topographical organization of spinal afferents to the lateral reticular nucleus of the cat. J. Comp. Neurol., **149:** 103–117.

1391. KÜNZLE, H. 1975. Autoradiographic tracing of the cerebellar projections from the lateral reticular nucleus in the cat. Exp. Brain Res., **22:** 255–266.

1392. KÜNZLE, H. 1975a. Bilateral projections from precentral motor cortex to the putamen and other parts of the basal ganglia: An autoradiographic study in *Macaca fascicularis.* Brain Res., **88:** 195–209.

1393. KÜNZLE, H. 1976. Thalamic projections from the precentral motor cortex in *Macaca fascicularis.* Brain Res., **105:** 253–267.

1394. KÜNZLE, H. 1978. An autoradiographic analysis of the efferent connections from premotor and adjacent prefrontal regions (areas 6 and 9) in *Macaca fascicularis.* Brain Behav. Evol., **15:** 185–234.

1395. KÜNZLE, H., AND AKERT, K. 1977. Efferent connections of cortical Area 8 (frontal eye field) in *Macaca fascicularis*: A reinvestigation using the autoradiographic technique. J. Comp. Neurol., **173:** 147–164.

1396. KÜNZLE, H., AKERT, K., AND WURTZ, R. H. 1976. Projections of area 8 (frontal eye field) to superior colliculus in the monkey: An autoradiographic study. Brain Res., **117:** 487–492.

1397. KUO, D., PILE, E., AND KRAUTHAMER, G. M. 1978. Projections of central medianum to caudate nucleus in the cat as demonstrated by retrograde transport of horseradish peroxidase. Neurosci Abstr., Soc. Neurosci., **4:** 45.

1398. KUO, J.-S., AND CARPENTER, M. B. 1973. Organization of pallidothalamic projections in the rhesus monkey. J. Comp. Neurol., **151:** 201–236.

1399. KUPFER, C. 1962. The projection of the macula in the lateral geniculate nucleus of man. Am. J. Ophthalmol., **54:** 597–609.

1400. KURIYAMA, K., HABER, B., SISKEN, B., AND ROBERTS, E. 1966. The γ-amino-butyric acid system in rabbit cerebellum. Proc. Natl. Acad. Sci. U. S. A., **55:** 846–852.

1401. KURU, M. 1949. *Sensory Paths in the Spinal Cord and Brain Stem of Man.* Sogenska, Tokyo, pp. 675–713.

1402. KUSAMA, T., AND MABUCHI, T. 1970. *Stereotaxic Atlas of the Brain of Macaca Fuscata.* University of Tokyo Press, Tokyo.

1403. Kusama, T., Mabuchi, M., and Sumino, T. 1971. Cerebellar projections to the thalamic nuclei in monkey. Proc. Jpn. Acad., **47**: 505–510.

1404. Kuypers, H. G. J. M. 1958. An anatomical analysis of cortico-bulbar connexions to the pons and lower brain stem in the cat. J. Anat., **92**: 198–218.

1405. Kuypers, H. G. J. M. 1958a. Corticobulbar connexions to the pons and lower brain-stem in man: An anatomical study. Brain, **81**: 364–388.

1406. Kuypers, H. G. J. M. 1958b. Some projections from the peri-central cortex to the pons and lower brain stem in monkey and chimpanzee. J. Comp. Neurol., **110**: 221–256.

1407. Kuypers, H. G. J. M. 1958c. Pericentral cortical projections to motor and sensory nuclei. Science, **128**: 662–663.

1408. Kuypers, H. G. J. M. 1960. Central cortical projections to motor and somato-sensory cell groups. Brain, **83**: 161–184.

1409. Kuypers, H. G. J. M., and Brinkman, J. 1970. Precentral projections to different parts of the spinal intermediate zone in the rhesus monkey. Brain Res., **24**: 29–481.

1410. Kuypers, H. G. J. M., Hoffman, A. L., and Beasley, R. M. 1961. Distribution of cortical "feedback" fibers in the nuclei cuneatus and gracilis. Proc. Soc. Exper. Biol. Med., **108**: 634–637.

1411. Kuypers, H. G. J. M., and Lawrence, D. G. 1967. Cortical projections to the red nucleus and the brain stem in the rhesus monkey. Brain Res., **4**: 151–188.

1412. Kuypers, H. G. J. M., and Maisky, V. A. 1975. Retrograde axonal transport of horseradish peroxidase from spinal cord to brain stem cell groups in the cat. Neuroscience Lett., **1**: 9–14.

1413. Kuypers, H. G. J. M., and Tuerk, J. D. 1964. The distribution of cortical fibres within the nuclei cuneatus and gracilis in the cat. J. Anat., **98**: 143–162.

1414. Ladpli, R., and Brodal, A. 1968. Experimental studies of commissural and reticular projections from the vestibular nuclei in the cat. Brain Res., **8**: 65–96.

1415. Laemle, L. K. 1975. Cell populations of the lateral geniculate nucleus of the cat as determined with horseradish peroxidase. Brain Res., **100**: 650–656.

1416. Laemle, L. K., and Noback, C. R. 1970. The visual pathways of the lorisid lemurs (*Nycticebus concang* and *Galago crassicaudatus*). J. Comp. Neurol., **138**: 49–62.

1417. Lammers, H. J. 1972. The neural connections of the amygdaloid complex in mammals. In B. E. Eleftheriou (Editor), *The Neurobiology of the Amygdala*. Plenum Press, New York, pp. 123–144.

1418. La Motte, C., Pert, C. B., and Snyder, S. H. 1976. Opiate receptor binding in primate spinal cord: Distribution and changes after dorsal root section. Brain Res., **112**: 407–412.

1419. La Motte, C. C., Snowman, A., Pert, C. B. and Snyder, S. H. 1978. Opiate receptor binding in rhesus monkey brain: Association with limbic structures. Brain Res., **155**: 374–379.

1420. Land, L. J. 1973. Localized projection of olfactory nerves to rabbit olfactory bulb. Brain Res., **63**: 153–166.

1421. Landgren, S., Nordwall, A., and Wengström, C. 1965. The location of the thalamus relay in the spino-cervico-lemniscal path. Acta physiol. Scand., **65**: 164–175.

1422. Landis, C., Zubin, J., and Mettler, F. A. 1950. The functions of the human frontal lobe. J. Psychol., **30**: 123–138.

1423. Lang, W., Büttner-Ennever, J. A., and Büttner, U. 1979. Vestibular projections to the monkey thalamus: An autoradiographic study. Brain Res., **177**: 3–17

1424. Langley, J. N. 1898. On the union of cranial autonomic (visceral) fibres with the nerve cells of the superior cervical ganglion. J. Physiol. (Lond.), **23**: 240.

1425. Langley, J. N. 1921. *The Autonomic Nervous System*, Vol. 1. W. Heffer and Sons, Cambridge.

1426. Langman, J. 1968. Histogenesis of the central nervous system. In G. H. Bourne (Editor), *The Structure and Function of Nervous Tissue*, Vol. 1. Academic Press, New York, pp. 33–65.

1427. Langman, J. 1969. *Medical Embryology*, Ed. 2. Williams & Wilkins, Baltimore, 386 pp.

1428. Langman, J. 1981. *Medical Embryology*. Ed. 4 Williams & Wilkins, Baltimore.

1429. Langman, J., Guerrant, R. L., and Freeman, B. G. 1966. Behavior of neuroepithelial cells during closure of the neural tube. J. Comp. Neurol., **127**: 399–411.

1430. Langman, J., and Haden, C. C. 1970. Formation and migration of neuroblasts in the spinal cord of the chick embryo. J. Comp. Neurol., **138**: 419–432.

1431. LaPorte, Y., Emonet-Denand, F., and Jami, L. 1981. The skeleto-fusimotor or β innervation of mammalian muscle spindles. Trends Neurosci., **4**: 97–99.

1432. Larsell, O. 1923. The cerebellum of the frog. J. Comp. Neurol., **36**: 89–122.

1433. Larsell, O. 1947. The cerebellum of myxinoids and petromyzonts, including developmental stages in the lampreys. J. Comp. Neurol., **86**: 395–446.

1434. Larsell, O. 1947a. The development of the cerebellum in man in relation to its comparative anatomy. J. Comp. Neurol., **87**: 85–129.

1435. Larsell, O. 1951. *Anatomy of the Nervous System*, Ed. 2. Appleton-Century-Crofts, Inc., New York, 520 pp.

1436. Larsell, O., and Dow, R. S. 1933. Innervation of the human lung. Am. J. Anat., **52**: 414–438.

1437. Larsell, O., and Jansen, J. 1972. *The Comparative Anatomy and Histology of the Cerebellum: The Human Cerebellum, Cerebellar Connections and Cerebellar Cortex*. University of Minnesota Press, Minneapolis, 264 pp.

1438. Larsen, K. D., and McBride, R. L. 1979. The organization of feline entopeduncular nucleus projections: Anatomical studies. J. Comp. Neurol., **184**: 293–308.

1439. Larsen, K. D., and Sutin J. 1978. Output organization of the feline entopeduncular and subthalamic nuclei. Brain Res., **157**: 21–31.

1440. Lasek, R. J. 1970. Protein transport in neurons. Int. Rev. Neurobiol., **13**: 289–324.

1441. Lasek, R. J. 1980. Axonal transport: A dynamic view of neuronal structures. Trends Neurosci., **3**: 87–91.

1442. Lassek, A. M. 1940. The human pyramidal tract. II. A numerical investigation of the Betz cells of the motor area. Arch. Neurol. Psychiatry, **44**: 718–724.

1443. Lassek, A. M. 1942. The human pyramidal tract. IV. A study of the mature, myelinated fibers of the pyramid. J. Comp. Neurol., **76**: 217–225.

1444. Lassek, A. M. 1942. The pyramidal tract. The effect of pre- and postcentral cortical lesions on the fiber components of the pyramids in monkey. J. Nerv. Ment. Dis., **95**: 721–729.

1445. Lassek, A. M. 1947. The pyramidal tract: Basic considerations of corticospinal neurons. Proc. Assoc. Res. Nerv. Ment. Dis., **27**: 106–128.

1446. Lassek, A. M. 1953. Potency of isolated brachial dorsal roots in controlling muscular physiology. Neurology (Minneap.), **3**: 53–57.

1447. Lassek, A. M. 1954. *The Pyramidal Tract: Its Status in Medicine*. Charles C Thomas, Publisher, Springfield, Ill., 166 pp.

1448. Lassek, A. M., and Evans, J. P. 1945. The human pyramidal tract. XII. The effect of hemispherectomies on the fiber components of the pyramids. J. Comp. Neurol., **83**: 113–119.

1449. Lassek, A. M., and Rasmussen, G. L. 1939. The human pyramidal tract: A fiber and numerical analysis. Arch. Neurol. Psychiatry, **42**: 872–876.

1450. Lassek, A. M., and Rasmussen, G. L. 1940. A comparative fiber and numerical analysis of the pyramidal tract. J. Comp. Neurol., 72: 417–428.

1451. LaVAIL, J. H. 1975. Retrograde cell degeneration and retrograde transport techniques. In W. M. COWAN AND M. CUÉNOD (Editors), *The Use of Axonal Transport for Studies of Neuronal Connectivity.* Elsevier Scientific Publishing Co., Amsterdam, pp. 217–247.

1453. LA VAIL, J. H., AND LAVAIL, M. M. 1972. Retrograde axonal transport in the central nervous system. Science, 176: 1416–1417.

1454. LaVAIL, J. H., AND LaVAIL, M. M. 1974. The retrograde intraaxonal transport of horseradish peroxidase in the chick visual system: A light and electron microscopic study. J. Comp. Neurol., 157: 303–358.

1455. LaVAIL, J. H., RAPISARDI, S., AND SUGINO, I. K. 1980. Evidence against the smooth endoplasmic reticulum as a continuous channel for the retrograde axonal transport of horseradish peroxidase. Brain Res., 191: 3–20.

1456. LaVAIL, J. H., WINSTON, K. R., AND TISH, A. 1973. A method based on retrograde intra-axonal transport of protein for identification of cell bodies of origin of axons terminating within the C.N.S. Brain Res., 58: 470–477.

1457. LAWRENCE, D. G., AND HOPKINS, D. A. 1976. The development of motor control in the rhesus monkey: Evidence concerning the role of corticomotorneuronal connections. Brain, 99: 235–254.

1458. LAWRENCE, D. G., AND KUYPERS, H. G. J. M. 1968. The functional organization of the motor system in the monkey. I. The effects of bilateral pyramidal lesions. Brain, 91: 1–14.

1459. LAZORTHES, G., GOUSZÉ, A., AND SALAMON, G. 1976. *Vascularization et Circulation de l'Encéphale,* Vol. 1 and 2. Masson et Cie, Paris.

1460. LAZORTHES, G., POULHES, J., BASTIDE, G., ROLLEAU, J., AND CHANCHOLLE, A. R. 1957. Récherches sur las vascularisation artérielle de la moëlle: Application à la pathologie médullaire. Bull. Acad. Natl. Med., 141: 464–477.

1461. LAZORTHES, G., AND SALAMON, G. 1971. The arteries of the thalamus: An anatomical and radiological study. J. Neurosurg., 34: 23–26.

1462. LEÃO, A. A. P. 1944. Spreading depression of activity in the cerebral cortex. J. Neurophysiol., 7: 359–390.

1463. LEE, J. C. Y. 1963. Electron microscopy of Wallerian degeneration. J. Comp. Neurol., 120: 65–79.

1464. LEIBOWITZ, S. F. 1976. Brain catecholaminergic mechanisms for control of hunger. In D. NOVIN, W. WYRWICKA, AND G. A. BRAY (Editors), *Hunger: Brain Mechanisms and Clinical Implications.* Raven Press, New York, pp. 1–18.

1465. LEICHNETZ, G. R., AND ASTRUC, J. 1976. The efferent projections of the medial prefrontal cortex in the squirrel monkey (*Samiri scuiresus*). Brain Res., 109: 455–472.

1466. LEMMEN, L. J., DAVIS, J. S., AND RADNOR, L. L. 1959. Observations on stimulation of the human frontal eye field. J. Comp. Neurol., 112: 163–168.

1467. LEONARD, C. M. 1972. The connections of the dorsomedial nuclei. Brain Behav. Evol., 6: 524–541.

1468. LEONARD, C. M., AND SCOTT, J. W. 1971. Origin and distribution of amygdalofugal pathways in the rat: An experimental neuroanatomical study. J. Comp. Neurol., 144: 313–330.

1469. LEUSEN, I. 1972. Regulation of cerebrospinal fluid composition with reference to breathing. Physiol. Rev., 52: 1–56.

1470. LeVAY, S., HUBEL, D., AND WIESEL, T. N. 1975. The pattern of ocular dominance columns in Macaque visual cortex revealed by reduced silver stain. J. Comp. Neurol., 159: 559–576.

1471. LeVAY, S. WIESEL, T. N., AND HUBEL, D. H. 1980. The development of ocular dominance columns in normal and visually deprived monkeys. J. Comp. Neurol., 191: 1–51.

1472. LEVI-MONTALCINI, R., AND ANGELETTI, P. V. 1961. Growth control of the sympathetic system by a specific protein factor. Q. Rev. Biol., 36: 99–108.

1473. LEVI-MONTALCINI, R., AND ANGELETTI, P. V. 1963. Essential role of the nerve growth factor in the survival and maintenance of dissociated sensory and sympathetic embryonic nerve cells *in vitro.* Dev. Biol., 7: 653–659.

1474. LEVI-MONTALCINI, R., AND BOOKER, B. 1960. Excessive growth of the sympathetic ganglia evoked by a protein isolated from mouse. Proc. Natl. Acad. Sci., U. S. A., 46: 373–391.

1475. LEVI-MONTALCINI, R., COHEN, S. 1960. Effects of the extract of the mouse submaxillary salivary glands on the sympathetic system of mammals. Ann. N. Y. Acad. Sci., 85: 324–341.

1476. LEVI-MONTALCINI, R., AND HAMBURGER, V. 1951. Selective growth stimulating effects of mouse sarcoma on the sensory and sympathetic nervous system of the chick embryo. J. Zool. (Lond.), 116: 321–362.

1477. LEVI-MONTALCINI, R., MEYER, H., AND HAMBURGER, V. 1954. *In vitro* experiments on the effects of mouse sarcomas 180 and 37 on the spinal and sympathetic ganglia of the chick embryo. Cancer Res., 14: 49–57.

1478. LEVIN, P. M. 1936. The efferent fibers of the frontal lobe of the monkey (*Macaca mulatta*). J. Comp. Neurol., 63: 369–419.

1479. LEVIN, P. M. 1949. Efferent fibers. In P. C. BUCY (Editor), *The Precentral Motor Cortex,* Ed. 2. University of Illinois Press, Urbana, Ch. 5, pp. 133–148.

1480. LEVIN, P. M., AND BRADFORD, F. K. 1938. The exact origin of the corticospinal tract in the monkey. J. Comp. Neurol., 68: 411–422.

1481. LEVITT, M., CARRERAS, M., CHAMBERS, W. W., AND LIU, C. N. 1960. Pyramidal influence on unit activity in posterior column nuclei of cat. Physiologist, 3: 103.

1482. LEVITT, P., AND MOORE, R. Y. 1979. Origin and organization of brainstem catecholamine innervation in the rat. J. Comp. Neurol., 186: 505–528.

1483. LEVITT, P., AND RAKIC, P. 1980. Immunoperoxidase localization of glial fibrillary acidic protein in radial glial cells and astrocytes of the developing rhesus monkey brain. J. Comp. Neurol., 193: 815–840.

1484. LEWIS, P. R., AND SHUTE, C. C. D. 1967. The cholinergic limbic system: Projections to hippocampal formation, medial cortex, nuclei of the ascending cholinergic reticular system, and the subfornical organ and supraoptic crest. Brain, 90: 521–540.

1485. LEWIS, P. R., SHUTE, C. C. D., AND SILVER, A. 1967. Confirmation of choline acetylase analyses of massive cholinergic innervation to the rat hippocampus. J. Physiol (Lond.), 191: 215–224.

1486. LEWY, F. H., AND KOBRAK, H. 1936. Neural projection of cochlear spirals on primary acoustic centers. Arch. Neurol. Psychiatry, 35: 839–852.

1487. LIDBRINK, P. 1974. The effects of lesions of ascending noradrenaline pathways on sleep and waking in the cat. Brain Res., 74: 19–40.

1488. LIDDELL, E. G. T., AND PHILLIPS, C. G. 1940. Experimental lesions in the basal ganglia of the cat. Brain, 63: 264–274.

1489. LIEDGREN, S. R. C., MILNE, A. C., RUBIN, A. M., SCHWARZ, D. W. F., AND TOMLINSEN, R. D. 1976. Representation of vestibular afferents in somatosensory thalamic nuclei of the squirrel monkey (*Saimiri sciureus*). J. Neurophysiol., 39: 601–612.

1490. LIGHT, A. R., AND PERL, E. R. 1979. Reexamination of the dorsal root projection to the spinal dorsal horn including observations on the differential termination of coarse and fine fibers. J. Comp. Neurol., 186: 117–132.

1491. LIGHT, A. R., AND PERL, E. R. 1979a. Spinal terminations of functionally identified primary afferent neurons with slowly conducting myelinated fibers. J. Comp. Neurol., 186: 133–150.

1492. LIGHT, A. R., TREVINO, D. L., AND PERL, E.

R. 1979. Morphological features of functionally defined neurons in the marginal zone and substantia gelatinosa of the spinal dorsal horn. J. Comp. Neurol., **186:** 151–172.

1493. LIM, R. 1980. Glia maturation factor. Curr. Top. Dev. Biol., **16:** 305–322.

1494. LIM, R. K. S., KRAUTHAMER, G., GUZMAN, F., AND FULP, R. R. 1969. Central nervous system activity associated with pain evoked by bradykinin and its alteration by morphine and aspirin. Proc. Natl. Acad. Sci. U. S. A., **63:** 705–712.

1495. LINDBLOM, U., AND LUND, L. 1966. The discharge from vibration-sensitive receptors in the monkey foot. Exp. Neurol., **15:** 401–417.

1496. LINDSLEY, D. B. 1960. Attention, consciousness, sleep and wakefulness. In J. FIELD (Editor), *Handbook of Physiology*, Sect. 1, Vol. III. American Physiological Society, Washington, D. C., pp. 1553–1593.

1497. LINDVALL, O., AND BJÖRKLUND, A. 1974. The glyoxylic acid fluorescence histochemical method: A detailed account of the methodology for the visualization of central catecholamine neurons. Histochemistry, **39:** 97–127.

1498. LINDVALL, O., AND BJÖRKLUND, A. 1974a. The organization of the ascending catecholamine neuron systems in the rat brain as revealed by the glyoxylic acid fluorescence method. Acta Physiol. Scand. (Suppl.), **412:** 1–48.

1498a. LINDVALL, O., AND BJÖRKLUND, A. 1978. Organization of catecholamine neurons in the rat central nervous system. In L. L. IVERSEN, S. D. IVERSEN AND S. H. SNYDER (Editors). *Handbook of Psychopharmacology*, Vol. 9, Plenum Press, N.Y., pp. 139–231.

1499. LIU, C. N. 1956. Afferent nerves to Clarke's and the lateral cuneate nuclei in the cat. Arch. Neurol. Psychiatry, **75:** 67–77.

1500. LIU, C. N., AND CHAMBERS, W. W. 1964. An experimental study of the corticospinal system in the monkey (*Macaca mulatta*): The spinal pathways and preterminal distribution of degenerating fibers following discrete lesions of the pre- and postcentral gyri and bulbar pyramid. J. Comp. Neurol., **123:** 257–284.

1501. LIVETT, B. G. 1978. Immunohistochemical localization of nervous system specific proteins and peptides. Int. Rev. Cytol. (Suppl.), **7:** 53–237.

1502. LIVINGSTON, R. B. 1964. Mechanics of cerebrospinal fluid. In T. C. RUCH AND H. D. PATTON (Editors), *Physiology and Biophysics*. W. B. Saunders Company, Philadelphia, Ch. 47, pp. 935–940.

1503. LLINÁS, R., BAKER, R., AND SOTELO, C. 1974. Electrotonic coupling between neurons in cat inferior olive. J. Neurophysiol., **37:** 560–571.

1504. LLOYD, D. P. C. 1943. Conduction and synaptic transmission of reflex response to stretch in spinal cats. J. Neurophysiol., **6:** 317–326.

1505. LLOYD, D. P. C., AND MCINTYRE, A. K. 1950. Dorsal column conduction of group I muscle afferent impulses and their relay through Clarke's column. J. Neurophysiol., **13:** 39–54.

1506. LOCKE, S., ANGEVINE, J. B., JR. AND YAKOVLEV, P. I. 1961. Limbic nuclei of thalamus and connections of limbic cortex. II. Thalamo-cortical projections of the lateral dorsal nucleus in man. Arch. Neurol., **4:** 355–364.

1507. LOCKE, S., ANGEVINE, J. B., JR., AND YAKOVLEV, P. I. 1964. Limbic nuclei of thalamus and connections of limbic cortex. VI. Thalamo-cortical projection of lateral dorsal nucleus in cat and monkey. Arch. Neurol., **11:** 1–12.

1508. LOEWENSTEIN, W. R. 1959. The generation of electric activity in a nerve ending. Ann. N. Y. Acad. Sci., **81:** 367–387.

1509. LOEWENSTEIN, W. R. 1960. Biological transducers. Sci. Am. **203:** 99–108.

1510. LOEWENSTEIN, W. R. 1971. Mechano-electric transduction in the Pacinian corpuscle: Initiation of sensory impulses in mechanoreceptors. In W. R. LOEWENSTEIN (Editor), *Principles of Receptor Physiology*. Springer-Verlag, Berlin. Ch. 9, pp. 269–290.

1511. LOEWENSTEIN, W. R., AND ALTAMIRANO-ORREGO, R. 1958. The refractory state of the generator and propagated potentials in a Pacinian corpuscle. J. Gen. Physiol., **41:** 805–824.

1512. LOEWENTHAL, M., AND HORSLEY, V. 1897. On the relations between the cerebellum and other centres (namely cerebral and spinal) with special reference to the action of antagonistic muscles. Proc. R. Soc. Ser. B, **61:** 20–25.

1513. LOEWI, O. 1921. Über humorale Übertragbarkeit der Herznervenwirkung. Arch. Gesamte Physiol., Menschen Tiere **189:** 239–242.

1514. LOEWI, O. 1945. Chemical transmission of nerve impulses. Sci. Prog. **4:** 98–119.

1515. LOEWY, A. D. 1981. Descending pathways to sympathetic and parasympathetic preganglionic neurons. J. Auton. Nerv. Syst., **3:** 265–275.

1516. LOEWY, A. D., ARAUJO, J. C., AND KERR, F. W. L. 1973. Pupillodilator pathways in the brain stem of the cat: Anatomical and electrophysiological identification of a central autonomic pathway. Brain Res., **60:** 65–91.

1517. LOEWY, A. D., AND BURTON, H. 1978. Nuclei of the solitary tract: Efferent projections to the lower brain stem and spinal cord of the cat. J. Comp. Neurol., **181:** 421–450.

1518. LOEWY, A. D., AND MCKELLAR, S. 1980. The neuroanatomical basis of central cardiovascular control. Fed. Proc., **39:** 2495–2503.

1519. LOEWY, A. D., AND SAPER, C. B. 1978. Edinger-Westphal nucleus: Projections to the brain stem and spinal cord in the cat. Brain Res., **150:** 1–27.

1520. LOEWY, A. D., SAPER, C. B., AND YAMODIS, N. D. 1978. Re-evaluation of the efferent projections of the Edinger-Westphal nucleus. Brain Res., **141:** 153–159.

1521. LOHMAN, A. H. M. 1963. The anterior olfactory lobe of the guinea pig. Acta Anat. (Basel), **53:** (suppl. 49): 1–109.

1522. LONG, D. M., AND HAGFORS, N. 1975. Electrical stimulation in the nervous system: The current status of electrical stimulation of the nervous system for the relief of pain. Pain, **1:** 109–124.

1523. LORÉN, I., ALUMETS, J., HÅKANSON, R., AND SUNDLER, F. 1979. Distribution of gastrin and CCK-like peptides in rat brain: An immunocytochemical study. Histochemistry, **59:** 249–257.

1524. LORÉN, I., BJÖRKLUND, A., FALK, B., AND LINDVALL, O. 1980. The aluminum-formaldehyde (alfa) histofluorescence method for improved visualization of catecholamines and indoleamines. I. A detailed account of the methodology for central nervous tissue using paraffin, cryostat or vibratome sections. J. Neurosci. Methods, **2:** 277–300.

1525. LORENTE DE NÓ, R. 1924. Études sur le cerveau postérieur. Trav. Lab. Rech. Biol. Univ. Madrid, **22:** 51–65.

1526. LORENTE DE NÓ, R. 1928. *Die Labyrinthreflexe auf die Augenmuskeln nach einseitiger Labyrinthextirpation nebst einer kurzen Angabe über den Nervenmechanismus der vestibulären Augenbewegungen.* Urban and Schwarzenberg, Vienna.

1527. LORENTE DE NÓ, R. 1931. Ausgewählte Kapitel aus der vergleichenden Physiologie des Labyrinthes: Die Augenmuskelreflexe beim Kaninchen und ihre Grundlagen. Ergebn. Physiol., **32:** 73–242.

1528. LORENTE DE NÓ, R. 1933. Studies on the structure of the cerebral cortex. I. The area entorhinalis. J. Psychol. Neurol., **45:** 381–438.

1529. LORENTE DE NÓ, R. 1933. Anatomy of the eighth nerve: The central projection of the nerve endings of the internal ear. Laryngoscope, **43:** 1–38.

1530. LORENTE DE NÓ, R. 1934. Studies on the structure of the cerebral cortex. II. Continuation of the study of the ammonic system. J. Psychol. Neurol., **46:** 113–177.

1531. LORENTE DE NÓ, R. 1949. The structure of the cerebral cortex. In J. F. FULTON (Editor), *Physiology of the Nervous System*, Ed. 3. Oxford University Press, New York, pp. 288–330.

1532. LORENTE DE NÓ, R. 1953. Symposium discussion. In J. L. MALCOLM AND J. A. B. GRAY (Editors), *The Spinal Cord*. Ciba Foundation Symposium. Little, Brown & Company, Boston, pp. 40–41.

1533. DE LORENZO, A. J. D. 1963. Studies on the ultrastructure and histophysiology of cell membranes, nerve fibers and synaptic junctions in chemoreceptors. In Y. ZOTTERMAN (Editor), *Olfaction and Taste*. Pergamon Press, New York, pp. 5–17.

1534. LOWENSTEIN, O. 1954. Clinical pupillary symptoms in lesions of the optic nerve, optic chiasm and optic tract. A. M. A. Arch. Ophthalmol., **52:** 385–403.

1535. LUK, G. D., MOREST, D. K., AND McKENNA, N. M. 1974. Origins of the crossed olivocochlear bundle shown by an acid phosphatase method in the cat. Ann. Otol. Rhinol. Laryngol., **83:** 382–391.

1536. LUND, J. S. 1973. Organization of neurons in the visual cortex, area 17, of the monkey. J. Comp. Neurol., **147:** 455–406.

1537. LUND, J. S., LUND, R. D., HENDRICKSON, A. E., BUNT, A. H., AND FUCHS, A. F. 1975. The origin of efferent pathays from the primary visual cortex, area 17, of the macaque monkey as shown by retrograde transport of horseradish peroxidase. J. Comp. Neurol., **164:** 287–304.

1538. LUNDBERG, A. 1958. Electrophysiology of the salivary glands. Physiol. Rev., **38:** 21–40.

1539. LUNDBERG, A. 1964. Ascending spinal hindlimb pathways in the cat. In J. C. ECCLES AND J. P. SCHADÉ (Editors), *Progress in Brain Research*, Vol. 12: *Physiology of Spinal Neurons*. Elsevier Publishing Company, Amsterdam, pp. 135–163.

1540. LUNDBERG, A., AND OSCARSSON, O. 1962. Functional organization of the ventral spino-cerebellar tract in the cat. IV. Identification of units by antidromic activation from the cerebellar cortex. Acta Physiol. Scand., **54:** 252–269.

1541. LUNDBERG, J. M., DAHLSTRÖM, A., LARSSON, I., PETTERSSON, G., AHLMAN, H., AND KEWENTER, J. 1978. Efferent innervation of the small intestine by adrenergic neurons from the cervical sympathetic and stellate ganglia, studied by retrograde transport of peroxidase. Acta Physiol. Scand., **104:** 33–42.

1542. LUSCHEI, E. S., AND FUCHS, A. F. 1972. Activity of brain stem neurons during eye movements of alert monkeys. J. Neurophysiol., **35:** 445–461.

1543. LUSE, S. A. 1956. Electron microscopic observations of central nervous system. J. Biophys. Biochem. Cytol., **2:** 531–542.

1544. LUSE, S. A. 1956a. Formation of myelin in the central nervous system of mice and rats, as studied with the electron microscope. J. Biophys. Biochem. Cytol., **2:** 777–783.

1545. LUSE, S. A. 1958. Ultrastructure of reactive and neoplastic astrocytes. Lab. Invest., **7:** 401–417.

1546. LUSE, S. A. 1968. Microglia: Neuroglia. In J. MINCKLER (Editor), *Pathology of the Nervous System*. McGraw-Hill Book Company, New York, pp. 531–553.

1547. LYSER, K. M. 1964. Early differentiation of motor neuroblasts in the chick embryo as studied by electron microscopy. Dev. Biol., **10:** 433–466.

1548. LYSER, K. M. 1968. Early differentiation of motor neuroblasts in the chick embryo as studied by electron microscopy. II. Microtubules and neurofilaments. Dev. Biol., **17:** 117–142.

1549. MACLEAN, P. D. 1952. Some psychiatric implications of physiological studies on frontotemporal portions of limbic system (visceral brain). Electroencephalogr. Clin. Neurophysiol., **4:** 407–418.

1550. MACLEAN, P. D. 1957. Chemical and electrical stimulation of the hippocampus in unrestrained animals. I. Methods and electroencephalographic findings.

A. M. A. Arch. Neurol. Psychiatry, **78:** 113–127.

1551. MACLEAN, P. D. 1957a. Chemical and electrical stimulation of the hippocampus in unrestrained animals. II. Behavioral findings. A. M. A. Arch. Neurol. Psychiatry, **78:** 128–142.

1552. MACLEAN, P. D., AND DELGADO, J. M. R. 1953. Electrical and chemical stimulation of fronto-temporal portion of limbic system in the waking animal. Electroencephalogr. Clin. Neurophysiol., **5:** 91–100.

1553. MACLUSKY, N. J., AND NAFTOLIN, F. 1981. Sexual differentiation of the central nervous system. Science, **211:** 1294–1302.

1554. McBRIDE, R. L., AND LARSEN, K. D. 1980. Projections of the feline globus pallidus. Brain Res., **198:** 3–14.

1555. McBRIDE, R. L., AND SUTIN, J. 1976. Projections of the locus coerulus and adjacent pontine tegmentum in the cat. J. Comp. Neurol., **165:** 265–284.

1556. McBRIDE, R. L., AND SUTIN, J. 1977. Amygdaloid and pontine projections to the ventromedial nucleus of the hypothalamus. J. Comp. Neurol., **174:** 377–396.

1557. McCOMAS, A. J. 1963. Responses of the rat dorsal column system to mechanical stimulation of the hind paw. J. Physiol. (Lond.), **166:** 435–445.

1558. McCREA, R. A., BISHOP, G. A., AND KITAI, S. T. 1976. Intracellular staining of Purkinje cells and their axons with horseradish peroxidase. Brain Res., **118:** 132–136.

1559. McCREA, R. A., BISHOP, G. A., AND KITAI, S. T. 1977. Electrophysiological and horseradish peroxidase studies of precerebellar afferents to the nucleus interpositus anterior. II. Mossy fiber system. Brain Res., **122:** 215–228.

1560. McCULLOCH, W. S. 1949. Cortico-cortical connections. In P. C. BUCY (Editor), *The Precentral Motor Cortex*, Ed. 2. University of Illinois Press, Urbana, Ch. 8, pp. 214–242.

1561. McCULLOCH, W. S., AND GAROL, H. W. 1941. Cortical origin and distribution of corpus callosum and anterior commissure in the monkey (*Macaca mulatta*). J. Neurophysiol., **4:** 555–563.

1562. McEWEN, B. S. 1981. Neural gonadal steroid actions. Science, **211:** 1303–1311.

1563. McGEER, P. L., FIBIGER, H. C., MALER, L., HATTORI, T., AND McGEER, E. G. 1974. Evidence for descending pallido-nigral GABA-containing neurons. Adv. Neurol., **5:** 153–160.

1564. McGEER, P. L., McGEER, E. G., WADA, J. A., AND JUNG, E. 1971. Effects of globus pallidus lesions and Parkinson's disease on brain glutamic acid decarboxylase. Brain Res., **32:** 425–431.

1565. McGUINNESS, C. M., AND KRAUTHAMER, G. M. 1980. The afferent projections to the centrum medianum of the cat as demonstrated by retrograde transport of horseradish peroxidase. Brain Res., **184:** 255–269.

1566. McKINLEY, W. A., AND MAGOUN, H. W. 1942. The bulbar projection of the trigeminal nerve. Am. J. Physiol., **137:** 217–224.

1567. McLARDY, T. 1948. Projection of the centromedian nucleus of the human thalamus. Brain, **71:** 290–303.

1568. McLARDY, T. 1950. The thalamic projection to frontal cortex in man. J. Neurol. Neurosurg. Psychiatry, **13:** 198–202.

1569. McLENNAN, H. 1963. *Synaptic Transmission*. W.B. Saunders Company, Philadelphia, pp. 3–15.

1570. McLENNAN, H. 1971. The pharmacology of inhibition of mitral cells in the olfactory bulb. Brain Res., **29:** 177–184.

1571. McLENNAN, H., AND YORK, D. H. 1967. The action of dopamine on neurons of the caudate nucleus. J. Physiol. (Lond.), **189:** 393–402.

1572. McMANUS, J. F. A., AND MOWRY, R. W. 1960. *Staining Methods: Histologic and Histochemical*. Paul B. Hoeber Inc., New York, pp. 324–357.

1573. McMASTERS, R. E., WEISS, A. H., AND CARPENTER, M. B. 1966. Vestibular projections to the nuclei of the extraocular muscles: Degeneration resulting from discrete partial lesions of the vestibular nuclei in the monkey. Am. J. Anat., **118**: 163–194.

1574. McMichael, J. 1945. Spinal tracts subserving micturition in a case of Erb's spinal paralysis. Brain., **68**: 162.

1575. McNeill, T. H., and Sladek, J. R., Jr. 1980. Simultaneous monoamine histofluorescence and neuropeptide immunocytochemistry. II. Correlative distribution of catecholamine varicosities and magnocellular neurosecretory neurons in the rat supraoptic and paraventricular nuclei. J. Comp. Neurol., **193**: 1023–1033.

1576. Macchi, G., Bentivoglio, M., Rossini, P., and Tempesta, E. 1978. The basolateral amygdaloid projections to the neocortex in the cat. Neurosci. Lett., **9**: 347–352.

1577. Machine, X., and Segundo, J. P. 1956. Unitary responses to afferent volleys in amygdaloid complex. J. Neurophysiol., **19**: 232–240.

1578. Maciewicz, R. J., Eagen, K., Kaneko, C. R. S., and Highstein, S. M. 1977. Vestibular and medullary brain stem afferents to the abducens nucleus in the cat. Brain Res., **123**: 229–240.

1579. Madigan, J. C., Jr., and Carpenter, M. B. 1971. *Cerebellum of the Rhesus Monkey: Atlas of Lobules, Laminae, and Folia, in Sections.* University Park Press, Baltimore, 137 pp.

1580. Madonick, M. J. 1957. Statistical control studies in neurology. VII. The cutaneous abdominal reflex. Neurology (Minneap.), **7**: 459–465.

1581. Maeda, T., Pin, C., Salvert, D., Ligier, M., and Jouvet, M. 1973. Les neurones contenant des catécholamines du tegmentum pontique et leurs voies de projection chez le chat. Brain Res., **57**: 119–152.

1582. Maeda, T., and Shimizu, N. 1972. Projections ascendantes du locus coeruleus et d'antres neurones aminergiques pontiques au niveau du prosencéphale du rat. Brain Res., **36**: 19–35.

1583. Maffel, L., and Pompeiano, O. 1962. Cerebellar control of flexor motoneurons. Arch. Ital. Biol., **100**: 476–509.

1584. Magnin, M., and Fuchs, A. F. 1977. Discharge properties of neurons in the monkey thalamus tested with angular acceleration, eye movement and visual stimuli. Exp. Brain Res., **28**: 293–299.

1585. Magoun, H. W. 1940. Descending connections from the hypothalamus. J. Nerv. Ment. Dis., **20**: 270–285.

1586. Magoun, H. W. 1952. An ascending reticular activating system in the brain stem. A. M. A. Arch. Neurol. Psychiatry, **67**: 145–154.

1587. Magoun, H. W. 1954. The ascending reticular system and wakefulness. J. B. In Delafresnaye (Editor), *Brain Mechanisms and Consciousness.* Blackwell Scientific Publications., Oxford, pp. 1–20.

1588. Magoun, H. W. 1963. *The Waking Brain*, Ed. 2. Charles C Thomas, Publisher, Springfield, Ill.

1589. Magoun, H. W., Atlas, D., Ingersoll, E. H., and Ranson, S. W. 1937. Associated facial, vocal and respiratory components of emotional expression. J. Neurol. Psychopathol., **17**: 241–255.

1590. Magoun, H. W., and Ranson, S. W. 1935. The central path of the light reflex: A study of the effect of lesions. Arch. Ophthalmol., **13**: 791–811.

1591. Magoun, H. W., and Ranson, S. W. 1935a. The afferent path of the light reflex: A review of the literature. Arch. Ophthalmol., **13**: 862–874.

1592. Magoun, H. W., Ranson, S. W., and Mayer, L. L. 1935. The pupillary light reflex after lesions of the posterior commissure in the cat. Am. J. Ophthalmol., **18**: 624–630.

1593. Magoun, H. W., and Rhines, R. 1946. An inhibitory mechanism in the bulbar reticular formation. J. Neurophysiol., **9**: 165–171.

1594. Magoun, H. W., and Rhines, R. 1947. *Spasticity: The Stretch-reflex and Extrapyramidal Systems.* Charles C Thomas, Publisher, Springfield, Ill.

1595. Malmförs, T. 1964. Release and depletion of the transmitter in adrenergic terminals produced by nerve impulses after the inhibition of noradrenalin synthesis or reabsorption. Life Sci., **3**: 1397–1402.

1596. Malone, E. F. 1910. Über die Kerne des menschlichen Diencephalon: Abhandlungen der königl. preuss. Akademie der Wissenschaften, p. 92.

1597. Malpeli, J. G., and Baker, F. H. 1975. The representation of the visual field in the lateral geniculate nucleus of the *Macaca mulatta.* J. Comp. Neurol., **161**: 569–594.

1598. Mannen, H., and Sugiura, Y. 1976. Reconstruction of neurons of dorsal horn proper using Golgistained sections. J. Comp. Neurol., **168**: 303–312.

1599. Manni, E., Bortolami, R., and Desole, C. 1966. Eye muscle proprioception in the semilunar ganglion. Exp. Neurol., **16**: 226–236.

1600. Marburg, O., and Warner, F. J. 1947. The pathways of the tectum (anterior colliculus) of the midbrain in cats. J. Nerv. Ment. Dis., **106**: 415–446.

1601. Marchi, V., and Algeri, G. 1885. Sulle degenerazioni discendenti consecutive a lesioni sperimentale in diverse zone della corteccia cerebrale. Riv. Sper. Freniat. Med. Leg. Alien. Ment., **11**: 492–494.

1602. Margolis, F. L. 1974. Carnosine in the primary olfactory pathway. Science, **84**: 909–911.

1603. Marle, P. 1906. Revision de la question de l'aphasie: La troisième circonvolution frontale gauche ne joue aucun rôle special dans la fonction du langage. Sem. Med **26**: 241–247.

1604. Mark, V. H., Ervin, F. R., and Sweet, W. H. 1972. Deep temporal lobe stimulation in man. In B. E. Eleftheriou (Editor), *The Neurobiology of the Amygdala.* Plenum Press, New York, pp. 485–507.

1605. Markee, J. E., Sawyer, C. H., and Hollinshead, W. H. 1946. Activation of the anterior hypophysis by electrical stimulation in the rabbit. Endocrinology, **38**: 345–357.

1606. Markham, C. H., Precht, W., and Shimazu, H. 1966. Effects of stimulation of interstitial nucleus of Cajal on vestibular unit activity in the cat. J. Neurophysiol., **29**: 493–507.

1607. Marlowe, W. B., Mancall, E. L., and Thomas, J. J. 1975. Complete Klüver-Bucy syndrome in man. Cortex, **11**: 53–59.

1608. Mars, H. 1973. Modification of levodopa effect by systematic decarboxylase inhibition. Arch. Neurol., **28**: 91–95.

1609. Marsden, C. D. 1961. Pigmentation in the nucleus substantiae nigrae of mammals. J. Anat., **95**: 256–261.

1610. Marshall, W. H. 1950. The relation of dehydration of the brain to the spreading depression of Leão. Electroencephalogr. Clin. Neurophysiol., **2**: 177–186.

1611. Marshall, W. H. 1959. Spreading cortical depression of Leão. Physiol. Rev., **39** (suppl. 3): 239–279.

1612. Marshall, W. H., and Essig, C. F. 1951. Relation of air exposure of cortex to spreading depression of Leão. J. Neurophysiol., **14**: 265–273.

1613. Marshall, W. H., Essig, C. F., and Dubroff, S. J. 1951. Relation of temperature of cerebral cortex to spreading depression of Leão. J. Neurophysiol., **14**: 153–166.

1614. Marshall, W. R., Woolsey, C. N., and Bard, P. 1941. Observations on cortical somatic sensory mechanisms of the cat and monkey. J. Neurophysiol., **4**: 1–24.

1615. Martin, G. F., and Dom, R. 1970. Rubrobulbar projections of the opossum (*Didelphia virginiana*). J. Comp. Neurol., **139**: 199–214.

1616. Martin, G. F., King, J. S., and Dom, R. 1974. The projections of the deep cerebellar nuclei of the opossum *Didelphis Marsupialis Virginiana.* J. Hirnforsch., **15**: 545–573.

1617. Martin, J. B., Reichlin, S., and Brown, G. M. 1977. *Clinical Neuroendocrinology.* F. A. Davis Company, Philadelphia, pp. 229–246.

1618. MARTIN, J. P. 1927. Hemichorea resulting from a local lesion of the brain. (The syndrome of body of Luys.) Brain, **50:** 637-651.

1619. MARTIN, J. P. 1959. Remarks on the functions of the basal ganglia. Lancet, **1:** 999-1005.

1620. MARTIN, J. P. 1960. Further remarks on the functions of the basal ganglia. Lancet, **1:** 1362-1365.

1621. MARTIN, J. P. 1967. *The Basal Ganglia and Posture.* Pitman Medical Publishing Company, Ltd., London, 152 pp.

1622. MARTIN, J. P., AND ALCOCK, N. S. 1934. Hemichorea associated with lesions of the corpus Luysii. Brain, **57:** 504-516.

1623. MARTIN, J. P., AND HURWITZ, L. J. 1962. Locomotion and the basal ganglia. Brain, **85:** 261-276.

1624. MARTIN, J. P., HURWITZ, L. J., AND FINLAYSON, M. H. 1962. The negative symptoms of basal gangliar disease: A survey of 130 postencephalitic cases. Lancet, **2:** 1-6, and 62-66.

1625. MARTIN, J. P., AND McCAUL, I. R. 1959. Acute hemiballismus treated by ventrolateral thalamolysis. Brain, **82:** 104-108.

1626. MARTIN, R. F., HABER, L. H., AND WILLIS, W. D. 1979. Primary afferent depolarization of identified cutaneous fibers following stimulation in medial brain stem. J. Neurophysiol., **42:** 779-790.

1627. MARTIN, R. G., GRANT, J. L., PEACE, D., THEISS, C., AND RHOTON, A. L. 1980. Microsurgical relationships of the anterior inferior cerebellar artery and the facial-vestibulocochlear nerve complex. Neurosurgery, **6:** 483-507.

1628. MARTINEZ-MILLÁN, L., AND HOLLÄNDER, H. 1975. Cortico-cortical projections from striate cortex of the squirrel monkey (*Saimiri sciureus*): A radioautographic study. Brain Res., **83:** 405-417.

1629. MASON, S. T., AND FIBIGER, H. C. 1978. Kainic acid lesions of the striatum: Behavioral sequelae similar to Huntington's chorea. Brain Res., **155:** 313-329.

1630. MASON, S. T., AND FIBIGER, H. C. 1979. Regional topography within noradrenergic locus coeruleus as revealed by retrograde transport of horseradish peroxidase. J. Comp. Neurol., **187:** 703-724.

1631. MASSERMAN, J. H. 1943. *Behavior and Neurosis.* University of Chicago Press, Chicago.

1632. MASSION, J. 1967. The mammalian red nucleus. Physiol. Rev., **47:** 383-436.

1633. MASUCCI, E. F. 1965. Bilateral ophthalmoplegia in basilar-vertebral artery disease, Brain, **88:** 97-106.

1634. MASUROVSKY, E. B., BUNGE, M. B., AND BUNGE, R. P. 1967. Cytological studies of organotypic cultures of rat dorsal root ganglia following X-irradiation in vitro. I. Changes in neurons and satellitè cells. J. Cell Biol., **32:** 467-496.

1635. MATSUSHITA, M., AND HOSOYA, Y. 1978. The location of spinal projection neurons in the cerebellar nuclei (cerebellospinal tract neurons) of the cat: A study with the horseradish peroxidase technique. Brain Res., **142:** 237-248.

1636. MATSUSHITA, M., HOSOYA, Y., AND IKEDA, M. 1979. Anatomical organization of the spinocerebellar system in the cat as studied by retrograde transport of horseradish peroxidase. J. Comp. Neurol., **184:** 81-106.

1637. MATSUSHITA, M., AND IKEDA, M. 1975. The central cervical nucleus as cell origin of a spinocerebellar tract arising from the cervical cord: A study in the cat using horseradish peroxidase. Brain Res., **100:** 412-417.

1638. MATSUSHITA, M., AND IKEDA, M. 1976. Projections from the lateral reticular nucleus to the cerebellar cortex and nuclei in the cat. Exp. Brain Res., **24:** 403-422.

1639. MATSUSHITA, M., IKEDA, M., AND HOSOYA, Y. 1979. The location of spinal neurons with long descending axons (long descending propriospinal tract neurons) in the cat: A study with the horseradish peroxidase technique. J. Comp. Neurol., **184:** 63-80.

1640. MATSUSHITA, M., AND IWAHORI, N. 1971. Structural organization of the fastigial nucleus. I. Dendrites and axonal pathways. Brain Res., **25:** 597-610.

1641. MATTHEWS, M. R., COWAN, W. M., AND POWELL, T. P. S. 1960. Transneuronal cell degeneration in the lateral geniculate nucleus of the macaque monkey. J. Anat., **94:** 145-169.

1642. MATTHEWS, P. B. C. 1964. Muscle spindles and their motor control. Physiol. Rev., **44:** 219-288.

1643. MATZKE, H. A. 1951. The course of fibers arising from the nucleus gracilis and cuneatus of the cat. J. Comp. Neurol., **94:** 439-452.

1644. MAXWELL, D. S., AND KRUGER, L. 1965. The fine structure of astrocytes in the cerebral cortex and their response to focal injury produced by heavy ionizing particles. J. Cell Biol., **25:** 141-157.

1645. MAXWELL, D. S., AND KRUGER, L. 1965a. Small blood vessels and the origin of phagocytes in the rat cerebral cortex following heavy particle irradiation. Exp. Neurol., **12:** 33-54.

1646. MAXWELL, D. S., AND KRUGER, L. 1966. The reactive oligodendrocyte: An electron microscopic study of cerebral cortex following Alpha particle irradiation. Am. J. Anat., **118:** 437-460.

1647. MAYNARD, C. W., LEONARD, R. B., COULTER, J. D., AND COGGESHALL, R. E. 1977. Central connections of ventral root afferents as demonstrated by the HRP method. J. Comp. Neurol., **172:** 601-608.

1648. MAYNARD, E. A., SCHULTZ, R. L., AND PEASE, D. C. 1957. Electron microscopy of the vascular bed of rat cerebral cortex. Am. J. Anat., **100:** 409-434.

1649. MEESEN, H., AND OLSZEWSKI, J. 1949. *A Cytoarchitectonic Atlas of the Rhombencephalon of the Rabbit.* S. Karger, Basel.

1650. MEHLER, W. R. 1962. The anatomy of the so-called "pain tract" in man: An analysis of the course and distribution of the ascending fibers of the fasciculus anterolateralis. In J. D. FRENCH AND R. W. PORTER (Editors), *Basic Research in Paraplegia.* Charles C Thomas, Springfield, Ill., pp. 26-55.

1651. MEHLER, W. R. 1966. Further notes on the center median nucleus of Luys. In D. P. PURPURA AND M. D. YAHR (Editors), *The Thalamus.* Columbia University Press, New York, pp. 109-127.

1652. MEHLER, W. R. 1966a. The posterior thalamic region. Confin. Neurol., **27:** 18-29.

1653. MEHLER, W. R. 1966b. Some observations on secondary ascending afferent systems in the central nervous system. In R. S. KNIGHTON AND P. R. DUMKE (Editors), *Pain.* Little, Brown & Company, Boston, Ch. 2, pp. 11-32.

1654. MEHLER, W. R. 1971. Idea of a new anatomy of the thalamus. J. Psychiatr. Res., **8:** 203-217.

1655. MEHLER, W. R. 1974. Central pain and the spinothalamic tract. Adv. Neurol., **4:** 127-146.

1656. MEHLER, W. R. 1980. Subcortical afferent connections of the amygdala in the monkey. J. Comp. Neurol., **190:** 733-762.

1657. MEHLER, W. R., FEFERMAN, M. E., AND NAUTA, W. J. G. 1956. Ascending axon degeneration following anterolateral chordotomy in the monkey. Anat. Rec., **124:** 332-333.

1658. MEHLER, W. B., FEFERMAN, M. E., AND NAUTA, W. J. H. 1960. Ascending axon degeneration following anterolateral cordotomy: An experimental study in the monkey. Brain, **83:** 718-750.

1659. MEHLER, W. R., AND NAUTA, W. J. H. 1974. Connections of the basal ganglia of the cerebellum. Confin. Neurol., **36:** 205-222.

1660. MEHLER, W. R., VERNIER, V. G., AND NAUTA, W. J. H. 1958. Efferent projections from the dentate and interpositus nuclei in primates. Anat. Rec., **130:** 430-431.

1661. MEIBACH, R. C., AND SIEGEL, A. 1975. The origin of fornix fibers which project to the mammillary bodies in the rat: A horseradish peroxidade study. Brain Res., **88:** 508-512.

1662. MEIBACH, R. C., AND SIEGEL. A. 1977. Efferent connections of the hippocampal formation in the rat. Brain Res., **124:** 197–224.

1663. MELLGREN, S. I., HARKMARK, W., AND SREBRO, B. 1977. Some enzyme histochemical characteristics of the human hippocampus. Cell Tissue Res., **181:** 459–471.

1664. MELTZER, S. J. 1906–1907. The factors of safety in animal structure and animal economy. Harvey Lect., pp. 139–169.

1665. MELZACK, R., AND WALL, P. D. 1965. Pain mechanisms: A new theory. Science, **150:** 971–979.

1666. MENAKER, M. 1974. Aspects of the physiology of circadian rhythmicity in the vertebrate central nervous system. In F. O. SCHMITT, AND F. G. WORDEN (Editors), *The Neurosciences: Third Study Program.* M.I.T. Press, Cambridge, Mass., pp. 479–489.

1667. MERKEL, F. 1875. Tastzellen und Tastkörperchen beiden Hausthieren und beim Menschen. Arch. Mikrosk. Anat., Entwick. Mech. **11:** 636–652.

1668. MERRILLEES, N. C. R. 1962. Some observations on the fine structure of a Golgi tendon organ of a rat. In D. BARKER (Editor), *Symposium on Muscle Receptors.* Hong Kong University Press, Hong Kong, pp. 199–206.

1669. MERRILLEES, N., SUNDERLAND, S., AND HAYHOW, W. 1950. Neuromuscular spindles in the extraocular muscles in man. Anat. Rec., **23:** 30.

1670. MERRITT, H. H. 1979. *A Textbook of Neurology.* Lea & Febiger, Philadelphia, 961 pp.

1671. MERTON, P. A. 1953. Speculations on the servo-control of movement. In G. E. W. WOLSTENHOLME (Editor), *The Spinal Cord.* J. B. A. Churchill, Ltd., London, pp. 247–255.

1672. MERZENICH, M. M., AND BRUGGE, J. F. 1973. Representation of the cochlear partition on the superior temporal plane of the Macaque monkey. Brain Res., **50:** 275–296.

1673. MERZENICH, M. M., KAAS, J. H., SUR, M., AND LIN, C. S. 1978. Double representation of the body surface within cytoarchitectonic Areas 3b and 1 in "S 1" in the owl monkey (*Aotus trivigatus*). J. Comp. Neurol., **181:** 41–74.

1674. MERZENICH, M. M., KNIGHT, P. L., AND ROTH, G. L. 1973. Cochleotopic organization of primary auditory cortex in the cat. Brain Res., **63:** 343–346.

1675. MERZENICH, M. M., KNIGHT, P. L., AND ROTH, G. L. 1975. Representation of cochlea within the primary auditory cortex in the cat. J. Neurophysiol., **38:** 231–249.

1676. MERZENICH, M. M., AND REID, M. D. 1974. Representation of the cochlea within the inferior colliculus of the cat. Brain Res., **77:** 397–415.

1677. MESTRES, P. 1978. Old and new concepts about circumventricular organs: An overview: Scan. Electron Micros., **2:** 137–143.

1678. MESULAM, M.-M. 1978. Tetramethylbenzidine for horseradish peroxidase neurohistochemistry: A non-carcinogenic blue reaction-product with superior sensitivity for visualizing neural afferents and efferents. J. Histochem. Cytochem., **26:** 106–117.

1679. MESULAM, M.-M., AND GESCHWIND, N. 1978. On the possible role of neocortex and its limbic connections in the process of attention and schizophrenia: Clinical cases of inattention in man and experimental anatomy in monkey. J. Psychiatr. Res., **14:** 249–260.

1680. MESULAM, M. M., AND ROSENE, D. L. 1977. Differential sensitivity between blue and brown reaction procedures for HRP neurohistochemistry. Neurosci. Lett., **5:** 7–14.

1681. METTLER, F. A. 1932. Connections of the auditory cortex of the cat. J. Comp. Neurol., **55:** 139–183.

1681a. METTLER, F. A. 1942. Relation between pyramidal and extrapyramidal function. Proc. Assoc. Res. Nerv. Ment. Dis., **21:** 150–227.

1682. METTLER, F. A. 1943. Extensive unilateral cerebral removals in the primate: Physiologic effects and resultant degeneration. J. Comp. Neurol., **79:** 185–243.

1683. METTLER, F. A. 1944. The tegmento-olivary and

central tegmental fasciculi. J. Comp. Neurol., **80:** 149–175.

1684. METTLER, F. A. 1944a. On the origin of the fibers in the pyramid of the primate brain. Proc. Soc. Exp. Biol. Med., **57:** 111–113.

1685. METTLER, F. A. 1947. The non-pyramidal motor projections from the frontal cerebral cortex. Proc. Assoc. Res. Nerv. Ment. Dis., **26:** 162–199.

1686. METTLER, F. A. 1947a. Extracortical connections of the primate frontal cerebral cortex. I. Thalamo-cortical connections. J. Comp. Neurol., **86:** 95–117.

1687. METTLER, F. A. 1947b. Extracortical connections of the primate frontal cerebral cortex. II. Corticofugal connections. J. Comp. Neurol., **86:** 119–154.

1688. METTLER, F. A. 1948. *Neuroanatomy.* C.V. Mosby Company, St. Louis, 536 pp.

1689. METTLER, F. A. 1949. *Selective Partial Ablation of the Frontal Cortex: A Correlative Study of the Effects on Human Psychotic Subjects.* Paul B. Hoeber, Inc., New York, 527 pp.

1690. METTLER, F. A. 1955. The experimental anatomo-physiologic approach to the study of diseases of the basal ganglia. J. Neuropathol. Exp. Neurol., **14:** 115–141.

1691. METTLER, F. A. 1968. Anatomy of the basal ganglia. In P. J. VINKEN AND G. W. BRUYN (Editors), *Handbook of Clinical Neurology,* Vol. 6. North-Holland Publishing Company, Amsterdam, pp. 1–55.

1692. METTLER, F. A., COOPER, I. S., LISS, H., CARPENTER, M. B., AND NOBACK, C. R. 1954. Patterns of vascular failure in the central nervous system. J. Neuropathol. Exp. Neurol., **13:** 528–539.

1693. METTLER, F. A., LISS, H. R., AND STEVENS, G. H. 1956. Blood supply of the primate striopallidum. J. Neuropathol. Exp. Neurol., **15:** 377–383.

1694. METTLER, F. A., AND LUBIN, A. J. 1942. Termination of the brachium pontis. J. Comp. Neurol., **77:** 391–397.

1695. METUZALS. J. 1965. Ultrastructure of the nodes of Ranvier and their surrounding structures in the central nervous system. Z. Zellforsch. Mikrosk. Anat., **65:** 719–759.

1696. MEYER, A. 1971. *Historical Aspects of Cerebral Anatomy.* Oxford University Press, London, 230 pp.

1697. MEYER, A., BECK, E., AND McLARDY, T. 1947. Prefontal leucotomy: A neuroanatomical report. Brain, **70:** 18–49.

1698. MEYER, D. R., AND WOOLSEY, C. N. 1952. Effects of localized cortical destruction upon auditory discriminative conditioning in the cat. J. Neurophysiol., **15:** 149–162.

1699. MEYERS, R. E. 1956. Function of corpus callosum in interocular transfer. Brain, **79:** 358–363.

1700. MIALE, I. L., AND SIDMAN, R. L. 1961. An autoradiographic analysis of histogenesis in the mouse cerebellum. Exp. Neurol., **4:** 277–296.

1701. MILLAR, J. 1973. Topography and receptive fields of ventroposterolateral thalamic neurones excited by afferents projecting through the dorsolateral funiculus of the spinal cord. Exp. Neurol., **41:** 303–313.

1702. MILLEN, J. W., AND WOOLLAM, D. H. M. 1961. Observations on the nature of the pia mater. Brain, **84:** 514–520.

1703. MILLEN, J. W., AND WOOLLAM, D. H. M. 1962. *The Anatomy of the Cerebrospinal Fluid.* Oxford University Press, New York, pp. 90–102.

1704. MILLER, J. J., RICHARDSON, T. L., FIBIGER, H. C., AND McLENNAN, H. 1975. Anatomical and electrophysiological identification of a projection from the mesencephalic raphe to the caudate putamen in the rat. Brain Res., **97:** 133–138.

1705. MILLER, M. R., RALSTON, H. J., AND KASAHARA, M. 1958. The pattern of cutaneous innervation of the human hand. Am. J. Anat., **102:** 183–218.

1706. MILLER, M. R., RALSTON, H. J., AND KASAHARA, M. 1960. The pattern of cutaneous innervation of the human hand, foot, and breast. In W. MONTAGNA (Editor), *Advances in Biology of Skin* Vol. I: *Cutaneous*

Innervation. Pergamon Press, New York, pp. 1–47.

1707. MILLER, R. A., AND STROMINGER, N. L. 1973. Efferent connections of the red nucleus in the brainstem and spinal cord of the rhesus monkey. J. Comp. Neurol., **152:** 327–346.

1708. MILLER, R. A., AND STROMINGER, N. L. 1977. An experimental study of the efferent connections of the superior peduncle in the rhesus monkey. Brain Res., **133:** 237–250.

1709. MILLER, S., AND OSCARSSON, O. 1970. Termination and functional organization of spino-olivocerebellar paths. In W. S. FIELDS AND W. D. WILLIS (Editors), *The Cerebellum in Health and Disease*. Warren H. Green, Inc., St. Louis, Ch. 6, pp. 172–200.

1710. MILLHOUSE, O. E. 1979. A Golgi anatomy of the rodent hypothalamus. In P. MORGANE, AND J. PANK-SEPP (Editors), *Handbook of the Hypothalamus*, Vol. I: *Anatomy of the Hypothalamus*. Marcel Dekker, New York, pp. 221–265.

1711. MINER, L. C., AND REED, D. J. 1972. Composition of fluid obtained from choroid plexus tissue isolated in a chamber in situ. J. Physiol. (Lond.), **227:** 127–139.

1712. MINKOWSKI, M. 1913. Experimentelle Untersuchungen über die Beziehungen der Grosshirnrinde und der Netzhaut zu den primären optischen Zentren, besonders zum Corpus geniculatum externum. Arb. Hirnanat. Inst. Zürich, **7:** 225–362.

1713. MINKOWSKI, M. 1920. Über den Verlauf, die Endigung und die zentrale Repräsentation von gekreuzten und ungekreuzten Sehnervenfastern bei einigen beim menschen. Schweiz. Arch. Neurol. Psychiatr., **6:** 201–252.

1714. MINKOWSKI, M. 1923–1924. Etude sur les connections anatomiques des circonvolutions rolandiques, parietales et frontales. Schweiz. Arch. Neurol. Psychiatr., **12:** 71–104 and 227–268; **14:** 255–278; **15:** 97–132.

1715. MINNEMAN, K. P., DIBNER, M. D., WOLFE, B. B., AND MOLINOFF, P. B. 1979. β_1- and β_2-adrenergic receptors in rat cerebral cortex are independently regulated. Science, **204:** 866–868.

1715a. MINNEMAN, K. P., PITTMAN, R. N., AND MOLINOFF, P. B. 1981. β-Adrenergic receptor subtypes; properties, distribution and regulation. Ann. Rev. Neurosci., **4:** 419–461.

1716. MISCOLCZY, D. 1931. Uber die Endigungsweise der spinocerebellaren Bahnen. Z. Anat. Entwickl.-Gesch., **96:** 537–542.

1717. MISCOLCZY, D. 1934. Die Endigungsweise der olivocerebellaren Faserung. Arch. Psychiatr. Nervenk., **102:** 197–201.

1718. MITCHELL, G. A. G. 1953. *Anatomy of the Autonomic Nervous System*. E. & S. Livingstone, Ltd., Edinburgh.

1719. MØLLER, M. 1978. Presence of a pineal nerve (nervus pinealis) in the human fetus: A light and electron microscopical study of the innervation of the pineal gland. Brain Res., **154:** 1–12.

1720. VON MONAKOW, C. 1895. Experimentelle und pathologisch-anatomische Untersuchungen über die Haubenregion, den Sehhügel und die Regio subthalamica. Arch. Psychiatr. Nervenkr., **27:** 1–219.

1721. VON MONAKOW, C. 1905. *Gehirnpathologie*, Ed. 2. Hölder, Wien, 1319 pp.

1722. MONIZ, E. 1931. *Diagnostic des Tumeurs Cérébrales et Épreuve de l'Encéphalographie Artérielle*. Mason et Cie, Paris, 512 pp.

1723. MONIZ, E. 1934. *L'Angiographie Cérébrale, ses Applications et Resultats en Anatomie, Physiologie et Clinique*. Mason et Cie, Paris, 327 pp.

1724. MONIZ, E. 1936. *Tentative Opératoire dans le Traitement de Certaines Psychoses*. Masson et Cie, Paris, 248 pp.

1725. MONRAD-KROHN, G. H. 1924. On the dissociation of voluntary and emotional innervation in facial paresis of central origin. Brain, **47:** 22–35.

1726. MONRAD-KROHN, G. H. 1939. On facial dissociation. Acta Psychiatr. Neurol. Scand., **14:** 557–566.

1727. MONTAGNA, W. 1977. Morphology of cutaneous sensory receptors. J. Invest. Dermatol., **69:** 4–7.

1728. MONTI GRAZIADEI, G. A., KARLAN, M. S., BERNSTEIN, J. J., AND GRAZIADEI, P. P. C. 1980. Reinnervation of the olfactory bulb after section of the olfactory nerve in monkey (*Saimiri Sciureus*). Brain Res., **189:** 343–355.

1729. MOON EDLEY, S. L. 1979. *A Neuroanatomical Study of the Nucleus Tegmenti Pedunculopontinus in the Cat*. Doctoral Dissertation, Massachusetts Institute of Technology, Cambridge, Mass.

1730. MOON EDLEY, S., AND GRAYBIEL, A. M. 1980. Connections of the nucleus tegmenti pedunculopontinus, pars compacta (TP_c) in cat. Anat. Rec., **196:** 129A.

1731. MOORE, B. W. 1973. Brain-specific proteins. In D. J. SCHNEIDER (Editor), *Proteins of the Nervous System*. Raven Press, New York, pp. 1–12.

1732. MOORE, R. Y. 1973. Retinohypothalamic projection in mammals: A comparative study. Brain Res., **49:** 403–409.

1733. MOORE, R. Y. 1978. The innervation of the mammalian pineal gland. In R. J. REITER (Editor), *The Pineal and Reproduction*. S. Karger, Basel, pp. 1–29.

1734. MOORE, R. Y., BHATNAGAR, R. K., AND HELLER, A. 1971. Anatomical and chemical studies of a nigroneostriatal projection in the cat. Brain Res., **30:** 119–135.

1735. MOORE, R. Y., AND GOLDBERG, J. M. 1963. Ascending projections of the inferior colliculus in the cat. J. Comp. Neurol., **121:** 109–136.

1736. MOORE, R. Y., AND GOLDBERG, J. M. 1966. Projections of the inferior colliculus in the monkey. Exp. Neurol., **14:** 429–438.

1737. MOORE, R. Y., HALARIS, A. E., AND JONES, B. E. 1978. Serotonin neurons of the midbrain raphe: Ascending projections. J. Comp. Neurol., **180:** 417–438.

1738. MOORE, R. Y., AND KLEIN, D. C. 1974. Visual pathways and the central neural control of a circadian rhythm in pineal serotonin N-acetyltransferase activity. Brain Res., **71:** 17–33.

1739. MOORE, R. Y., AND LENN, N. J. 1972. A retinohypothalamic projection in the rat. J. Comp. Neurol., **146:** 1–14.

1740. MOORE, R. Y., AND RAPPORT, R. L. 1970. Pineal and gonadal function in the rat following cervical sympathectomy. Neuroendocrinology, **7:** 361–374.

1741. MOREL, F. 1947. La massa intermedia ou commissure grise. Acta Anat. (Basel), **4:** 203–207.

1742. MOREST, D. K. 1960. A study of the structure of the area postrema with Golgi methods. Am. J. Anat., **107:** 291–303.

1743. MOREST, D. K. 1964. The neuronal architecture of the medial geniculate body of the cat. J. Anat., **98:** 611–638.

1744. MOREST, D. K. 1965. The laminar structure of the medial geniculate body of the cat. J. Anat., **99:** 143–159.

1745. MOREST, D. K. 1965a. The lateral tegmental system of the midbrain and the medial geniculate body: Study with Golgi and Nauta methods in the cat. J. Anat., **99:** 611–634.

1746. MOREST, D. K. 1967. Experimental study of the projections of the nucleus of the tractus solitarius and the area postrema in the cat. J. Comp. Neurol., **130:** 277–299.

1747. MORGAN, L. R. 1927. The corpus striatum. Arch. Neurol. Psychiatry, **18:** 495–549.

1748. MORIN, F. 1955. A new spinal pathway for cutaneous impulses. Am. J. Physiol., **183:** 245–252.

1749. MORIN, F., AND CATALANO, J. V. 1955. Central connections of a cervical nucleus (nucleus cervicalis lateralis of the cat). J. Comp. Neurol., **103:** 17–32.

1750. MORIN, F., AND GARDNER, E. D. 1953. Spinal pathways for cerebellar projections in the monkey (*Macaca mulatta*). Am. J. Physiol., **174:** 155–161.

1751. MORIN, F., SCHWARTZ, H. G., AND O'LEARY, J. L. 1951. Experimental study of the spinothalamic and related tract. Acta Psychiatr. Neurol. Scand., **26:** 371–396.

1752. MORISON, R. S., AND DEMPSEY, E. W. 1942. A study of thalamocortical relations. Am. J. Physiol., **135:** 281–292.

1753. MORISON, R. S., AND DEMPSEY, E. W. 1942a. Mechanisms of thalamocortical augmentation and repetition. Am. J. Physiol., **138:** 297–308.

1754. MORRIS, R., SALT, T. E., SOFRONIEW, M. W., AND HILL, R. G. 1980. Actions of microiontophoretically applied oxytocin, and immunohistochemical localization of oxytocin, vasopressin and neurophysin in the rat caudal medulla. Neurosci. Lett., **18:** 163–168.

1755. MORUZZI, G. 1963. Active processes in the brain stem during sleep. Harvey Lect., ser. **58:** 233–297.

1756. MORUZZI, G., AND MAGOUN, H. W. 1949. Brain stem reticular formation and activation of the EEG. Electroencephalogr. Clin. Neurophysiol., **1:** 455–473.

1756a. MORUZZI, G., AND POMPEIANO, O. 1956. Crossed fastigial influence on decerebrate rigidity. J. Comp. Neurol., **106:** 371–392.

1757. MOSCONA, A. A., AND HAUSMAN, R. E. 1977. Biological and biochemical studies on embryonic cell recognition. In J. W. LASH AND M. M. BURGER (Editors), *Cell and Tissue Interactions.* Raven Press, New York, pp. 173–186.

1758. MOSKO, S. S., AND MOORE, R. Y. 1979. Neonatal suprachiasmatic nucleus lesions: Effects on the development of circadian rhythms in the rat. Brain Res., **164:** 17–38.

1759. MOSKOWITZ, N., AND LIU, J.-C. 1972. Central projections of the spiral ganglion of the squirrel monkey. J. Comp. Neurol., **144:** 335–344.

1760. MOSS, M., MAHUT, H., AND ZOLA-MORGAN, S. 1981. Concurrent discrimination learning of monkeys after hippocampal, entorhinal, or fornix lesions. J. Neurosci., **1:** 227–240.

1761. MOTT, F. W., AND SHERRINGTON, C. S. 1895. Experiments upon the influence of sensory nerves upon movement and nutrition of the limbs. Proc. R. Soc., **57:** 481–488.

1762. MOULTON, D. G., AND BEIDLER, L. M. 1967. Structure and function in the peripheral olfactory system. Physiol. Rev., **47:** 1–52.

1763. MOUNTCASTLE, V. B. 1957. Modality and topographic properties of single neurons of cat's somatic sensory cortex. J. Neurophysiol., **20:** 408–434.

1764. MOUNTCASTLE, V. B. 1962. *Interhemispheric Relations and Cerebral Dominance.* Johns Hopkins University Press, Baltimore, 294 pp.

1765. MOUNTCASTLE, V. B. 1974. Sensory receptors and neural encoding: Introduction to sensory processes. In V. B. MOUNTCASTLE (Editor), *Medical Physiology,* Vol. I. C. V. Mosby Company, St. Louis, pp. 285–306 and 348–381.

1766. MOUNTCASTLE, V. B., AND HENNEMAN, E. 1949. Pattern of tactile representation in thalamus of cat. J. Neurophysiol., **12:** 85–100.

1767. MOUNTCASTLE, V. B., AND HENNEMAN, E. 1952. The representation of tactile sensibility in the thalamus of the monkey. J. Comp. Neurol., **97:** 409–440.

1768. MOUNTCASTLE, V. B., LYNCH, J. C., GEORGOPOULOS, A., SAKATA, H., AND ACUNA, C. 1975. Posterior parietal association cortex of the monkey: Command functions for operation within extrapersonal space. J. Neurophysiol., **38:** 871–908.

1769. MOUNTCASTLE, V. B., AND POWELL, T. P. S. 1959. Central nervous mechanisms subserving position sense and kinesthesis. Bull. Johns Hopkins Hosp., **105:** 173–200.

1770. MOUNTCASTLE, V. B., AND POWELL, T. P. S. 1959a. Neural mechanisms subserving cutaneous sensibility with special reference to the role of afferent inhibition in sensory perception and discrimination. Bull. Johns Hopkins Hosp., **105:** 201–232.

1771. MOUNTCASTLE, V. B., TALBOT, W. H., DARIAN-SMITH, I., AND KORNHUBER, H. H. 1967. The neural base for the sense of flutter vibration. Science, **155:** 597–600.

1772. MOZELL, M. M. 1964. Olfactory discrimination: Electrophysiological spatio-temporal basis. Science, **143:** 1336–1337.

1773. MROZ, E. A., BROWNSTEIN, M. J., AND LEEMAN, S. 1977. Distribution of immunoassayable substance P in the rat brain: Evidence for the existence of substance P-containing tracts. In U. S. VON EULER AND B. PERNOW (Editors), *Substance P.* Raven Press, New York, pp. 147–154.

1774. MUGNAINI, E. 1972. The histology and cytology of the cerebellar cortex. In O. LARSELL AND J. JANSEN (Editors), *The Comparative Anatomy and Histology of the Cerebellum. The Human Cerebellum, Cerebellar Connections, and Cerebellar Cortex.* University of Minnesota Press, Minneapolis, pp. 201–262.

1775. MUGNAINI, E., AND WALBERG, F. 1964. Ultrastructure of neuroglia. Ergeb. Anat. Entwickl.-Gesch., **37:** 194–236.

1776. MUGNAINI, E., AND WALBERG, F. 1967. An experimental electron microscopical study on the mode of termination of cerebellar corticovestibular fibres in the cat lateral vestibular nucleus (Deiters' nucleus). Exp. Brain Res., **4:** 212–236.

1777. MUGNAINI, E., WALBERG, F., AND BRODAL, A. 1967. Mode of termination of primary vestibular fibres in the lateral vestibular nucleus: An experimental electron microscopical study in the cat. Exp. Brain Res., **4:** 187–211.

1778. MUGNAINI, E., WALBERG, F., AND HAUGLIE-HANSSEN, E. 1967. Observations on the fine structure of the lateral vestibular nucleus (Deiters' Nucleus) in the cat. Exp. Brain Res., **4:** 146–186.

1779. MULLAN, S., AND PENFIELD, W. 1959. Illusions of comparative interpretation and emotion. A. M. A. Arch. Neurol. Psychiatry, **81:** 269–284.

1780. MÜLLER-PREUSS, P., AND JÜRGENS, U. 1975. Projections from the "cingular" vocalization area in the squirrel monkey. Brain Res., **103:** 29–43.

1781. MUNGER, B. L. 1965. The intraepidermal innervation of the snout skin of the opossum: A light and electron microscope study, with observations of the nature of Merkel's Tastzellen. J. Cell Biol., **26:** 79–97.

1782. MUNGER, B. L. 1966. Discussion of: Fine structure of the receptor organs and its probable functional significance. In A. V. S. DE REUCK AND J. KNIGHT (Editors), *Touch, Heat, and Pain.* Ciba Foundation Symposium. Little, Brown and Company, Boston, pp. 129–130.

1783. MURPHY, M. G., O'LEARY, J. L., AND CORNBLATH, D. 1973. Axoplasmic flow in cerebellar mossy and climbing fibers. Arch. Neurol., **28:** 118–123.

1784. MURRAY, E. A., AND COULTER, J. D. 1976. Origins of cortical projections to cervical and lumbar spinal cord in monkey. Neurosci. Abstr. Soc. Neurosci., **2:** 917.

1785. MURRAY, E. A., AND COULTER, J. D. 1977. Corticospinal projections from the medial cerebral hemisphere in monkey. Neurosci. Abstr. Soc. Neurosci., **3:** 275.

1786. MURRAY, M. R. 1957. Tissue culture studies of neural tissue. In W. F. WINDLE (Editor), *New Research Techniques of Neuroanatomy.* Charles C Thomas, Publisher, Springfield, Ill., Ch. 5, pp. 40–50.

1787. MURRAY, M. R. 1958. Response of oligodendrocytes to serotonin. In W. F. WINDLE (Editor), *Biology of Neuroglia.* Charles C Thomas, Publisher, Springfield, Ill., pp. 176–180.

1788. MURRAY, M. R. 1965. Nervous tissue *in vitro.* In E. N. WILMER (Editor), *Cells and Tissues in Culture,* Vol. 2: *Methods, Biology and Physiology,* Academic Press, New York, pp. 373–455.

1789. MURRAY, M. R., AND STOUT, A. P. 1947. Adult human sympathetic ganglion cells cultivated *in vitro.* Am. J. Anat., **80:** 225–273.

1790. MUSSEN, A. T. 1927. Experimental investigations on the cerebellum. Brain, **50:** 313–349.

1791. MYTILINEOU, C., ISSIDORIDES, M., AND SHANKLIN, W. M. 1963. Histochemical reactions of human autonomic ganglia. J. Anat., **97:** 533–542.

1792. NAGEOTTE, J. 1906. The pars intermedia or nervus intermedius of Wrisberg, and the bulbo-pontine gustatory nucleus in man. Rev. Neurol. Psychiatry, **4:** 473–488.

1793. NAKAI, Y., AND TAKAORI, S. 1974. Influence of norepinephrine-containing neurons derived from the locus coeruleus on lateral geniculate neuronal activities of cats. Brain Res., **71:** 47–60.

1794. NAKAMURA, S., AND SUTIN, J. 1972. The pattern of termination of pallidal axons upon cells of the subthalamic nucleus. Exp. Neurol., **35:** 254–264.

1795. NAKAO, H. 1958. Emotional behavior produced by hypothalamic stimulation. Am. J. Physiol., **194:** 411–418.

1796. VON NAMBA, M. 1957. Cytoarchitektonische Untersuchungen am Striatum. J. Hirnforsch., **3:** 24–48.

1797. NAMBA, T., NAKAMURA, T., AND GROB, D. 1968. Motor nerve endings in human extraocular muscle. Neurology (Minneap.), **18:** 403–407.

1798. NANDY, K. 1968. Histochemical study of chromatolytic neurons. Arch. Neurol., **18:** 425–434.

1799. NARABAYASHI, H. 1972. Stereotaxic amygdalotomy. In B. E. ELEFTHERIOU (Editor), *The Neurobiology of the Amygdala*. Plenum Press, New York, pp. 459–483.

1800. NARABAYASHI, H., NAGAO, T., SAITO, Y., YOSHIDA, M., AND NAGAHATA, M. 1963. Stereotaxic amygdalotomy for behavior disorders. Arch. Neurol., **9:** 1–16.

1801. NARABAYASHI, H., OKUMA, T., AND SHIKIBA, S. 1956. Procaine oil blocking of the globus pallidus. A. M. A. Arch. Neurol. Psychiatry, **75:** 36–48.

1802. NARKIEWICZ, O. 1964. Degenerations in the claustrum after regional neocortical ablations in the cat. J. Comp. Neurol., **123:** 335–356.

1803. NAROTZKY, R. A., AND KERR, F. W. L. 1978. Marginal neurons of the spinal cord. Brain Res., **139:** 1–20.

1804. NATHAN, P. W., AND SMITH, M. C. 1951. The centripetal pathway from the bladder and urethra within the spinal cord. J. Neurol. Neurosurg. Psychiatry, **14:** 262–280.

1805. NATHAN, P. W., AND SMITH, M. C. 1955. Spinocortical fibres in man. J. Neurol. Neurosurg. Psychiatry, **18:** 181–190.

1806. NATHAN, P. W., AND SMITH, M. C. 1955a. Long descending tracts in man. I. Review of present knowledge. Brain, **78:** 248–303.

1807. NATHAN, P. W., AND WALL, P. D. 1974. Treatment of post-herpetic neuralgia by prolonged electric stimulation. Br. Med. J., **3:** 645–647.

1808. NATHANIEL, E. J. H., AND NATHANIEL, D. R. 1966. The ultrastructural features of the synapses in the posterior horn of the spinal cord in the rat. J. Ultrastruct. Res., **14:** 540–555.

1809. NATHANIEL, E. J. H., AND PEASE, D. C. 1963. Degenerative changes in rat dorsal roots during Wallerian degeneration. J. Ultrastruct. Res., **9:** 511–532.

1810. NATHANIEL, E. J. H., AND PEASE, D. C. 1963a. Regenerative changes in rat dorsal roots following Wallerian degeneration. J. Ultrastruct. Res., **9:** 533–549.

1811. NAUTA, H. J. W. 1974. Evidence of a pallidohabenular pathway in the cat. J. Comp. Neurol., **156:** 19–28.

1812. NAUTA, H. J. W, AND COLE, M. 1978. Efferent projections of the subthalamic nucleus: An autoradiographic study in monkey and cat. J. Comp. Neurol., **180:** 1–16.

1813. NAUTA, H. J. W., KAISERMAN-ABRAMOF, I. R., AND LASEK, R. J. 1975. Electron microscopic observations of horseradish peroxidase transported from the caudoputamen to the substantia nigra in the rat: Possible involvement of the granular reticulum. Brain Res., **85:** 373–384.

1814. NAUTA, H. J. W., PRITZ, M. B., AND LASEK, R. J. 1974. Afferents to the rat caudoputamen studied with horseradish peroxidase: An evaluation of a retrograde neuroanatomical research method. Brain Res., **67:** 219–238.

1815. NAUTA, W. J. H. 1956. An experimental study of the fornix in the rat. J. Comp. Neurol., **104:** 247–272.

1816. NAUTA, W. J. H. 1958. Hippocampal projections and related neural pathways to the midbrain in the cat. Brain, **81:** 319–340.

1817. NAUTA, W. J. H. 1961. Fibre degeneration following lesions of the amygdaloid complex in the monkey. J. Anat., **95:** 515–531.

1818. NAUTA, W. J. H. 1962. Neural associations of the amygdaloid complex in the monkey. Brain, **85:** 505–520.

1819. NAUTA, W. J. H. 1964. Some efferent connections of the prefrontal cortex in the monkey. In J. M. WARREN AND K. AKERT (Editors), *The Frontal Granular Cortex and Behavior.* McGraw-Hill, New York, pp. 397–409.

1820. NAUTA, W. J. H. 1972. The central visceromotor system: A general survey. In C. H. HOCKMAN (Editor), *Limbic System Mechanisms and Autonomic Function.* Charles C Thomas, Publisher, Springfield, Ill., Ch. 2, pp. 21–33.

1821. NAUTA, W. J. H., AND GYGAX, P. A. 1951. Silver impregnation of degenerating axon terminals in the central nervous system. I. Technic; II. Chemical notes. Stain Technol., **26:** 5–11.

1822. NAUTA, W. J. H., AND GYGAX, P. A. 1954. Silver impregnation of degenerating axons in the central nervous system: A modified technic. Stain Technol., **29:** 91–93.

1823. NAUTA, W. J. H., AND HAYMAKER, W. 1969. Hypothalamic nuclei and fiber connections. In W. HAYMAKER et al. (Editors), *The Hypothalamus.* Charles C. Thomas Publisher, Springfield, Ill., Ch. 4, pp. 136–209.

1824. NAUTA, W. J. H., AND KUYPERS, H. G. J. M. 1958. Some ascending pathways in the brain stem reticular formation. In H. H. JASPER et al. (Editors), *Reticular Formation of the Brain.* Henry Ford Hospital International Symposium. Little, Brown and Company, Boston, Ch. 1, pp. 3–30.

1825. NAUTA, W. J. H., AND MEHLER, W. R. 1966. Projections of the lentiform nucleus in the monkey. Brain Res., **1:** 3–42.

1826. NAUTA, W. J. H., SMITH, G. P., FAULL, R. L. M., AND DOMESICK, V. B. 1978. Efferent connections and nigral afferents of the nucleus accumbens septi in the rat. Neuroscience, **3:** 385–401.

1827. NAUTA, W. J. H., AND WHITLOCK, D. G. 1954. An anatomical analysis of the non-specific thalamic projection system. In J. F. DELAFRESNAYE (Editor), *Brain Mechanisms and Consciousness* (Symposium), Blackwell Scientific Publications, Oxford, pp. 81–98.

1828. NEFF, W. D. 1961. Neural mechanisms of auditory discrimination. In W. A. ROSENBLITH (Editor), *Sensory Communications.* M. I. T. Press and John Wiley & Sons, New York.

1829. NEFF, W. D., AND DIAMOND, I. T. 1958. The neural basis of auditory discrimination. In H. F. HARLOW AND C. N. WOOLSEY (Editors), *Biological and Biochemical Bases of Behavior.* University of Wisconsin Press, Madison, pp. 101–126.

1830. NEFF, W. D., FISHER, J. F., DIAMOND, I. T., AND YELA, M. 1956. Role of auditory cortex in discrimination requiring localization of sound in space. J. Neurophysiol., **19:** 500–512.

1831. NEUTRA, M., AND LEBLOND, C. P. 1969. The Golgi apparatus. Sci. Am., **220:** 100–107.

1832. NEW, P. F. J., AND SCOTT, W. R. 1975. *Computed Tomography of the Brain and Orbit (EMI Scanning).* Williams & Wilkins, Baltimore.

1833. NGAI, S. H., AND WANG, S. C. 1957. Organization of central respiratory mechanisms in the brain stem of the cat: Localization by stimulation and destruction. Am. J. Physiol., **190:** 343–349.

1834. NICKERSON, M. 1970. Drugs inhibiting adrenergic nerves and structures innervated by them. In L. S. GOODMAN AND A. GILMAN (Editors), *The Pharmacological Basis of Therapeutics.* The Macmillan Company, New York, Ch. 26, pp. 549–584.

1835. NIEMER, W. T., AND MAGOUN, H. W. 1947.

Reticulospinal tracts influencing motor activity. J. Comp. Neurol., **87**: 367–379.

1836. NIIMI, K., AND INOSHITA, H. 1971. Cortical projections of the lateral thalamic nuclei in the cat. Proc. Jpn. Acac., **47**: 664–669.

1837. NIIMI, K., KATAYAMA, K., KANASEKI, T., AND MORIMOTO, K. 1960. Studies on the derivation of the centre median nucleus of Luys. Tokushima J. Exp. Med., **6**: 261–268.

1838. NIIMI, K., AND MATSUOKA, H. 1979. Thalamo-cortical organization of the auditory system in the cat studied by retrograde axonal transport of horseradish peroxidase. Adv. Anat. Embryol. Cell Biol., **57**: 1–56.

1839. NIIMI, K., NIIMI, M., AND OKADA, Y. 1978. Thalamic afferents to the limbic cortex in the cat studied with the method of retrograde axonal transport of horseradish peroxidase. Brain Res., **145**: 225–238.

1840. NIIMI, K., AND SPRAGUE, J. M. 1970. Thalamo-cortical organization of the visual system in the cat. J. Comp. Neurol., **138**: 219–250.

1841. NIIMI, M. 1978. Cortical projections of the anterior thalamic nuclei in the cat. Exp. Brain Res., **31**: 403–416.

1842. NILAVER, G., ZIMMERMAN, E. A., WILKINS, J., MICHAELS, J., HOFFMAN, D., AND SILVERMAN, A.-J. 1980. Magnocellular hypothalamic projections to the lower brain stem and spinal cord of the rat. Neuroendocrinology, **30**: 150–158.

1843. NOBACK, C. R., AND LAEMLE, L. K. 1970. Structural and functional aspects of the visual pathways of primates. In C. R. NOBACK AND W. MONTAGNA (Editors), *Advances in Primatology*, Vol. 1: *The Primate Brain*. Appleton-Century-Crofts, New York, Ch. 3, pp. 55–81.

1843a. NOBACK, C. R., AND DEMAREST, R. J. 1981. *The Human Nervous System*, 3rd Ed., McGraw-Hill Book Co., New York, 591 pp.

1844. NOMURA, S., MIZUNO, N., AND SUGIMOTO, T. 1980. Direct projections from the pedunculopontine tegmental nucleus to the subthalamic nucleus in the cat. Brain Res., **196**: 223–227.

1845. NORBERG, K. A. 1967. Transmitter histochemistry of the sympathetic adrenergic nervous system. Brain Res., **5**: 125–170.

1846. NORGREN, R. 1974. Gustatory afferents to ventral forebrain. Brain Res., **81**: 285–295.

1847. NORGREN, R., AND LEONARD, C. M. 1973. Ascending central gustatory pathways. J. Comp. Neurol., **150**: 217–238.

1848. NORGREN, R., AND PFAFFMAN, C. 1975. The pontine taste area in the rat. Brain Res., **91**: 99–117.

1849. NORGREN, R., AND WOLF, G. 1975. Projection of thalamic gustatory and lingual areas in the rat. Brain Res., **92**: 123–129.

1850. NORITA, M. 1977. Demonstration of bilateral claustro-cortical connections in the cat with the method of retrograde axonal transport of horseradish peroxidase. Arch. Histol. Jpn., **40**: 1–10.

1851. NORRSELL, U., AND VOORHOEVE, P. 1962. Tactile pathways from the hindlimb to the cerebral cortex in cat. Acta Physiol. Scand., **54**: 9–17.

1852. NOVAK, J., AND SALAFSKY, B. 1967. Early electrophysiological changes after denervation of slow skeletal muscle. Exp. Neurol., **19**: 388–400.

1853. NYBERG-HANSEN, R. 1964. Origin and termination of fibers from the vestibular nuclei descending in the medial longitudinal fasciculus: An experimental study with silver impregnation methods in the cat. J. Comp. Neurol., **122**: 355–368.

1854. NYBERG-HANSEN, R. 1965. Sites and mode of termination of reticulospinal fibers in the cat: An experimental study with silver impregnation methods. J. Comp. Neurol., **124**: 71–99.

1855. NYBERG-HANSEN, R. 1966. Functional organization of descending supraspinal fibre systems to the spinal cord: Anatomical observations and physiological correlations. Ergeb. Anat. Entwickl.-Gesch., **39**: 1–48.

1856. NYBERG-HANSEN, R., AND BRODAL, A. 1964. Sites and mode of termination of rubrospinal fibres in the cat:

An experimental study with silver impregnation methods. J. Anat., **98**: 235–253.

1857. NYBERG-HANSEN, R., AND MASCITTI, T. A. 1964. Sites and mode of termination of fibers of the vestibulospinal tract in the cat: An experimental study with silver impregnation methods. J. Comp. Neurol., **122**: 369–387.

1858. NYBY, O., AND JANSEN, J. 1951. An experimental investigation of the corticopontine projection in *Macaca mulatta*. Norsk. Vidensk. Akad. Avh. Mat.-Naturv., **3**: 1–47.

1859. NYGREN, L. G., AND OLSON, L. 1977. A new major projection from the locus coeruleus: The main source of noradrenergic nerve terminals in the ventral and dorsal columns of the spinal cord. Brain Res., **132**: 85–93.

1860. OBATA, K., ITO, M., OCHI, R., AND SATO, N. 1967. Pharmacological properties of the postsynaptic inhibition by Purkinje cell axons and the action of γ-aminobutyric acid on Deiters neurones. Exp. Brain Res., **4**: 43–57.

1861. OCHS, S. 1972. Rate of fast axoplasmic transport in mammalian nerve fibers. J. Physiol. (Lond.), **227**: 627–645.

1862. OCHS, S., AND RANISH, N. 1969. Characteristics of the fast transport system in mammalian nerve fibers. J. Neurobiol., **1**: 247–261.

1863. ÖDKVIST, L. M., SCHWARZ, D. W. F., FREDRICKSON, J. M., AND HASSLER, R. 1974. Projection of the vestibular nerve to the area 3a arm field in the squirrel monkey (Saimiri sciureus). Exp. Brain Res., **21**: 97–105.

1864. OGREN, M. P., AND HENDRICKSON, A. E. 1976. Pathways between striate cortex and subcortical regions in *Macaca mulatta* and *Saimiri sciureus*: Evidence for a reciprocal pulvinar connection. Exp. Neurol., **53**: 780–800.

1865. OKADA, Y., NITCH-HASSLER, C., KIM, J. S., BAK, I. J., AND HASSLER, R. 1971. The role of δ-aminobutyric acid (GABA) in the extrapyramidal motor system. I. Regional distribution of GABA in rabbit, rat and guinea pig brain. Exp. Brain Res., **13**: 514–518.

1866. O'KEEFE, J., AND CONWAY, D. H. 1978. Hippocampal place units in the freely moving rat: Why they fire where they fire. Exp. Brain Res., **31**: 573–590.

1867. O'KEEFE, J., AND NADEL, L. 1978. *The Hippocampus as a Cognitive Map*. Oxford University Press, Oxford.

1868. OKON, E., AND KOCH, Y. 1976. Localization of gonadotropin-releasing and thyrotropin-releasing hormones in human brain by radioimmunoassay. Nature, **263**: 345–347.

1869. OLDENDORF, W. H. 1961. Isolated flying spot detection of radiodensity discontinuities-displaying the internal structural pattern of a complex object. IRE Trans. Biomed. Electron., **8**: 68–72.

1870. OLDS, J. 1960. Differentiation of reward systems in the brain by self-stimulation technics. In S. R. RAMEY AND D. S. O'DOHERTY (Editors), *Electrical Studies on the Unanesthetized Brain*. Paul B. Hoeber, Inc., New York, Ch. 2, pp. 17–51.

1871. OLDS, J., AND MILNER, P. 1954. Positive reinforcement produced by electrical stimulation of septal area and other regions of the rat brain. J. Comp. Physiol. Psychol., **47**: 419–427.

1872. O'LEARY, J. L., KERR, F. W. L., AND GOLDRING, S. 1958. The relation between spinoreticular and ascending cephalic systems. In H. H. JASPERS et al. (Editors), *Reticular Formation of the Brain*. Henry Ford Hospital International Symposium. Little, Brown and Company, Boston, Ch. 8, pp. 187–201.

1873. OLIVECRONA, H. 1957. Paraventricular nucleus and the pituitary gland. Acta Physiol. Scand., **40**: (suppl 136): 1–178.

1874. OLIVER, D. L., AND HALL, W. C. 1978. The medial geniculate body of the tree shrew, *Tupaia glis*. I. Cytoarchitecture and midbrain connections. J. Comp. Neurol., **182**: 423–458.

1875. OLIVER, D. L., AND HALL, W. C. 1978a. The medial

geniculate body of the tree shrew, *Tapaia glis*. II. Connections with the neocortex. J. Comp. Neurol., **182:** 459–494.

1876. OLIVERAS, J. L., HOSOBUCHI, Y., GUILBAUD, G., AND BESSON, J. M. 1978. Analgesic electrical stimulation of the feline nucleus raphe magnus: Development of tolerance and its reversal by 5-HTP. Brain Res., **146:** 404–409.

1877. DE OLMOS, J. S. 1972. The amygdaloid projection field in the rat as studied with the cupric-silver method. In B. E. ELEFTHERIOU (Editor), *The Neurobiology of the Amygdala.* Plenum Press, New York, pp. 145–204.

1878. OLPE, H-R., AND KOELLA, W. P. 1977. The response of striatal cells upon stimulation of the dorsal and median raphe nuclei. Brain Res., **122:** 357–360.

1879. OLSEN, L., AND FUXE, K. 1971. On the projections from the locus coeruleus noradrenalin neurons: The cerebellar innervation. Brain Res., **28:** 165–171.

1880. OLSON, C. R., AND GRAYBIEL, A. M. 1980. Sensory maps in the claustrum of the cat. Nature, **288:** 479–481.

1881. OLSSON, Y., AND REESE, T. S. 1971. Permeability of vasa nervorum and perineurium in mouse sciatic nerve studied by fluorescence and electron microscopy. J. Neuropathol. Exp. Neurol., **30:** 105–119.

1882. OLSZEWSKI, J. 1950. On the anatomical and functional organization of the spinal trigeminal nucleus. J. Comp. Neurol., **92:** 401–413.

1883. OLSZEWSKI, J. 1952. *The Thalamus of the Macaca Mulatta.* S. Karger, Basel, 93 pp.

1884. OLSEWSKI, J. 1954. Cytoarchitecture of the human reticular formation. In J. F. DELAFRESNAYE (Editor), *Brain Mechanisms and Consciousness* (Symposium). Blackwell Scientific Publications, Oxford, pp. 54–80.

1885. OLSZEWSKI, J., AND BAXTER, D. 1954. *Cytoarchitecture of the Human Brain Stem.* J. B. Lippincott Company, Philadelphia.

1886. OMMAYA, A. K., CORRAO, P., AND LETCHER, F. S. 1973. Head injury in the chimpanzee. I. Biodynamics of traumatic unconsciousness. J. Neurosurg., **39:** 152–166.

1887. ONO, T., NICHINO, H., SASAKA, K., MURAMOTO, K., YANO, I., AND SIMPSON, A. 1978. Paraventricular nucleus connections to spinal cord and pituitary. Neurosci. Lett., **10:** 141–146.

1888. ONO, T., OOMURA, Y., SUGIMORI, M., NAKAMURA, T., SHIMIZU, N., KITA, H., AND ISHIBASHI, S. 1976. Hypothalamic unit activity related to lever pressing and eating in the chronic monkey. In D. NOVIN, W. R. WYRWICKA, AND G. A. BRAY (Editors), *Hunger: Basic Mechanisms and Clinical Implications.* Raven Press, New York, pp. 159–170.

1889. OOMURA, Y., ONO, T., AND OOYAMA, H. 1970. Inhibitory action of the amygdala on the lateral hypothalamic area in rats. Nature, **228:** 1108–1110.

1890. OPPENHEIMER, D. R., PALMER, E., AND WEDELL, G. 1958. Nerve endings in the conjunctiva. J. Anat., **92:** 321–352.

1891. ORBACH, J., AND CHOW, K. L. 1959. Differential effects of resection of somatic areas I and II in monkeys. J. Neurophysiol., **22:** 195–203.

1892. ORBACH, J., MILNER, B., AND RASMUSSEN, T. 1960. Learning and retention in monkeys after amygdala-hippocampus resection. Arch. Neurol., **3:** 230–251.

1893. ORIOLI, F. L., AND METTLER, F. A. 1956. The rubrospinal tract in *Macaca mulatta.* J. Comp. Neurol., **106:** 299–318.

1894. ORKAND, R. K. 1977. Glial cells. In E. R. KANDEL (Volume Editor), *Handbook of Physiology,* Sect. I: *The Nervous System,* Vol. 1, Part 2. American Physiological Society, Washington, D. C., pp. 855–876.

1895. ORLOVSKY, G. N. 1972. Activity of vestibulospinal neurons during locomotion. Brain Res., **46:** 85–98.

1896. ORLOVSKY, G. N. 1972a. Activity of rubrospinal neurons during locomotion. Brain Res., **46:** 99–112.

1897. ORTMANN, R. 1960. Neurosecretion. In J. FIELD (Editor), *Handbook of Physiology, Neurophysiology,* Vol. II. American Physiological Society, Washington, D. C., Ch. 40, pp. 1039–1065.

1898. OSCARSSON, O. 1964. Three ascending tracts activated from group I afferents in forelimb nerves of the cat. Prog. Brain Res., **12:** 179–196.

1899. OSCARSSON, O. 1964a. Integrative organization of the rostral spinocerebellar tract in the cat. Acta Physiol. Scand., **64:** 154–166.

1900. OSCARSSON, O. 1965. Functional organization of the spino- and cuneocerebellar tracts. Physiol. Rev., **45:** 495–522.

1901. OSCARSSON, O. 1967. Termination and functional organization of a dorsal spino-olivocerebellar path. Brain Res., **5:** 531–534.

1902. OSCARSSON, O. 1967a. Functional significance of information channels from the spinal cord to the cerebellum. In M. D. YAHR AND D. P. PURPURA (Editors), *Neurophysiological Basis of Normal and Abnormal Motor Activities.* Raven Press, New York, pp. 93–113.

1903. OSCARSSON, O. 1973. Functional organization of spinocerebellar paths. In A. IGGO(Editor), *Handbook of Sensory Physiology,* Vol. 2. Springer-Verlag, Berlin, pp. 339–380.

1904. OSCARSSON, O., AND ROSÉN, I. 1966. Short-latency projections to the cat's cerebral cortex from skin and muscle afferents in the contralateral forelimb. J. Physiol. (Lond.), **182:** 164–184.

1905. OSCARSSON, O, AND SJÖLUND, B. 1977. The ventral spino-olivocerebellar system in the cat. I. Identification of five paths and their terminations in the cerebellar anterior lobe. Exp. Brain Res., **28:** 469–486.

1906. OSCARSSON, O., AND UDDENBERG, N. 1964. Identification of a spinocerebellar tract activated from forelimb afferents in the cat. Acta Physiol. Scand. **62:** 125–136.

1907. OSEN, K. K. 1969. The intrinsic organization of the cochlear nuclei in the cat. Acta Otolaryngol. (Stockh.), **67:** 352–359.

1908. OSEN, K. K. 1969a. Cytoarchitecture of the cochlear nuclei in the cat. J. Comp. Neurol., **136:** 453–484.

1909. OSTROWSKI, A. Z., WEBSTER, J. E., AND GURDJIAN, E. S. 1960. The proximal anterior cerebral artery: An anatomic study. Arch. Neurol., **3:** 661–664.

1910. OTSUKA, R., AND HASSLER, R. 1962. Über Aufbau und Gliederung der corticalen Sehsphäre bei der Katze. Arch Psychiatr. Nervenk., **203:** 212–234.

1911. OTTERSEN, O. P., AND BEN-ARI, Y. 1978. Pontine and mesencephalic afferents to the central nucleus of the amygdala of the rat. Neurosci. Lett., **8:** 329–334.

1912. OZEKI, M., AND SATO, M. 1964. Initiation of impulses at the non-myelinated terminal in Pacinian corpuscles. J. Physiol. (Lond.), **170:** 167–185.

1913. OZEKI, M., AND SATO, M. 1965. Changes in the membrane potential and the membrane conductance associated with a sustained compression of the non-myelinated nerve terminal in Pacinian corpuscles. J. Physiol. (Lond.), **180:** 186–208.

1914. PAGE, R. B., ROSENSTEIN, J. M., DOVEY, B. J., AND LEURE-DUPREE, A. E. 1979. Ependymal changes in experimental hydrocephalus. Anat. Rec., **194:** 83–104.

1915. PAGE, R. B., ROSENSTEIN, J. M., AND LEURE-DUPREE, A. E. 1979. The morphology of extrachoroidal ependyma overlying gray and white matter in the rabbit lateral ventricle. Anat. Rec., **194:** 67–82.

1916. PALAY, S. L. 1945. Neurosecretion. VII. The preoptico-hypophysial pathway in fishes. J. Comp. Neurol., **82:** 129–143.

1917. PALAY, S. L. 1957. The fine structure of the neurohypophysis. In H. WAELSCH (Editor), *Ultrastructure and Cellular Chemistry of Neural Tissue.* Paul B. Hoeber, Inc., New York, pp. 31–44.

1918. PALAY, S. L. 1958. An electron microscopical study of neuroglia. In W. F. WINDLE (Editor), *Biology of Neuroglia.* Charles C Thomas, Publisher, Springfield, Ill., pp. 24–38.

1919. PALAY, S. L. 1966. The role of neuroglia in the organization of the central nervous system. In K. RODAHL AND B. ISSEKUTZ, JR. (Editors), *Nerve as A Tissue.* Harper & Row Publishers, Inc., New York, pp. 3–10.

1920. PALAY, S. L., AND CHAN-PALAY, V. 1974. *Cerebellar Cortex: Cytology and Organization.* Springer-Verlag, Berlin.

1921. PALAY, S. L., AND PALADE, G. E. 1955. The fine structure of neurons. J. Biophys. Biochem. Cytol., **1:** 69–88.

1922. PALKOVITS, M. 1981. Catecholamines in the hypothalamus: An anatomical review. Neuroendocrinology, **33:** 123–128.

1923. PALKOVITZ, M., BROWNSTEIN, M., AND SAAVEDRA, J. M. 1974. Serotonin content of the brain stem nuclei in the rat. Brain Res., **80:** 237–249.

1924. PANDYA, D. N., VAN HOESEN, G. W., AND DOMESICK, V. B. 1973. A cingulo-amygdaloid projection in the rhesus monkey. Brain Res., **61:** 369–373.

1925. PANDYA, D. N., AND VIGNOLO, L. A. 1971. Intra- and interhemispheric projections of the precentral, premotor and arcuate areas in the rhesus monkey. Brain Res., **26:** 217–233.

1926. PANNETON, W. M., AND LOEWY, A. D. 1980. Projections of the carotid sinus nerve to the nucleus of the solitary tract in the cat. Brain Res., **191:** 239–244.

1927. PAPEZ, J. W. 1927. Subdivisions of the facial nucleus. J. Comp. Neurol., **43:** 159–191.

1928. PAPEZ, J. W. 1936. Evolution of the medial geniculate body. J. Comp. Neurol., **64:** 41–61.

1929. PAPEZ, J. W. 1937. A proposed mechanism of emotion. Arch. Neurol. Psychiatry, **38:** 725–743.

1930. PAPEZ, J. W. 1938. Thalamic connections in a hemidecorticate dog. J. Comp. Neurol., **69:** 103–119.

1931. PAPEZ, J. W. 1942. A summary of fiber connections of the basal ganglia with each other and with other portions of the brain. Proc. Assoc. Res. Nerv. Ment. Dis., **21:** 21–68.

1932. PAPEZ, J. W. 1956. Central reticular path to intralaminar and reticular nuclei of thalamus for activating EEG related to consciousness. Electroencephalogr. Clin. Neurophysiol., **8:** 117–128.

1933. PAPEZ, J. W. 1956a. Path for projection of non-specific diffuse impulses to cortex for EEG, related to consciousness. Dis. Nerv. Syst., **17:** 3–8.

1934. PAPEZ, J. W., BENNETT, A. E., AND CASH, P. T. 1942. Hemichorea (Hemiballismus): Association with a pallidal lesion involving afferent and efferent connections of the subthalamic nucleus: Curare therapy. Arch. Neurol. Psychiatry, **47:** 667–676.

1935. PAPEZ, J. W., AND FREEMAN, G. L. 1930. Superior colliculi and their fiber connections in the rat. J. Comp. Neurol., **51:** 409–439.

1936. PAPEZ, J. W., AND RUNDLES, W. 1937. The dorsal trigeminal tract and the centre median nucleus of Luys. J. Nerv. Ment. Dis., **85:** 509–519.

1937. PAPPAS, G. D. 1966. Electron microscopy of neuronal junctions involved in transmission in the central nervous system. In K. RODAHL AND B. ISSEKUTZ, JR. (Editors), *Nerve as a Tissue.* Harper & Row Publishers, Inc., New York, pp. 49–87.

1938. PAPPAS, G. D., AND TENNYSON, J. M. 1962. An electron microscopic study of the passage of colloidal particles from the blood vessels of the ciliary processes and choroid plexus of the rabbit. J. Cell Biol., **15:** 227–239.

1939. PARDRIDGE, W. M., FRANK, H. J. L., CORNFORD, E. M., BRAUN, L. D., CRANE, P. D., AND OLDENDORF, W. H. 1981. Neuropeptides and the blood brain barrier. Adv. Biochem. Psychopharmacol., **28:** 321–328.

1940. PARIZEK, J., HASSLER, R., AND BAK, I. J. 1971. Light and electron microscopic autoradiography of substantia nigra of rat after intraventricular administration of tritium labelled norepinephrine, dopamine, serotonin and the precursors. Z. Zellforsch. Mikrosk. Anat., **115:** 137–148.

1941. PARTLOW, G. D., COLONNIER, M., AND SZABO, J. 1977. Thalamic projections of the superior colliculus in the rhesus monkey, *Macaca mulatta*: A light and electron microscopic study. J. Comp. Neurol., **171:** 285–318.

1942. PARTRIDGE, M. 1950. *Prefrontal Leucotomy: A Survey of 300 Cases Personally Followed over 1½–3 Years.* Blackwell Scientific Publications, Oxford, 496 pp.

1943. PASIK, P., PASIK, T., AND DI FIGLIA, M. 1976. Quantitative aspects of neuronal organization in the neostriatum of the Macaque monkey. Proc. Assoc. Res. Nerv. Ment. Dis., **55:** 57–89.

1944. PASIK, P., PASIK, T., AND HÁMORI, J. 1976. Synapses between interneurons in the lateral geniculate nucleus of monkeys. Exp. Brain Res., **25:** 1–13.

1945. PASIK, P., PASIK, T., HÁMORI, J., AND SZENTÁGOTHAI, J. 1973. Golgi type II interneurons in the neuronal circuit of the monkey lateral geniculate nucleus. Exp. Brain Res., **17:** 18–34.

1946. PASS, I. J. 1933. Anatomic and functional relationship of nuc. dorsalis (Clarke's column). Arch. Neurol. Psychiatry, **30:** 1025–1045.

1947. PATTERSON, P. H. 1978. Environmental determination of autonomic neurotransmitter functions. Annu. Rev. Neurosci., **1:** 1–17.

1948. PATTON, H. D. 1961. Reflex regulation of movement and posture. In T. C. RUCH *et al.* (Editors), *Neurophysiology.* W. B. Saunders Company, Philadelphia, Ch. 6, pp. 167–198.

1949. PATTON, H. D. 1961a. Special properties of nerve trunks and tracts. In T. C. RUCH *et al.* (Editors), *Neurophysiology.* W. B. Saunders Company, Philadelphia, Ch. 3, pp. 66–95.

1950. PATTON, H. D., AND RUCH, T. C. 1946. The relation of the foot of the pre- and postcentral gyrus to taste in the monkey and chimpanzee. Fed. Proc., **5:** 79.

1951. PATTON, H. D., RUCH, T. C., AND WALKER, A. E. 1944. Experimental hypogeusia from Horsley-Clarke lesions of the thalamus in *Macaca mulatta.* J. Neurophysiol., **7:** 171–184.

1952. PAYNE, F. 1924. General description of a 7-somite human embryo. Contrib. Embryol., **16:** 115–124.

1953. PEARSON, A. A. 1949. The development and connections of the mesencephalic root of the trigeminal nerve in man. J. Comp. Neurol., **90:** 1–46.

1954. PEARSON, A. A. 1949a. Further observations on the mesencephalic root of the trigeminal nerve. J. Comp. Neurol., **91:** 147–194.

1955. PEARSON, A. A. 1952. Role of gelatinous substance of spinal cord in conduction of pain. A. M. A. Arch. Neurol. Psychiatry, **68:** 515–529.

1956. PEARSON, A. A., SAUTER, R. W., AND BUCKELY, T. W. 1966. Further observations on the cutaneous branches of the dorsal primary rami of the spinal nerves. Am. J. Anat., **118:** 891–904.

1957. PEARSON, R. C., BRODAL, P., AND POWELL, T. P. S. 1978. The projection of the thalamus upon the parietal lobe in the monkey. Brain Res., **144:** 143–148.

1958. PEASE, D. C., AND SCHULTZ, R. L. 1958. Electron microscopy of rat cranial meninges. Am. J. Anat., **102:** 301–313.

1959. PEELE, T. L. 1942. Cytoarchitecture of individual parietal areas in the monkey (*Macaca mulatta*) and distribution of the efferent fibers. J. Comp. Neurol., **77:** 693–737.

1960. PEELE, T. L. 1961. *The Neuroanatomical Basis for Clinical Neurology.* McGraw Hill Book Company, New York.

1961. PENFIELD, W. 1932. Neuroglia, normal and pathological. In W. G. PENFIELD (Editor), *Cytology and Cellular Pathology of the Nervous System,* Vol. II. Paul B. Hoeber, Inc., New York, pp. 423–479.

1962. PENFIELD, W. 1957. Vestibular sensation and the cerebral cortex. Ann. Otol. Rhinol. Laryngol., **66:** 691–698.

1963. PENFIELD, W., AND BOLDREY, E. 1937. Somatic motor and sensory representation in the cerebral cortex of man as studied by electrical stimulation. Brain, **60:** 389–443.

1964. PENFIELD, W., AND EVANS, J. 1934. Functional defects produced by cerebral lobectomies. Proc. Assoc. Res. Nerv. Ment. Dis., **13:** 352–377.

1965. PENFIELD, W., AND JASPER, H. H. 1954. *Epilepsy and the Functional Anatomy of the Human Brain.* Little Brown & Company, Boston, 896 pp.

1966. PENFIELD, W., AND McNAUGHTON, F. 1940. Dural headache and innervation of the dura mater. Arch. Neurol. Psychiatry, **44:** 43–75.

1967. PENFIELD, W., AND MILNER, B. 1958. Memory deficit produced by bilateral lesions in the hippocampal zone. A. M. A. Arch. Neurol. Psychiatry, **79:** 475–497.

1968. PENFIELD, W., AND RASMUSSEN, T. 1950. *The Cerebral Cortex of Man: A Clinical Study of Localization of Function.* MacMillan Company, New York, 248 pp.

1969. PENFIELD, W., AND ROBERTS, L. 1959. *Speech and Brain Mechanisms.* Princeton University Press, Princeton, N. J.

1970. PENFIELD, W., AND WELCH, K. 1951. The supplementary motor area of the cerebral cortex. A clinical and experimental study. A. M. A. Arch. Neurol. Psychiatry, **66:** 289–317.

1971. PERCHERON, G. 1977. The thalamic territory of cerebellar afferents and the lateral region of the thalamus of the macaque in stereotaxic ventricular coordinates. J. Hirnforsch., **18:** 375–400.

1972. PERL, E. R., AND WHITLOCK, D. G. 1961. Somatic stimuli exciting spinothalamic projections in thalamic neurons in the cat and monkey. Exp. Neurol., **3:** 256–296.

1973. PERL, E. R., WHITLOCK, D. G., AND GENTRY, J. R. 1962. Cutaneous projection to second-order neurons of the dorsal column system. J. Neurophysiol., **25:** 337–353.

1974. PERLMUTTER, D., AND RHOTON, A. L. 1976. Microsurgical anatomy of the anterior cerebral-anterior communicating-recurrent artery complex. J. Neurosurg., **45:** 259–272.

1975. PERLMUTTER, D., AND RHOTON, A. L. 1978. Microsurgical anatomy of the distal anterior cerebral artery. J. Neurosurg., **49:** 204–228.

1976. PERT, C. 1978. Opiate receptors and pain pathways. Neurosci. Res. Program Bull., **16:** 133–141.

1977. PERT, C. B., KUHAR, M. J., AND SNYDER, S. H. 1975. Autoradiographic localization of the opiate receptor in rat brain. Life Sci., **16:** 1849–1854.

1978. PERT, C. B., SNOWMAN, A. M., AND SNYDER, S. H. 1974. Localization of opiate receptor binding in synaptic membranes of rat brain. Brain Res., **70:** 184–188.

1979. PETERS, A. 1960. The formation and structure of myelin sheaths in the central nervous system. J. Biophys. Biochem. Cytol., **8:** 431–446.

1980. PETERS, A. 1966. The node of Ranvier in the central nervous system. Q. J. Exp. Physiol., **51:** 229–236.

1981. PETERS, A., AND PALAY, S. L. 1965. An electron microscopy study of the distribution and patterns of astroglial processes in the central nervous system. J. Anat., **99:** 419.

1982. PETERS, A., PALAY, S. L., AND WEBSTER, H. DE F. 1976. *The Fine Structure of the Nervous System: The Neurons and Supporting Cells.* W. B. Saunders Co., Philadelphia.

1983. PETERS, A., PROSKAUER, C. C., AND KAISERMAN-ABRAMOF, I. R. 1968. The small pyramidal neuron of the rat cerebral cortex: The Axon hillock and initial segment. J. Cell Biol., **39:** 604–619.

1984. PETERS, A., AND VAUGHN, J. E. 1967. Microtubules and filaments in the axons and astrocytes of early postnatal rat optic nerve. J. Cell Biol., **32:** 113–119.

1985. PETERSON, B. W. 1979. Reticulo-motor pathways: Their connections and possible roles in motor behavior. In H. ASANUMA AND V. J. WILSON (Editors), *Integration in the Nervous System.* Igaku Shoin, Ltd., Tokyo, pp. 185–200.

1986. PETERSON, B. W. 1979a. Reticulospinal projections to spinal motor nuclei. Annu. Rev. Physiol., **41:** 127–140.

1987. PETERSON, E. R., AND MURRAY, M. R. 1955. Myelin

sheath formation in cultures of avian spinal ganglia. Am. J. Anat., **96:** 319–355.

1988. PETRAS, J. M. 1964. Some fiber connections of the precentral cortex (areas 4 and 6) with the diencephalon in the monkey (*Macaca mulatta*). Anat. Rec., **148:** 322.

1989. PETRAS, J. M. 1965. Some fiber connections of the precentral and postcentral cortex with the basal ganglia, thalamus and subthalamus. Trans. Am. Neurol. Assoc., **90:** 274–275.

1990. PETRAS, J. M. 1966. Fiber degeneration in the basal ganglia and diencephalon following lesions in the precentral and postcentral cortex of the monkey (*Macaca mulatta*): with additional observations in the chimpanzee, In *Proceedings of the VII International Congress on Anatomy,* Wiesbaden,

1991. PETRAS, J. M. 1967. Cortical, tectal and tegmental fiber connections in the spinal cord of the cat. Brain Res., **6:** 275–324.

1992. PETRAS, J. M. 1969. Some efferent connections of the motor and somatosensory cortex of simian primates and Felid, Canid and Procyonid carnivores. Ann. N. Y. Acad. Sci., **167:** 469–505.

1993. PETRAS, J. M. 1971. Connections of the parietal lobe. J. Psychiatr. Res., **8:** 189–201.

1994. PETRAS, J. M., AND CUMMINGS, J. F. 1972. Autonomic neurons in the spinal cord of the Rhesus monkey: A correlation of the findings of cytoarchitectonics and sympathectomy with fiber degeneration following dorsal rhizotomy. J. Comp. Neurol., **146:** 189–218.

1995. PETRAS, J. M., AND CUMMINGS, J. F. 1977. The origin of spinocerebellar pathways. II. The nucleus centrobasalis of the cervical enlargement and the nucleus dorsalis of the thoracolumbar spinal cord. J. Comp. Neurol., **173:** 693–716.

1996. PFAFF, D. W., AND KEINER, M. 1972. Estradiol-concentrating cells in the rat amygdala as part of a limbic-hypothalamic hormone-sensitive system. In B. E. ELEFTHERIOU (Editor), *The Neurobiology of the Amygdala,* Plenum Press, New York, pp. 775–785.

1997. PFAFF, D. W., AND KEINER, M. 1973. Atlas of estradiol concentrating cells in the central nervous system of the female rat. J. Comp. Neurol., **151:** 121–159.

1998. PFAFFMANN, C. 1939. Afferent impulses from the teeth resulting from a vibratory stimulus. J. Physiol. (Lond.), **97:** 220–232.

1999. PHALEN, G. S., AND DAVENPORT, H. A. 1937. Pericellular end-bulbs in the central nervous system of vertebrates. J. Comp. Neurol., **68:** 67–81.

2000. PHILLIPS, C. G., POWELL, T. P. S., AND WIESENDANGER, M. 1971. Projection from low-threshold muscle afferents of hand and forearm to area 3a of baboons cortex. J. Physiol. (Lond.), **217:** 419–446.

2001. PHILLIPS, M. I., FELIX, D., HOFFMAN, W. E., AND GANTEN, A. 1977. Angiotensin-sensitive sites in the brain ventricular system. Neurosci. Symp., **2:** 308–339.

2002. PICK, J. 1970. *The Autonomic Nervous System.* J. B. Lippincott Company, Philadelphia, 483 pp.

2003. PICK, J., AND SHEEHAN, D. 1946. Sympathetic rami in man. J. Anat., **80:** 12–20.

2004. PICKEL, V. M. 1979. Immunocytochemical localization of neuronal antigens: Tyrosine hydroxylase, substance P, [Met⁵]-enkephalin. Fed. Proc., **38:** 2374–2380.

2005. PICKEL, V. M., REIS, D. J., AND LEEMAN, S. E. 1977. Ultrastructural localization of substance P in neurons of rat spinal cord. Brain Res., **122:** 534–540.

2006. PICKEL, V. M., SEGAL, M., AND BLOOM, F. E. 1974. A radioautographic study of the efferent pathways of the nucleus locus coeruleus. J. Comp. Neurol., **155:** 15–42.

2007. PICKFORD, M. 1969. Neurohypophysis-antidiuretic (vasopressor) and oxytocic hormones. In W. HAYMAKER *et al.* (Editors), *The Hypothalamus.* Charles C Thomas Publisher, Springfield, Ill., Ch. 13, pp. 463–505.

2008. PICTET, R. L., RALL, L. B., PHELPS, P., AND RUTTER, W. J. 1976. The neural crest and the origin of the insulin-producing and other gastrointestinal hormone-producing cells. Science, **191:** 191–192.

2009. PIERSON, R. J., AND CARPENTER, M. B. 1974. Anatomical analysis of pupillary reflex pathways in the rhesus monkey. J. Comp. Neurol., **158:** 121–143.

2010. PIN, C., JONES, B., AND JOUVET, M. 1968. Topographie des neurones monoaminergiques du tronc cérébral du chat: Étude par histofluorescence. C. R. Soc. Biol. (Paris), **162:** 2137–2141.

2011. PINDER, R. M. 1973. The pharmacology of Parkinsonism. Prog. Med. Chem., **9:** 191–274.

2012. PINEDA, A., MAXWELL, D. S., AND KRUGER, L. 1967. The fine structure of neurons and satellite cells in the trigeminal ganglion of cat and monkey. Am. J. Anat., **121:** 461–488.

2013. PINES, I. L. 1925. Über die Innervation der Hypophysis cerebri. II. Mitteilung. Über die Innervation des Mittel- und Hinterlappens der Hypophyse. Z. Gesamte Neurol. Psychiatry, **100:** 123–138.

2014. PITTS, R. F. 1940. The respiratory center and its descending pathways. J. Comp. Neurol., **72:** 605–625.

2015. PITTS, R. F. 1946. Organization of the respiratory center. Physiol Rev., **26:** 609–630.

2016. PITTS, R. F., MAGOUN, H. W., AND RANSON, S. W. 1939. Localization of the medullary respiratory centers in the cat. Am. J. Physiol., **126:** 673–688.

2017. PLUM, F., GJEDDE, A., AND SAMSON, F. E. 1976. Neuroanatomical functional mapping by radioactive 2-deoxy-d-glucose method. Neurosci. Res. Program Bull., **14:** 457–518.

2018. PLUM, F., AND POSNER, J. B. 1966. *The Diagnosis of Stupor and Coma.* F. A. Davis Company, Philadelphia.

2019. POGGIO, G. F., AND MOUNTCASTLE, V. B. 1960. A study of the functional contributions of the lemniscal and spinothalamic systems to somatic sensibility. Bull. Johns Hopkins Hosp., **106:** 266–316.

2020. POGGIO, G. F., AND MOUNTCASTLE, V. B. 1963. The functional properties of ventrobasal thalamic neurons studied in unanesthetized monkeys. J. Neurophysiol., **26:** 775–806.

2021. POIRIER, L. 1952. Anatomical and experimental studies on the temporal pole of the macaque. J. Comp. Neurol., **96:** 209–248.

2022. POIRIER, L. J., AND BERTRAND, C. 1955. Experimental and anatomical investigation of the lateral spino-thalamic and spinotectal tracts. J. Comp. Neurol., **102:** 745–757.

2023. POIRIER, L. J., AND BOUVIER, G. 1966. The red nucleus and its efferent nervous pathways in the monkey. J. Comp. Neurol., **128:** 223–244.

2024. POIRIER, L. J., SINGH, P., BOUCHER, R., BOUVIER, G., OLIVER, A., AND LAROCHELLE, P. 1957. Effect of brain lesions on striatal monoamines in the cat. A. M. A. Arch. Neurol., **17:** 601–608.

2025. POIRIER, L. J., AND SOURKES, T. L. 1965. Influence of the substantia nigra on catecholamine content of the striatum. Brain, **88:** 181–192.

2026. POITRAS, D., AND PARENT, A. 1978. Atlas of the distribution of monoamine-containing nerve cell bodies in the brain stem of the cat. J. Comp. Neurol., **179:** 699–718.

2027. VAN DEN POL, A. N., AND POWLEY, T. 1979. A fine-grained anatomical analysis of the role of the rat suprachiasmatic nucleus in circadian rhythms of feeding and drinking. Brain Res., **160:** 307–326.

2028. POLAK, M. 1965. Morphological and functional characteristics of the central and peripheral neuroglia. (light microscopic observations). Prog. Brain Res., **15:** 12–34.

2029. POLIAK, S. 1924. Die Struktureigentümlichkeiten des Rückenmarkes bei den Chiroptern. Zugleich ein Beitrag zu der Frage über die spinalen Zentren des Sympatheticus. Z. Anat. Entwickl.-Gesch., **74:** 509–576.

2030. POLLAY, M., AND CURL, F. 1967. Secretion of cerebrospinal fluid by the ventricular ependyma of the rabbit. Am. J. Physiol., **213:** 1031–1038.

2031. POLYAK, S L. 1957. *The Vertebrate Visual System.* University of Chicago Press, Chicago, 1390 pp.

2032. POMERAT, C. M. 1958. Functional concepts based on tissue culture studies of neuroglia cells. In W. F. WINDLE (Editor), *Biology of Neuroglia.* Charles C Thomas, Publisher, Springfield, Ill., pp. 162–175.

2033. POMPEIANO, O. 1956. Sulle risposte posturali alla stimolazione elettrica del nucleo rosso nel gatto decerebrato. Boll. Soc. Ital. Biol. Sper., **32:** 1450–1451.

2034. POMPEIANO, O. 1957. Analisi degli effetti della stimolazione elettrica del nucleo rosso nel gatto decerebrato. Rend. Accad. Naz. Lincei, Cl. Sci. Fis. Mat. Nat., **22:** 100–103.

2035. POMPEIANO, O. 1959. Organizzazione somatotopica delle risposte flessorie alla stimolazione elettrica del nucleo interposito nel gatto decerebrato. Arch. Sci. Biol. (Bologna), **43:** 163–176.

2036. POMPEIANO, O. 1960. Organizzazione somatotopica delle risposte posturali alla stimolazione elettrica del nucleo di Deiters nel Gatto cerebrato. Arch. Sci. Biol. (Bologna), **44:** 497–511.

2037. POMPEIANO, O. 1960a. Localizzazione delle risposte estensorie alla stimolazione elettrica del nucleo interposito nel gatto decerebrato. Arch. Sci. Biol. (Bologna), **44:** 473–496.

2038. POMPEIANO, O. 1967. The neurophysiological mechanisms of the postural and motor events during desynchronized sleep. Proc. Assoc. Res. Nerv. Ment. Dis., **45:** 351–423.

2039. POMPEIANO, O., AND BRODAL, A. 1957. Experimental demonstration of a somatotopical origin of rubrospinal fibers in the cat. J. Comp. Neurol., **108:** 225–251.

2040. POMPEIANO, O., AND BRODAL, A. 1957a. Spinovestibular fibers in the cat: An experimental study. J. Comp. Neurol., **108:** 353–382.

2041. POMPEIANO, O., AND BRODAL, A. 1957b. The origin of the vestibulospinal fibres in the cat: An experimental-anatomical study, with comments on the descending medial longitudinal fasciculus. Arch. Ital. Biol., **95:** 166–195.

2042. POMPEIANO, O., AND MORRISON, A. R. 1965. Vestibular influences during sleep. I. Abolition of rapid eye movements of desynchronized sleep following vestibular lesions. Arch. Ital. Biol., **103:** 569–595.

2043. POMPEIANO, O., AND WALBERG, F. 1957. Descending connections to the vestibular nuclei: An experimental study in the cat. J. Comp. Neurol., **108:** 465–502.

2044. POOL, J. L. 1954. Neurophysiological symposium: Visceral brain of man. J. Neurosurg., **11:** 45–63.

2045. POPA, G. T., AND FIELDING, U. 1930. A portal circulation from the pituitary to the hypothalamic region. J. Anat., **65:** 88–91.

2046. PORRINO, L. J., CRANE, A. M., AND GOLDMAN-RAKIC, P. S. 1981. Direct and indirect pathways from the amygdala to the frontal lobe in rhesus monkeys. J. Comp. Neurol., **198:** 121–136.

2047. PORTER, J. C., AND JONES, J. C. 1956. Effect of plasma from hypophyseal-portal vessel blood on adrenal ascorbic acid. Endocrinology, **58:** 62–67.

2048. PORTER, J. C., ONDON, J. G, AND CRAMER, O. M. 1974. Nervous and vascular supply of the pituitary gland. In R. O. GREEP AND E. B. ASTWOOD (Editors), *Handbook of Physiology,* Sect. 7., Vol. IV: *Endocrinology.* American Physiological Society, Washington, D. C., Chap. 2, pp. 33–43.

2049. POTTER, H., AND NAUTA, W. J. H. 1979. A note on the problem of olfactory associations of the orbitofrontal cortex in the monkey. Neuroscience, **4:** 361–369.

2050. POTTS, T. K. 1924. The main peripheral connections of the human sympathetic nervous system. J. Anat., **59:** 129–135.

2051. POWELL, D., LEEMAN, S. E., TREGEAR, G. W., NIALL, H. D., AND POTTS, J. T. 1973. Radioimmunoassay for substance P. Nature, **241:** 252–254.

2052. POWELL, E. W., AND HATTON, J. B. 1969. Projections of the inferior colliculus in the cat. J. Comp. Neurol., **136:** 183–192.

2053. POWELL, E. W., AND ROBINSON, P. F. 1975. Cinguloseptal projections in the squirrel monkey. Brain

Res., **96:** 310–316.

2054. POWELL, T. P. S. 1952. Residual neurons in the human thalamus following hemidecortication. Brain, **75:** 571–584.

2055. POWELL, T. P. S., AND COWAN, W. M. 1956. A study of thalamo-striate relations in the monkey. Brain, **79:** 364–390.

2056. POWELL, T. P. S., AND COWAN, W. M. 1962. An experimental study of the projection of the cochlea. J. Anat., **96:** 269–284.

2057. POWELL, T. P. S., AND COWAN, W. M. 1963. Centrifugal fibers in the lateral olfactory tract. Nature, **199:** 1296–1297.

2058. POWELL, T. P. S., AND COWAN, W. M. 1967. The interpretation of the degenerative changes in the intralaminar nuclei of the thalamus. J. Neurol. Neurosurg. Psychiatry, **30:** 140–153.

2059. POWELL, T. P. S., COWAN, W. M., AND RAISMAN, G. 1963. Olfactory relationship of the diencephalon. Nature, **199:** 710–712.

2060. POWELL, T. P. S., COWAN, W. M., AND RAISMAN, G. 1965. The central olfactory connexions. J. Anat., **99:** 791–813.

2061. POWELL, T. P. S., AND ERULKAR, S. D. 1962. Transneuronal cell degeneration in the auditory relay nuclei of the cat. J. Anat., **96:** 249–268.

2062. POWELL, T. P. S., GUILLERY, R. W., AND COWAN, W. M. 1957. A quantitative study of the fornix-mammillo-thalamic system. J. Anat., **91:** 419–432.

2063. POWELL, T. P. S., AND MOUNTCASTLE, V. B. 1959. The cytoarchitecture of the postcentral gyrus of the monkey *Macaca mulatta*. Bull. Johns Hopkins Hosp., **105:** 108–131.

2064. POWELL, T. P. S., AND MOUNTCASTLE, V. B. 1959a. Some aspects of the functional organization of the cortex of the postcentral gyrus of the monkey: A correlation of findings obtained in a single unit analysis with cytoarchitecture. Bull. Johns Hopkins Hosp., **105:**133–162.

2065. POWERS, J. B., FIELDS, R. B., AND WINANS, S. S. 1979. Olfactory and vomeronasal system participation in male hamsters attraction to female vaginal secretions. Physiol. Behav., **22:** 77–84.

2066. PRENTISS, C. W., AND AREY, L. B. 1920. *A Laboratory Manual and Textbook of Embryology*. W. B. Saunders Company, Philadelphia, Ch. XII, pp. 321–352.

2067. PRESTON, J. B., AND WHITLOCK, D. G. 1960. Precentral facilitation and inhibition of spinal motoneurons. J. Neurophysiol., **23:** 154–170.

2068. PRESTON, J. B., AND WHITLOCK, D. G. 1961. Intracellular potentials recorded from motoneurons following precentral gyrus stimulation in primate. J. Neurophysiol., **24:** 91–100.

2069. PRIBRAM, K. H., AND BAGSHAW, M. 1953. Further analysis of the temporal lobe syndrome utilizing frontotemporal ablations. J. Comp. Neurol., **99:** 347–375.

2070. PRIBRAM, K. H., ROSNER, B. S., AND ROSENBLITH, W. A. 1954. Electrical response to acoustic clicks in monkey: Extent of neocortex activated. J. Neurophysiol., **17:** 336–344.

2071. PRICE, D. D., DUBNER, R., AND HU, J. W. 1976. Trigeminothalamic neurons in nucleus caudalis responsive to tactile, thermal and nociceptive stimulation of monkeys face. J. Neurophysiol., **39:** 936–953.

2072. PRICE, D. D., AND MAYER, D. J. 1974. Physiological laminar organization of dorsal horn of *M. Mulatta*. Brain Res., **79:** 321–325.

2073. PRICE, J. L., AND POWELL, T. P. S. 1970. The morphology of the granule cells of the olfactory bulb. J. Cell Sci., **7:** 91–124.

2074. PRICE, J. L., AND POWELL, T. P. S. 1970a. The mitral and short axon cells of the olfactory bulb. J. Cell Sci., **7:** 631–652.

2075. PROUDFIT, H. K., AND ANDERSON, E. G. 1975. Morphine analgesia: Blockade by raphe magnus lesions. Brain Res., **98:** 612–618.

2076. PUBOLS, B. H. 1977. The second somatic sensory

area (Sm II) of opossum neocortex. J. Comp. Neurol., **174:** 71–78.

2077. PURPURA, D. P. 1970. Operations and processes in thalamic and synaptically related neural subsystems. In F. O. SCHMITT (Editor), *The Neurosciences. Second Study Program*. Rockefeller University Press, New York, Ch. 42, pp. 458–470.

2078. PURPURA, D. P. 1972. Intracellular studies of synaptic organization in the mammalian brain. In G. D. PAPPAS AND D. P. PURPURA (Editors), *Structure and Function of Synapses*. Raven Press, New York, pp. 257–302.

2079. PURPURA, D. P., AND COHEN, B. 1962. Intracellular synaptic activities of thalamic neurons during evoked recruiting responses. In *22nd International Congress of Physiological Sciences*, Excerpta Medica International Congress Series 48, Leiden.

2079a. PURPURA, D. P., AND GRUNDFEST, H. 1956. Nature of dendritic potentials and synoptic mechanisms in cerebral cortex of cat. J. Neurophysiol., **19:** 573–595.

2080. PURPURA, D. P., AND SHOFER, R. 1963. Intracellular recordings from thalamic neurons during reticulocortical activation. J. Neurophysiol., **26:** 494–505.

2081. PURVES, D., AND LICHTMAN, J. W. 1978. Formation and maintenance of synaptic connections in autonomic ganglia. Physiol. Rev., **58:** 821–862.

2082. PYCOCK, C., HORTON, R. W., AND MARSDEN, C. D. 1976. The behavioural effects of manipulating GABA function in the globus pallidus. Brain Res., **116:** 353–359.

2083. QUAY, W. B. 1974. *Pineal Chemistry in the Cellular and Physiological Mechanisms*. Charles C Thomas Publisher, Springfield, Ill.

2084. QUENSEL, F. 1910. Über den Stabkranz des menschlichen Stirnhirns. Folia Neuro-biol. **4:** 319–334.

2085. QUENSEL, F. 1944. Über die Faserspezifität in sensiblen Hautnerven. Pflügers Arch. Gesamte Physiol. Menschen Tiere, **248:** 1–20.

2086. QUILLIAM, T. A. 1966. Unit design and array patterns in receptor organs. In A. V. S. DE REUCK AND J. KNIGHT (Editors), *Touch, Heat and Pain*. Ciba Foundation Symposium. Little, Brown & Company, Boston, pp. 86–112.

2087. RACZKOWSKI, D., DIAMOND, I. T., AND WINER, J., JR. 1976. Organization of thalamocortical auditory system in the at studied with horseradish peroxidase. Brain Res., **101:** 345–354.

2088. RADEMAKER, G. G. T. 1926. *Die Bedeutung der roten Kerne und des übrigen Mittelhirns für Muskeltonus, Körperstellung, und Labyrinthreflexe*. Julius Springer, Berlin, pp. 64–222.

2089. RAFOLS, J., AND FOX, C. S. 1976. The neurons of the primate subthalamic nucleus: A Golgi and electron microscopic study. J. Comp. Neurol., **168:** 75–112.

2090. RAISMAN, G. 1966. Neural connexions of hypothalamus. Br. Med. Bull., **22:** 197–201.

2091. RAISMAN, G. 1966a. The connexions of the septum. Brain, **89:** 317–348.

2092. RAISMAN, G. 1970. An evaluation of the basic pattern of connections between the limbic system and the hypothalamus. Am. J. Anat., **129:** 197–202.

2093. RAISMAN, G. 1972. An experimental study of the projection of the amygdala to the accessory olfactory bulb and its relationship to the concept of a dual olfactory system. Exp. Brain Res., **14:** 395–408.

2094. RAISMAN, G., COWAN, W. M., AND POWELL, T. P. S. 1965. The extrinsic afferent, commissural and association fibres of the hippocampus. Brain, **88:** 963–996.

2095. RAISMAN, G., COWAN, W. M., AND POWELL, T. P. S. 1966. An experimental analysis of the efferent projections of the hippocampus. Brain, **89:** 83–108.

2096. RAISMAN, G., AND FIELD, P. M. 1973. Sexual dimorphism in the neuropil of the preoptic area of the rat and its dependence on neonatal androgen. Brain Res., **54:** 1–29.

2097. RALSTON, H. J., III. 1965. The organization of the

substantia gelatinosa Rolandi in the cat lumbosacral spinal cord. Z. Zellforsch. Mikrosk. Anat., **67:** 1–23.

2098. RALSTON, H. J., III. 1968. The fine structure of neurons in the dorsal horn of the cat spinal cord. J. Comp. Neurol., **132:** 275–302.

2099. RALSTON, H. J., III. 1968a. Dorsal root projections to the dorsal horn neurons in the cat spinal cord. J. Comp. Neurol., **132:** 303–330.

2100. RALSTON, H. J., III. 1979. The fine structure of laminae I, II, and III of the macaque spinal cord. J. Comp. Neurol., **184:** 619–642.

2101. RALSTON, H. J., III., AND RALSTON, D. D. 1979. The distribution of dorsal root axons in laminae I, II and III of the macaque spinal cord: A quantitative electron microscope study. J. Comp. Neurol., **184:** 643–684.

2102. RALSTON, H. J., III., MILLER, M. R., AND KASAHARA, M. 1960. Nerve endings in human fasciae, tendons, ligaments, periosteum, and joint synovial membrane. Anat. Rec., **136:** 137–148.

2103. RAMON-MOLINER, E. 1958. A tungstate modification of the Golgi-Cox method. Stain Technol., **33:** 19–29.

2104. RAMON-MOLINER, E. 1977. The reciprocal synapses of the olfactory bulb: Questioning the evidence. Brain Res., **128:** 1–20.

2105. RANSON, S. W. 1912. The structure of the spinal ganglia and of the spinal nerves. J. Comp. Neurol., **22:** 159–175.

2106. RANSON, S. W. 1913. The course within the spinal cord of the non-medullated fibers of the dorsal roots: A study of Lissauer's tract in the cat. J. Comp. Neurol., **23:** 259–281.

2107. RANSON, S. W. 1914. The tract of Lissauer and the substantia gelatinosa Rolandi. Am. J. Anat., **16:** 97–126.

2108. RANSON, S. W. 1939. Somnolence caused by hypothalamic lesions in the monkey. Arch. Neurol. Psychiatry, **41:** 1–23.

2109. RANSON, S. W., AND BILLINGSLEY, P. R. 1918. The superior cervical ganglion and the cervical portion of the sympathetic trunk. J. Comp. Neurol., **29:** 313–358.

2110. RANSON, S. W., AND INGRAM, W. R. 1932. The diencephalic course and termination of the medial lemniscus and brachium conjunctivum. J. Comp. Neurol., **56:** 257–275.

2111. RANSON, S. W., AND MAGOUN, H. W. 1933. The central path of the pupillo-constrictor reflex in response to light. Arch. Neurol. Psychiatry, **30:** 1193–1204.

2112. RANSON, S. W., AND RANSON, S. W., JR. 1942. Efferent fibers of the corpus striatum. Proc. Assoc. Res. Nerv. Ment. Dis., **21:** 69–76.

2113. RANSON, S. W., RANSON, S. W., JR., AND RANSON, M. 1941. Corpus striatum and thalamus of a partially decorticate monkey. Arch. Neurol. Psychaitry, **46:** 402–415.

2114. RAPOPORT, S. I. 1976. *Blood-Brain Barrier in Physiology and Medicine.* Raven Press, New York, 316 pp.

2115. RASMINSKY, M., MAURO, A. J., AND ALBE-FESSARD, D. 1973. Projections of medial thalamic nuclei to putamen and cerebral frontal cortex in the cat. Brain Res., **61:** 69–77.

2116. RASMUSSEN, A. T. 1936. Tractus tecto-spinalis in the cat. J. Comp. Neurol., **63:** 501–525.

2117. RASMUSSEN, A. T., AND PEYTON, W. T. 1948. The course and termination of the medial lemniscus in man. J. Comp. Neurol., **88:** 411–424.

2118. RASMUSSEN, G. L. 1946. The olivary peduncle and other fiber projections of the superior olivary complex. J. Comp. Neurol., **84:** 141–219.

2119. RASMUSSEN, G. L. 1953. Further observations of the efferent cochlear bundle. J. Comp. Neurol., **99:** 61–74.

2119a. RASMUSSEN, G. L. 1957. Selective silver impregnations of synaptic endings. In, W. F. WINDLE (Editor), *New Research Techniques in Neuroanatomy.* Charles C Thomas, Publisher, Springfield, Ill., pp. 27–39.

2120. RASMUSSEN, G. L. 1960. Efferent fibers of the cochlear nerve and cochlear nucleus. In G. L. RASMUSSEN AND W. F. WINDLE (Editors), *Neural Mechanisms of the Auditory and Vestibular Systems.* Charles C

Thomas Publisher, Springfield, Ill., Ch. 8, pp. 105–115.

2121. RASMUSSEN, G. L. 1964. Anatomic relationships of the ascending and descending auditory systems. In W. S. FIELD AND B. R. ALFORD (Editors), *Neurological Aspects of Auditory and Vestibular Disorders.* Charles C Thomas Publisher, Springfield, Ill., Ch. 1, pp. 1–14.

2122. RAKIC, P., AND YAKOVLEV, P. I. 1968. Development of the corpus callosum and cavum septi in man. J. Comp. Neurol., **132:** 45–72.

2123. RAYMOND, J., SANS, A., AND MARTY, R. 1974. Projections thalamiques des noyaux vestibulaires etude histologique chez le chat. Exp. Brain Res., **20:** 273–283.

2124. REESE, T. S., AND KARNOVSKY, M. J. 1967. Fine structural localization of a blood-brain barrier to exogenous peroxidase. J. Cell Biol., **34:** 207–217.

2125. REESE, T. S., AND SHEPHERD, G. M. 1972. Dendrodendritic synapses in the central nervous system. In G. D. PAPPAS AND D. P. PURPURA (Editors), *Structure and Function of Synapses.* Raven Press, New York, pp. 121–136.

2126. REGER, J. F. 1955. Electron microscopy of the motor end plate in rat intercostal muscle. Anat. Rec., **122:** 1–10.

2127. REGER, J. R. 1957. The ultrastructure of normal and denervated neuromuscular synapses in mouse gastrocnemius muscle. Exp. Cell Res., **12:** 661–665.

2128. REID, J. M., GWYN, D. G., FLUMERFELT, B. A. 1975. A cytoarchitectonic and Golgi study of the red nucleus of the rat. J. Comp. Neurol., **162:** 337–362.

2129. REIS, D. J., AND OLIPHANT, M. C. 1964. Bradycardia and tachycardia following electrical stimulation of the amygdaloid region in monkey. J. Neurophysiol., **27:** 893–912.

2130. RELKIN, R. 1976. *The Pineal.* Eden Press, Montreal.

2131. RENAUD, L. P., AND HOPKINS, D. A. 1977. Amygdala afferents from the mediobasal hypothalamus: An electrophysiological and neuroanatomical study in the rat. Brain Res., **121:** 201–213.

2132. RENSHAW, B. 1940. Activity in the simplest spinal reflex pathways. J. Neurophysiol., **3:** 370–387.

2133. RENSHAW, B. 1941. Influence of discharge of motoneurons upon excitation of neighboring motoneurons. J. Neurophysiol., **4:** 167–183.

2134. RENSHAW, B. 1946. Central effects of centripetal impulses in axons of spinal ventral roots. J. Neurophysiol., **9:** 191–204.

2135. REXED, B. 1952. The cytoarchitectonic organization of the spinal cord in the cat. J. Comp. Neurol., **96:** 415–495.

2136. REXED, B. 1954. A cytoarchitectonic atlas of the spinal cord in the cat. J. Comp. Neurol., **100:** 297–379.

2137. REXED, B. 1964. Some aspects of the cytoarchitectonics and synaptology of the spinal cord. In J. C. ECCLES AND J. P. SCHADÉ (Editors), *Progress in Brain Research,* Vol. II: *Organization of the Spinal Cord.* Elsevier Publishing Company, Amsterdam, pp. 58–92.

2138. REXED, B., AND BRODAL, A. 1951. The nucleus cervicalis lateralis: A spinocerebellar relay nucleus. J. Neurophysiol., **14:** 399–407.

2139. REZAK, M., AND BENEVENTO, L. A. 1979. A comparison of the organization of the projections of the dorsal lateral geniculate nucleus, the inferior pulvinar and adjacent lateral pulvinar to primary visual cortex (area 17) in the macaque monkey. Brain Res., **167:** 19–40.

2140. RHINES, R., AND MAGOUN, H. W. 1946. Brainstem facilitation of cortical motor response. J. Neurophysiol., **9:** 219–229.

2141. RHOTON, A. L., O'LEARY, J. L., AND FERGUSON, J. P. 1966. The trigeminal, facial, vagal and glosspharyngeal nerves in the monkey. Arch. Neurol., **14:** 530–540.

2142. RIBAK, C. E., AND PETERS, A. 1975. An autoradiographic study of the projections from the lateral geniculate body of the rat. Brain Res., **92:** 341–368.

2143. RIBAK, C. E., VAUGHN, J. E., SAITO, K., BARBER, R., AND ROBERTS, E. 1977. Glutamate decarboxylase in neurons of the olfactory bulb. Brain Res., **126:** 1–18.

2144. RICARDO, J. A. 1980. Efferent connections of the subthalamic region in the rat. I. The subthalamic nucleus of Luys. Brain Res., **202:** 257-271.

2145. RICARDO, J. A., AND KOH, E. T. 1978. Anatomical evidence of direct projections from the nucleus of the solitary tract to the hypothalamus, amygdala and other forebrain structures in the rat. Brain Res., **153:** 1-26.

2146. RICHE, D., AND LANOIR, J. 1978. Some claustro-cortical connections in the cat and baboon as studied by retrograde horseradish peroxidase transport. J. Comp. Neurol., **177:** 434-444.

2147. RICHTER, C. P., AND HINES, M. 1932. Experimental production of the grasp reflex in adult monkeys by lesions of the frontal lobe. Am. J. Physiol., **101:** 87-88.

2148. RICHTER, C. P., AND WOODRUFF, B. G. 1945. Lumbar sympathetic dermatomes in man determined by the electrical skin resistance method. J. Neurophysiol., **8:** 323-338.

2149. RICHTER, E. 1965. *Die Entwicklung des Globus Pallidus und des Corpus Subthalamicum.* Springer-Verlag, Berlin.

2150. RIES, E. A., AND LANGWORTHY, O. R. 1937. A study of the surface structure of the brain of the whale (*Balaenoptera physolus* and *Physter catadon*). J. Comp. Neurol., **68:** 1-47.

2151. RILEY, C. M. 1952. Familial autonomic dysfunction. J. A. M. A., **149:** 1532-1535.

2152. RILEY, C. M. 1957. Familial dysautonomia. Adv. Pediatr., **9:** 157-190.

2153. RILEY, C. M., DAY, R. L., GREELEY, D. M., AND LANGFORD, W. S. 1949. Central autonomic dysfunction with defective lacrimation. Pediatrics, **3:** 468-481.

2154. RILEY, C. M., AND MOORE, R. H. 1966. Familial dysautonomia differentiated from related disorders. Pediatrics, **37:** 435-446.

2155. RILEY, H. A. 1943. *An Atlas of the Basal Ganglia, Brain Stem and Spinal Cord.* Williams & Wilkins, Baltimore, 708 pp.

2156. RINVIK, E. 1966. The cortico-nigral projection in the cat: An experimental study with silver impregnation methods. J. Comp. Neurol., **126:** 241-254.

2157. RINVIK, E. 1968. The corticothalamic projection from the pericruciate and coronal gyri in the cat: An experimental study with silver-impregnation methods. Brain Res., **10:** 79-119.

2158. RINVIK, E. 1975. Demonstration of nigro-thalamic connections in the cat by retrograde axonal transport of horseradish peroxidase. Brain Res., **90:** 313-318.

2159. RINVIK, E., AND GROFOVÁ, I. 1970. Observations on the fine structure of the substantia nigra in the cat. Exp. Brain Res., **11:** 229-248.

2160. RINVIK, E., AND GROFOVÁ, I. 1974. Cerebellar projections to the nuclei ventralis lateralis and ventralis anterior thalami. Anat. Embryol. (Berl.), **146:** 95-111.

2161. RINVIK, E., GROFOVÁ, I., HAMMOND, C., FÉGER, J., AND DENIAU, J. M. 1979. A study of the afferent connections of the subthalamic nucleus in the monkey and cat using the HRP technique. In L. J. PIORIER, T. L. SOURKES, AND P. J. BÉDARD (Editors), *Advances in Neurology.* Raven Press, New York, pp. 53-70.

2162. RINVIK, E., GROFOVÁ, I., AND PETTER OTTERSEN, O. 1976. Demonstration of the nigrotectal and nigroreticular projections in the cat by axonal transport of protein. Brain Res., **112:** 388-394.

2163. RINVIK, E., AND WALBERG, F. 1963. Demonstration of a somatotopically arranged cortico-rubral projection in the cat: An experimental study with silver methods. J. Comp. Neurol., **120:** 393-407.

2164. RINVIK, E., AND WALBERG, F. 1969. Is there a cortico-nigral tract? A comment based on experimental electron microscopic observations in the cat. Brain Res., **14:** 742-744.

2165. RINVIK, E., AND WALBERG, F. 1975. Studies on the cerebellar projections from the main and external cuneate nuclei in the cat by means of retrograde axonal transport of horseradish peroxidase. Brain Res., **95:** 371-381.

2166. DEL RIO-HORTEGA, P. 1919. El "tercer elemento" de los centros nerviosus. Bol. Soc. Espan. Biol., **9:** 69-120.

2167. DEL RIO-HORTEGA, P. 1921. El Tercer elemento de los centros nerviosus. Histogenesis y evolucion normal; exoda y distribucion regional de microglia. Mem. R. Soc. Espan. Hist. Nat., **11:** 213-268.

2168. DEL RIO-HORTEGA, P. 1921*a*. Estudios sobre la neuroglia. La glía de escasas radiaciones (oligodendroglia). Bol. R. Soc. Espan. Hist. Nat., **21:** 63-92.

2169. DEL RIO-HORTEGA, P. 1932. Microglia. In W. G. PENFIELD (Editor), *Cytology and Cellular Pathology of the Nervous System,* Vol. II. Paul B. Hoeber, Inc., New York, pp. 483-534.

2170. RISPAL-PADEL, L., MASSION, J., AND GRANGETTO, A. 1973. Relations between the ventrolateral thalamic nucleus and motor cortex and their possible role in the central organization of motor control. Brain Res., **60:** 1-20.

2171. RIVERA-DOMINGUEZ, M., AGATE, F. J., JR., AND NOBACK, C. R. 1973. Scanning electron microscopy of the spiral organ of Corti of the adult rhesus monkey. Brain Res., **65:** 159-164.

2172. DE ROBERTIS, E. D. P. 1965. Some new electron microscopical contributions to the biology of neuroglia. In E. D. P. DE ROBERTIS AND R. CARREA (Editors), *Progress in Brain Reserach,* Vol. 15: *Biology of Neuroglia.* Elsevier Publishing Company, Amsterdam, pp. 1-11.

2173. DE ROBERTIS, E. 1959. Submicroscopic morphology of the synapse. Int. Rev. Cytol., **8:** 61-96.

2174. DE ROBERTIS, E. 1966. Synaptic complexes and synaptic vesicles as structural and biochemical units of the central nervous system. In K. RODAHL AND B. ISSEKUTZ, JR. (Editors), *Nerve as a Tissue.* Hoeber Med. Div., Harper & Row, New York, pp. 88-115.

2175. DE ROBERTIS, E. 1967. Ultrastructure and cytochemistry of the synaptic region. Science, **156:** 907-914.

2176. DE ROBERTIS, E., AND BENNETT, H. S. 1954. Submicroscopic vesicular component in the synapse. Fed. Proc., **13:** 35.

2177. DE ROBERTIS, E., DE IRALDI, A. P., DE LORES, R., ARNAIZ, G., AND SALGANICOFF, L. 1962. Cholinergic and non-cholinergic nerve endings in rat brain. I. Isolation and subcellular distribution of acetylcholine and acetylcholinesterase. J. Neurochem., **9:** 23-35.

2178. ROBERTS, T. S., AND AKERT, K. 1963. Insular and opercular cortex and its thalamic projection in *Macaca mulatta.* Schweiz. Arch. Neurol. Neurochir. Psychiatr., **92:** 1-43.

2179. ROBERTSON, A., AND GINGLE, A. R. 1977. Axial bending in the early chick embryo by a cyclic adenosine monophosphate source. Science, **197:** 1078-1079.

2180. ROBERTSON, D. M., AND VOGEL, F. S. 1962. Concentric lamination of glial processes in oligodendrogliomas. J. Cell Biol., **15:** 313-334.

2181. ROBERTSON, J. D. 1955. Ultrastructure of adult vertebrate peripheral myelinated nerve fibers in relation to myelinogenesis. J. Biophys. Biochem. Cytol., **1:** 271-278.

2182. ROBERTSON, J. D. 1956. The ultrastructure of a reptilian myoneural junction. J. Biophys. Biochem. Cytol., **2:** 381-394.

2183. ROBERTSON, J. D. 1958. The ultrastructure of Schmidt-Lantermann clefts and related shearing defects of the myelin sheath. J. Biophys. Biochem. Cytol., **4:** 39-46.

2184. ROBERTSON, J. D. 1959. Preliminary observations on the ultrastructure of nodes of Ranvier. Z. Zellforsch. Mikrosk. Anat., **50:** 553-560.

2185. ROBERTSON, J. D. 1960. Electron microscopy of the motor end-plate and the neuromuscular spindle. Am. J. Phys. Med., **39:** 1-43.

2186. ROBERTSON, R. T., AND RINVIK, E. 1973. The corticothalamic projections from parietal regions of the cerebral cortex: Experimental degeneration studies in the cat. Brain Res., **51:** 61-79.

2187. ROBERTSON, R. T., AND TRAVERS, J. T. 1975. Brain stem projections to the striatum: Experimental morphological studies in the rat. Exp. Neurol., **48:** 447–459.

2188. ROBINSON, B. W., AND MISHKIN, M. 1962. Alimentary responses evoked from forebrain structures in *Macaca mulatta*. Science, **136:** 260–261.

2189. ROBINSON, B. W., AND MISHKIN, M. 1968. Alimentary responses to forebrain stimulation in monkeys. Exp. Brain Res., **4:** 330–366.

2190. ROBINSON, C. J., AND BURTON, H. 1980. Somatotopographic organization in the second somatosensory area of *M. fascicularis*. J. Comp. Neurol., **192:** 43–67.

2191. ROBINSON, C. J., AND BURTON, H. 1980a. The organization of somatosensory receptive fields in cortical area 7b, retroinsular, postauditory and granular insular of *M. fascicularis*. J. Comp. Neurol., **192:** 69–92.

2192. ROBINSON, C. J., AND BURTON, H. 1980b. Somatic submodality distribution within the second somatosensory (S II), 7b, retroinsular, postauditory and granular insular cortical areas of *M. fascicularis*. J. Comp. Neurol., **192:** 93–108.

2193. ROBINSON, D. A. 1972. Eye movements evoked by collicular stimulation in the alert monkey. Vision Res., **12:** 1795–1808.

2194. ROCKEL, A. J., AND JONES, E. G. 1973. The neuronal organization of the inferior colliculus of the adult cat. I. The central nucleus. J. Comp. Neurol., **147:** 11–60.

2195. ROCKEL, A. J., AND JONES, E. G. 1973a. The neuronal organization of the inferior colliculus of the adult cat. II. The pericentral nucleus. J. Comp. Neurol., **149:** 301–334.

2196. RODIECK, R. W. 1979. Visual pathways. Annu. Rev. Neurosci., **2:** 193–225.

2197. ROEDER, F., AND ORTHNER, H. 1956. Erfahrungen mit stereotaktischen Eingriffen. I. Mitteilung: Zur Pathogenese und Therapie extrapyramidal-motorischer Bewegungsstörungen. Erfolgreiche Behandlung eines Falles schweren Hemiballismus mit gezielter Electrokoagulation des Globus pallidus. Dtsch. Z. Nervenh., **175:** 419–434.

2198. ROGER, A., ROSSI, G. F., AND ZIRONDOLI, A. 1956. Le rôle des nerfs craniens dans le maintein de l'état vigile de la preparation "encéphale isolé." Electroencephalogr. Clin. Neurophysiol., **8:** 1–13.

2199. ROGERS, D. C., AND BURNSTOCK, G. 1966. Multiaxonal autonomic junctions in smooth muscle of the toad (*Bufo marinus*). J. Comp. Neurol., **126:** 625–652.

2200. ROGERS, F. T. 1922. Studies of the brain stem. VI. An experimental study of the corpus striatum of the pigeon as related to various instinctive types of behavior. J. Comp. Neurol., **35:** 21–59.

2201. ROMANES, G. J. 1951. The motor cell columns of the lumbosacral spinal cord of the cat. J. Comp. Neurol., **94:** 313–363.

2202. ROMANSKY, K. V., USUNOFF, K. G., IVANOV, D. P., AND GALABOV, G. P. 1979. Corticosubthalamic projection in the cat: An electron microscopic study. Brain Res., **163:** 319–322.

2203. ROPPER, A. H., FISHER, C. M., AND KLEINMAN, G. M. 1979. Pyramidal infarction in the medulla: A cause of pure motor hemiplegia sparing the face. Neurology (Minneap.), **29:** 91–95.

2204. ROOT, W. S. 1969. Physiology of micturition: A specific autonomic function. In V. B. MOUNTCASTLE (Editor), *Medical Physiology*, Ed. 12. C. V. Mosby Company, St. Louis, Ch. 79, pp. 1831–1838.

2205. ROSE, J. 1975. Response properties and anatomical organization of pontine and medullary units responsive to vaginal stimulation in the cat. Brain Res., **97:** 79–93.

2206. ROSE, J., AND SUTIN, J. 1973. Responses of single units in the medulla to genital stimulation in estrous and anestrous cats. Brain Res., **50:** 87–99.

2207. ROSE, J. E. 1952. The cortical connections of the reticular complex of the thalamus. Proc. Assoc. Res. Nerv. Ment. Dis., **30:** 454–479.

2208. ROSE, J. E. 1960. Organization of frequency sensitive neurons in the cochlear complex of the cat. In G. L. RASMUSSEN AND W. R. WINDLE (Editors), *Neural Mechanisms of the Auditory and Vestibular Systems*.

Charles C Thomas Publisher, Springfield, Ill., Ch. 9, pp. 116–136.

2209. ROSE, J. E., GALAMBOS, R., AND HUGHES, J. R. 1959. Microelectrode studies of the cochlear nuclei of the cat. Bull. Johns Hopkins Hosp., **104:** 211–251.

2210. ROSE, J. E., GALAMBOS, R., AND HUGHES, J. R. 1960. Organization of frequency sensitive neurons in the cochlear complex of the cat. In G. RASMUSSEN AND W. WINDLE (Editors), *Mechanisms of the Auditory and Vestibular Systems*. Charles C Thomas Publisher, Springfield, Ill., pp. 116–136.

2211. ROSE, J. E., GREENWOOD, D. B., GOLDBERG, J. M., AND HIND, J. E. 1963. Some discharge characteristics of single neurons in the inferior colliculus of the cat. I. Tonotopical organization, relation of spike-counts to tone intensity, and firing patterns of single elements. J. Neurophysiol., **26:** 293–320.

2212. ROSE, J. E., GROSS, N. B., GEISLER, C. D., AND HIND, J. E. 1966. Some neural mechanisms in the inferior colliculus of the cat which may be relevant to localization of a sound source. J. Neurophysiol., **29:** 288–314.

2213. ROSE, J. E., AND MALIS, L. I. 1965. Geniculostriate connections in the rabbit. II. Cytoarchitectonic structure of the striate region and of the dorsal lateral geniculate body: Organization of the geniculo-striate projections. J. Comp. Neurol., **125:** 121–140.

2214. ROSE, J. E., AND MOUNTCASTLE, V. B. 1952. The thalamic tactile region in rabbit and cat. J. Comp. Neurol., **97:** 441–490.

2215. ROSE, J. E., AND MOUNTCASTLE, V. B. 1959. Touch and kinesthesis. In J. FIELDS (Editor), *Handbook of Physiology*, Section I, Vol. I: *Neurophysiology*. American Physiological Society, Washington, D. C., Ch. 17, pp. 387–429.

2216. ROSE, J. E., AND WOOLSEY, C. N. 1943. A study of thalamocortical relations in the rabbit. Bull. Johns Hopkins Hosp., **72:** 65–128.

2217. ROSE, J. E., AND WOOLSEY, C. N. 1943a. Potential changes in the olfactory brain produced by electrical stimulation of the olfactory bulb. Fed. Proc., **2:** 42.

2218. ROSE, J. E., AND WOOLSEY, C. N. 1958. Cortical connections and functional organization of the thalamic auditory system of the cat. In H. F. HARLOW AND C. N. WOOLSEY (Editors), *Biological and Biochemical Bases of Behavior*. University of Wisconsin Press, Madison, pp. 127–150.

2219. ROSE, M. 1935. Cytoarchitektonik und Myeloarchitektonik der Grosshirnrinde. In O. BUMKE AND O. FOERSTER (Editors), *Handbuch der Neurologie*, Vol. 1. Springer-Verlag, Berlin, pp. 588–778.

2220. ROSEGAY, H. 1944. An experimental investigation of the connections between the corpus striatum and the substantia nigra in the cat. J. Comp. Neurol., **80:** 293–310.

2221. ROSÉN, I., AND ASANUMA, H. 1972. Peripheral afferent inputs to the forelimb area of the monkey motor cortex: input-output relations. Exp. Brain Res., **14:** 257–273.

2222. ROSÉN, I., AND SCHEID, P. 1973. Patterns of afferent input to the lateral reticular nucleus of the cat. Exp. Brain Res., **18:** 242–255.

2223. ROSENE, D. L., AND VAN HOESEN, G. W. 1977. Hippocampal efferents reach widespread areas of cerebral cortex and amygdala in the rhesus monkey. Science, **198:** 315–317.

2224. ROSENQUIST, A. C., EDWARDS, S. B., AND PALMER, L. A. 1974. An autoradiographic study of the projections of the dorsal lateral geniculate nucleus and the posterior nucleus in the cat. Brain Res., **80:** 71–93.

2225. ROSENZWEIG, M. R. 1954. Cortical correlates of auditory localization and of related perceptual phenomena. J. Comp. Physiol. Psychol., **47:** 269–276.

2226. ROSS, L. L., BORNSTEIN, M. B., AND LEHRER, G. 1962. Electron microscope observations of rat and mouse cerebellum in tissue culture. J. Cell Biol., **14:** 19–30.

2227. ROSSI, G. F., AND BRODAL, A. 1956. Corticofugal fibers to the brain stem reticular formation: An experimental study in the cat. J. Anat., **90:** 42–62.

2228. ROSSI, G. F., AND BRODAL, A. 1956*a*. Spinal afferents to the trigeminal sensory nuclei and the nucleus of the solitary tract. Confin. Neurol., **16:** 321–332.

2229. ROSSI, G. F., AND BRODAL, A. 1957. Terminal distribution of spinoreticular fibers in the cat. A. M. A. Arch. Neurol. Psychiatry, **78:** 439–453.

2230. ROSSI, G. F., AND ZANCHETTI, A. 1957. The brain stem reticular formation: Anatomy and physiology. Arch. Ital. Biol., **95:** 199–435.

2231. ROSSI, G. F., AND ZIRONDOLI, A. 1955. On the mechanism of the cortical desynchronization elicited by volatile anesthetics. Electroencephalogr. Clin. Neurophysiol., **7:** 383–390.

2232. ROTH, G. L., AITKIN, L. M., ANDERSON, R. A., AND MERZENICH, M. M. 1978. Some features of the spatial organization of the central nucleus of the inferior colliculus of the cat. J. Comp. Neurol., **182:** 661–680.

2233. ROUDOMIN, P., MALLIANI, A., BARLONE, M., AND ZANCHETTI, A. 1965. Distributuion of electrical responses to somatic stimuli in the diencephalon of the cat, with special reference to the hypothalamus. Arch. Ital. Biol., **103:** 60–89.

2234. RUBINSTEIN, L. J., KLATZO, I., AND MIQUEL, J. 1962. Histochemical observations on oxidative enzyme activity of glial cells in a local brain injury. J. Neuropathol. Exp. Neurol., **21:** 116–136.

2235. RUFFINI, A. 1894. Sur un nouvel Organe nerveux terminal et sur la présence des corpuscles Golgi-Mazzoni dans le conjunctif sous-cutane de la pulpe des doigts de l'homme. Arch. Ital. Biol., **21:** 249–265.

2236. RUGGIERO, D., BATTON, R. R., III., JAYARAMAN, A., AND CARPENTER, M. B. 1977. Brainstem afferents to the fastigial nucleus in the cat demonstrated by transport of horseradish peroxidase. J. Comp. Neurol., **172:** 189–210.

2237. RUNDLES, R. W., AND PAPEZ, J. W. 1937. Connections between the striatum and the substantia nigra in a human brain. Arch. Neurol. Psychiatry, **38:** 550–563.

2238. RUSSELL, G. V. 1954. The dorsal trigemino-thalamic tract in the cat: Reconsidered as a lateral reticulo-thalamic system of connections. J. Comp. Neurol., **101:** 237–264.

2239. RUSSELL, G. V. 1955. The nucleus locus coeruleus (dorsolateralis tegmenti). Tex. Rep. Biol. Med., **13:** 939–988.

2240. RUSSELL, G. V. 1955*a*. A schematic presentation of thalamic morphology and connections. Tex. Rep. Biol. Med., **13:** 989–992.

2241. RUSSELL, J. R., AND DEMYER, W. 1961. The quantitative cortical origin of pyramidal axons of *Macaca rhesus*. Neurology (Minneap.), **11:** 96–108.

2242. RUSSELL, W. R. 1948. Functions of the frontal lobes. Lancet, **254:** 356–360.

2243. RYLANDER, G. 1948. Personality analysis before and after frontal lobotomy. Proc. Assoc. Nerv. Ment. Dis., **27:** 691–705.

2244. SACHS, E. JR., BRENDLER, S. J., AND FULTON, J. F. 1949. The orbital gyri. Brain, **72:** 227–240.

2245. SADUN, A. A., AND PAPPAS, G. D. 1978. Development of distinct cell types in the feline red nucleus: A Golgi-Cox and electron microscopic study. J. Comp. Neurol., **182:** 315–366.

2246. SAHAR, A. 1972. Choroidal origin of cerebrospinal fluid. Isr. J. Med. Sci., **8:** 594–596.

2247. SAIGAL, R. P., KARAMANLIDIS, A. N., VOOGD, J., MICHALOUD, H., AND MANGANA, O. 1980. Cerebellar afferents from motor nuclei of cranial nerves, the nucleus of the solitary tract and nuclei coeruleus and parabrachialis in sheep, demonstrated with retrograde transport of horseradish peroxidase. Brain Res., **197:** 200–206.

2248. SAINT-CYR, J. A., AND COURVILLE, J. 1979. Projection from the vestibular nuclei to the inferior olive in the cat: An autoradiographic and horseradish peroxidase study. Brain Res. **165:** 189–201.

2249. SAINT-CYR, J. A., AND COURVILLE, J. 1981. Sources of descending afferents to the inferior olive from the upper brain stem in the cat as revealed by the retrograde transport of horseradish peroxidase. J. Comp. Neurol., **198:** 567–581.

2250. SALAFSKY, B., AND JASINSKI, D. 1967. Early electrophysiological changes after denervation of fast skeletal muscle. Exp. Neurol., **19:** 375–387.

2251. SALAMON, G., AND LAZORTHES, G. 1971. *Atlas of the Arteries of the Human Brain.* Sandoz, Paris.

2252. SANIDES, D. 1975. The retinal projection to the ventral lateral geniculate nucleus of the cat. Brain Res., **85:** 313–316.

2253. VON SANTHA, K. 1928. Zur Klinik und Anatomie des Hemiballismus. Arch Psychiatr. Nervenkr., **84:** 664–678.

2254. VON SANTHA, K. 1932. Hemiballismus und Corpus Luysi: (Anatomische und pathophysiologische Beiträge zur Frage des Hemiballismus nebst Versuch einer somatotopischen Lokalisation im Corpus Luysi.) Z. Gesamte. Neurol. Psychiatr., **141:** 321–342.

2255. SAPER, C. B., LOEWY, A. D., SWANSON, L. W., AND COWAN, W. M. 1976. Direct hypothalamo-autonomic connections. Brain Res., **117:** 305–312.

2256. SASA, M., AND TAKAORI, S. 1973. Influence of the locus coeruleus on transmission in the spinal trigeminal nucleus neurons. Brain Res., **55:** 203–208.

2257. SASAKI, K., NAMIKAWA, A., AND HASHIRAMOTO, S., 1960. The effect of midbrain stimulation upon alpha motoneurons in lumbar spinal cord. Nippon Seirugaku Zassi, **3:** 303–316.

2258. SASAKI, K., TANAKA, T., AND MORI, K. 1962. Effects of stimulation of pontine and bulbar reticular formation upon spinal motoneurons of the cat. Jpn. J. Physiol., **12:** 45–62.

2259. SATO, O., AND BERING, E. A. 1967. Extra-ventricular formation of cerebrospinal fluid. Brain Nerve (Tokyo), **19:** 883–885.

2260. SATOMI, H., YAMAMOTO, T., ISE, H., AND TAKATAMA, H. 1978. Origins of the parasympathetic preganglionic fibers to the cat intestine, as demonstrated by the horseradish peroxidase method. Brain Res., **151:** 571–578.

2261. SAWYER, C. H. 1959. Nervous control of ovulation. In C. W. LLOYD (Editor), *Endocrinology of Reproduction.* Academic Press, New York, pp. 1–18.

2262. SAWYER, C. H. 1969. Regulatory mechanisms of secretion of gonadotrophic hormones. In W. HAYMAKER *et al.* (Editors), *The Hypothalamus.* Charles C Thomas Publisher, Springfield, Ill., Ch. 11, pp.. 389–430.

2263. SCALIA, F. 1972. The termination of retinal axons in the pretectal region of mammals. J. Comp. Neurol., **145:** 223–257.

2264. SCALIA, F., AND WINANS, S. S. 1975. The differential projections of the olfactory bulb and accessory olfactory bulb in mammals. J. Comp. Neurol., **161:** 31–56.

2265. SCARFF, J. E. 1940. Primary cortical centers for movement of upper and lower limbs in man. Arch. Neurol. Psychiatry, **44:** 243–299.

2266. SCARFF, J. E. 1949. Unilateral prefrontal lobotomy for relief of intractable pain and termination of narcotic addiction. Surg. Gynecol. Obstet., **89:** 385–392.

2267. SCHALLY, A. V., KASTIN, A. J., AND ARIMURA, A. 1977. Hypothalamic hormones: The link between brain and body. Am. Sci., **65:** 712–719.

2268. SCHALTENBRAND, G. 1955. Plexus and Meningen. Saccus vasculosus. In W. VON MÖLLENDORFF (Editor), *Handbuch der mikroskopisch. Anatomie des Menschen,* Vol. IV, part 2. Springer-Verlag, Berlin, pp. 94–98.

2269. SCHARRER, B. 1965. Recent progress in the study of neuroendocrine mechanisms in insects. Arch. Anat. Microscop. Morphol. Exp., **54:** 331–342.

2270. SCHARRER, E. 1944. The blood vessels of the nervous tissue. Q. Rev. Biol., **19:** 308–318.

2271. SCHARRER, E., AND SCHARRER, B. 1940. Secretory cells within the hypothalamus. Proc. Assoc. Res. Nerv. Ment. Dis., **20:** 170–194.

2272. SCHARRER, E., AND SCHARRER, B. 1945. Neurosecretion. Physiol. Rev., **25:** 171–181.

2273. SCHEIBEL, M. E., AND SCHEIBEL, A. B. 1954. Observations on the intracortical relations of the climbing fibers of the cerebellum: A Golgi study. J. Comp. Neurol., 101: 733–764.

2274. SCHEIBEL, M. E., AND SCHEIBEL, A. B. 1958. Structural substrates for integrative patterns in the brain stem reticular core. In H. H. JASPER et al. (Editors), Reticular Formation of the Brain. Little Brown & Company, Boston, Ch. 2, pp. 31–55.

2275. SCHEIBEL, M. E., AND SCHEIBEL, A. B. 1958a. Neurons and neuroglial cells as seen with the light microscope. In W. F. WINDLE (Editor), Biology of Neuroglia. Charles C Thomas Publisher, Springfield, Ill., pp. 5–23.

2276. SCHEIBEL, M. E., AND SCHEIBEL, A. B. 1966. The organization of the nucleus reticularis thalami: A Golgi study. Brain Res., 1: 43–62.

2277. SCHEIBEL, M. E., AND SCHEIBEL, A. B. 1966 a. The organization of the ventral anterior nucleus of the thalamus: A Golgi study. Brain Res., 1: 250–268.

2278. SCHEIBEL, M. E., AND SCHEIBEL, A. B. 1966b. Spinal motoneurons, interneurons and Renshaw cells. Arch. Ital. Biol., 104: 328–353.

2279. SCHEIBEL, M. E., AND SCHEIBEL, A. B. 1967. Structural organization of nonspecific thalamic nuclei and their projection toward cortex. Brain Res., 6: 60–94.

2280. SCHILLER, P. H., AND STRYKER, M. 1972. Single-unit recording and stimulation in superior colliculus of the alert rhesus monkey. J. Neurophysiol., 35: 915–924.

2281. SCHLAG, J., AND WASZAK, M. 1970. Characteristics of unit responses in nucleus reticularis thalami. Brain Res., 21: 286–288.

2282. SCHLESINGER, B. 1939. Venous drainage of the brain, with special reference to Galenic system. Brain, 62: 274–291.

2283. SCHMIDT, C. F. 1960. Central nervous system circulation, fluids and barriers—introduction. In J. FIELD (Editor), Handbook of Physiology, Section I, Vol. III: Neurophysiology. American Physiological Society, Washington, D. C., Ch. 70, pp. 1745–1760.

2284. SCHMITT, F. O., BEAR, R. S. AND PALMER, K. J. 1941. X-ray diffraction studies on the structure of the nerve myelin sheath. J. Cell. Comp. Physiol., 18: 31–42.

2285. SCHNITZLEIN, H. N., HOFFMAN, H. H., HAMLETT, D. M., AND HOWELL, E. M. 1963. A study of the sacral parasympathetic nucleus. J. Comp. Neurol., 120: 477–493.

2286. SCHOULTZ, T. W., AND SWETT, J. E. 1972. The fine structure of the Golgi tendon organ. J. Neurocytol., 1: 1–26.

2287. SCHREINER, L. H., AND KLING, A. 1954. Effects of castration on hypersexual behavior induced by rhinencephalic injury in cat. A. M. A. Arch. Neurol. Psychiatry, 72: 180–186.

2288. SCHRÖDER, K. F., HOPF, A., LANGE, H., AND THÖRNER, G. 1975. Morphometrisch-statische Strukturanalysen des Striatum, Pallidum und Nucleus subthalamicus beim Menschen. J. Hirnforsch., 16: 333–350.

2289. SCHULTZ, R. L., MAYNARD, E. A., AND PEASE, D. C. 1957. Electron microscopy of neurons and neuroglia of cerebral cortex and corpus callosum. Am. J. Anat., 100: 369–407.

2290. SCHULTZ, R. L., AND PEASE, D. C. 1959. Cicatrix formation in rat cerebral cortex as revealed by electron microscopy. Am. J. Pathol., 35: 1017–1041.

2291. SCHÜTZ, H. 1891. Anatomische Untersuchungen über den Faserverlauf im zentralen Höhlengrau und den Nervenfaserschwund in demselben bei der progressiven Paralyse der Irren. Arch. Psychiatr. Nervenkr., 22: 527–587.

2292. SCHWARCZ, R., AND COYLE, J. T. 1977. Striatal lesions with kainic acid: Neurochemical characteristics. Brain Res., 127: 235–249.

2293. SCHWARTZ, J. H. 1979. Axonal transport: Components, mechanisms and specificity. Annu. Rev. Neurosci., 2: 467–504.

2294. SCHWARTZ, P., AND FINK, L. 1926. Morphologie und Entstehung der geburtstraumatischen Blutungen im Gehirn und Schädel des Neugeborenen. Z. Kinder heilk., 40: 427–474.

2295. SCHWARTZMAN, R. J. 1978. A behavioral analysis of complete unilateral section of the pyramidal tract at the medullary level in Macaca mulatta. Ann. Neurol., 4: 234–244.

2296. SCHWARZ, D. W. F., AND FREDRICKSON, J. M. 1971. Rhesus monkey vestibular cortex: A bimodal primary projection field. Science, 171: 280–281.

2297. SCHWYN, R. C. 1967. An autoradiographic study of satellite cells in autonomic ganglia. Am. J. Anat., 121: 727–740.

2298. SCHWYN, R. C., AND FOX, C. A. 1974. The primate substantia nigra: A Golgi and electron microscopic study. J. Hirnforsch., 15: 95–126.

2299. SCOLLO-LAVIZZARI, G., AND AKERT, K. 1963. Cortical area 8 and its thalamic projection in Macaca mulatta. J. Comp. Neurol., 121: 259–267.

2300. SCOTT, D., JR., 1963. Influence of nerve growth factor on spinal regeneration in kittens. Anat. Rec., 145: 283.

2301. SCOTT, D. JR., AND CLEMENTE, C. D. 1952. Mechanism of spinal cord regeneration in the cat. Fed. Proc., 11: 143–144.

2302. SCOTT, D. E., AND KROBISCH-DUDLEY, G. 1975. Ultrastructural analysis of the mammalian median eminence. In K. M. KNIGGE, D. E. SCOTT, H. KOBAYASHI, AND S. ISHII (Editors), Brain-Endocrine Interaction II. S. Karger, Basel, pp. 29–39.

2303. SCOTT, J. W., MCBRIDE, R. L., AND SCHNEIDER, S. P. 1980. The organization of projections from the olfactory bulb to the piriform cortex and olfactory tubercle in the rat. J. Comp. Neurol., 194: 519–534.

2304. SCOVILLE, W. B. 1954. Neurophysiological symposium: Limbic lobe in man. J. Neurosurg., 11: 64–66.

2305. SCOVILLE, W. B., AND MILNER, B. 1957. Loss of recent memory after bilateral hippocampal lesions. J. Neurol., Neurosurg. Psychiatry, 20: 11–21.

2306. SEDDON, H. J. 1943. Three types of nerve injury. Brain, 66: 237–288.

2307. SELZER, M. E., MYERS, R. E., AND HOLSTEIN, S.B. 1972. Maturational changes in brain water and electrolytes in rhesus monkey with some implications for electrogenesis. Brain Res., 45: 193–204.

2308. SHANER, R. F. 1932. Development of nuclei and tracts of mid-brain. J. Comp. Neurol., 55: 493–512.

2309. SHANER, R. F. 1936. Development of the finer structure and fiber connections of the globus pallidus, corpus of Luys and substantia nigra in the pig. J. Comp. Neurol., 64: 213–233.

2310. SHANTHAVEERAPPA, T. R., AND BOURNE, G. H. 1964. Arachnoid villi in the optic nerve of man and the monkey. Exp. Eye Res., 3: 31–35.

2311. SHANZER, S., WAGMAN, I. H., AND BENDER, M. B. 1959. Further observations on the median longitudinal fasciculus. Trans. Am. Neurol. Assoc., 84: 14–17.

2312. SHEALY, C. N., AND PEELE, T. L. 1957. Studies on amygdaloid nucleus of cat. J. Neurophysiol., 20: 125–139.

2313. SHEARD, M. H. 1969. The effect of PCPA in behavior in rats: Relation to brain serotonin and 5-hydroxyindoleacetic acid. Brain Res., 15: 524–528.

2314. SHEARD, M. H., AND FLYNN, J. P. 1967. Facilitation of attack behavior by stimulation of the midbrain of cats. Brain Res., 4: 324–333.

2315. SHEEHAN, D. 1936. Discovery of the autonomic nervous system. Arch. Neurol. Psychiatry, 35: 1081–1115.

2316. SHEEHAN, D. 1941. Spinal autonomic outflows in man and monkey. J. Comp. Neurol., 75: 341–370.

2317. SHEEHAN, D. 1941 a. The autonomic nervous system. Annu. Rev. Physiol., 3: 399–448.

2318. SHEPS, J. G. 1945. The nuclear configuration and

cortical connections of the human thalamus. J. Comp. Neurol., **83:** 1–56.

2319. SHERIDAN, M. N., AND SLADEK, J. R. JR. 1975. Histofluorescence and ultrastructural analysis of hamster and monkey pineal. Cell Tissue Res., **164:** 145–152.

2320. SHERK, H. 1978. Visual response properties and visual field topography in the cats parabigeminal nucleus. Brain Res., **145:** 375–379.

2321. SHERK, H., AND LEVAY, S. 1981. Visual claustrum: topography and receptive field properties in the cat. Science, **212:** 87–89.

2322. SHERRINGTON, C. S. 1893. Experiments in examination of the peripheral distribution of the fibers of the posterior roots of some spinal nerves. Philos. Trans. R. Soc. Lond. (Biol.), **184:** 641–763.

2323. SHERRINGTON, C. S. 1893 a. Note on the spinal portion of some ascending degenerations. J. Physiol. (Lond.), **14:** 255–302.

2324. SHERRINGTON, C. S. 1898. Decerebrate rigidity, and reflex co-ordination of movements. J. Physiol. (Lond.), **22:** 319–332.

2325. SHERRINGTON, C. S. 1906. *The Integrative Action of the Nervous System.* Charles Scribner's Sons, New York. (Reprinted, Yale University Press, New Haven, 1947.)

2326. SHILANSKI, M. 1974. Methods for the neurochemical study of microtubules. In N. MARKS AND R. RODNIGHT (Editors), *Research Methods in Neurochemistry*, Vol. 2. Plenum Press, New York, p. 281.

2327. SHIMAZU, H., AND PRECHT, W. 1966. Inhibition of central vestibular neurons from the contralateral labyrinth and its mediating pathway. J. Neurophysiol., **29:** 467–492.

2328. SHINODA, Y., ZARZECKI, P., AND ASANUMA, H. 1979. Spinal branching of pyramidal tract neurons in the monkey. Exp. Brain Res., **34:** 59–72.

2329. SHOLL, D. A. 1956. *The Organization of the Cerebral Cortex.* John Wiley & Sons, Inc., New York.

2330. SHOULSON, I., AND CHASE, T. N. 1975. Huntington's disease. Annu. Rev. Med., **26:** 419–426.

2331. SHOULSON, I., KARTZINEL, R., AND CHASE, T. N. 1976. Huntington's disease: Treatment with dipropylacetic acid and gamma-aminobutyric acid. Neurology (Minneap.), **26:** 61–63.

2332. SHOWERS, M. J. C. 1958. Correlation of medial thalamic nuclear activity with cortical and subcortical neuronal arc. J. Comp. Neurol., **109:** 261–315.

2333. SHRIVER, J. E., STEIN, B. M., AND CARPENTER, M. B. 1968. Central projections of spinal dorsal roots in the monkey. I. Cervical and upper thoracic dorsal roots. Am. J. Anat., **123:** 27–74.

2334. SHUANGSHOTI, S., AND NETSKY, M. G. 1966. Histogenesis of choroid plexus in man. Am. J. Anat., **118:** 283–316.

2335. SHUANGSHOTI, S., AND NETSKY, M. G. 1970. Human choroid plexus: Morphologic and histochemical alterations with age. Am. J. Anat., **128:** 73–96.

2336. SHUTE, C. C. D., AND LEWIS, P. R. 1963. Cholinesterase-containing systems of the brain of the rat. Nature, **199:** 1160–1163.

2337. SIDMAN, R. L. 1970. Cell proliferation, migration and interaction in the developing mammalian central nervous system. In F. O. SCHMITT (Editor), *The Neurosciences.* Second Study Program. Rockefeller University Press, New York, pp. 100–116.

2338. SIEGEL, A., EDINGER, H., AND LOWENTHAL, H. 1974. Effects of electrical stimulation on the medial aspect of the prefrontal cortex upon attack behavior in cats. Brain Res. **66:** 467–479.

2339. SIEGEL, A., EDINGER, H., AND TROIANO, R. 1973. The pathways from the mediodorsal nucleus of the thalamus to the hypothalamus in the cat. Exp. Neurol. **38:** 202–217.

2340. SIGGINS, G. R., HOFFER, B. J., BLOOM, F. E., AND UNGERSTEDT, U. 1976. Cytochemical and electrophysiological studies of dopamine in the caudate nu-

cleus. In M. D. YAHR (Editor), *The Basal Ganglia.* Proc. Assoc. Res. Nerv. Ment. Dis., **55:** 227–247.

2341. SIMANTOV, R., KUHAR, M. J., PASTERNAK, G. W., AND SNYDER, S. H. 1976. The regional distribution of a morphine-like factor enkephalin in monkey brain. Brain Res., **106:** 189–197.

2342. SIMPSON, D. A. 1952. The projection of the pulvinar to the temporal lobe. J. Anat., **86:** 20–28.

2343. SINCLAIR, D. C. 1967. *Cutaneous Sensation.* Oxford University Press, New York, pp. 35–80.

2344. SINCLAIR, D. C., WEDDELL, G., AND FEINDEL W. H. 1948. Referred pain and associated phenomena. Brain, **71:** 184–211.

2345. SIQUEIRA, E. B. 1971. The cortical connections of the nucleus pulvinaris of the dorsal thalamus in the rhesus monkey. J. Hirnforsch. **10:** 487–498.

2346. SJÖQVIST, O. 1938. Studies on pain conduction in the trigeminal nerve: A contribution to surgical treatment of facial pain. Acta Psychiat. Neurol., Scand, **17:** (suppl.) 1–139.

2347. SJÖSTRAND, F. S. 1963. The structure and formation of the myelin sheath. In A. S. ROSE AND C. M. PEARSON (Editors), *Mechanisms of Demyelination.* McGraw-Hill, Book Company, New York, pp. 1–43.

2348. SJÖSTRAND, J. 1966. Morphological changes in glial cells during nerve regeneration. Acta. Physiol. Scand. (Suppl.), **270:** 19–43.

2349. SKEEN, L. C., AND HALL, W. C. 1977. Efferent projections of the main and the accessory olfactory bulb in the tree shrew (*Tupaia glis*). J. Comp. Neurol., **172:** 1–36.

2350. SKINNER, J. E., AND LINDSLEY, D. B. 1967. Electrophysiological and behavioral effects of blockage on the nonspecific thalamocortical system. Brain Res., **6:** 95–117.

2351. SLADEK, J. R., JR., AND BOWMAN, J. P. 1975. The distribution of catecholamines within the inferior olivary complex of the cat and rhesus monkey. J. Comp. Neurol., **163:** 203–214.

2352. SLOAN, N., AND JASPER, H. 1950. The identity of spreading depression and "suppression." Electroencephalogr. Clin. Neurophysiol., **2:** 59–78.

2353. SLOPER, J. C. 1966. Hypothalamic neurosecretion: The validity of the concept of neurosecretion and its physiological and pathological implications. Br. Med. Bull., **22:** 209–215.

2354. SMIRNOW, A. 1895. Über die sensiblen Nervenendigungen im Herzen bei Amphibien und Saügetieren. Anat. Anz., **10:** 737–749.

2355. SMITH, A. M., MASSION, J., GAHÉRY, Y., AND ROUMIEU, J. 1978. Unitary activity of ventrolateral nucleus during placing movement and associated postural adjustment. Brain Res., **149:** 329–346.

2356. SMITH, C. A. 1967. Innervation of the organ of Corti. In S. IURATO (Editor) *Submicroscopic Structure of the Inner Ear*, Pergamon Press Ltd., Oxford., pp. 107–131.

2357. SMITH, C. A., AND RASMUSSEN, G. L. 1963. Recent observations on the olivo-cochlear bundle. Ann. Otol., Rhinol. Laryngol., **72:** 489–507.

2358. SMITH, C. A., AND RASMUSSEN, G. L. 1965. Degeneration in the efferent nerve endings in the cochlea after axonal section. J. Cell Biol., **26:** 63–77.

2359. SMITH, M. C. 1951. The use of Marchi staining in the later stages of human tract degeneration. J. Neurol. Neurosurg. Psychiatry, **14:** 222–225.

2360. SMITH, M. C. 1956. The recognition and prevention of artefacts of the Marchi method. J. Neurol. Neurosurg. Psychiatry, **19:** 74–83.

2361. SMITH, M. C. 1957. The anatomy of the spino-cerebellar fibers in man. I. The course of the fibers in the spinal cord and brain stem. J. Comp. Neurol., **108:** 285–352.

2362. SMITH, M. C. 1961. The anatomy of the spino-cerebellar fibers in man. II. The distribution of the fibers in the cerebellum. J. Comp. Neurol., **117:** 329–354.

2363. SMITH, M. C. 1967. Stereotaxic operations for Par-

kinson's disease—Anatomical observations. In D. WIL-
LIAMS (Editor), *Modern Trends in Neurology*, Vol. 4.
Butterworths & Company, London, pp. 21–52.

2364. SMITH, O. A., JR., AND CLARKE, N. P. 1964. Central
autonomic pathways: A study in functional neuroanatomy. J. Comp. Neurol., **122:** 399–406.

2365. SMITH, W. K. 1945. The functional significance of
the rostral cingular cortex as revealed by its responses
to electrical excitation. J. Neurophysiol., **8:** 241–255.

2366. SMYTH, G. E. 1939. The systemization and central
connections of the spinal tract and nucleus of the trigeminal nerve. Brain, **62:** 41–87.

2367. SNIDER, R. S. 1936. Alterations which occur in
mossy terminals of the cerebellum following transection
of the brachium pontis. J. Comp. Neurol., **64:** 417–435.

2368. SNIDER, R. S. 1940. Morphology of the cerebellar
nuclei in rabbit and cat. J. Comp. Neurol., **72:** 399–415.

2369. SNIDER, R. S. 1950. Recent contributions to the
anatomy and physiology of the cerebellum. Arch. Neurol. Psychiatry, **64:** 196–219.

2370. SNIDER, R. S., AND ELDRED, E. 1952. Cerebro-cerebellar relationships in the monkey. J. Neurophysiol., **15:**
27–40.

2371. SNIDER, R. S., AND STOWELL, A. 1944. Receiving
areas of the tactile, auditory, and visual systems in the
cerebellum. J. Neurophysiol., **7:** 331–357.

2372. SNIDER, M., HALL, W. C., AND DIAMOND, I.
T. 1966. Vision in tree shrews after removal of striate
cortex. Psychonomic. Sci., **6:** 243–244.

2373. SNYDER, R. L. 1977. The organization of dorsal root
entry zone in cats and monkeys. J. Comp. Neurol., **174:**
47–69.

2374. SNYDER, R. L., JR., AND SUTIN, J. 1961. Effect of
lesions of the medulla oblongata on electrolyte and
water metabolism in the rat. Exp. Neurol., **4:** 424–435.

2375. SNYDER, S. H. 1980. Brain peptides as neurotransmitters. Science, **209:** 976–983.

2376. SOFRONIEW, M. V., AND WEINDL, A. 1980.
Identification of parvocellular vasopressin and neurophysin neurons in the suprachiasmatic nucleus of a
variety of mammals including primates. J. Comp. Neurol., **193:** 659–676.

2377. SOKOLOFF, L. 1977. Relation between physiological
function and energy metabolism in the central nervous
system. J. Neurochem., **29:** 13–26.

2378. SOMANA, R., KOTCHABHAKDI, N., AND WALBERG,
F. 1980. Cerebellar afferents from the trigeminal sensory nuclei in the cat. Exp. Brain Res., **38:** 57–64.

2379. SOMANA, R., AND WALBERG, F. 1978. Cerebellar afferents from the paramedian reticular nucleus studied
with retrograde transport of horseradish peroxidase.
Anat. Embryol. (Berl.), **154:** 353–368.

2380. SOMANA, R., AND WALBERG, F. 1978 a. The cerebellar projection from locus coeruleus as studied with retrograde transport of horseradish peroxidase in the cat.
Anat. Embryol. (Berl.), **155:** 87–94.

2381. SOMANA, R., AND WALBERG, F. 1979. Cerebellar afferents from the nucleus of the solitary tract. Neurosci.
Lett., **11:** 41–47.

2382. SOMANA, R., AND WALBERG, F. 1980. A re-examination of the cerebellar projections from the gracile, main
and external cuneate nuclei in the cat. Brain Res., **186:**
33–42.

2383. SOSA, J. M., AND DEZORRILLA, N. B. 1966. Spinal
ganglion cytological responses to axon and to dendrite
sectioning. Acta Anat. (Basel), **65:** 236–255.

2384. SOTELO, C. 1967. Cerebellar neuroglia: Morphological and histochemical aspects. In C. A. FOX AND R. S.
SNIDER (Editors), *Progress in Brain Research*, Vol. 25:
The Cerebellum. Elsevier Publishing Company, Amsterdam, pp. 226–250.

2385. SOTELO, C., LLINAS, R., AND BAKER, R. 1974.
Structural study of inferior olivary nucleus of the cat:
Morphological correlates of electrotonic coupling. J.
Neurophysiol., **37:** 541–559.

2386. SOTELO, C., AND PALAY, S. L. 1968. The fine structure of the lateral vestibular nucleus in the rat. I. Neu-

rons and neurological cells. J. Cell Biol., **36:** 151–179.

2387. SOUSA-PINTO, A. 1970. The cortical projection onto
the paramedian reticular and perihypoglossal nuclei of
the medulla oblongata of the cat: An experimental anatomical study. Brain Res., **18:** 77–91.

2388. SOUSA-PINTO, A. 1973. Cortical projections of the
medial geniculate body in the cat. Adv. Anat. Embryol.
Cell Biol., **48:** 1–42.

2389. SPARKS, D. L., HOLLAND, R., AND GUTHRIE, B.
L. 1976. Size and distribution of movement fields in
the monkey superior colliculus. Brain Res., **113:** 21–34.

2390. SPECTOR, I., HASSMANNOVA, J., AND ALBE-FESSARD,
D. 1974. Sensory properties of single neurons of cat's
claustrum. Brain Res., **66:** 39–65.

2391. SPECTOR, I., HASSMANNOVA, J., AND ALBE-FESSARD,
D. 1978. A macrophysiological study of functional
organization of the claustrum. Exp. Neurol., **29:** 31–51.

2392. SPEIDEL, C. G. 1919. Gland cells of internal secretion
in the spinal coard of the skates. Carnegie Inst. Wash.
Publ., **13:** 1–31.

2393. SPENCER, H. J. 1976. Antagonism of cortical excitation of striatal neurons by glutamic acid diethyl ester:
Evidence for glutamic acid as an excitatory transmitter
in the rat striatum. Brain Res., **102:** 91–101.

2394. SPENCER, R. F., AND STERLING, P. 1977. An electron
microscopic study of motoneurones and interneurones
in the cat abducens nucleus identified by retrograde
intraaxonal transport of horseradish peroxidase. J.
Comp. Neurol., **176:** 65–86.

2395. SPERRY, R. W. 1961. Cerebral organization and behavior. Science, **133:** 1749–1757.

2396. SPERRY, R. W. 1962. Some general aspects of interhemispheric integration. In V. B. MOUNTCASTLE (Editor), *Inter hemispheric Relations and Cerebral Dominance.* Johns Hopkins (University) Press, Baltimore,
Ch. 3, pp. 43–49.

2397. SPERRY, R. W. 1963. Chemoaffinity in the orderly
growth of nerve fiber patterns and connections. Proc.
Natl. Acad. Sci. U. S. A., **50:** 703–710.

2398. SPERRY, R. W. 1974. Lateral specialization in the
surgically separated hemispheres. In F. O. SCHMITT AND
F. G. WORDEN (Editors), *The Neurosciences.* Third
Study Program, M. I. T. Press, Cambridge, Mass., pp.
5–19.

2399. SPIEGEL, E. A. 1929. Experimentalstudien am Nervensystem: XV. Der Mechanismus des labyrinthären
Nystagmus. Z. Hals- Nasen- Ohrenheilk., **25:** 200–217.

2400. SPIEGEL, E. A., KLETZKIN, M., AND SZEKELY, E.
G. 1954. Pain reactions upon stimulation of the tectum mesencephali. J. Neuropathol. Exp. Neurol., **13:**
212–220.

2401. SPIEGEL, E. A., AND SOMMER, I. 1944. *Neurology of
the Eye, Ear, Nose and Throat.* Grune & Stratton, Inc.,
New York, 667 pp.

2402. SPIEGEL, E. A., AND WYCIS, H. T. 1950.
Pallidothalamotmy in chorea. Arch. Neurol. Psychiatry, **64:** 295–296.

2403. SPIEGEL, E. A., AND WYCIS, H. T. 1954. Ansotomy
in paralysis agitans. A. M. A. Arch. Neurol. Psychiatry,
71: 598–614.

2404. SPIEGEL, E. A., AND WYCIS, H. T. 1958. Pallido-an-
sotomy: Anatomic-physiologic foundation and histo-
pathologic control. In W. S. FIELDS (Editor), *Pathogenesis and Treatment of Parkinsonism.* Charles C
Thomas Publisher, Springfield, Ill., Ch. 3, pp. 86–105.

2405. SPILLER, W. G. 1924. Ophthalmoplegia internu-
clearis anterior: A case with necropsy. Brain, **47:** 345–
357.

2406. SPOENDLIN, H. H. 1966. The organization of the
cochlear receptor. Adv. Otorhinolaryngol. **13:** 1–227.

2407. SPOENDLIN, H. H. 1972. Innervation densities of the
cochlea. Acta Otolaryngol. (Stockh.), **73:** 235–248.

2408. SPOENDLIN, H. H. 1973. The innervation of the cochlear receptor. In A. R. MØLLER (Editor), *Basic Mechanisms in Hearing.* Academic Press, Inc., New York, pp.
185–234.

2409. SPOENDLIN, H. H., AND GACEK, R. R. 1963.

Electronmicroscopic study of the efferent and afferent innervation of the organ of Corti in the cat. Ann. Otol. Rhinol. Laryngol. **72:** 660–686.

2410. SPRAGUE, J. M. 1951. Motor and propriospinal cells in the thoracic and lumbar ventral horn of the Rhesus monkey. J. Comp. Neurol., **95:** 103–124.

2411. SPRAGUE, J. M. 1958. The distribution of dorsal root fibers on motor cells in the lumbosacral spinal cord of the cat, and the site of excitatory and inhibitory terminals in monosynaptic pathways. Proc. R. Soc. Lond. (Biol), **149:** 534–556.

2412. SPRAGUE, J. M. 1972. The superior colliculus and pretectum in visual behavior. Invest. Ophthalmol., **11:** 473–482.

2412a. SPRAGUE, J. M., AND CHAMBERS, W. W. 1953. Regulation of posture in intact and decerebrate cat; I. Cerebellum, reticular formation, vestibular nuclei. J. Neurophysiol., **16:** 451–463.

2413. SPRAGUE, J. M., AND CHAMBERS, W. W. 1954. Control of posture by reticular formation and cerebellum in the intact, anesthetized, unanesthetized and in the decerebrated cat. Am. J. Physiol., **176:** 52–64.

2414. SPRAGUE, J. M., AND HA, H. 1964. The terminal fields of dorsal root fibers in the lumbosacral spinal cord of the cat, and the dendritic organization of the motor nuclei. In J. C. ECCLES AND J. P. SCHADE (Editors), *Progress in Brain Research*, Vol. 2.: *Organization of the Spinal Cord.* Elsevier Publishing Company, Amsterdam, pp. 120–152.

2415. SPRAGUE, J. M., LEVITT, M., ROBSON, K., LIU, C. N., STELLER, E., AND CHAMBERS, W. W. 1963. A neuroanatomical and behavioral analysis of the syndromes resulting from midbrain lemniscal and reticular lesions in the cat. Arch. Ital. Biol., **101:** 225–295.

2416. SPRAGUE, J. M., AND MEIKLE, T. H., JR. 1965. The role of the superior colliculus in visually guided behavior. Exp. Neurol., **11:** 115–146.

2417. STAAL, A. 1961. *Subcortical Projections on the Spinal Gray Matter of the Cat.* Koninkl. Druk., Lankhout-Immig N. V., The Hague, 164 pp.

2418. STANDAERT, F. G., AND DRETCHEN, K. L. 1979. Cyclic nucleotides and neuromuscular transmission. Fed. Proc., **38:** 2183–2192.

2419. STANTON, G. B. 1980. Topographical organization of ascending cerebellar projections from the dentate and interposed nuclei in *Macaca mulatta:* An anterograde degeneration study. J. Comp. Neurol., **190:** 699–731.

2420. STANTON, G. B. 1980 *a.* Afferents to oculomotor nuclei from area "Y" in *Macaca* mulatta: An anterograde degeneration study. J. Comp. Neurol., **192:** 377–385.

2421. STARZL, T. E., AND MAGOUN, H. W. 1951. Organization of the diffuse thalamic projection system. J. Neurophysiol., **14:** 133–146.

2422. STARZL, T. E., TAYLOR, C. W., AND MAGOUN, H. W. 1951. Ascending conduction in reticular activating system, with special reference to the diencephalon. J. Neurophysiol., **14:** 461–477.

2423. STARZL, T. E., TAYLOR, C. W., AND MAGOUN, H. W. 1951 *a.* Collateral afferent excitation of the reticular formation of the brain stem. J. Neurophysiol., **14:** 479–496.

2424. STARZL, T. E. AND WHITLOCK, D. G. 1952. Diffuse thalamic projection system in monkey. J. Neurophysiol., **15:** 449–468.

2425. STEIGER, H.-J., AND BÜTTNER-ENNEVER, J. 1978. Relationship between motoneurons and internuclear neurons in the abducens nucleus: A double retrograde tracer study in the cat. Brain Res., **148:** 181–188.

2426. STEIGER, H.-J., AND BÜTTNER-ENNEVER, J. A. 1979. Oculomotor nucleus afferents in the monkey demonstrated with horseradish peroxidase. Brain Res., **160:** 1–15.

2427. STEIN, B. E., MAGALHAES-CASTRO, B., AND KRUGER, L. 1976. Relationships between visual and tactile representation in cat superior colliculus. J. Neurophysiol., **39:** 401–419.

2428. STEIN, B. M., AND CARPENTER, M. B. 1965. Effects of dorsal rhizotomy upon subthalamic dyskinesia in the monkey. Arch. Neurol., **13:** 567–583.

2429. STEIN, B. M., AND CARPENTER, M. B. 1967. Central projections of portions of the vestibular ganglia innervating specific parts of the labyrinth in the rhesus monkey. Am. J. Anat., **120:** 281–318.

2430. STEINBUSCH, H. W. M. 1981. Distribution of serotonin-immunoreactivity in the central nervous system of the rat—cell bodies and terminals. Neuroscience, **6:** 577–618.

2431. STENGEL, E. 1926. Über den Ursprung der Nervenfasern der Neurohypophyse im Zwischenhirn. Arb. Neurol. Inst. Wiener Univ., **28:** 25–37.

2432. STENSAAS, L. J. 1968. The development of hippocampal and dorsolateral pallial regions of the cerebral hemisphere in fetal rabbits. J. Comp. Neurol., **132:** 93–108.

2433. STEPHENS, R. B., AND STILWELL, D. L. 1969. *Arteries and Veins of the Human Brain.* Charles C Thomas, Springfield, Ill.

2434. STEPIEN, L. S., CORDEAU, J. P. AND RASMUSSEN, T. 1960. The effect of temporal lobe and hippocampal lesions on auditory and visual recent memory in monkeys. Brain, **83:** 470–489.

2435. STERLING, P., AND KUYPERS, H. G. J. M. 1967. Anatomical organization of the brachial spinal cord of the cat II. The motoneuron plexus. Brain Res. **4:** 16–32.

2436. STERLING, P., AND WICKELGREN, B. G. 1969. Visual receptive fields in the superior colliculus of the cat. J. Neurophysiol., **32:** 1–15.

2437. STERN, K. 1938. Note on the nucleus ruber magnocellularis and its efferent pathway in man. Brain, **61:** 284–289.

2438. STEVENSON, J. A. F. 1949. Effects of hypothalamic lesions on water and energy metabolism in the rat. Recent Prog. Horm. Res., **4:** 363–394.

2439. STEVENSON, J. A. F. 1969. Neural control of food and water intake. In W. HAYMAKER *et al.* (Editors), *The Hypothalamus.* Charles C Thomas Publisher, Springfield, Ill., Ch. 15, pp. 524–621.

2440. STONE, J., AND FUKUDA, Y. 1974. Properties of cat retinal ganglion cells: A comparison of W cells with X and Y cells. J. Neurophysiol., **37:** 722–748.

2441. STOOKEY, B., AND SCARFF, J. 1943. Injuries of peripheral nerves. In *Neurosurgery and Thoracic Surgery.* National Research Council Committee on Surgery. W. B. Saunders Company, Philadelphia, pp. 81–184.

2442. STOPFORD, J. S. B. 1915. The arteries of the pons and medulla oblongata. Part I. J. Anat. Physiol., **50:** 131–164.

2443. STOPFORD, J. S. B. 1916. The arteries of the pons and medulla oblongata. Part II. J. Anat. Physiol., **51:** 255–280.

2444. STOTLER, W. A. 1953. An experimental study of the cells and connections of the superior olivary complex of the cat. J. Comp. Neurol., **98:** 401–423.

2445. STRICK, P. L. 1976. Anatomical analysis of ventrolateral thalamic input to primate motor cortex. J. Neurophysiol., **39:** 1020–1031.

2446. STRICK, P. L. 1976 *a.* Activity of ventrolateral thalamic neurons during arm movement. J. Neurophysiol., **39:** 1032–1044.

2447. STRICK, P. L., BURKE, R. E., KANDA, K., KIM, C.C., AND WALMSLEY, B. 1976. Differences between alpha and gamma motoneurons labeled with horseradish peroxidase by retrograde transport. Brain Res., **113:** 582–588.

2448. STRICK, P. L., AND KIM, C. C. 1978. Input to primate motor cortex from posterior parietal cortex (area 5). I. Demonstration by retrograde transport. Brain Res., **157:** 325–330.

2449. STRICK, P. L., AND PRESTON, J. B. 1978. Multiple representation in the primate motor cortex. Brain Res., **154:** 366–370.

2450. STRICK, P. L., AND STERLING, P. 1974. Synaptic terminations of afferents from the ventrolateral nucleus of the thalamus in the cat motor cortex: A light and electron microscope study. J. Comp. Neurol., **153:** 77–

106.

2451. STROMINGER, N. L. 1969. Subdivisions of auditory cortex and their role in localization of sound in space. Exp. Neurol., **24**: 348–362.

2452. STROMINGER, N. L. 1973. The origins, course and distribution of the dorsal and intermediate acoustic striae in the Rhesus monkey. J. Comp. Neurol., **147**: 209–234.

2453. STROMINGER, N. L. 1978. The anatomical organization of the primate auditory pathways. In C. R. NOBACK (Editor), *Sensory Systems of Primates*. Plenum Publishing Co., New York, pp. 53–91.

2454. STROMINGER, N. L., AND CARPENTER, M. B. 1965. Effects of lesions in the substantia nigra upon subthalamic dyskinesia in the monkey. Neurology (Minneap.), **15**: 587–594.

2455. STROMINGER, N. L., AND HURWITZ, J. L. 1976. Anatomical aspects of the superior olivary complex. J. Comp. Neurol., **170**: 485–498.

2456. STROMINGER, N. L., NELSON, L. R., AND DOUGHTERTY, W. J. 1977. Second order auditory pathways in the chimpanzee. J. Comp. Neurol., **172**: 349–366.

2457. STROMINGER, N. L., AND STROMINGER, A. I. 1971. Ascending brain stem projections of the anteroventral cochlear nucleus in the rhesus monkey. J. Comp. Neurol., **143**: 217–242.

2458. STRONG, O. S. 1915. A case of unilateral cerebellar agenesia. J. Comp. Neurol., **25**: 361–391.

2459. STRYKER, M. P., AND SCHILLER, P. H. 1975. Eye and head movements evoked by electrical stimulation of monkey superior colliculus. Exp. Brain Res., **23**: 103–112.

2460. STUMPF, W. E. 1970. Estrogen-neurons and estrogen-neuron systems in the periventricular brain. Am. J. Anat., **129**: 207–217.

2461. STUMPF, W. E. 1972. Estrogen, androgen and glucocorticosteroid concentrating neurons in the amygdala, studied by dry autoradiography. In B. E. ELEFTHERIOU (Editor), *The Neurobiology of the Amygdala*. Plenum Press, New York, pp. 763–774.

2462. SUGAR, O., AMADOR, L. V., AND GRIPONISSIOTES, B. 1950. Corticocortical connections of the walls of the superior temporal sulcus in the monkey (*Macaca mulatta*). J. Neuropathol. Exp. Neurol., **9**: 179–185.

2463. SUGAR, O., FRENCH, J. D. AND CHUSID, J. G. 1948. Corticocortical connections of the superior surface of the temporal operculum in the monkey (*Macaca mulatta*). J. Neurophysiol., **11**: 175–184.

2464. SUGAR, O., AND GERARD, R. W. 1940. Spinal cord regeneration in the rat. J. Neurophysiol., **3**: 1–19.

2465. SUGIMOTO, T., ITOH, K. AND MIZUNO, H. 1978. Direct projections from the Edinger-Westphal nucleus to the cerebellum and spinal cord in the cat: A HRP study. Neurosci. Lett., **9**: 17–22.

2466. SUH, T. H., AND ALEXANDER, L. 1939. Vascular system of the human spinal cord. Arch. Neurol. Psychiatry, **41**: 659–677.

2467. SULKIN, N. M. 1953. Histochemical studies of the pigments in the human autonomic ganglion cells. J. Gerontol., **8**: 435–445.

2468. SULKIN, N. M., AND SRIVANIJ, P. 1960. The experimental production of senile pigments in the nerve cells of young rats. J. Gerontol., **15**: 2–9.

2469. SUMMY-LONG, J. Y., KEIL, L. C., AND SEVERS, W. B. 1978. Identification of vasopressin in the subfornical organ region: Effects of dehydration. Brain Res., **140**: 241–250.

2470. SUNDERLAND, S. 1950. Capacity of reinnervated muscles to function efficiently after prolonged denervation. Arch. Neurol. Psychiatry, **64**: 755–771.

2471. SUNDERLAND, S. 1952. Factors influencing the course of regeneration and the quality of the recovery after nerve suture. Brain, **75**: 19–54.

2472. SUTIN, J. 1966. The periventricular structures of the hypothalamus. Int. Rev. of Neurobiology, **9**: 263–300.

2473. SUTIN, J. 1973. Neural factors in the control of food intake. In G. A. BRAY, (Editor), *Obesity in Perspective*, DHEW Publication No. (NIH) 75-708, U.S. Government Printing Office, Washington, D. C., pp. 1–11.

2474. SUTIN, J., AND MCBRIDE, R. L. 1977. Anatomical analysis of neuronal connectivity. In R. D. MYERS (Editor), *Methods in Psychobiology*, Vol. 3. Academic Press, New York, pp. 1–26.

2475. SUTIN, J., AND MCBRIDE, R. L. 1979. Limbic and brainstem connections of the hypothalamus. In P. J. MORGANE AND J. PANKSEPP (Editors), *Handbook of the Hypothalamus*, Vol. 1: *Anatomy of the Hypothalamus*. Marcel Dekker, Inc., New York, pp. 555–592.

2476. SWANN, H. G. 1934. The function of the brain in olfaction. II. The results of destruction of olfactory and other nervous structures upon the discrimination of odors. J. Comp. Neurol., **59**: 175–201.

2477. SWANN, H. G. 1935. The function of the brain in olfaction. III. The effects of large cortical lesions on olfactory discrimination. Am. J. Physiol., **111**: 257–262.

2478. SWANSON, L. W., AND COWAN, W. M. 1975. A note on the connections and development of the nucleus accumbens. Brain Res., **92**: 324–330.

2479. SWANSON, L. W., AND COWAN, W. M. 1975a. The efferent connections of the suprachiasmatic nucleus of the hypothalamus. J. Comp. Neurol., **160**: 1–12.

2480. SWANSON, L. W., AND COWAN W. M. 1975b. Hippocampal-hypothalamic connections: Origin in subicular cortex, not Ammon's horn. Science, **189**: 303–304.

2481. SWANSON, L. W., AND COWAN, W. M. 1977. An autoradiographic study of the organization of the efferent connections of the hippocampal formation in the rat. J. Comp. Neurol., **172**: 49–84.

2482. SWANSON, L. W., COWAN, W. M., AND JONES, E. G. 1974. An autoradiographic study of the efferent connections of the ventral lateral geniculate nucleus in the albino rat and the cat. J. Comp. Neurol., **156**: 143–163.

2483. SWANSON, L. W., AND KUYPERS, H. G. J. M. 1980. The paraventricular nucleus of the hypothalamus: Cytoarchitectonic subdivisions and organization of projections to the pituitary, dorsal vagal complex, and spinal cord as demonstrated by retrograde fluorescence double-labeling methods. J. Comp. Neurol., **194**: 555–570.

2484. SWANSON, L. W., AND MCKELLAR, S. 1979. The distribution of oxytocin and neurophysin stained fibers in the spinal cord of the rat and monkey. J. Comp. Neurol., **188**: 87–106.

2485. SWANSON, L. W., AND SAWCHENKO, P. E. 1980. Paraventricular nucleus: A site for the integration of neuroendocrine and autonomic mechanisms. Neuroendocrinology, **31**: 410–417.

2486. SWANSON, L. W., SAWCHENKO, P. E., AND COWAN, W. M. 1981. Evidence for collateral projections by neurons in Ammon's horn, the dentate gyrus and the subiculum: A multiple retrograde labeling study in the rat. J. Neurosci., **1**: 548–559.

2487. SWEET, W. H., TALLAND, G. A., AND ERVIN, F. R. 1959. Loss of recent memory following section of the fornix. Trans. Am. Neurol., Assoc., **84**: 76–82.

2488. SYMONDS, C. 1966. Disorders of memory. Brain, **89**: 625–644.

2489. SZABO, J. 1962. Topical distribution of the striatal efferents in the monkey. Exp. Neurol., **5**: 21–36.

2490. SZABO, J. 1967. The efferent projections of the putamen in the monkey. Exp. Neurol., **19**: 463–476.

2491. SZABO, J. 1970. Projections from the body of the caudate nucleus in the rhesus monkey. Exp. Neurol., **27**: 1–15.

2492. SZABO, J. 1980. Distribution of striatal afferents from the mesencephalon in the cat. Brain Res., **188**: 3–21.

2493. SZABO, J. 1980a. Organization of the ascending striatal afferents in monkeys. J. Comp. Neurol., **189**: 307–321.

2494. SZENTÁGOTHAI, J. 1950. The elementary vestibulo-ocular reflex arc. J. Neurophysiol., **13**: 395–407.

2495. SZENTÁGOTHAI, J. 1950a. Recherches experimentales sur les voies oculogyres. Sem. Hop. Paris, **26:** 2989–2995.

2496. SZENTÁGOTHAI, J. 1964. Neuronal and synaptic arrangement in the substantia gelatinosa Rolandi. J. Comp. Neurol., **122:** 219–239.

2497. SZENTÁGOTHAI, J. 1970. Glomerular synapses, complex synaptic arrangements, and their operational significance. In F. O. SCHMITT (Editor), *The Neurosciences.* Second Study Program. Rockefeller University Press, New York, Ch. 40, pp. 427–443.

2498. SZENTÁGOTHAI, J. 1973. Neuronal and synaptic architecture of the lateral geniculate nucleus. In R. JUNG (Editor), *Handbook of Sensory Physiology,* Vol 7: *Central Processing of Visual Information,* Part B; *Morphology and Function of Visual Centers in the Brain.* Springer-Verlag, Berlin, pp. 141–176.

2499. SZENTÁGOTHAI, J. 1978. The neuron network of the cerebral cortex: A functional interpretation. Proc. R. Soc. Lond. (Biol.), **201:** 219–248.

2500. SZENTÁGOTHAI, J., AND ALBERT, A. 1955. The synaptology of Clarke's column. Acta Morphol. Acad. Sci. Hung., **5:** 43–51.

2501. SZENTÁGOTHAI, J., FLERKO, B., MESS, B., AND HALASZ, B. 1968. *Hypothalamic Control of the Anterior Pituitary: An Experimental-Morphological Study.* Akademiai Kiado, Budapest.

2502. SZENTÁGOTHAI, J., AND RAJKOVITS, K. 1959. Über den Ursprung der Kletterfasern des Kleinhirn. Z. Anat. Entwickl.-Gesch., **121:** 130–141.

2503. SZENTÁGOTHAI-SCHIMERT, J. 1941. Die Endigungsweise der absteigenden Rückenmarksbahnen. Z. Anat. Entwickl.-Gesch., **111:** 322–330.

2504. TABER, E. 1961. The cytoarchitecture of the brain stem of the cat. I. Brain stem nuclei of cat. J. Comp. Neurol., **116:** 27–70.

2505. TABER, E., BRODAL, A., AND WALBERG, F. 1960. The raphe nuclei of the brain stem in the cat. I. Normal topography and cytoarchitecture and general discussion. J. Comp. Neurol., **114:** 161–187.

2506. TABER-PIERCE, E., HODDEVIK, G. H., AND WALBERG, F. 1977. The cerebellar projection from the raphe nuclei in the cat as studied with the method of retrograde transport of horseradish peroxidase. Anat. Embryol. (Berl.), **152:** 73–87.

2507. TAKAHASHI, T., AND OTSUKA, M. 1975. Regional distribution of substance P in the spinal cord and nerve roots of the cat and the effects of dorsal root section. Brain Res., **87:** 1–11.

2508. TAKEUCHI, Y., UEMURA, M., MATSUDA, K., MATSUSHIMA, R., AND MIZUNO, N. 1980. Parabrachial nucleus neurons projecting to the lower brain stem and the spinal cord: A study in the cat by the Fink-Heimer and the horseradish peroxidase methods. Exp. Neurol., **70:** 403–413.

2509. TALAAT, M. 1937. Afferent impulses in the nerves supplying the urinary bladder. J. Physiol. (Lond.), **89:** 1–13.

2510. TALAIRACH, J., PAILLAS, J. E., AND DAVID, M. 1950. Dyskinésie de type hémiballique traitée par cortectomie frontale limitée, puis par coagulation de l'anse lenticulaire et de la portion interne du globus pallidus. Rev. Neurol. (Paris), **83:** 440–451.

2511. TALBOT, S. A., AND MARSHALL, W. H. 1941. Physiological studies on neuronal mechanisms of visual localization and discrimination. Am. J. Ophthalmol., **24:** 1255–1263.

2512. TANABE, T., YARITA, H., IINO, M., OOSHIMA, Y., AND TAKAGI, S. F. 1975. An olfactory projection area in orbitofrontal cortex of the monkey. J. Neurophysiol., **38:** 1269–1283.

2513. TANG, P. C., AND RUCH, T. C. 1956. Localization of brain stem and diencephalic areas controlling the micturition reflex. J. Comp. Neurol., **106:** 213–246.

2514. TARKHAN, A. A., AND ABD-EL-MALEK, S. 1950. On the presence of sensory nerve cells on the hypoglossal nerve. J. Comp. Neurol., **93:** 219–228.

2515. TARLOV, E. C., AND MOORE, R. Y. 1973. The tecto-thalamic connections in the brain of the rabbit. J. Comp. Neurol., **126:** 403–422.

2516. TASAKI, I. 1954. Nerve impulses in individual auditory nerve fibers of guinea pig. J. Neurophysiol., **17:** 97–122.

2517. TAUB, A. 1964. Local, segmental and supraspinal interaction with a dorsolateral spinal cutaneous afferent system. Exp. Neurol., **10:** 357–374.

2518. TAUB, A., AND BISHOP, P. O. 1965. The spinocervical tract: Dorsal column linkage, conduction velocity, primary afferent spectrum. Exp. Neurol., **13:** 1–21.

2519. TAVERAS, J. 1961. Angiographic observation in occlusive cerebrovascular disease. Neurology (Minneap.), **11:** 86–90.

2520. TAVERAS, J. M., AND WOOD, E. H. 1976. *Diagnostic Neuroradiology,* Ed. 2. Williams & Wilkins, Baltimore.

2521. TAYLOR, A. C., AND WEISS, P. 1965. Demonstration of axonal flow by the movement of tritium-labeled protein in mature optic nerve fibers. Proc. Natl. Acad. Sci. U. S.A., **54:** 1521–1527.

2522. TAYLOR, J., GREENFIELD, J. G., AND MARTIN, J. P. 1922. Two cases of syringomyelia and syringobulbia, observed clinically over many years and examined pathologically. Brain, **45:** 323–356.

2523. TELLO, J. F. 1922. Die Entstehungen der motorischen und sensiblen Nervenendigungen. Z. Gesamte Anat., **64:** 348–440.

2524. TENNYSON, V. M. 1965. Electron microscopic study of the developing neuroblast of the dorsal root ganglion of the rabbit embryo. J. Comp. Neurol., **124:** 267–318.

2525. TENNYSON, V. M. 1971. The differences in fine structure of the myelencephalic and telencephalic choroid plexuses in the fetuses of man and rabbit, and a comparison with the mature stage. In A. E. WALKER and R. ARANA-IÑIGUEZ (Editors), *Cerebrospinal Fluid in Health and Disease.* Acta Neurol. Lát. Am., **17:** (suppl. 1,): 11–52.

2526. TENNYSON, V. M., BARRETT, R. E., COHEN, G., CÔTÉ, L., HEIKKILA, R., AND MYTILINEOU, C. 1973. Correlation of anatomical and biochemical development of the rabbit neostriatum. In D. FORD (Editor), *Neurobiological Aspects of Maturation and Aging. Progress in Brain Research,* Vol. 40. Elsevier Publishing Company, Amsterdam, pp. 203–217.

2527. TENNYSON, V. M., AND PAPPAS, G. D. 1961. Electron microscope studies of the developing telencephalic choroid plexus in normal and hydrocephalic rabbits. In W. FIELDS AND M. DESMOND (Editors), *Disorders of the Developing Nervous System.* Charles C Thomas Publishing, Springfield, Ill., Ch. 12, pp. 267–318.

2528. TENNYSON, V. M., AND PAPPAS, G. D. 1964. Fine structure of the developing telencephalic and myelencephalic choroid plexus of the rabbit. J. Comp. Neurol., **123:** 379–412.

2529. TENNYSON, V. M., AND PAPPAS, G. D. 1968. Some aspects of the fine structure of the ependyma. In J. MINCKLER (Editor), *Pathology of the Nervous System.* Vol. 1. McGraw-Hill Book Company, New York. pp. 518–531.

2530. TENNYSON, V. M., AND PAPPAS, G. D. 1968a. The fine structure of the choroid plexus: Adult and developmental stages. In A. LAJTHA AND D. H. FORD (Editors), *Progress in Brain Research,* Vol. 29: *Brain Barrier Systems.* Elsevier Publishing Company, Amsterdam, pp. 63–86.

2531. TERAYAMA, Y., AND YAMAMOTO, K. 1971. Olivocochlear bundle in the guinea pig cochlea after central transection of the crossed bundle: Electron microscopic study on origin and distribution of unmyelinated efferent fibers by axonal degeneration. Acta Otolaryngol. (Stockh.), **72:** 385–396.

2532. TERNAUX, J. P., HÉRY, F., BOURGOIN, S., ADRIEN, J., GLOWINSKI, J. , AND HAMON, M. 1977. The topographical distribution of serotoninergic terminals in the neostriatum of the rat and the caudate nucleus of the cat. Brain Res., **121**: 311–326.

2533. TERRY, R. D.   1968.   Electron microscopy of the central nervous system. In O. T. BAILEY AND D. E. SMITH (Editors). *The Central Nervous System*, Williams & Wilkins, Baltimore, pp. 335–347.

2534. TERZIAN, H.   1958.   Observations on the clinical symptomatology of bilateral partial or total removal of the temporal lobe in man. In M. BALDWIN AND P. BAILEY (Editors), *Temporal Lobe Epilepsy*. Charles C Thomas Publishing, Springfield, Ill., pp. 510–529.

2535. TERZIAN, H., AND ORE, G. D.   1955.   Syndrome of Klüver and Bucy reproduced in man by bilateral removal of the temporal lobes. Neurology (Minneap.), **5**: 373–380.

2536. TERZUOLO, C., AND TERZIAN, H.   1953.   Cerebellar increase of postural tonus after deafferentation and labyrinthectomy. J. Neurophysiol., **16**: 551–561.

2537. THACH, W. T.   1970.   The behavior of Purkinje and cerebellar nuclear cells during two types of voluntary arm movement in the monkey. In W. S. FIELDS AND W. D. WILLIS (Editors), *The Cerebellum in Health and Disease*. Warren H. Green, Inc., St. Louis, Ch. 8, pp. 217–230.

2538. THACH, W. T., AND JONES, E. G.   1979.   The cerebellar dentatothalamic connection: Terminal field, lamellae, rods and somatotopy. Brain Res., **169**: 168–172.

2539. THAEMERT, J. C.   1966.   Ultrastructural interrelationships of nerve processes and smooth muscle cells in three dimensions. J. Cell Biol., **28**: 37–49.

2540. THAEMERT, J. C.   1966a.   Ultrastructure of cardiac muscle and nerve contiguities. J Cell Biol., **29**: 156–162.

2541. THOMAS, D. M., KAUFMAN, R. P., SPRAGUE, J. M. AND CHAMBERS, W. W.   1956.   Experimental studies of the vermal cerebellar projections in the brain stem of the cat (fastigiobulbar tract). J. Anat., **90**: 371–385.

2542. THOMAS, P. K.   1963.   The connective tissue of peripheral nerve: An electron microscope study. J. Anat., **97**: 35–44.

2543. THOMPSON, J. M., WOOLSEY, C. N., AND TALBOT, S. A.   1950.   Visual areas I and II of cerebral cortex of rabbit. J. Neurophysiol., **13**: 277–288.

2544. THOMSON, A. F., AND WALKER, A. E.   1951.   Behavioral alterations following lesions of the medial surface of the temporal lobe. A. M. A. Arch. Neurol. Psychiatry, **65**: 251–252.

2545. TIGGES, J., AND O'STEEN, W. K.   1974.   Terminations of retinofugal fibers in squirrel monkey: A re-investigation using autoradiographic methods. Brain Res., **79**: 489–495.

2546. TIGGES, M., AND TIGGES, J.   1970.   The retinofugal fibers and their terminal nuclei in *Galago crassicaudatus* (Primates). J. Comp. Neurol., **138**: 87–102.

2547. TINDALL, G. T. AND MCLANAHAN, C. S.   1980.   Hyperfunctional pituitary tumors: Pre- and postoperative management considerations. Clin Neurosurg., **27**: 48–82.

2548. TOBIAS, T. J.   1975.   Afferents to prefrontal cortex from the thalamic mediodorsal nucleus in the rhesus monkey. Brain Res., **83**: 191–212.

2549. TOHYAMA, M., SAKAI, M., SLAVERT, D., TOURET, M., AND JOUVET, M.   1979.   Spinal projections from the lower brain stem in the cat as demonstrated by the horseradish peroxidase technique. I. Origins of the reticulospinal tracts and their funicular trajectories. Brain Res., **173**: 383–403.

2550. TOLBERT, D. L., AND BANTLI, H.   1979.   An HRP and autoradiographic study of cerebellar corticonuclear-nucleocortical reciprocity in the monkey. Exp. Brain Res., **36**: 563–571.

2551. TOLBERT, D. L., BANTLI, H., AND BLOEDEL, J. R.   1976.   Anatomical and physiological evidence for a cerebellar nucleocortical projection in the cat. Neuroscience, **1**: 205–217.

2552. TOLBERT, D. L., BANTLI, H., AND BLOEDEL, J. R.   1977.   The intracerebellar nucleocortical projection in a primate. Exp. Brain Res., **30**: 425–434.

2553. TOLBERT, D. L., BANTLI, H., AND BLOEDEL, J. R.   1978.   Multiple branching of cerebellar efferent projections in cats. Exp. Brain Res., **31**: 305–316.

2554. TOLBERT, D. L., BANTLI, H., AND BLOEDEL, J. R.   1978a.   Organization features of the cat and monkey cerebellar nucleocortical projection. J. Comp. Neurol., **182**: 39–56.

2555. TOLBERT, D. L., MASSOPUST, L. C., MURPHY, M. G., AND YOUNG, P. A.   1976.   The anatomical organization of the cerebello-olivary projection in the cat. J. Comp. Neurol., **170**: 525–544.

2556. TOMASCH, J.   1969.   The numerical capacity of the human cortico-ponto-cerebellar system. Brain Res., **13**: 476–484.

2557. TONCRAY, J. E., AND KRIEG, W. J. S.   1946.   The nuclei of the human thalamus: A comparative approach. J. Comp. Neurol., **85**: 421–459.

2558. TORVIK, A.   1956.   Afferent connections to the sensory trigeminal nuclei, the nucleus of the solitary tract and adjacent structures: An experimental study in the rat. J. Comp. Neurol., **106**: 51–142.

2559. TORVIK, A.   1957.   The ascending fibers from the main trigeminal sensory nucleus: An experimental study in the cat. Am. J. Anat., **100**: 1–15.

2560. TORVIK, A., AND BRODAL, A.   1954.   The cerebellar projection of the peri-hypoglossal nuclei (nuclei intercalatus, nucleus praepositus hypoglossi and nucleus of Roller) in the cat. J. Neuropathol. Exp. Neurol., **13**: 515–527.

2561. TORVIK, A., AND BRODAL, A.   1957.   The origin of reticulospinal fibers in the cat: An experimental study. Anat. Rec., **128**: 113–137.

2562. TOWER, D. B.   1960.   Chemical architecture of the central nervous system. In J. FIELD (Editor), *Handbook of Physiology*, Section I, Vol. III. American Physiological Society, Washington, D.C., pp. 1793–1813.

2563. TOWER, S. S.   1937.   Function and structure in the chronically isolated lumbosacral spinal cord of the dog. J. Comp. Neurol., **67**: 109–131.

2564. TOWER, S. S.   1940.   Pyramidal lesion in the monkey. Brain, **63**: 36–90.

2565. TOWER, S. S.   1949.   The pyramidal tract. In P. C. BUCY (Editor), *The Precentral Motor Cortex*, Ed. 2. University of Illinois Press, Urbana, Ch. 6, pp. 149–172.

2566. TOYAMA, K., TSUKAHARA, N., AND UDO, M.   1968.   Nature of the cerebellar influences upon the red nucleus neurons. Exp. Brain Res., **4**: 292–309.

2567. TRACEY, D. J., ASANUMA, C., JONES, E. G., AND PORTER, R.   1980.   Thalamic relay to moter cortex: Afferent pathways from brain stem, cerebellum, and spinal cord in monkeys. J. Neurophysiol., **44**: 532–553.

2568. TRAVIS, A. M.   1955.   Neurological deficiencies after ablation of the precentral motor area in *Macaca mulatta*. Brain, **78**: 155–173.

2569. TRAVIS, A. M.   1955a.   Neurological deficiencies following supplementary motor area lesions in *Macaca mulatta*. Brain, **78**: 174–198.

2570. TRAVIS, A. M., AND WOOLSEY, C. N.   1956.   Motor performance of monkeys after bilateral partial and total cerebral decortications. Am. J. Phys. Med., **35**: 273–303.

2571. TREGEAR, G. W., NIALL, H. D., POTTS, J. T., LEEMAN, S. E., AND CHANG, M. M.   1971.   Synthesis of substance P. Nature, **232**: 87–89.

2572. TRETIAKOFF, C.   1919.   Contribution à l'étude de l'anatomopathologie du locus niger de Sommering. Thèse, Université de Paris, Number 293. Jouve et Cie, Paris.

2573. TREVINO, D. L.   1976.   The origin and projections of a spinal nociceptive and thermoreceptive pathway. In Y. Zotterman (Editor), *Sensory Functions in the Skin*. Pergamon Press, New York, pp. 367–377.

2574. TREVINO, D. L., AND CARSTENS, E.   1975.   Confirmation of the location of spinothalamic neurons in the cat and monkey by the retrograde transport of horseradish peroxidase. Brain Res., **98**: 177–182.

2575. TREVINO, D. L., COULTER, J. D., AND WILLIS, W.

D. 1973. Location of cells of origin of spinothalamic tract in lumbar enlargement of the monkey. J. Neurophysiol., **36**: 750–761.

2576. TROJANOWSKI, J., AND JACOBSON, S. 1974. Medial pulvinar afferents to frontal eye fields in rhesus monkey demonstrated by horseradish peroxidase. Brain Res., **80**: 395–411.

2577. TROJANOWSKI, J. J., AND JACOBSON, S. 1975. A combined horseradish peroxidase-autoradiographic investigation of reciprocal connections between superior temporal gyrus and pulvinar in squirrel monkey. Brain Res., **85**: 347–353.

2578. TRUEX, R. C. 1939. Observations on the chicken Gasserian ganglion with special reference to the bipolar neurons. J. Comp. Neurol., **71**: 473–486.

2579. TRUEX, R. C. 1940. Morphological alterations in the Gasserian ganglion cells and their association with senescence in man. Am. J. Pathol., **16**: 255–268.

2580. TRUEX, R. C. 1941. Degenerate versus multipolar neurons in sensory ganglia. Am. J. Pathol., **17**: 211–218.

2581. TRUEX, R. C. 1951. The sympathetic ganglions of hypertensive patients. A. M. A. Arch. Pathol., **51**: 186–191.

2582. TRUEX, R. C., AND KELLNER, C. E. 1948. *Detailed Atlas of the Head and Neck.* Oxford University Press, New York.

2583. TRUEX, R. C., AND TAYLOR, M. 1968. Gray matter lamination of the human spinal cord. Anat. Rec., **160**: 502.

2584. TRUEX, R. C., TAYLOR, M. J., SMYTHE, M. Q., AND GILDENBERG, P. L. 1970. The lateral cervical nuclei of cat, dog and man. J. Comp. Neurol., **139**: 93–104.

2585. TSCHIRGI, R. D. 1960. Chemical environment of the central nervous system. In J. FIELD (Editor), *Handbook of Physiology,* Section I, Vol. III. American Physiological Society, Washington, D.C., Ch. 78, 1865–1890.

2586. TSUBOKAWA, T., AND SUTIN, J. 1972. Pallidal and tegmental inhibition of oscillatory slow waves and unit activity in the subthalamic nucleus. Brain Res., **41**: 101–118.

2587. TSUKAHARA, N., TOYAMA K., AND KOSAKA, K. 1964. Intracellular recorded responses of the red nucleus neurons during antidromic and orthodromic activation. Experientia, **20**: 632–637.

2588. TSUKAHARA, N., TOYAMA, K., AND KOSAKA, K. 1967. Electrical activity of red nucleus neurones investigated with microelectrodes. Exp. Brain Res., **4**: 18–33.

2589. TUCHMANN-DUPLESSIS, H., AURONX, M., AND HAEGEL, P.. 1974. *Illustrated Human Embryology. Vol. 3, Nervous System and Endocrine Glands* (translated from French). Springer-Verlag, New York, 143 pp.

2590. TURNBULL, I. M. 1972. Blood supply of the spinal cord. In P. J. VINKEN AND G. W. BRUYN (Editors), *Handbook of Clinical Neurology,* Vol. 12. North-Holland Publishing Company, Amsterdam, pp. 478–491.

2591. TURNBULL, I. M. 1973. Blood supply of the spinal cord: Normal and pathological considerations. Clin. Neurosurg., **20**: 56–84.

2592. TUSA, R. J., ROSENQUIST, A. C., AND PALMER, L. A. 1979. Retinotopic organization of areas 18 and 19 in the cat. J. Comp. Neurol., **185**: 657–678.

2593. TWITCHELL, T. E. 1954. Sensory factors in purposive movement. J. Neurophysiol., **17**: 239–252.

2594. TYLER, D. B., AND BARD, P. 1949. Motion sickness. Physiol. Rev., **29**: 311–369.

2595. UEMURA, T., AND COHEN, B. 1973. Effects of vestibular nuclei lesions on vestibulo-ocular reflexes and posture in monkeys. Acta Otolaryngol [Suppl] (Stockh.), **315**: 1–71.

2596. UHL, G. R., GOODMAN, R. R., KUHAR, M. J., CHILDERS, S. R. AND SNYDER, S. H. 1979. Immunohistochemical mapping of enkephalin containing cell bodies, fibers and nerve terminals in the brain stem of the rat. Brain Res., **166**: 75–94.

2597. UHL, G. R., GOODMAN, R. R., AND SNYDER, S. H. 1979. Neurotensin-containing cell bodies, fibers and nerve terminals in the brain stem of the rat: Im-

munohistochemical mapping. Brain Res., **167**: 77–91.

2598. UNGERSTEDT, U. 1971. Stereotaxic mapping of the monoamine pathways in the rat brain. Acta Physiol. Scand. (Suppl.), **367**: 1–48.

2599. UNO, M., YOSHIDA, M., AND HIROTA, I. 1970. The mode of cerebello-thalamic relay transmission investigated with intracellular recordings from cells of the ventrolateral nucleus of cat's thalamus. Exp. Brain Res., **10**: 121–139.

2600. URSIN, H., AND KAADA, B. R. 1960. Functional localization within the amygdaloid complex in the cat. Electroencephalogr. Clin. Neurophysiol., **12**: 1–20.

2601. UZMAN, B. G., AND NOGUEIRA-GRAF, G. 1957. Electron microscope studies of the formation of nodes of Ranvier in mouse sciatic nerves. J. Biophys. Biochem. Cytol., **3**: 589–598.

2602. UZMAN, L. L. 1960. The histogenesis of the mouse cerebellum as studied by its tritiated thymidine uptake. J. Comp. Neurol., **114**: 137–159.

2603. VALENSTEIN, E. S., AND NAUTA, W. J. H. 1959. A comparison of the distribution of the fornix system in the rat, guinea pig, cat and monkey. J. Comp. Neurol., **113**: 337–363.

2604. VALVERDE, F. 1965. *Studies on the Piriform Lobe.* Harvard University Press, Cambridge, 131 pp.

2605. VANDESANDE, F., AND DIERICKX, K. 1979. The activated hypothalamic magnocellular neurosecretory system and the one neuron—one neurohypophysial hormone concept. Cell Tissue Res., **200**: 29–33.

2606. VATES, T. S., BONTING, S. L., AND OPPELT, W. W. 1964. Na-K activated adenosine triphosphatase formation of cerebrospinal fluid in the cat. Am. J. Physiol., **206**: 1165–1172.

2607. VAUGHN, J. E., AND PETERS, A. 1968. A third neuroglial cell type: An electron microscopic study. J. Comp. Neurol., **133**: 269–288.

2608. VEENING, J. G. 1978. Subcortical afferents of the amygdaloid complex in the rat: An HRP study. Neurosci. Lett., **8**: 197–202.

2609. VEHARA, Y., AND BURNSTOCK, G. 1970. Demonstration of "gap junctions" between smooth muscle cells. J. Cell Biol., **40**: 215–217.

2610. VELASCO, M., AND LINDSLEY, D. B. 1965. Role of orbital cortex in regulation of thalamo-cortical electrical activity. Science, **149**: 1375–1377.

2611. VELASCO, M. E., AND TALEISNIK, S. 1969. Release of gonadotropins induced by amygdaloid stimulation in the rat. Endocrinology, **84**: 132–139.

2612. VERHAART, W. J. C. 1935. Die aberrierenden Pyramidenfasern bei Menschen und Affen. Schweiz. Arch. Neurol. Neurochir. Psychiatr. **36**: 170–190.

2613. VERHAART, W. J. C. 1950. Fiber analysis of the basal ganglia. J. Comp. Neurol., **93**: 425–440.

2614. VERHAART, W. J. C. 1954. The tractus trigeminalis of Wallenberg. Acta Psychiat. Neurol. Scand., **290**: 269–279.

2615. VERHAART, W. J. C., AND KENNARD, M. A. 1940. Corticofugal degeneration following thermocoagulation of areas 4, 6, and 4S in *Macaca mulatta.* J. Anat., **74**: 239–254.

2616. VERHAART, W. J. C., AND KRAMER, W. 1952. The uncrossed pyramidal tract. Acta Psychiat. Neurol. Scand., **27**: 181–200.

2617. VERNEY, E. B. 1947. The antidiuretic hormone and factors which determine its release. Proc. R. Soc., Lond. (Biol.), **135**: 25–106.

2618. VICTOR, M. 1964. Functions of memory and learning in man and their relationship to lesions in the temporal lobe and diencephalon. In M. A. B. BRAZIER (Editor), *Brain Function,* Vol. III: *RNA in Brain Function; Memory and Learning,* American Institute of Biological Sciences, Washington, D. C.

2619. VICTOR, M., ANGEVINE, J. B., Jr., MANCALL, E. L., AND FISHER, C. M. 1961. Memory loss with lesions of hippocampal formation. Arch. Neurol., **5**: 244–263.

2620. VIGIER, D., AND ROUVIÈRE, A. 1979. Afferent and efferent connections of the area postrema demonstrated by the horseradish peroxidase method. Arch. Ital. Biol., **117:** 325–339.

2621. VIRCHOW, R. 1860. *Cellular Pathology.* Translated from the second German edition by F. Chance. Churchill, Ltd., London.

2622. VIZOSO, A. D., AND YOUNG, J. Z. 1948. Internode length and fibre diameter in developing and regenerating nerves. J. Anat., **82:** 110–134.

2623. VOGT, B. A., AND PANDYA, D. N. 1978. Cortico-cortical connections of somatic sensory cortex (areas 3, 1, and 2) in the rhesus monkey. J. Comp Neurol., **177:** 170–192.

2624. VOGT, B. A., ROSENE, D. L., AND PANDYA, D. N. 1979. Thalamic and cortical afferents differentiate anterior from posterior cingulate cortex in the monkey. Science, **204:** 205–207.

2625. VOGT, C., AND VOGT, O. 1919. Allgemeine Ergebnisse unserer Hirnforschung. Vierte Mitteilung: Die physiologische Bedeutung der architektonischen Rindenreizungen. J. Psychol. Neurol., **25:** 279–462.

2626. VONEIDA, T. J. 1960. An experimental study of the course and destination of fibers arising in the head of caudate nucleus in the cat and monkey. J. Comp Neurol., **115:** 75–87.

2627. VOOGD, J. 1964. *The Cerebellum of the Cat. Structure and Fibre Connexions.* Gorcum & Co. N. V., Assen, The Netherlands.

2628. VOSS, H. 1956. Zahl und Anordnung der Muskelspindeln in den oberen Zungenbeinmuskeln, im M. trapezius und M. latissimus dorsi. Anat. Anz., **103:** 443–446.

2629. VRAA-JENSEN, G. F. 1942. *The Motor Nucleus of the Facial Nerve, with a Survey of the Efferent Innervation of the Facial Muscles,* Thesis. Ejnar Munksgaard, Copenhagen 157pp.

2630. WAKSMAN, B. H. 1961. Experimental study of diphtheritic polyneuritis in the rabbit and guinea pig. III. The blood nerve barrier in the rabbit. J. Neuropathol. & Exp. Neurol., **20:** 35–77.

2631. WALBERG, F. 1952. Lateral reticular nucleus in medulla oblongata in mammals: Comparative-anatomical study. J. Comp. Neurol., **96:** 283–343.

2632. WALBERG, F. 1956. Descending connections to the inferior olive: An experimental study in the cat. J. Comp. Neurol., **104:** 77–173.

2633. WALBERG, F. 1957. Corticofugal fibres to the nuclei of the dorsal columns: An experimental study in the cat. Brain, **80:** 273–287.

2634. WALBERG, F. 1957*a.* Do the motor nuclei of the cranial nerves receive corticofugal fibres? An experimental study in the cat. Brain, **80:** 597–605.

2635. WALBERG, F. 1958. On the termination of rubrobulbar fibers: Experimental observations in the cat. J. Comp. Neurol., **110:** 66–73.

2636. WALBERG, F. 1958*a.* Descending connections to the lateral reticular nucleus: An experimental study in the cat. J. Comp. Neurol., **109:** 363–389.

2637. WALBERG, F. 1972. Cerebellovestibular relations: Anatomy. Prog. Brain Res., **37:** 361–376.

2638. WALBERG, F. 1974. Descending connections from the mesencephalon to the inferior olive: An experimental study in the cat. Exp. Brain Res., **21:** 145–156.

2639. WALBERG, F. 1974*a.* Crossed reticulo-reticular projections in the medulla, pons and mesencephalon: An autoradiographic study in the cat. Z. Anat. Entwickl. Gesch., **143:** 127–134.

2640. WALBERG, F., BOWSHER, D., AND BRODAL, A. 1958. The termination of primary vestibular fibers in the vestibular nuclei in the cat: An experimental study with silver methods. J. Comp. Neurol., **110:** 391–419.

2641. WALBERG, F., AND BRODAL, A. 1953. Spinopontine fibers in the cat: An experimental study. J. Comp. Neurol., **99:** 251–288.

2642. WALBERG F., HOLLÄNDER, H., AND GROFOVÁ, I. 1976. An autoradiographic identification of Purkinje axon terminals in the cat. J. Neurocytol., **5:** 157–169.

2643. WALBERG, F., AND JANSEN, J. 1961. Cerebellar corticovestibular fibers in the cat. Exp. Neurol., **3:** 32–52.

2644. WALBERG, F., KOTCHABHAKDI, N., AND HODDEVIK, G.

H. 1979. The olivocerebellar projections to the flocculus and paraflocculus in the cat, compared to the rabbit: A study using horseradish peroxidase as a tracer. Brain Res., **161:** 389–398.

2645. WALBERG, F., AND POMPEIANO, O. 1960. Fastigiofugal fibers to the lateral reticular nucleus. An experimental study in the cat. Exp. Neurol., **2:** 40–53.

2646. WALBERG, F., POMPEIANO, O., BRODAL, A., AND JANSEN, J. 1962. The fastigiovestibular projection in the cat: An experimental study with silver impregnation methods. J. Comp. Neurol., **118:** 49–75.

2646a. WALBERG, F., POMPEIANO, O., WESTRUM, L. E., AND HAUGLIE-HANSSEN, E. 1962. Fastigioreticular fibers in the cat. An experimental study with silver methods. J. Comp. Neurol., **119:** 187–199.

2647. WALD, G. 1968. Molecular basis of visual excitation. Science, **162:** 230–239.

2648. WALDEYER, W. 1891. Ueber einige neuere Forschungen im Gebiete der Antomie des Centralnervensystems. Dtsch. Med. Wochenschr., **17:** 1213–1218, 1244–1246, 1267–1269, 1287–1289, 1331–1332, 1352–1356.

2649. WALKER, A. E. 1936. An experimental study of the thalamocortical projection of the macaque monkey. J. Comp. Neurol., **64:** 1–39.

2650. WALKER, A. E. 1938. The thalamus of the chimpanzee. IV. Thalamic projections to the cerebral cortex. J. Anat., **73:** 37–93.

2651. WALKER, A. E. 1938*a. The Primate Thalamus.* University of Chicago Press, Chicago.

2652. WALKER, A. E. 1939. The origin, course and terminations of the secondary pathways of the trigeminal nerve in primates. J. Comp. Neurol., **71:** 59–89.

2653. WALKER, A. E. 1939*a.* Anatomy, physiology and surgical considerations of the spinal tract of the trigeminal nerve. J. Neurophysiol., **2:** 234–248.

2654. WALKER, A. E. 1942. Somatotopic localization of spinothalamic and secondary trigeminal tracts in mesencephalon. Arch. Neurol. Psychiatry, **48:** 884–889.

2655. WALKER, A. E. 1949. Afferent connections. In P. C. BUCY (Editor), *The Precentral Motor Cortex,* Ed. 2. University of Illinois, Urbana, Ch. 4, pp. 112–132.

2656. WALKER, A. E. 1959. Normal and pathological physiology of the thalamus. In G. SCHALTENBRAND AND P. BAILEY (Editors), *Introduction to Stereotaxis with an Atlas of the Human Brain,* Vol. I. Georg Thieme Verlag, Stuttgart, pp. 291–330.

2657. WALKER, A. E. 1966. Internal structure and afferent-efferent relations of the thalamus. In D. P. PURPURA AND M. D. YAHR (Editors), *The Thalamus.* Columbia University Press, New York, pp. 1–12.

2658. WALKER, A. E., AND FULTON, J. F. 1938. Hemidecortication in chimpanzee, baboon, macaque, potto, cat and coati: A study in encephalization. J. Nerv. Ment. Dis., **87:** 677–700.

2659. WALKER, A. E, AND WEAVER, T. A., JR. 1940. Ocular movements from the occipital lobe in the monkey. J. Neurophysiol., **3:** 353–357.

2660. WALKER, A. E., AND WEAVER, T. A., JR. 1942. The topical organization and termination of fibers in the posterior columns in *Macaca mulatta.* J. Comp. Neurol., **76:** 145–158.

2661. WALL, P. D. 1967. The laminar organization of dorsal horn and effects of descending impulses. J. Physiol. (Lond.), **188:** 403–423.

2662. WALL, P. D. 1978. The gate control theory of pain mechanisms: A re-examination and re-statement. Brain, **101:** 1–18.

2663. WALL, P. D., AND SWEET, W. H. 1967. Temporary abolition of pain in man. Science, **155:** 108–109.

2664. WALL, P. D., AND TAUB, A. 1962. Four aspects of the trigeminal nucleus and a paradox. J. Neurophysiol., **25:** 110–126.

2665. WALLENBERG, A. 1905. Die secondären Bahnen aus dem frontalen sensiblen Trigeminus Kerne des Kaninchens. Anat. Anz., **26:** 145–155.

2666. WALLS, G. L. 1963. *The Vertebrate Eye and Its Adaptive Radiation.* Hafner Publishing Company, New York (reprinted from 1942).

2667. WALSHE, F. M. R. 1942. The anatomy and physiology of cutaneous sensibility: A critical review. Brain, **65**: 48–114.

2668. WALTHER, J. B., AND RASMUSSEN, G. L. 1960. Descending connections of auditory cortex and thalamus of the cat. Fed. Proc., **19**: 291.

2669. WAMSLEY, J. K., LEWIS, M. S., YOUNG, W. S. III, AND KUHAR, M. J. 1981. Autoradiographic localization of muscarinic cholinergic receptors in rat brainstem. J. Neurosci., **I**: 176–191.

2670. WANG, S. C. 1955. Bulbar regulation of cardiovascular activity. In *Proceedings of the Annual Meeting of the Council for High Blood Pressure Research.* American Heart Association, New York, pp. 145–158.

2671. WARD, A. A., JR. 1948. The cingular gyrus: Area 24. J. Neurophysiol., **11**: 13–24.

2672. WARD, A. A., JR., AND MCCULLOCH, W. S. 1947. The projection of the frontal lobe on the hypothalamus. J. Neurophysiol., **10**: 309–314.

2673. WARR, W. B. 1966. Fiber degeneration following lesions in the anterior ventral cochlear nucleus of the cat. Exp. Neurol., **14**: 453–474.

2674. WARR, W. B. 1969. Fiber degeneration following lesions in the posteroventral cochlear nucleus of the cat. Exp. Neurol., **23**: 140–155.

2675. WARR, W. B. 1975. Olivocochlear and vestibular efferent neurons of the feline brain stem: Their location, morphology and number determined by retrograde axonal transport and acetylcholinesterase histochemistry. J. Comp. Neurol., **161**: 159–182.

2676. WARRINGTON, W. B., AND GRIFFITH, F. 1904. On the cells of the spinal ganglia and on the relationship of their histological structure to axonal distribution. Brain, **27**: 297–326.

2677. WARWICK, R. 1953. Representation of the extraocular muscles in the oculomotor nuclei of the monkey. J. Comp. Neurol., **98**: 449–504.

2678. WARWICK, R. 1953a. The identity of the posterocentral nucleus of Panegrossi. J. Comp. Neurol., **99**: 599–612.

2679. WARWICK, R. 1954. The ocular parasympathetic nerve supply and its mesencephalic sources. J. Anat., **88**: 71–93.

2680. WARWICK, R. 1955. The so-called nucleus of convergence. Brain, **78**: 92–114.

2681. WEBSTER, H. D. 1962. Transient, focal accumulation of axonal mitochondria during the early stages of Wallerian degeneration. J. Cell Biol., **12**: 361–377.

2682. WEBSTER, K. E. 1961. Cortico-striate interrelations in the albino rat. J. Anat., **95**: 532–544.

2683. WEBSTER, K. E. 1965. The cortico-striatal projection in the cat. J. Anat., **99**: 329–337.

2684. WEDDELL, G. 1941. The pattern of cutaneous innervation in relation to cutaneous sensibility. J. Anat., **75**: 346–367.

2685. WEDDELL, G., TAYLOR D. A., WILLIAMS, C. M. 1955. Studies on the innervation of skin. III. The patterned arrangement of the spinal sensory nerves to the rabbit ear. J. Anat., **89**: 317–342.

2686. WEIL, A., AND LASSEK, A. 1929. A quantitative distribution of the pyramidal tract in man. Arch. Neurol. Psychiatry, **22**: 495–510.

2687. WEINBERG, C., SANES, J. R., AND HALL, Z. 1981. Formation of neuromuscular junctions in adult rats: Accumulation of acetylcholine receptors, acetylcholinesterase, and components of the synaptic basal lamina. Dev. Biol., **84**: 255–266.

2688. WEINBERGER, L. M., AND GRANT, F. C. 1942. Experiences with intramedullary tractotomy. III. Studies in sensation. Arch. Neurol. Psychiatry, **48**: 355–381.

2689. WEINDL, A., AND SOFRONIEW, M. V. 1981. Relation of neuropeptides to mammalian circumventricular organs. In J. B. MARTIN, S. REICHLIN, AND K. L. BICK (Editors), *Advances in Biochemical Psychopharmacology*, Vol. 28: *Neurosecretion and Brain Peptides.* Raven Press, New York, pp. 303–320.

2690. WEISS, P. 1970. Neuronal dynamics and neuroplasmic flow. In F. D. Schmidt (Editor), *The Neurosci-*ences. Second Study Program. Rockfeller University Press, New York, pp. 840–850.

2691. WEISS, P., AND HISCOE, H. B. 1948. Experiments on the mechanism of nerve growth. J. Exp. Zool., **107**: 315–396.

2692. WEISS, P., AND WANG, H. 1936. Neurofibrils in living ganglion cells of the chick, cultivated *in vitro.* Anat. Rec., **67**: 105–117.

2693. WELCH, K. 1963. Secretion of cerebrospinal fluid by choroid plexus of the rabbit. Am. J. Physiol., **205**: 617–624.

2694. WELCH, K., AND FRIEDMAN, J. 1960. The cerebrospinal fluid valves. Brain, **83**: 454–469.

2695. WELCH, W. K., AND KENNARD, M. A. 1944. Relation of cerebral cortex to spasticity and flaccidity. J. Neurophysiol., **7**: 255–268.

2696. WERNER, G. W., AND WHITSEL, B. L. 1968. The topology of the body representation in somotosensory area I of primates. J. Neurophysiol., **31**: 856–869.

2697. WERNER, G. W., AND WHITSEL, B. L. 1973. Functional organization of the somatosensory cortex. In A. IGGO (Editor), *Handbook of Sensory Physiology*, Vol. 2. Springer-Verlag, Berlin, pp. 621–700.

2698. WESTERGAARD, E., AND BRIGHTMAN, M. W. 1973. Transport of proteins across normal cerebral arterioles. J. Comp. Neurol., **152**: 17–44.

2699. WHEATLEY, M. D. 1944. Hypothalamus and affective behavior in cats. Arch. Neurol. Psychiatry, **52**: 296–316.

2700. WHEATON, J. E., KRULICH, L., AND MCCANN, S. M. 1975. Localization of luteinizing hormone releasing hormone in the pre-optic area and hypothalamus of the rat using radioimmunoassay. Endocrinology, **97**: 30–38.

2701. WHITE, J. C., OKELBERRY, A. M., AND WHITELAW, G. P. 1936. Vasomotor tonus of the denervated artery. Arch. Neurol. α Psychiatry, **36**: 1251–1276.

2702. WHITE, L. E. 1965. Olfactory bulb projections of the rat. Anat. Rec., **152**: 465–480.

2703. WHITFIELD, I. C. 1967. *The Auditory Pathway.* Williams & Wilkins, Baltimore.

2704. WHITLOCK, D. G. 1952. A neurohistological and neurophysiological investigation of the afferent fiber tracts and the receptive areas of the avian cerebellum. J. Comp. Neurol., **97**: 567–636.

2705. WHITLOCK, D. G., AND NAUTA, W. J. H. 1956. Subcortical projections from the temporal neocortex in the *Macaca mulatta.* J. Comp. Neurol., **106**: 183–212.

2706. WHITLOCK, D. G., AND PERL, E. R. 1959. Afferent projections through ventrolateral funiculi to thalamus of cat. J. Neurophysiol., **22**: 133–148.

2707. WHITLOCK, D. G., AND PERL, E. R. 1961. Thalamic projections of spinothalamic pathways in monkey. Exp. Neurol., **3**: 240–255.

2708. WHITSEL, B. L., PETRUCELLI, L. M., AND WERNER, G. 1969. Symmetry and connectivity in the map of the body surface in somatosensory area II of primates. J. Neurophysiol., **32**: 170–183.

2709. WHITTAKER, V. P. 1965. The application of subcellular fractionation techniques to the study of brain function. Prog. Biophys. Chem., **15**: 39–96.

2710. WHITTIER, J. R. 1947. Ballism and the subthalamic nucleus (nucleus hypothalamicus; corpus Luysi). Arch. Neurol. Psychiatry, **58**: 672–692.

2711. WHITTIER, J. R., AND METTLER, F. A. 1949. Studies on the subthalamus of the rhesus monkey. I. Anatomy and fiber connections of the subthalamic nucleus of Luys. J. Comp. Neurol., **90**: 281–317.

2712. WHITTIER, J. R., AND METTLER, F. A. 1949a. Studies on the subthalamus of the rhesus monkey. II. Hyperkinesia and other physiologic effects of subthalamic lesions with special reference to the subthalmic nucleus of Luys. J. Comp. Neurol., **90**: 319–372.

2713. WICHMANN, R. 1900. *Die Rückenmarksnerven und ihre Segmentbezüge*, part 2. Viotto Salle, Berlin, pp. 151–279.

2714. WICKELGREN, B. G., AND STERLING, P. 1969. Influence of visual cortex on receptive fields in the superior colliculus of the cat. J. Neurophysiol., **32:** 16–32.

2715. DE WIED, D. 1980. Behavioral actions of neurohypophyseal peptides. Proc. R. Soc. Lond. (Biol.), **210:** 183–195.

2716. WIESEL, T. N., AND HUBEL, D. H. 1963. Effects of visual deprivation on morphology and physiology of cells in the cat's lateral geniculate body. J. Neurophysiol., **26:** 978–993.

2717. WIESEL, T. N., AND HUBEL, D. H. 1974. Ordered arrangement of orientation columns in monkeys lacking visual experience. J. Comp. Neurol., **158:** 307–318.

2718. WIESEL, T. N., HUBEL, D. H., AND LAM, D. M. K. 1974. Autoradiographic demonstration of ocular-dominance columns in the monkey striate cortex by means of transneuronal transport. Brain Res., **79:** 273–279.

2719. WIESENDANGER, M. 1973. Input from muscle and cutaneous nerves of the hand and forearm to neurones of the precentral gyrus of baboons and monkeys. J. Physiol. (Lond.), **228:** 203–219.

2720. WIESENDANGER, M. J., SÉGUIN, J. J., AND KÜNZLE, H. 1974. The supplementary motor area—a control system for posture. Adv. Behav. Biol., **7:** 331–346.

2721. WHITANEN, J. T. 1969. Selective silver impregnation of degenerating axons and axon terminals in the central nervous system of the monkey (*Macaca mulatta*). Brain Res., **14:** 546–548.

2722. WILLIAMS, T. H. 1967. Electron microscopic evidence for an autonomic interneuron. Nature, **214:** 309–310.

2723. WILLIAMS, T. H., BLACK, A. C., CHIBA, T., AND JEW, J. Y. 1977. Species differences in mammalian SIF cells. In E. COSTA AND G. L., GESSA, (Editors), *Advances in Biochemical Psychopharmacology.* Vol. 16, Raven Press, New York, pp. 505–511.

2724. WILLIS, W. 1977. Visceral pain. In F. P. BROOKS, AND P. W. EVERS (Editors), *Nerves and the Gut,* Charles B. Slack, Inc., Thorofare, N. J., pp. 350–364.

2725. WILLIS, W. D., AND COGGESHALL, R. E. 1978. *Sensory Mechanisms of the Spinal Cord.* Plenum Press, New York.

2725a. WILLIS, W. D., JR., AND GROSSMAN, R. G. 1981. *Medical Neurobiology,* 3rd Edition, The C. V. Mosby Company, St. Louis, 593 pp.

2726. WILLIS, W. D., HABER, L. H., AND MARTIN, R. F. 1977. Inhibition of spinothalamic tract cells and interneurons by brainstem stimulation in the monkey. J. Neurophysiol., **40:** 968–981.

2727. WILLIS, W. D., LEONARD, R. B., AND KENSHALO, D. R., JR. 1978. Spinothalamic tract neurons in the substantia gelatinosa. Science, **202:** 986–988.

2728. WILLIS, W. D., TREVINO, D. L., COULTER, J. D., AND MAUNZ, R. A. 1974. Responses of primate spinothalamic tract neurons to natural stimulation of hindlimb. J. Neurophysiol., **37:** 358–372.

2729. WILLIS, W. D., AND WILLIS, J. C. 1964. Location of Renshaw Cells. Science, **204:** 1214–1215.

2730. WILLIS, W. D., AND WILLIS, J. C. 1966. Properties of interneurons in the ventral spinal cord. Arch Ital. Biol., **104:** 354–386.

2731. WILSON, M. E., AND CRAGG, B. G. 1967. Projection from the lateral geniculate nucleus in the cat and monkey. J. Anat., **101:** 677–692.

2732. WILSON, M. E., AND TOYNE, M. J. 1970. Retino-tectal and cortico-tectal projections in *Macaca mulatta.* Brain Res., **24:** 395–406.

2733. WILSON, R. C., LEVY, W. B., AND STEWARD, O. 1979. Functional effects of lesion-induced plasticity: Long term potentiation in normal and lesion-induced temporodentate connections. Brain Res., **176:** 65–78.

2734. WILSON, R. C., AND STEWARD, O. 1978. Polysynaptic activation of the dentate gyrus of the hippocampal formation: An olfactory input via the lateral entorhinal cortex. Exp. Brain Res., **33:** 523–534.

2735. WILSON, S. A. K. 1912. Progressive lenticular degeneration: A familial nervous disease associated with cirrhosis of the liver. Brain, **34:** 295–509.

2736. WILSON, S. A. K. 1914. An experimental research into the anatomy and physiology of the corpus striatum. Brain, **36:** 427–492.

2737. WILSON, S. A. K. 1925. Disorders of motility and muscle tone with special reference to the corpus striatum (Croonian Lectures). Lancet, **2:** 215–291.

2738. WILSON, S. A. K. 1928. *Modern Problems in Neurology.* Edward Arnold Publishers, Ltd., London.

2739. WILSON, V. J., AND PETERSON, B. W. 1978. Peripheral and central substrates of vestibulospinal reflexes. Physiol. Rev., **58:** 80–105.

2740. WILSON, V. J., UCHINO, Y., MAUNZ, R. A., SUSSWEIN, A., AND FUKUSHIMA, K. 1978. Properties and connections of cat fastigiospinal neurons. Exp. Brain Res., **32:** 1–17.

2741. WILSON, V. J., UCHINO, Y., SUSSWEIN, A., AND FUKUSHIMA, K. 1977. Properties of direct fastigiospinal fibers in the cat. Brain Res., **126:** 543–546.

2742. WILSON, V. J., AND YOSHIDA, M. 1969. Monosynaptic inhibition of neck motoneurons by the medial vestibular nucleus. Exp. Brain Res., **9:** 365–380.

2743. WILSON, W. S., SCHULZ, R. A., AND COOPER, J. R. 1973. The isolation of cholinergic synaptic vesicles from bovine superior cervical ganglion and estimations of their acetylcholine content. J. Neurochem., **20:** 659–667.

2744. WINDLE, W. F. 1926. Non-bifurcating nerve fibers of the trigeminal nerve. J. Comp. Neurol., **40:** 229–240.

2745. WINDLE, W. F. 1931. Neurons of the sensory type in the ventral roots of man and of other mammals. Arch. Neurol. Psychiatry, **26:** 791–800.

2746. WINDLE, W. F. (Editor). 1955. *Regeneration in the Central Nervous System.* Charles C Thomas, Publisher, Springfield, Ill., 311 pp.

2747. WINDLE, W. F. (Editor). 1957. *New Research Techniques of Neuroanatomy.* Charles C Thomas, Publisher, Springfield, Ill.

2748. WINDLE, W. F. (Editor). 1958. *Biology of Neuroglia.* Charles C Thomas, Publisher, Springfield, Ill., 340 pp.

2749. WINDLE, W. F., AND CHAMBERS, W. W. 1950. Regeneration in the spinal cord of the cat and dog. J. Comp. Neurol., **93:** 241–257.

2750. WINER, J. A., DIAMOND, I. T., AND RACZKOWSKI, D. Subdivisions of the auditory cortex in the cat: The retrograde transport of horseradish peroxidase to the medial geniculate body and posterior thalamic nuclei. J Comp. Neurol., **176:** 387–418.

2751. WINKLER, C. 1918–1933. *Opera omnia,* Vols. 1 to 10. E. F. Bohn, Haarlem, the Netherlands.

2752. WINTER, D. L. 1965. N. gracilis of cat: Functional organization and corticofugal effects. J. Neurophysiol., **28:** 48–70.

2753. WISCHNITZER, S. 1960. The ultrastructure of the nucleus and nucleocytoplasmic relations. Int. Rev. Cytol., **10:** 137–162.

2754. WISE, S. P., AND TANJI, J. 1981. Supplementary and precentral motor cortex: Contrast in responsiveness to peripheral input in the hindlimb area of the unanesthetized monkey. J. Comp. Neurol., **195:** 433–451.

2755. WISLOCKI, G. B., AND LEDUC, E. 1953. The cytology and histochemistry of the subcommissural organ and Reissner's fibers in rodents. J. Comp. Neurol., **97:** 515–543.

2756. WITELSON, S. F., AND POLLIE, W. 1973. Left hemisphere specialization for language in the newborn: Neuroanatomical evidence of asymmetry. Brain, **96:** 641–646.

2757. WOLF, G., AND SUTIN, J. 1966. Fiber degeneration after lateral hypothalamic lesions in the rat. J. Comp. Neurol., **127:** 137–156.

2758. WOLF, G. A., JR. 1941. The ratio of preganglionic neurons to postganglionic neurons in the visceral nervous system. J. Comp. Neurol., **75:** 235–243.

2759. WOLFE, D. E., POTTER, L. T., RICHARDSON, K. C., AND AXELROD, J. 1962. Localizing tritiated norepinephrine in sympathetic axons by electron microscopic autoradiography. Science, **138:** 440–442.

2760. WONG-RILEY, M. T. T. 1972. Changes in the dorsal lateral geniculate nucleus of the squirrel monkey after unilateral ablation of the visual cortex. J. Comp. Neurol., **146:** 519–548.

2761. WONG-RILEY, M. T. T. 1974. Demonstration of geniculocortical and callosal projection neurons in the squirrel monkey by means of retrograde axonal transport of horseradish peroxidase. Brain Res., **79:** 267–272.

2762. WONG-RILEY, M. T. T. 1976. Projections from the dorsal lateral geniculate nucleus to prestriate cortex in the squirrel monkey as demonstrated by retrograde transport of horseradish peroxidase. Brain Res., **109:** 595–600.

2763. WONG-RILEY, M. T. T. 1979. Columnar cortico-cortical interconnections within the visual system of the squirrel and macaque monkeys. Brain Res., **162:** 201–217.

2764. WOODBURNE, R. T. 1936. A phylogenetic consideration of the primary and secondary centers and connections of the trigeminal complex in a series of vertebrates. J. Comp. Neurol., **65:** 403–501.

2765. WOODBURNE, R. T., CROSBY, E. C., AND MCCOTTER, R. E. 1946. The mammalian midbrain and isthmus regions. Part II. The fiber connections. A. The relations of the tegmentum of the midbrain with the basal ganglia in *Macaca mulatta.* J. Comp. Neurol., **85:** 67–92.

2766. WOODBURY, D. M. 1958. Symposium discussion. In W. F. WINDLE, (Editor), *Biology of Neuroglia.* Charles C. Thomas, Publisher, Springfield, Ill., pp. 120–127.

2767. WOOLEY, D. W., AND SHAW, E. 1954. A biochemical and pharmacological suggestion about certain mental disorders. Proc. Natl. Acad. Sci. U. S. A., **40:** 228–231.

2768. WOOLLARD, H. H. 1935. Observations on the terminations of cutaneous nerves. Brain, **58:** 352–367.

2769. WOOLLARD, H. H., AND HARPMAN, J. A. 1940. The connections of the inferior colliculus and dorsal nucleus of the lateral lemniscus. J. Anat. **74:** 441–458.

2770. WOOLSEY, C. N. 1947. Patterns of sensory representation in the cerebral cortex. Fed. Proc., **6:** 437–441.

2771. WOOLSEY, C. N. 1958. Organization of somatic sensory and motor areas of the cerebral cortex. In H. F. HARLOW AND C. N. WOOLSEY (Editors), *Biological and Biochemical Bases of Behavior.* University of Wisconsin, Madison, pp. 63–81.

2772. WOOLSEY, C. N. 1960. Organization of cortical auditory system: A review and synthesis. In G. L. RAMUSSEN AND W. F. WINDLE (Editors), *Neural Mechanisms of the Auditory and Vestibular Systems.* Charles C Thomas, Publisher, Springfield, Ill., pp. 165–180.

2773. WOOLSEY, C. N. 1971. Tonotopic organization of the auditory cortex. In M. B. SACHS (Editor), *Physiology of the Auditory System.* A Workshop. National Consultants, Inc., Baltimore, pp. 271–282.

2774. WOOLSEY, C. N. 1975. Cortical motor map of *Macaca mulatta* after chronic section of the medullary pyramid. In K. J. ZULCH, O. CREUTZFELDT, AND G. C. GALBRAITH (Editors), *Cerebral Localization.* Springer-Verlag, Berlin, pp. 19–31.

2775. WOOLSEY, C. N., AND FAIRMAN, D. 1946. Contralateral, ipsilateral and bilateral representation of cutaneous receptors in somatic areas I and II of the cerebral cortex of pigs, sheep and other mammals. Surgery, **19:** 684–702.

2776. WOOLSEY, C. N., GORSKA, T., WETZEL, A., ERICKSON, T. C., EARLS, F. J., AND ALLMAN, J. M. 1972. Complete unilateral section of the pyramidal tract at the medullary level in *Macaca mulatta.* Brain Res., **40:** 119–124.

2777. WOOLSEY, C. N., SETTLAGE, P. H., MEYER, D. R., SENCER, W., HAMUY, T. P., AND TRAVIS, A. M. 1951. Patterns of localization in precentral and "supplementary" motor areas and their relation to the concept of a premotor area. Proc. Assoc. Nerv. Ment. Dis., **30:** 238–264.

2778. WOOLSEY, C. N., AND WALZL, E. M. 1942. Topical projection of nerve fibers from local regions of the cochlea to the cerebral cortex of the cat. Bull. Johns Hopkins Hosp., **71:** 315–344.

2779. WURTMAN, R. J. 1971. Brain monamines and endocrine function. Neurosci. Res. Program Bull., **9:** 177–297.

2780. WYBURN, G. M. 1958. The capsule of spinal ganglion cells. J. Anat., **92:** 528–533.

2781. WYCIS, H. T., AND SPIEGEL, E. A. 1952. Ansotomy in paralysis agitans. Confin. Neurol., **12:** 245–246.

2782. WYSOCKI, C. J. 1979. Neurobehavioral evidence for the involvement of the vomeronasal system in mammalian reproduction. Neurosci. Behav. Rev., **3:** 301–341.

2783. YAKOVLEV, P. I., LOCKE, S., AND ANGEVINE, J. B. JR. 1966. The limbus of the cerebral hemisphere, limbic nuclei of the thalamus and the cingulum bundle. In D. P. PURPURA AND M. D. YAHR (Editors), *The Thalamus.* Columbia University Press, New York, pp. 77–97.

2784. YOSHIDA, M., YAJIMA, K., AND UNO, M. 1966. Different activation of the two types of the pyramidal tract neurons through the cerebello-thalamocortical pathway. Experientia, **22:** 331–332.

2785. YOUNG, J. Z. 1942. The functional repair of nervous tissue. Physiol. Rev., **23:** 318–374.

2786. YOUNG, J. Z. 1949. Factors influencing the regeneration of nerves. Adv. Surg., **1:** 165–220.

2787. ZABORSKY, I., FEMINGER, A., AND PALKOVITS, M. 1979. Afferent brain stem connections of the central amygdaloid nucleus. Verh. Anat. Ges., **73:** 1117–1120.

2788. ZACKS, S. I. 1964. *The Motor Endplate.* W. B. Saunders, Philadelphia, pp. 1–83.

2789. ZACZEK, R., SCHWARCZ, R., AND COYLE, J. T. 1978. Long term sequelae of striatal kainate lesion. Brain Res., **152:** 626–632.

2790. ZANGWILL, O. L. 1969. *Cerebral Dominance and Its Relation to Psychological Function.* Charles C Thomas Publisher, Springfield, Ill., 31 pp.

2791. ZARZECKI, P., STRICK, P. L., AND ASANUMA, H. 1978. Input to primate motor cortex from posterior parietal cortex (area 5). II. Identification by antidromic activation. Brain Res., **157:** 331–335.

2792. ZBROŻYNA, A. W. 1972. The organization of the defence reaction elicited from amygdala and its connections. In B. E. ELEFTHERIOU (Editor), *The Neurobiology of the Amygdala,* Plenum Press, New York, p. 597–606.

2793. ZEAL, A. A., AND RHOTON, A. L. 1978. Microsurgical anatomy of the posterior cerebral artery. J. Neurosurg., **48:** 534–559.

2794. ZEKI, S. M. 1971. Interhemispheric connections of prestriate cortex in monkeys. Brain Res., **19:** 63–75.

2795. ZEMLAN, F. P., AND PFAFF, D. W. 1979. Topographical organization in medullary reticulospinal systems as demonstrated by the horseradish peroxidase technique. Brain Res., **174:** 161–166.

2796. ZIMMERMAN, E. A., CHAMBERS, W. W., AND LIU, C. N. 1964. An experimental study of the anatomical organization of the cortico-bulbar system in the albino rat. J. Comp. Neurol., **123:** 301–324.

2797. ZIMMERMAN, H. M. 1969. Brain tumors: Their incidence and classification in man and their experimental production. Ann. N. Y. Acad. Sci., **159:** 337–359.

2798. ZIMMERMAN, H. M. 1971. The ten most common types of brain tumor. Semin. Roentgenol., **6:** 48–58.

2799. ZIMMERMAN, H. 1979. Vesicle recycling and transmitter release. Neuroscience, **4:** 1773–1804.

2800. ZOLOVICK, A. J. 1972. Effects of lesions and electrical stimulation of the amygdala on hypothalamic-hypophyseal regulation. In B. E. ELEFTHERIOU (Editor), *The Neurobiology of the Amygdala.* Plenum Press, New York, pp. 643–683.

2801. ZOTTERMAN, Y. 1939. Touch, pain and tickling: An electrophysiological investigation on cutaneous sensory nerves. J. Physiol. (Lond.), **95:** 1–28.

2802. ZÜLCH, K. J. 1954. Mangeldurchblutung an der Grenzzone zweier Gefässgebiete als Ursache bisher ungeklärter Rückenmarksschädigungen. Dtsch. Z. Nervenheilk., **172:** 81–101.

Atlas of Brain and Brain Stem

SECTION I
Transverse sections of Brain Stem (A–1 to A–13).

SECTION II
Frontal sections cut transverse to the longitudinal axis of the diencephalon (A–14 to A–18).

SECTION III
Frontal sections of diencephalon and basal ganglia (A–19 to A–24).

SECTION IV
Sagittal sections of brain and brain stem (A–25 to A–32).

The following series of drawings of transverse sections of the brain stem taken at critical levels are reproduced in colors that faithfully reveal the definition of fiber tracts and cellular groupings characteristic of the original preparations. These sections, stained with luxol fast blue and counterstained with cresyl violet (1334), appear particularly appropriate for laboratory instruction since the student is presented with a complete picture of cellular configurations in relationship with the myelinated fiber tracts in a single microscopic slide. The outline drawing of the brain stem indicates the levels and planes of section of the individual figures and should be used as a key. The magnification of the figures is noted in the legends.

Illustrations used in Sections I, II and III were prepared by Miss Marjorie Stodgell, Medical Artist, of the Hahnemann Medical College and Hospital of Philadelphia. Photographs used in Section IV were made from original Weigert preparations of the late Professor Andrew T. Rasmussen of the University of Minnesota.

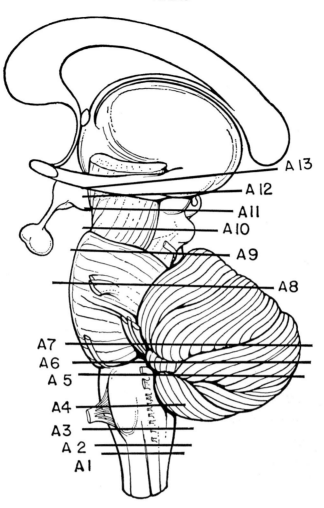

Brain Stem Atlas

Drawing of the brain stem indicating the level and plane of sections A-1 through A-13.

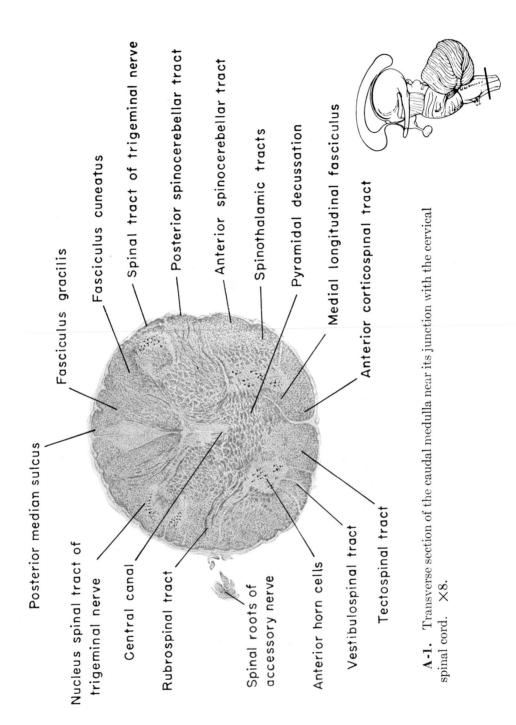

Posterior median sulcus

Fasciculus gracilis

Fasciculus cuneatus

Spinal tract of trigeminal nerve

Posterior spinocerebellar tract

Anterior spinocerebellar tract

Spinothalamic tracts

Pyramidal decussation

Medial longitudinal fasciculus

Anterior corticospinal tract

Nucleus spinal tract of trigeminal nerve

Central canal

Rubrospinal tract

Spinal roots of accessory nerve

Anterior horn cells

Vestibulospinal tract

Tectospinal tract

A-1. Transverse section of the caudal medulla near its junction with the cervical spinal cord. ×8.

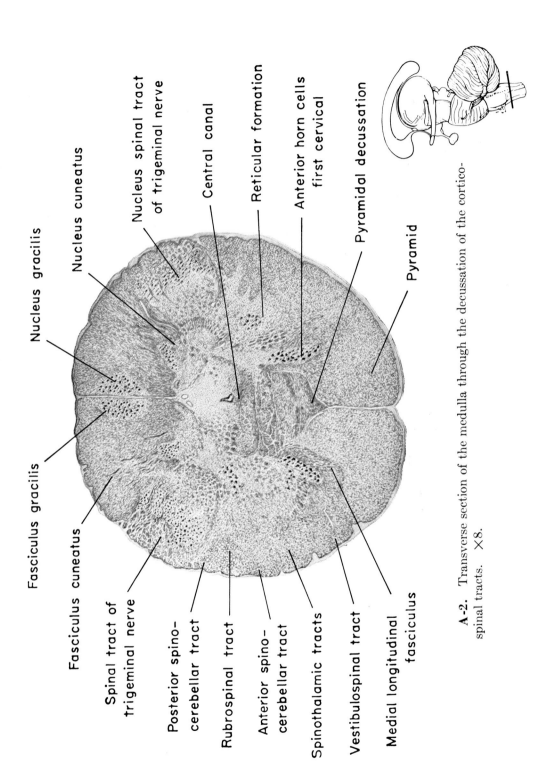

Nucleus gracilis

Nucleus cuneatus

Nucleus spinal tract of trigeminal nerve

Central canal

Reticular formation

Anterior horn cells first cervical

Pyramidal decussation

Pyramid

Fasciculus gracilis

Fasciculus cuneatus

Spinal tract of trigeminal nerve

Posterior spino-cerebellar tract

Rubrospinal tract

Anterior spino-cerebellar tract

Spinothalamic tracts

Vestibulospinal tract

Medial longitudinal fasciculus

A-2. Transverse section of the medulla through the decussation of the cortico-spinal tracts. ×8.

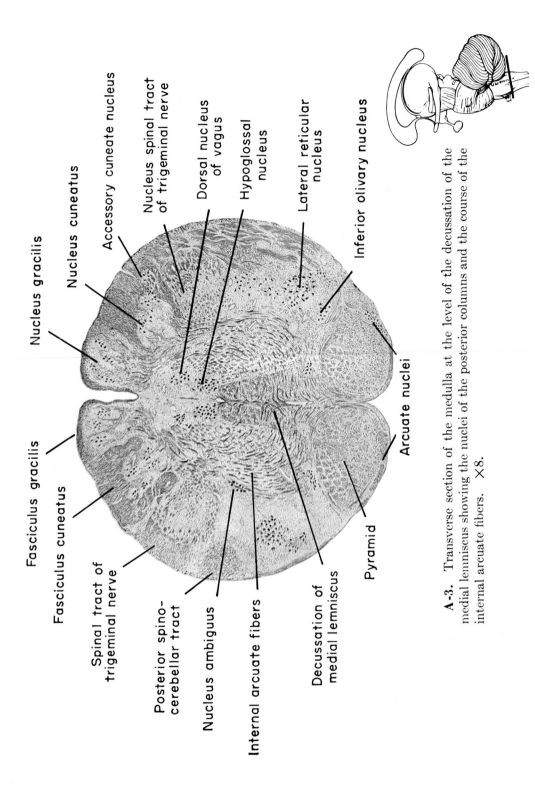

A-3. Transverse section of the medulla at the level of the decussation of the medial lemniscus showing the nuclei of the posterior columns and the course of the internal arcuate fibers. ×8.

Labels:
Nucleus gracilis
Nucleus cuneatus
Accessory cuneate nucleus
Nucleus spinal tract of trigeminal nerve
Dorsal nucleus of vagus
Hypoglossal nucleus
Lateral reticular nucleus
Inferior olivary nucleus
Fasciculus gracilis
Fasciculus cuneatus
Spinal tract of trigeminal nerve
Posterior spino-cerebellar tract
Nucleus ambiguus
Internal arcuate fibers
Decussation of medial lemniscus
Pyramid
Arcuate nuclei

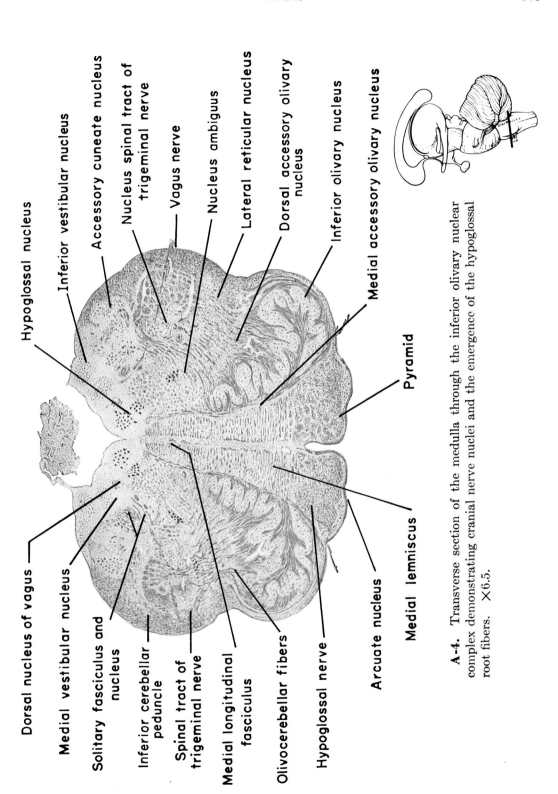

Dorsal nucleus of vagus

Medial vestibular nucleus

Solitary fasciculus and nucleus

Inferior cerebellar peduncle

Spinal tract of trigeminal nerve

Medial longitudinal fasciculus

Olivocerebellar fibers

Hypoglossal nerve

Arcuate nucleus

Medial lemniscus

Hypoglossal nucleus

Inferior vestibular nucleus

Accessory cuneate nucleus

Nucleus spinal tract of trigeminal nerve

Vagus nerve

Nucleus ambiguus

Lateral reticular nucleus

Dorsal accessory olivary nucleus

Inferior olivary nucleus

Medial accessory olivary nucleus

Pyramid

A-4. Transverse section of the medulla through the inferior olivary nuclear complex demonstrating cranial nerve nuclei and the emergence of the hypoglossal root fibers. ×6.5.

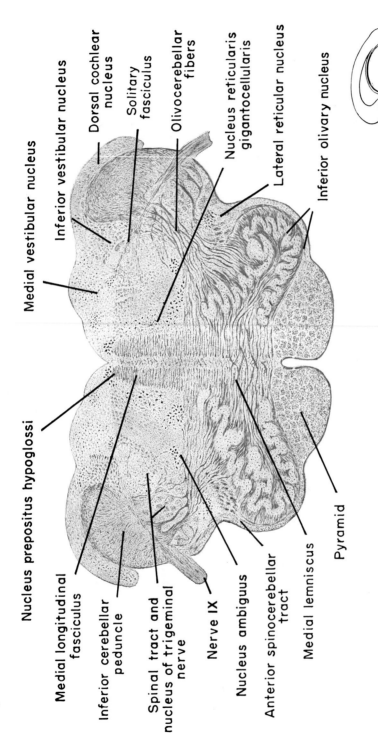

Nucleus prepositus hypoglossi

Medial vestibular nucleus

Inferior vestibular nucleus

Dorsal cochlear nucleus

Solitary fasciculus

Olivocerebellar fibers

Nucleus reticularis gigantocellularis

Lateral reticular nucleus

Inferior olivary nucleus

Medial longitudinal fasciculus

Inferior cerebellar peduncle

Spinal tract and nucleus of trigeminal nerve

Nerve IX

Nucleus ambiguus

Anterior spinocerebellar tract

Medial lemniscus

Pyramid

A-5. Transverse section of the full development of the medulla showing the glossopharyngeal nerve, the vestibular nuclei in the floor of the fourth ventricle, and the dorsal cochlear nuclei. ×6.5

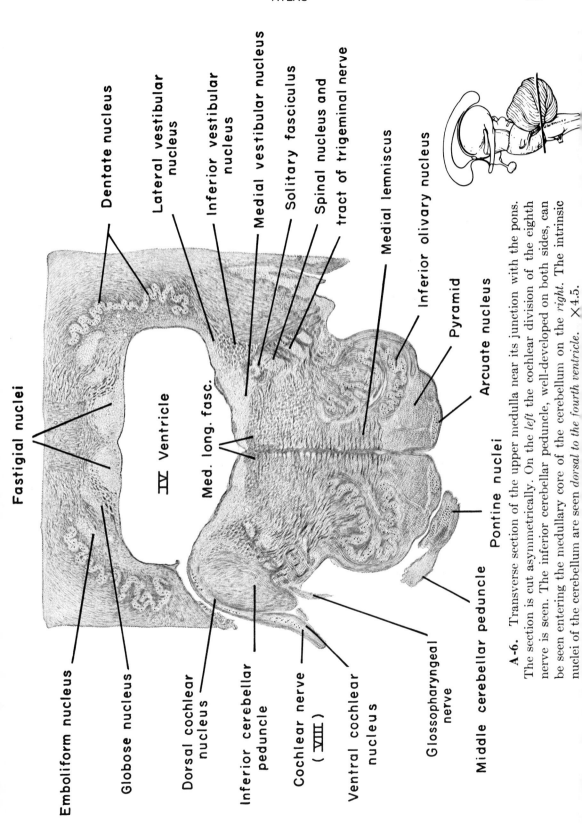

Fastigial nuclei

Emboliform nucleus

Globose nucleus

Dentate nucleus

Lateral vestibular nucleus

Inferior vestibular nucleus

Medial vestibular nucleus

Solitary fasciculus

Spinal nucleus and tract of trigeminal nerve

Medial lemniscus

Inferior olivary nucleus

Ventricle

Med. long. fasc.

IV Ventricle

Dorsal cochlear nucleus

Inferior cerebellar peduncle

Cochlear nerve (VIII)

Ventral cochlear nucleus

Glossopharyngeal nerve

Middle cerebellar peduncle

Pontine nuclei

Arcuate nucleus

Pyramid

A-6. Transverse section of the upper medulla near its junction with the pons. The section is cut asymmetrically. On the *left* the cochlear division of the eighth nerve is seen. The inferior cerebellar peduncle, well-developed on both sides, can be seen entering the medullary core of the cerebellum on the *right*. The intrinsic nuclei of the cerebellum are seen *dorsal to the fourth ventricle*. ×4.5.

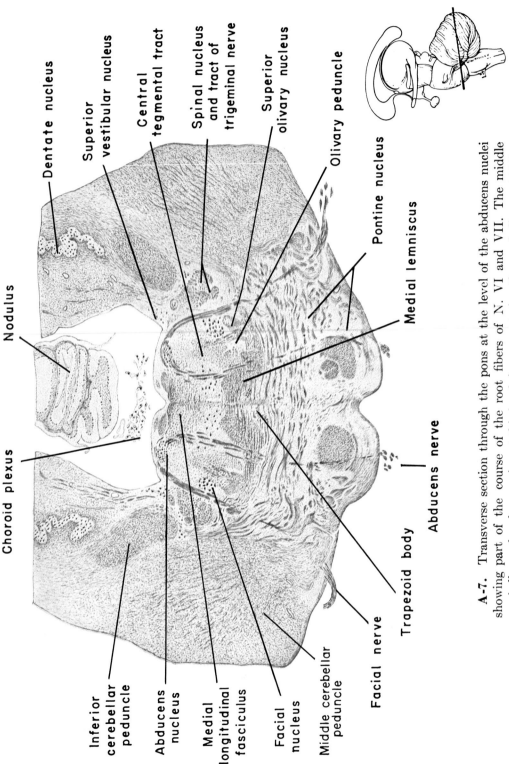

Dentate nucleus

Superior vestibular nucleus

Central tegmental tract

Spinal nucleus and tract of trigeminal nerve

Superior olivary nucleus

Olivary peduncle

Pontine nucleus

Medial lemniscus

Nodulus

Choroid plexus

Abducens nerve

Inferior cerebellar peduncle

Abducens nucleus

Medial longitudinal fasciculus

Facial nucleus

Middle cerebellar peduncle

Facial nerve

Trapezoid body

A-7. Transverse section through the pons at the level of the abducens nuclei showing part of the course of the root fibers of N. VI and VII. The middle cerebellar peduncle, massive at this level, is seen entering the cerebellum. ×4.5.

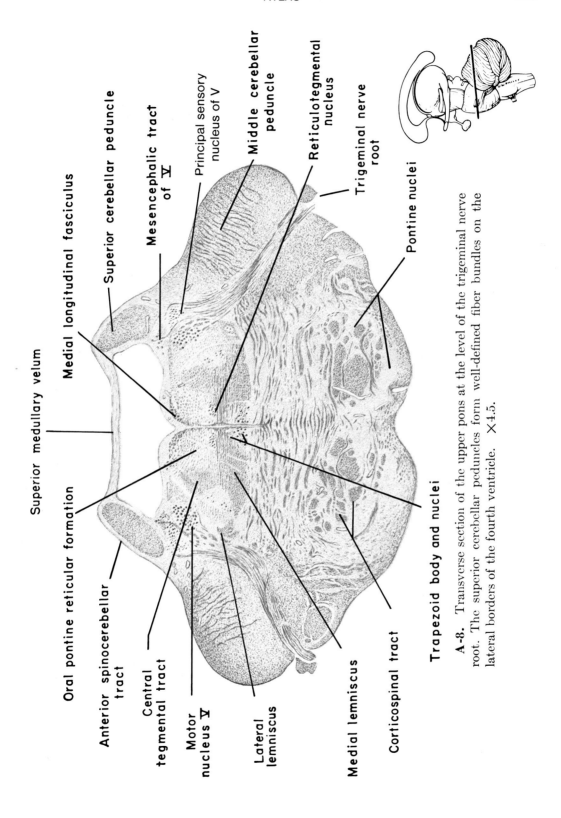

Superior medullary velum

Medial longitudinal fasciculus

Superior cerebellar peduncle

Mesencephalic tract of Ⅴ

Principal sensory nucleus of V

Middle cerebellar peduncle

Reticulotegmental nucleus

Trigeminal nerve root

Pontine nuclei

Oral pontine reticular formation

Anterior spinocerebellar tract

Central tegmental tract

Motor nucleus Ⅴ

Lateral lemniscus

Medial lemniscus

Corticospinal tract

Trapezoid body and nuclei

A-8. Transverse section of the upper pons at the level of the trigeminal nerve root. The superior cerebellar peduncles form well-defined fiber bundles on the lateral borders of the fourth ventricle. ×4.5.

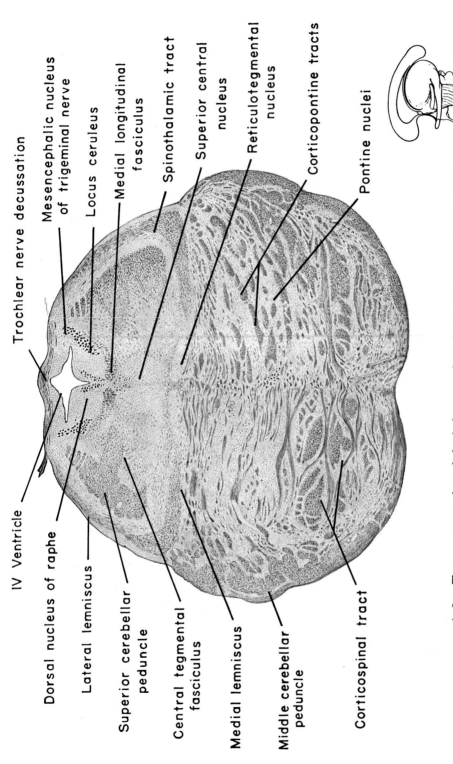

Trochlear nerve decussation

Mesencephalic nucleus of trigeminal nerve

Locus ceruleus

Medial longitudinal fasciculus

Spinothalamic tract

Superior central nucleus

Reticulotegmental nucleus

Corticopontine tracts

Pontine nuclei

IV Ventricle

Dorsal nucleus of raphe

Lateral lemniscus

Superior cerebellar peduncle

Central tegmental fasciculus

Medial lemniscus

Middle cerebellar peduncle

Corticospinal tract

A-9. Transverse section of the isthmus region of the brain stem. Root fibers of the trochlear nerves can be seen decussating in the superior medullary velum. ×4.5.

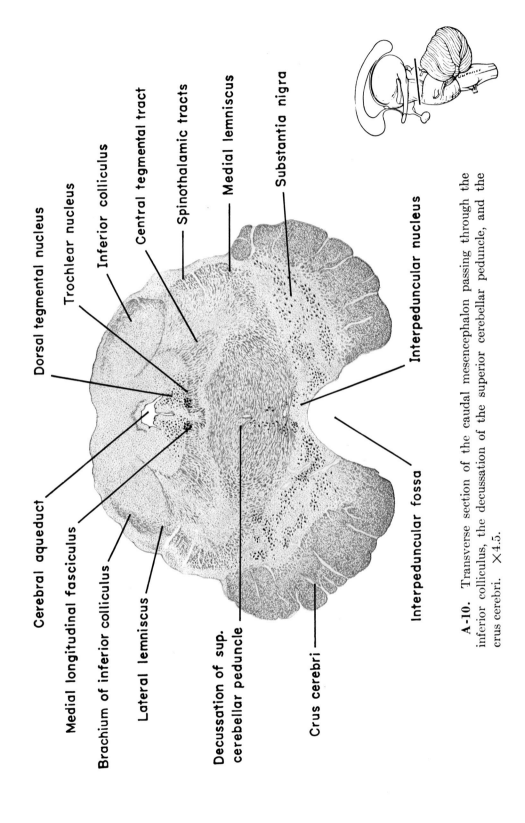

Dorsal tegmental nucleus

Trochlear nucleus

Inferior colliculus

Central tegmental tract

Spinothalamic tracts

Medial lemniscus

Substantia nigra

Cerebral aqueduct

Medial longitudinal fasciculus

Brachium of inferior colliculus

Lateral lemniscus

Decussation of sup. cerebellar peduncle

Crus cerebri

Interpeduncular fossa

Interpeduncular nucleus

A-10. Transverse section of the caudal mesencephalon passing through the inferior colliculus, the decussation of the superior cerebellar peduncle, and the crus cerebri. ×4.5.

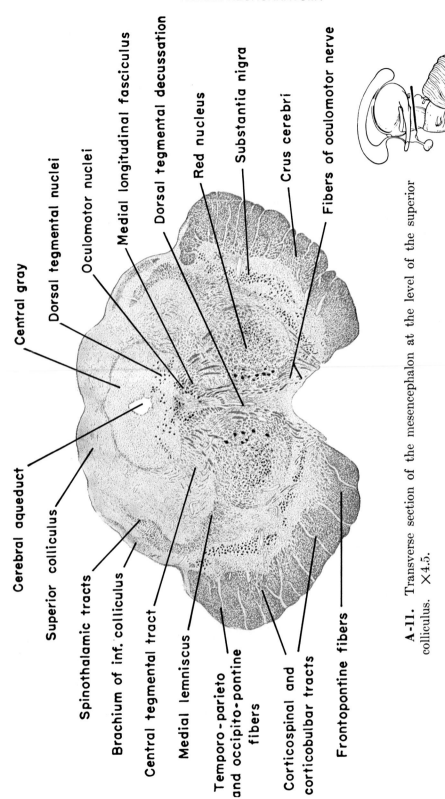

Central gray

Cerebral aqueduct

Superior colliculus

Spinothalamic tracts

Brachium of inf. colliculus

Central tegmental tract

Medial lemniscus

Temporo-parieto
and occipito-pontine
fibers

Corticospinal and
corticobulbar tracts

Frontopontine fibers

Dorsal tegmental nuclei

Oculomotor nuclei

Medial longitudinal fasciculus

Dorsal tegmental decussation

Red nucleus

Substantia nigra

Crus cerebri

Fibers of oculomotor nerve

A-11.   Transverse section of the mesencephalon at the level of the superior colliculus. ×4.5.

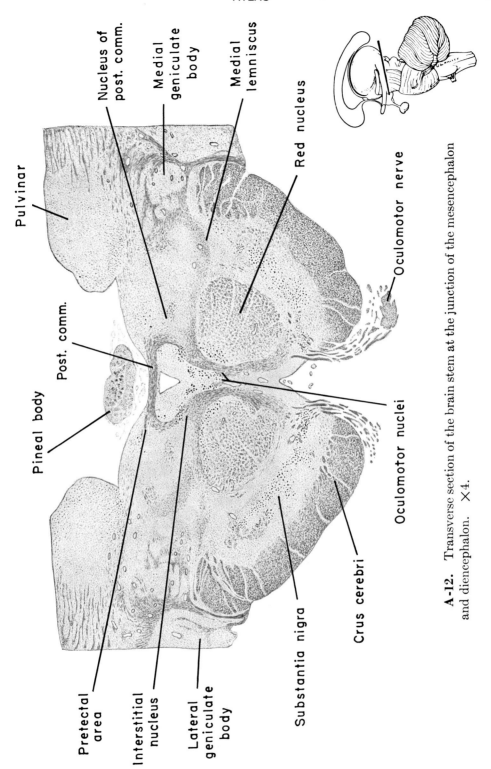

Pulvinar

Nucleus of post. comm.

Medial geniculate body

Medial lemniscus

Red nucleus

Oculomotor nerve

Post. comm.

Pineal body

Oculomotor nuclei

Pretectal area

Interstitial nucleus

Lateral geniculate body

Substantia nigra

Crus cerebri

A-12. Transverse section of the brain stem at the junction of the mesencephalon and diencephalon. ×4.

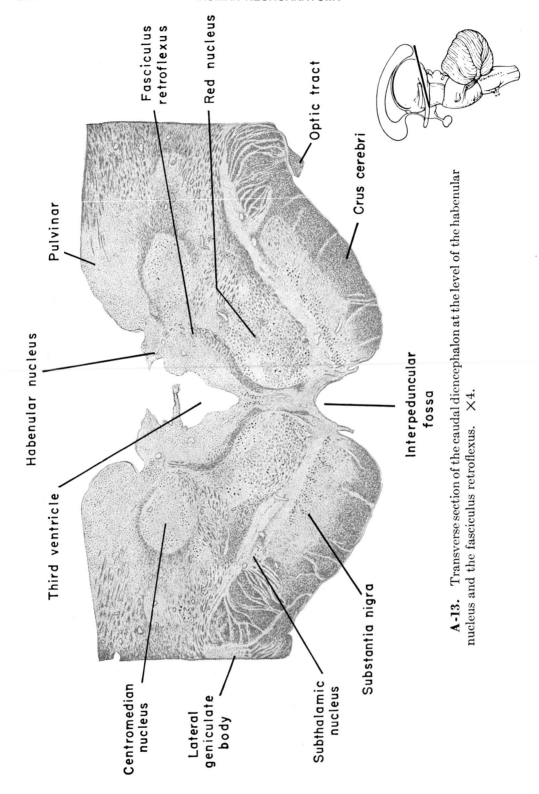

A-13. Transverse section of the caudal diencephalon at the level of the habenular nucleus and the fasciculus retroflexus. ×4.

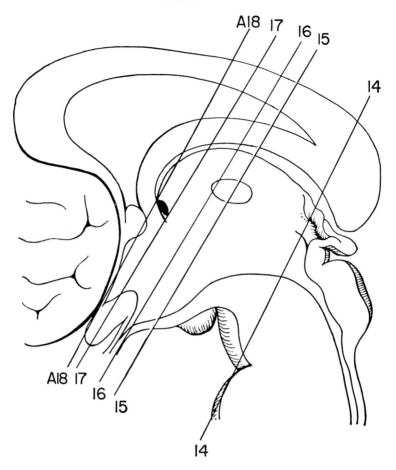

Outline of median sagittal surface of brain indicating level and plane of frontal sections A–14 to A–18.

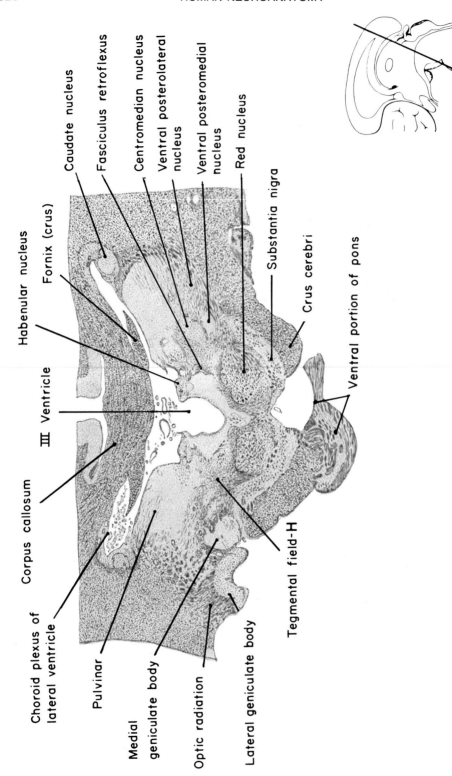

Caudate nucleus

Fasciculus retroflexus

Centromedian nucleus

Ventral posterolateral nucleus

Ventral posteromedial nucleus

Red nucleus

Habenular nucleus

Fornix (crus)

Substantia nigra

III Ventricle

Crus cerebri

Corpus callosum

Ventral portion of pons

Choroid plexus of lateral ventricle

Pulvinar

Medial geniculate body

Optic radiation

Lateral geniculate body

Tegmental field-H

A–14. Frontal section through the junction of the midbrain and the diencephalon at the level of the habenular nucleus. ×2.5.

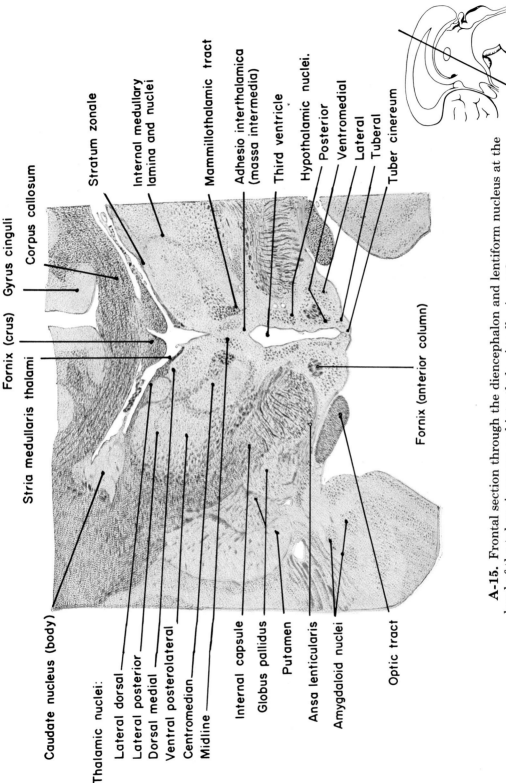

Corpus callosum

Gyrus cinguli

Stratum zonale

Internal medullary
lamina and nuclei

Mammillothalamic tract

Adhesio interthalamica
(massa intermedia)

Third ventricle

Hypothalamic nuclei.

Posterior

Ventromedial

Lateral

Tuberal

Tuber cinereum

Fornix (crus)

Stria medullaris thalami

Caudate nucleus (body)

Thalamic nuclei:

Lateral dorsal

Lateral posterior

Dorsal medial

Ventral posterolateral

Centromedian

Midline

Internal capsule

Globus pallidus

Putamen

Ansa lenticularis

Amygdaloid nuclei

Optic tract

Fornix (anterior column)

A-15. Frontal section through the diencephalon and lentiform nucleus at the
level of the tuber cinereum and interthalamic adhesion. ×3.

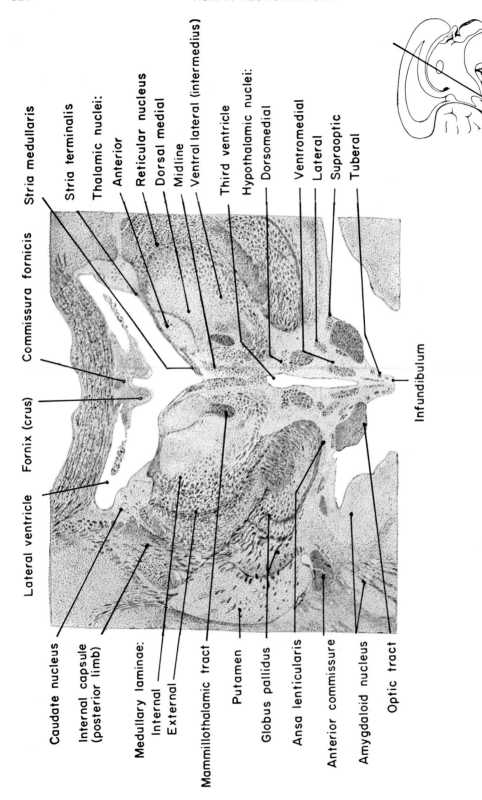

Stria medullaris

Stria terminalis

Thalamic nuclei:
  Anterior
  Reticular nucleus
  Dorsal medial
  Midline
  Ventral lateral (intermedius)

Third ventricle

Hypothalamic nuclei:
  Dorsomedial
  Ventromedial
  Lateral
  Supraoptic
  Tuberal

Commissura fornicis

Fornix (crus)

Lateral ventricle

Caudate nucleus

Internal capsule (posterior limb)

Medullary laminae:
  Internal
  External

Mammillothalamic tract

Putamen

Globus pallidus

Ansa lenticularis

Anterior commissure

Amygdaloid nucleus

Optic tract

Infundibulum

A-16. Frontal section through the diencephalon and lentiform nucleus at the level of the infundibulum and interthalamic adhesion. ×3.

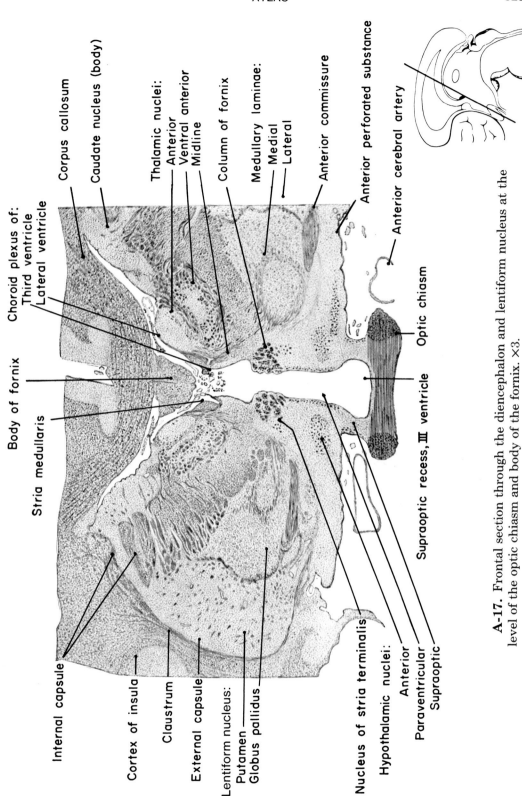

Corpus callosum

Caudate nucleus (body)

Thalamic nuclei:
Anterior
Ventral anterior
Midline

Column of fornix

Medullary laminae:
Medial
Lateral

Anterior commissure

Anterior perforated substance

Anterior cerebral artery

Optic chiasm

Supraoptic recess, III ventricle

Hypothalamic nuclei:
Anterior
Paraventricular
Supraoptic

Nucleus of stria terminalis

Lentiform nucleus:
Putamen
Globus pallidus

External capsule

Claustrum

Cortex of insula

Internal capsule

Stria medullaris

Body of fornix

Choroid plexus of:
Third ventricle
Lateral ventricle

A-17. Frontal section through the diencephalon and lentiform nucleus at the level of the optic chiasm and body of the fornix. ×3.

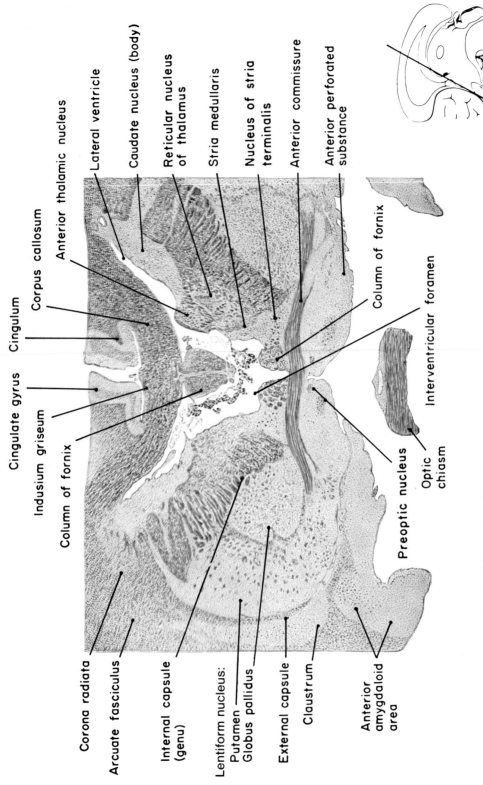

A–18. Frontal section through the rostral diencephalon at the level of the optic chiasm and interventricular foramen. ×3.

Anterior thalamic nucleus

Lateral ventricle

Caudate nucleus (body)

Reticular nucleus of thalamus

Stria medullaris

Nucleus of stria terminalis

Anterior commissure

Anterior perforated substance

Corpus callosum

Cingulum

Cingulate gyrus

Indusium griseum

Column of fornix

Corona radiata

Arcuate fasciculus

Internal capsule (genu)

Lentiform nucleus:
Putamen
Globus pallidus

External capsule

Claustrum

Anterior amygdaloid area

Preoptic nucleus

Optic chiasm

Interventricular foramen

Column of fornix

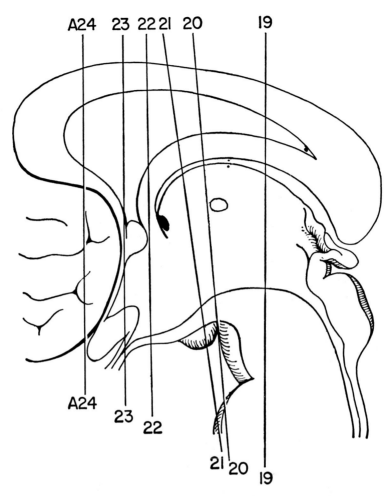

Outline of median sagittal surface of brain indicating level and plane of frontal sections A–19 to A–24.

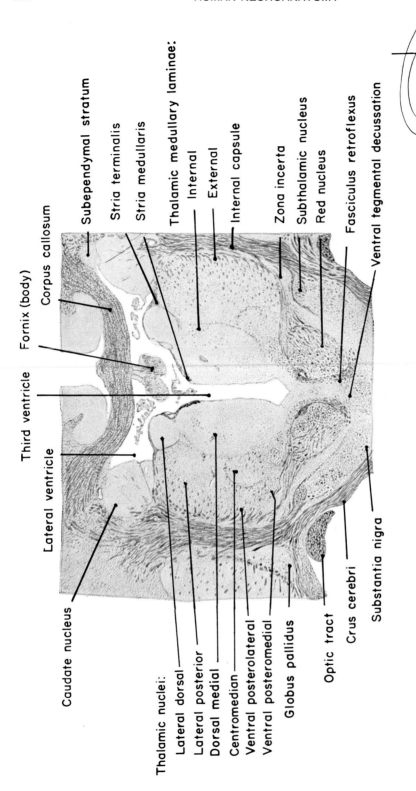

A-19. Frontal section through midbrain and diencephalon at the level of red nucleus and posterior thalamic nuclei. ×2.5.

Corpus callosum

Fornix (body)

Subependymal stratum

Stria terminalis

Stria medullaris

Thalamic medullary laminae:
  Internal
  External

Internal capsule

Zona incerta

Subthalamic nucleus

Red nucleus

Fasciculus retroflexus

Ventral tegmental decussation

Third ventricle

Lateral ventricle

Caudate nucleus

Thalamic nuclei:
  Lateral dorsal
  Lateral posterior
  Dorsal medial
  Centromedian
  Ventral posterolateral
  Ventral posteromedial

Globus pallidus

Optic tract

Crus cerebri

Substantia nigra

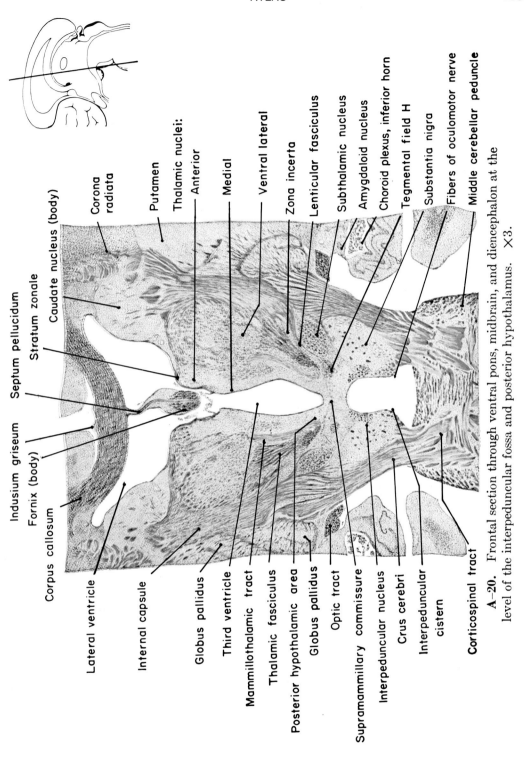

Indusium griseum
Septum pellucidum
Fornix (body)
Corpus callosum
Lateral ventricle
Internal capsule
Globus pallidus
Third ventricle
Mammillothalamic tract
Thalamic fasciculus
Posterior hypothalamic area
Globus pallidus
Optic tract
Supramammillary commissure
Interpeduncular nucleus
Crus cerebri
Interpeduncular cistern
Corticospinal tract

Caudate nucleus (body)
Stratum zonale
Corona radiata
Putamen
Thalamic nuclei:
Anterior
Medial
Ventral lateral
Zona incerta
Lenticular fasciculus
Subthalamic nucleus
Amygdaloid nucleus
Choroid plexus, inferior horn
Tegmental field H
Substantia nigra
Fibers of oculomotor nerve
Middle cerebellar peduncle

A–20. Frontal section through ventral pons, midbrain, and diencephalon at the level of the interpeduncular fossa and posterior hypothalamus. ×3.

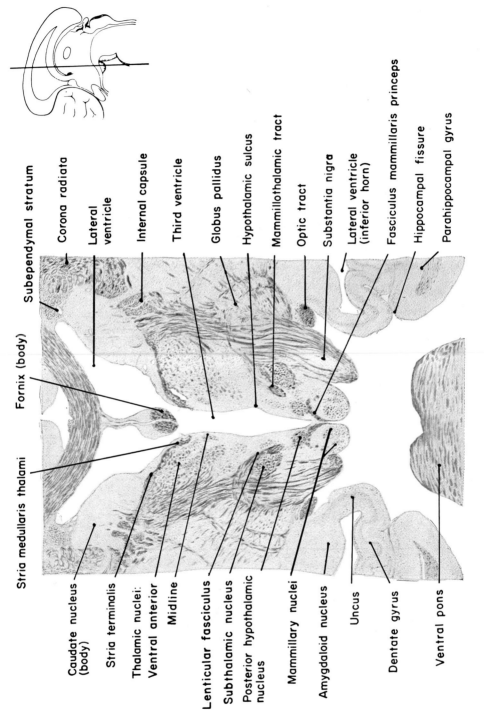

A-21. Frontal section through diencephalon at the level of the mammillary body. ×3.

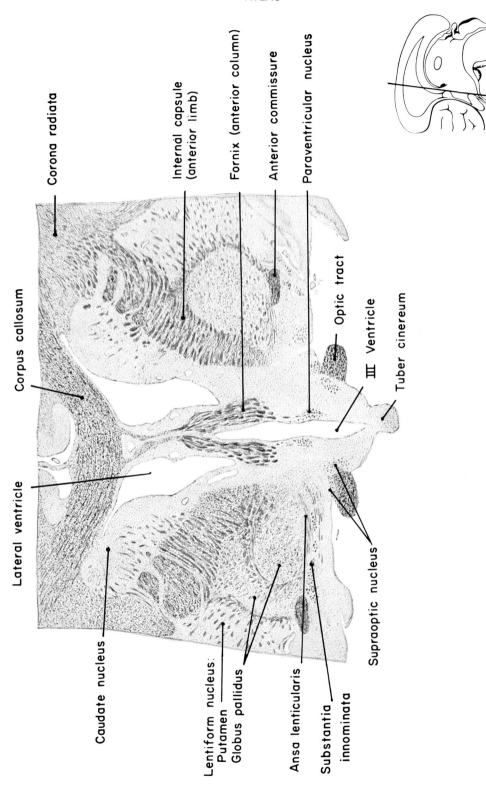

A-22. Frontal section through rostral hypothalamus and lentiform nucleus at the level of the tuber cinereum and columns of the fornix. ×3.

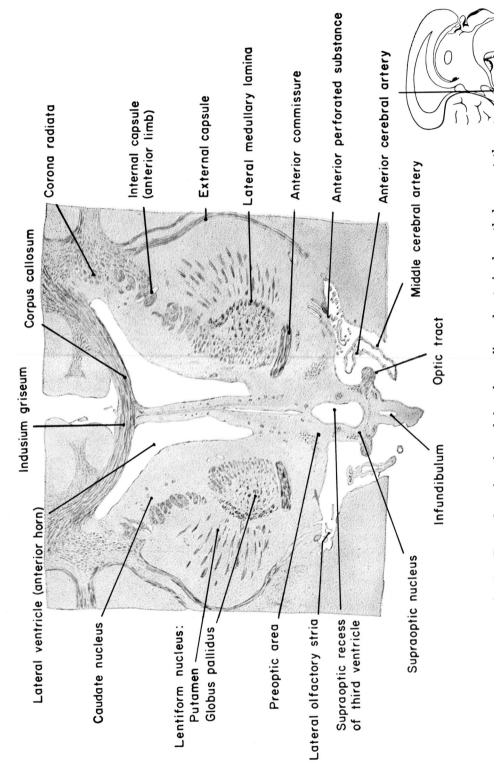

Corona radiata

Internal capsule (anterior limb)

External capsule

Lateral medullary lamina

Anterior commissure

Anterior perforated substance

Anterior cerebral artery

Corpus callosum

Indusium griseum

Middle cerebral artery

Lateral ventricle (anterior horn)

Optic tract

Caudate nucleus

Infundibulum

Lentiform nucleus:
Putamen
Globus pallidus

Preoptic area

Lateral olfactory stria

Supraoptic recess
of third ventricle

Supraoptic nucleus

A–23. Frontal section through basal ganglia and anterior hypothalamus at the level of the infundibulum and anterior limb of the internal capsule. ×3.

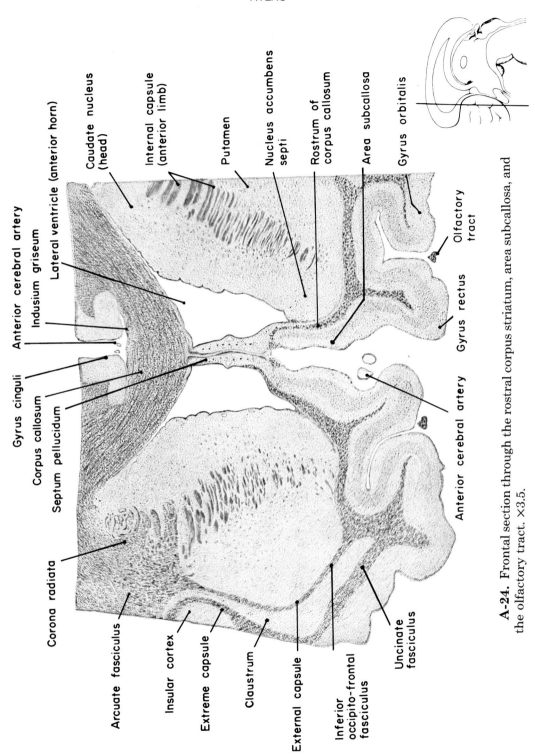

A-24. Frontal section through the rostral corpus striatum, area subcallosa, and the olfactory tract. ×3.5.

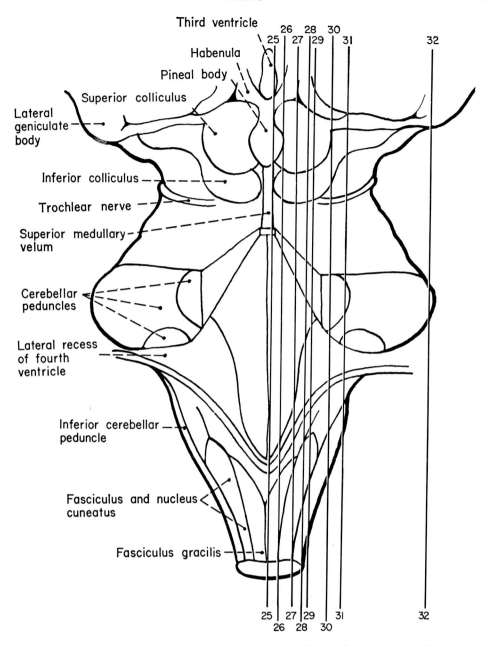

Outline of dorsal surface of brain indicating level and plane of sagittal sections A-25 to A-32.

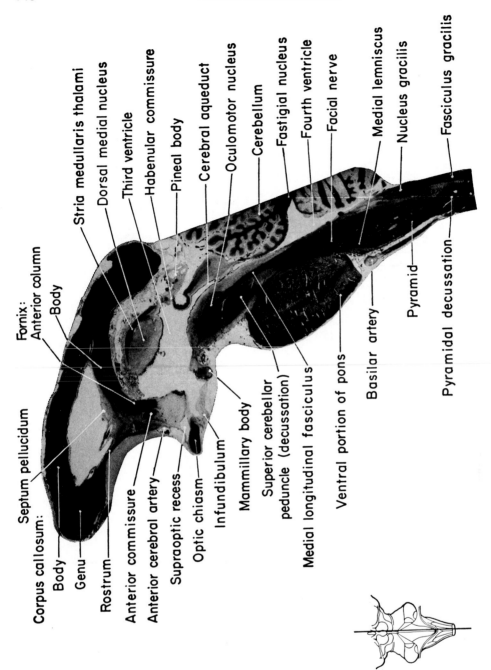

A-25. Sagittal section through the ventricular system and brain stem at the level of the pineal body. ×15.

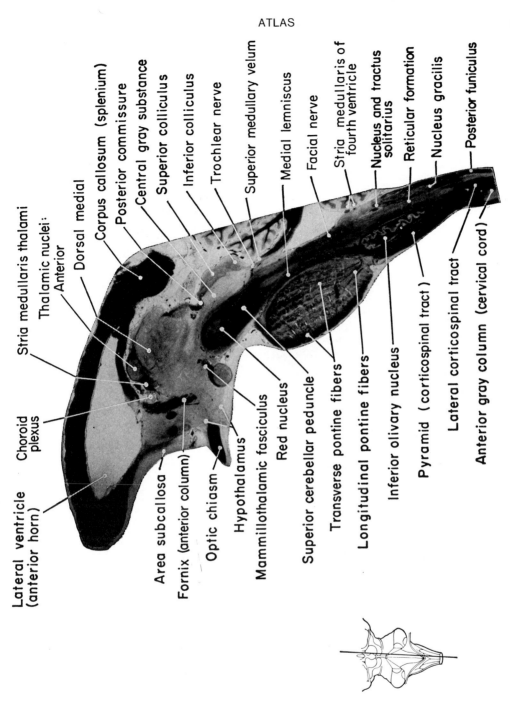

A-26. Sagittal section through brain stem at the level of the nucleus gracilis and emergence of the trochlear nerve. ×1.3.

Lateral ventricle (anterior horn)

Choroid plexus

Stria medullaris thalami

Thalamic nuclei: Anterior

Dorsal medial

Corpus callosum (splenium)

Posterior commissure

Central gray substance

Superior colliculus

Inferior colliculus

Trochlear nerve

Superior medullary velum

Medial lemniscus

Facial nerve

Stria medullaris of fourth ventricle

Nucleus and tractus solitarius

Reticular formation

Nucleus gracilis

Posterior funiculus

Area subcallosa

Fornix (anterior column)

Optic chiasm

Hypothalamus

Mammillothalamic fasciculus

Red nucleus

Superior cerebellar peduncle

Transverse pontine fibers

Longitudinal pontine fibers

Inferior olivary nucleus

Pyramid (corticospinal tract)

Lateral corticospinal tract

Anterior gray column (cervical cord)

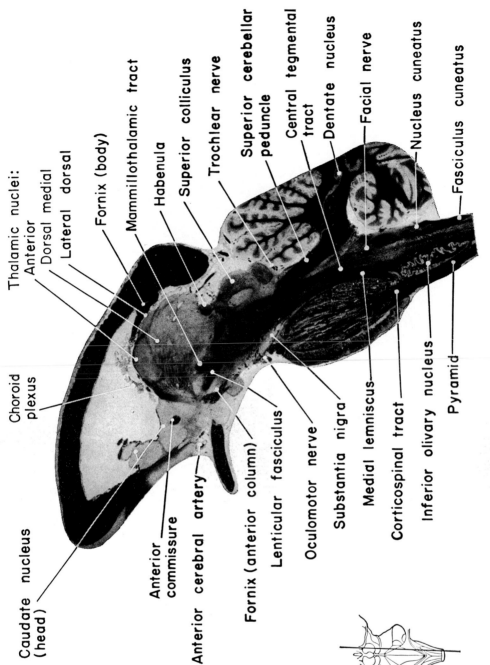

Thalamic nuclei:
Anterior
Dorsal medial
Lateral dorsal
Fornix (body)
Mammillothalamic tract
Habenula
Superior colliculus
Trochlear nerve
Superior cerebellar peduncle
Central tegmental tract
Dentate nucleus
Facial nerve
Nucleus cuneatus
Fasciculus cuneatus

Choroid plexus
Caudate nucleus (head)
Anterior commissure
Anterior cerebral artery
Fornix (anterior column)
Lenticular fasciculus
Oculomotor nerve
Substantia nigra
Medial lemniscus
Corticospinal tract
Inferior olivary nucleus
Pyramid

A-27. Sagittal section through the brain stem at the level of the nucleus cuneatus and habenula. ×1.3.

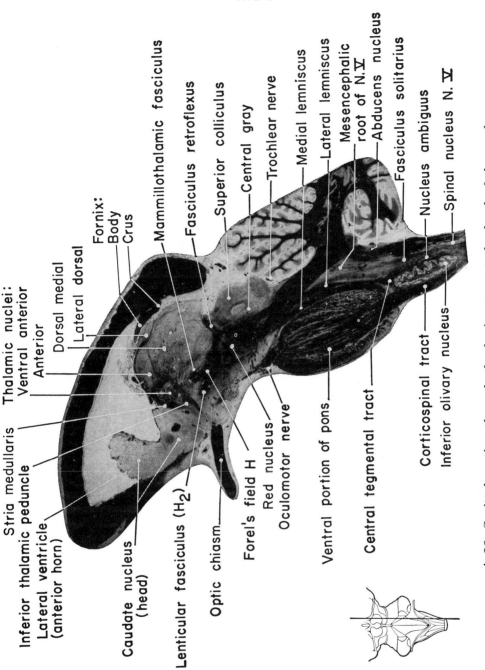

Thalamic nuclei:
Ventral anterior
Anterior
Dorsal medial
Lateral dorsal

Fornix:
Body
Crus

Mammillothalamic fasciculus
Fasciculus retroflexus
Superior colliculus
Central gray
Trochlear nerve
Medial lemniscus
Lateral lemniscus
Mesencephalic root of N. V
Abducens nucleus
Fasciculus solitarius
Nucleus ambiguus
Spinal nucleus N. V

Stria medullaris
Inferior thalamic peduncle
Lateral ventricle (anterior horn)
Caudate nucleus (head)
Lenticular fasciculus (H₂)
Optic chiasm
Forel's field H
Red nucleus
Oculomotor nerve
Ventral portion of pons
Central tegmental tract
Corticospinal tract
Inferior olivary nucleus

A-28. Sagittal section through the brain stem at the level of the nucleus ambiguus, lateral lemniscus, and fasciculus retroflexus. ×1.3.

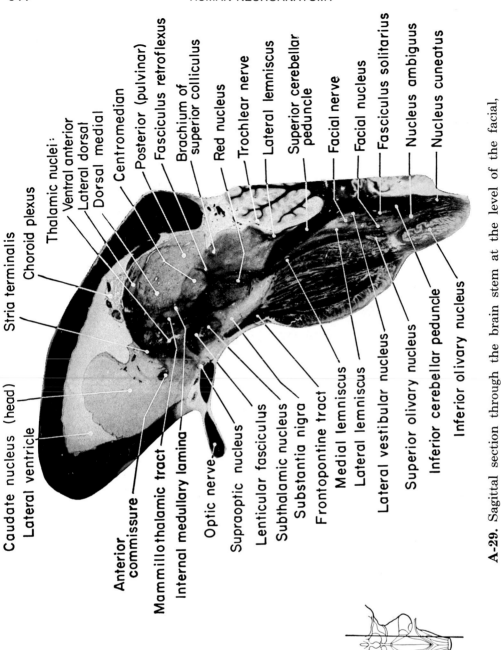

Caudate nucleus (head)
Lateral ventricle

Stria terminalis
Choroid plexus

Thalamic nuclei:
Ventral anterior
Lateral dorsal
Dorsal medial
Centromedian
Posterior (pulvinar)
Fasciculus retroflexus
Brachium of superior colliculus
Red nucleus
Trochlear nerve
Lateral lemniscus
Superior cerebellar peduncle
Facial nerve
Facial nucleus
Fasciculus solitarius
Nucleus ambiguus
Nucleus cuneatus

Anterior commissure
Mammillothalamic tract
Internal medullary lamina
Optic nerve
Supraoptic nucleus
Lenticular fasciculus
Subthalamic nucleus
Substantia nigra
Frontopontine tract
Medial lemniscus
Lateral lemniscus
Lateral vestibular nucleus
Superior olivary nucleus
Inferior cerebellar peduncle
Inferior olivary nucleus

A-29. Sagittal section through the brain stem at the level of the facial, subthalamic and centromedian nuclei. ×1.3.

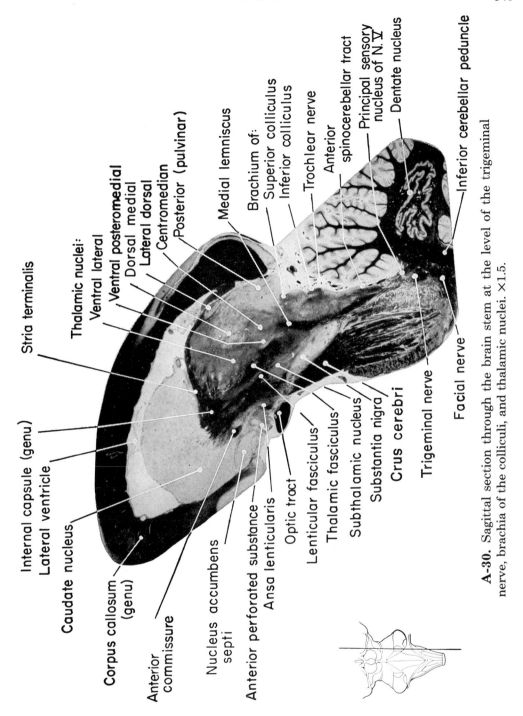

Internal capsule (genu)
Lateral ventricle
Stria terminalis

Caudate nucleus

Thalamic nuclei:
Ventral lateral
Ventral posteromedial
Dorsal medial
Lateral dorsal
Centromedian
Posterior (pulvinar)

Medial lemniscus

Brachium of:
Superior colliculus
Inferior colliculus

Trochlear nerve

Anterior
spinocerebellar tract

Principal sensory
nucleus of N.Ⅴ

Dentate nucleus

Inferior cerebellar peduncle

Corpus callosum
(genu)

Anterior
commissure

Nucleus accumbens
septi

Anterior perforated substance
Ansa lenticularis

Optic tract

Lenticular fasciculus

Thalamic fasciculus

Subthalamic nucleus

Substantia nigra

Crus cerebri

Trigeminal nerve

Facial nerve

A-30. Sagittal section through the brain stem at the level of the trigeminal nerve, brachia of the colliculi, and thalamic nuclei. ×1.5.

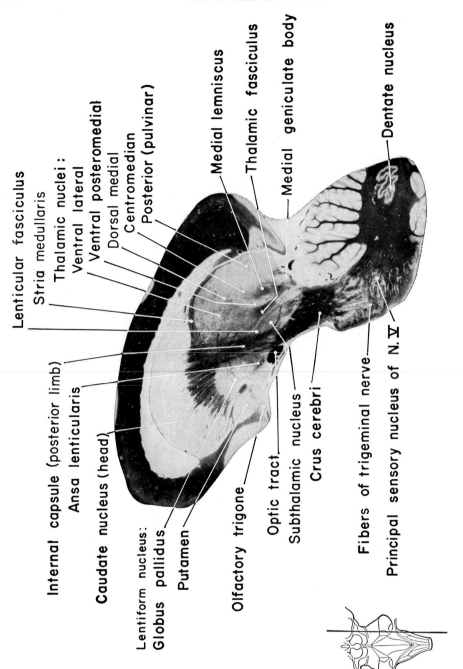

Lenticular fasciculus
Stria medullaris
Thalamic nuclei :
Ventral lateral
Ventral posteromedial
Dorsal medial
Centromedian
Posterior (pulvinar)
Medial lemniscus
Thalamic fasciculus
Medial geniculate body
Dentate nucleus

Internal capsule (posterior limb)
Ansa lenticularis

Caudate nucleus (head)

Lentiform nucleus:
Globus pallidus
Putamen

Olfactory trigone

Optic tract
Subthalamic nucleus
Crus cerebri

Fibers of trigeminal nerve
Principal sensory nucleus of N. V

A-31. Sagittal section through upper brain stem at the level of the trigeminal nerve and the medial geniculate body. ×1.3.

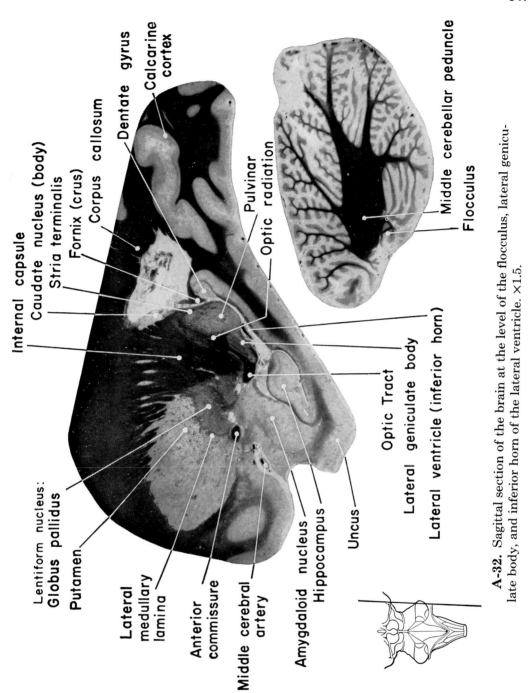

A-32. Sagittal section of the brain at the level of the flocculus, lateral geniculate body, and inferior horn of the lateral ventricle. ×1.5.

Internal capsule

Caudate nucleus (body)

Stria terminalis

Fornix (crus)

Corpus callosum

Dentate gyrus

Calcarine cortex

Pulvinar

Optic radiation

Middle cerebellar peduncle

Flocculus

Lentiform nucleus:
Globus pallidus

Putamen

Lateral medullary lamina

Anterior commissure

Middle cerebral artery

Amygdaloid nucleus

Hippocampus

Uncus

Optic Tract

Lateral geniculate body

Lateral ventricle (inferior horn)

Index

Boldface numbers indicate principal references. *Italic* numbers refer to illustrations.